SEVENTH EDITION

The MD Anderson Surgical Oncology Manual

SEVENTH EDITION

The MD Anderson Surgical Oncology Manual

Senior Editor

Barry W. Feig, MD

Professor, Surgical Oncology
Department of Surgical Oncology
The University of Texas MD Anderson Cancer Center
Houston, Texas

Associate Editors

Michael G. White, MD, MSc

Assistant Professor
Department of Colon and Rectal Surgery
The University of Texas MD Anderson
   Cancer Center
Houston, Texas

Anai N. Kothari, MD, MS, FSSO

Assistant Professor of Surgical Oncology
Department of Surgery
Medical College of Wisconsin
Milwaukee, Wisconsin

Cameron E. Gaskill, MD, MPH

Assistant Professor of Surgical Oncology
Department of Surgery
UC Davis Medical Center
Sacramento, California

Sandra R. DiBrito, MD, PhD

Assistant Professor of Surgery
Hepatobiliary and Surgical Oncology
Albany Medical College
Albany, New York

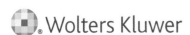. Wolters Kluwer

Philadelphia • Baltimore • New York • London
Buenos Aires • Hong Kong • Sydney • Tokyo

Senior Acquisitions Editor: Keith Donnellan
Senior Development Editor: Ashley Fischer
Editorial Coordinator: Sunmerrilika Baskar
Marketing Manager: Kirsten Watrud
Senior Production Project Manager: Alicia Jackson
Manager, Graphic Arts & Design: Stephen Druding
Senior Manufacturing Coordinator: Beth Welsh
Prepress Vendor: Aptara, Inc.

7th edition

9 8 7 6 5 4 3 2 1

Printed in Mexico

Library of Congress Cataloging-in-Publication Data available upon request.

978-1-9751-9263-1

To our friends and families, for their support, enthusiasm, and patience through our many years of training and continued long hours spent in the care of patients with cancer.

CONTRIBUTORS

Jack R. Andrews, MD
Urologic Oncology Fellow
Department of Urologic Oncology
The University of Texas MD Anderson Cancer Center
Houston, Texas

Natalia Paez Arango, MD, MS
Department of Surgical Oncology/
   Hepatobiliary Surgery
Trihealth Cancer Institute
Cincinnati, Ohio

Scott Atay, MD
Assistant Professor of Surgery
Surgical Director Lung Transplantation
University of Southern California, Keck School
   of Medicine
Los Angeles, California

Brian D. Badgwell, MD, MS
Professor of Surgery
Department of Surgical Oncology
The University of Texas MD Anderson
   Cancer Center
Houston, Texas

Donald P. Baumann, MD
Professor
Department of Plastic Surgery
The University of Texas MD Anderson
   Cancer Center
Houston, Texas

Neal Bhutiani, MD, PhD
Complex General Surgical Oncology Fellow
Department of Surgical Oncology
The University of Texas MD Anderson
   Cancer Center
Houston, Texas

Ian C. Bostock, MD, MS
Assistant Professor
Department of Cardiothoracic Surgery
Medical University of South Carolina
Charleston, South Carolina

Adrienne Cobb, MD, MS
Assistant Profssor
Department of Surgery
Medical College of Wisonsin
Milwaukee, Wisconsin

Seth J. Concors, MD
Complex General Surgical Oncology Fellow
Department of Surgical Oncology
The University of Texas MD Anderson Cancer Center
Houston, Texas

Brandon M. Cope, MD
Research Resident
Department of Surgical Oncology
The University of Texas MD Anderson Cancer Center
Houston, Texas

Christopher Crane, MD
Chief, Gastrointestinal Service
Department of Radiation Oncology
Memorial Sloan Kettering Cancer Center
New York, New York

Han T. Cun, MD, MS
Fellow
Department of Gynecologic Oncology and
   Reproductive Medicine
The University of Texas MD Anderson Cancer Center
Houston, Texas

Prajnan Das, MD, MS, MOH
Professor
Department of Radiation Oncology
The University of Texas MD Anderson Cancer Center
Houston, Texas

Sandra R. DiBrito, MD, PhD
Assistant Professor of Surgery
Hepatobiliary and Surgical Oncology
Albany Medical College
Albany, New York

Chibawanye I. Ene, MD, PhD
Assistant Professor
Department of Neurological Surgery
The University of Texas MD Anderson Cancer Center
Houston, Texas

Derek J. Erstad, MD
Assistant Professor of Surgery
Division of Surgical Oncology
Baylor College of Medicine
Houston, Texas

Rachel Feig, MPAS, PA-C
Physician Assistant
Department of Surgical Oncology
Parkland Health & Hospital System
Dallas, Texas

Keith F. Fournier, MD
Associate Professor
Department of Surgical Oncology
The University of Texas MD Anderson Cancer Center
Houston, Texas

Cameron E. Gaskill, MD, MPH
Assistant Professor of Surgical Oncology
Department of Surgery
UC Davis Medical Center
Sacramento, California

Jeffrey E. Gershenwald, MD
Professor
Department of Surgical Oncology and
  Cancer Biology
The University of Texas MD Anderson Cancer Center
Houston, Texas

Ryan P. Goepfert, MD
Assistant Professor
Department of Head and Neck Surgery
The University of Texas MD Anderson Cancer Center
Houston, Texas

Elizabeth G. Grubbs, MD, MS
Professor
Department of Surgical Oncology
The University of Texas MD Anderson Cancer Center
Houston, Texas

Matthew M. Hanasono, MD
Professor
Department of Plastic Surgery
The University of Texas MD Anderson Cancer Center
Houston, Texas

Caitlin A. Hester, MD
Assistant Professor of Surgery
Department of Surgery
University of Miami
Miami, Florida

Wayne L. Hofstetter, MD
Professor
Department of Thoracic and Cardiovascular Surgery
The University of Texas MD Anderson Cancer Center
Houston, Texas

Ryan Huey, MD
Assistant Professor
Department of Gastrointestinal Medical Oncology
The University of Texas MD Anderson Cancer Center
Houston, Texas

Kelly K. Hunt, MD
Chair and Professor
Department of Breast Surgical Oncology
The University of Texas MD Anderson Cancer Center
Houston, Texas

Naruhiko Ikoma, MD
Assistant Professor
Department of Surgical Oncology
The University of Texas MD Anderson Cancer Center
Houston, Texas

Yelda Jozaghi, MD, FRCSC
Fellow
Department of Head and Neck Surgical Oncology
The University of Texas MD Anderson Cancer Center
Houston, Texas

Jose A. Karam, MD, FACS
Associate Professor of Urology and Translational
  Molecular Pathology
The University of Texas MD Anderson Cancer Center
Houston, Texas

Matthew H.G. Katz, MD
Professor of Surgery
Department of Surgical Oncology
The University of Texas MD Anderson Cancer Center
Houston, Texas

Emily Z. Keung, MD
Assistant Professor
Department of Surgical Oncology
The University of Texas MD Anderson Cancer Center
Houston, Texas

Bradford J. Kim, MD, MHS
Associate Professor of Surgical Oncology
Department of Surgical Oncology
City of Hope
Duarte, California

Michael P. Kim, MD
Associate Professor
Department of Surgical Oncology
The University of Texas MD Anderson Cancer Center
Houston, Texas

Anai N. Kothari, MD, MS, FSSO
Assistant Professor of Surgical Oncology
Medical College of Wisconsin
Milwaukee, Wisconsin

Hun Ju Lee, MD
Associate Professor
Department of Lymphoma and Myeloma
The University of Texas MD Anderson Cancer Center
Houston, Texas

Jeffrey E. Lee, MD
Professor and VP Medical and Academic Affairs,
 Cancer Network
Department of Surgical Oncology
The University of Texas MD Anderson Cancer Center
Houston, Texas

Harufumi Maki, MD, PhD
Postdoctoral Fellow
Department of Surgical Oncology
The University of Texas MD Anderson Cancer Center
Houston, Texas

Naveen V. Manisundaram, MD
Surgery Resident
Department of Surgical Oncology
The University of Texas MD Anderson Cancer Center
Houston, Texas

Allison N. Martin, MD, MPH
Fellow, Complex General Surgical Oncology
Department of Surgical Oncology
The University of Texas MD Anderson Cancer Center
Houston, Texas

Meredith C. Mason, MD
Assistant Professor of Surgery
Department of Surgery
Division of Surgical Oncology
Emory University School of Medicine
Atlanta, Georgia

Jessica E. Maxwell, MD, MBA
Assistant Professor
Department of Surgical Oncology
The University of Texas MD Anderson Cancer Center
Houston, Texas

Ian E. McCutcheon, MD
Professor
Department of Neurosurgery
The University of Texas MD Anderson Cancer Center
Houston, Texas

Shalini Moningi, MD
Attending Physician
Department of Radiation Oncology
Brigham and Women's Hospital/Dana Farber
 Cancer Institute
Boston, Massachusetts

Andrew D. Newton, MD
Staff Surgeon
Oschner Health
New Orleans, Louisiana

Elizabeth C. Poli, MD
Assistant Professor
Northshore University Health
Evanston, Illinois

Geoffrey L. Robb, MD, FACS
Professor
Department of Plastic Surgery
The University of Texas MD Anderson Cancer Center
Houston, Texas

Christina L. Roland, MD, MS
Associate Professor
Department of Surgical Oncology
The University of Texas MD Anderson Cancer Center
Houston, Texas

Michael K. Rooney, MD
Resident Physician
Department of Radiation Oncology
The University of Texas MD Anderson Cancer Center
Houston, Texas

Margaret S. Roubaud, MD
Assistant Professor
Department of Plastic and Reconstructive Surgery
The University of Texas MD Anderson Cancer Center
Houston, Texas

Aysegul A. Sahin, MD
Professor
Department of Pathology
The University of Texas MD Anderson Cancer Center
Houston, Texas

David Santos, MD, MS
Associate Professor of Surgery
Department of Surgical Oncology
The University of Texas MD Anderson Cancer Center
Houston, Texas

Boris Sepesi, MD
Associate Professor
Department of Thoracic Surgery
The University of Texas MD Anderson Cancer Center
Houston, Texas

Aditya S. Shirali, MD
Assistant Professor
Department of Surgery
University of Florida
Gainesville, Florida

Puneet Singh, MD, FACS
Assistant Professor
Department of Breast Surgical Oncology
The University of Texas MD Anderson Cancer Center
Houston, Texas

Rebecca A. Snyder, MD, MPH
Assistant Professor
Department of Surgical Oncology
The University of Texas MD Anderson Cancer Center
Houston, Texas

Pamela T. Soliman, MD, MPH
Professor
Department of Gynecologic Oncology &
    Reproductive Medicine
The University of Texas MD Anderson Cancer Center
Houston, Texas

Douglas Swords, MD
Staff Surgeon
Genesis Care
Asheville, North Carolina

Mediget Teshome, MD, MPH
Associate Professor
Department of Breast Surgical Oncology
The University of Texas MD Anderson Cancer Center
Houston, Texas

Abhineet Uppal, MD
Assistant Professor
Department of Colorectal Surgery
The University of Texas MD Anderson Cancer Center
Houston, Texas

Jean-Nicolas Vauthey, MD
Professor of Surgery
Department of Surgical Oncology
The University of Texas MD Anderson Cancer Center
Houston, Texas

Mark T. Villa, MD
Professor of Plastic Surgery
Department of Plastic Surgery
The University of Texas MD Anderson Cancer Center
Houston, Texas

Rachel K. Voss, MD, MPH
Assistant Professor
Department of Sarcoma Oncology
H. Lee Moffitt Cancer Center
Department of Oncologic Science
Morsani College of Medicine, University of Florida
Tampa, Florida

Steven Wei, EdD, MPH, MS, PA-C
Supervisor, Advanced Practice Providers
Department of Surgical Oncology
The University of Texas MD Anderson Cancer Center
Houston, Texas

Michael G. White, MD, MSc
Assistant Professor
Department of Colon and Rectal Surgery
The University of Texas MD Anderson
    Cancer Center
Houston, Texas

Russell G. Witt, MD, MAS
Complex General Surgical Oncology Fellow
Department of Surgical Oncology
The University of Texas MD Anderson Cancer Center
Houston, Texas

Christopher G. Wood, MD[†]
Professor and Deputy Chairman
Department of Urology
The University of Texas MD Anderson Cancer Center
Houston, Texas

Y. Nancy You, MD
Professor
Department of Colon and Rectal Surgery
The University of Texas MD Anderson Cancer Center
Houston, Texas

Mark E. Zafereo, MD
Professor
Department of Head and Neck Surgery
The University of Texas MD Anderson Cancer Center
Houston, Texas

[†]Deceased.

PREFACE

Never say never....

I was pretty sure that there was not going to be a seventh edition of the *The MD Anderson Surgical Oncology Handbook*, and I was even more sure of the fact that if there was a seventh edition that I would not be participating in the process. My skepticism was based on two recent observations that I have had; one sprung on me unexpectedly and the other something that I have observed multiple times over the almost 30 years that I have been editing this book. The first is that due to my failing health, which has resulted in my surgical career being interrupted slightly earlier than I had planned, I was not sure that I would be available to see the project through to completion. The second is that despite numerous genuine offers from a multitude of people offering to "help" with the book, it has pretty much remained a solo project of mine, and mine alone.

Two events proved my prophecies to be incorrect. When my daughter who was in Physician Assistant school just shortly after the sixth edition came out, called me to ask why she could not find any information in the book on Merkel Cell carcinoma, followed shortly thereafter by four new fellows asking to meet with me to discuss how they thought we could "improve" the handbook, I determined that my fate was sealed. I went back to see what I had written in the preface of the sixth edition and fortunately I had said that the sixth edition would "most likely" be the last edition of the handbook that I would be involved with... I never said "never"!

Although the objectives of *The Handbook* remain unchanged ("to document the philosophies...and outline basic management approaches based on the complex surgical oncology fellow's experience...at the MD Anderson Cancer Center") the seventh edition has been enhanced with clinical case scenarios for almost every disease site as well as with case-based multiple-choice questions. These questions are intended to serve as an opportunity for the trainees using the handbook to become more comfortable with, the thought processes that the complex surgical oncology fellows at the MD Anderson Cancer Center feel are representative of the key points in each disease site.

I am now comfortable leaving future editions of The MD Anderson Surgical Oncology Handbook in the hands of the four new editors that have undertaken the task of bringing this seventh edition to completion. I hope that the readers will find this edition to be even more valuable than previous editions and that this trend will continue for a long into future editions.

I am grateful to have been part of this incredible team of talented individuals that have made The MD Anderson Surgical Oncology handbook a valuable resource for students, surgical trainees, and anyone taking care of cancer patients.

Barry W. Feig, MD

CONTENTS

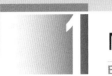

Noninvasive Breast Cancer

Elizabeth C. Poli, Aysegul A. Sahin, and Kelly K. Hunt

INTRODUCTION

Ductal carcinoma in situ (DCIS) is noninvasive carcinoma of the breast and is defined as the proliferation of malignant epithelial cells confined to the mammary ducts and without evidence of invasion through the basement membrane. Because it is noninvasive, DCIS does not pose a risk of metastasis. Lobular carcinoma in situ (LCIS) was previously considered a form of noninvasive carcinoma, but is now understood to be a benign entity that is a pathologic marker of increased breast cancer risk in either breast. Atypical lobular hyperplasia (ALH) and LCIS are both forms of lobular neoplasia and, together with atypical ductal hyperplasia (ADH), represent proliferative nonmalignant breast lesions.

Ductal Carcinoma In Situ

Epidemiology

One in eight women in the United States (US) will be diagnosed with breast cancer in her lifetime, and 20% to 25% of these newly diagnosed cases will be DCIS. In 2019, an estimated 48,100 cases of DCIS were diagnosed in US. Widespread use of screening mammography has resulted in a 10-fold increase in the reported incidence of DCIS since the mid-1980s. However, since 2003, the incidence of DCIS has declined in women aged 50 years and older—possibly due to decreased use of hormone replacement therapy—while the incidence in women aged under 50 years continues to increase. Approximately 1 in every 1,300 mammography examinations performed in US will lead to a diagnosis of DCIS, representing 17% to 34% of all mammographically detected breast cancers. Before the introduction of screening mammography, most cases of DCIS were not detected until a palpable mass formed, but today, 80% to 85% of DCIS cases are detected on screening. The incidence of DCIS in autopsy studies is higher than in the general population, suggesting that not all DCIS lesions are clinically significant and supporting concerns that most of the increase in DCIS incidence is due to the detection of nonaggressive subtypes that are unlikely to progress to invasive cancer.

The median age reported for patients with DCIS ranges from 47 to 63 years, similar to that reported for patients with invasive carcinoma. However, the age of peak incidence for DCIS—96.7 per 100,000 women—occurs between the ages of 65 and 69 years, which is younger than for invasive breast cancer, for which peak incidence—453.1 per 100,000 women—occurs between the ages of 75 and 79 years. The frequency of first-degree relatives having breast cancer (10% to 35%) as well as rates of deleterious mutations in the breast cancer–associated (BRCA) genes are similar for patients with DCIS as for women with invasive breast cancer. Other risk factors for DCIS—including older age, proliferative breast disease, increased breast density, nulliparity, older age at primiparity, history of breast biopsy, early menarche, late menopause, long-term use of postmenopausal hormone replacement therapy, and elevated body mass index in postmenopausal women—are the same as those for invasive breast cancer.

Pathology

DCIS is a proliferation of malignant cells that have not breached the ductal basement membrane. They arise from ductal epithelium in the region of the terminal ductal–lobular unit. DCIS had previously been considered one stage in the continuum of histologic progression from ADH to invasive carcinoma. It is now understood that DCIS comprises a heterogeneous group of lesions with variable histologic architecture, molecular and cellular characteristics, and clinical behavior (Fig. 1.1). Malignant cells proliferate until the ducts is obliterated, and there may be associated breakdown of the myoepithelial cell layer of the basement membrane surrounding the ductal lumen. DCIS has also been linked with changes in the surrounding stroma resulting in fibroblast proliferation, lymphocyte infiltration, and angiogenesis. Thus, although the process is poorly understood, most—but not all—invasive ductal carcinomas are believed to arise from DCIS. Therefore, DCIS is considered a nonobligate precursor of invasive breast carcinoma with a variable risk of progression, depending on a combination of pathologic factors. These factors include growth pattern, histologic grade, presence or absence of necrosis, size of the lesion, margin status, and expression of tumor biomarkers (estrogen and progesterone receptors).

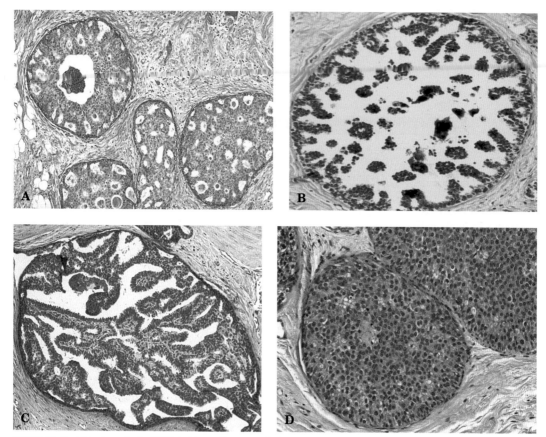

FIGURE 1.1 Ductal carcinoma in situ (DCIS). Architectural heterogeneity is a common feature of DCIS. Even in the same lesion, DCIS may show different growth patterns. The most common patterns include (**A**) Cribiform, (**B**) Micropapillary, (**C**) Papillary and (**D**) Solid.

Common growth patterns of DCIS include solid, cribriform, micropapillary, and papillary. Cribriform, solid, and micropapillary are the more common subtypes, and two or more patterns coexist in up to 50% of cases. Nuclear grading is based on the size, texture, and nucleoli. Similar to invasive carcinoma, three grades are recognized for DCIS. Low-grade lesions are characterized by a proliferation of monotonous cells with well-defined cell borders. Uniformity of nuclear features is the key feature. High-grade DCIS is composed of pleomorphic cells with variable nuclear size and shape. Mitoses are frequent in individual cells and comedonecrosis is common. Intermediate grade is used when nuclear features are in between low and high grade. Central (comedo) necrosis is most frequently associated with high-grade lesions, less frequently found in intermediate lesions and very rarely present in low-grade lesions. Both the World Health Organization (WHO) and the College of American Pathologists (CAP) recommend that architectural and nuclear features and the presence of comedonecrosis should be evaluated independently of one another and all of these features should be included in pathology reports.

Since DCIS only rarely forms a grossly visible mass, measurement of lesion size is typically done by microscopic evaluation. The pathologist must be able to reconstruct the specimen to estimate size of the lesion. This is a difficult task and requires that the histologic sections be submitted in orderly fashion to permit such reconstruction. Even so, it is sometimes difficult to assess lesion size when small foci of DCIS are scattered throughout the resected specimen. As most recurrences of DCIS probably represent persistence of DCIS following incomplete removal, the evaluation of margins is not trivial. Routine specimen mammography and careful sectioning of the specimen are required. The most common approach involves the application of different colored inks to the surfaces of a specimen that has been oriented by the surgeon. The specimen is then submitted for histologic examination in serial sections and the shortest distance between DCIS and the inked margin is reported as the margin width. In a joint consensus statement, the Society of Surgical Oncology (SSO), the American Society for Radiation Oncology (ASTRO), and the American Society of Clinical Oncology (ASCO) recommended the margin width for breast-conserving surgery for DCIS to be 2 mm based on data from patients treated with adjuvant whole-breast radiation. A 2-mm margin was determined after comparison to narrower margin widths demonstrated a significant decrease in in-breast recurrence. However, the panel recommended exercising clinical judgment based on other clinical and imaging factors when determining the need for reoperation for re-excision for patients with margins <2 mm.

In addition to tumor factors, stromal features have also been found to be prognostic in DCIS lesions. The presence of periductal fibrosis has been associated with increased likelihood of recurrence. Stromal tumor-infiltrating lymphocytes (TILs) have been found to be associated with younger age, larger tumor size, higher nuclear grade, comedonecrosis, and estrogen receptor negative status.

Given all of these considerations, the pathology report in cases of DCIS should include a large amount of data. The College of American Pathologists (CAP) has recommended use of a template form to ensure that all histopathologic data are reported. Such a form would typically include histologic pattern, nuclear grade, presence of necrosis, distance to margin, size, presence of calcifications, and status of estrogen and progesterone receptor expression.

Microinvasion

The eighth edition of the American Joint Committee on Cancer (AJCC) staging system defines microinvasion as invasion of breast cancer cells through the basement membrane at one or more foci, none of which exceeds a dimension of 1 mm. DCIS is a Tis lesion and is classified as stage 0 cancer; DCIS with microinvasion is considered T1mi and upstages DCIS from stage 0 to stage I disease. By definition, DCIS without microinvasion does not have the ability to metastasize to axillary lymph nodes or distant sites, whereas DCIS with microinvasion does. Axillary metastases have been reported in 0% to 20% of patients with DCIS with microinvasion.

The incidence of microinvasion in DCIS varies according to the size and extent of the index lesion. Lagios et al. reported a 2% incidence of microinvasion in patients with DCIS measuring less than 25 mm in diameter, compared with a 29% incidence of microinvasion in those with lesions larger than 26 mm. The incidence of microinvasion is also higher in patients with high-grade or comedo-type DCIS with necrosis and in patients with DCIS who present with a palpable mass or nipple discharge.

There is conflicting data in the literature on the prognosis of DCIS with microinvasion compared to DCIS without microinvasion. Historically, studies have shown that patients with DCIS with microinvasion have a worse prognosis compared with those who have DCIS alone. In a retrospective study of 1,248 serially sectioned DCIS tumors, de Mascarel et al. reported a 10.1% incidence of axillary metastases in cases of DCIS with microinvasion. Patients with DCIS alone had a better 10-year distant metastasis-free survival rate than patients with DCIS with microinvasion (98% and 91%, respectively). The overall survival rate was also better in patients with DCIS alone (96.5% vs. 88.4%). However, the metastasis-free and overall survival rates were worse in patients with invasive ductal carcinoma compared with those with DCIS with microinvasion. In a retrospective review of the SEER database from Champion et al., 134,569 women with DCIS alone, DCIS with microinvasion, and T1a intraductal carcinoma were compared. They found that the disease-specific survival of DCIS with microinvasion was significantly different from the other two groups (DCIS alone: hazard ratio [HR] 0.59, confidence interval [CI] 0.43–0.80; invasive: HR 1.43, CI 1.04–1.96) but the overall survival of DCIS with microinvasion was similar to early invasive disease. Patients with DCIS alone had an improved overall survival compared to DCIS with microinvasion (HR 0.83, CI 0.75–0.93). These results suggest that DCIS with microinvasion should be characterized as an early invasive tumor with a good outcome and that the therapeutic approach for these patients should be similar to that for patients with invasive cancer.

However, some studies have pointed toward DCIS with microinvasion as having a more similar natural history to DCIS alone than to early-stage invasive disease. In a review of 393 patients treated at Yale between 1973 and 2004, there was no significant difference between patients with DCIS alone and those with DCIS with microinvasion with regard to the presence of axillary metastases (in those who had axillary staging) or the likelihood of recurrence (locoregional and distant) or overall survival. In a more recent study from Zheng et al., 308 cases of DCIS alone were compared to 92 cases of DCIS with microinvasion and 111 cases of T1a tumors. With a 25-month median follow-up, their analysis demonstrated no difference in disease-free survival and overall survival among the three groups.

Diagnosis
Clinical Presentation

Before the implementation of routine screening mammography, most patients with DCIS presented with a palpable mass, nipple thickening, discharge, or Paget's disease of the nipple. Occasionally, DCIS was an incidental finding in an otherwise benign breast biopsy specimen. In patients with palpable lesions, up to 25% demonstrated foci of invasive disease. Now that screening mammography is more prevalent, most cases of DCIS are

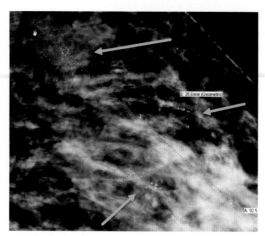

FIGURE 1.2 Calcifications seen on diagnostic mammography associated with ductal carcinoma in situ (DCIS). Magnification view is shown to demonstrate calcifications spanning approximately 9 cm.

diagnosed when the tumor is clinically occult. Patients with abnormalities detected by screening mammography should always undergo diagnostic imaging of the bilateral breasts because 0.5% to 3.0% of patients have synchronous occult abnormalities or cancers in the contralateral breast. Mammographic images should be compared with previous images, if available, to establish interval changes.

Mammographic Features

On a mammogram, DCIS can present as microcalcifications, a soft tissue density, or both (Fig. 1.2). Microcalcifications are the most common (80% to 90%) mammographic manifestation of DCIS, which accounts for 80% of all breast carcinomas presenting with calcifications. Any interval change from a previous mammogram is associated with malignancy in 15% to 20% of cases and most often indicates in situ disease. Holland et al. described two different classes of microcalcifications: (a) linear branching-type microcalcifications, which are more often associated with high nuclear-grade, comedo-type lesions; and (b) fine, granular calcifications, which are primarily associated with micropapillary or cribriform lesions of lower nuclear grade and that do not show necrosis. Although the morphology of microcalcifications suggests the architectural type of DCIS, it is not always reliable. Holland et al. also demonstrated that the mammographic findings significantly underestimated the pathologic extent of disease, particularly in cases of micropapillary DCIS. Lesions were more than 2 cm larger by histologic examination than by mammographic estimation in 44% of cases of micropapillary lesions, compared with only 12% of cases of the pure comedo subtype. However, when magnification views were used in diagnostic mammographic examination, the extent of disease was underestimated in only 14% of cases of micropapillary tumors. Hence, magnification views increase the image resolution and are better able to delineate the shape, number, and extent of microcalcifications when compared with mammography alone and should be used routinely in the evaluation of suspicious mammographic findings.

Magnetic Resonance Imaging

Mammography remains the standard for radiographic evaluation of DCIS. The cost and accessibility of magnetic resonance imaging (MRI) make it less feasible as an effective screening method. However, there is evidence that patients at high risk for breast cancer or those with very dense breasts may benefit from screening with MRI. Contrast-enhanced MRI is more sensitive than mammography in the detection of both DCIS and invasive cancer. However, fibrocystic changes and other benign findings can mimic DCIS on MRI, leading to unnecessary biopsies. MRI is increasingly being utilized after initial diagnosis in the preoperative evaluation to identify multicentric and contralateral lesions because presence of either of these may change the surgical treatment strategy. Hollingsworth et al. reported that MRI detected multicentric disease, defined as a separate focus of cancer more than 5 cm away from the index lesion or discontinuous growth in another breast quadrant, in 4.3% of 149 patients who presented with DCIS. Lehman et al. reported the utility of MRI in detecting contralateral breast cancer in a group of 969 patients with unilateral breast cancer, 196 of whom had DCIS. Of the patients with DCIS, MRI prompted additional biopsies in 18 patients. Contralateral breast cancer was detected in five patients (28% of those biopsied and 2.6% of those with DCIS). The sensitivity of detecting contralateral breast cancer was 71% and the specificity was 90%. While MRI is associated with increased likelihood of change in the surgical plan for a patient with unilateral breast cancer, it is unclear whether these altered (and usually more extensive) surgical plans are actually treating clinically significant disease that might have otherwise decreased disease-free or overall survival. In a review of over 2,300 patients with breast-conserving therapy (BCT, i.e., lumpectomy and radiation) for DCIS at Memorial Sloan Kettering between 1997 and 2010, there was no association between receipt of preoperative MRI and risk of locoregional recurrence or contralateral breast cancer, regardless of whether the patient received adjuvant radiation.

Diagnostic Biopsy

Stereotactic core-needle or vacuum-assisted biopsy is the preferred method for diagnosing DCIS. Calcifications that appear faint on mammogram or that are deep in the breast and close to the chest wall may be difficult to target with stereotactic biopsy. In addition, use of stereotactic biopsy in patients above the weight limit of the stereotactic system (approximately 150 kg) and in patients with very small breasts may be difficult. Patients who cannot remain prone or who cannot cooperate for the duration of the procedure are also not appropriate candidates for stereotactic biopsy. Bleeding disorders and the concomitant use of anticoagulants are relative contraindications. Biopsy specimens should be radiographed to document the sampling of suspicious microcalcifications. Care should be taken to mark the biopsy site with a metallic clip in the event that all microcalcifications are removed with the biopsy procedure. In the final biopsy procedure report, it is important to report the needle gauge used, how many cores were obtained, and an estimate as to what percentage of the calcifications was removed.

Because stereotactic core-needle and vacuum-assisted biopsy specimens represent only a sample of an abnormality observed on mammography, the results are subject to sampling error. Invasive carcinoma is found on excision in 20% of patients in whom DCIS was diagnosed by a stereotactic core-needle biopsy. Thus, if the core-needle biopsy results are discordant with the findings of imaging studies, a wire- or seed-localized excisional biopsy can be performed to establish the diagnosis. After diagnosis using stereotactic core-needle biopsy, approximately 20% to 30% of patients with ADH, up to 20% of patients with radial scar, and approximately 5% to 10% of patients with flat epithelial atypia (FEA) are found to have a coexistent carcinoma near the site of the biopsy when complete excision is performed. Therefore, when the final pathologic studies from core-needle biopsy procedures indicate any of these diagnoses, consideration should be made for excisional biopsy, though in the case of pure FEA, there is some evidence to suggest that surgical excision is not necessary if all calcifications are removed at the time of biopsy. Patients who are not candidates for stereotactic biopsy or who have stereotactic biopsy results that are inconclusive or discordant with the mammographic findings should undergo excisional biopsy. This technique is performed with the assistance of preoperatively performed wire or seed localization of the mammographic abnormality in conjunction with the previously placed metallic clip marking the biopsy site. Postexcision specimen radiography is essential to confirm the removal of microcalcifications or targeted lesion in addition to the marking clip if present. The excisional biopsy should be performed with the aim of obtaining a margin-negative resection that can serve as a definitive surgery.

Treatment

The diagnosis of DCIS is followed by surgical treatment with breast-conserving surgery (also referred to as segmental mastectomy, partial mastectomy, lumpectomy, or wide local excision) or mastectomy. Most patients who undergo breast-conserving surgery receive postoperative radiation therapy to improve local control. Postoperative endocrine therapy with tamoxifen or an aromatase inhibitor should also be considered for those patients whose tumors are hormone (estrogen and/or progesterone) receptor positive.

Mastectomy Versus Breast-Conserving Therapy

Historically, DCIS was treated with mastectomy. The rationale for performing total mastectomy in patients with DCIS was based on the high incidence of multifocality and multicentricity, as well as on the risk of occult invasion associated with the disease. Thus, mastectomy remains the standard against which other proposed therapeutic modalities are compared. However, in patients with DCIS, there are no prospective trials comparing outcomes after mastectomy with those after breast-conserving surgery.

In one study comparing breast-conserving therapy with mastectomy, Silverstein et al. examined 227 cases of DCIS without microinvasion. In this nonrandomized study, patients with tumors smaller than 4 cm with microscopically clear margins underwent breast-conserving surgery and radiation therapy, whereas patients with tumors larger than 4 cm or with positive margins underwent mastectomy. The rate of disease-free survival at 7 years was 98% in the mastectomy group compared with 84% in the breast-conserving surgery group

($p = .04$), with no difference in overall survival rates. In a meta-analysis from 1999, Boyages et al. reported a recurrence rate of 22.5%, 8.9%, and 1.4% following breast-conserving surgery alone, breast-conserving surgery with radiation therapy, and mastectomy, respectively. In patients who underwent breast-conserving surgery alone, approximately 50% of the recurrences were invasive cancers. These older studies are of historical interest as there have been significant improvements in imaging techniques and pathologic assessment with overall lower rates of local recurrence with breast-conserving surgery.

A more recent meta-analysis from 2015 by Stuart et al. included 9,404 cases of DCIS with 10-year follow-up and demonstrated a local recurrence rate (LRR) for mastectomy to be 2.6% (CI 0.8–4.5), while the LRR for breast-conserving surgery with radiotherapy was 13.6% (CI 9.8–17.4), and breast-conserving therapy with radiation and tamoxifen was 9.7% (CI 4.4–15.0). Although recurrence rates are higher in patients who undergo breast-conserving surgery than in patients who undergo mastectomy, no survival advantage has been shown for patients treated with mastectomy.

Technique of Breast-Conserving Surgery

The goal of breast-conserving surgery is to remove all suspicious calcifications or radiographic abnormalities and obtain negative surgical margins. Because DCIS is usually nonpalpable, breast-conserving surgery can be performed with mammographically or sonographically guided placement of a localizing wire or seed. Seed localization of nonpalpable breast lesions is increasingly used in the US and—through multidisciplinary collaboration with surgeons, radiologists, and pathologists—has the advantage of allowing a marker to be placed at a time that is uncoupled from the time of surgery. At most centers where seed localization is performed, the seed is placed by a radiologist within the area of disease in much the same way wire localization has historically been performed. The seed is localized intraoperatively using a probe to detect the signal from the seed, and the surrounding tissue is excised. Resection of the seed, lesion, and previously placed clip are confirmed intraoperatively by pathologic and radiologic review. There are numerous methods of seed localization including radioactive and nonradioactive technologies.

Data from Piotrowski et al. has shown that labeling a breast specimen on three surfaces (e.g., superior, lateral and posterior) for pathologic assessment was superior to only labeling two surfaces and resulted in a 65% reduction in need for reorientation by the surgeon in the pathology suite (OR 0.35 CI 0.16–0.75). In addition, specimen radiography is essential to confirm the removal of all microcalcifications or other radiographic abnormalities. In patients with extensive calcifications, bracketing of the calcifications with two or more seeds or wires may assist in the excision of all suspicious calcifications.

After whole-specimen radiography, the specimen should be inked and then serially sectioned for pathologic examination to evaluate the margin status and extent of disease. Chagpar et al. demonstrated that intraoperative margin assessment with the use of sectioned-specimen radiography enabled re-excisions to be performed at the same surgery if the microcalcifications extended to the cut edge of the specimen, minimizing the need for second procedures for margin control. After margins are deemed adequate intraoperatively, the boundary of the resection cavity is marked with radiopaque clips to aid in the planning of postoperative radiation therapy and to facilitate mammographic follow-up.

The goal of breast-conserving surgery is to obtain tumor-free margins. A detailed pathologic study of DCIS, reported in 1990 by Holland et al., demonstrated that up to 44% of lesions extended more than 2 cm further on histologic examination than that estimated by mammography. However, in most women, a 1- to 2-cm margin around a lesion is not feasible in breast conservation as this may result in a poor cosmetic result. National consensus guidelines dictate that close (<1-mm) margins are inadequate for DCIS and should be re-excised, but for patients in whom the border of disease is the fibroglandular boundary such as the chest wall or skin, radiation with a boost to the surgical scar is an acceptable alternative to re-excision. As noted above, SSO, ASTRO, and ASCO convened a panel to review literature concerning margin width and ipsilateral breast tumor recurrence (IBTR) in patients with DCIS undergoing breast-conserving therapy. The meta-analysis included 20 studies with 7,883 patients and 865 IBTRs with a median follow-up of 78.3 months. The panel reported that positive margins were associated with a twofold increased risk of IBTR compared with patients who had negative margins. They also reported that margins of at least 2 mm were associated with a lower risk of IBTR compared with narrower margins. Patients treated with wide local excision alone without radiation therapy had substantially higher rates of IBTR compared with patients undergoing wide local excision and whole-breast irradiation (WBI) regardless of the margin width. Rates of IBTR and contralateral breast cancer were reduced in patients who received tamoxifen, however, there was no significant impact on IBTR in patients with negative margins when compared with patients receiving placebo. The panel concluded that a 2-mm margin was adequate in patients undergoing breast-conserving surgery and WBI for DCIS. Clinical judgment should be utilized in deciding on the need for re-excision in patients with margins <2 mm on final pathology.

Radiation Therapy

Most patients with DCIS who undergo breast-conserving surgery should receive postoperative radiation therapy to reduce IBTR. Five prospective randomized studies have evaluated the role of radiation therapy following breast-conserving surgery for DCIS. In the National Surgical Adjuvant Breast and Bowel Project (NSABP) B-17 trial, 818 women with localized DCIS enrolled from 1985 to 1990 and were randomized to breast-conserving surgery or breast-conserving surgery plus radiation therapy after margin-negative resections. At a follow-up time of 12 years, radiation therapy was associated with a reduction in the cumulative incidence of noninvasive ipsilateral breast tumors from 14.6% to 8% and with a reduction in the incidence of invasive ipsilateral breast tumors from 16.8% to 7.7%. After 15 years, radiation therapy was associated with a reduction in the cumulative incidence of noninvasive ipsilateral breast tumors from 15.7% to 8.8% (HR 0.53, CI 0.35–0.80) and a reduction in the incidence of invasive ipsilateral breast tumors from 19.4% to 8.9% (HR 0.48, CI 0.33–0.69). There was no difference in the 15-year overall survival rate in the two groups.

The overall benefit of radiation therapy for patients with DCIS was also observed in the European Organization for Research and Treatment of Cancer (EORTC) 10853 trial. In this trial, 1,010 women with DCIS treated between 1986 and 1996 were randomized to breast-conserving surgery or breast-conserving surgery plus radiation therapy. Initially, at a median follow-up time of 4.25 years, radiation therapy was associated with a reduction in the incidence of noninvasive ipsilateral breast tumors from 8.8% to 5.8% and with a reduction in the incidence of invasive ipsilateral breast tumors from 8.0% to 4.8%. The lower recurrence rates in this trial when compared with those in NSABP B-17 were attributed to the shorter follow-up time. However, at 15 years, radiation therapy was associated with a reduction in noninvasive recurrence from 16% to 8% (HR 0.49, CI 0.33–0.73) and in invasive recurrence from 16% to 10% (HR 0.61, CI 0.42–0.87), demonstrating rates of recurrence and magnitudes of risk reduction similar to those observed in long-term follow-up of patients in the NSABP B-17 trial. Likewise, there was no difference in the 15-year overall survival rate between the two groups.

A third trial, conducted by the United Kingdom (UK) Coordinating Committee on Cancer Research, enrolled 1,701 women from the UK, Australia, and New Zealand, between 1990 and 1998. This trial confirmed the benefits of radiation therapy for local control. After margin-negative lumpectomy, patients were randomized to one of three arms: (1) no adjuvant treatment, (2) adjuvant radiation therapy or tamoxifen, or (3) adjuvant radiation therapy plus tamoxifen. After a median follow-up time of 4.4 years, there was a reduction in the incidence of noninvasive ipsilateral breast tumors from 7% to 3% (HR 0.36, CI 0.19–0.66) and a reduction in the incidence of invasive ipsilateral tumors from 6% to 3% (HR 0.45, 0.24 to 0.85) when those who received radiation were compared to those who did not. After a median follow-up of 12.7 years, radiation continued to be associated with a reduced incidence of both ipsilateral DCIS (HR 0.38, CI 0.22–0.63) and ipsilateral invasive disease (HR 0.32, CI 0.19–0.56).

The Radiation Therapy Oncology Group (RTOG) 9804 trial was a US and Canadian trial that randomized patients with low- or intermediate-grade DCIS less than 25 mm and excised with margins of at least 3 mm to postoperative radiation therapy or observation with the option of tamoxifen use in each group. The trial was closed early due to poor accrual, with only 636 patients enrolled between 1998 and 2006 instead of the 1,790 participants that had been planned. In a recent update, the 15-year cumulative incidence of ipsilateral breast tumor recurrence (IBTR) was 7.1% in the cohort that had radiation and 15.1% in the observation group ($p <$ .001). The 15-year cumulative incidence for invasive local recurrence was 5.6% in the radiation group versus 9.5% in the observation group ($p =$ .03).

Finally, in the SweDCIS trial, 1,046 women diagnosed with DCIS between 1987 and 1999 were randomized to either be observed or to receive adjuvant radiation therapy after lumpectomy. At 20-year follow-up, radiation therapy reduced the risk of local recurrence by 37.5%, though breast cancer–specific death and overall survival were the same between the irradiated and observed cohorts.

Taken together, these five prospective randomized trials demonstrate that the addition of radiation therapy following breast-conserving therapy for DCIS results in an approximately 50% relative reduction in breast cancer recurrence but does not impact disease-specific or overall survival.

WBI has been the standard for patients undergoing breast-conserving surgery and is generally well tolerated. The most common morbidity is radiation-induced skin change including discoloration, fibrosis, and telangiectasia. Rare, severe side effects include damage to the heart and lungs, and development of angiosarcoma, a radiation-associated secondary malignancy.

Partial Breast Irradiation

In patients not receiving radiation therapy, local recurrences in the breast tend to occur in the immediate vicinity of the surgical resection cavity. Hence, the main effect of WBI is likely the reduction of local recurrence in the immediate area surrounding the original tumor bed. Therefore, some have suggested that equivalent local control can be achieved by using partial breast irradiation, which focuses the treatment on the tissue surrounding the surgical resection cavity. Accelerated partial breast irradiation (APBI) is a technique where high-dose radiation is delivered over a shorter period of time to a limited region of the breast surrounding the primary tumor site. The treatment is completed over 4 to 5 days, whereas conventional whole-breast external beam radiation therapy typically requires 4 to 6 weeks. Several methods of partial breast irradiation have been described, including brachytherapy via multiple catheters placed in the breast parenchyma, localized conformal three-dimensional external beam radiation therapy (3D-XRT), brachytherapy via bead or seed implants, single-dose intraoperative radiation therapy, and brachytherapy via a balloon catheter inserted into the cavity after breast-conserving surgery.

In 2010, Jeruss et al. presented results from the American Society of Breast Surgeons (ASBS) APBI Registry Trial. Of 194 enrolled patients with DCIS, 63 had at least 5 years of follow-up and of these, 92% had favorable cosmetic results. The 5-year locoregional recurrence rate of 3.39% compared favorably with the rate of 7.5% reported using whole-breast radiation in the NSABP B-17 trial. The NSABP B-39/RTOG 0413 trial, which opened in 2005, was a randomized phase III multicenter trial developed to determine whether patients who received APBI via 3D-XRT, brachytherapy, or single-entry intracavitary delivery had rates of local control comparable to those of patients who received conventional WBI. Enrollment was limited to women with no more than 3 cm of DCIS or invasive stage I or II breast cancer and limited nodal disease (≤3 lymph nodes) who underwent margin-negative lumpectomy with endocrine therapy and chemotherapy administered at the discretion of their treating physician. There were 2,109 patients assigned to the WBI group (513 with DCIS) and 2,107 assigned to the APBI group (518 with DCIS). The primary endpoint was invasive and noninvasive IBTR, and the secondary endpoints were disease-free and overall survival, cosmetic results, and treatment toxicity. There were 90 (4%) women in the APBI group that developed an IBTR compared to 71 (3%) women in the WBI group (HR 1.22, 90% CI 0.94–1.58). Based on this finding, the authors concluded that APBI did not meet equivalence criteria to WBI in controlling IBTR for breast-conserving therapy. There were no significant differences between APBI and WBI for distant disease-free interval or overall survival. The authors also concluded that the trial was not designed to test equivalence in patient subgroups, but did report that 5.8% of patients with DCIS in the WBI group had an IBTR compared to 6.2% of patients with DCIS in the APBI group (HR 1.01, 95% CI 0.61–1.68).

Omitting Radiation Therapy

A survey by Jagsi et al. demonstrated that 95% of women with breast cancer and strong indications for post-lumpectomy radiation went on to receive it, but rates of postlumpectomy radiation therapy use have been shown to vary, depending on the region of the country in which the patient lives, the age of the patient, and the disease being treated. Among patients who undergo breast-conserving surgery for DCIS, only 50% are estimated to receive adjuvant radiation.

Some patients choose mastectomy over breast-conserving surgery for DCIS because they are not able or willing to complete adjuvant radiation therapy secondary to social or health considerations. Other patients who are candidates for breast-conserving surgery choose to undergo a mastectomy because of concerns about postradiation complications. Breast-conserving surgery alone (without radiation therapy) may be sufficient in a select subgroup of patients with DCIS. Initial data that supported the use of breast-conserving surgery alone in the treatment of DCIS came from a study by Lagios et al. in 1989 in which 79 patients with mammographically detected DCIS underwent margin-negative excision alone. After a follow-up time of 124 months, the local recurrence rate was 16% overall, specifically, 33% for the subgroup of patients with high-grade lesions and comedonecrosis versus only 2% for the patients with low- or intermediate-grade lesions. In a retrospective analysis of 469 patients with DCIS who underwent breast conservation with margins that were at least 10 mm, Silverstein et al. did not detect a lower recurrence rate when postoperative radiation therapy was employed.

In contrast, even on reanalysis of the NSABP B-17 data, all patient cohorts benefited from radiation therapy, regardless of the clinical or mammographic tumor characteristics. Furthermore, Wong et al. reported the early termination of a prospective single-arm trial conducted at the Dana-Farber/Harvard Cancer Center in 2014 in which radiation therapy was omitted in patients with grade 1 or 2 DCIS that was no more than 25-mm and excised with 10-mm or greater margins. At a median follow-up of 3.3 years, the number of local recurrences observed was 2.5% per patient-year, corresponding to a 5-year rate of 12.5%.

In 2010, Rudloff and colleagues at Memorial Sloan Kettering published a multivariable nomogram to estimate risk for local recurrence in women with DCIS treated with breast-conserving surgery. The nomogram incorporates commonly available factors that have previously been shown to affect risk of IBTR. These include age at diagnosis, family history, type of patient presentation (radiologic or clinical), nuclear grade, necrosis, margins, number of excisions, and receipt of radiation and/or adjuvant endocrine therapy. The nomogram calculates an actual, individualized estimate of absolute risk of IBTR at 5 and 10 years, which can be weighed against the use of available adjuvant treatment options.

In addition to the five clinical trials discussed earlier, there are two large, prospective, observational studies designed to investigate the role of observation versus radiation therapy after breast-conserving therapy in patients with DCIS. As mentioned earlier, Wong and colleagues at Harvard conducted a single-arm, phase III observational study examining long-term outcomes in women with small (≤25-mm), low- and intermediate-grade DCIS who were treated with lumpectomy and margins ≥10 mm and did not receive adjuvant tamoxifen or radiation. With a median follow-up of 11 years, 13% (19 of 143) of patients experienced local recurrence, approximately two-thirds of which were DCIS. In the Eastern Cooperative Oncology Group–American College of Radiology Imaging Network (ECOG-ACRIN; formerly known as the Eastern Cooperative Oncology Group) Cancer Research Group E5194 study, patients with low- or intermediate-grade DCIS smaller than 25 mm (cohort 1), or high-grade DCIS smaller than 10 mm (cohort 2), with excisional margins of at least 3 mm, underwent breast-conserving surgery without radiation therapy; 30% of patients received tamoxifen. At 12 years, 14.4% of the participants in cohort 1 experienced an in-breast event, while 24.6% of those in cohort 2 experienced an in-breast event ($p < .001$), and this overall effect was driven by a significant difference in noninvasive recurrence ($p = .02$). In addition, patients in cohort 2 with a larger tumor size had an increased likelihood of recurrence.

Endocrine Therapy

Two prospective randomized trials have evaluated the effect of tamoxifen on outcome in patients with DCIS treated with breast-conserving therapy. In the NSABP B-24 trial, 1,804 women with DCIS were randomly assigned to breast-conserving surgery and radiation therapy followed by either tamoxifen at 20 mg/day or a placebo for 5 years. Sixteen percent of the women in this study had positive resection margins. At 7 years of follow-up, women who received tamoxifen had fewer breast cancer events than did the placebo group (10.0% vs. 16.9%). Among those who received tamoxifen, the rate of ipsilateral invasive breast cancer was 2.6% at 7 years compared with 5.3% in the control group. Tamoxifen also decreased the 7-year cumulative incidence of contralateral breast neoplasms (invasive and noninvasive) to 2.3% compared with 4.9% in the control group. The benefit of tamoxifen therapy also extended to patients with positive margins or margins of unknown status. There was no difference in the 7-year overall survival rate, which was 95% in both the tamoxifen and the placebo groups. Most deaths occurred before recurrence developed and were not necessarily related to breast cancer. A subgroup analysis based on retrospectively determined estrogen receptor (ER) status, indicated that women with ER-positive (ER+) DCIS who received tamoxifen had over 50% reduction in their relative risk of subsequent breast cancer at 10 years when compared with those who received placebo. Among patients with ER-negative (ER−) DCIS, there was no added benefit from tamoxifen.

In the United Kingdom Coordinating Committee on Cancer Research trial, radiation therapy had the greatest impact on reducing ipsilateral breast cancer events after approximately 4 years of follow-up, whereas tamoxifen added to radiation therapy did not result in significant additional benefit. However, the relatively short follow-up time and complex design of this trial made direct comparison of the initial results to those of the NSABP B-24 trial difficult. In a subsequent analysis of the UK trial for which median follow-up was 12.7 years, tamoxifen was found to have reduced the incidence of all new breast events (HR 0.71, CI 0.58–0.88), a finding that was driven by a significant reduction in both recurrent ipsilateral DCIS (HR 0.70, CI 0.51–0.86) and contralateral invasive and noninvasive tumors (HR 0.44, CI 0.25–0.77); there was no effect on ipsilateral invasive disease (HR 0.95, CI 0.66–1.38).

Endocrine therapy should be reserved for patients with ER+ tumors. The use of tamoxifen has been associated with vasomotor symptoms, deep vein thrombosis, pulmonary embolism, and increased cataract formation. The risk of endometrial cancer is increased two to seven times among patients who receive the drug. Tamoxifen is also associated with increased rates of stroke and benign ovarian cysts. Accordingly, although tamoxifen plays an important role in the adjuvant treatment of DCIS, better-tolerated alternatives have been the subject of ongoing investigation.

Aromatase inhibitors have been shown to be beneficial in the adjuvant treatment of invasive breast cancer in postmenopausal women with ER+ disease. These agents have fewer cardiovascular side effects than tamoxifen and may be beneficial in the adjuvant treatment of patients with DCIS following breast-conserving surgery. Two randomized prospective clinical trials opened in 2003—NSABP B-35 and the International Breast Cancer Intervention Study (IBIS-II)—to compare the adjuvant use of tamoxifen versus the aromatase inhibitor anastrozole (Arimidex) following breast-conserving surgery in patients with a diagnosis of DCIS.

NSABP-35 was a phase III, double-blinded controlled trial that randomized over 3,000 patients with DCIS from 333 US and Canadian centers treated between 2003 and 2006 to receive either 20 mg of tamoxifen every day or 1 mg anastrozole every day for 5 years. After a median follow-up of 9 years, there were 122 interval events (defined as local, regional, or distant recurrence, or contralateral breast cancer, invasive disease, or DCIS) in the tamoxifen cohort and 90 events among those who received anastrozole (HR 0.73, CI 0.56–0.96), with anastrozole being superior to tamoxifen only in women younger than 60. Rates of venous thromboembolic events were higher among those who received tamoxifen.

IBIS-II was a phase III, double-blinded randomized controlled trial that enrolled postmenopausal women aged 40 to 70 years old from 18 countries over the course of 9 years, from 2003 to 2012. Participants were randomized to receive either daily anastrozole 1 mg or placebo for 5 years. After a median follow-up of 5 years, 40 women in the anastrozole group (2%) and 85 in the placebo group (4%) developed breast cancer (HR 0.47, CI 0.32–0.68), representing a >50% reduction in risk for those taking anastrozole.

These two trials demonstrate that anastrozole is a reasonable alternative to tamoxifen for adjuvant treatment of ER+ DCIS in postmenopausal women, though additional investigation is warranted to assess the safety and efficacy of other aromatase inhibitors in this setting.

Active Surveillance

As previously discussed, much of the increased incidence in DCIS is likely due to increased detection of DCIS subtypes of unclear long-term significance. Given the speculation that we may be overtreating low-risk DCIS, there are two ongoing trials and one closed trial designed to examine whether some patients with DCIS can be spared any form of locoregional or systemic treatment. LORD (LOw Risk DCIS) is a multicenter, international, noninferiority trial launched by the European Organisation for Research and Treatment of Cancer (EORTC) in January 2017. The trial compares two strategies for management of low-grade DCIS: for the experimental arm, patients only receive active surveillance with annual mammography and do not receive any locoregional or endocrine therapy, while in the comparator arm, patients receive standard surgical treatment—which can consist of breast-conserving surgery only, breast-conserving surgery and radiation, or mastectomy—with or without endocrine therapy. The Comparing an Operation to Monitoring, With or Without Endocrine Therapy (COMET) Trial For Low Risk DCIS (COMET) is based in the US and received federal funding in 2016. Participants are randomized to either undergo standard of care treatment (including surgery and radiation) or active surveillance, with participants in both arms free to choose endocrine therapy. The LORIS (Low Risk DCIS) trial was a similar phase III trial in the UK comparing active surveillance with surgery for low- and intermediate-grade DCIS. The trial completed accruing patients in March 2020 and results are still pending.

It will be several years before data from these trials are available. In the interim, retrospective cohort studies have been performed to evaluate the outcomes in patients with DCIS undergoing active surveillance. Ryser et al. used the US National Cancer Institute's Surveillance, Epidemiology, and End Results (SEER) program database to identify 1,286 patients with DCIS who did not undergo locoregional therapy from 1992 to 2014. This study demonstrated that among women with low-grade (1/2) DCIS, the 10-year net risk of ipsilateral invasive breast cancer was 12.2%. Women with high-grade (3) DCIS had a 10-year net risk for ipsilateral invasive breast cancer of 17.6%. Sun et al. also used the SEER database to compare the risk of developing ipsilateral invasive breast cancer in patients with low-risk DCIS who had no treatment versus surgical excision with or without radiation. They found that in women <50 years old, having breast-conserving surgery only (HR 0.21, CI 0.10–0.44) or breast-conserving surgery with radiation (HR 0.13, CI 0.07–0.27) was associated with decreased risk of invasive cancer compared with no treatment. Results were similar for the women who were 50 to 69 years old (BCS only: HR 0.38, CI 0.21–0.69; BCS and RT: HR 0.1, CI 0.08–0.27). However, in women aged 70 years or older, there was no statistically significant difference between the no treatment group and surgery groups, suggesting that active surveillance may not increase the risk of ipsilateral invasive cancer in older women.

Nodal Staging

Because DCIS is a noninvasive disease, lymph node involvement is not expected. Indeed, if a patient presents with DCIS in the breast but is found to have cancer in the lymph nodes preoperatively, the patient has, by definition, invasive breast cancer and not DCIS alone. In cases where patients have large tumors (>4 cm) or extensive microcalcifications, a focus of invasion can be missed because of limited pathologic sampling (as discussed earlier, a 20% to 30% rate of concomitant invasive cancers has been reported on final pathology in patients who were diagnosed with DCIS on stereotactic core needle biopsy). Such patients, as well as those with high-grade or palpable disease, are at higher risk for lymph node metastasis and may also warrant sentinel lymph node (SLN) mapping, particularly if they are undergoing mastectomy or if breast-conserving surgery is to be followed by oncoplastic tissue rearrangement. The risk of missing disease in the lymph nodes must be weighed against the risk of lymphedema associated with SLN dissection in each patient. In a study by Cox et al., the combination of hematoxylin–eosin staining and immunohistochemistry revealed that 6% of patients with newly diagnosed DCIS had metastatic disease in the sentinel nodes. Klauber-DeMore et al. found that SLNs were positive for cancer in 12% of patients with DCIS considered to be at high risk for invasion and in 10% of patients who had DCIS with microinvasion. In a study from the MD Anderson Cancer Center, Francis et al. examined the incidence of positive nodes and the clinical significance of these findings in 1,234 patients with an initial diagnosis of DCIS planned for SLN dissection. There were positive findings in the SLNs in 132 (10.7%) patients. The findings included isolated tumor cells in 66 (5.4%) patients, micrometastases in 36 (2.9%), and macrometastases in 30 (2.4%). There was upstaging of the primary tumor in 327 (26.5%) patients to microinvasion or invasive cancer. Factors predicting a positive SLN were diagnosis by excisional biopsy, papillary histology, DCIS >2 cm, more than three interventions prior to SLN dissection (needle biopsy, excisional biopsy, etc.), microinvasion, or invasive cancer. It was noted that with increasing numbers of preoperative interventions (biopsy, needle localization, etc.), there was a higher likelihood of positive SLN findings with the majority being isolated tumor cells (44/907, 4.2%) or micrometastases (12/907, 1.3%). There were no macrometastases identified in the SLNs of patients with DCIS alone. The high incidence of isolated tumor cells in SLNs of patients with increasing preoperative interventions supports the concept of benign mechanical transport of epithelial cells during manipulation of the primary tumor. At a median follow-up of 61.7 months, there was no difference in disease-free survival outcomes in the patients with DCIS alone with or without positive SLN findings. In general terms, SLN dissection should be limited to patients who undergo mastectomy for large, high-grade DCIS because it is difficult to perform lymphatic mapping (discussed along with sentinel node biopsy in Chapter 2) after a mastectomy if invasive cancer is found on final pathology in the mastectomy specimen.

Predictors of Local Recurrence

Several features of DCIS are associated with a less favorable clinical course. Pathologic variables, such as large tumor size (>3 cm), high nuclear grade, comedo-type necrosis, and positive margins are associated with a greater risk of local recurrence. Involved margins of resection constitute the most important independent prognostic variable for predicting local recurrence. Molecular markers, such as overexpression of HER-2/*neu*, nm23, heat shock protein, and metallothionein; low expression of p21, Waf1, and Bcl2; and DNA aneuploidy have been reported to be associated with high-grade comedo lesions, but their importance as independent prognostic variables in DCIS has not been clarified.

In 2011, Solin et al. presented the results of a study examining the prognostic efficacy of Oncotype Dx DCIS, a 12-gene molecular assay modeled on Oncotype DX, which is a 21-gene assay used to assess the likelihood that a given patient's ER+ invasive breast cancer will recur within 10 years of diagnosis and to what extent said patient might be expected to benefit from receiving adjuvant chemotherapy in addition to endocrine therapy. As with Oncotype DX, Oncotype Dx DCIS stratifies patients into three score-based tiers: low risk (<39); intermediate risk (39 to 54); and high risk (≥55). Using a new, prespecified algorithm that had been optimized for DCIS gene expression, tissue samples from 650 women in the ECOG-ACRIN E5194 trial were tested, and higher Oncotype Dx DCIS Score™ was found to be associated with increased likelihood of both overall (invasive and noninvasive, HR 2.34, CI 1.15–4.59) and invasive-only (HR 3.73, CI 1.34–9.82) ipsilateral breast events at 10 years. However, since the E5194 cohort was, by design, biased toward low-risk DCIS phenotypes, additional validation was sought. Rakovitch and colleagues subsequently validated Oncotype Dx DCIS in a cohort of 2,720 women with a more diverse distribution of DCIS clinicopathologic characteristics and who had been treated with breast-conserving surgery +/− radiation therapy. The DCIS score was associated with increased risk of both invasive (HR 1.78, CI 1.03–3.05) and noninvasive (HR 2.43, CI 1.31–4.42) local recurrence regardless of ER status, though, notably, 94.7% of participants had ER+ disease. Oncotype Dx DCIS holds promise as a clinical decision-making tool in the management of DCIS, but further prospective validation is warranted.

Another biosignature, DCISionRT (PreludeDx), was developed to prognosticate the 10-year total and invasive recurrence risk after breast-conserving surgery for DCIS and then predict an individual patient's benefit from radiation therapy. The decision score from the DCISionRT test is calculated from seven IHC-evaluated biomarkers and four clinicopathologic factors. In a validation study from Bremer et al, higher "decision scores" were calculated from tissue blocks of women treated for DCIS from 1986 to 2008. The authors demonstrated that an "Elevated Risk Group" based on their decision score received significant radiation therapy benefit (invasive breast event HR 0.3, P = .003; ipsilateral breast event HR 0.3, P < .001). Again, prospective validation of this tool is needed to determine if the DCISionRT test can identify a subset of women that would not benefit from radiation therapy.

Treatment and Outcome of Local Recurrence

The overall survival rate in patients with DCIS is excellent. In the NSABP B-17 trial, only 27 deaths (3.3%) attributed to breast cancer occurred after a median follow-up time of 12 years. In the NSABP B-24 trial, 0.8% of the patients died as a consequence of their breast cancer after 7 years of follow-up. In both trials and in several other studies, approximately 50% of all local recurrences were invasive cancers, and risk of recurrence was greatest within the first 5 years after treatment. The management of local recurrence depends on the therapy the patient received for the primary cancer. In cases of local recurrence in patients who underwent breast-conserving surgery without radiation therapy, re-excision with negative margins and postoperative radiation therapy are recommended. For patients who have recurrent breast cancer after receiving breast-conserving surgery and radiation therapy, mastectomy is the preferred treatment. If the recurrent tumor is invasive, staging of the axillary nodes is performed with lymphatic mapping and SLN dissection.

The prognosis after treatment of local recurrence depends on whether the recurrence is invasive or noninvasive. Silverstein et al. found that among patients with invasive recurrences, the 8-year disease-specific mortality rate was 14.4%, and the distant disease probability was 27.1%. In a follow-up study, Romero et al. reported a 10-year disease-specific mortality rate of 15% in patients with invasive recurrence. Although most patients with recurrent disease after DCIS do survive, an invasive recurrence is a serious event. In a retrospective study from MD Anderson, Roses et al. followed 2,449 patients with a diagnosis of DCIS to determine the incidence of the development of metastatic disease. There were 16 patients who developed an invasive local–regional recurrence who also had synchronous or subsequent metastatic disease. There were nine patients who did not have a local or regional recurrence but developed metastatic disease. Given the small sample size of the patients that developed metastatic disease, the authors were not able to find factors associated with the risk of metastatic disease after a diagnosis of DCIS. Patients with DCIS should undergo long-term follow-up for both recurrent disease and development of new ipsilateral or contralateral primary tumors.

Surveillance

Guidelines from the ASCO recommend that a mammogram be obtained 6 months after the completion of radiation therapy to establish a new baseline. Follow-up of patients after breast-conserving surgery with or without radiation therapy should include annual or biannual physical examination and annual mammography for the first 5 years, with an annual physical examination and mammogram thereafter. The most recent national treatment guidelines recommend a physical examination every 6 months for 5 years and annually thereafter. Whether these measures improve the detection of recurrence and outcome is not known. Both patients who undergo breast-conserving therapy and those who undergo mastectomy should be monitored for the development of new primary cancers in the contralateral breast. The risk of development of a new primary cancer in the contralateral breast after treatment of DCIS is two to five times greater than the risk of development of a first primary breast cancer and is approximately the same as the risk of development of a new contralateral primary cancer after invasive cancer.

Current Management of DCIS at The University of Texas MD Anderson Cancer Center

An algorithm for the current treatment of DCIS at MD Anderson Cancer Center is outlined in Figure 1.3. Annual updates can be found at https://www.mdanderson.org/for-physicians/clinical-tools-resources/clinical-practice-algorithms/cancer-treatment-algorithms.html. Patients diagnosed with a mammographic abnormality undergo bilateral diagnostic mammography, and the mammograms are compared with previous images, if available. Magnification views are routinely used to delineate the abnormality in the index breast. Ultrasound can also be used to assess tumor size, multicentricity, and nodal status. Diagnostic biopsy is performed by using a vacuum-assisted stereotactic core-needle biopsy technique. When DCIS is diagnosed, the pathologic evaluation details the tumor type and grade, any evidence of microinvasion, and the status of both the estrogen and the progesterone receptors. HER2/*neu* amplification or overexpression is not routinely assessed, as its presence has unknown clinical significance in noninvasive breast cancer. MRI is not routinely employed in the preoperative evaluation of patients with DCIS. The decision to use MRI is based on the density of the breasts, findings on mammographic and sonographic imaging, and clinical judgment.

The choice of surgical therapy for an individual patient is based on several factors, including tumor size and grade, margin width, mammographic appearance, and patient preference. The benefits and risks of breast-conserving surgery and mastectomy should be discussed in detail with each patient. Most patients with DCIS are candidates for breast-conserving therapy, and this tends to be the preferred method of local treatment since it offers similar overall survival outcomes compared with mastectomy. Mastectomy is indicated in patients with diffuse, malignant-appearing calcifications in the breast and/or persistent positive

Note: Consider Clinical Trials as treatment options for eligible patients.

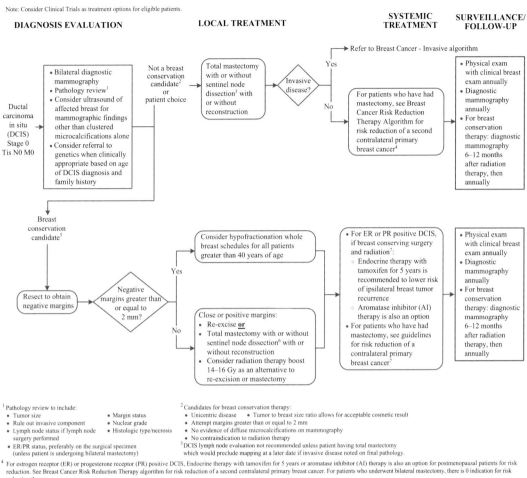

FIGURE 1.3 Management algorithm of ductal carcinoma in situ (DCIS) at MD Anderson Cancer Center. Pathology review includes tumor size, histologic type, margin status, nuclear grade, and estrogen and progesterone receptor status, as well as ruling out an invasive component and lymph node status if lymph node surgery is performed. Candidates for breast-conserving surgery are those with unicentric disease, whose ratio of tumor size to breast size allows for an acceptable cosmetic result with resection margins greater than or equal to 2 mm, no evidence of diffuse microcalcifications on mammography, and no contraindications to radiotherapy. Lymph node evaluation for patients with DCIS is not recommended unless patients are planned for total mastectomy which would preclude mapping at a later date if invasive disease noted on final pathology. When available, clinical trials are the preferred option for eligible patients. (Copyright 2020 The University of Texas MD Anderson Cancer Center.)

margins after attempts at surgical excision, and those with a contraindication to postoperative radiation therapy. Although tumor size is not an absolute indication for mastectomy, mastectomy is often preferred for patients with large (>4 cm in diameter), high-grade DCIS depending on the breast-to-tumor size ratio. There are few data available on the efficacy of breast-conserving surgery for DCIS with index lesions greater than 4 cm in diameter. Mastectomy may also be a better choice when a patient's anxiety over the possibility of recurrence outweighs the impact a mastectomy would have on her quality of life. Immediate breast reconstruction should be considered for all patients who require or elect mastectomy. Intraoperative margin assessment with sectioned-specimen radiography is used in patients undergoing breast-conserving surgery and for patients with extensive calcifications undergoing skin-sparing or nipple-sparing mastectomy. Re-excision is usually recommended for patients who have margins less than 2 mm on final pathologic examination after breast-conserving surgery.

Patients who undergo mastectomy for DCIS routinely undergo intraoperative lymphatic mapping and SLN dissection. In patients who undergo breast-conserving surgery, SLN dissection is performed on an individual basis and primarily reserved for cases where the DCIS is palpable, very large or is high grade, or exhibits comedo-type necrosis.

Adjuvant radiation therapy is recommended to reduce the risk of local recurrence in patients who undergo breast-conserving surgery. Breast-conserving surgery alone (without radiation therapy) is considered for select patients with small (<1 cm in diameter), low-grade lesions that have been excised with margins of at least 5 to 10 mm, occur in women of advanced age with short (<15-year) life expectancy, and can be observed diligently for recurrence. Partial breast irradiation and hypofractionated regimens are offered for selected patients. Endocrine therapy is offered for 5 years to women with ER+ DCIS who do not have a history of venous thromboembolism or stroke.

Following surgical resection, patients undergo annual physical and clinical breast examinations. Patients who undergo breast-conserving surgery and radiation therapy are recommended to have a diagnostic mammogram 6 months after the completion of radiation therapy and annual bilateral mammograms thereafter. If a mastectomy is performed, the patient is followed with an annual diagnostic mammogram of the contralateral breast.

High-Risk Premalignant Conditions

The multistep model for breast carcinogenesis suggests that invasive carcinomas arise from preinvasive hyperplastic and neoplastic proliferations. These early proliferative lesions have taken on greater significance as a result of mammographic screening and detection programs. Pathologists are encountering these proliferative lesions with increasing frequency, and this has highlighted deficiencies in classification systems as well as a lack of data on natural history, making clinical management a challenge.

Lobular Neoplasia: Lobular Carcinoma In Situ and Atypical Lobular Hyperplasia

LCIS was first described in 1941. During the era that followed, the treatment of LCIS was the same as that of invasive carcinoma which included radical mastectomy. Haagensen et al. is credited with altering the treatment philosophy for LCIS. In a review of 211 cases, a 17% incidence of subsequent invasive carcinoma was found among women with LCIS treated with observation alone (without surgery). The risk of developing a subsequent carcinoma was equal for both breasts, and only six patients died of breast cancer. Haagensen concluded that close observation for LCIS allowed for early detection of subsequent malignancy with associated high cure rates. Haagensen's rationale for observation of LCIS was based on his view that patients with LCIS were at increased risk for invasive breast cancer but that LCIS itself did not progress into a malignancy.

Today, LCIS is not considered a preinvasive lesion but rather an indicator for increased breast cancer risk of approximately 1% per year, or approximately 20% to 30% at 15 years. The cancer that develops may be invasive ductal or lobular and may occur in either breast. It is, in many instances, multicentric or multifocal as well as bilateral, with LCIS identified in the contralateral breast in anywhere from 30% to 90% of cases.

Epidemiology

The incidence of LCIS is difficult to estimate because the diagnosis is most often made as an incidental finding. LCIS is often not detectable by palpation, gross pathologic examination, or mammography. On evaluation of mammographic abnormalities, LCIS is found in 0.5% to 1.3% of breast core-needle biopsy specimens and 0.5% to 3.9% of excisional breast biopsy specimens. Traditionally, LCIS was more commonly reported in premenopausal women than in postmenopausal women. In Haagensen's series, 90% of the patients were premenopausal. However, in a review of the Surveillance, Epidemiology, and End Results program database, Li et al. reported that from 1978 to 1998, the incidence of LCIS increased in all age groups, but it increased the most in women 50 to 79 years old. The reason for this increase in LCIS seen in women 50 years of age or older is multifactorial. Increased use of screening mammography led to an increased number of biopsies performed, which increased the identification rate of LCIS. Furthermore, as estrogen is hypothesized to play a role in the pathogenesis of LCIS, hormone replacement therapy in postmenopausal women may also have accounted for the increased incidence of LCIS in this age group.

The theory that LCIS represents a marker of increased risk of invasive breast carcinoma is supported by the fact that the mean age at diagnosis is 10 to 15 years younger than that for invasive cancer. However, in women 50 years of age or older, as the incidence of LCIS has increased, the incidence of infiltrating lobular carcinoma has increased concurrently in this age group, whereas women younger than 50 years old have not experienced an increase in invasive lobular carcinoma.

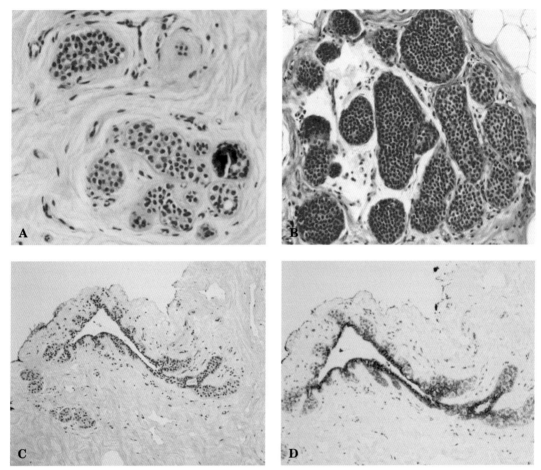

FIGURE 1.4 Lobular neoplasia. Lobular neoplasia cells are characterized by small round nuclei with diffuse chromatin pattern and scant cytoplasm. The classification into atypical lobular hyperplasia (ALH) versus lobular carcinoma in situ (LCIS) is based on the extent of involvement and expansion of lobular units. In ALH, lobular units are not expanded (**A**) in contrast LCIS expands lobular units (**B**). Lobular neoplasia cells typically show pagetoid extension into adjacent ducts (**C**). Immunohistochemical staining shows lack of E-cadherin staining in lobular neoplasia cells (**D**).

Pathology

LCIS is characterized by intraepithelial proliferation of the terminal ductal–lobular unit, but the proliferating cells do not penetrate the basement membrane. Lobular architecture is maintained in LCIS, but all acini are distended and the cells are monomorphic with uniform nuclei containing evenly dispersed chromatin and are only loosely cohesive with a high nucleus-to-cytoplasmic ratio. Calcifications, mitoses, and necrosis are rare. In ALH, as opposed to LCIS, not all of the acini are abnormal or all of the acini are involved but not all of them are distended, and there may be residual lumina (Fig. 1.4).

Pleomorphic LCIS—which has larger, polymorphic nuclei, central necrosis, more abundant, eosinophilic cytoplasm, and calcifications on histologic examination—is a more aggressive variant that is more likely to progress to invasive disease and is treated more like DCIS.

Molecular analysis of LCIS and invasive lobular carcinoma has revealed decreased expression or complete loss of the cell surface adhesion molecule E-cadherin, which can be stained to distinguish between borderline DCIS and LCIS. LCIS and invasive ductal carcinoma have in common a similar loss of heterozygosity.

The diagnosis of LCIS involves the differentiation of LCIS from other forms of benign disease and from invasive lesions. Papillomatosis in the terminal ducts may resemble LCIS but lacks the characteristic involvement of the acini. DCIS may extend retrograde into the acini, but it has a more characteristic anaplastic cell morphology and cells generally express E-cadherin. LCIS is contained within the basement membrane and is thus distinguished from invasive lobular carcinoma. In the absence of complete replacement of the lobular unit, ALH is the designated pathologic term.

Taken together, ALH and LCIS constitute a pathologic spectrum known as lobular neoplasia. Historically, ALH was thought to have a weaker association with malignancy, but a recent study suggested that both ADH and ALH confer equal levels of risk, with both markers being associated with an approximately 4.5× increased risk of invasive breast cancer. In contrast, LCIS increases the risk of invasive breast cancer by a factor of 7 to 12.

Diagnosis

Clinical Presentation

Because LCIS and ALH are usually not detectable on physical examination or mammography, they are most commonly diagnosed as incidental findings in a breast biopsy specimen. Therefore, the clinical presentation of patients with lobular neoplasia is similar to that of patients requiring breast biopsy for fibroadenoma, benign ductal disease, DCIS, or invasive breast cancer. Patients diagnosed with lobular neoplasia should undergo bilateral diagnostic mammography to exclude other abnormalities in the breast. Ultrasound is also useful in evaluating suspicious findings.

Treatment

Treatment options are (1) lifelong surveillance, (2) bilateral total mastectomies with immediate reconstruction for selected women with a strong family history after appropriate counseling, or (3) pharmacologic risk reduction with an antiestrogen treatment.

Surgery

In the past, many surgeons opted to observe such patients because a diagnosis of LCIS was considered a marker for increased risk of breast cancer rather than a precursor of invasive cancer. Patients with LCIS that is extensive, an aggressive variant (pleomorphic, signet cell, macroacinar, or necrotic), or associated with other high-risk features may require surgical excision with negative margins in order to rule out and potentially treat synchronous invasive cancer and DCIS. ALH and low-risk LCIS that is well sampled—as indicated by the number of vacuum-assisted cores obtained, the gauge of the needle used, and what percentage of any associated calcifications are no longer visible on postbiopsy imaging—do not necessarily warrant surgical excision. At MD Anderson, it is our practice to discuss proliferative benign lesions such as ALH and LCIS in a weekly conference attended by surgeons, pathologists, radiologists, and internists/medical oncologists with expertise in cancer prevention and risk reduction. After multidisciplinary discussion and review, it is often determined that asymptomatic, low-risk lesions can either be observed closely with high-risk surveillance (e.g., mammogram and MRI annually or mammogram and MRI obtained in an alternating fashion every 6 months) or treated with antiestrogen therapy. If incidentally discovered lobular neoplasia has not been well sampled or is associated with a residual mass, calcifications, or symptoms, excisional biopsy is appropriate.

Endocrine Therapy and Risk Reduction

A reasonable treatment option for patients with a diagnosis of lobular neoplasia is pharmacologic risk reduction (previously known as chemoprevention) with hormonal (endocrine) therapy. In the NSABP P-1 breast cancer prevention trial, which was implemented in 1992, Fisher et al. observed a 56% decrease in the incidence of invasive breast cancers in a subset of women with LCIS who received tamoxifen as compared with women with LCIS who underwent observation (placebo) alone (RR 0.44, $P < .01$) and an 86% reduction in invasive breast cancer risk among women with atypia who took tamoxifen (RR 0.14, $P < .01$). In the NSABP P-2 trial, postmenopausal women with LCIS and atypical hyperplasia were eligible to be randomized to either tamoxifen or raloxifene. Vogel et al. reported that the two agents offered an equivalent risk reduction for invasive breast cancer (incidence 4.30 per 1,000, vs. 4.41 per 1,000, for tamoxifen and raloxifene, respectively). Patients receiving raloxifene had a lower risk of thromboembolic events and cataracts. There was no statistical difference in risk of other cancers, fractures, ischemic heart disease, and stroke for the two drugs. Updates in 2010 and 2015 revealed that raloxifene was 78% and 81%, respectively, as effective as tamoxifen over time at preventing invasive disease in patients with LCIS and atypical hyperplasia, but had far fewer toxicities, with significantly fewer endometrial cancers. Vogel et al. concluded that depending on an individual's personal risk factors, both raloxifene and tamoxifen are valuable for breast cancer risk reduction in patients with lobular neoplasia and ADH. Raloxifene may be particularly beneficial to a postmenopausal woman with an intact uterus who also faces a risk of osteoporosis; tamoxifen would be an appropriate choice for high-risk postmenopausal women.

The NCIC Clinical Trials Group Mammary Prevention.3 trial (NCIC CTG MAP.3) was an international, randomized, double-blind, placebo-controlled trial designed to detect a 65% reduction in risk of breast cancer among postmenopausal women with a Gail risk score of 1.7% or higher (at least a 1.7% risk of breast cancer in the subsequent 5 years) through use of the aromatase inhibitor exemestane with or without the COX-2 inhibitor celecoxib. Patients were enrolled between 2004 and 2010 and were initially randomized to one of three arms: 25 mg of exemestane plus placebo daily, 25 mg of exemestane plus celecoxib daily, or placebo plus placebo pills daily. After an unexpectedly high number of cardiovascular events, celecoxib was removed from the protocol, leaving just two arms: exemestane versus placebo. Exemestane provided a 65% reduction in risk of invasive breast cancer (RR 0.35, $P = .002$) but did not provide a significant reduction in risk of noninvasive breast cancer. As a result, exemestane, in addition to raloxifene, is now considered an acceptable choice for pharmacologic risk reduction among postmenopausal women with proliferative breast lesions that put them at higher risk for breast cancer.

Atypical Ductal Hyperplasia

ADH is a proliferative lesion that lies on the spectrum between usual ductal hyperplasia and low-grade DCIS and is associated with an elevated risk of breast cancer.

Epidemiology

ADH is found in approximately 5% to 10% of benign breast biopsies and increases the likelihood of future breast cancer by a factor of 4 to 5. Although ADH has long been assumed to be a direct precursor of DCIS and subsequently invasive ductal carcinoma, a recent longitudinal study from the Mayo Clinic suggests the role of ADH in breast cancer development is more akin to that of ALH. In the study, subsequent ipsilateral breast cancer occurred at twice the rate of contralateral breast cancer for both ADH and ALH, pointing toward the likelihood that both forms of atypia not only serve as precursors of invasive disease but may also be pathologic biomarkers representing the premalignant potential of the surrounding tissue bed and of both breasts in an affected individual. Atypical ductal hyperplasia is associated with a 30% 25-year cumulative incidence of either invasive or noninvasive breast cancer.

Pathology

On pathologic assessment, ADH fulfills some, but not all, of the criteria for a diagnosis of low-grade DCIS (Fig. 1.5). Quantitatively, ADH is defined as involving fewer than two terminal ductal–lobular units and occupying an area of less than 2 mm in diameter. It consists of monotonous, round, cuboidal, or polygonal cells arranged in a regular pattern, with rare mitoses and evenly distributed nuclei. However, in contrast to DCIS, there is retention of normal epithelium in parts of the duct. Cribriform-like secondary lumens, micropapillary formations, and necrotic patterns may be observed. It tends to be strongly ER+ and PR+, like lobular neoplasia and low-grade DCIS, and is rarely HER2/*neu*-amplified.

Diagnosis
Clinical Presentation
As with lobular neoplasia, ADH is often diagnosed as an incidental finding in the specimen from a breast biopsy performed for symptoms or as part of the workup of an abnormal finding on mammographic screening. If not already performed, bilateral diagnostic mammogram and, if necessary, ultrasound should be performed once ADH is found.

Treatment
Because one of the pathologic criteria for differentiating ADH from DCIS is size, formal exclusion of DCIS cannot be confirmed on core-needle biopsy. Furthermore, an estimated 25% to 30% of cases of ADH are found

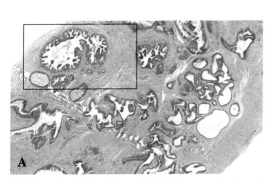
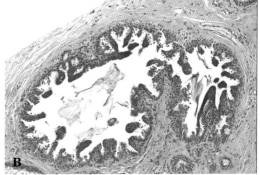

FIGURE 1.5 Atypical ductal hyperplasia (ADH). Intraductal proliferation of monotonous cells with cribriform and micropapillary features involving a single duct (**A**). Higher magnification of the duct within the frame showing uniformity of the proliferating cells with cytologic features consistent with low-grade ductal carcinoma in situ (**B**). Based on focal involvement and small size of the lesion (less than 1 mm) it is classified as ADH.

to be associated with DCIS on surgical excision. Accordingly, excisional biopsy is often warranted for ADH found on core-needle biopsy.

As discussed before, proliferative benign lesions such as ADH are discussed at MD Anderson in a weekly multidisciplinary conference at which it is sometimes determined that asymptomatic, well-sampled, low-risk lesions can either be observed with imaging surveillance or treated with antiestrogen therapy. As discussed above, NSABP P-1 demonstrated an 86% reduction in risk of future invasive breast cancer among women with atypia (including ALH and ADH) who took tamoxifen, while NSABP P-2 and MAP.3 demonstrated the efficacy of raloxifene and exemestane, respectively, as risk-reducing agents in postmenopausal women with ADH and ALH.

The most recent guidelines from the ASCO recommend consideration of pharmacologic risk reduction with tamoxifen for premenopausal women and raloxifene or exemestane for postmenopausal women in women with a 5-year absolute risk of breast cancer greater than or equal to 1.7%, a criterion that is met by women with ADH, ALH, and LCIS. However, only a minority of women who meet these criteria are counseled about these medications and an even smaller proportion are ever prescribed or initiated on these treatments. Surgeons are critical in this risk-prevention strategy and should seek opportunities to counsel appropriate patients with high-risk proliferative lesions and to encourage their enrollment in clinical trials as appropriate and available.

CASE SCENARIO

Case Scenario 1: Ductal Carcinoma In Situ

Presentation

A 52-year-old postmenopausal female presents after her annual screening mammogram detected clustered microcalcifications in her left breast. She has an unremarkable medical and family history and has not had any previous breast biopsies. She has been told that she has dense breasts on her mammogram reports. Her breast examination reveals symmetric breasts without any skin changes, dimpling, nipple inversion, or masses. She has no axillary, infraclavicular, supraclavicular, or cervical adenopathy. A diagnostic mammogram is obtained, which demonstrates a 4-cm area of fine, granular microcalcifications in the upper-outer quadrant of her left breast. No mass was seen on ultrasound. A stereotactic core-needle biopsy of the center of the calcifications was obtained, and the pathology demonstrated ductal carcinoma in situ (DCIS), nuclear grade 1, estrogen receptor positive and progesterone receptor positive by immunohistochemistry.

Additional Workup

If mammography is limited by the density of the patient's breast tissue, a contrast-enhanced breast MRI should be obtained to further characterize the extent of disease and determine if there are any areas suspicious for multicentric or contralateral disease that would necessitate an additional biopsy. MRI with contrast has a very small risk of contrast-induced nephropathy and therefore use should be limited in patients with pre-existing renal disease.

Approach to Treatment

The patient in this scenario undergoes a contrast-enhanced MRI which demonstrates a 4-cm area of nonmass enhancement in the upper-outer quadrant of her left breast, in concordance with the mammographic findings. The approach to DCIS treatment is multimodal and includes surgery, possibly radiation, and endocrine therapy. Currently, there are clinical trials in process for patients with grade 1 and 2, hormone receptor-positive DCIS undergoing active surveillance along with treatment with a selective estrogen receptor modulator, such as tamoxifen or aromatase inhibitors. However, results from these trials will not be available for several years and the current standard of care for these patients would be surgical resection.

Surgical Management

The patient in this scenario is potentially eligible for breast-conserving surgery or mastectomy. If the patient's breast size and extent of disease is favorable for good cosmesis after partial mastectomy with negative margins and there are no contraindications to radiation, then breast-conserving surgery is an appropriate option. Preoperative review of the radiologic images in a multidisciplinary setting with a dedicated radiologist will help determine the best intraoperative localization method, including wires or seeds, and to determine if a bracketing technique of the lesion will be necessary.

If there is multicentric or multifocal disease, or if resection of the disease with negative margins would significantly impact cosmesis relative to the patient's breast size, total mastectomy should be considered. Mastectomy is also indicated in cases of DCIS recurrence after previous segmental mastectomy and radiation, or in patients with persistently positive margins after segmental mastectomy. Some patients may simply prefer mastectomy over breast conservation. These patients should be counseled that there is no survival benefit to having a mastectomy compared to breast conservation. For patients who are undergoing a mastectomy and desire reconstruction, patient's breast size, ptosis, and relation of the disease to the nipple–areolar complex can help determine if a skin-sparing or nipple-sparing approach should be considered.

Sentinel lymph node dissection with breast-conserving surgery is not typically performed for DCIS, unless there is high suspicion for upstaging on final pathology or microinvasion is seen on the biopsy. It is possible to perform a sentinel lymph node dissection as a second surgery if invasive disease is found on the final pathology. Sentinel lymph node dissection should be considered if mastectomy is used to treat DCIS.

Postoperative Management and Surveillance

The patient in this scenario underwent breast-conserving surgery. She was seen at her postoperative visit and her incision was healing well with no evidence of infection, hematoma, or seroma. The final pathology demonstrated 4.5 cm of DCIS, grade 2, estrogen and progesterone receptor positive, with all margins greater than 3 mm. She was referred to radiation oncology to complete her adjuvant radiation and was started on an aromatase inhibitor with a plan to continue endocrine therapy for 5 years. She had a bilateral diagnostic mammogram 6 months after the completion of radiation to establish a new baseline. If no further findings are discovered at that time, she can then continue with standard annual screening mammography.

Take Home Points

- DCIS is frequently diagnosed on mammography as suspicious calcifications. Rarely, it can present as a palpable mass or a mass seen on mammography.
- Contrast-enhanced MRI can be obtained to evaluate the extent of ipsilateral disease and to detect contralateral disease, but may lead to additional findings that require biopsy and ultimately benign findings.
- The multimodal treatment of DCIS includes breast-conservation surgery with radiation versus mastectomy with no radiation, and endocrine therapy for patients with hormone receptor positive disease.
- The surgical approach is based on extent of disease in relation to the patient's breast size, ability to tolerate postoperative radiation, and patient preference. There is no survival advantage when comparing breast-conserving surgery and mastectomy for DCIS.
- Sentinel lymph node dissection should be considered in patients with high-risk features, including high-grade disease and microinvasion, or in patients who are undergoing a mastectomy.

CASE SCENARIO 1 REVIEW

Case Scenario 1 Questions

1. Which of the following physical and pathologic features on the initial presentation of DCIS would be worrisome for upstaging to invasive disease?

   A. Palpable mass
   B. Microinvasion
   C. High grade
   D. All of the above

2. A 45-year-old woman was found to have a 3-cm area of pleomorphic branching calcifications in the right breast on screening mammogram. Stereotactic biopsy demonstrated ductal carcinoma in situ (DCIS), intermediate grade, estrogen and progesterone receptor positive. She underwent breast-conserving surgery, and on final pathology, DCIS was within 0.5 mm of the superior margin. All other margins were negative. What is the most reasonable next step in her management?

   A. Observation
   B. Whole-breast radiation
   C. Re-excision of the superior margin
   D. Mastectomy

3. Which of the following patients would be appropriate to enroll in the Comparing an Operation to Monitoring, With or Without Endocrine Therapy (COMET) Trial For Low Risk DCIS (COMET)?

A. A 68-year-old female with a 2-cm invasive ductal carcinoma of the right breast that is grade 1 and estrogen and progesterone receptor positive.

B. A 76-year-old female with a history of DCIS of the left breast, who is status post breast-conserving surgery and radiation 4 years ago, now presenting with intermediate-grade DCIS in the ipsilateral breast.

C. A 62-year-old female with high-grade DCIS that is estrogen and progesterone receptor positive and has microinvasion on biopsy.

D. A 42-year-old female with intermediate-grade DCIS that has comedonecrosis and is estrogen receptor positive.

4. A 52-year-old female with scleroderma presents after a screening mammogram detects a cluster of calcifications in her left breast. Stereotactic biopsy demonstrates high-grade DCIS with comedonecrosis that is estrogen and progesterone receptor negative. What is the appropriate management of this patient?

A. Enroll in a trial of active surveillance

B. Wire-localized breast-conserving surgery with whole-breast irradiation

C. Seed-localized breast-conserving surgery, sentinel lymph node dissection, whole-breast irradiation.

D. Skin-sparing mastectomy and sentinel lymph node dissection

5. A 52-year-old postmenopausal woman was found to have a 5-cm span of calcifications on mammography. Biopsy demonstrated intermediate-grade ductal carcinoma in situ (DCIS). In which of the following scenarios would it be appropriate to avoid adjuvant radiation?

A. Skin-sparing mastectomy with final pathology demonstrating 5-cm DCIS, intermediate-grade, 0/2 sentinel lymph nodes positive

B. Breast-conserving surgery with final pathology demonstrating 5-cm DCIS, intermediate-grade, with <1-mm margins

C. Breast-conserving surgery with final pathology demonstrating 5-cm DCIS, intermediate-grade, negative margins

D. Skin-sparing mastectomy with final pathology demonstrating 5-cm DCIS, high grade, with 1.0 cm of invasive ductal carcinoma with 2/3 sentinel lymph nodes positive

Case Scenario 1 Answers

1. **The correct answer is D.** *Rationale:* Several studies have shown the upstaging rate of DCIS to invasive cancer can range from 8 to 59%. The majority of these tumors are upstaged to small invasive cancers. Several factors can help physicians anticipate which DCIS tumors may be upstaged. DCIS that presents with a palpable mass, is >2 cm on preoperative imaging, and demonstrates microinvasion or high-grade features on biopsy is more likely to be upstaged after resection.

2. **The correct answer is C.** *Rationale:* The Society of Surgical Oncology (SSO), American Society for Radiation Oncology (ASTRO), and the American Society of Clinical Oncology (ASCO) developed consensus guidelines on margins after segmental mastectomy for DCIS. Based on a meta-analysis, it was determined that 2-mm margins minimize the risk of breast tumor recurrence compared to narrower margins. Therefore, this patient would require re-excision to achieve adequate margins in the superior aspect.

3. **The correct answer is D.** *Rationale:* Inclusion criteria for the COMET for Low-Risk DCIS include women aged 40 years or older; a diagnosis of unilateral, bilateral, unifocal, multifocal, or multicentric DCIS; grade 1 or 2 (respective of necrosis/comedonecrosis); the absence of invasion or microinvasion; and estrogen and/or progesterone receptor positivity.

4. **The correct answer is D.** *Rationale:* Scleroderma is a relative contraindication to breast-conserving therapy, as radiation can cause radiation-induced fibrosis of the skin and lung. Therefore, this patient would not be a candidate for breast conservation and would require a mastectomy. A sentinel lymph node dissection should be performed in the same procedure given the histologic features of the DCIS and the limited ability to perform sentinel lymph node localization following mastectomy.

5. **The correct answer is A.** *Rationale:* Several prospective randomized trials, including the NSABP B-17 trial, have demonstrated a 50% risk reduction in local recurrence when comparing patients who did and did not receive radiation after breast-conserving surgery for DCIS. Therefore, most patients receiving breast-conserving surgery should undergo postoperative radiation.

CASE SCENARIO

Case Scenario 2: Atypical Ductal Hyperplasia

Presentation

A 42-year-old G2P2 premenopausal female presents to clinic after a screening mammogram detected a small (4-mm) cluster of calcifications in her right breast. She reports no history of masses, skin changes, or nipple discharge. She is otherwise healthy and takes no medications. Her family history is significant for breast cancer in her mother at age 52 and in her maternal aunt at age 60. Her physical examination demonstrates symmetric breasts, with no palpable masses or skin changes, and no lymphadenopathy.

Additional Workup

A bilateral diagnostic mammogram was ordered with spot views of the area of concern in the right breast. This re-demonstrated the 4-mm area of clustered calcifications. There was no mass associated with this area on ultrasound. A stereotactic vacuum-assisted biopsy was obtained. Six cores were removed, three of which contained calcifications. A clip was placed at the biopsy site. A postprocedure mammogram was obtained, which demonstrated a clip in the correct location, but 1 mm of remaining calcifications. Biopsy of the cores demonstrated atypical ductal hyperplasia (ADH).

Approach to Treatment

The patient in this scenario has a diagnosis of atypical ductal hyperplasia, and has some high-risk features, including remaining calcifications on mammography. Therefore, she should undergo excisional breast biopsy. Given she has no palpable findings on examination, the area for excisional biopsy can be localized preoperatively with a wire or seed, depending on available technology and surgeon preference. After excisional biopsy, a radiograph of the specimen should be obtained to confirm that it contains both the biopsy clip and remaining calcifications. This surgery can be performed under monitored anesthesia care or general anesthesia.

Final pathology of the biopsy specimen demonstrates atypical ductal hyperplasia involving one terminal duct–lobular unit and a focus of lobular carcinoma in situ (LCIS).

Next Steps and Surveillance

The patient in this scenario had an excisional biopsy which demonstrated ADH and LCIS, both of which are markers of increased risk for the development of invasive breast cancer in the ipsilateral or contralateral breast. In addition, she has a family history of breast cancer in her mother and aunt. She should be referred to a genetic counselor. She should be counseled on risk reduction strategies, including lifestyle modifications, high-risk screening, and pharmacologic risk reduction. Lifestyle modifications to reduce the risk of developing invasive breast cancer include maintaining a healthy body mass index (BMI) through diet and exercise, avoiding smoking and smoke exposure, and avoiding alcohol in excess. High-risk screening for this patient may include yearly clinical breast examination with yearly screening mammogram and MRI performed at 6-month intervals. This patient is premenopausal and is appropriate for treatment with tamoxifen.

While nonsurgical methods of risk reduction are preferred, the option of prophylactic bilateral mastectomies can be discussed. This option should be discussed in the context of her family history and any available results from genetic testing.

Take Home Points

- Atypical ductal hyperplasia and lobular carcinoma in situ are markers of increased risk and nonobligate precursors of invasive disease.
- ADH found on biopsy is associated with a rate of upstage to noninvasive or invasive breast cancer in 18% to 31% of cases following excision.
- ADH is associated with a four- to fivefold increased lifetime risk of breast cancer; LCIS is associated with an 8- to 10-times increased lifetime risk of breast cancer.
- Women with high-risk pathology should be counseled on risk reduction methods, including lifestyle modifications, enhanced screening, pharmacologic risk reduction with tamoxifen (20 mg for 5 years) for premenopausal women or raloxifene (60 mg daily for 5 years) or exemestane for postmenopausal women.

CASE SCENARIO 2 REVIEW

Case Scenario 2 Questions

1. A 52-year-old female with no significant past medical history presents after a screening mammogram detected a cluster of calcifications in the right breast. After core needle biopsy, for which of the following pathologic results should an excisional biopsy be recommended?

   A. Atypical lobular hyperplasia
   B. Pleomorphic lobular carcinoma in situ (PLCIS)
   C. Flat epithelial atypia
   D. Florid ductal hyperplasia

2. A 58-year-old postmenopausal woman with an intact uterus and osteopenia presents to clinic to discuss pharmacologic risk reduction after a recent biopsy demonstrated lobular carcinoma in situ in her left breast. Which of the following medications would be recommended?

   A. Tamoxifen
   B. Anastrozole
   C. Exemestane
   D. Raloxifene

3. A 65-year-old female underwent core needle biopsy of a cluster of calcifications seen on mammogram. Pathologic examination demonstrated atypical ductal hyperplasia (ADH) involving two terminal ductal–lobular units, and >95% of the calcifications were removed with the biopsy. What is the most appropriate next step in her management?

   A. Observation with risk-reducing strategies
   B. Excisional biopsy
   C. Breast-conserving surgery and radiation
   D. Unilateral mastectomy

4. What is the most common presentation of LCIS?

   A. A palpable mass
   B. Incidental finding seen on biopsy for another lesion
   C. Calcifications seen on mammography
   D. Asymmetry seen on mammography

5. Of the following choices, what is the lowest 5-year absolute risk of breast cancer at which women should be offered pharmacologic risk reduction?

   A. 1%
   B. 2%
   C. 5%
   D. 8%

Case Scenario 2 Answers

1. **The correct answer is B.** *Rationale:* PLCIS is a phenotypic variant of LCIS that is found to have a higher rate of progression to noninvasive or invasive carcinoma. Therefore, surgical excision with negative margins is recommended. If DCIS or invasive carcinoma is found in the excised specimen, negative margins should be achieved, and adjuvant radiation is recommended. Atypical lobular hyperplasia, flat epithelial atypia, and florid ductal hyperplasia on core needle biopsy do not typically need an excisional biopsy, unless the pathology is discordant with imaging findings.

2. **The correct answer is D.** *Rationale:* The NSABP P-2 breast cancer prevention trial demonstrated an equivalent invasive cancer risk reduction in women with LCIS when comparing those prescribed tamoxifen to those prescribed raloxifene. However, tamoxifen carries a higher risk of the development of uterine cancer in postmenopausal women with an intact uterus. Aromatase inhibitors, such as anastrozole and exemestane, are another option for pharmacologic risk reduction but have a higher risk of osteoporosis. Therefore, in a postmenopausal woman with an intact uterus and osteopenia, raloxifene would be the best option.

3. **The correct answer is A.** *Rationale:* Several studies have shown features of ADH that are predictive of upstage to noninvasive or invasive carcinoma, including involvement of three or more terminal ductal–lobular units,

presence of significant atypia, presence of necrosis, and <95% of calcifications removed on biopsy. In the scenario described above, there are no high-risk features of the biopsy demonstrating ADH, so further surgical management would not be indicated. The patient should be counseled that she is at a four- to fivefold higher risk of developing invasive breast cancer and should consider risk-reducing strategies.

4. **The correct answer is B.** *Rationale:* LCIS is frequently diagnosed after excisional biopsy for a different lesion. It does not typically present with a palpable mass, calcifications, or asymmetry.

5. **The correct answer is B.** *Rationale:* Guidelines from the American Society of Clinical Oncology (ASCO) recommend consideration of pharmacologic risk reduction with tamoxifen for premenopausal women and raloxifene or an aromatase inhibitor, such as exemestane, for postmenopausal women, in women with a 5-year absolute risk of breast cancer greater than or equal to 1.7%. All women with a diagnosis of ADH or LCIS will have a 5-year relative risk of breast cancer greater than 1.7% and should be offered pharmacologic risk reduction.

Recommended Readings

Allegra CJ, Aberle DR, Ganschow P, et al. National Institutes of Health state-of-the-science conference statement: diagnosis and management of ductal carcinoma in situ. *J Natl Cancer Inst.* 2010;102(3):161–169.

Alvarado R, Lari SA, Roses RE, et al. Biology, treatment, and outcome in very young and older women with DCIS. *Ann Surg Oncol.* 2012;19(12):3777–3784.

Anderson BO, Calhoun KE, Rosen EL. Evolving concepts in the management of lobular neoplasia. *J Natl Compr Canc Netw.* 2006; 4(5):511–522.

Arpino G, Allred DC, Mohsin SK, Weiss HL, Conrow D, Elledge RM. Lobular neoplasia on core-needle biopsy—clinical significance. *Cancer.* 2004;101(2):242–250.

Bayraktar S, Elsayegh N, Gutierrez Barrera AM, et al. Predictive factors for BRCA1/BRCA2 mutations in women with ductal carcinoma in situ. *Cancer.* 2012;118(6):1515–1522.

Boyages J, Delaney G, Taylor R. Predictors of local recurrence after treatment of ductal carcinoma in situ: a meta-analysis. *Cancer.* 1999;85(3):616–628.

Bremer T, Whitworth PW, Patel R, et al. A biological signature for breast ductal carcinoma in situ to predict radiotherapy benefit and assess recurrence risk. *Clin Cancer Res.* 2018;24(23):5895–5901.

Brinton LA, Sherman ME, Carreon JD, Anderson WF. Recent trends in breast cancer among younger women in the United States. *J Natl Cancer Inst.* 2008;100(22):1643–1648.

Calhoun BC, Sobel A, White RL, et al. Management of flat epithelial atypia on breast core biopsy may be individualized based on correlation with imaging studies. *Mod Pathol.* 2015;28(5):670–676.

Calle C, Kuba MG, Brogi E. Non-invasive lobular neoplasia of the breast: morphologic features, clinical presentation, and management dilemmas. *Breast J.* 2020;26(6):1148–1155.

Chagpar A, Yen T, Sahin A, et al. Intraoperative margin assessment reduces re-excision rates in patients with ductal carcinoma in situ treated with breast-conserving surgery. *Am J Surg.* 2003;186(4):371–377.

Champion CD, Ren Y, Thomas SM, et al. DCIS with Microinvasion: is it in situ or invasive disease? *Ann of Surg Onc.* 2019;26(10):3124–3132.

Ciocca RM, Li T, Freedman GM, Morrow M. Presence of lobular carcinoma in situ does not increase local recurrence in patients treated with breast-conserving therapy. *Ann Surg Oncol.* 2008;15(8):2263–2271.

Cox CE, Pendas S, Cox JM, et al. Guidelines for sentinel node biopsy and lymphatic mapping of patients with breast cancer. *Ann Surg.* 1998;227(5):645–651; discussion 651–653.

Cuzick J, Sestak I, Forbes JF, et al. Anastrozole for prevention of breast cancer in high-risk postmenopausal women (IBIS-II): an international, double-blind, randomised placebo-controlled trial. *Lancet.* 2014;383:1041–1048.

Cuzick J, Sestak I, Pinder SE, et al. Effect of tamoxifen and radiotherapy in women with locally excised ductal carcinoma in situ: long-term results from the UK/ANZ DCIS trial. *Lancet Oncol.* 2011;12:21–29.

de Mascarel I, MacGrogan G, Mathoulin-Pélissier S, Soubeyran I, Picot V, Coindre JM. Breast ductal carcinoma in situ with microinvasion: a definition supported by a long-term study of 1248 serially sectioned ductal carcinomas. *Cancer.* 2002;94(8):2134–2142.

DeSantis CE, Ma J, Gaudet MM, et al. Breast Cancer Statistics, 2019. *CA Cancer J Clin.* 2019;69:438–451.

Donker M, Litière S, Werutsky G, et al. Breast-conserving treatment with or without radiotherapy in ductal carcinoma in situ: 15-year recurrence rates and outcome after a recurrence, from the EORTC 10853 randomized phase III trial. *J Clin Oncol.* 2013;31(32):4054–4059.

Early Breast Cancer Trialists' Collaborative Group (EBCTCG); Correa C, McGale P, Taylor C, et al. Overview of the randomized trials of radiotherapy in ductal carcinoma in situ of the breast. *J Natl Cancer Inst Monogr.* 2010;2010(41):162–177.

El-Tamer M, Chun J, Gill M, et al. Incidence and clinical significance of lymph node metastasis detected by cytokeratin immunohistochemical staining in ductal carcinoma in situ. *Ann Surg Oncol.* 2005;12(3):254–259.

Eng-Wong J, Costantino JP, Swain SM. The impact of systemic therapy following ductal carcinoma in situ. *J Natl Cancer Inst Monogr.* 2010;2010(41):200–203.

Fisher ER, Costantino J, Fisher B, Palekar AS, Redmond C, Mamounas E. Pathologic findings from the National Surgical Adjuvant Breast Project (NSABP) Protocol B-17. Intraductal carcinoma (ductal carcinoma in situ). The National Surgical Adjuvant Breast and Bowel Project Collaborating Investigators. *Cancer.* 1995;75(6):1310–1319.

Fisher B, Costantino J, Redmond C, et al. Lumpectomy compared with lumpectomy and radiation therapy for the treatment of intraductal breast cancer. *N Engl J Med.* 1993;328(22):1581–1586.

Fisher B, Costantino JP, Wickerham DL, et al. Tamoxifen for prevention of breast cancer: report of the National Surgical Adjuvant Breast and Bowel Project P-1 Study. *J Natl Cancer Inst.* 1998;90(18):1371–1388.

Fisher B, Dignam J, Wolmark N, et al. Lumpectomy and radiation therapy for the treatment of intraductal breast cancer: findings from the National Surgical Adjuvant Breast and Bowel Project B-17. *J Clin Oncol.* 1998;16(2):441–452.

Fisher B, Dignam J, Wolmark N, et al. Tamoxifen in treatment of intraductal breast cancer: National Surgical Adjuvant Breast and Bowel Project B-24 randomised controlled trial. *Lancet.* 1999;353(9169):1993–2000.

Fisher ER, Land SR, Fisher B, Mamounas E, Gilarski L, Wolmark N. Pathologic findings from the National Surgical Adjuvant Breast and Bowel Project: twelve-year observations concerning lobular carcinoma in situ. *Cancer.* 2004;100(2):238–244.

Fisher B, Land S, Mamounas E, Dignam J, Fisher ER, Wolmark N. Prevention of invasive breast cancer in women with ductal carcinoma in situ: an update of the National Surgical Adjuvant Breast and Bowel Project experience. *Semin Oncol.* 2001;28(4):400–418.

Francis AM, Haugen CE, Grimes LM, et al. Is sentinel node dissection warranted for patients with a diagnosis of ductal carcinoma in situ? *Ann Surg Oncol.* 2015;22(13):4270–4279.

Gill JK, Maskarinec G, Pagano I, Kolonel LN. The association of mammographic density with ductal carcinoma in situ of the breast: the Multiethnic Cohort. *Breast Cancer Res.* 2006;8(3):R30.

Goss PE, Ingle JN, Alés-Martínez JE; NCIC CTG MAP.3 Study Investigators. Exemestane for breast-cancer prevention in postmenopausal women. *N Engl J Med.* 2011;364(25):2381–2391.

Haagensen CD, Lane N, Lattes R, Bodian C. Lobular neoplasia (so-called lobular carcinoma in situ) of the breast. *Cancer.* 1978;42(2):737–769.

Hartmann LC, Degnim AC, Santen RJ, Dupont WD, Ghosh K. Atypical hyperplasia of the breast—risk assessment and management options. *N Engl J Med.* 2015;372:78–89

Hartmann LC, Radisky DC, Frost MH, et al. Understanding the premalignant potential of atypical hyperplasia through its natural history: a longitudinal cohort study. *Cancer Prev Res.* 2014;7:211–217.

Hollingsworth AB, Stough RG, O'Dell CA, Brekke CE. Breast magnetic resonance imaging for preoperative locoregional staging. *Am J Surg.* 2008;196(3):389–397.

Houghton J, George WD, Cuzick J, Duggan C, Fentiman IS, Spittle M; UK Coordinating Committee on Cancer Research, Ductal Carcinoma in situ Working Party, DCIS trialists in the UK, Australia, and New Zealand. Radiotherapy and tamoxifen in women with completely excised ductal carcinoma in situ of the breast in the UK, Australia, and New Zealand: randomised controlled trial. *Lancet.* 2003;362(9378):95–102.

Hughes LL, Wang M, Page DL, et al. Local excision alone without irradiation for ductal carcinoma in situ of the breast: a trial of the Eastern Cooperative Oncology Group. *J Clin Oncol.* 2009;27(32):5319–5324.

Jagsi R, Abrahamse P, Morrow M, et al. Patterns and correlates of adjuvant radiotherapy receipt after lumpectomy and after mastectomy for breast cancer. *J Clin Oncol.* 2010;28:2396–2403.

Jeruss JS, Kuerer HM, Beitsch PD, Vicini FA, Keisch M. Update on DCIS outcomes from the American Society of Breast Surgeons accelerated partial breast irradiation registry trial. *Ann Surg Oncol.* 2011;18(1):65–71.

Julien JP, Bijker N, Fentiman IS, et al. Radiotherapy in breast-conserving treatment for ductal carcinoma in situ: first results of the EORTC randomised phase III trial 10853. EORTC Breast Cancer Cooperative Group and EORTC Radiotherapy Group. *Lancet.* 2000;355(9203):528–533.

Kerlikowskie K. Epidemiology of ductal carcinoma in situ. *J Natl Cancer Inst Monogr.* 2010(41):139–141.

Kerlikowske K, Molinaro AM, Gauthier ML, et al. Biomarker expression and risk of subsequent tumors after initial ductal carcinoma in situ diagnosis. *J Natl Cancer Inst.* 2010;102(9):627–637.

Klauber-DeMore N, Tan LK, Liberman L, et al. Sentinel lymph node biopsy: is it indicated in patients with high-risk ductal carcinoma-in-situ and ductal carcinoma-in-situ with microinvasion? *Ann Surg Oncol.* 2000;7(9):636–642.

Kuerer HM, Albarracin CT, Yang WT, et al. Ductal carcinoma in situ: state of the science and roadmap to advance the field. *J Clin Oncol.* 2009;27(2):279–288.

Lagios MD, Margolin FR, Westdahl PR, Rose MR. Mammographically detected duct carcinoma in situ. Frequency of local recurrence following tylectomy and prognostic effect of nuclear grade on local recurrence. *Cancer.* 1989;63(4):618–624.

Land SR, Wickerham DL, Costantino JP, et al. Patient-reported symptoms and quality of life during treatment with tamoxifen or raloxifene for breast cancer prevention: the NSABP Study of Tamoxifen and Raloxifene (STAR) P-2 trial. *JAMA.* 2006;295(23):2742–2751.

Lari SA, Kuerer HM. Biological markers in DCIS and risk of breast recurrence: a systematic review. *J Cancer.* 2011;2:232–261.

Lehman CD, Gatsonis C, Kuhl CK, et al; ACRIN Trial 6667 Investigators Group. MRI evaluation of the contralateral breast in women with recently diagnosed breast cancer. *N Engl J Med.* 2007;356(13):1295–1303.

Lester SC, Bose S, Chen YY, et al; Members of the Cancer Committee, College of American Pathologists. Protocol for the examination of specimens from patients with ductal carcinoma in situ of the breast. *Arch Pathol Lab Med.* 2009;133(1):15-25.

Li CI, Anderson BO, Daling JR, Moe RE. Changing incidence of lobular carcinoma in situ of the breast. *Breast Cancer Res Treat.* 2002;75(3):259–268.

Margolese RG, Cecchini RS, Julian TB, et al. Anastrozole versus tamoxifen in postmenopausal women with ductal carcinoma in situ undergoing lumpectomy plus radiotherapy (NSABP B-35): a randomised, double-blind, phase 3 clinical trial. *Lancet.* 2016;387:849–856.

McCormick B, Winter KA, Woodward W, et al. Randomized phase III trial evaluating radiation following surgical excision for good-risk ductal carcinoma in situ: long-term report from NRG Oncology/RTOG 9804. *J Clin Oncol.* 2021;39:3574–3582.

Morrow M, Van Zee KJ, Solin LJ, et al. Society of Surgical Oncology-American Society for Radiation Oncology-American Society of Clinical Oncology Consensus guideline on margins for breast-conserving surgery with whole-breast irradiation in ductal carcinoma in situ. *J Clin Oncol.* 2016;34(33):4040–4046.

Neuschatz AC, DiPetrillo T, Steinhoff M, et al. The value of breast lumpectomy margin assessment as a predictor of residual tumor burden in ductal carcinoma in situ of the breast. *Cancer.* 2002;94(7):1917–1924.

Nielsen M, Thomsen JL, Primdahl S, Dyreborg U, Andersen JA. Breast cancer and atypia among young and middle-aged women: a study of 110 medicolegal autopsies. *Br J Cancer.* 1987;56(6):814–819.

Oppong BA, King TA. Recommendations for women with lobular carcinoma in situ (LCIS). *Oncology (Williston Park).* 2011;25(11):1051–1056, 1058.

Ottesen GL, Graversen HP, Blichert-Toft M, Christensen IJ, Andersen JA. Carcinoma in situ of the female breast. 10 year follow-up results of a prospective nationwide study. *Breast Cancer Res Treat.* 2000;62(3):197–210.

Page DL, Dupont WD, Rogers LW, Jensen RA, Schuyler PA. Continued local recurrence of carcinoma 15–25 years after a diagnosis of low grade ductal carcinoma in situ of the breast treated only by biopsy. *Cancer.* 1995;76(7):1197–1200.

Parikh RR, Haffty BG, Lannin D, Moran MS. Ductal carcinoma in situ with microinvasion: prognostic implications, long-term outcomes, and role of axillary evaluation. *Int J Radiat Oncol Biol Phys.* 2012;82(1):7–13.

Pilewskie M, Olcese C, Eaton A, et al. Perioperative breast MRI is not associated with lower locoregional recurrence rates in DCIS patients treated with or without radiation. *Ann Surg Oncol.* 2014;21(5):1552–1560.

Piotrowski MJ, Yi M, Contreras A, et al. Optimization of intraoperative lumpectomy specimen labeling improves concordance between surgeon and pathology. The American Society of Breast Surgeons [ASBrS] Volume XXI, 5/2020.

Rakovitch E, Nofech-Mozes S, Hanna W, et al. A population-based validation study of the DCIS Score predicting recurrence risk in individuals treated by breast-conserving surgery alone. *Breast Cancer Res Treat.* 2015;152(2):389–398.

Romero L, Klein L, Ye W, et al. Outcome after invasive recurrence in patients with ductal carcinoma in situ of the breast. *Am J Surg.* 2004;188(4):371–376.

Roses RE, Arun BK, Lari SA. Ductal carcinoma-in-situ of the breast with subsequent distant metastasis and death. *Ann Surg Oncol.* 2011;18:2873–2878.

Rudloff U, Jacks LM, Goldberg JI, et al. Nomogram for predicting the risk of local recurrence after breast-conserving surgery for ductal carcinoma in situ. *J Clin Oncol.* 2010;28(23):3762–3769.

Ryser MD, Weaver DL, Zhao F, et al. Cancer outcomes in DCIS patients without locoregional treatment. *J Natl Cancer Inst.* 2019;111(9):952–960.

Siegel RL, Miller KD, Jemal A. Cancer statistics, 2016. *CA Cancer J Clin.* 2016;66(1):7–30.

Silverstein MJ, Lagios MD, Groshen S, et al. The influence of margin width on local control of ductal carcinoma in situ of the breast. *N Engl J Med.* 1999;340(19):1455–1461.

Silverstein MJ, Lagios MD, Martino S, et al. Outcome after invasive local recurrence in patients with ductal carcinoma in situ of the breast. *J Clin Oncol.* 1998;16(4):1367–1373.

Smart CE, Furnival CM, Lakhani SR. High-risk lesions: ALH/LCIS/ADH. In: Kuerer HM, ed. *Kuerer's Breast Surgical Oncology.* McGraw-Hill Medical; 2010:179–187.

Solin LJ, Gray R, Baehner FL, et al. A quantitative multigene RT-PCR assay for predicting recurrence risk after surgical excision alone without irradiation for ductal carcinoma in situ (DCIS): a prospective validation study of the DCIS Score from ECOG E5194. *Cancer Res.* 2011;71(suppl 24):S4–S6.

Solin LJ, Gray R, Hughes LL, et al. Surgical excision without radiation for ductal carcinoma in situ of the breast: 12-year results from the ECOG-ACRIN E5194 study. *J Clin Oncol.* 2015;33:3938–3944.

Stuart KE, Houssami N, Taylor R, Hayen A, Boyages J. Long-term outcomes of ductal carcinoma in situ of the breast: a systematic review, meta-analysis and meta-regression analysis. *BMC Cancer.* 2015;15:890.

Sun SX, Suk R, Kuerer HM, Cantor SB, Raber BM, Deshmukh AA. No treatment versus partial mastectomy plus radiation for ductal carcinoma in situ. *Ann Surg Oncol.* 2022;29(1):39–41. doi: 10.1245/s10434-021-10758-9. Epub 2021 Sep 1.

Tan PH, Ellis I, Allison K, et al; WHO Classification of Tumours Editorial Board. The 2019 World Health Organization classification of tumours of the breast. *Histopathology.* 2020;77(2):181–185.

Vicini FA, Cecchini RS, White JR, et al. Long-term primary results of accelerated partial breast irradiation after breast-conserving surgery for early-stage breast cancer: a randomized, phase 3, equivalence trial. *Lancet.* 2019;394(10215):2155–2164.

Vigeland E, Klaasen H, Klingen TA, Hofvind S, Skaane P. Full-field digital mammography compared to screen film mammography in the prevalent round of a population-based screening programme: the Vestfold County Study. *Eur Radiol.* 2008;18(1):183–191.

Vogel VG, Costantino JP, Wickerham DL, et al; National Surgical Adjuvant Breast and Bowel Project (NSABP). Effects of tamoxifen vs raloxifene on the risk of developing invasive breast cancer and other disease outcomes: the NSABP Study of Tamoxifen and Raloxifene (STAR) P-2 trial. *JAMA.* 2006;295(23):2727–2741.

Vogel VG, Costantino JP, Wickerham DL, et al; National Surgical Adjuvant Breast and Bowel Project. Update of the National Surgical Adjuvant Breast and Bowel Project Study of Tamoxifen And Raloxifene (STAR) P-2 trial: preventing breast cancer. *Cancer Prev Res (Phila Pa).* 2010;3(6):696–706.

Wapnir IL, Dignam JJ, Fisher B, et al. Long-term outcomes of invasive ipsilateral breast tumor recurrences after lumpectomy in NSABP B-17 and B-24 randomized clinical trials for DCIS. *J Natl Cancer Inst.* 2011;103:478–488.

Wärnberg F, Garmo H, Emdin S, et al. Effect of radiotherapy after breast-conserving surgery for ductal carcinoma in situ: 20 years follow-up in the randomized SweDCIS trial. *J Clin Oncol.* 2014;32:3613–3618.

Wong JS, Chen YH, Gadd MA, et al. Eight-year update of a prospective study of wide excision alone for small low- or intermediate-grade ductal carcinoma in situ (DCIS). *Breast Cancer Res Treat.* 2014;143:343–350.

Yi M, Meric-Bernstam F, Kuerer HM, et al. Evaluation of a breast cancer nomogram for predicting risk of ipsilateral breast tumor recurrences in patients with ductal carcinoma in situ after local excision. *J Clin Oncol.* 2012;30(6):600–607.

Zheng J, Zhou T, Li F, Shi J, Zhang L. Clinic-pathological features of breast ductal carcinoma in situ with micro-invasion. *Cancer Invest.* 2020;38(2):113–121.

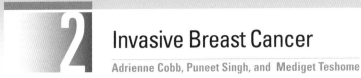

Invasive Breast Cancer

Adrienne Cobb, Puneet Singh, and Mediget Teshome

INTRODUCTION

Invasive breast malignancy is a systemic disease. Over the past several decades, breast cancer management has changed dramatically, evolving from primarily surgical therapy to a multidisciplinary approach with improved understanding of tumor biology and emphasis on personalized care and specialized techniques. Surgical therapy and decision making are embedded within the context of multidisciplinary care. This chapter will comprehensively review contemporary practice, diagnosis, and management of invasive breast cancer.

Epidemiology

Breast cancer remains the most common cancer diagnosed and the second most common cause of cancer-related mortality among women in the United States. The American Cancer Society estimates that in 2022, approximately 287,850 new cases of invasive breast cancer will be diagnosed in women and approximately 2,710 cases will be diagnosed in men. Of those, nearly 43,250 breast cancer–related deaths will occur. Currently, the lifetime risk of invasive breast cancer among women is 1 in 8 or 13% compared to 1 in 11 for women in the 1970s. This increase in risk over the past four decades is attributed to longer life expectancy, changes in reproductive patterns, hormone use, the rising prevalence of obesity, as well as increased detection through screening mammography. Although the incidence of breast cancer has risen, breast cancer mortality has decreased. Breast cancer death rates have decreased 40% from 1989 to 2017, after slowly increasing (0.4% per year) since 1975. This likely reflects the increased use of screening mammography beginning in the early 1980s leading to detection of earlier stage disease, as well as continued improvements in systemic adjuvant therapy.

Breast cancer incidence rates are highest in non-Hispanic White women, followed by African American women and are lowest among Asian/Pacific Islander women. Contrastingly, breast cancer death rates are highest for African American women, followed by non-Hispanic White women, and are lowest for Asian/Pacific Islander women. Furthermore, the difference in long-term breast cancer mortality by race/ethnicity persists and is increasing with breast cancer death rates being 40% higher in African American than Caucasian women in 2017. This disparity reflects a combination of factors, including differences in stage at diagnosis, tumor characteristics, screening, access, and response to treatment. Unfortunately, this disparity has persisted despite other advancements in systemic and targeted therapies for breast cancer.

Risk Factors

Contemporary breast cancer care increasingly relies on a personalized multidisciplinary approach to treatment. In order to provide individual counseling of risk, several risk assessment models are available. The most important risk factor for the development of breast cancer is gender. The female-to-male ratio for breast cancer is 100:1. Therefore, this section focuses on risk factors among women.

Multiple additional factors are associated with an increased risk of developing breast cancer, including age, genetic predisposition, a history of proliferative breast disease, prior radiation exposure, a personal or family history of breast cancer, obesity, and hormone exposure. A simplified version of previously summarized risk factors for breast cancer is provided in Table 2.1.

Age
According to the National Cancer Institute's Surveillance, Epidemiology, and End Results (SEER) Program, the incidence of breast cancer increases rapidly during the fourth decade of life. After menopause, the incidence continues to increase but at a much slower rate, peaking in the fifth and sixth decades of life and slowly leveling off during the sixth and seventh decades. Approximately one out of eight invasive breast cancers will be found in women younger than 45 years and approximately two-thirds of invasive breast cancers are found in women older than 55 years.

Personal and Family History of Breast Cancer
A strong family history of breast cancer has been recognized to increase a woman's risk of breast cancer. The overall risk depends on the number of relatives with breast cancer, their ages at diagnosis, and whether the

Risk Factors for Breast Cancer and Associated Relative Risks

Risk Factor	Category at Risk	Relative Risk
Germline mutations	*BRCA1* and younger than 40 yrs old	200
	BRCA1 and 60–69 yrs old	15
Proliferative breast disease	Lobular carcinoma in situ	16.4
	Ductal carcinoma in situ	17.3
Personal history of breast cancer	Invasive breast cancer	6.8
Ionizing radiation exposure	Hodgkin disease	5.2
Family history	First-degree relative with premenopausal breast cancer	3.3
	First-degree relative with postmenopausal breast cancer	1.8
Age at first childbirth	Older than 30 yrs	1.7–1.9
Hormone replacement therapy with estrogen and progesterone	Current user for at least 5 yrs	1.3
Early menarche	Younger than 12 yrs	1.3
Late menopause	Older than 55 yrs	1.2–1.5

From Singletary SE. Rating the risk factors for breast cancer. *Ann Surg.* 2003;237:474–482, with permission.

disease was unilateral or bilateral. The highest risk is associated with a young first-degree relative with bilateral breast cancer. Overall, the risk of developing breast cancer is increased approximately 1.5- to 3-fold if a woman has a first-degree relative (mother or sister) with breast cancer. A personal history of breast cancer is a significant risk factor for the development of cancer in the contralateral breast with an estimated risk of approximately 0.5% to 1% per year of follow-up.

Genetic Predisposition
Hereditary breast cancer secondary to genetic mutations accounts for 5% to 10% of all breast cancer. Several mutations have been identified to have an increased association with breast cancer risk although to varying degrees. These include BRCA1, BRCA2, PALB2, CHEK2, p53 (Li–Fraumeni syndrome), PTEN (Cowden disease), ATM, CDH1, STK11 (Peutz–Jeghers syndrome), and Lynch syndrome. Expanded panel genetic testing is becoming increasingly common although the penetrance of these mutations and relative risk of breast cancer may vary. Testing of an affected family member is recommended to identify and direct testing for a specific genetic loci mutation in unaffected family members. Genetic testing should be preceded by genetic counseling (Table 2.2).

The most widely studied and known mutations are in the BRCA1 and 2 genes. BRCA1 mutations have an estimated lifetime risk of breast cancer of 57% to 65%, and are also associated with risk of ovarian (lifetime risk of approximately 10% to 40%), fallopian tube, peritoneal, pancreatic cancers, and melanoma. BRCA2 mutation carriers have an estimated breast cancer lifetime risk of 45% to 55% in addition to the risk of ovarian (lifetime risk of approximately 10% to 20%), pancreatic, prostate, and higher association with male breast cancers (lifetime risk approximately 5% to 10%) in addition to Fanconi anemia, a syndrome that is associated with childhood solid tumors and development of acute myeloid leukemia. BRCA1 and 2 mutation carriers are encouraged to undergo high-risk screening with annual mammogram alternating with breast MRI or prophylactic mastectomy for risk-reduction.

Proliferative Breast Disease
Nonproliferative breast diseases such as adenosis, fibroadenomas, apocrine changes, duct ectasia, and mild hyperplasia are not associated with an increased risk of breast cancer. However, proliferative breast diseases are associated with breast cancer to various degrees (RR is 1.5 to 2). Moderate or florid hyperplasia without atypia, papilloma, and sclerosing adenosis carry a slightly increased risk of breast cancer, 1.5 to 2 times that of the general population. Atypical ductal hyperplasia (ADH) or atypical lobular hyperplasia (ALH) is associated with a four- to fivefold increased risk of developing breast cancer in either breast. Lobular carcinoma in situ (LCIS) is associated with up to an 8- to 10-fold risk of breast cancer. Risk factor modification with chemoprevention in the setting of high-risk lesions is highly effective as evidenced by the findings of the NSABP P2 trial. This study found chemoprevention with tamoxifen or raloxifene was associated with a significant decrease in the incidence of invasive and noninvasive breast cancer in the setting of ADH and LCIS. Therefore, consideration of chemoprevention and risk assessment strategies for patients with high-risk lesions should be strongly encouraged.

Gene mutation	Syndrome	Associated Risk
High penetrance		
BRCA1	Hereditary breast and ovarian cancer (HBOC)	Malignancies of the breast, ovaries, and possibly prostate and colon
BRCA2	HBOC	Malignancies of the breast (including male), ovaries, prostate, larynx, and pancreas
TP53	Li–Fraumeni	Malignancies of the breast, brain, and adrenal glands; soft tissue sarcomas
PTEN	Cowden disease	Malignancies of the breast, colon, uterus, thyroid, lung, and bladder; hamartomatous polyps in gastrointestinal tract
STK11	Peutz–Jeghers	Malignancies of the breast and pancreas; mucocutaneous melanin deposition, hamartomas of the GI tract
CDH1	Hereditary diffuse gastric cancer	Malignancies of the breast (lobular carcinoma) and stomach
Moderate penetrance		
CHEK2		Malignancies of the breast, prostate, kidney, colon, thyroid (*CHEK2*1100delC is most common mutation associated with breast cancer risk*)
PALB2	Fanconi anemia	Malignancies of the breast and pancreas Biallelic loss leads to Fanconi anemia
ATM	Ataxia-telangiectasia	Malignancies of the breast Biallelic loss leads to Ataxia-telangiectasia

TABLE 2.2 Common Genetic Mutations Associated With Breast Cancer

Radiation Exposure

Therapeutic radiation exposure to treat disease can be a significant cause of radiation-induced carcinogenesis. The highest associated risk is seen with higher doses of radiation and radiation treatment given at a young age, particularly before age 30 (relative risk is 5.2). This has been observed in women receiving mantle irradiation for treatment of Hodgkin disease. Given the elevated lifetime risk of breast cancer in this population, high-risk screening with annual mammography and breast MRI is recommended.

Endogenous Hormone Exposure

The hormonal milieu at different times in a woman's life may affect her risk of breast cancer and the total duration of exposure to endogenous estrogen is an important factor in breast cancer risk. Increased risk has been associated with early age at menarche, establishment of regular ovulatory cycles, nulliparity, advanced age at first childbirth, and late menopause. Interestingly, women who have their first child between ages 30 and 34 have the same risk as nulliparous women whereas women older than 35 years have a greater risk than nulliparous women. Obesity can also contribute to endogenous estrogen exposure, given higher rates of conversion of androgenic precursors through peripheral aromatization in adipose tissue. Lifestyle modification with healthy diet and regular physical activity is beneficial.

Exogenous Hormone Exposure

Exogenous hormone replacement therapy is a known risk factor for breast cancer. The Women's Health Initiative, a large-scale prospective study, was abruptly halted in 2002 after interim analysis indicated hormonal replacement therapy (HRT) was associated with a 26% increase in the risk of breast cancer over a 5-year period as well as an increased risk of stroke and coronary artery disease. HRT was found to be associated with increased bone density and fewer menopausal symptoms, which makes the ongoing use of HRT attractive to many woman. A meta-analysis from the Mayo Clinic by Benkhadra et al. looked at 43 randomized controlled trials and found no association between the use of HRT and cardiac death or stroke. Estrogen plus progesterone use was associated with a likely increase in breast cancer mortality (relative risk [RR] 1.96 [95% confidence interval (CI) 0.98–3.94]), whereas the use of estrogen alone did not increase this risk. In women who started HRT at less than 60 years of age, there was a reduction in all-cause mortality including cardiovascular and cancer deaths. Overall, the current evidence suggests that HRT does not affect the risk of death from all causes, cardiac death, and death from stroke or cancer. Therefore, treating physicians should thoroughly discuss the risks and benefits of this therapy with their patients.

Risk Assessment Tools

Multiple models exist that assess the risk of developing breast cancer. The Breast Cancer Risk Assessment Tool (http://www.cancer.gov/bcrisktool/) is a publicly available resource that was developed by scientists at the National Cancer Institute (NCI) and the National Surgical Adjuvant Breast and Bowel Project (NSABP). It is based on a statistical model known as the Gail model. This model incorporates a woman's personal medical history (number of previous breast biopsies and the presence of atypia in those biopsies), reproductive history (age at the start of menstruation and age at the first live birth), and the history of breast cancer among her first-degree relatives (mother, sisters, daughters) to estimate her risk of developing invasive breast cancer over a 5-year period and over her lifetime.

The appropriate risk assessment tool should be chosen based on a patient's specific risk factors. For example, while the Gail model is appropriate for women with a history of atypia, it is not applicable to women with a BRCA mutation. In these patients, the BRCAPRO model is more informative. The Tyrer–Cuzick model can better predict risk in patients with an extensive family history that would be underestimated by other models.

Pathology

Invasive carcinomas of the breast tend to be histologically heterogeneous tumors. The vast majority are adenocarcinomas that arise from the terminal ductal lobular units. There are five common histologic variants of mammary adenocarcinoma.

1. *Invasive ductal carcinoma* accounts for 75% of all breast cancers. This lesion is characterized by the absence of special histologic features. It is firm on palpation and gritty when transected. It is associated with various degrees of fibrotic response. Often there is associated ductal carcinoma in situ (DCIS) within the specimen. Invasive ductal carcinomas may metastasize to axillary lymph nodes. The prognosis for patients with these tumors is poorer than that for patients with some of the other histologic subtypes (i.e., mucinous, colloid, tubular, and medullary). Distant metastases are found most often in the bones, lungs, liver, and brain.

2. *Invasive lobular carcinoma* accounts for 15% of breast cancers. Clinically, this lesion often has an area of ill-defined thickening within the breast. Microscopically, small cells in a single-file pattern are characteristically seen. Invasive lobular cancers tend to grow around ducts and lobules and have the tendency to present with a radiographically occult infiltrative pattern. Multicentricity and bilaterality are observed more frequently in invasive lobular carcinoma than in invasive ductal carcinoma. The prognosis for invasive lobular carcinoma is similar to that for invasive ductal carcinoma. In addition to metastasizing to axillary lymph nodes, invasive lobular carcinoma is known to metastasize to unusual sites (e.g., meninges and serosal surfaces) more often than other forms of breast cancer.

3. *Tubular carcinoma* accounts for only 2% of breast carcinomas. The diagnosis of tubular carcinoma is made only when more than 75% of the tumor demonstrates tubule formation. Axillary nodal metastases are uncommon with this type of tumor. The prognosis for patients with tubular carcinoma is more favorable than that for patients with other types of breast cancer.

4. *Medullary carcinoma* accounts for 5% to 7% of breast cancers. Histologically, the lesion is characterized by poorly differentiated nuclei, a syncytial growth pattern, a well-circumscribed border, intense infiltration with small lymphocytes and plasma cells, and little or no associated DCIS. The prognosis for patients with pure medullary carcinoma is favorable, however, mixed variants with invasive ductal components will have prognoses similar to invasive ductal carcinoma. Medullary carcinoma occurs more frequently in BRCA mutation carriers.

5. *Mucinous or colloid carcinoma* constitutes approximately 3% of breast cancers. It is characterized by an abundant accumulation of extracellular mucin surrounding clusters of tumor cells. Colloid carcinoma is slow growing and tends to be bulky. These tumors are associated with a favorable prognosis.

6. *Rare histologic types* of breast malignancy include papillary, apocrine, secretory, squamous cell and spindle cell carcinomas, and metaplastic carcinoma. Invasive ductal carcinomas occasionally have small areas containing one or more of these special histologic types. Tumors with these mixed histologic appearances behave similarly to pure invasive ductal carcinomas.

Breast Cancer Molecular Subtypes

Perhaps one of the most striking advances in breast cancer management and understanding came with the molecular profiling of breast cancer characterizing four distinct subtypes based on the landmark paper by Perou et al., in 2000. These define tumor biology and correlate with outcome and are broadly described as

TABLE 2.3	Breast Cancer Molecular Subtypes
Subtype[a]	Typical Histopathologic Features
Luminal A	ER positive and/or PR positive HER2 negative Low Ki-67
Luminal B	ER positive and/or PR positive HER2 positive (or HER2 negative with high Ki-67)
Basal-like	ER negative PR negative HER2 negative
HER2 enriched	ER negative PR negative HER2 positive

[a]Not all tumors within each subtype contain all features. ER, estrogen receptor; PR, progesterone receptor; HER2, human epidermal growth factor receptor 2.

luminal A, luminal B, human epidermal growth factor receptor 2 (HER2)-enriched, and basal like according to the most common profiles for each subtype. However, not all tumors within each subtype contain all features. The estrogen receptor (ER), progesterone receptor (PR), and HER2 receptor are used as surrogates to approximate these subtypes and guide clinical care and management decisions (Table 2.3).

Luminal A: most (74%) of breast cancers express the estrogen receptor (ER-positive) and/or the progesterone receptor (PR+) but not HER2. These cancers tend to be more indolent than other subtypes. Luminal A tumors are associated with the most favorable prognosis, particularly in the short term, in part because expression of hormone receptors is predictive of a favorable response to hormonal therapy.

Luminal B: these breast cancers are ER-positive and/or PR+ and are further defined by either HER2 amplification, or high Ki-67 (an indicator of cellular proliferation). They tend to have higher grade and more aggressive features than luminal A breast cancers.

HER2-enriched: these breast cancers produce excess HER2 and do not express hormone receptors. These cancers tend to grow and spread more aggressively than other breast cancers and are associated with poorer short-term prognosis compared to ER-positive breast cancers. However, the recent widespread use of targeted therapies for HER2-positive cancers has reversed much of the adverse prognostic impact of HER2 overexpression, with 40% to 70% of women achieving a pathologic complete response to combination chemotherapy and targeted anti-HER2 therapies.

Basal like: these tumors are more biologically aggressive and are typically characterized by the lack of the ER, PR, and HER2 receptor. These cancers are often found in premenopausal women, those with a BRCA1 gene mutation, and are nearly two times more common in Black women than White women in US. The majority (>70%) of triple negative breast cancers fall into the basal-like subtype. Triple negative breast cancers have a poorer short-term prognosis than other breast cancer types, in part because there are currently no targeted therapies for these tumors. However, a proportion of these tumors are very chemosensitive, exhibiting a pathologic complete response in up to a third of patients. Furthermore, several molecular subtypes of triple negative breast cancer have been described. These may provide further insights into the varying biologic response and assist in development of therapeutic targets in addition to chemotherapy.

Diagnosis and Evaluation

The diagnosis of breast cancer has undergone a dramatic evolution over the past 25 years. Previously, most breast cancers were detected by self-examination however, with implementation of mammographic screening, there has been a greater shift toward the diagnosis of nonpalpable lesions. Evaluation of breast cancer relies on comprehensive history and physical examination, radiographic, and tissue diagnosis.

History and Physical Examination

The history is directed at assessing cancer risk and establishing the presence or absence of symptoms indicative of breast disease. It should include age at menarche, menopausal status, previous pregnancies, and use of oral contraceptives or postmenopausal replacement estrogens. A personal history of breast cancer and the age at diagnosis, as well as a personal history of other cancers treated with radiation (e.g., Hodgkin disease) is important. In addition, the family history of breast cancer or ovarian cancer in first-degree relatives should be established. Any significant prior breast history should be elucidated including previous breast biopsies, especially if done for atypical disease, breast augmentation/reduction, breast problems, and any imaging history. After the risk for breast cancer has been determined, the patient should be assessed for specific symptoms. Breast pain and nipple discharge are often, but not always, associated with benign processes such as fibrocystic disease and intraductal papilloma. Malaise, bony pain, and weight loss are rare but may indicate potential metastatic disease.

Physical examination by the health care provider should take into consideration the comfort and emotional well-being of the patient. Examination should include careful visual inspection with the patient in the upright and supine positions. Nipple changes, breast size, degree of ptosis, breast asymmetry, and obvious masses are all noted. The skin must be inspected for subtle changes; these can range from slight dimpling/flattening to the more dramatic *peau d'orange* (an erythematous and thickened appearance associated with locally advanced or inflammatory breast cancer [IBC]). In large or ptotic breasts, the breasts should be lifted to facilitate inspection of the inferior portion of the breast and the inframammary fold. After careful inspection and with the patient remaining in the sitting position, the cervical, occipital, and periclavicular nodal basins are examined for potential disease. Both axillae are then carefully palpated. If palpable, nodes should be characterized as to their number, size, and mobility. Examination of the axilla always includes palpation of the axillary tail of the breast as assessment of this area is often overlooked once the patient is placed in a supine position. Palpation of the breast parenchyma itself is accomplished with the patient supine and the ipsilateral arm placed over the head. The subareolar tissues and each quadrant of both breasts are systematically palpated. Masses are noted with respect to their size, shape, location, consistency, and mobility. If patients are evaluated after the completion of diagnostic biopsy, documentation of ecchymoses or associated hematoma should be noted as well.

Critical analysis of the breast physical examination has shown limitations in differentiating benign and malignant disease, even among experienced examiners. Because of the high rate of inaccuracy, any persistent breast concern requires additional evaluation.

Diagnostic Imaging

The choice of initial diagnostic evaluation after the detection of a breast mass should be individualized for each patient according to age, perceived cancer risk, and characteristics of the lesion. For most patients, mammographic evaluation is the essential initial step, followed by ultrasound.

The American College of Radiology developed the breast imaging reporting and data system (BIRADS), which categorizes findings as follows:

- BIRADS 0, incomplete or further imaging needed
- BIRADS 1, negative (no findings)
- BIRADS 2, benign appearance
- BIRADS 3, probably benign appearance, short interval follow-up recommended (<2% chance of malignancy)
- BIRADS 4, findings suspicious for breast cancer (2% to 94% chance of malignancy)
  - 4a low suspicion (2% to 9%)
  - 4b moderate suspicion (10% to 49%)
  - 4c high suspicion (50% to 94%)
- BIRADS 5, findings highly suspicious for breast cancer (>95% chance of malignancy)
- BIRADS 6, known biopsy-proven malignancy

Based on these findings, recommendations are made for either short- or long-term surveillance versus further immediate workup. For lesions interpreted as "probably benign" (BIRADS 3) such as well-defined, solitary masses, careful counseling, and short-term follow-up with repeat radiographic studies in 6 months may be undertaken in patients at low risk for breast cancer, whereas a BIRADS 4 reading usually recommends further evaluation with biopsy as indicated. However, if a stellate or spiculated mass typical of malignancy (BIRADS 5) is identified, immediate evaluation with biopsy is required.

Mammography should evaluate both breasts for evaluation of the palpable lesion as well as identifying nonpalpable lesions. Bilateral synchronous cancers occur in approximately 3% of all cases and at least half of these lesions are nonpalpable. Mammographic signs of malignancy include microcalcifications and density changes such as a discrete masses, architectural distortion, and focal asymmetry. The most predictive mammographic findings of malignancy are spiculated masses with associated architectural distortion, clustered microcalcifications in a linear or branching array, and microcalcifications associated with a mass. Additional suspicious findings on mammogram include nipple changes and axillary adenopathy. The presence or absence of these mammographic findings can predict malignancy with an accuracy of 70% to 80%. Mammography is least accurate in younger patients with dense breasts and for this reason, it is not commonly used in patients younger than the age of 35 years for screening.

Breast ultrasound is an important adjunct to mammography and assists in clinical decision making. Particularly in young women with dense breast tissue, ultrasound is often used to further evaluate suspicious areas or palpable lesions. For all ages, it is regularly included in the initial evaluation and workup of mammographically indeterminate lesions, solid and cystic lesions, as well as regional nodal evaluation. Ultrasound is routinely used at the University of Texas MD Anderson Cancer Center (MDACC) to evaluate the axillary nodal basin and any suspicious infraclavicular, supraclavicular, or internal mammary adenopathy. Any suspicious nodes are sampled at that time by ultrasound-guided fine-needle aspiration (FNA) or core-needle biopsy with or without placement of a marker clip. Marking the biopsy-proven axillary lymph node has increasing importance in the current era of evaluating lymph nodes after neoadjuvant chemotherapy (NAC).

Breast MRI has been gaining in popularity for the diagnosis and surgical planning of breast cancer though its utility remains controversial. The increased sensitivity of MRI can lead to overdiagnosis, more benign biopsies and is associated with an increased conversion from breast conservation to mastectomy. However, MRI is indicated in the following circumstances:

- As an adjunct for evaluating inconclusive findings on conventional imaging (mammogram and ultrasound)
- For determining the extent of cancer or presence of multifocal tumor or contralateral cancer in patients with a proven breast cancer
- In the case of nodal or metastatic breast cancer with an unknown primary
- A diagnosis of Paget disease, without mammographically or sonographically identified mass
- To evaluate suspected chest wall invasion of a tumor
- Assessment for eligibility and response to neoadjuvant endocrine therapy or chemotherapy before during or after treatment

MRI is also indicated for high-risk screening in women with a history of mantle radiation, BRCA1 or BRCA2 gene mutation or a documented lifetime risk of breast cancer greater than 20% to 25%. Studies evaluating high-risk patients with an overall cumulative lifetime risk of developing breast cancer of approximately 30% show that MRI is able to detect cancer in approximately 1% to 3% of patients.

Tissue Biopsy

Biopsy for diagnosis should follow radiographic evaluation of suspicious breast lesions. FNA is unable to distinguish between *in situ* and invasive disease and therefore core-needle biopsy is preferred for initial diagnosis. Image guidance is recommended. Palpable lesions may be amenable to ultrasound-guided biopsy whereas nonpalpable lesions identified only by mammography are more suitable for stereotactic biopsy. Placement of a marking clip at the time of biopsy is necessary for several reasons; to confirm that the intended lesion was biopsied, to assist in long-term follow-up of benign masses and to identify the location of any malignant lesion for future excision and/or to follow response to neoadjuvant therapy. A postbiopsy mammogram should be performed to ensure proper placement of the marker clip. Biopsy should be deferred until after radiographic examination is completed as a postbiopsy hematoma can obscure subsequent radiographic evaluation. It is imperative that the imaging findings and final pathology are evaluated for concordance in regard to the suspicion of malignancy. In the setting of discordance, additional evaluation is necessary to rule out a malignancy.

Excisional Biopsy

Excisional biopsy for the diagnosis of breast cancer has fallen out of favor as the importance of preoperative histopathology increasingly dictates multidisciplinary care and operative planning. Furthermore, advances in radiologic interventions including ultrasound- and stereotactic-guided biopsy and MRI-guided biopsies mean that it is rare that a tissue diagnosis cannot be reached percutaneously, and excisional biopsy may be needed in only a handful of circumstances. Appropriate indications for excisional biopsy are shown in Table 2.4.

When core-needle biopsy or FNA is impossible or inappropriate, excisional breast biopsy may be performed and serves both diagnostic and local treatment objectives. The location and orientation of the incision for an excisional biopsy must take into consideration potential future breast-conserving therapy (BCT) or mastectomy incisions. Preoperative needle localization with a self-retaining hook wire or seed technology under image guidance is required, as is careful communication between the radiologist and the surgeon. Postlocalization mammograms are reviewed to confirm placement of the wire or seed within the targeted area. Excision is then performed by removing breast tissue around the marker with incisions placed preferentially overlying the lesion (not necessarily at the wire entry site if utilizing wire localization). Postexcision specimen radiographs

TABLE 2.4	Indications for Excisional Biopsy in the Evaluation of a Breast Lesion Suspicious for Cancer (*percutaneous biopsy is preferred method of diagnosis*)

Indications for Excisional Biopsy

Inability to obtain radiographic-guided biopsy

Discordance of clinical radiographic and core biopsy pathologic features

Presence of a high-risk lesion (ADH, ALH, LCIS) and associated mass lesion to rule out associated cancer

Removal of growing or suspicious fibroadenoma or fibroepithelial lesion to rule out phyllodes tumor

Patient preference due to distortion, pain, or psychological distress

ADH, atypical ductal hyperplasia; ALH, atypical lobular hyperplasia; LCIS, lobular carcinoma in situ.

are essential to confirm excision of the target lesion and that the marker clip and localization wire or seed are in the specimen as well.

Meticulous orientation and handling of the specimen is critical. The specimen should be oriented such that the margins are clearly identified (e.g., short stitch superior, long stitch lateral, ink deep with breast laterality clearly labeled) and when possible, hand delivered to the pathology department for further assessment.

Staging

Following a breast cancer diagnosis, the patient is clinically staged using the American Joint Committee on Cancer (AJCC) guidelines. The AJCC TNM breast cancer staging system was updated in 2017 and published in the eighth edition of the *AJCC Cancer Staging Manual.* Three major changes were incorporated into the most recent AJCC edition. First, LCIS was removed from the staging system, asserting the belief that it is not a breast malignancy, but a risk factor. This includes exclusion of pleomorphic LCIS. In disease identified to be a mix of LCIS and DCIS, the case is classified as pTis. Second, biologic factors including hormone receptor expression, HER2 amplification, and genomic panels were determined to be as equally important as anatomic descriptors of disease in defining prognosis. Therefore, these factors have been incorporated into the AJCC staging, specifically with multigene panel results being identified as stage modifiers. Finally, immunohistochemically detected tumor markers (ER/PR/HER2) are now incorporated into the staging system. With incorporation of these additional factors, the AJCC eighth edition is able to define a clinical prognostic stage for all patients with breast cancer and a pathologic prognostic stage for patients treated with upfront surgery.

Early-Stage Breast Cancer

The majority of patients with breast cancer present with tumors less than 5 cm in diameter and no evidence of fixed or matted nodes consistent with clinical stage I or II disease. Workup for patients with clinical stage I or stage II breast cancer is usually limited to a complete history and physical examination, dedicated breast imaging, a chest radiograph, and evaluation of serum liver chemistries. The routine use of systemic staging examinations in asymptomatic patients is not generally indicated.

The treatment approach consists of locoregional therapy with surgery and radiation therapy when indicated. Surgical options include breast conservation therapy including segmental mastectomy followed by radiation therapy or total mastectomy with or without reconstruction. Sentinel lymph node dissection (SLND) is standard practice for axillary staging in clinically node-negative breast cancer. Systemic therapy in the neoadjuvant or adjuvant setting is indicated as many patients may harbor micrometastatic disease. The systemic therapy options are formulated based on patient- and tumor-related factors including receptor status, final pathologic stage, and genomic assays in the adjuvant setting.

Locally Advanced Breast Cancer

Locally advanced breast cancers are typically large and/or have extensive regional lymph nodal involvement without evidence of distant metastatic disease at initial presentation. Approximately 10% to 20% of all patients with breast cancer have stage III disease with one-quarter of these patients initially inoperable at the time of diagnosis.

Many locally advanced breast cancers are discovered by self-examination or routine physical examination. Occasionally, a discrete mass may not be present and diffuse infiltration of the breast tissue is apparent. Seventy-five percent of patients with stage III disease will have clinically palpable axillary or supraclavicular lymph nodes at the time of diagnosis. This clinical finding is confirmed on pathologic examination in 66% to 90% of patients. Of the patients with positive nodes, 50% will have more than four nodes involved. Metastatic workup should be performed in the setting of stage III disease as 20% of patients are found to have distant metastases at presentation and are often asymptomatic. Distant metastases are also the most frequent form of treatment failure and usually appear within 2 years of the initial diagnosis.

The standard of care in patients with locally advanced breast cancer is a neoadjuvant systemic therapy approach followed by surgery and adjuvant radiation therapy. Adjuvant hormonal therapy is routinely offered to all patients with hormone receptor–positive tumors. In addition, in the setting of residual disease after NAC, additional systemic therapy is indicated and guided by the tumor subtype.

Surgical options include breast conservation (if limited disease in the breast) and mastectomy. If contralateral mastectomy is desired or planned, a delayed or staged approach should be considered as the majority of risk is determined by the index malignancy. Axillary dissection is the standard for surgical management of the axilla, however, the clinical landscape is changing in the setting of node-positive disease after NAC. In selected cases with limited nodal involvement and demonstration of clinical response to NAC, SLND or targeted axillary dissection (TAD) for axillary staging may be appropriate.

Inflammatory Breast Cancer

IBC, denoted within the AJCC staging system as T4d disease, is a rare, aggressive form of locally advanced breast cancer. It represents 1% to 6% of all breast cancers and presents as rapid onset of erythema, warmth, and edema involving greater than one-third of the breast skin. Onset of symptoms within 3 months is required to make the diagnosis of IBC and distinguishes it from locally advanced breast cancer with secondary lymphatic invasion (T4b disease), which usually progresses slowly over more than 3 months. Distinct from the majority of breast cancers, pain is also present in half of patients with IBC. Initial diagnosis of these physical findings as sequelae of an infectious process often delays diagnosis and treatment. The characteristic pathologic finding is dermal lymphatic invasion by carcinoma on skin punch biopsy. Ultimately, the diagnosis of IBC is based on the clinical evaluation and the absence of dermal lymphatic invasion pathologically does not exclude the diagnosis.

Inflammatory breast carcinoma, like other forms of locally advanced breast cancer, is a systemic disease. Systemic staging evaluating for distant metastatic disease is indicated even in asymptomatic patients presenting with IBC. In a study of inflammatory carcinoma, local therapy as the only treatment modality resulted in poor outcomes; the median survival was less than 2 years, and the 5-year overall survival (OS) rate was 5%. The use of multimodality therapy in these patients has improved local control and overall survival over local therapy alone. Standard-of-care treatment is NAC with targeted therapy in the setting of HER2-positive disease, followed by modified radical mastectomy and adjuvant radiation therapy. With the addition of chemotherapy to the treatment regimen, the 5-year overall survival rate is approximately 40%, although this number has not improved since the 1970s. However, with a dedicated multidisciplinary treating team utilizing contemporary systemic therapy regimens and comprehensive locoregional therapy, 5-year overall survival can approach 69% for patients with stage III disease as reported by MD Anderson. Patients with disease progression during chemotherapy can proceed to preoperative radiation therapy or in the setting of operable disease, surgery with modified radical mastectomy. BCT and sentinel lymph node (SLN) dissection are not appropriate in these patients as dermal involvement extends beyond the tumor and precludes reliable drainage of tracer or dye to the lymph node basins. Breast reconstruction should be delayed, as nearly all patients will require chest wall and regional nodal radiation, to include axillary, infraclavicular, supraclavicular, and internal mammary nodes. In addition, contralateral prophylactic mastectomy (CPM) is not recommended.

Multidisciplinary Evaluation

Once the diagnosis of breast cancer has been made, the optimization of treatment decisions is best coordinated in a multidisciplinary fashion. The collaborative efforts of surgical oncologists with medical oncology, radiation oncologists, geneticists, plastic and reconstructive surgeons, and cancer care coordinators can direct the choice of surgery, systemic therapy, radiation options, and reconstructive choices (Figure 2.1). For reference, updated MD Anderson breast cancer treatment algorithms are available at https://www.mdanderson.org/for-physicians/clinical-tools-resources/clinical-practice-algorithms/cancer-treatment-algorithms.html.

Local/Regional Therapy

Surgery

Management of the Breast Primary

Surgical management of the breast primary has evolved over time from the Halsted radical mastectomy which included resection of the breast, axillary nodes, and pectoralis muscle. This evolution has been influenced by several landmark randomized, prospective clinical trials which have changed clinical practice as well as an understanding of the biology of breast cancer. In the United States, the majority of these were performed by the NSABP. A summary of selected trials is presented in Table 2.5.

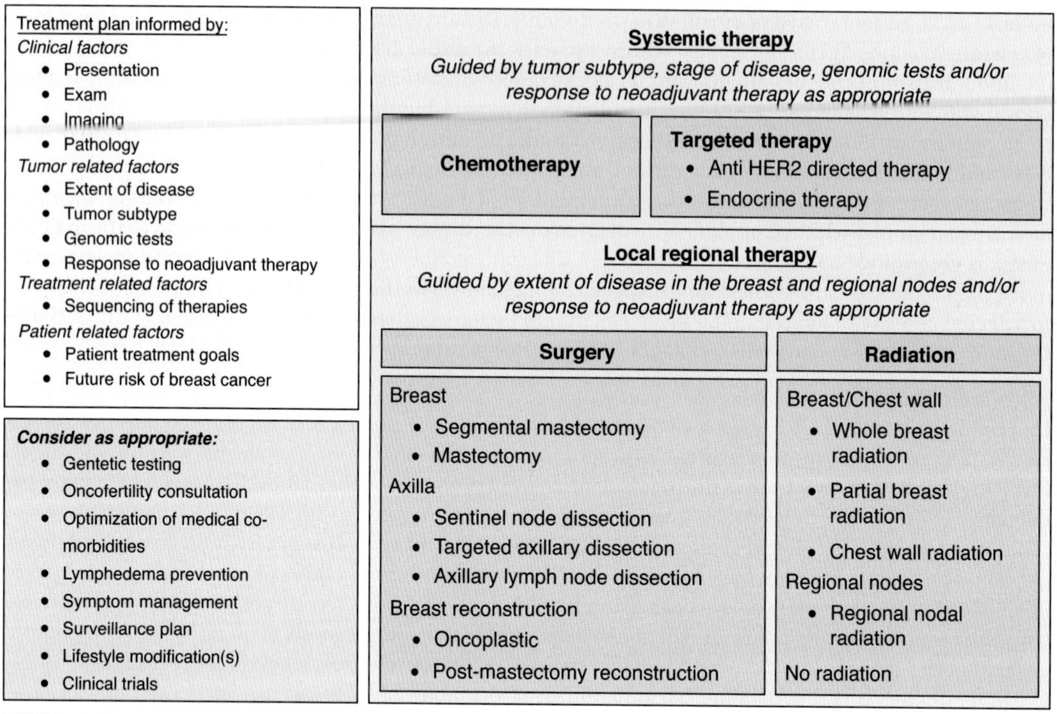

Treatment plan informed by:
Clinical factors
- Presentation
- Exam
- Imaging
- Pathology

Tumor related factors
- Extent of disease
- Tumor subtype
- Genomic tests
- Response to neoadjuvant therapy

Treatment related factors
- Sequencing of therapies

Patient related factors
- Patient treatment goals
- Future risk of breast cancer

Consider as appropriate:
- Gentetic testing
- Oncofertility consultation
- Optimization of medical co-morbidities
- Lymphedema prevention
- Symptom management
- Surveillance plan
- Lifestyle modification(s)
- Clinical trials

Systemic therapy
Guided by tumor subtype, stage of disease, genomic tests and/or response to neoadjuvant therapy as appropriate

Chemotherapy

Targeted therapy
- Anti HER2 directed therapy
- Endocrine therapy

Local regional therapy
Guided by extent of disease in the breast and regional nodes and/or response to neoadjuvant therapy as appropriate

Surgery

Breast
- Segmental mastectomy
- Mastectomy

Axilla
- Sentinel node dissection
- Targeted axillary dissection
- Axillary lymph node dissection

Breast reconstruction
- Oncoplastic
- Post-mastectomy reconstruction

Radiation

Breast/Chest wall
- Whole breast radiation
- Partial breast radiation
- Chest wall radiation

Regional nodes
- Regional nodal radiation

No radiation

FIGURE 2.1 Creation of a multidisciplinary treatment plan after diagnosis of invasive breast cancer.

TABLE 2.5 Summary of Selected NSABP Therapeutic Trials for Invasive Breast Cancer

Trial	Treatment	Outcome
NSABP B-04	Total mastectomy vs. total mastectomy with XRT vs. radical mastectomy	No significant difference in disease-free or overall survival rates
NSABP B-06	Total mastectomy vs. lumpectomy vs. lumpectomy with XRT	No significant difference in disease-free or overall survival rates; addition of XRT to lumpectomy reduced local recurrence rate from 39% to 10%
NSABP B-13	Surgery alone vs. surgery plus adjuvant chemotherapy in node-negative patients with estrogen receptor-negative tumors	Improved disease-free survival rate for adjuvant chemotherapy group
NSABP B-14	Surgery alone vs. surgery plus adjuvant tamoxifen in node-negative patients with estrogen receptor-positive tumors	Improved disease-free survival rate for adjuvant tamoxifen group
NSABP B-18	Neoadjuvant chemotherapy with doxorubicin, cyclophosphamide, or both for 4 cycles vs. the same regimen given postoperatively	No significant difference in overall survival or disease-free survival rates (53–70% at 9 yrs in the postoperative group and 69% and 55% in the preoperative group)
NSABP B-21	Lumpectomy plus tamoxifen vs. lumpectomy plus tamoxifen plus XRT vs. lumpectomy plus XRT for node-negative tumors <1 cm	Combination of XRT and tamoxifen was more effective than either alone in reducing ipsilateral breast tumor recurrence
NSABP B-27	Neoadjuvant chemotherapy comparing AC × 4 cycles than surgery vs. AC × 4 cycles, docetaxel × 4 cycles than surgery vs. surgery between 4 cycles of AC and 4 cycles of docetaxel	Groups I and III were combined and compared with group II; clinical and pathologic complete response rates increased significantly among patients who received preoperative AC and docetaxel
NSABP B-32	SLN biopsy followed by axillary dissection vs. SLN biopsy alone for clinically node-negative patients	SLN identification rate was similar in both groups, accuracy was high for both, negative predictive value was high for both

NSABP, National Surgical Adjuvant Breast and Bowel Project; XRT, radiation therapy; AC, doxorubicin (Adriamycin), cyclophosphamide; SLN, sentinel lymph node.

Breast-Conserving Therapy Many patients with early-stage breast cancer can be treated effectively with BCT, which entails complete removal of the tumor with negative histologic margins in combination with adjuvant radiation therapy. Six prospective randomized trials comparing breast conservation with radical or modified radical mastectomy have shown no survival advantage to mastectomy.

In the United States, the trial establishing survival equivalence of breast conservation with mastectomy was the NSABP B-06. This trial included women with primary tumors up to 4 cm and clinical N0 or N1 nodal status. Patients were randomly assigned to modified radical mastectomy, lumpectomy with axillary lymph node dissection (ALND), or lumpectomy with ALND and radiation therapy. Histologically, negative margins were required in the breast conservation groups. Disease-free and overall survival rates did not differ significantly among the three groups, but the local recurrence rate was markedly reduced at 10 years by radiation therapy in the breast-conserving groups such that 12% recurred after lumpectomy and radiation therapy versus 53% with lumpectomy alone. These results supported breast conservation as an appropriate treatment strategy for patients with clinical stage I or II breast cancer and cemented radiation therapy as an integral part of BCT.

No significant differences in local control, disease-free survival (DFS), or overall survival have been observed, even after 20 years of follow-up, indicating that survival in these patients is not dependent on the choice of mastectomy versus BCT.

Given the oncologic equivalence with respect to outcome, the decision for BCT should include the patient's motivation and commitment to conserving the natural breast. Inappropriate candidates for BCT include patients who are unable to receive radiation, diffuse disease, or persistent positive margins. Also, relative contraindications include patients with small breast volume or high tumor-to-breast ratio, where the cosmetic result may be unacceptable following BCT. Increasingly, incorporation of oncoplastic technique or coordination with a plastic surgeon for oncoplastic reconstruction in conjunction with contralateral surgery for symmetry can yield excellent oncologic results without aesthetic compromise. Patients with large tumors may benefit from neoadjuvant systemic therapy to downstage the breast primary thereby facilitating breast conservation. Although the use of BCT has increased during the past 14 years, nonclinical factors including socioeconomic demographics, insurance, and travel distance to the treatment facility persist as key barriers to BCT. Other factors that must be considered in making the choice between mastectomy and breast conservation surgery, are outlined in Table 2.6.

Margin assessment is critical in BCT. Positive margins require re-excision or conversion to mastectomy. Determination of an appropriate negative margin has been controversial with national re-excision rates of 20% to 40%. Given this, in 2014, the SSO in collaboration with the American Society for Radiation Oncology (ASTRO) published national guidelines to address this clinical concern. These guidelines have defined a negative margin to be "no ink on tumor" and noted that wider margins did not significantly lower the risk of ipsilateral breast tumor recurrence. In cases with invasive disease "no tumor on ink" references both the invasive tumor and DCIS margin. Furthermore, cases should be reviewed in a multidisciplinary fashion with consideration for re-excision in selected cases including extensive involvement by DCIS, discrepancy with clinical and radiographic tumor size, and multiple close margins.

TABLE 2.6	Absolute and Relative Contraindications to Breast-Conserving Therapy

Absolute Contraindications

Widespread disease that cannot achieve negative margins with a satisfactory aesthetic result

Radiotherapy use during pregnancy

Diffuse suspicious or malignant-appearing microcalcifications

Diffuse positive margins or positive margins after multiple excisions

Relative Contraindications

Active connective tissue disease involving the skin (including scleroderma and lupus)

Large tumor to breast size ratio

Prior radiation therapy to the chest wall or breast (knowledge of doses and volumes prescribed is essential)

Women with a known or suspected genetic predisposition to breast cancer, who may have an increased risk of ipsilateral breast recurrence or contralateral breast cancer. Prophylactic bilateral mastectomy for risk reduction may be considered

Based on national consensus guidelines.

The standard for BCT at MDACC is excision of the tumor with negative margins followed by radiation therapy. An oncoplastic approach with reconstruction of the segmental defect is favored in the majority of cases. This is further discussed in Chapter 26, Reconstructive Surgery in Cancer Patients. An extensive intra-operative assessment of margins is standard practice. This includes a multidisciplinary effort by radiology, pathology, and surgery. The specimen is oriented by the surgeon and taken to the pathology suite where a specimen radiograph is performed to confirm excision of the lesion. The specimen is then inked and sectioned followed by an additional radiographic assessment to determine any close or involved margins. The specimen is also evaluated grossly for margins. Frozen section or additional margin excision is performed based on this assessment. Typically, surgical clips are placed within the segmental cavity to delineate the tumor bed and guide radiation treatment. In the adjuvant setting, radiation planning is initiated approximately 3 to 4 weeks after surgery. A dose of 50 Gy is given to the whole breast, and then 10 Gy is given to the operative site as a boost using tangential ports and computerized dosimetry in selected patients. Long-term mammographic surveillance of the preserved breast is necessary to detect potential in-breast recurrence.

The local recurrence rates following BCT, as documented in the Milan study, NSABP B-06, and the Danish Breast Cancer Cooperative Group study range from 2.6% to 18%, which is slightly higher than the range quoted for mastectomy (2.3% to 13%). However, there was no significant difference in overall survival between BCT and mastectomy in any of these studies. Furthermore, this data does not account for the major advancements in diagnosis, risk assessment, adjuvant hormonal therapy, chemotherapy, or targeted therapy. The influence of tumor biopsy on recurrence rates among patients treated with BCT has been shown to have no impact on outcomes in both the neoadjuvant and adjuvant systemic therapy settings. The ultimate goal of BCT for patients with early-stage breast cancer is to provide an optimal cosmetic result without compromising local control. Clearly, a multidisciplinary effort coupled with careful patient selection is critical for the successful outcome of BCT.

Mastectomy The mastectomy has evolved greatly over time since the Halsted radical mastectomy, which included resection of the breast glandular tissue (including skin, nipple, and areola), pectoralis major and minor muscles, and regional axillary nodes (level I to III). The NSABP B-04 trial demonstrated equivalence of the modified radical mastectomy preserving the pectoralis muscle as compared to the radical mastectomy. With the advent of the SLN technique allowing more precise axillary nodal evaluation, not all patients will require axillary dissection. The simple or total mastectomy removes the breast tissue with the majority of over-lying skin, nipple, and areola, but preserves the majority of the axillary nodal contents and pectoralis muscles.

In 1991, popularization of the skin-sparing mastectomy (SSM) transformed breast oncologic surgery allowing for immediate breast reconstruction. SSM consists of a total mastectomy with resection of the nipple–areola complex, while allowing access to the axilla as indicated. It preserves a significant amount of the native skin envelope along with the inframammary fold, thus enhancing the aesthetic results of immediate breast reconstruction. Several retrospective reviews have documented the oncologic safety of this procedure, and in early-stage breast cancer, the added benefit of immediate reconstruction can reduce the psychological impact of the surgery and improve body image without compromise of local, regional, or systemic recurrence rates when compared to conventional mastectomy.

Nipple-sparing mastectomy (NSM), which allows for preservation of the nipple and areolar complex is accepted as an oncologically safe procedure when there is no evidence of nipple involvement. Conventional indications for NSM include women with early-stage tumors located more than 2 cm from the nipple with a clinically negative axilla. For aesthetic and technical reasons, very large or ptotic breasts may be relative contraindications. Particular care must be taken in women with central DCIS as preoperative imaging can underestimate the extent of disease; therefore, careful attention to the final pathology is imperative in all cases. NSM is increasingly being performed for risk reduction in BRCA and other high-risk patients undergo-ing prophylactic mastectomy, with excellent oncologic and aesthetic results. In a recent multicenter Italian trial of 1,006 procedures, NSM failure rate, with NAC removal for any reason was 11.5%, with a NAC necrosis rate of 4.8%, and large skin-flap necrosis occurring in 2.3%. All NSM must be performed in close consultation with a plastic surgeon and patient selection and surgeon comfort remain important considerations.

Prophylactic mastectomy is utilized in high-risk patients as a risk-reduction strategy resulting in 90% to 95% relative risk reduction. Among average-risk women, rates of CPM in the United States have increased dramatically over the past 10 years. This is in contrast to declining rates of contralateral breast cancer (CBC), particularly in patients with ER-positive breast cancer. Furthermore, the risk of a CBC in women with spo-radic breast cancer is low and estimated at 0.5% to 0.75% per year among women with early-stage disease. Several studies have not shown a survival advantage to CPM, even among the highest risk individuals. When

Summary of Selected Clinical Trials Guiding Current Axillary Management

Trial	Intervention	Outcome
ACOSOG Z0010	cT1-2 N0 M0 invasive breast cancer treated with upfront BCT and SLN dissection. IHC performed on negative SLNs to evaluate for incidence and prognostic impact of occult micrometastatic disease.	Occult micrometastasis by IHC was identified 10.5% of SLNs. No significant difference in OS or DFS based on presence of occult micrometastatic SLN disease at 6.3 yrs follow-up.
ACOSOG Z0011	cT1-2 N0 M0 invasive breast cancer treated with upfront BCT and SLN dissection. Patients with 1–2 positive SLNs randomized to ALND vs. omission of ALND.	No significant difference in OS or locoregional recurrence at 10 yrs follow-up.
AMAROS	cT1-2 N0 M0 invasive breast cancer treated with upfront surgery (BCT or mastectomy) including SLN dissection. Patients with positive SLNs randomized to ALND vs. axillary radiation	No significant difference in axillary recurrence at 5 yrs follow-up. Lower rates of lymphedema following axillary radiation compared with ALND.
IBCSG 23-01	cT1-2 N0 M0 invasive breast cancer treated with upfront surgery (BCT or mastectomy) including SLN dissection. Patients with micrometastic (0.2–2 mm) positive SLNs were randomized to ALND vs. omission of ALND.	No significant difference in 5-yr and 10-yr DFS.
ACOSOG Z1071	cT0-4 N1-2* M0 invasive breast cancer treated with neoadjuvant chemotherapy. All patients received SLN dissection and ALND to determine false-negative rate (FNR) of SLND in this population. (*analysis included N1 patients only)	FNR for SLN following chemotherapy was 12.6%. FNR improved when 3 or more SLNs were evaluated (9.1%) and when dual tracer technique was used (10.8%). Further analysis showed further improvement in FNR with excision of the clipped node (6.8%) and IHC evaluation classifying ITCs as node-positive (8.7%).
SENTINA (Arm C)	cN1-2 invasive breast cancer treated with neoadjuvant chemotherapy. All patients in Arm C received SLN dissection followed by ALND.	FNR of SLN dissection was 14.2%. FNR improved when 3 or more SLNs were examined (<10%) and when dual tracer technique was used (8.6%).
SN-FNAC	cT0-3 N1-2 M0 invasive breast cancer treated with neoadjuvant chemotherapy. All patients received SLN dissection and ALND to determine false-negative rate of SLND in this population. Metastasis of any size, including ITCs identified on IHC, was considered positive.	FNR of SLN dissection was 8.4%. FNR improved when 2 or more SLNs were examined (4.9%) and when dual tracer technique was used (5.2%).

BCT, breast conserving therapy; SLN, sentinel lymph node; IHC, immunohistochemistry; OS, overall survival; DFS, disease-free survival; ALND, axillary lymph node dissection; ITC, isolated tumor cells.

discussing CPM, it is important to note the absolute benefit in risk reduction may be modest in addition to comparing the risk of systemic recurrence and death from the index malignancy and medical comorbidities against the risk of a future contralateral breast cancer.

Management of the Axilla

Axillary staging is indicated in patients with invasive breast cancer, as identifying patients with nodal metastases impacts prognosis and multidisciplinary local, regional, and systemic treatment recommendations. Axillary surgery for breast cancer is one of the most rapidly evolving areas in breast cancer treatment guided by several landmark clinical trials (Table 2.7). Management algorithms for patients with clinically node-negative and clinically node-positive disease are outlined in Figure 2.2.

Clinically Node-Negative Disease ALND was once considered the gold standard for evaluating the draining nodal basin for lymph node metastases. However, lymphatic mapping with SLN dissection is now the standard of care for axillary staging in clinically node-negative patients with breast cancer. The SLN is defined as the first lymph node or group of nodes that receive lymphatic drainage from a primary breast cancer and as such are most likely to contain metastatic disease. Several randomized clinical trials have demonstrated the feasibility and oncologic safety of SLN dissection including the NSABP B-32 clinical trial. Most studies report successful

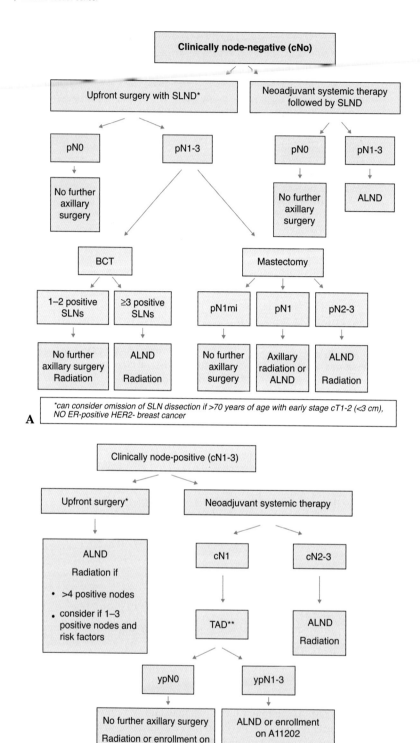

FIGURE 2.2 Management of the axilla in (**A**) clinically node-negative (cN0) and (**B**) clinically node-positive (cN1-3) invasive breast cancer.

SLN detection in 94% to 98% of patients, an accuracy rate of 97% to 100%, and a false-negative rate of 0% to 15%. Furthermore, it is well documented that SLN dissection results in reduced morbidity including pain, paresthesia, decreased range of motion, seroma, and lymphedema.

At MDACC, lymphatic mapping is performed with preoperative or intraoperative injection of Technetium-99 followed by transcutaneous localization of increased radioactivity performed with a handheld gamma probe, with or without the addition of isosulfan blue dye. Use of dual tracer has been shown to decrease false-negative rates and should strongly be considered, particularly in patients who may have impaired lymphatic drainage to the axilla, such as in cases of prior breast and/or axillary surgery or radiation and after receipt of NAC. Preoperative lymphoscintigraphy, although not mandatory, can also be used to identify the SLN and document patterns of lymphatic drainage. Once the SLN(s) are removed, the axilla is examined to confirm a reduction in radioactivity to less than 10% of the highest lymph node count identified. A residual high level of radioactivity indicates that additional sentinel nodes remain in the nodal basin.

Studies have shown that approximately 24% of patients with early-stage clinically node-negative breast cancer will have a positive sentinel node. The incidence of finding a positive SLN correlates with primary tumor size.

Management of SLN-Positive Patients Traditionally, ALND was performed in the setting of a positive SLN. A paradigm shift occurred in 2010 following results of the ACOSOG Z0011 trial which challenged the traditional approach. This trial definitively changed the management of SLN-positive axillary metastases in patients with early-stage clinically node-negative breast cancer.

The Z0011 trial enrolled patients with clinically node-negative, T1 or T2 early-stage breast cancer undergoing BCT and SLN dissection, with two or fewer positive SLNs as detected by hematoxylin and eosin (H&E) staining. Critically important to this study was the requirement that all patients received postoperative whole-breast radiation and chemotherapy as indicated. Patients were randomized to completion axillary dissection versus no further axillary surgery. At a median follow-up of 6.3 years, there was no difference in overall survival (ALND 91.9% vs. 92.5% in SLN-only; $P = .24$) or DFS (ALND 82.2% vs. 83.8% in SLN-only; $P = .13$) at 5 years. There was no significant difference in local recurrence reported (3.6% of the ALND group vs. 1.8% of the SLND-only group). After ALND alone, ipsilateral axillary recurrence was identified in 0.5% of patients versus 0.9% in the SLN dissection-only arm. Although this study closed early due to poor accrual, results suggest that in clinically node-negative patients with early-stage breast cancer who are found to have up to two histologically positive SLN's and will receive whole-breast radiotherapy and systemic adjuvant therapy as indicated by standerd of care, that ALND does not confer an improved survival advantage. In this setting, SLN dissection alone for appropriate staging with completed adjuvant therapy may offer excellent regional control with decreased morbidity.

Since the publication of these practice-changing results, the Z0011 findings have been rapidly and widely adopted and are now considered standard practice. It is important to note that these findings are not applicable to all patients including those with locally advanced (T3 or T4) disease, those who received NAC or those undergoing mastectomy.

Furthermore, these findings were supported by other similar clinical trials evaluating axillary management in the setting of limited pN1 disease identified on SLN dissection after upfront surgery for early-stage breast cancer. The AMAROS trial randomized patients with T1-2, N0 invasive breast cancer and positive SLNs (that are not clincally palpable, to ALND versus axillary radiation. Interestingly, approximately 17% to 18% of patients in both arms received mastectomy as the definitive breast operation thereby possibly allowing for extrapolation of these findings to that population. Although the planned noninferiority test was underpowered due to a low overall event rate, at 6 years median follow-up, radiotherapy provided comparable regional control compared to ALND with no significant difference in axillary recurrence between the groups (0.43% after ALND and 1.19% after axillary radiation). Importantly, the rate of lymphedema at 1, 3, and 5 years was markedly lower in the axillary radiotherapy arm.

The IBCSG 23-01 trial evaluated patients with early-stage node-negative breast cancer found to have micrometastatic disease in the SLNs (less than or equal to 2 mm). Patients were randomized to ALND or omission of ALND. Approximately 9% of patients in each treatment arm were treated with mastectomy. The investigators report that 5- and 10-year DFS is noninferior after omission of ALND as compared to ALND (87.8% and 76.8% vs. 84.4% and 74.9%, respectively) in this patient population.

Clinically Node-Positive Disease In the setting of clinical nodal involvement at presentation, axillary dissection is the standard of care. This is evolving in the setting of NAC in selected patients where repeat axillary staging after completion of neoadjuvant treatment, may be appropriate.

ALND consists of en bloc removal of the level I and II axillary nodal tissue. When level III nodes are grossly or pathologically involved, removal of these nodes may be indicated, however, removal of clinically negative level III lymph nodes is of little benefit with respect to staging because only 1% to 3% of stage I or II patients show level III involvement in the absence of level I or level II disease. Level III dissections carry a substantially higher risk of subsequent lymphedema, particularly when used in conjunction with radiation therapy. ALND should preserve the long thoracic and thoracodorsal nerves and avoid stripping of the axillary vein. A closed-suction drain is typically placed and removed once the drainage has sufficiently decreased.

Management of Clinical N1 Disease After Neoadjuvant Chemotherapy Following NAC, pathologic complete response (pCR) in the axillary nodes is found in 40% of patients presenting with biopsy-proven node-positive disease. This observation led to several clinical trials including ACOSOG Z1071, SENTINA (Arm C), and SN FNAC, evaluating the feasibility and accuracy of SLN dissection as axillary staging after NAC in clinical N1 (cN1) disease. Although the false-negative rate of SLN dissection in this setting was above the predetermined threshold, several important factors associated with and impacting the false-negative rate were described. This included use of dual-agent mapping technique, evaluation of at least 2 to 3 SLNs, immunohistochemistry (IHC) evaluation in addition to H&E staining, and documented excision of the clipped (biopsy-proven) axillary node.

The results of these findings led to the refined technique termed TAD. This procedure involves SLN dissection and selective targeted excision of the clipped (biopsy-proven) axillary node. At MDACC, at the time of initial evaluation, patients undergo an axillary ultrasound with biopsy of any suspicious nodes. In the setting of N1 disease, a clip is placed to mark the biopsy-proven axillary node. Patients with advanced nodal involvement by ultrasound or examination (matted nodes, internal mammary, infraclavicular, or supraclavicular nodes) are not candidates for this approach and will undergo axillary dissection. Response is documented during chemotherapy with ultrasound and clinical examination. In selected patients planned for TAD, the clipped node is preoperatively localized with a seed. Intraoperatively, dual lymphatic mapping for SLN identification is employed and targeted excision of the clipped node is performed. Excision is confirmed with specimen radiograph. In approximately 23% of cases, the clipped node will not be a sentinel node. Compared with ALND, the false-negative rate of this approach was 10.1% with sentinel node biopsy alone, 4.2% for excision of the clipped node alone, and 2.0% for TAD. In carefully selected patients, TAD alone may offer an accurate approach to axillary staging and assessment of residual disease with limited morbidity.

Radiation Therapy

The role of radiation therapy in breast cancer has been well established as an adjunct to surgery in the management of locoregional recurrence (LRR). In early-stage breast cancer, BCT with whole-breast radiation has been associated with equivalent long-term survival results versus mastectomy alone; recurrence rates are improved in all subsets of patients and radiation therapy to the nodal basin helps achieve long-term regional control.

The addition of a radiation boost to the primary tumor site after whole-breast radiation to reduce the risk of local recurrence has been validated in two prospective randomized trials. In the European Organization for Research and Treatment of Cancer (EORTC) 10981–22023 trial, patients were randomly assigned to receive whole-breast irradiation of 50 Gy plus a boost dose of 16 Gy compared with no boost in patients with negative surgical margins. The 10-year rate of local recurrence was reduced from 10.2% without a boost to 6.2% with a boost ($P < .0001$), with a hazard ratio of 0.59 in favor of a boost; the benefit in reducing local recurrence was maintained through 16 years of follow-up. Furthermore, contemporary management includes consideration of hypofractionated regimens shortening the treatment course without compromising therapeutic effectiveness.

For tumor recurrence with BCT, the majority of relapses occur at or near the original tumor bed, rarely extending beyond 1 to 2 cm of the prior cavity. This has led to the rationale that accelerated partial breast irradiation (APBI) could be used to deliver a homogeneous dose of radiation within a confined space. Advantages of APBI include shorter treatment (5 days vs. 6 weeks), less scatter radiation to the lungs, heart, and coronary vessels, and less skin burning and desquamation. Preliminary studies of APBI suggest that rates of local control in highly selected patients with early-stage breast cancer may be comparable to those treated with standard whole-breast radiation therapy. However, follow-up is limited and studies are ongoing; compared to standard whole-breast radiation, several recent studies document an inferior cosmetic outcome with APBI. Currently, the consensus statement from ASTRO states that possible candidates for APBI include women older than 60 years with unifocal T1 N0 M0 ER-positive breast cancer, who are not BRCA1/BRCA2 mutation carriers, and who have infiltrating ductal or a favorable ductal subtype, with negative margins not associated with an extensive intraductal component or LCIS.

Postmastectomy radiation therapy (PMRT) may reduce the risk of locoregional failure. Traditionally, the greatest benefit of PMRT is seen in patients at highest risk for locoregional failure with greater than four positive lymph nodes, tumor size greater than or equal to 5 cm, T4 disease, or positive margins. Other factors associated with locoregional failure include age, histologic grade of tumors, presence of lymphovascular invasion, and extracapsular spread seen in the lymph nodes. There has been considerable debate whether patients with one to three positive axillary lymph nodes benefit from PMRT. There seems to be more data suggesting better outcomes with this subset population who undergo PMRT, but it has been unclear whether it is the effect of PMRT itself, or the improved delivery and efficacy of systemic therapy or better surgical technique that contribute to these results. Little prospective data exists on present-day LRR rates after mastectomy without PMRT. Sharma et al. examined women with early-stage breast cancer and one to three positive axillary lymph nodes treated with mastectomy showing that the 10-year risk of LRR was not significantly different between patients without lymph node metastases and patients with one positive lymph node. They concluded that in this era of improved systemic therapy, any potential absolute LRR reduction and survival advantage that may be gained from the use of PMRT must be balanced against possible morbidities associated with radiation.

Radiotherapy is also highly effective for treatment of axillary disease, with locoregional control rates comparable to axillary surgery as evidenced by the AMAROS trial findings.

Breast Reconstruction

For the majority of patients treated with mastectomy, breast reconstruction should be offered. Immediate reconstruction is contraindicated in the setting of IBC. Breast reconstruction may involve autologous tissue, synthetic implants, or both. The options, patient selection, decision making, and technical details of breast reconstruction are discussed in Chapter 26.

Although satisfactory results can be obtained with either immediate or delayed reconstruction, an important consideration is the likelihood of PMRT. Acute and chronic complications and poor aesthetic outcomes have been identified in patients who undergo immediate reconstruction with placement of a permanent breast implant followed by PMRT. For this reason, close multidisciplinary discussion with a radiation oncologist is important to ensure that optimal oncologic delivery of radiation is not compromised by an underlying implant or tissue expander. In cases where receipt of PMRT is unknown or planned, a delayed immediate approach may be employed whereby the patient undergoes SSM with insertion of a saline-filled tissue expander. This serves as an adjustable scaffolding to preserve a three-dimensional contour of the breast skin envelope. Based on pathologic evaluation, if the patient requires PMRT, the tissue expander can be deflated to allow radiation delivery followed by delayed reconstruction typically with autologous tissue. If no PMRT is required, then the patient can undergo definitive reconstruction once the desired breast size and symmetry have been achieved.

Systemic Therapy

Chemotherapy

As our knowledge of the complexity of breast cancer grows, it is clear that breast cancer is no longer a single disease entity, but rather a group of molecularly distinct subtypes each with different prognoses, natural histories, and chemotherapeutic sensitivities. The decision to receive chemotherapy is becoming highly individualized and is based on a combination of hormone receptor status, HER2 amplification, tumor size, tumor grade, lymph node status, and Ki-67 proliferation index. Systemic treatment decisions should be made within a multidisciplinary setting. Typical regimens include anthracycline and taxane-based therapy with the addition of targeted therapy where indicated. Detailed discussion of specific chemotherapy regimens and current guidelines are available through a variety of national and international resources

Adjuvant chemotherapy is directed at treating occult micrometastatic disease, thereby reducing the risk of local and systemic recurrence. Chemotherapy works most effectively when tumor volume is small and still in its linear growth phase. This rationale led to some of the first adjuvant clinical trials of polychemotherapy versus observation in lymph node–positive breast cancer that showed improved disease-free and overall survival with chemotherapy.

Neoadjuvant Chemotherapy

Several phase II studies and eight randomized controlled trials have observed no difference in DFS or overall survival between adjuvant (chemotherapy following surgery) and neoadjuvant (chemotherapy preceding surgery) therapy. Adjuvant chemotherapy is equally effective up to 12 weeks after definitive surgery but may be compromised by delays of more than 12 weeks after definitive surgery.

These trials, however, uncovered multiple benefits to NAC including facilitation of BCT, conversion of tumors from inoperable to operable, and the ability to gain prognostic information at an individual patient level based on response to therapy. In addition, response to systemic therapy for triple negative and HER2-positive breast cancers impacts recommendations for adjuvant systemic therapy, thereby impacting oncologic outcomes. The CREATE-X trial demonstrated that patients with residual triple negative breast cancer after NAC and surgery had improved disease-free and overall survival when treated with capecitabine postoperatively. For patients with HER2-positive tumors and residual disease after NAC, the KATHERINE trial showed improved invasive DFS in patients treated with T-DMI1 (trastuzumab conjugated with a cytotoxic agent emtansine) over trastuzumab alone after surgery.

Increasingly, NAC may allow for downstaging of disease in the axilla, providing an opportunity to limit the extent of axillary surgery, and may allow for less radiotherapy if axillary nodal disease is cleared after receiving NAC. The neoadjuvant approach also allows for modification of systemic treatment if there is no or poor preoperative therapy response or progression of disease. Finally, NAC provides an excellent research platform to investigate novel therapies, continue clinical trials, and test predictive biomarkers for ongoing evolution in the treatment of breast cancer.

Possible disadvantages to NAC include possible overtreatment with systemic therapy if clinical stage is overestimated, and the rare possibility of disease progression during preoperative systemic therapy (in 2% to 3% of cases), though this is usually an indicator of aggressive tumor biology and poor oncologic outcome and allows for a better understanding of the tumor biology and subsequent changes to the chemotherapy regimen. For these reasons, treatment within a multidisciplinary conference with ongoing reassessment and communication among treatment teams is critical.

Candidates for NAC include those with IBC, N2/N3 nodal disease, or T4 tumors as well as patients with a large primary tumor relative to breast size in a patient who desires breast conservation and those in whom adjuvant chemotherapy is planned (e.g., triple negative, HER2-positive, node-positive patients). Patients with inoperable breast cancer are typically treated with chemotherapy and may become operative candidates based on favorable tumor response. Patients who are not appropriate for NAC include patients with extensive in situ disease in whom the extent of invasive carcinoma is not well defined or patients with a poorly delineated extent of tumor preoperatively, either by radiologic or physical examination. It is critical to note that definitive tissue diagnosis both of the primary tumor and nodal disease is required, with placement of radiologically confirmed localizing clips prior to the initiation of chemotherapy to ensure proper ocalization of the tumor and, in certain cases, of the histologically positive axillary lymph node, during surgery in the event that NAC produces a complete clinical and radiographic response.

Tumor Biology and Choice of Systemic Therapy

Important differences in the clinical behavior of ER-positive and ER-negative breast cancers have long been recognized. Gene expression profiling studies have identified at least four distinct molecular subtypes of breast cancer: basal-like, HER2-enriched, luminal A, and luminal B. (Table 2.3) In addition to differing biologic and clinical behaviors, they also have unique chemosensitivities. While gene expression profiling is not routinely performed, immunohistochemical surrogates are commonly used to determine subtype. In general, the basal-like and HER2-positive subtypes are predominately ER-negative, while the luminal subtypes are ER-positive. Clinically, the triple negative phenotype is used to identify basal-like cancers, however, this misclassifies up to 30% of basal-like cancers. Tumor biology is one of the most significant factors in determining the need for systemic therapy and whether it should be given in the neoadjuvant versus the adjuvant setting.

Hormone Receptor–Positive Breast Cancer Hormone receptor–positive breast cancer comprises about 75% of all invasive breast cancers. Substantial molecular differences exist between high- and low-risk ER-positive tumors and genomic assays are routinely used to characterize these tumors as high or low risk. The most widely used commercially available test in the United States is Oncotype DX® Breast Recurrence Score (Genomic Health Inc, Redwood City, CA). This reverse-transcriptase polymerase chain reaction (RT-PCR) assay is intended for use in Hormone Receptor (HR)–positive node-negative breast cancer patients who will receive 5 years of endocrine therapy. It measures the gene expression of 16 cancer-related genes (including ER, PR, HER2, and Ki-67) and 5 reference genes in paraffin-embedded tumor tissue and uses a regression model to calculate a recurrence score (RS) that is an estimate of the risk of developing distant metastases at 10 years. Two suggested cut-off points categorize patients into low (RS <18), intermediate (RS ≥18 < 31), and high (RS ≥31) risk groups corresponding to 6.8%, 14.3%, and 30.5% risk of distant recurrence at 10 years after 5 years of tamoxifen therapy, respectively. Similarly, these subgroups by RS also correlate with risk of LRR. Furthermore, analysis using the population studied in NSABP B20 trial (ER positive, node negative) suggested the predictive power of this genomic assay regarding the benefit of chemotherapy within this subset of patients such that in the high-RS group, chemotherapy in addition to tamoxifen resulted in increased survival whereas in the low-RS group there was no survival advantage with chemotherapy over tamoxifen. The benefit in the intermediate RS group was less clear.

The TAILORx (Trial Assigning Individualized Options for Treatment) study was designed to answer the question regarding benefit of chemotherapy within the intermediate RS group. This trial randomized patients with HR-positive, node-negative breast cancer and an intermediate RS to chemotherapy and endocrine therapy versus endocrine therapy only. Patients with a score of 0 to 10 were assigned to receive endocrine therapy alone, and those with a score of 26 or higher were assigned to receive chemotherapy plus endocrine therapy. Patients with a midrange score of 11 to 25 were randomly assigned to receive chemotherapy plus endocrine therapy or endocrine therapy alone. To minimize the potential for undertreatment of the enrolled participants, investigators used lower thresholds for low-, intermediate-, and high-risk individuals from the originally defined scores. At 9 years, in the intermediate group, invasive DFS was 83.3% in the endocrine therapy group versus 84.3% in the chemotherapy and endocrine-therapy group, distant recurrence-free survival was 94.5% versus 95.0%, and overall survival was 93.9% versus 93.8%. In a subgroup analysis of women 50 years or younger with a score of 16 to 20, distant recurrence was lower in the chemotherapy and endocrine-therapy group though overall survival was similar. The study also confirmed survival rates in the low-risk and high-risk groups. The study indicated that up to 85% of women with early-stage breast cancer can safely omit adjuvant chemotherapy.

The recently presented RxPonder trial randomly assigned over 5,000 patients with HR-positive, HER2-negative breast cancer, one to three positive lymph nodes, and an RS of 25 or less to endocrine therapy alone versus chemotherapy and endocrine therapy. Initial results demonstrated similar invasive DFS of 91.9% in the endocrine therapy group versus 91.6% in the chemotherapy and endocrine therapy group for postmenopausal patients. Chemotherapy provided a benefit in premenopausal women who had an invasive DFS of 89.0% versus 94.2% in patients who received endocrine therapy alone. The mechanism of benefit in the premenopausal group is being investigated further and longer-term follow-up remains to be reported.

The FDA-approved 70-gene signature MammaPrint (Agendia) was developed at the Netherlands Cancer Institute from a retrospective series of 78 patients younger than 55 years who received no adjuvant systemic therapy and had T1/T2, node-negative breast cancer. This assay stratifies patients into low and high-risk groups with respect to development of distant metastasis. The results of the prospective multicenter randomized MINDACT (microarray in node-negative disease may avoid chemotherapy) trial evaluating the clinical utility of MammaPrint in selecting patients with node-negative, HR-positive breast cancer for adjuvant chemotherapy showed that MammaPrint low-risk patients had a 94.7% 5-year distant metastasis-free survival without chemotherapy, even in the presence of high-risk clinical factors such as node positivity, high grade, large tumor size, and age <50 years. The absolute difference in 5-year survival rate was 1.5% lower in those receiving no chemotherapy, with no difference in distant metastasis in the subgroup of patients with ER-positive, HER2-negative, and either node-negative or node-positive disease. The authors suggested that the use of MammaPrint can therefore reduce overtreatment of patients in this group by 46%. These findings validate changes in clinical practice and help avoid unnecessary treatment with chemotherapy in selected patients limiting long-term side effects of cardiac toxicity, secondary cancers, early menopause, and psychosocial harm.

The molecular subtypes often align with the genomic assay profile. Luminal A cancers (Oncotype DX® "low RS," MammaPrint "low risk") are characterized by high expression of ER and ER-related genes and have low expression of proliferative markers such as Ki-67 and are typically low grade. These patients have a favorable prognosis and high likelihood of benefit from endocrine therapy. In contrast, luminal B (Oncotype DX® "high RS," MammaPrint "high-risk") cancers are characterized by lower expression of ER and ER-related genes, and high expression of proliferation markers. These are typically high-grade tumors and have a poorer prognosis. Standard chemotherapeutic regimens in addition to endocrine therapy should be considered for these patients in line with the clinical trials presented previously.

Recently, there has been a focus to develop more targeted therapies that enhance endocrine sensitivity, can be potential alternatives to chemotherapy, and are better tolerated by patients. CDK 4/6 inhibitors have emerged as one such class and in conjunction with endocrine therapy have shown promising results in the metastatic and adjuvant settings. The PALOMA clinical trials program demonstrated improved efficacy of endocrine therapy (ET) combined with palbociclib, a CDK 4/6 inhibitor, for advanced breast cancer demonstrated by a longer progression-free survival. Another CDK 4/6 inhibitor abemaciclib was evaluated in the adjuvant setting in the monarchE trial and found to improve invasive DFS when combined with endocrine therapy versus endocrine therapy alone for high risk, early-stage ER-positive, HER2-negative breast cancer. These drugs continue to be investigated along with the development of novel targeted therapies for this subtype.

HER2-Positive Breast Cancer Between 20% and 25% of breast cancers are HER2-positive which is predictive of a response to anti-HER2 agents such as trastuzumab (Herceptin; Genentech, South San Francisco, CA), a humanized monoclonal antibody that targets the extracellular domain of the HER2 receptor. In the preoperative setting, pathologic complete response rates of up to 65% have been reported with trastuzumab in combination with chemotherapy. The administration of chemotherapy in combination with 1 year of trastuzumab is associated with a 50% reduction in the risk of recurrence and about a 30% reduction in the risk of death. This has been confirmed in a Cochrane meta-analysis of randomized controlled trials (RCTs), including six adjuvant and two neoadjuvant studies (NSABP B-31, NCCTG N9831, BCIRG 006, HERA, FinHer, PACS-04, Buzdar, and NOAH), and 1 year of adjuvant trastuzumab has become standard of care in HER2-positive breast cancers.

Pertuzumab (Perjeta, Genentech, South San Francisco, CA) was initially an FDA-approved treatment for HER2-positive metastatic breast cancer. It is a HER2 dimerization inhibitor that is currently used in combination with Herceptin (trastuzumab) and docetaxel as first-line treatment of HER2-positive metastatic breast cancer. The CLEOPATRA trial published in 2012 studied the safety and efficacy of pertuzumab plus trastuzumab plus docetaxel, as compared with placebo plus trastuzumab plus docetaxel in patients with HER2-positive metastatic breast cancer. Median progression-free survival was 18.5 months versus 12.4 months in the pertuzumab groups and control groups, respectively. The APHINITY trial was a randomized trial evaluating 4,805 women with early breast cancer assigned to receive standard adjuvant chemotherapy for 18 weeks plus 1 year of either trastuzumab and placebo or trastuzumab and pertuzumab in the adjuvant setting. Modest benefits in 3-year invasive DFS were seen in the group receiving pertuzumab with trastuzumab (94.1%) versus the placebo/trastuzumab group (93.2%). Slightly greater benefits were seen with the use of pertuzumab in patients with node-positive disease.

Given the results of these trials, in current practice, most HER2-positive cancers are treated with neoadjuvant systemic therapy including dual anti-HER2 therapy especially for larger tumors (>2 cm) and/or positive nodes. However, there are also opportunities to treat patients in the adjuvant setting and potentially with fewer drugs. The APT trial was a single-arm study of predominately stage I HER2-positive breast cancers measuring up to 3 cm in size and showed a 3-year invasive DFS of 98.7% with adjuvant paclitaxel and trastuzumab. These results indicate that it may be reasonable to de-escalated systemic therapy for smaller HER2-positive, node-negative tumors. For this reason, upfront surgery to clarify the pathologic stage and candidacy for this approach may be considered in clinical stage I HER2-positive breast cancer.

Triple Negative Breast Cancer Triple negative cancers are highly proliferative and carry a worse prognosis than other breast cancer subtypes but are uniquely sensitive to standard chemotherapy. Distinct molecular subtypes of triple negative breast cancer have been described, basal-like 1, basal-like 2, mesenchymal-like, mesenchymal stem-like, immunomodulatory, and luminal AR, and may explain the heterogeneous nature of this subtype in response to conventional chemotherapy and identify opportunities for targeted therapy. Recently, several new targeted therapies and immunotherapies have shown promise in this subtype. These include the following:

PARP inhibitors. Homologous recombination, a high-fidelity DNA repair pathway, relies on a functioning BRCA1 gene. When this pathway is dysfunctional, the poly (ADP-ribose) polymerase (PARP) DNA repair mechanisms take over. PARP has been identified as an important drug target in order to bring about so-called "synthetic lethality" of BRCA-mutated tumors. The OlympiA trial enrolled women with BRCA1/2 gene mutations and high-risk, HER2-negative breast cancer treated with local therapy and neoadjuvant or adjuvant chemotherapy and randomly assigned them to a year of adjuvant olaparib or placebo. Three-year invasive DFS was 85.9% in the olaparib group versus 77.1% in the placebo group and 3-year distant DFS was significantly higher with olaparib.

Immunotherapy. Immunotherapy has also been investigated in triple negative breast cancer. Pembrolizumab, a monoclonal antibody against programmed death 1 (PD-1), and atezolizumab, a monoclonal antibody inhibiting programmed death ligand 1 (PD-L1) initially were shown to have benefit in metastatic triple negative breast cancer. The phase III KEYNOTE-522 trial randomly assigned patients with stage II to III triple negative breast cancer to NAC plus pembrolizumab versus NAC plus placebo followed by adjuvant pembrolizumab versus placebo for up to nine cycles. There was a higher rate of pathologic complete response in the pembrolizumab arm, 63%, versus 56% in the placebo arm and improved event-free survival. These results led to FDA approval of pembrolizumab for triple negative breast cancer. Sacituzumab govitecan, an anti–Trop-2 antibody conjugated to a chemotherapeutic agent, has been shown to improve progression-free and overall survival in patients with metastatic or unresectable locally advanced triple negative breast cancer leading to its approval in this group of patients.

Epothilones, antiangiogenic agents, EGFR inhibitors, mTOR inhibitors, PI3 kinase inhibitors, and agents that induce DNA double-strand breaks such as platinum agents continue to be tested in clinical trials particular in the advanced and metastatic settings.

Endocrine Therapy

Endocrine therapy has been associated with significant reductions in the risk of local recurrence, distant metastasis, and contralateral breast cancer. Tamoxifen, which was originally recommended for the treatment of postmenopausal women with ER-positive breast cancer, is now indicated for a much broader range of patients. Tamoxifen therapy is considered standard of care for premenopausal women with tumors expressing ER or PR hormone receptors, regardless of age or nodal status. Tamoxifen therapy is generally well tolerated with treatment-limiting adverse effects in less than 5% of patients. In addition to its antitumor properties, tamoxifen increases bone density and reduces serum cholesterol levels. However, tamoxifen also increases the incidence of endometrial cancer and thromboembolic events. Standard treatment with tamoxifen is 5 years based on data from NSABP B-14 indicating that 10 years of tamoxifen use offer no survival advantage over 5 years, however, there is ongoing research in this area and national consensus guidelines now recommend consideration of 5 to 10 years of endocrine therapy.

In 2014, results of the long-awaited TEXT and SOFT trials for premenopausal patients looked at 4,690 patients from the two phase III trials comparing combined therapy with exemestane and ovarian suppression versus tamoxifen and ovarian suppression for 5 years. At a median follow-up of 68 months, DFS and rate of freedom from breast cancer at 5 years were significantly improved with exemestane and ovarian suppression and side effect profiles were similar to those in postmenopausal women. However, overall survival was no different among the groups. In the SOFT trial, premenopausal patients who received adjuvant chemotherapy due to increased risk, in the exemestane/ovarian suppression group, were found to have a significantly improved freedom from breast cancer at 5 years (85.7%). This led to the conclusion that adjuvant treatment with exemestane plus ovarian suppression, as compared with tamoxifen plus ovarian suppression, significantly reduced recurrence in premenopausal women with hormone receptor–positive early breast cancer.

Current national consensus guideline recommendations for postmenopausal women include aromatase inhibitors as a component of adjuvant endocrine therapy. The aromatase inhibitors anastrozole, letrozole, and exemestane work by inhibiting aromatase, an enzyme that catalyzes the conversion of adrenal corticosteroids to estrogens and therefore decreases the conversion of precursor hormones to estrogen in adipose tissue. In the ATAC (Arimidex, Tamoxifen Alone or in Combination) trial, the efficacy and side effect profiles of anastrozole and tamoxifen were compared in postmenopausal women. For postmenopausal patients with early-stage breast cancer, anastrozole resulted in a higher DFS rate (86.9% vs. 84.5%) than tamoxifen, longer time to recurrence, and lower incidence of contralateral breast cancer. The results also demonstrated that the incidence of endometrial cancer, vaginal bleeding and discharge, cerebrovascular events, venous thromboembolic events, and hot flashes occurred significantly less frequently with anastrozole, whereas musculoskeletal disorders and fractures occurred less frequently with tamoxifen. As a result of the ATAC trial, anastrozole is now the preferred hormone therapy for postmenopausal patients with receptor-positive breast cancer. For patients who have already been taking tamoxifen, studies have shown that switching to an aromatase inhibitor is safe, and results in improvements in DFS rates in postmenopausal women.

Ovarian suppression with LHRH-agonists (e.g., leuprolide, triptorelin, or goserelin) or ovarian ablation is another effective adjuvant endocrine treatment in premenopausal women. American Society of Clinical Oncology (ASCO) now recommends that women with stage II or III breast cancers who are advised to receive adjuvant chemotherapy should receive ovarian suppression in combination with either tamoxifen or an aromatase inhibitor. In addition, women with stage I or II breast cancers at higher risk of recurrence who are considered for chemotherapy may be offered ovarian suppression with endocrine therapy. Women with stage I breast cancers not warranting chemotherapy, such as those with node-negative cancers 1 cm or less, should not receive ovarian suppression.

Neoadjuvant Endocrine Therapy

Endocrine therapy in the neoadjuvant setting has been utilized in HR-positive breast cancer, particularly in postmenopausal women. This is largely based on the significant impact on survival and recurrence outcome seen in the adjuvant setting. Although not associated with high rates of pCR, neoadjuvant endocrine therapy has been documented to facilitate increasing rates of breast conservation in this population. Furthermore, response to therapy may be followed by change in Ki-67 percentage or evaluation of the preoperative endocrine prognostic index (PEPI) score though these have mostly been used as endpoints in clinical trials. Several trials have shown superior response to aromatase inhibitors as compared to tamoxifen in the neoadjuvant setting in postmenopausal women. Moreover, the ACOSOG Z1031 trial which compared therapy with exemestane, letrozole, and anastrozole in the preoperative setting is currently finding similar rates of BCT conversion among the therapies and similar biologic effect. Management paradigms for neoadjuvant endocrine therapy and the implications for surgical planning are an increasing focus of ongoing clinical research.

Surveillance

After primary therapy for invasive breast cancer, patients must be made aware of the long-term risk for recurrent or metastatic disease. Although most studies report that the majority of recurrences occur within 5 years after primary therapy, recurrences can occur more than 20 years after primary therapy.

The published ASCO guidelines for follow-up recommend scheduled visits that include a detailed cancer-related history and physical examination every 3 to 6 months for years 1 through 3, every 6 to 12 months for years 4 through 5, and every 12 months thereafter. Mammography is done 6 months after the completion of BCT to allow surgery- and radiation-induced changes to stabilize, and then yearly. Alternating mammograms and MRI can be considered for patients with germline mutations or dense breasts. For patients who have undergone mastectomy, a contralateral mammogram is obtained yearly. Clinicians should counsel patients to adhere to adjuvant endocrine therapy. Routine bone scans, skeletal surveys, laboratory tests, and computed tomographic scans yield an extremely low rate of occult metastases in otherwise asymptomatic patients and are not cost-effective for patients with early-stage breast cancer.

Locally Recurrent Breast Cancer

Local recurrence may occur in the breast after BCT (in-breast tumor recurrence), chest wall after mastectomy (chest wall recurrence) or involving the axillary and/or regional nodes. Given this is a heterogeneous population with varied disease presentation, there are limited randomized clinical trials which guide current management. Risk factors include young age at diagnosis, positive final surgical margins, advanced tumor stage, poor response to neoadjuvant systemic therapy, and aggressive tumor biology. Several contemporary studies have demonstrated that the tumor subtype and response to neoadjuvant systemic therapy (if received) are significant drivers of LRR rather than the type of surgery received. Multidisciplinary evaluation is paramount as patients will benefit from systemic therapy, surgery, and radiation (if feasible).

Any patient with a local recurrence should undergo complete restaging after detection of the recurrence. Initial workup should also include bilateral diagnostic mammogram for patients with an intact breast, ultrasound evaluation of affected breast and nodal basins, consideration of breast MRI, core-needle biopsy with assessment of hormone receptor and HER2-neu status, and consideration of NAC. For patients with a purely local recurrence, surgical excision plus radiation therapy, if eligible, provides better local control than does either modality alone. In the case of prior BCT, mastectomy is typically performed, however, repeat breast conservation surgery may be considered in some cases after multidisciplinary discussion. In ER-negative disease patients with isolated in-breast tumor recurrence, chemotherapy has been shown to improve 5-year DFS over those not treated with chemotherapy, based on the CALOR trial. In patients with ER-positive recurrence, hormonal therapy may be considered as it has been shown to reduce second local failures at 5 years, although overall survival was not significantly changed.

Metastatic Breast Cancer

Patients with metastatic breast cancer are unlikely to be cured of their disease. Complete remissions from systemic chemotherapy are uncommon, and only a fraction of complete responders remain progression free for a prolonged period. The median survival for patients with stage IV breast cancer is 18 to 24 months, though a subset of patients can live for many years, especially with the improvement in multimodality treatments, particularly systemic treatments. The typical approach to the evaluation of metastatic disease is to perform a core biopsy of the tumor for histologic and biomarker confirmation of the diagnosis, stage with laboratory tests, bone scan, and CT or PET/CT to understand the full extent of the disease, then to proceed directly to systemic therapy.

Chemotherapy rarely prolongs survival and is directed at improving tumor-related symptoms and slowing the spread of the tumor. The most common site of distant metastatic spread is the bone with other common sites including the lungs, pleura, brain, liver, soft tissues, adrenal glands, and lymph nodes. Different patterns of metastases have been observed by subtype. For example, patients with rapidly growing, hormone receptor–negative, and poorly differentiated tumors are likely to have metastases to visceral organs (e.g., liver, lungs, and brain), whereas patients with slowly growing, hormone receptor–positive, and well-differentiated tumors are likely to develop metastases to bone and soft tissues and are less likely to exhibit early life-threatening manifestations. Therapy is directed by tumor subtype and enrollment in clinical trials is always encouraged as novel targeted agents are actively under investigation.

Most oncologists agree that once metastases have occurred, there is no survival benefit to aggressive local therapy and surgery for stage IV breast cancer was historically reserved for palliation of symptoms including pain, bleeding, ulceration, and infection. However, in de novo stage IV disease, surgical resection of the intact primary and involved nodes remains controversial. While several retrospective studies have shown a survival benefit to aggressive local therapy, RCTs have shown mixed results and two of the trials have not shown an overall survival benefit. For this reason, the decision for local therapy in stage IV setting should be reserved for selected cases following a multidisciplinary discussion. Patients who may benefit most include those with oligo-metastatic disease and favorable response to systemic therapy. In these cases, surgical resection and radiotherapy of the primary as well as definitive therapy to the metastatic site(s) may render the patient with no evidence of disease (NED) status, which is associated with improved survival outcomes, particularly in patients with a durable response to treatment.

Special Considerations
Male Breast Cancer
Approximately 1% of all breast cancers occur in men. Diagnosis, staging, and treatment strategies parallel that for women with breast cancer, given the lack of randomized trials in this population. In comparison to women, men with breast cancer typically present at an older age with more advanced disease and higher nodal tumor burden. This may be because of lack of screening or awareness. The majority of tumors are located in the subareolar position presenting as a mass or nipple inversion. Diagnosis includes history, physical examination, dedicated breast imaging with mammography, and ultrasound as well as core-needle biopsy. The pathology typically shows ductal histology with approximately 90% of cases ER-positive. Traditionally, men diagnosed with breast cancer have been treated with total mastectomy although breast conservation with segmental mastectomy and adjuvant radiation therapy may be an appropriate strategy with the addition of mammographic surveillance. Sentinel node dissection has been shown to be accurate for axillary staging in men with clinically node-negative disease. Axillary dissection is recommended in patients with node-positive disease. Adjuvant (or neoadjuvant) systemic therapy recommendations are guided by stage of disease and receptor status. Patients with hormone receptor–positive breast cancer are recommended treatment with tamoxifen in the adjuvant setting. A personal or family history of male breast cancer is an indication for genetic counseling as there is a higher frequency of BRCA mutation positivity in this population, particularly BRCA2 mutations.

Breast Cancer and Pregnancy
The definition of pregnancy-associated breast cancer is described as any breast carcinoma diagnosed during pregnancy, lactation, or during the first postpartum year. There is a low incidence of pregnancy-associated breast cancer, accounting for 2.8% of all breast malignancies, but breast cancer is one of the most common pregnancy-associated malignancies. Historically, the incidence is estimated at 1 in 3,000 pregnancies. These breast cancers are often identified in women at an earlier age, present as more advanced stage, and are often ER-negative, suggesting these tumors have other biologically distinct characteristics.

The diagnosis of pregnancy-associated breast cancer is typically more difficult due to a low level of suspicion based on a comparatively young patient age, the relative frequency of nodular changes in the breast associated with pregnancy, and the increase in breast density during pregnancy. These difficulties in the physical examination and hormonal changes associated with pregnancy help account for a 2.5-fold increased risk for diagnosis at an advanced stage.

Both the safety and efficacy of mammography during pregnancy have been supported, with sensitivity rates from 78% to 90% in detecting suspicious features of malignancy. When the fetus is shielded adequately, the estimated fetal dose of radiation from a standard two-view mammogram is well below the threshold exposure associated with risk of fetal harm as published by the International Commission of Radiological Protection. Breast ultrasound is highly sensitive and specific in diagnosis during pregnancy and lactation and is considered a standard method for the evaluation of a palpable breast mass. In addition, all persistent and suspicious breast masses should undergo evaluation by FNA, core-needle biopsy, or in rare cases, excisional biopsy. Excisional biopsy under local anesthesia is safe at any time during pregnancy.

Once a diagnosis of malignancy is established, treatment decisions are influenced by the specific trimester of pregnancy. The goal should be curative treatment of the breast cancer and preservation of pregnancy without injury to the fetus. The approach to each patient must be individualized, considering gestational age at presentation, stage of disease, and patient preference. Termination of pregnancy in the hope of minimizing hormonal stimulation of the tumor does not alter maternal survival and is not recommended. Genetic counseling is also recommended for all women with breast cancer during pregnancy.

Surgical treatment of gestational breast cancer is generally identical to that of nongestational breast cancer. There is no evidence that extra-abdominal surgical procedures are associated with premature labor or that the typically used anesthetic agents are teratogenic. Modified radical mastectomy or breast-conserving surgery with SLND or ALND as primary therapy can be undertaken at any point during pregnancy without undue risk to the mother or fetus. SLN dissection in pregnant breast cancer patients is safe and accurate using 99-Tc and can be safely used in conjunction with lymphoscintigraphy. Isosulfan blue and methylene blue dye are contraindicated in pregnancy.

The safety of surgical intervention during pregnancy is well supported, but patients may defer until the 12th gestational week to avoid the risk of spontaneous abortion, which is highest in the first trimester. For cancer detected during the third trimester, delaying primary treatment for up to 4 weeks to allow for delivery before surgery is acceptable. If modified radical mastectomy is undertaken during pregnancy, breast reconstruction should not be performed simultaneously as reconstruction options, especially rectus or other myocutaneous flaps, are limited during pregnancy and the postpartum appearance of the contralateral breast is unknown until after pregnancy.

For women desiring breast conservation, treatment is complicated by the fact that radiation therapy is contraindicated during pregnancy during all trimesters. For cancers detected during the third trimester, lumpectomy and axillary dissection can be performed safely using general anesthesia, and radiation therapy can be delayed until after delivery. Longer delays may be detrimental to maternal outcome, although the time limit within which radiation therapy must be carried out to minimize the risk of local recurrence is unknown.

The decision to administer neoadjuvant or adjuvant chemotherapy is difficult, as fears of congenital malformations are a serious concern for the pregnant patient. Most studies have demonstrated a safety profile and no increased risk of fetal malformation associated with chemotherapy administered during the second and third trimesters. In contrast, chemotherapy administration during the first trimester is associated with an increased incidence of spontaneous abortion, teratogenesis, or fetal malformations. Anthracycline-based chemotherapy regimens are preferred and data on taxane safety is limited. HER2-targeted therapies, including trastuzumab and pertuzumab, are contraindicated.

The role of endocrine therapy is contraindicated secondary to teratogenicity and possible fetal malformation. There have been reports of up to a 20% incidence of fetal abnormalities, including craniofacial malformations and ambiguous genitalia, leading to the recommendation that endocrine therapy be delayed until after delivery.

Published studies have found that stage-for-stage patients with pregnancy-associated breast cancer have similar survivals compared to those with nonpregnancy-associated breast cancer. These findings emphasize that definitive treatment and local control of breast cancer during pregnancy is not only feasible but also effective. Safe and effective treatment is available for many of these women with pregnancy-associated breast cancer.

Phyllodes Tumor

Phyllodes tumor represents an uncommon fibroepithelial breast neoplasm and accounts for only 0.5% to 1% of breast carcinomas. These tumors can occur in women of all ages, including adolescents and the elderly, but most arise in women between 35 and 55 years of age. Phyllodes tumors may be quite large and have a mean diameter of 4 to 5 cm. Because phyllodes tumors and fibroadenomas are mammographically indistinguishable, core-needle biopsy should precede any surgical intervention, however, they may still be indistinguishable on biopsy and more generally characterized as a fibroepithelial lesion recommended for surgical excision. The decision to perform excisional biopsy is usually based on large tumor size, history of rapid growth, patient age, and inability to rule out an associated or obscured cancer.

Phyllodes tumors are classified as benign, borderline/low-grade malignant, or malignant based on mitotic activity, type of margin, stromal overgrowth, and cellular pleomorphism similar to other soft tissue sarcomas. More than 70% of these tumors are benign, and approximately 10% are malignant. Common sites of metastases from malignant phyllodes are lung, bone, and mediastinum.

Appropriate treatment for phyllodes tumors is complete surgical excision with a negative margin, and breast conservation surgery with appropriate margins is the preferred primary therapy. Traditionally, a 1-cm margin was recommended, however, in patients with benign or borderline phyllodes tumor, complete excision with a negative margin is adequate. The incidence of local recurrence ranges from 5% to 20% for benign tumors and 20% to 40% for malignant tumors. Local recurrences are typically salvageable with total mastectomy and do not affect the overall survival rate. For all phyllodes tumors, the low incidence of axillary nodal metastases (less than 1%) obviates the need for lymphadenectomy. The reported rates of distant metastasis for patients with malignant tumors range from 25% to 40%, with the most common site of distant metastasis being the lung. The presence of stromal overgrowth may be the strongest predictor of distant metastasis and ultimate outcome, though 5- and 10-year overall survival rates are 75% to 88%, and 57% to 80%, respectively. To date, no role for chemotherapy or hormonal therapy has been established for this disease and there may be a limited role for radiation therapy in select cases of malignant phyllodes tumors.

CASE SCENARIO

Case Scenario 1: Hormone Receptor–Positive Breast Cancer

Presentation

A 72-year-old woman presents to the clinic with a screening mammogram detected 0.5-cm area of microcalcifications in the right breast. Workup includes bilateral diagnostic mammogram confirming the focus of macrocalcifications in the lower inner right breast and nodal ultrasound confirms presence of 0.7-cm mass in the 4 o'clock position, 5 cm from the nipple, with one abnormal-appearing axillary level I lymph node. Core needle biopsy of the breast mass demonstrates invasive ductal carcinoma, grade 2, ER positive, PR positive, HER2 negative, Ki-67 8%. Fine-needle aspiration of the index axillary lymph node is negative for metastatic carcinoma. She has a past medical history significant for hypertension, diabetes, and hyperlipidemia. She lives independently and is functional in all her activities of daily living. She denies family history of malignancy and underwent menopause at age 55.

Additional Workup

A thorough history and physical are imperative to delineate the possibility of metastatic disease which would necessitate further staging workup. Given patient's low likelihood for metastatic disease, additional imaging, such as staging CT scan or bone scan, is not needed. There is no role for breast MRI in this case scenario, but in other circumstances, it may be appropriate to determine extent of disease, or to clarify discordant imaging. Genetic counseling with panel testing can be omitted in this older patient with no family history of breast cancer. A 21-gene RT-PCR assay (Oncotype DX®) should be considered as this patient's tumor is between 0.5 and 5 cm on final pathology, to determine the benefit of chemotherapy. If the recurrence score (RS) is less than or equal to 25, adjuvant endocrine therapy would be sufficient. If the recurrence score is greater than or equal to 26, adjuvant chemotherapy should be considered in patients that can tolerate therapy.

Approach to Treatment

The key features to recognize in this patient's presentation include that she is postmenopausal with a small, early-stage, clinically node-negative breast malignancy that is hormone receptor positive and HER2 negative. This patient does not meet the criteria for neoadjuvant chemotherapy and would proceed with up front surgery. Given that she is postmenopausal, she will benefit from adjuvant endocrine therapy with an aromatase inhibitor for 5 to 10 years. She should be followed while on endocrine therapy to assess for medication tolerance and side effects. Patients treated with breast-conserving surgery receive adjuvant whole-breast radiation as the standard of care. However, in patients older than 70, with T1 or T2 (<3 cm) N0 hormone receptor–positive breast cancer treated with breast-conserving surgery and planned for adjuvant endocrine therapy, sentinel node staging and radiation may be omitted. In addition, partial breast radiation may be considered in postmenopausal women with small tumors and >3-mm margins and negative sentinel lymph nodes (SLNs).

Surgical Management

All older adults undergoing surgery should undergo an assessment for components of frailty including comorbidities, cognition, mobility, functional status, and nutrition. Patients with early-stage breast cancer are eligible for breast conservation surgery or mastectomy, given the survival equivalence. This patient is an ideal candidate for breast-conserving therapy given the small tumor size, but shared surgical decision making should include discussions of breast to tumor volume, plan for radiation therapy, and patient preference. Reconstruction options also should be discussed with the patient and referral to Plastic Surgery as appropriate. In clinically node-negative disease, sentinel node dissection is recommended for nodal staging. However, it has been shown that sentinel lymph node biopsy can safely be omitted in patients over 70 years of age with early-stage, node-negative, hormone receptor–positive, HER2-negative cancers that are treated with endocrine therapy. The rates of locoregional recurrence and breast cancer mortality are not negatively impacted. Axillary staging should be individually considered if the results will impact radiation therapy recommendations or systemic therapy decisions.

Take Home Points

- Patients with early-stage, hormone receptor–positive, HER2-negative breast cancer benefit from up front surgical resection.
- In patients with tumors 0.5 to 5 cm, with pN0 or pN1 disease (1 to 3 positive axillary nodes), the need for chemotherapy is largely determined by the 21 gene RT-PCR assay results.
- Elderly patients (>70 years old) with early-stage, node-negative, hormone receptor–positive, HER2-negative tumors that receive endocrine therapy can consider omission of sentinel node biopsy and radiation therapy.

CASE SCENARIO 1 REVIEW

Case Scenario 1 Questions

1. What is the next best step in management for an 87-year-old woman with 4-mm, ER-positive, PR-positive, HER2-negative invasive ductal carcinoma with negative margins after segmental mastectomy and negative sentinel lymph node biopsy?

   A. Chemotherapy
   B. Tamoxifen therapy
   C. Radiation therapy
   D. Aromatase inhibitor therapy
   E. None of the above

2. A 67-year-old woman has 2.2-cm, grade 2, ER-positive, PR-positive, HER2-negative invasive ductal carcinoma treated with segmental mastectomy with negative margins and two negative sentinel lymph nodes. The next step in management is:

   A. Endocrine therapy
   B. Genetic expression profile of the tumor
   C. Chemotherapy
   D. Chemotherapy and endocrine therapy
   E. None of the above

3. A 46-year-old woman has 2.2-cm, grade 2, ER-positive, PR-positive, HER2-negative invasive ductal carcinoma treated with segmental mastectomy with negative margins and one of two positive sentinel lymph nodes. The next step in management is:

   A. Axillary lymph node dissection
   B. No further axillary surgery
   C. Adjuvant radiation therapy
   D. Adjuvant systemic therapy
   E. B, C, and D

4. What factors must be considered to safely omit sentinel lymph node biopsy and radiation therapy in patients with early-stage breast cancer?

   A. Age >70 years old
   B. Clinically node negative
   C. Tumor size
   D. Receipt of endocrine therapy
   E. All of the above

5. A 55-year-old postmenopausal woman presents with a 5-cm breast mass with no associated axillary adenopathy. Biopsy demonstrates invasive ductal carcinoma, grade 2, ER-positive, PR-positive, HER2-negative with Ki-67 10%. Preoperative endocrine therapy in this patient:

   A. Is associated with lower response rates than with neoadjuvant chemotherapy
   B. Is typically given for 6 weeks
   C. Will not affect the chance for lumpectomy
   D. Is less toxic than neoadjuvant chemotherapy
   E. Should include tamoxifen

Case Scenario 1 Answers

1. **The correct answer is D.** *Rationale:* Elderly patients with breast cancer pose unique challenges to long-term management. Patient fitness and frailty should always be considered when deciding on a treatment plan. The Cancer and Leukemia Group B (CALGB) 9343 study evaluated women >70 years old who underwent segmental mastectomy for clinical T1 N0 ER-positive breast cancer. CALGB 9343 trial randomized to either to hormone therapy alone or hormone therapy plus radiation. Interestingly, a large proportion of patients in both groups did not undergo axillary surgery. It showed that the addition of radiation therapy in elderly patients decreased the risk of ipsilateral recurrence, but did not increase overall survival, disease-free survival, or breast preservation. In addition, even though the study did not specifically look at axillary surgery, there were low rates of axillary recurrence even among those not randomized to radiation therapy. Chemotherapy may be required in patients with triple negative breast cancers, but in patients with HR+ cancers, hormonal therapy is key to treatment. This patient has a <0.5-cm tumor, so endocrine therapy alone is sufficient. One would consider 21-gene PCR testing if the mass was greater than 0.5 cm. Postmenopausal women should receive aromatase inhibitors over tamoxifen. The ATAC trial compared anastrozole to tamoxifen and found an absolute improvement in disease-free survival of 3% for anastrozole compared with tamoxifen.

2. **The correct answer is B.** *Rationale:* For a patient with a node-negative, hormone receptor–positive, HER2-negative, >0.5-cm breast cancer, national consensus guidelines recommend multianalyte genetic expression profiles to predict outcomes and assist in making decisions about adjuvant therapy. The 21-gene RT-PCR assay (Oncotype DX®) helps to estimate the likelihood of recurrence and the benefit of chemotherapy. It can also be used in select patients with one to three involved ipsilateral nodes to guide the addition of chemotherapy to standard endocrine therapy.

3. **The correct answer is E.** *Rationale:* This patient meets criteria outlined in the ACOSOG Z11 trial. This trial defined that women with early-stage cT1-2 N0 invasive breast cancer treated with breast-conserving surgery and SLN dissection may omit ALND in the setting of limited (1 to 2) positive SLNs. These findings apply to patients treated with upfront surgery and exclude those treated after neoadjuvant therapy, mastectomy or gross extranodal extension. In addition, in this premenopausal patient with pathologically node-positive breast cancer, adjuvant systemic therapy is indicated with chemotherapy and endocrine therapy. In the postmenopausal setting, the RxPonder trial defined that in patients with ER-positive, PR-positive, HER2-negative breast cancer with one to three nodes involved, Oncotype ≤25 is associated with no additional benefit from chemotherapy in addition to endocrine therapy.

4. **The correct answer is E.** *Rationale:* We have made progress in de-escalating both surgical and systemic treatments in elderly patients. However, each patient case should be evaluated individually to ensure that all of the aforementioned criteria are met to avoid inadequate oncologic treatment. Studies including CALGB 9343 (discussed above) as well as the PRIME II trial

have contributed to this treatment paradigm. The PRIME II study examined patients >65 years old with T1/T2 tumors up to 3 cm that were node negative and ER positive who underwent lumpectomy with axillary evaluation and adjuvant endocrine therapy. Patients were randomized to receive whole-breast radiation therapy or not. They found no difference in overall survival, regional recurrence, distant metastasis, or new breast cancers. The Choosing Wisely guidelines from the Society of Surgical Oncology recommend against routine use of SLN dissection in clinically node-negative women >70 years of age who are hormone receptor positive. If these women are treated with hormonal therapy, there is no significant difference in the rate of locoregional recurrence and there is no impact on breast cancer mortality.

5. **The correct answer is D.** *Rationale:* In the NEOCENT trial, a meta-analysis of 20 prospective, randomized clinical trials, neoadjuvant endocrine therapy with aromatase inhibitors had a similar overall response rate but less toxicity compared with neoadjuvant chemotherapy. The trial showed that the radiologic response to neoadjuvant endocrine therapy was similar to that seen in neoadjuvant chemotherapy in postmenopausal women with ER-positive breast cancer. ACOSOG Z1031 demonstrated an overall response rate of 69%. There were statistically significant differences in alopecia, nausea, vomiting, stomatitis, and anemia between the treatment groups as well. The duration of treatment varied between studies, but the mean duration of treatment was 12 to 24 weeks, with the highest response rates seen in patient who received more than 3 months. Aromatase inhibitors had a better overall response rate in postmenopausal women than tamoxifen. Neoadjuvant endocrine therapy is a well-tolerated option for ER-positive breast cancer patients. In many patients, neoadjuvant chemotherapy is still preferred, however, neoadjuvant endocrine therapy is a safe and feasible alternative. Future studies should more clearly establish its role in good risk postmenopausal women.

CASE SCENARIO

Case Scenario 2: Triple Negative Breast Cancer

Presentation

A 30-year-old woman presents to the clinic with a self-palpated right breast mass. Workup includes bilateral diagnostic mammogram showing axillary adenopathy and right breast and nodal ultrasound demonstrates a 2.6-cm mass in the upper outer quadrant of the breast with normal-appearing axillary level I lymph nodes. Core-needle biopsy of the breast mass demonstrates invasive ductal carcinoma, grade 3, ER negative, PR negative, HER2 negative, Ki-67 80%. She is premenopausal, healthy, and takes no medications. She has a family history of breast cancer in her mother at age 45, maternal grandmother at age 50, and paternal aunt at age 55. There is also a history of ovarian cancer in her maternal aunt.

Additional Workup

Given her young age at diagnosis and strong family history of breast and ovarian cancer, extended panel genetic testing was performed. This showed a deleterious BRCA1 mutation. Breast MRI was performed showing a 4.2-cm mass in the right upper outer breast with nonmass enhancement spanning 7 cm to the base of the nipple. There were no suspicious findings in the left breast or bilateral axillary nodes. She is interested in potentially having children in the future and is referred to an oncofertility specialist.

Approach to Treatment

After thorough evaluation to characterize the extent of the breast malignancy and clarify the clinical stage, neoadjuvant chemotherapy is recommended. Standard chemotherapy typically includes Adriamycin Cytoxan (AC) given for 4 cycles and Taxol given for 12 cycles. In patients where there is a poor response to AC, the addition of carboplatin with the taxane may be considered, however, this may be associated with increased toxicity. In addition, the current standard of care landscape is shifting after the Keynote 522 trial showing improved benefit with pembrolizumab in the neoadjuvant setting. Close monitoring of tumor response with breast and nodal ultrasound is recommended during chemotherapy.

Surgical Management

Following the completion of chemotherapy, surgery is recommended. Given the extent of disease in the breast, mastectomy is recommended. This strategy will treat the breast malignancy and reduce the risk for future breast malignancy given her high-risk status secondary to the BRCA mutation. Postmastectomy reconstruction should be discussed with referral to plastic surgery. Consideration for contralateral pro-phylactic mastectomy for risk reduction whether at the time of definitive cancer surgery or staged at a later date should be discussed as well. Sentinel node staging of the axilla is recommended. If the sentinel node dissection is positive, completion axillary dissection should be performed followed by adjuvant radiation.

In the setting of residual disease identified at surgical pathology, this patient may benefit from olapa-rib therapy showing improved outcomes in women with BRCA-associated breast cancer as evidenced by the OlympiA trial. Ovarian cancer screening should be initiated with consideration for risk-reducing oophorectomy between ages 35 and 40.

Take Home Points

- Patients with triple negative breast cancer benefit from the use of anthracycline-taxane–based systemic therapy. The neoadjuvant approach often is preferred to facilitate BCT, downstage disease in the axilla, provide an understanding of the tumor response to therapy in order to better predict prognosis and guide adjuvant systemic therapy decision making.
- Neoadjuvant systemic therapy approaches may utilize immunotherapy with pembrolizumab given improved pCR rates and event-free survival at 3 years.
- Genetic testing is indicated in women with triple negative breast cancer diagnosed under the age of 60 as well as those with strong family history of breast cancer, or family history of ovarian cancer.
- In premenopausal women with breast cancer, consider oncofertility consultation prior to initiation of chemotherapy if future fertility is desired.

CASE SCENARIO 2 REVIEW

Case Scenario 2 Questions

1. Which of the following are indications for genetic testing in a patient with breast cancer?

  A. Family history of breast cancer in three maternal aunts
  B. Family history of male breast cancer and/or ovarian cancer
  C. Age <45 years at diagnosis
  D. Personal history of triple negative breast cancer
  E. All of the above

2. Which of the following best describes the management for patients with a BRCA mutation and no personal history of breast cancer?

  A. Chemoprevention with tamoxifen to reduce cancer risk
  B. Annual mammogram alone
  C. Annual mammogram and MRI (alternating every 6 months)
  D. Risk-reducing bilateral mastectomy
  E. C and D

3. In patients with triple negative breast cancer who receive neoadjuvant chemotherapy and have residual disease identified on final pathology, which of the following describes the adjuvant treatment options? Select all that apply.

  A. No additional systemic therapy
  B. Leuprolide
  C. Pembrolizumab (if received preoperatively)
  D. Olaparib (if BRCA positive)
  E. C and D

4. All of the following are advantages of neoadjuvant chemotherapy EXCEPT:

  A. Down-staging of disease, facilitating breast-conserving surgery
  B. Reduced likelihood for axillary lymph node dissection in cN0 disease or limited cN1 disease
  C. Tumor response aiding in prognostication
  D. Improved survival
  E. Response informs decision making for adjuvant systemic therapy

Case Scenario 2 Answers

1. **The correct answer is E.** *Rationale:* After a breast cancer diagnosis, national consensus guidelines recommend genetic counseling and testing for high-penetrance genes (BRCA1, BRCA2, CDH1, PALB2, PTEN, TP53) in the following patients:

Diagnosed at age 45 or younger
Triple negative breast cancer
Personal history of invasive lobular breast cancer or gastric cancer
Ashkenazi Jewish ancestry
Blood relative with known pathogenic mutation
Family history of breast cancer in first-, second-, or third-degree relative (in ≥1 relative if patient is 46 to 50 years of age; in ≥1 relative diagnosed at ≤50 years of age or ≥2 relatives if patient is ≥51 years old)
Family history of ovarian, pancreatic, prostate, or male breast cancer
Diagnosed at age 50 or younger with unknown/limited family history or multiple primary breast cancers
Knowledge of high-penetrance gene status will influence clinical decision making regarding the use of PARP inhibitors in the metastatic or adjuvant setting

2. **The correct answer is E.** *Rationale:* In women with known BRCA mutation with no personal history of breast cancer, appropriate management approaches include early detection of malignancy with high-risk screening (annual mammogram and MRI, alternating every 6 months) with clinical breast examination every 6 months or risk reduction with bilateral prophylactic mastectomy. Several studies have demonstrated the oncologic safety of nipple-sparing mastectomy in this patient population and this approach may be considered in selected patients who meet anatomic criteria. Chemoprevention with tamoxifen or aromatase inhibitors has been shown to reduce the risk of breast cancer in high-risk postmenopausal women, however, the data is limited in women with BRCA mutations. Gynecology consultation for ovarian cancer screening and/or risk-reducing salpingo-oophorectomy (between ages 35 and 40) should also be considered.

3. **The correct answer is E.** *Rationale:* The clinical landscape for patients with triple negative breast cancer is rapidly evolving. While a high proportion of patients may achieve pathologic complete response (pCR) with neoadjuvant chemotherapy, treatment of patients with chemoresistant or residual disease remains a clinical challenge. The Keynote 522 trial demonstrated higher rates of pCR as well as improved recurrence-free survival at 36 months with the addition of pembrolizumab to neoadjuvant anthracycline-taxane-carboplatin–based chemotherapy followed by adjuvant pembrolizumab. The OlympiA trial evaluated therapy with olaparib (a PARP inhibitor) in patients with high-risk BRCA-associated HER2-negative breast cancer, showing improved 3-year invasive disease-free survival and 3-year distant disease-free survival and thus is now standard of care in this patient population. Tamoxifen is contraindicated in ER/PR-negative disease. In the setting of residual triple negative disease, additional systemic therapy should be considered based on the neoadjuvant treatment received and BRCA status.

4. **The correct answer is D.** *Rationale:* Several landmark clinical trials have demonstrated no survival advantage of chemotherapy when delivered in the neoadjuvant or adjuvant setting. However, these studies clearly identified the utility of neoadjuvant chemotherapy in down-staging disease in the breast, which allows for breast-conserving surgery in approximately 25% of patients. Studies also demonstrate the prognostic value of tumor response, with longer survival observed in patients with pCR and pathologically negative axillary nodes. Further studies have shown decreased likelihood of positive SLNs and lower risk for ALND in patients with clinically node-negative disease, as well as enabling targeted axillary dissection in patients with limited cN1 disease, reducing the need for ALND in selected patients with no residual disease in the SLNs and clipped node. Furthermore, several clinical trials (CREATE-X, KATHERINE trial, monarchE, OlympiA) have shown that for patients with residual disease after neoadjuvant chemotherapy, oncologic outcomes can be improved with adjuvant therapies as directed by the tumor subtype and patient population treated.

CASE SCENARIO

Case Scenario 3: HER2-positive Breast Cancer

Presentation

A 37-year-old 26-week pregnant female presents to the clinic with self-palpated left breast mass. Workup including bilateral diagnostic mammogram, left breast and nodal ultrasound demonstrates a 3.8-cm mass in the upper outer quadrant with four abnormal-appearing level I axillary lymph nodes. Core-needle biopsy of the breast mass demonstrates invasive ductal carcinoma, grade 3, ER negative, PR negative, HER2 positive, Ki-67 60%. Fine-needle aspiration of the index axillary lymph node confirms metastatic carcinoma consistent with breast primary. She is otherwise healthy and has had no complications associated with the pregnancy.

Additional Workup

Breast MRI cannot be performed during pregnancy, as gadolinium is contraindicated. Typically, imaging for systemic staging is performed for Stage II or III breast cancer. For pregnant patients, imaging includes US or MRI of the liver without contrast, CXR with abdominal shielding, and MRI spine without contrast. A thorough review of systems will direct the clinician toward further imaging as needed, based on symptoms. The patient should also be referred to a maternal–fetal medicine specialist to coordinate care. This includes verification of fetal age and determination of a safe delivery window. Genetic counseling with panel testing is appropriate in this patient due to her young age (<45 years) regardless of family history.

Approach to Treatment

The key features to recognize in this patient's presentation include that she presents with a node-positive, HER2-positive breast cancer and is pregnant. Neoadjuvant systemic therapy is recommended in this scenario, however, trastuzumab and pertuzumab, the HER2-targeted therapies that are part of the standard regimen, are contraindicated in pregnancy. Anthracycline-based regimens are the preferred chemotherapy for pregnant patients and can be given safely to patients in the second trimester. Ultrasound imaging to monitor tumor response to therapy is standard.

Following delivery, continued systemic therapy with taxane and dual HER2-targeted therapy would be recommended. Surgery is performed after completion of systemic therapy. Adjuvant radiotherapy is also recommended in this case due to axillary nodal involvement and completion of 1 year of HER2 therapy. Based on the results of the KATHERINE trial showing improvement in invasive disease-free survival, any residual disease on surgical pathology would lead to switching her adjuvant therapy to trastuzumab emtansine (T-DM1).

Surgical Management

She is potentially eligible for breast conservation surgery or mastectomy. Important factors to include in the shared surgical decision-making process are tumor response to therapy as well as tumor-to-breast volume ratio, genetic-testing results, and patient preference. For patients who must undergo breast surgery during early pregnancy, mastectomy is the preferred approach, as radiotherapy is contraindicated. Reconstruction options also should be discussed with the patient with referral to plastic and reconstructive surgery as appropriate and available. Multidisciplinary discussion with radiation oncology and plastic surgery specialists is important when determining the best approach to immediate versus delayed reconstruction.

Axillary surgery is dependent on the initial nodal burden as seen on the axillary ultrasound. In the clinical N1 setting, patients who have limited axillary nodal burden, that is, fewer than four abnormal lymph nodes, may be eligible for de-escalation of axillary surgery with a targeted axillary dissection. This patient does not qualify, as her initial axillary ultrasound demonstrated four suspicious lymph nodes and therefore, axillary lymph node dissection (ALND) is indicated. A complete ALND requires removal of the axillary contents in levels I and II with identification of the key structures in the axilla: latissimus dorsi defining the lateral border, axillary vein, at the superior border, medial border defined by the pectoralis minor muscle, subscapularis muscle as the posterior extent as well as all of the fibroareolar tissue along the thoracodorsal neurovascular bundle and the long thoracic nerve. Anatomical understanding and awareness of critical axillary structures allow for a safe and oncologically complete ALND.

Take Home Points

■ Patients with HER2-positive breast cancer benefit from the use of systemic chemotherapy including HER2-targeted therapy. The neoadjuvant approach often is preferred in patients who have larger tumors and positive lymph nodes. The response to therapy impacts adjuvant treatment recommendations based on the KATHERINE trial.

■ Management of HER2-positive breast cancer during pregnancy requires an understanding of which imaging and therapies are safe. Anthracycline-based chemotherapy regimens are recommended, while HER2-targeted therapies and gadolinium contrast are contraindicated.

■ Patients with limited number of clinically positive nodes (less than four) who undergo neoadjuvant systemic therapy may be eligible for de-escalation of axillary surgery and should be considered for targeted axillary dissection. This technique involves sentinel lymph node dissection, including resection of the initially biopsied lymph node marked with a biopsy clip.

CASE SCENARIO 3 REVIEW

Case Scenario 3 Questions

1. When performing imaging to evaluate a palpable breast mass in a pregnant patient, which of the following is contraindicated?

   A. MRI spine without gadolinium
   B. Breast ultrasound
   C. Breast MRI with gadolinium
   D. Diagnostic mammogram
   E. None of the above

2. The following are key components of a level I and II axillary lymph node dissection EXCEPT:

   A. Identification of the long thoracic nerve
   B. Removal of all lymph nodes medial to the pectoralis minor muscle
   C. Definition of the latissimus dorsi muscle as the lateral border
   D. Identification of the thoracodorsal neurovascular bundle
   E. None of the above

3. What factor should the surgeon prioritize the most when making a surgical recommendation to a young patient with smaller breast size and HER2-positive multicentric breast cancer as demonstrated by a 4-cm mass with surrounding malignant-appearing calcifications measuring up to 7 cm?

   A. Genetic testing results
   B. Patient preference
   C. Tumor response to neoadjuvant therapy
   D. Extent of disease
   E. None of the above

4. Which of the following is true with regard to treatment of HER2-positive breast cancer with neoadjuvant systemic therapy?

   A. There is no role for de-escalation of axillary surgery in clinically node-positive patients
   B. Patients who have a radiographically complete response do not require surgery
   C. For breast conservation surgery, extent of resection is based on the initial volume of disease on imaging prior to systemic therapy
   D. Based on the KATHERINE trial, patients with residual disease on surgical resection are recommended adjuvant trastuzumab emtansine (T-DM1) instead of trastuzumab and pertuzumab
   E. None of the above

5. For a patient with biopsy-proven node-positive, HER2-positive breast cancer and two suspicious lymph nodes on initial axillary ultrasound who undergoes neoadjuvant systemic therapy, all of the following are true EXCEPT:

   A. For residual disease identified on targeted axillary dissection, radiotherapy can be performed instead of completion axillary lymph node dissection
   B. The biopsied lymph node should have a biopsy clip placed so that it can be localized at the time of surgery

    C. Dual tracer technique, including technetium sulfur colloid and blue dye, is recommended for sentinel lymph node mapping after neoadjuvant systemic therapy

    D. Use of blue dye is contraindicated in pregnancy

    E. None of the above

Case Scenario 3 Answers

1. **The correct answer is C.** *Rationale:* Gadolinium is contraindicated in pregnancy. Diagnostic mammogram and ultrasound are standard imaging techniques that are safe in pregnancy. MRI of the spine and liver without contrast can be performed safely and used in systemic staging. CXR is a component of systemic imaging and liver ultrasound is an option instead of contrast MRI of the liver or CT.

2. **The correct answer is B.** *Rationale:* A level I to II axillary lymph node dissection involves complete removal of the tissue within the defined borders of the axilla which include the latissimus dorsi laterally, axillary vein superiorly, medial border defined by the pectoralis minor muscle, and the subscapularis muscle posteriorly. Critical structures to identify and preserve include the long thoracic nerve and the thoracodorsal neurovascular bundle. Intercostobrachial nerves should also be identified and preserved as appropriate. The level III axilla is defined as the region medial to the pectoralis minor and is not a standard part of an axillary lymph node dissection in breast cancer.

3. **The correct answer is D.** *Rationale:* All four of the answer choices are important to consider when discussing surgical options with a patient in clinic. However, in this case, the patient has multicentric disease with a large area of calcifications and a small breast size. The extent of disease is the most important criterion and while it is likely the tumor size will decrease with neoadjuvant therapy, the initial area of calcifications necessitates a larger area of resection. Mastectomy would be the appropriate option to ensure a margin-negative surgery.

4. **The correct answer is D.** *Rationale:* Patients with biopsy-proven axillary nodal disease and fewer than four abnormal lymph nodes on ultrasound may be eligible for a targeted axillary dissection as opposed to a standard axillary lymphadenectomy. Particularly high rates of nodal pathologic complete response (pCR) in HER2-positive breast cancer patients allow surgeons to potentially avoid much of the morbidity of ALND in certain patients. Ongoing trials are evaluating the feasibility of omitting surgery in patients with a radiologic complete response and a biopsy of the tumor bed demonstrating pathologic complete response after neoadjuvant systemic therapy, favoring local treatment with only whole-breast radiotherapy. However, currently, the standard of care is surgical resection, even in the setting of a high likelihood of pCR. Because of high rates of pCR and predictably good response to neoadjuvant systemic therapy, the area of excision is dependent on both imaging prior to and after neoadjuvant therapy. The size of the partial mastectomy is not solely based on the size of disease on the initial imaging. For patients with HER2-positive breast cancer, the KATHERINE trial significantly impacted the recommendations for adjuvant therapy in patients who do not achieve a pCR. These patients should be switched to T-DM1 therapy to benefit from an improvement in invasive disease-free survival when compared to trastuzumab alone.

5. **The correct answer is A.** *Rationale:* Ongoing trials are evaluating whether radiotherapy is an appropriate alternative for ALND, however, the current standard of care for positive lymph nodes on targeted axillary dissection after neoadjuvant systemic therapy is a completion axillary lymph node dissection. In order to perform a targeted axillary dissection, the initially biopsied lymph node must be removed, since in approximately 20% to 25% of cases, this is not a sentinel node. By placing a larger, more visible clip in this lymph node using radiologic guidance prior to start of neoadjuvant therapy, the tumor response in this lymph node can be monitored with ultrasound and it can be localized for removal at the time of surgery. To perform a sentinel lymph node dissection after neoadjuvant systemic therapy, dual tracer use is recommended to ensure the highest likelihood of successful lymphatic mapping. Blue dye is contraindicated during pregnancy, however, sentinel lymph node dissection can be safely performed during pregnancy with technetium sulfur colloid alone.

Recommended Readings

Akay CL, Meric-Bernstam F, Hunt KK, et al. Evaluation of the MD Anderson Prognostic Index for local-regional recurrence after breast conserving therapy in patients receiving neoadjuvant chemotherapy. *Ann Surg Oncol.* 2012;19(3):901–907.

Arthur DW, Winter KA, Kuerer HK, et al. Effectiveness of breast-conserving surgery and 3-dimensional conformal partial breast reirradiation for recurrence of breast cancer in the ipsilateral breast: the NRG Oncology/RTOG 1014 phase 2 clinical trial. *JAMA Oncol.* 2020;6(1):75–82.

Badwe R, Hawaldar R, Nair N, et al. Locoregional treatment versus no treatment of the primary tumour in metastatic breast cancer: an open-label randomised controlled trial. *Lancet Oncol.* 2015;16(13):1380–1388.

Bateni SB, Davidson AJ, Arora M, et al. Is breast-conserving therapy appropriate for male breast cancer patients? A National Cancer Database analysis. *Ann Surg Oncol.* 2019;26(7):2144–2153.

Bedrosian I, Hu CY, Chang GJ. Population-based study of contralateral prophylactic mastectomy and survival outcomes of breast cancer patients. *J Natl Cancer Inst.* 2010;102(6):401–409.

Bishop AJ, Ensor J, Moulder SL, et al. Prognosis for patients with metastatic breast cancer who achieve a no-evidence-of-disease status after systemic or local therapy. *Cancer.* 2015;121(24):4324–4332.

Boileau JF, Poirier B, Basik M, et al. Sentinel node biopsy after neoadjuvant chemotherapy in biopsy-proven node-positive breast cancer: the SN FNAC study. *J Clin Oncol.* 2015;33(3):258–264.

Boughey JC, Suman VJ, Mittendorf EA et al; Alliance for Clinical Trials in Oncology. Sentinel lymph node surgery after neoadjuvant chemotherapy in patients with node-positive breast cancer: the ACOSOG Z1071 (Alliance) clinical trial. *JAMA.* 2013;310(14):1455–1461.

Boughey JC, Ballman KV, Le-Petross HT, et al. Identification and resection of clipped node decreases the false-negative rate of sentinel lymph node surgery in patients presenting with node-positive breast cancer (T0-T4, N1-N2) who receive neoadjuvant chemotherapy: results from ACOSOG Z1071 (Alliance). *Ann Surg.* 2016;263(4):802–807.

Boughey JC, Attai DJ, Chen SL, et al. Contralateral prophylactic mastectomy (CPM) consensus statement from the American Society of Breast Surgeons: data on CPM outcomes and risks. *Ann Surg Oncol.* 2016;23(10):3100–3105.

Boughey JC, Ballman KV, McCall LM, et al. Tumor biology and response to chemotherapy impact breast cancer-specific survival in node-positive breast cancer patients treated with neoadjuvant chemotherapy: long-term follow-up from ACOSOG Z1071 (Alliance). *Ann Surg.* 2017;266(4):667–676.

Brunt AM, Haviland JS, Wheatley DA, et al; FAST-Forward Trial Management Group. Hypofractionated breast radiotherapy for 1 week versus 3 weeks (FAST-Forward): 5-year efficacy and late normal tissue effects results from a multicentre, non-inferiority, randomised, phase 3 trial. *Lancet.* 2020;395(10237):1613–1626.

Brunt AM, Haviland JS, Sydenham M, et al. Ten-year results of FAST: a randomized controlled trial of 5-fraction whole-breast radiotherapy for early breast cancer. *J Clin Oncol.* 2020;38(28):3261–3272.

Buchholz TA, Ali S, Hunt KK. Multidisciplinary management of locoregional recurrent breast cancer. *J Clin Oncol.* 2020;38(20):2321–2328.

Cardoso F, van't Veer LJ, Bogaerts J, et al; MINDACT Investigators. 70-gene signature as an aid to treatment decisions in early-stage breast cancer. *N Engl J Med.* 2016;375(8):717–729.

Carter SA, Lyons GR, Kuerer HM, et al. Operative and oncologic outcomes in 9861 patients with operable breast cancer: single-institution analysis of breast conservation with oncoplastic reconstruction. *Ann Surg Oncol.* 2016;23(10):3190–3198.

Cataliotti L, Buzdar AU, Nogushi S, et al. Comparison of anastrozole versus tamoxifen as preoperative therapy in postmenopausal women with hormone receptor-positive breast cancer: the Pre-Operative "Arimidex" Compared to Tamoxifen (PROACT) trial. *Cancer.* 2006;106(10):2095–2103.

Caudle AS, Yang WT, Krishnamurthy S, et al. Improved axillary evaluation following neoadjuvant therapy for patients with node-positive breast cancer using selective evaluation of clipped nodes: implementation of targeted axillary dissection. *J Clin Oncol.* 2016;34(10):1072—1078.

Cortazar P, Zhang L, Untch M, et al. Pathological complete response and long-term clinical benefit in breast cancer: the CTNeoBC pooled analysis. *Lancet.* 2014;384(9938):164–172.

Donker M, van Tienhoven G, Straver ME, et al. Radiotherapy or surgery of the axilla after a positive sentinel node for breast cancer (EORTC 10981–22023 AMAROS): a randomized, multicentre, open label, phase 3 non-inferiority trial. *Lancet Oncol.* 2014;15(12):1303–1310.

Early Breast Cancer Trialists' Collaborative Group (EBCTCG). Effects of chemotherapy and hormonal therapy for early breast cancer on recurrence and 15-year survival: an overview of the randomised trials. *Lancet.* 2005;365(9472):1687–1717.

EBCTCG (Early Breast Cancer Trialists' Collaborative Group); McGale P, Taylor C, Correa C, et al. Effect of radiotherapy after mastectomy and axillary surgery on 10-year recurrence and 20-year breast cancer mortality: meta-analysis of individual patient data for 8135 women in 22 randomised trials. *Lancet.* 2014;383(9935):2127–2135.

Elmore LC, Dietz JR, Myckatyn TM, Margenthaler JA. The landmark series: mastectomy trials (skin-sparing and nipple-sparing and reconstruction landmark trials). *Ann Surg Oncol.* 2021(1):273–280.

Fisher B, Jeong JH, Anderson S, Bryant J, Fisher ER, Wolmark N. Twenty-five-year follow-up of a randomized trial comparing radical mastectomy, total mastectomy and total mastectomy followed by irradiation. *N Engl J Med.* 2002;347(8):567–575.

Fisher CS, Margenthaler JA, Hunt KK, Schwartz T. The landmark series: axillary management for breast cancer. *Ann Surg Oncol.* 2020; 27(3):724–729.

Galimberti V, Cole BF, Viale G, et al; International Breast Cancer Study Group Trial 23-01. Axillary dissection versus no axillary dissection in patients with breast cancer and sentinel-node micrometastases (IBCSG 23-01): 10-year follow up of a randomized, controlled phase 3 trial. *Lancet Oncol.* 2018;19(10):1385–1393.

Giuliano AE, Ballman K, McCall L, et al. Locoregional recurrence after sentinel lymph node dissection with or without axillary dissection in patients with sentinel lymph node metastases: long-term follow-up from the American College of Surgeons Oncology Group (Alliance) ACOSOG Z0011 randomized trial. *Ann Surg.* 2016;264(3):413-420.

Gropper AB, Calvillo KZ, Dominici L, et al. Sentinel lymph node biopsy in pregnant women with breast cancer. *Ann Surg Oncol.* 2014;21(8):2506–2511.

Hassett MJ, Somerfield MR, Baker ER, et al. Management of male breast cancer: ASCO guideline. *J Clin Oncol.* 2020;38(16):1849–1863.

Houssami N, Macaskill P, von Minckwitz G, Marinovich ML, Mamounas E. Meta-analysis of the association of breast cancer subtype and pathologic complete response to neoadjuvant chemotherapy. *Eur J Cancer.* 2012;48(18):3342–3354.

Johnston SRD, Harbeck N, Hegg R, et al; monarchE Committee Members and Investigators. Abemaciclib combined with endocrine therapy for the adjuvant treatment of HR+, HER2-, node-positive, high-risk, early breast cancer (monarchE). *J Clin Oncol.* 2020;38(34):3987–3998.

Kalinsky K, Barlow WE, Gralow JR, et al. 21-gene assay to inform chemotherapy benefit in node-positive breast cancer. *N Engl J Med.* 2021;385(25):2336–2347.

Khan SA, Zhao F, Goldstein LJ, et al. Early local therapy for the primary site in de novo stage IV breast cancer: results of a randomized clinical trial (EA2108). *J Clin Oncol.* 2022;40(9):978–987.

King TA, Lyman JP, Gonen M, et al. Prognostic impact of 21-gene recurrence score in patients with stage IV breast cancer: TBCRC 013. *J Clin Oncol.* 2016 Jul;34(20):2359–2365.

Kuehn T, Bauerfeind I, Fehm T, et al. Sentinel-lymph-node biopsy in patients with breast cancer before and after neoadjuvant chemotherapy (SENTINA): a prospective, multicentre cohort study. *Lancet Oncol.* 2013;14(7):609–618.

Kunkler IH, Williams LJ, Jack WJL, Cameron DA, Dixon JM; PRIME II investigators. Breast-conserving surgery with or without irradiation in women aged 65 years or older with early breast cancer (PRIME II): a randomised controlled trial. *Lancet Oncol.* 2015; 16:266–273.

Lautner M, Lin H, Shen Y, et al. Disparities in the use of breast-conserving therapy among patients with early-stage breast cancer. *JAMA Surg.* 2015;150(8):778–786.

Leon-Ferre RA, Hieken TJ, Boughey JC. The landmark series: neoadjuvant chemotherapy for triple negative breast cancer and HER2-positive breast cancer. *Ann Surg Oncol.* 2021;28(4):2111–2119.

Manahan ER, Kuerer HM, Sebastian M, et al. Consensus guidelines on genetic testing for hereditary breast cancer from the American Society of Breast Surgeons. *Ann Surg Oncol.* 2019;26(10):3025–3031.

Margenthaler JA, Dietz JR, Chatterjee A. The landmark series: breast conservation trials (including oncoplastic breast surgery). *Ann Surg Oncol.* 2021;28(4):2120–2127.

Masuda N, Lee SJ, Ohtani S, et al. Adjuvant capecitabine for breast cancer after preoperative chemotherapy. *N Engl J Med.* 2017;376(22):2147–2159.

Mittendorf EA, Vila J, Tucker SL, et al. The neo-bioscore update for staging breast cancer treated with neoadjuvant chemotherapy: incorporation of prognostic biologic factors into staging after treatment. *JAMA Oncol.* 2016;2(7):929–936.

Moran MS, Schnitt SJ, Giuliano AE, et al; Society of Surgical Oncology, American Society for Radiation Oncology. Society of Surgical Oncology-American Society for Radiation Oncology consensus guideline on margins for breast-conserving surgery with whole breast irradiation in stages I and II invasive breast cancer. *J Clin Oncol.* 2014;32(14):1507–1515.

Newman LA, Kaljee LM. Health disparities and triple-negative breast cancer in African American women: a review. *JAMA Surg.* 2017;152(5):485–493.

Pagani O, Regan MM, Walley BA, et al; TEXT and SOFT Investigators, International Breast Cancer Study Group. Adjuvant exemestane with ovarian suppression in premenopausal breast cancer. *N Engl J Med.* 2014;371(2):107–118.

Paik S, Shak S, Tang G, et al. A multigene assay to predict recurrence of tamoxifen-treated, node-negative breast cancer. *N Engl J Med.* 2004;351(27):2817–2826.

Parker PA, Peterson SK, Bedrosian I, et al. Prospective study of surgical decision-making processes for contralateral prophylactic mastectomy in women with breast cancer. *Ann Surg.* 2016;263(1):178–183.

Partain N, Postlewait LM, Teshome M, et al. The role of mastectomy in de novo stage IV inflammatory breast cancer. *Ann Surg Oncol.* 2021;28(8):4265–4274.

Rosenberger LH, Thomas SM, Nimbkar SN, et al. Contemporary multi-institutional cohort of 550 cases of phyllodes tumors (2007–2017) demonstrates a need for more individualized margin guidelines. *J Clin Oncol.* 2021;39(3):178–189.

Rosso KJ, Tadros AB, Weiss A, et al. Improved locoregional control in a contemporary cohort of nonmetastatic inflammatory breast cancer patients undergoing surgery. *Ann Surg Oncol.* 2017;24(10):2981–2988.

Schmid P, Cortes J, Dent R, et al. Event-free survival with Pembrolizumab in early triple-negative breast cancer. *N Engl J Med.* 2022; 386 (6):556–567.

Schmid P, Cortes J, Pusztai L, et al; KEYNOTE-522 Investigators. Pembrolizumab for early triple-negative breast cancer. *N Engl J Med.* 2020;382(9):810–821.

Shaitelman SF, Lei X, Thompson A, et al. Three-year outcomes with hypofractionated versus conventionally fractionated whole-breast irradiation: results of a randomized, noninferiority clinical trial. *J Clin Oncol.* 2018;36(35):3495–3503.

Singletary SE. Rating the risk factors for breast cancer. *Ann Surg.* 2003;237(4):474–482.

Smith BD, Bellon JR, Blitzblau R, et al. Radiation therapy for the whole breast: executive summary of an American Society for Radiation Oncology (ASTRO) evidence-based guideline. *Pract Radiat Oncol.* 2018;8(3):145–152.

Soran A, Ozmen V, Ozbas S, et al; MF07-01 Study Group. Primary surgery with systemic therapy in patients with de novo stage IV breast cancer: 10-year follow-up; Protocol MF07-01 randomized clinical trial. *J Am Coll Surg.* 2021;233(6):742–751.

Soran A, Ozmen V, Ozbas S, et al. Randomized trial comparing resection of primary tumor with no surgery in stage IV breast cancer at presentation: Protocol MF07-01. *Ann Surg Oncol.* 2018;25(11):3141–3149.

Spanheimer PM, Murray MP, Zabor EC, et al. Long-Term Outcomes After Surgical Treatment of Malignant/Borderline Phyllodes Tumors of the Breast. *Ann Surg Oncol.* 2019;26(7):2136–2143.

Sparano JA, Gray RJ, Makower DF, et al. Prospective validation of a 21-gene expression assay in breast cancer. *N Engl J Med.* 2015;373(21):2005–2014.

Sparano JA, Gray RJ, Makower DF, et al. Adjuvant chemotherapy guided by a 21-gene expression assay in breast cancer. *N Engl J Med.* 2018;379(2):111–121.

Swisher SK, Vila J, Tucker SL, et al. Locoregional control according to breast cancer subtype and response to neoadjuvant chemotherapy in breast cancer patients undergoing breast-conserving therapy. *Ann Surg Oncol.* 2016;23(3):749–756.

Tolaney SM, Guo H, Pernas S, et al. Seven-year follow-up analysis of adjuvant paclitaxel and trastuzumab trial for node-negative human epidermal growth factor receptor 2-positive breast cancer. *J Clin Oncol.* 2019;37(22):1868–1875.

Tung NM, Boughey JC, Pierce LJ, et al. Management of hereditary breast cancer: American Society of Clinical Oncology, American Society of Radiation Oncology and Society of Surgical Oncology Guideline. *J Clin Oncol.* 2020;38(18):2080–2106.

Tutt ANJ, Garber JE, Kaufman B, et al; OlympiA Clinical Trial Steering Committee and Investigators. Adjuvant olaparib for patients with BRCA1- or BRCA2- mutated breast cancer. *N Engl J Med.* 2021;384(25):2394–2405.

Ueno NT, Fernandez JRE, Cristofanilli M, et al. International consensus on the clinical management of inflammatory breast cancer from the Morgan Welch Inflammatory Breast Cancer Research Program 10th Anniversary Conference. *J Cancer.* 2018;9(8):1437–1447.

Valente SA, Shah C. The landmark series: adjuvant radiation therapy for breast cancer. *Ann Surg Oncol.* 2020;27(7):2203–2211.

Valero MG, Muhsen S, Moo TA, et al. Increase in utilization of nipple-sparing mastectomy for breast cancer: indications, complications, and oncologic outcomes. *Ann Surg Oncol.* 2020;27(2):344–351.

Vogel VG, Costantino JP, Wickerham DL, et al; National Surgical Adjuvant Breast and Bowel Project. Update of the National Surgical Adjuvant Breast and Bowel Project Study of Tamoxifen and Raloxifene (STAR) P-2 Trial: preventing breast cancer. *Cancer Prev Res (Phila).* 2010;3(6):696–706.

Von Minckwitz G, Huang CS, Mano MS, et al; KATHERINE Investigators. Trastuzumab emtansine for residual invasive HER2-positive breast cancer. *N Engl J Med.* 2019;380(7):617–628.

Wapnir IL, Price KN, Anderson SJ, et al; International Breast Cancer Study Group, NRG Oncology, GEICAM Spanish Breast Cancer Group, BOOG Dutch Breast Cancer Trialists' Group, Breast International Group. Efficacy of chemotherapy for ER-negative and ER-positive isolated locoregional recurrence of breast cancer: final analysis of the CALOR trial. *J Clin Oncol.* 2018;36(11):1073–1079.

Weiss A, King TA, Mittendorf EA. The landmark series: neoadjuvant endocrine therapy for breast cancer. *Ann Surg Oncol.* 2020;27(9):3393–3401.

Whelan TJ, Olivotto IA, Parulekar WR, et al; MA.20 Study Investigators. Regional nodal irrradiation in early-stage breast cancer. *N Engl J Med.* 2015;373(4):307–316.

Melanoma

Rachel K. Voss and Jeffrey E. Gershenwald

INTRODUCTION

The melanoma treatment landscape continues to rapidly evolve. The development and subsequent U.S. Food and Drug Administration (FDA) approval of targeted, immune, and intralesional therapies has significantly expanded treatment options for many patients with advanced disease. It is therefore important that surgical oncologists stay abreast of these developments. In this chapter, we provide a primer on the multidisciplinary care of patients with melanoma; new to this edition are two melanoma case studies with associated multiple-choice questions.

Epidemiology

The incidence of invasive cutaneous melanoma continues to be a major public health concern in the United States and has been increasing faster than that of nearly any other cancer over the last 30 years. An estimated 99,780 cases of invasive melanoma will be diagnosed in the United States in 2022, and approximately 7,650 will die from the disease. Despite the significant number of deaths from melanoma, this is a decrease, likely reflective of the evolving impact of recent significant advances in the treatment of advanced disease. Overall, the lifetime risk of being diagnosed with melanoma is about 2.5% (1 in 40) for whites, 0.1% (1 in 1,000) for blacks, and 0.5% (1 in 200) for Hispanics. The major environmental risk factor, exposure to ultraviolet (UV) radiation, is reflected in geographic and ethnic patterns of melanoma rates. There have also been changes in the distribution and stage of melanoma at diagnosis, with an overall trend toward thinner T1/T2 melanomas.

Risk Factors

Estimating an individual's risk of developing melanoma can be clinically useful in determining primary prevention strategies and in directing the level of screening. Patients identified as being at high risk for melanoma may also be recruited to prevention trials.

Multiple factors are associated with risk for developing melanoma. Some factors are modifiable while others are inherent to the individual.

1. *Skin type:* Caucasians have at least 20 times the melanoma incidence of African Americans and five times the melanoma incidence of American Hispanics. In addition, white patients with red or blond hair, fair complexion, or blue eyes are at increased risk for melanoma.
2. *Age and Gender:* The incidence of melanoma increases with age. The incidence of melanoma is 1.7-fold higher for women than men before 49 years of age. Over age 70, the incidence of melanoma is 2.4-fold higher for men than women. In general, the incidence of melanoma is higher in men than in women. Specifically, a man's lifetime risk of melanoma development is approximately 1.5 times greater than a woman's risk.
3. *Overexposure to ultraviolet radiation (UVR) from the sun:* Overexposure of UVR from the sun has been associated with an increased risk of melanoma. Genetic sequencing data also support the role of UV *melanomagenesis.* Known to be a tumor with one of the highest mutational loads, a seminal report of the melanoma effort within The Cancer Genome Atlas Program revealed that most somatic mutations in melanoma indeed have a "UV signature." Data support that damage from sunburns in childhood or even in adulthood are associated with increased risk. A correlation has been identified between the number of severe and painful sunburn episodes and the risk of melanoma; individuals who have a history of more than 10 severe sunburns are more than twice as likely to develop a melanoma compared those who have no history of sunburns.
4. *Use of indoor tanning devices:* Multiple studies support that indoor tanning device use is strongly associated with increased risk of melanoma. A systematic review by the International Agency for Research on Cancer (IARC) demonstrated a 15% increased relative risk of melanoma in individuals who had ever used a sunbed versus those who had never (RR 1.15; 95% CU 1.00 to 1.31); the dangers of indoor tanning have been corroborated by subsequent U.S. and Australian groups. Young age of onset and higher frequency of use are key risk factors that are associated with even greater risk of melanoma. Indeed, a well-designed

Minnesota case–control study showed increased risk with number of years, hours, and sessions of indoor tanning, independent of outdoor sun exposure. These researchers also found that 97% of women diagnosed with melanoma before age 30 had indoor tanned. Young patients who use indoor tanning devices more than 10 times annually have more than 7 times the melanoma risk compared to individuals who do not indoor tan. A meta-analysis estimated a 1.8% increased melanoma risk for each additional tanning bed session. Since 2009, the World Health Organization lists tanning beds as a Class I carcinogen.

5. *Previous melanoma:* Individuals with a personal history of melanoma have an increased risk of developing a second melanoma of approximately 3% to 7%.

6. *Benign nevi:* Although a benign nevus is most likely not a precursor of melanoma, the presence of large numbers of nevi has been consistently associated with an increased risk of melanoma. Persons with ≥50 nevi, all of which are >2 mm in diameter, have 5 to 17 times the melanoma risk of persons with fewer nevi. Individuals who tend to develop freckles also have an increased risk of melanoma.

7. *Family history:* Approximately 10% of individuals diagnosed with melanoma have a family member with a history of melanoma. A family history of melanoma increases an individual's risk of melanoma three- to eightfold. Furthermore, persons who have two or more family members with melanoma are also at a particularly high risk. When available, these patients should be referred to genetic counseling.

8. *Genetic predisposition:* Approximately 8% to 12% of melanomas occur in individuals with a genetic predisposition. Specific genetic alterations have been implicated in the pathogenesis of melanoma.

9. *Atypical mole and melanoma syndrome:* Previously known as dysplastic nevus syndrome, atypical mole and melanoma syndrome is characterized by the presence of multiple, large (>5 mm) atypical dysplastic nevi generally in nonexposed areas of skin that represent a distinct clinicopathologic type of melanocytic lesion. Melanomas can originate from either normal skin or from a dysplastic nevus. Since the actual frequency of an atypical mole progressing to melanoma is small, resection of all dysplastic nevi is not indicated. However, new, changing, or symptomatic lesions that appear suspicious for melanoma on clinical and/or dermoscopic examination should be evaluated histologically.

Clinical Presentation

Clinical features of melanoma often include variegated color, irregular raised surface, and/or irregular perimeter. A biopsy should be performed on a pigmented lesion that changes in size, configuration, or color. The so-called *ABCDE*s are a mnemonic device to help clinicians and laypersons remember potential early signs of melanoma. *A* denotes lesion asymmetry, *B* border irregularity, *C* color variegation, *D* diameter greater than 6 mm, and *E* a lesion that is elevating, evolving, or enlarging.

When a patient presents with a lesion suggestive of melanoma, in addition to biopsy, a thorough physical examination must be performed, with particular emphasis on the skin (including the scalp, interdigit webspace, and intertriginous areas), nodal basins, and subcutaneous tissues (see Staging section that follows).

Diagnosis

The choice of biopsy technique varies according to the anatomical site as well as the size and shape of the lesion. Particular attention should be placed on the impact of the biopsy on definitive surgical treatment. Either an excisional biopsy or an incisional biopsy using a scalpel or punch is acceptable. Punch biopsies can be performed for most lesions and should generally be performed at the most raised or darkest area of the lesion to sample the most aggressive area of the potential melanoma. Full-thickness biopsy into the subcutaneous tissue should be performed to ensure accurate staging of the lesion (see the T Category section later in this chapter). An excisional biopsy allows the pathologist to accurately determine the thickness of the lesion, since the entire lesion is available for evaluation. Excisional biopsies should be performed when the lesion is too large for a punch but still can be removed without excessive surgical intervention. For excisional biopsies, a narrow margin of normal-appearing skin (1 to 2 mm) is generally taken with the specimen. An elliptical incision is often used to facilitate closure. The biopsy incision should be oriented to facilitate later wide excision (e.g., axially on extremities) and minimize the need for a skin graft to provide wound closure at the time of wide excision.

Shave biopsy is generally discouraged if a diagnosis of melanoma is being considered since incomplete assessment of tumor thickness may result if the deep margin is not cleared. If a shave biopsy is performed, a deep shave/saucerization is preferable to obtain full-thickness biopsy of the suspect lesion.

In general, we submit all pigmented lesions for permanent section examination and perform definitive surgery later. We generally prefer image-guided fine-needle aspiration or core biopsy as an initial diagnostic maneuver to document nodal or other melanoma metastases, but not to diagnose primary melanomas.

Pathology

An experienced dermatopathologist is an important member of the multidisciplinary melanoma team and contributes to the accurate diagnosis and staging of patients with melanoma. It is our practice to have outside biopsies reviewed by our pathology staff upon referral to confirm diagnosis. Although the pathologic analysis primarily consists of microscopic examination of hematoxylin- and eosin (H&E)-stained tumor, several melanocytic cell markers may also be useful to confirm the diagnosis. Two antibodies that have been widely used in immunohistochemical evaluations are S-100 and HMB-45. S-100 is expressed not only by more than 90% of melanomas, but also by several other tumors and some normal tissues, including dendritic cells. In contrast, the monoclonal antibody HMB-45 is relatively specific (yet not as sensitive) for proliferative melanocytic cells and melanoma. It is therefore often used as a confirmatory stain when the diagnosis of melanoma is being considered. Anti–MART-1 staining has also been shown to be useful in the diagnosis of melanoma, and anti-tyrosinase and Sox10 may also be used.

The major histopathologic components that should be included in a primary melanoma pathology report include Breslow thickness, ulceration status, peripheral and deep margin status, and mitotic rate (the latter using the dermal hot spot approach with units of mitoses per mm^2). Other features that are often recorded include presence of microsatellites, histologic subtype, lymphovascular invasion, tumor-infiltrating lymphocytes (TIL), regression, neurotropism, growth phase, and the absence of epidermal component (as the latter may represent an uncommon dermal primary or a metastatic deposit).

The major histopathologic types of melanoma are outlined below. While melanoma has been traditionally described using these categories, prognosis is more dependent upon staging than by these histopathologic types.

1. *Superficial spreading melanomas* constitute the majority of melanomas (approximately 70%) and generally arise in a pre-existing nevus.
2. *Nodular melanomas* are the second most common type (15% to 30%). Nodular melanomas progress to invasiveness more quickly than other types. When depth of the melanoma is controlled for, nodular melanomas are generally associated with the same prognosis as other lesions, although at least one recent study suggests that a thin (i.e., T1 [see below]) nodular melanoma may be associated with worse prognosis than T1 superficial spreading-type melanoma.
3. *Lentigo maligna melanomas* constitute a small percentage of melanomas (4% to 10%). These lesions occur in sun-exposed areas. Lentigo maligna melanomas are classically located on the faces of older white women. In general, lentigo maligna melanomas are large (>3 cm at diagnosis), flat lesions and are uncommon in individuals younger than 50 years. Given their often-ill-defined appearance, margin control can sometimes be challenging at the time of wide excision.
4. *Acral lentiginous melanomas* occur on the palms (palmar), soles (plantar), or beneath the nail beds (subungual), although not all palmar, plantar, and subungual melanomas are acral lentiginous melanomas. These melanomas account for only 2% to 8% of melanomas in white patients but for a substantially higher proportion of melanomas (35% to 60%) diagnosed in darker-skinned patients; their clinical extent at the primary site may be difficult to define, and scouting biopsies are sometimes employed to facilitate clinical assessment of the extent of disease.
5. *Amelanotic melanomas* are relatively uncommon melanomas that occur without pigmentation changes. They are often more difficult to diagnose because of their lack of pigmentation. Factors such as change in size, asymmetry, and irregular borders may suggest malignancy and prompt a biopsy, but delays in diagnosis may sometimes be observed.

Morphogenetic Correlates and Mutations in Melanoma

In addition to the classical descriptions of melanomas, the ability to perform molecular profiling on tumors has added to our understanding of this complex and often heterogeneous disease. Although currently not generally reported as part of the primary staging of melanoma, genetic profiling has been employed in advanced disease. With advances in technology, mutational analysis is routinely performed from formalin-fixed paraffin-embedded archival tissue. This has identified actionable treatment strategies against specific molecular aberrations especially in the setting of unresectable and advanced disease, and more recently in the adjuvant setting. Studies also demonstrate that most melanomas have one or more mutations in essential kinase signaling pathways.

Important in melanoma is the RAS-RAF-MEK-ERK kinase-signaling pathway; 40% to 50% of cutaneous melanomas (particularly superficial spreading melanoma) harbor mutations in a particular member of the RAF family known as BRAF. Although multiple BRAF mutations have been identified, approximately 90% consist of a point mutation at V600E that leads to an approximately 400-fold increase in the activity of the BRAF protein. Interestingly, 70% to 80% of benign nevi also harbor BRAF mutations, suggesting that genetic alterations alone cannot fully explain the aggressive biology of melanoma. In the same kinase pathway, approximately 15% to 26% of melanomas are found to have an activating NRAS mutation. A comprehensive molecular analysis of cutaneous melanoma by The Cancer Genome Atlas (TCGA) melanoma project has provided insights into the roles and frequency of mutated cancer genes and other genomic signatures. These findings helped to establish that cutaneous melanoma can be grouped into one of four subtypes: BRAF mutant (most common), RAS mutant, NF1 mutant, and triple-WT (wild type). Interestingly, BRAF and NRAS mutations are rarely identified simultaneously in the same melanoma tumor. While MAP kinase signaling pathway mutations have been commonly found in cutaneous melanomas arising in sun-exposed areas, they are infrequent in mucosal and acral lentiginous melanomas. A missense mutation in the c-KIT gene has been found in more than 20% of mucosal melanomas and more than 10% of acral lentiginous melanomas.

More recently, gene expression profiling (GEP) has been proposed and deployed to aid in decisions around the performance of sentinel lymph node biopsies. A meta-analysis by Marchetti et al., however, demonstrated that these adjuncts varied by AJCC stage and provided limited clinical utility. These sentiments have also been echoed by the Melanoma Prevention Working Group that called for more evidence and stated that discussions around the utilization of GEP with patients should be made in the context of testing limitations. Ultimately, as this technology continues to mature, it will benefit by continued investigation and thoughtful inclusion into clinical practice, where appropriate (see also Current Practice Guidelines for the Use of Sentinel Lymph Node Biopsy that follow).

Staging

The 8th Edition AJCC melanoma staging system was published in 2017 and implemented in 2018. Some key features of the 8th Edition staging system include modifications to the T1 subcategory, more granular incorporation of satellite, in-transit, and microsatellite disease into the N category, refinement and expansion of the M1 subcategories, and the addition of primary tumor thickness in stage III stage groups (described below).

T Category

Breslow tumor thickness and tumor ulceration remain the dominant prognostic factors in the T category. The AJCC Melanoma Expert Panel continues to use Breslow tumor thickness cut-points of 1, 2, and 4 mm for the T categories (Table 3.1). However, in the 8th Edition of the AJCC staging system, a tumor thickness stratum of

 TABLE 3.1   Definition of T Category—8th Edition AJCC Melanoma Staging System

| T Category | Primary Tumor | |
	Thickness	Ulceration Status
TX: Primary tumor thickness cannot be assessed	Not applicable	Not applicable
T0: No evidence of primary tumor	Not applicable	Not applicable
Tis (melanoma *in situ*)	Not applicable	Not applicable
T1	≤1.0 mm	Unknown or unspecified
T1a	<0.8 mm	Without ulceration
T1b	<0.8 mm	With ulceration
	0.8–1.0 mm	With or without ulceration
T2	>1.0–2.0 mm	Unknown or unspecified
T2a	>1.0–2.0 mm	Without ulceration
T2b	>1.0–2.0 mm	With ulceration
T3	>2.0–4.0 mm	Unknown or unspecified
T3a	>2.0–4.0 mm	Without ulceration
T3b	>2.0–4.0 mm	With ulceration
T4	>4.0 mm	Unknown or unspecified
T4a	>4.0 mm	Without ulceration
T4b	>4.0 mm	With ulceration

From Gershenwald JE, Scolyer RA, Hess KR, et al. Melanoma of the skin. In: Amin MB, Edge SB, Greene FL, et al., eds. *AJCC Cancer Staging Manual.* 8th ed. Springer; 2017:563–585. Used with permission of the American Joint Committee on Cancer (AJCC), Chicago, IL. The original and primary source for this information is the AJCC Cancer Staging Manual, Eighth Edition (2017) published by Springer International Publishing.

0.8 mm plays a key prognostic role in subcategorizing T1 tumors. Specifically, in the 8th Edition, primary melanomas with a tumor thickness <0.8 mm without ulceration are designated T1a, whereas primary melanomas 0.8 to 1.0 mm or those <0.8 mm with ulceration are categorized as T1b. Despite its removal from the T category for thin melanomas, the AJCC recognizes the prognostic importance of mitotic rate in all T1-4 lesions and notes that this important covariate should be recorded (as number of mitoses/mm^2), as it will likely be included in the development of clinical tools and contemporary prognostic models.

When there is no evidence of a primary tumor (i.e., unknown primary or completely regressed melanoma) or when thickness cannot be assessed, the AJCC (8th Ed.) categorizes these as T0 and TX, respectively.

Primary tumor ulceration is histopathologically defined as the absence of an intact epidermis overlying a portion of the primary tumor. Importantly, ulcerated melanomas are associated with a significantly worse prognosis than nonulcerated melanomas of the same thickness. In the T category, ulcerated tumors are designated by *b* following the numerical T. An exception to this rule is for a nonulcerated primary melanoma with a tumor thickness 0.8 to 1 mm; it is also designated by a "b" (T1b).

N Category

The N category refers to melanoma metastases to regional lymph node basins and non-nodal regional metastases (e.g., in-transit, satellite, and microsatellite disease) (Table 3.2). Regional nodal tumor burden is the most important predictor of survival in patients without distant disease. Overall, there is significant heterogeneity in prognosis among patients with regional disease.

Multiple studies have demonstrated that the number of pathologically involved lymph nodes is an independent predictor of outcome in patients with melanoma. The 8th Edition AJCC staging system N category continues to use 1, 2 to 3, and 4 or more regional lymph nodes to generate N subcategories.

Aside from the number of tumor-involved lymph nodes, it is important to distinguish the burden of nodal disease. Patients who have clinically negative regional lymph nodes but pathologically documented nodal metastases (i.e., a positive sentinel node) are defined as having "clinically occult" nodal metastases (designated by the letter *a* in the N category). In contrast, patients with clinical evidence of regional nodal metastases that is confirmed on pathologic examination are defined as having "clinically detected" nodal metastases (designated by the letter *b* in the N category). Overall, survival for patients with clinically detected nodal disease is worse than for patients with clinically occult nodal disease.

Additional components of the N category include satellite, in-transit, or microsatellite disease. Presence of at least one of these types of metastasis is coded by a suffix "c" in the 8th Edition N category and further stratified

TABLE 3.2 Definition of N Category—8th Edition AJCC Melanoma Staging System

N Category	No. of Involved Lymph Nodes (LN)	Presence of In-transit, Satellite, and/or Microsatellite Metastases (ITM/SAT/MICRO)
NX	Regional nodes not assessed[a]	No
N0	No regional LN disease	No
N1	**1 or ITM/SAT/MICRO** with no tumor involved LNs	
N1a	1 clinically occult	No
N1b	1 clinically detected	No
N1c	No regional LN disease	Yes
N2	**2–3 or ITM/SAT/MICRO** with 1 tumor involved LN	
N2a	2–3 clinically occult	No
N2b	2–3, 1 of which was clinically detected	No
N2c	1 clinically occult or detected	Yes
N3	**≥4 or ITM/SAT/MICRO** with ≥2 tumor involved LN **or** any number of matted LNs ± **ITM/SAT/MICRO**	
N3a	≥4 clinically occult	No
N3b	≥4, at least 1 which is clinically detected, <u>or</u> presence of any number of matted LNs	No
N3c	≥2 clinically occult or detected and/or presence of any number of matted LNs	Yes

[a]Pathologic N not required for T1 melanomas, use cN if sentinel node biopsy not performed.
From Gershenwald JE, Scolyer RA, Hess KR, et al. Melanoma of the skin. In: Amin MB, Edge SB, Greene FL, et al., eds. *AJCC Cancer Staging Manual.* 8th ed. Springer; 2017:563–585. Used with permission of the American Joint Committee on Cancer (AJCC), Chicago, IL. The original and primary source for this information is the AJCC Cancer Staging Manual, Eighth Edition (2017) published by Springer International Publishing.

according to the number of tumor-involved regional lymph nodes (i.e., N1c, N2c, or N3c). Satellite and in-transit metastases are classically and somewhat arbitrarily defined as skin or subcutaneous lesions within 2 cm of the primary tumor or more than 2 cm from the primary melanoma, respectively, but generally not beyond the regional nodal basin, and are types of non-nodal regional metastasis. Microsatellites are defined as any foci of metastatic tumor cells adjacent or deep to, and discontinuous from the primary tumor. It is important that there be an element of normal interposition tissue; that is, if only fibrosis and/or inflammation separate a suspected microsatellite from its primary, one should query whether this represents regression of this intervening region. Microsatellites are also included in the N category staging system (see also Management of Locoregional Non-Nodal Disease section) (Table 3.2).

M Category

The M category refers to melanoma distant metastasis and is classified as stage IV. For patents with distant metastasis, there is only one stage, M1, and four subcategories, M1a through M1d (Table 3.3). Distant metastases to the skin, subcutaneous tissue, or distant lymph nodes are designated M1a; they are associated with a better prognosis than metastases to other anatomical sites. Metastases to the lungs are associated with an intermediate prognosis and are designated M1b. Visceral metastases are associated with a worse prognosis and are designated M1c. New to the 8th Edition is the addition of a subcategory for CNS metastasis (i.e., brain, spinal cord, and/or leptomeningeal disease), designated M1d. This category of disease is generally associated with worse survival compared to the other M categories.

Serum lactate dehydrogenase (LDH) level also continues to be included in the M category; an elevated LDH has been shown to adversely influence survival across patients with stage IV disease. LDH level is denoted with the suffix (0) in patients without elevation, or (1) for those with an elevated LDH (e.g., M1a(1)). In patients in whom LDH level is unknown or unspecified, no suffix is added (Table 3.3).

Clinical (c) and Pathologic (p) Staging (cTNM and pTNM) and Stage Groups

Clinical staging includes above-noted features of the primary tumor and clinical and/or radiologic studies. Pathologic staging involves incorporating all variables of microstaging of the primary tumor, as well as information from the surgical specimen, including treatment effect and margin status. Lymph node status is confirmed by both identification and quantification of sentinel and/or regional nodal basin involvement. Formal pathologic staging is crucial to both proper classification and prognostication of patient outcome. Stage groups are summarized in Table 3.4. A grid to facilitate assignment of stage III subgroups based on T

TABLE 3.3 Definition of M Category—8th Edition AJCC Melanoma Staging System

	M Criteria	
M Category	Anatomic Site	LDH Level
M0	No evidence of distant metastasis	Not applicable
M1	Evidence of distant metastasis	See below
M1a	Distant metastasis to skin, soft tissue incl. muscle and/or nonregional LN	Not recorded or unspecified
M1a(0)		Not elevated
M1a(1)		Elevated
M1b	Distant metastasis to lung with or without M1a sites of disease	Not recorded or unspecified
M1b(0)		Not elevated
M1b(1)		Elevated
M1c	Distant metastasis to non-CNS visceral sites with or without M1a or M1b sites of disease	Not recorded or unspecified
M1c(0)		Not elevated
M1c(1)		Elevated
M1d	Distant metastasis to CNS with or without M1a, M1b or M1c sites of disease	Not recorded or unspecified
M1d(0)		Not elevated
M1d(1)		Elevated

From Gershenwald JE, Scolyer RA, Hess KR, et al. Melanoma of the skin. In: Amin MB, Edge SB, Greene FL, et al., eds. *AJCC Cancer Staging Manual*. 8th ed. Springer; 2017:563–585. Used with permission of the American Joint Committee on Cancer (AJCC), Chicago, IL. The original and primary source for this information is the AJCC Cancer Staging Manual, Eighth Edition (2017) published by Springer International Publishing.

TABLE 3.4 Stage Groups—8th Edition AJCC Melanoma Staging System

	Clinical Staging[a]			Pathologic Staging[b]		
	T	N	M	T	N	M
0	Tis	N0	M0	Tis	N0	M0
IA	T1a	N0	M0	T1a/b	N0	M0
IB	T1b	N0	M0	T2a	N0	M0
	T2a	N0	M0			
IIA	T2b	N0	M0	T2b	N0	M0
	T3a	N0	M0	T3a	N0	M0
IIB	T3b	N0	M0	T3b	N0	M0
	T4a	N0	M0	T4a	N0	M0
IIC	T4b	N0	M0	T4b	N0	M0
III	Any T, Tis	≥ N1	M0			
IIIA				T1a/b-T2a	N1a or N2a	M0
IIIB				T0	N1b, N1c	M0
				T1a/b-T2a	N1b/c or N2b	M0
				T2b/T3a	N1a-N2b	M0
IIIC				T0	N2b, N2c, N3b or N3c	M0
				T1a-T3a	N2c or N3a/b/c	M0
				T3b/T4a	Any N ≥ N1	M0
				T4b	N1a-N2c	M0
IIID				T4b	N3a/b/c	M0
IV	Any T	Any N	M1	Any T, Tis	Any N	M1

[a]Clinical staging includes microstaging of the primary melanoma and clinical and/or radiologic evaluation for metastases. By convention, it should be used after complete excision of the primary melanoma with clinical assessment for regional and distant metastases.
[b]Pathologic staging includes microstaging of the primary melanoma and pathologic information about the regional lymph nodes gained after partial (i.e., sentinel node biopsy) or complete lymphadenectomy.
From Gershenwald JE, Scolyer RA, Hess KR, et al. Melanoma of the skin. In: Amin MB, Edge SB, Greene FL, et al., eds. *AJCC Cancer Staging Manual*. 8th ed. Springer; 2017:563–585. Used with permission of the American Joint Committee on Cancer (AJCC), Chicago, IL. The original and primary source for this information is the AJCC Cancer Staging Manual, Eighth Edition (2017) published by Springer International Publishing.

and N categories is presented in Figure 3.1. Kaplan-Meier melanoma-specific survival curves for stages I to II and stage III according to AJCC 8th edition stage groups are detailed in Figures 3.2 and 3.3, respectively.

Extent of Disease Evaluation

In addition to physical examination, several adjuncts are used to determine the extent of disease. National consensus guidelines provide recommendations to evaluate for possible metastatic melanoma with imaging. For melanoma in situ, imaging studies are not recommended. For stages I to II melanoma, imaging is generally currently recommended only if there are specific signs or symptoms that need evaluation, although imaging is often considered in the absence of signs or symptoms for patients with a T4 primary. For stage III melanoma, it is our general practice at MD Anderson to obtain baseline imaging with a chest x-ray, CT of the chest, abdomen, and pelvis or PET/CT, often accompanied by MRI of the brain. Ultrasonography with fine-needle aspiration +/− core biopsy of the associated lymph node basin or in-transit site may be useful in detecting metastatic disease in lymph nodes or non-nodal regional sites; excisional biopsy and/or formal resection of suspicious nodes solely for diagnostic purposes is discouraged. Patients who present with suspected stage IV are generally staged with CT of the chest, abdomen, and pelvis, or PET/CT, as well as MRI of the brain. When imaging is planned for patients with extremity-based primaries, we also often also include the relevant extremity. Image-guided percutaneous biopsy of concerning lesions can be used to confirm disease (excisional biopsy is rarely indicated).

Management of Primary Melanoma

Treatment of a primary melanoma includes wide excision with a radial margin of skin down to, but generally not including the underlying muscular fascia (Fig. 3.4). The surgical margin is measured from the edge of the biopsy site or residual intact component of the lesion. The risk of local recurrence correlates with tumor

AJCC Eighth Edition
Melanoma Stage III Subgroups

N Category	T Category								
	T0	T1a	T1b	T2a	T2b	T3a	T3b	T4a	T4b
N1a	N/A	A	A	A	B	B	C	C	C
N1b	B	B	B	B	B	B	C	C	C
N1c	B	B	B	B	B	B	C	C	C
N2a	N/A	A	A	A	B	B	C	C	C
N2b	C	B	B	B	B	B	C	C	C
N2c	C	C	C	C	C	C	C	C	C
N3a	N/A	C	C	C	C	C	C	C	D
N3b	C	C	C	C	C	C	C	C	D
N3c	C	C	C	C	C	C	C	C	D

Legend	
A	Stage IIIA
B	Stage IIIB
C	Stage IIIC
D	Stage IIID

FIGURE 3.1 American Joint Committee on Cancer (AJCC) eighth edition stage III subgroups based on T and N categories. To determine stage group: (1) Select patient's N category at left of chart. (2) Select patient's T category at top of chart. (3) Note letter at the intersection of T&N on grid. (4) Determine patient's AJCC stage using legend. N/A = Not assigned, please see AJCC eighth edition staging manual for details. A, Stage IIIA; B, Stage IIIB; C, Stage IIIC; D, Stage IIID. (Reprinted from Gershenwald JE, Scolyer RA, Hess KR, et al. Melanoma Staging: Evidence-based Changes in the American Joint Committee on Cancer Eighth Edition Cancer Staging Manual. *CA Cancer J Clin* 2017;67(6):472–492, with permission.)

thickness. Thus, it is rational to incorporate surgical margins according to tumor thickness based on the results of numerous clinical trials over the past few decades.

Margin of Excision

The first randomized study involving surgical margins for melanomas less than 2 mm thick was reported by the WHO Melanoma Group. In an update of the study including 612 patients randomly assigned to a 1- or 3-cm margin of excision, there were no local recurrences among patients with primary melanomas thinner than 1 mm. There were four local recurrences among the 100 patients with melanomas 1 to 2 mm thick, and all four occurred in patients with 1-cm margins. There was no significant difference in survival between the 1- and 3-cm surgical margin groups. These results demonstrate that a 1-cm excision margin is safe for thin (<1 mm thick) melanomas. A multi-institutional prospective randomized trial from France compared 2- and 5-cm excisional margins in 362 patients with melanomas less than 2 mm thick. There were no differences in local recurrence rate or survival between the two groups. Similarly, a randomized trial from Sweden compared

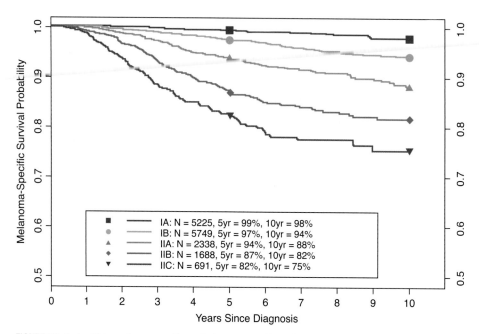

FIGURE 3.2 Kaplan-Meier melanoma-specific survival curves according to T category stage group for patients with stage I and II melanoma from the eighth edition International Melanoma Database. Patients with N0 melanoma were filtered, so that patients with T2 or thicker melanoma were included only if they had negative sentinel lymph nodes, whereas those with T1N0 melanoma were included regardless of whether they underwent SLNB. (Reprinted from Gershenwald JE, Scolyer RA, Hess KR, et al. Melanoma Staging: Evidence-based Changes in the American Joint Committee on Cancer Eighth Edition Cancer Staging Manual. *CA Cancer J Clin* 2017;67(6):472–492, with permission.)

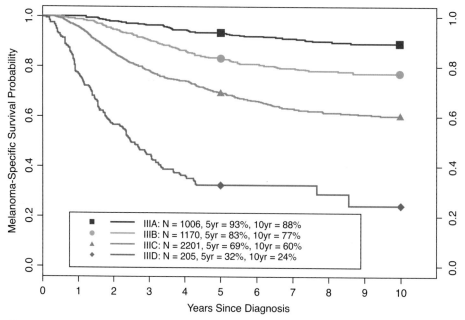

FIGURE 3.3 Kaplan-Meier melanoma-specific survival curves according to Stage III subgroups from the eighth edition International Melanoma Database. (Reprinted from Gershenwald JE, Scolyer RA, Hess KR, et al. Melanoma Staging: Evidence-based Changes in the American Joint Committee on Cancer Eighth Edition Cancer Staging Manual. *CA Cancer J Clin* 2017;67(6): 472–492, with permission.)

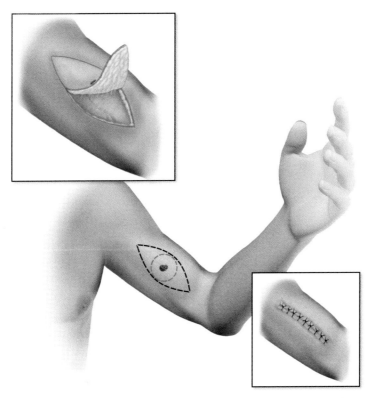

FIGURE 3.4 Wide excision of melanoma. Appropriate radial margin marked schematically (center image, *light gray dotted line*) along with properly axially oriented elliptical incision to facilitate primary closure (inset, bottom right) after wide excision (inset, top left). (Courtesy of Gershenwald JE, Houston, TX. Copyright retained by Gershenwald and the University of Texas MD Anderson Cancer Center.)

989 melanomas patients with lesions less than 2 mm thick excised with 2- and 5-cm margins. The results were similar. With regard to thicker lesions, a randomized clinical trial from the United Kingdom, the United Kingdom Melanoma Study Group (UKMSG) Trial, compared 1- and 3-cm excisional margins in 900 patients with melanomas at least 2 mm thick. With a median follow-up time of 60 months, a 1-cm margin was associated with a significantly increased risk of locoregional recurrence (37% vs. 32% for 3-cm margins); however, overall survival (OS) was similar in the two groups. For intermediate-thickness lesions, a randomized prospective study conducted by the Intergroup Melanoma Committee compared 2- and 4-cm radial margins of excision for 1- to 4-mm thickness melanomas. There was no difference in local recurrence rate between the two groups. Forty-six percent of patients in the 4-cm group required skin grafts, whereas only 11% of patients in the 2-cm group did ($P < .001$). Of note, however, a trend for improved 10-year disease-specific survival was seen in 4-cm margins (77%) versus 2-cm margins (70%). A clinical trial directly comparing 1- and 2-cm margins for 1- to 2-mm melanomas has not been performed. Based upon data from the WHO Trial and the Intergroup Melanoma Trial, 2-cm margins are recommended when the anatomic location is favorable and primary closure can be achieved. Since there is no demonstrable survival advantage for a 2-cm margin over a 1-cm margin in 1- to 2-mm melanomas, a 1-cm margin can be justified in cases in which a 2-cm margin is not easily achievable.

The optimal margin width for thick melanomas (>4 mm) is still unknown. A retrospective review of 278 patients with thick primary melanomas from MD Anderson and Moffitt Cancer Center demonstrated that the width of the excision margin (≤2 cm vs. >2 cm) did not significantly affect local recurrence, disease-free survival, or OS rates after a median follow-up of 27 months. In addition, based upon data from the UKMSG Trial (investigators concluded that a 3-cm margin is better than 1-cm margin for melanomas 2 to 4 mm thick) and the Intergroup Melanoma Trial (4-cm margin is not superior to a 2-cm margin for same tumor thickness), a margin greater than 2 cm is not necessary for these thick melanomas.

Based in large part on data from randomized, prospective trials, several recommendations can be made for margins of excision (Table 3.5). For patients with melanoma in situ, a 0.5-cm margin is generally adequate.

TABLE 3.5	Summary of Recommendations for Primary Melanoma Excision Margins

Tumor Thickness	Excision Margin
Melanoma in situ	0.5 cm–1 cm[a]
<1 mm	1 cm
1–2 mm	1 cm–2 cm
2–4 mm	2 cm
>4 mm	2 cm[a]

[a]No randomized prospective trials have specifically addressed this cohort. [a]See text for additional discussion.

Additional excision can be performed if the margin is inadequate. A 1-cm margin may sometimes be considered for melanoma in situ of large and/or ill-defined lesions for which it is difficult to discern the clinical extent of the lesion or if there is concern for possible occult invasive melanoma. Patients with invasive melanoma less than 1 mm in tumor thickness can be treated with a 1-cm margin. Based on clinical trials that included patients with melanomas with a tumor thickness of 1 to 2 mm, a 2-cm margin is generally preferred if anatomically and functionally feasible. In regions of anatomical constraint (e.g., the face), a 1-cm margin can be utilized, based on the observation that OS was similar for patients with 1- and 3-cm margins in the WHO Trial. Patients with melanomas 2 to 4 mm thick can be treated with a 2-cm margin. In patients with a melanoma thicker than 4 mm, a 2-cm margin is also recommended. These clinical trials were mostly conducted prior to the era of SLN biopsy. Given the interest in further reducing the extent of surgical resection margins for patients with melanoma, the ongoing Melanoma Margins Trial (MelMarT, NCT03860883) is assessing 1-cm versus 2-cm wide excision margins for primary invasive cutaneous melanomas with Breslow thickness >2 mm without ulceration or >1 mm with ulceration to determine if margin width can be further reduced for thicker tumors. The primary endpoint of this noninferiority trial is disease-free survival; secondary endpoints include local recurrence, distant-disease-free survival, melanoma-specific survival, OS, as well as quality of life, neuropathic pain assessments, surgery-related and other adverse events, and health economic evaluation.

Wound Closure

If there is concern regarding the ability to achieve suitable wound closure, a plastic or reconstructive surgeon may be consulted, ideally in the preoperative setting. Options for closure include primary closure, skin grafting, and local and distant flaps.

Primary closure is the method of choice for most lesions, but it should be avoided when it will distort the appearance of a mobile facial feature or interfere with function. Many defects can be closed using an advancement flap, undermining the skin and subcutaneous tissues to permit primary closure. Primary closure may be facilitated with the longitudinal axis of an elliptical incision to be approximately three times the length of the short axis; lesser extension of the longitudinal axis can also sometimes be employed. The skin and subcutaneous tissue are removed down to, but generally not including the underlying muscular fascia. Closure of the wound edges is usually performed in two layers—a dermal layer of 3-0 undyed absorbable sutures and either interrupted skin closure using 2-0, 3-0, or 4-0 nonabsorbable sutures and/or a running subcuticular skin closure using 4-0 monofilament absorbable sutures. Three layers are sometimes used, particularly for primary melanomas of the back, with approximation of Scarpa's fascia. After excision, the specimen should be oriented for permanent assessment of histologic margins.

Application of a skin graft is one of the simplest reconstructive methods used for wound closure. Split-thickness skin grafts are most commonly used. For lower extremity primary lesions, split-thickness grafts can be harvested from the contralateral extremity. In general, skin grafts should be harvested from an area remote from the primary melanoma and outside the zone of potential in-transit metastasis. A full-thickness skin graft can provide a result that is both more durable and of higher aesthetic quality than a split-thickness graft. Full-thickness grafts have most commonly been used on the face, where aesthetic considerations are most significant, but can also be used elsewhere. Donor sites for full-thickness skin graft to the face should be chosen from locations that are likely to match the color of the face, such as the postauricular or preauricular skin or the supraclavicular portion of the neck.

Local flaps offer numerous advantages for repair of defects that cannot be closed primarily, especially on the distal extremities and on the head and neck. Color match is excellent, durability of the skin is essentially normal, and normal sensation is usually preserved. Transposition flaps and rotation flaps of many varieties have been used, although for patients with high risk of in-transit metastasis, extensive flap reconstruction may significantly alter regional lymphatics.

Distant flaps may be considered when sufficient tissue for a local flap is not available and when a skin graft would not provide adequate wound coverage. Use of a wound VAC to facilitate granulation tissue that serves as a healthy tissue bed for subsequent skin graft can often obviate the need for complex reconstructive options (e.g., melanoma arising on the heel of the foot). Further discussion of such complex methods is beyond the scope of this chapter, but these techniques are familiar to plastic and reconstructive surgeons and are discussed in greater detail in Chapter 26.

Special Anatomic Considerations

Fingers and Toes

Most subungual melanomas involve either the great toe or the thumb, but the subungual region of any digit may be affected. A melanoma located on the skin of a digit is managed with wide excision, with distal digit lesions generally approached by concomitant partial digit amputation, the level of which is determined by extent of tumor and location. Invasive melanomas located beneath the nail bed (i.e., subungual) generally require amputation. For melanomas of the thumb or great toe, the amputation can generally be performed at the level of the interphalangeal joint. In general, amputations are performed at the distal or middle interphalangeal joint of the fingers, sparing a portion of the digit. More proximal amputations are not associated with improved survival. Melanoma arising between two digits can usually be treated by wide excision with the defect reconstructed with a local flap or skin graft. Phalanx-preserving procedures can sometimes be achieved for melanoma in situ.

Sole of the Foot

Excision of a melanoma on the plantar surface of the foot may result in a sizable defect in a weight-bearing area. When oncologically possible, deep fascia over the extensor tendons should be preserved as a base for skin graft coverage. A plantar flap, which can be raised either laterally or medially, can provide well-vascularized local tissue for weight-bearing areas, while also providing some sensation. Staged closure of some plantar melanomas, particularly of the heel, has been performed with initial use of a vacuum-assisted closure device to stimulate granulation tissue followed by staged skin graft application. This latter approach often obviates the need for complex reconstruction and has essentially eliminated the need for extensive flap reconstruction of the heel.

Face

Because of numerous functional and cosmetic considerations, facial lesions often cannot be excised with more than a 1-cm margin. Tumor diameter, tumor thickness, and tumor location must all be considered when margin width is planned. Radiation therapy can be considered as an adjunct when margins are closer than desired. Mohs micrographic surgery (MMS) has been proposed by some dermatologic surgeons, particularly for lentigo maligna–type melanoma in situ, particularly of the face or ears, as a means to excise melanoma with a minimal surgical margin. With this technique, resection occurs with serial histologic evaluations until the entire lesion is removed. Currently, there is a paucity of data to support MSS in place of standard surgical approach.

Breast

Wide excision with primary closure is the treatment of choice for primary melanoma on the skin of the breast; mastectomy is not generally recommended.

Umbilicus

Melanomas near or in the umbilicus may require resection of the umbilicus. In these cases, if desired, rotational flaps can be used to reconstruct the umbilicus.

Mucosal Melanoma

Historically, patients with true mucosal melanoma—including melanoma of the mucosa of the respiratory tract, vagina, and anal canal—have a poor prognosis. Because of their relative scarcity, few clinical trials have evaluated treatment options. We usually do not recommend an aggressive surgical approach to patients with clinically localized disease. In particular, we generally recommend local excision of anal melanomas rather than abdominoperineal resection. Abdominoperineal resection is associated with greater morbidity, leaves the patient with a permanent colostomy, offers no survival advantage, and does not treat at-risk inguinal nodes unless the procedure is combined with groin dissection. Adjuvant radiation therapy may be administered to decrease the risk of locoregional recurrence.

Management of Regional Disease

Regional lymph nodes are the most common site of melanoma metastasis. Lymph node involvement is categorized as clinically occult (i.e., detected by sentinel lymph node biopsy [SLNB]) or clinically detected (e.g., palpable and/or radiographically detected nodes). Fine-needle aspiration or core biopsy can usually yield a diagnosis in patients who develop clinically enlarged regional nodes. Incisional or excisional biopsy is rarely indicated for diagnostic purposes.

Intraoperative Lymphatic Mapping and Sentinel Lymph Node Biopsy

Beginning in the 1990s after its introduction by Morton and colleagues, several investigators proposed intraoperative lymphatic mapping and SLNB as a minimally invasive procedure for identifying approximately 15% to 20% of patients offered the procedure who harbor occult microscopic disease. This approach is sometimes termed *selective lymphadenectomy.* From a historical standpoint as initially proposed by Morton, the SLNB approach facilitates identification of patients for whom completion lymph node dissection would be recommended.

Several studies have demonstrated that the SLNs are the first nodes to contain metastases, if metastases are present, and thus the pathologic status of the SLNs reflects that of the entire regional nodal basin. If the SLN lacks metastasis, the rest of the regional lymph nodes are unlikely to contain disease, and a completion lymphadenectomy (CLND) would therefore be unnecessary. Multiple studies have demonstrated that the immediate false-negative rate for SLNB is less than 5%. Other studies have confirmed the validity of the SLN concept and the accuracy of SLNB as a staging procedure. It is imperative, however, that the surgeon employing SLNB has adequate pathology and nuclear medicine support.

Sentinel Lymph Node Biopsy Technique

It is strongly preferred that lymphatic mapping and SLNB be performed at the time of wide excision of the primary melanoma. If a wide excision has already been performed, SLNB can still generally be performed with equivalent accuracy; however, prior extensive reconstruction of the primary melanoma wide excision site (e.g., by extensive rotational flap reconstruction) that alters lymphatic pathways in the region may significantly reduce the accuracy of this technique if performed after wide excision in such patients. Since the introduction of lymphatic mapping and SLNB, the technique has undergone several refinements that have resulted in improved detection of SLNs. Use of a vital blue dye to identify SLNs has been part of the technique since its introduction. We typically use isosulfan blue 1% or *Lymphazurin* at our institution. If a patient is noted to have a significant history of allergic reactions, we may substitute methylene blue and anecdotally note overall similar results and a favorable side effect profile. Some surgeons prefer to give prophylaxis to prevent allergic reactions and routinely use a cocktail of I.V. diphenhydramine, I.V. hydrocortisone, and I.V. famotidine administered prior to injection of isosulfan blue.

The blue dye is injected intradermally around the residual intact tumor or biopsy site. It is taken up by the lymphatic system and carried via afferent lymphatics to the SLN(s). The draining nodal basin is explored, and the afferent lymphatic channels and first draining lymph nodes (the SLNs) are identified by the uptake of the blue dye. With the use of blue dye alone, an approach utilized mostly in the early 1990s, an SLN was identified in approximately 85% of cases. Although this initial approach was promising, 15% of patients were unable to benefit from the procedure because no SLN was identified.

Subsequently, additional techniques were incorporated that have significantly improved SLN localization: (a) preoperative lymphoscintigraphy and (b) intradermal injection of technetium-99 (^{99}Tc)-labeled sulfur colloid accompanied by intraoperative use of a handheld gamma probe. Preoperative lymphoscintigraphy using ^{99}Tc-labeled sulfur colloid facilitates the identification of patients with multiple draining nodal basins and patients with lymphatic drainage to SLNs located outside standard nodal basins, including epitrochlear, popliteal, and ectopic/interval/in-transit sites (Fig. 3.5). In 2013, Tc 99m tilmanocept (Lymphoseek) was approved by the FDA as a receptor-targeted lymphatic mapping agent (whose mechanism of action is to bind to mannose receptors on lymphatic tissue). It accumulates in lymphatic tissue within minutes and facilitates localization of SLNs; it can be used in place of ^{99}Tc-labeled sulfur colloid for both lymphoscintigraphic imaging as well as for intraoperative management.

In patients with melanomas that drain to multiple regional nodal basins, the histologic status of one draining basin does not predict the status of other basins. Therefore, it is particularly important to identify and assess all at-risk regional nodal basins to properly stage the patient. An advance from traditional nuclear imaging is the use of single-photon emission computed tomography (SPECT) imaging merged with CT. SPECT/CT facilitates localization of SLNs by overlaying radiotracer uptake activity onto the noncontrast CT image and is particularly

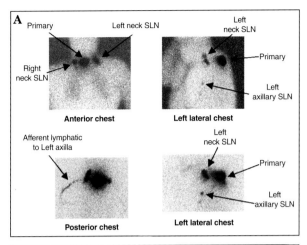

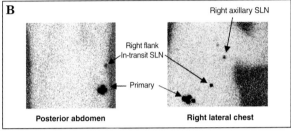

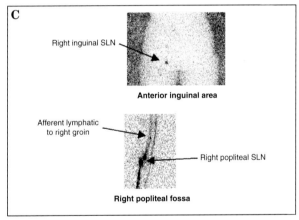

FIGURE 3.5 Preoperative lymphoscintigraphy. After injection of ^{99}Tc-labeled sulfur colloid at the primary cutaneous melanoma site (upper midline back), preoperative lymphoscintigraphy revealed (**A**) drainage to multiple nodal basins (bilateral neck and left axilla), (**B**) "in-transit"/ectopic sentinel lymph nodes (SLNs) in the right flank region and right axilla from a primary tumor of the right lateral back, and (**C**) SLNs in a right lower-extremity popliteal fossa lymph node basin and a right inguinal lymph node basin from a primary tumor of the heel. (Photos courtesy of Gershenwald JE. Copyright retained by Gershenwald and the University of Texas MD Anderson Cancer Center.)

helpful in the head and neck region. In one study, the surgical approach was revised because of SPECT/CT imaging in up to 30% of cases.

Perhaps the most important development in the SLNB technique has been the introduction of intraoperative lymphatic mapping using a handheld gamma probe. In this approach, 0.5-mCi ^{99}Tc-labeled sulfur colloid, or Lymphoseek is injected intradermally prior to surgery, either in nuclear medicine prior to arrival in the operating room (sometimes in concert with preoperative lymphoscintigraphy) or after induction of general anesthesia. During surgery, a handheld gamma probe is used to transcutaneously identify SLNs to facilitate their removal. The use of both blue dye and radiotracer increases the surgeon's ability to identify the SLN (>96% to 99% sensitivity) compared to the use of blue dye alone (≈84% sensitivity). Although most clinicians use a combined modality approach, some favor the single-agent strategy of radiotracer alone, and some have reported similarly excellent sensitivity compared to a combination strategy.

Incidence and Predictors of Positive Sentinel Lymph Nodes

Knowledge of the factors predictive of a positive SLN is useful for counseling patients regarding treatment options. In most studies, the overall incidence of a positive SLN among patients undergoing SLNB ranges from 15% to 20%. Multivariable analyses have revealed several factors associated with an increased risk of positive SLNs: increasing tumor thickness, ulceration, lymphovascular invasion, high mitotic rate, young age, and melanoma subtype. The overall incidence of SLN metastases by AJCC clinical substage among patients who had SLNB from one institutional study for stages IA, IB, IIA, IIB, and IIC was 2%, 9%, 24%, 34%, and 53%, respectively. Based on a published risk prediction model, investigators at Melanoma Institute Australia recently developed an SLN metastasis risk prediction tool that was validated with data from The University of Texas MD Anderson Cancer Center (MD Anderson) to serve as a general guide to estimate individual risk of harboring a tumor involved SLN (https://www.melanomarisk.org.au/index). (See also "Current Practice Guidelines for the Use of Sentinel Lymph Node Biopsy," below).

Prognostic Value of Sentinel Lymph Node Status

The prognostic significance of the pathologic status of the SLN has been convincingly demonstrated. Data from MD Anderson demonstrated that SLN status was the most significant clinicopathologic prognostic factor with respect to survival in patients with melanoma. In an analysis of 1,487 patients who underwent SLNB (median tumor thickness, 1.5 mm), the 5-year survival rate for patients with positive SLNs was 73.3%, compared to 96.8% for patients with negative SLNs (Fig. 3.6). Several other multivariate regression analyses have shown that regional lymph node status is the most powerful predictor of recurrence (both regional and distant) and survival, even among patients with thick melanomas. Taken together with patients who have clinical regional disease, according to analysis done by the International Melanoma Database and Discovery Platform (IMDDP) that provided revisions to the 8th edition AJCC melanoma staging system, 5-year melanoma-specific survival rates for patients with stage III disease range from 93% for patients with IIIA disease to 32% for patients with IIID disease (Figs. 3.1 and 3.3).

The prognostic importance of distinguishing between clinically occult and clinically detected lymph nodes has been emphasized by incorporation of this criterion into the 8th edition AJCC melanoma staging system. The concept of tumor burden has become important in the era of SLNB as accurate microscopic staging of SLNs allows patients to be better stratified into similar risk subgroups. Several studies have shown that the diameter of the largest SLN tumor nodule and the total SLN tumor volume are significant predictors of

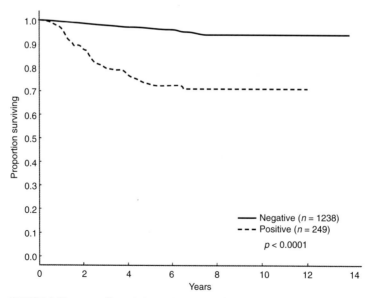

FIGURE 3.6 Disease-specific survival by sentinel lymph node (SLN) status in 1,487 patients. SLN status was the most significant clinicopathologic prognostic factor with respect to survival. The 5-year disease-specific survival rate was 73.3% for patients with positive SLNs, compared to 96.8% for patients with negative SLNs.

recurrence and survival. The prognostic significance of sentinel node tumor burden continues to be an active area of investigation worldwide.

The landmark prospective Multicenter Selective Lymphadenectomy Trial-I (MSLT-I) was designed in 1994 to assess whether a selective approach to regional lymphadenectomy—limiting completion lymph node dissection to patients with microscopic disease in SLNs—confers a survival benefit compared to wide excision of the primary melanoma and observation of the regional nodal basin. Patients with primary cutaneous melanomas at least 1 mm thick or with Clark level IV or V tumors with any Breslow thickness were eligible for the trial. Two thousand and one patients were randomly assigned to wide excision alone and observation of the regional nodal basin(s) (40%) or wide excision and lymphatic mapping and SLNB (60%), with subsequent CLND if any SLNs were positive.

In 2014, the final trial report was published with 10 years of follow-up data. Ten-year disease-free survival rates were significantly higher in the SLNB group than in the observation group among patients with intermediate-thickness melanomas: $71.3 \pm 1.8\%$ in the SLNB group compared to $64.7 \pm 2.3\%$ in the observation group (hazard ratio for recurrence or metastasis, 0.76; 95% CI 0.62 to 0.94; $P = .01$). When the SLNB group was further explored, it was noted that patients who had evidence of microscopic SLN involvement did worse than patients with a negative SLNB. For patients with intermediate-thickness primary melanoma (defined in MSLT-I as 1.2 to 3.5 mm), the melanoma-specific survival at 10 years was significantly worse in patients with a positive SLNB compared to those who had a negative SLNB (62% vs. 85%, HR 3.09, 95% CI 2.12 to 4.49). For patients with thick melanoma (defined in MSLT-I as >3.50 mm), the melanoma-specific survival rate at 10 years was again significantly worse in patients with lymph node involvement compared to those who had a negative lymph node biopsy (48.0% vs. 64.6%, HR 1.75, 95% CI 1.07 to 2.87). Interestingly, when applied to the study cohort, a statistical approach called latent-subgroup analysis (a technique that accounts for the observation that nodal status was initially only known in the SLNB group) showed a clear benefit of SLNB. Among patients who had SLNB and a positive SLN compared to those who developed clinical regional melanoma metastasis after wide excision alone, there was doubling of melanoma-specific and distant disease–free survival and a tripling of disease-free survival.

Pathologic Evaluation of Sentinel Lymph Nodes

Pathologists have traditionally examined lymph nodes obtained from a lymphadenectomy by examining an H&E-stained section from each paraffin block. This conventional approach, however, can miss disease in SLNs, primarily because of sampling error. In an MD Anderson study, 8 of 10 patients who underwent SLNB and subsequently developed regional nodal failure in nodal basins that were negative for disease according to conventional histologic examination of SLNs had microscopic disease detected when the SLNs were reassessed using specialized pathologic techniques. Data from this and other studies suggest that failure to use specialized techniques, rather than failure to correctly identify SLNs, accounts for many cases of false-negative findings on SLNB. These studies helped to define the current standards of SLN assessment using more enhanced pathologic evaluation than had been previously performed.

With the SLNB technique, fewer lymph nodes are submitted for analysis than are submitted with formal lymphadenectomy, and the pathologist can therefore focus on only those nodes that are at the highest risk. Currently, the combination of H&E assessment of several levels (i.e., serial sectioning) and immunohistochemical analysis is generally considered a standard practice in assessing SLNs. Several antibodies directed against melanoma-associated antigens (S-100, HMB-45, tyrosinase, MAGE3, and MART-1) are routinely used for immunohistochemical evaluation. Because certain antibodies have low specificity (S-100) and others have low sensitivity (HMB-45, MAGE3, and tyrosinase), a panel of antibodies is commonly used. At MD Anderson Cancer Center, this panel includes an antimelanocytic cocktail (HMB45, anti-MART1 and anti-tyrosinase).

The use of frozen section for immediate evaluation of SLNs has been controversial in melanoma. Frozen sections usually provide suboptimal morphology and may lack the subcapsular region of the lymph node (an area likely involved in SLN metastases). Also, processing of the frozen tissue requires additional sectioning and micrometastases may be lost in the discarded unexamined sections. We feel strongly that the use of frozen section risks a lower accuracy of detection of SLN metastases. We had historically employed this approach for the rare clinical scenario if a grossly suspicious SLN was identified and if a formal preoperative discussion of possible concomitant CLND was considered. Given the infrequent use of CLND following results of the Multicenter Selective Lymphadenectomy Trial-II (MSLT-II) trial (see below), this approach has been further rendered obsolete.

Identifying Additional Disease in Nonsentinel Nodes

Historically, patients who have a melanoma-positive SLN identified by SLNB had CLND. Pathologic evaluation of CLND specimens often reveals no additional disease. It is important to remember that CLND specimens are routinely assessed with standard histologic techniques rather than the more rigorous approach employed for SLNB specimens. As a result, there may be additional disease in the completion node dissection specimen that goes undetected. This disease, in theory, represents a potential source of subsequent recurrence if it were not removed. CLND performed for microscopic disease provides the potential for improved regional control. In addition, identifying patients with minimal disease burden by using the SLN approach may help identify the group of patients who may derive an improved survival benefit from early CLND. Furthermore, knowledge of the pathologic status of the SLNs allows proper staging and thus facilitates decision making regarding adjuvant treatment. In several studies, when the non-SLNs in a CLND specimen were evaluated by H&E staining and immunohistochemistry, only 8% to 25% of CLND specimens contained additional nodes with metastatic disease. Since most patients have metastatic disease identified only in SLNs, there has been interest in identifying patients who, despite having a positive SLN, have a low probability of metastatic disease in non-SLNs. In an analysis of primary tumor and SLN characteristics, the number of SLNs harvested, the Breslow thickness of the primary tumor, and SLN burden (largest focus of metastasis, total area of metastases, number of metastatic foci, and extracapsular extension) most accurately predicted the presence of tumor in non-SLNs.

Role of CLND for Patients With a Melanoma-Involved SLN

The Multicenter Selective Lymphadenectomy Trial-II (MSLT-II) sought to answer whether CLND was necessary following a positive SLN by randomizing patients with at least one positive SLN to nodal observation (with nodal basin ultrasound, termed active surveillance) or immediate CLND after a positive SLN. Overall, the trial accrued >1,900 patients and at a median follow-up of 43 months, in the per-protocol analysis, the 3-year melanoma-specific survival (primary endpoint) was similar in both the CLND group and the observation group. Disease control in the regional nodes at 3 years was also increased in the dissection group compared to the observation group (92% vs. 77%; $P < .001$). Nonsentinel node metastases (identified in 11.5% of the patients in the dissection group) were a strong and independent predictor of recurrence (hazard ratio, 1.78; $P = .005$). Taken together, these initial data support that immediate CLND increased regional disease control and provided prognostic information but did not increase MSS in these patients with SLN metastases.

In the German multicenter, randomized, phase III DeCOG-SLT clinical trial, 483 patients with a positive SLNB were randomly assigned to immediate surgery (i.e., CLND following a positive SLNB) or to regional node observation. Of note, 66% of patients had an SLN metastasis of 1 mm or less. At a median follow-up of 72 months, among 483 included, the authors found that there was no significant difference in their primary endpoint of 5-year distant metastasis-free survival: 67.6% versus 64.9% for the observation versus immediate complete dissection groups, respectively (HR 1.08, 95% CI 0.83 to 1.39). Furthermore, there were no significant differences in RFS and OS. Of note, the study did not reach its target accrual of 556 patients, thus reducing the power of the study.

Taken together, these trials have contributed to a significant paradigm shift in clinical practice for the patient with a positive SLN. As two clinical trials demonstrated that CLND provided no recurrence free survival (RFS) or OS benefit in melanoma patients with a positive sentinel node, the vast majority of melanoma surgical oncologists have integrated nodal observation (with active surveillance) rather than CLND as a preferred strategy into their practice. While CLND is still considered an option for these patients according to national consensus melanoma guidelines (e.g., in the setting of patient preference related to availability to be surveilled, when adjuvant therapy cannot be considered, particularly in the setting of high-risk disease with increased associated risk of non-SLN involvement), these situations are in clinical practice rather infrequent. With this change in practice, new questions have arisen, including the optimal screening algorithm for patients undergoing observation with a positive sentinel node. In the post MSLT-II era, CLND is generally recommended in the context of multidisciplinary team-based care for regional recurrence discovered during active surveillance/nodal observation post SLN biopsy.

Current Practice Guidelines for the Use of Sentinel Lymph Node Biopsy

Candidates for SLN biopsy include patients with newly diagnosed clinically node-negative primary cutaneous melanoma who are predicted to be at intermediate or high risk of harboring occult regional nodal disease based on primary tumor characteristics. Many melanoma clinicians consider a threshold risk of a positive SLN of at least 5% to be sufficient in an otherwise healthy individual to offer lymphatic mapping and sentinel node biopsy. Although uniform risk thresholds have not been completely resolved, a tumor thickness threshold for SLN of at least 0.8 mm or for tumors <0.8 mm with ulceration or other high-risk features, including lymphovascular invasion or high mitotic rate, particularly when associated with young age, can be considered for SLNB. The Melanoma Institute Australia SLN metastasis risk prediction tool may also be referenced as a useful guide to estimate individual risk of harboring a tumor-involved SLN (https://www.melanomarisk.org.au/index). While detailed discussion is beyond the scope of this chapter, one helpful source of information for this important clinical question that is also generally reflective of the ongoing debate can be found in national consensus guidelines. As introduced in the previous section, the use of primary melanoma GEP to aide clinical decision making on the use of SLN biopsy remains an area of active investigation and has not yet been integrated into our clinical practice or current national consensus guidelines. Of note, the presence of clinically evident lymphadenopathy at the time of diagnosis obviates the need for SLNB; management of such patients (in the absence of synchronous distant metastasis) is discussed in the section that follows.

Management of Clinically Detectable Lymph Node Disease at Presentation

For patients who present with clinically apparent or detectable disease in the regional lymph node basin, a staging work up is recommended. Physical examination should be performed to identify lesions suspicious for additional primary melanoma, as well as to identify satellite disease and/or in-transit metastases; a thorough nodal examination should also be performed to exclude clinically suspicious nodal disease in other regional basins. Staging evaluation typically includes baseline imaging with CT chest/abdomen/pelvis or PET/CT, and MRI of the brain. This approach allows the surgeon to identify disease beyond the regional basin that may preclude a recommendation for lymphadenectomy. If not already excised at the time of referral, image-guided biopsy (generally fine-needle aspiration biopsy or core) is preferred over excision to confirm regional disease; a similar approach may be used to document other patterns of metastasis, such as distant disease, that would alter treatment planning. Mutation testing for BRAF should also be performed. In the absence of distant metastasis, regional nodal disease has generally been approached with a recommendation for formal therapeutic lymphadenectomy followed by consideration of adjuvant therapy (see below).

Technical Considerations

Axillary Dissection

General Axillary dissection includes levels I, II, and III lymph nodes (Fig. 3.7). The arm, shoulder, and chest are prepped and included in the surgical field.

Incision We generally use a slightly S-shaped incision beginning anteriorly along the superior portion of the lateral edge of the pectoralis major muscle, traversing the axilla over the fourth rib, and extending inferiorly along the anterior border of the latissimus dorsi muscle. The incision should be constructed so that previous scars can be excised en bloc with the specimen.

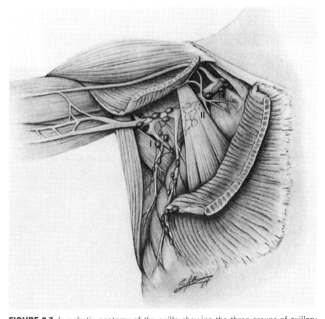

FIGURE 3.7 Lymphatic anatomy of the axilla showing the three groups of axillary lymph nodes defined by their relationship to the pectoralis minor muscle. The highest axillary nodes (level III) medial to the pectoralis minor muscle should be included in an axillary lymph node dissection for melanoma. (From Balch CM, Milton GW, Shaw HM, et al., eds. *Cutaneous Melanoma.* Lippincott; 1985, with permission.)

Skin Flaps Skin flaps are raised anteriorly to the lateral border of the pectoralis muscle and the midclavicular line, inferiorly to the sixth rib, posteriorly to the anterior border of the latissimus dorsi muscle, and superiorly to just below the pectoralis major insertion. The medial side of the latissimus dorsi muscle is dissected free from the specimen, exposing the thoracodorsal vessels and nerve. The lateral edge of the dissection then proceeds cephalad to the axillary vein. In a lateral to medial fashion, the thoracodorsal neurovascular bundle is skeletonized and preserved. These maneuvers generally allow the next portion of the dissection to proceed from medial to lateral. The fatty and lymphatic tissue adjacent to the pectoralis major muscle is dissected free around to its undersurface, where the pectoralis minor muscle is encountered. The interpectoral groove is exposed.

Lymph Node Dissection The medial pectoral nerve is generally preserved. The interpectoral nodes are dissected free and lymphoareolar tissue swept from Rotter's space. At this point, the dissection generally proceeds in a lateral to medial fashion, with lymph node bearing tissue swept medially; the thoracodorsal bundle is again visualized, and the long thoracic nerve is identified and preserved. The fatty tissue between the two nerves is separated from the subscapularis muscle and included with the specimen. The upper axilla is exposed by bringing the patient's arm over the chest by adduction and internal rotation. If nodes are bulky, the pectoralis minor muscle may be divided to facilitate exposure. Dissection of the upper axillary lymph nodes should be sufficiently complete that the thoracic outlet beneath the clavicle, Halsted's ligament, and subclavius muscle are seen (Fig. 3.8). Fatty and lymphatic tissues are dissected downward over the axillary vein. The apex of the dissected specimen may be tagged. The specimen is removed from the lateral chest wall.

Wound Closure One 15 French closed-suction drain is usually placed percutaneously through the inferior flap into the axilla. An additional drain may be inserted through the inferior flap depending on body habitus. The skin is closed with interrupted 3-0 undyed absorbable sutures and running 4-0 subcuticular absorbable sutures.

Postoperative Management Suction drainage is generally continued until output is less than 30 mL per day for 2 consecutive days. By approximately 4 weeks, the suction catheters are usually removed, regardless of the

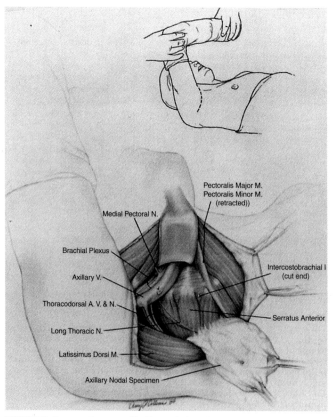

FIGURE 3.8 Access to the upper axilla. The arm is draped so that it can be brought over the chest wall during the operation. This facilitates retraction of the pectoralis muscles upward to reveal the level III axillary lymph nodes. (From Balch CM, Milton GW, Shaw HM, et al., eds. *Cutaneous Melanoma.* Lippincott; 1985, with permission.)

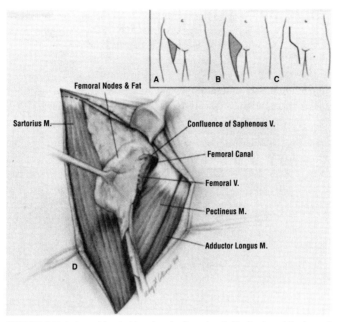

FIGURE 3.9 Technique of inguinal lymph node dissection. **A:** The borders of the femoral triangle are the inguinal ligament superiorly, the sartorius laterally, and the adductor longus medially. **B:** The lymphatic contents removed during a superficial inguinal lymphadenectomy include the lymphatic contents of the femoral triangle as well as nodal tissue that lies superficial to the external oblique superior to the inguinal ligament. **C:** The lazy-S incision used for an inguinal lymphadenectomy. **D:** The anatomy visualized during an inguinal lymphadenectomy. (From Balch CM, Milton GW, Shaw HM, et al., eds. *Cutaneous Melanoma.* Lippincott; 1985, with permission.)

amount of drainage, to reduce the likelihood of infection. Subsequent fluid collections are removed by needle aspiration, or on occasion by percutaneous drainage.

Superficial (Inguinal) Groin Dissection
General For groin dissection, the patient is placed in a slight frog-leg position with hip externally rotated and the knee partially flexed.

Incision A lazy-S incision is made from superomedial to the anterior superior iliac spine, vertically down to the inguinal crease, obliquely across the crease, and then vertically down to the apex of the femoral triangle. Previous SLNB incisions and underlying cavities should be excised en bloc with the specimen.

Skin Flaps The limits of the skin flaps are medially to the pubic tubercle and the midbody of the adductor magnus muscle, laterally to the lateral edge of the sartorius muscle, superiorly to approximately 5 cm above the inguinal ligament, and inferiorly to the apex of the femoral triangle.

Lymph Node Dissection Dissection is carried down to the muscular fascia superiorly (Fig. 3.9). All fatty, node-bearing tissue is swept down to the inguinal ligament and off the external oblique fascia. Medially, the spermatic cord or round ligament is exposed, and nodal tissue is swept laterally. Nodal tissue is swept off the adductor fascia to the femoral vein. At the apex of the femoral triangle, the saphenous vein is identified. If the saphenous vein can be preserved, nodal tissue is removed from the vessel circumferentially; otherwise, it is sacrificed. Laterally, nodal tissue is dissected off the sartorius muscle and the femoral nerve. With dissection in the plane of the femoral vessels, the nodal tissue is elevated up to the level of the fossa ovalis, where the saphenous vein is suture-ligated at the saphenofemoral junction if it is sacrificed. The specimen is dissected to the inguinal ligament. Although excision of Cloquet node (the lowest iliac node), accompanied by intraoperative frozen-section examination, has historically sometimes been employed to inform concomitant iliac-obturator node dissection in patients without clinically apparent or suspicious deep groin metastasis, this approach is uncommonly employed currently (Fig. 3.10).

Sartorius Muscle Transposition If the sartorius muscle is to be transposed, it is divided at its origin on the anterior superior iliac spine (Fig. 3.11). The lateral femoral cutaneous nerve is preserved if possible. The proximal

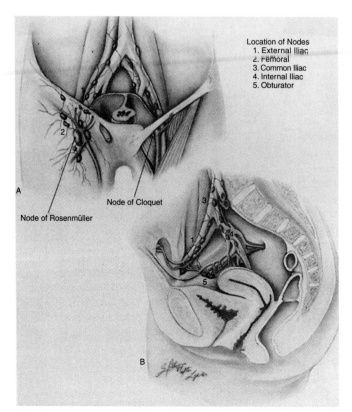

FIGURE 3.10   A: Lymphatic anatomy of the inguinal and iliac-obturator area demonstrating the superficial and deep lymphatic chains. Cloquet node lies at the transition between the superficial and deep inguinal nodes. It is located beneath the inguinal ligament in the femoral canal. **B:** The iliac-obturator nodes include those distal to the common iliac bifurcation, and around the external and internal iliac vessels, and the obturator nodes. Obturator nodes should be excised as part of an iliac-obturator nodal dissection. (From Balch CM, Milton GW, Shaw HM, et al., eds. *Cutaneous Melanoma.* Lippincott; 1985, with permission.)

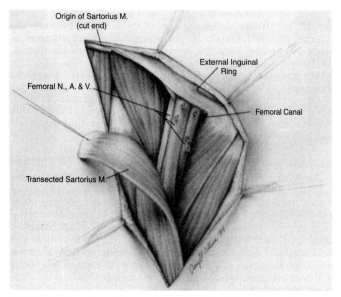

FIGURE 3.11 Transection of the sartorius muscle at its origin on the anterior superior iliac spine in preparation for transposition over the femoral vessels and nerves. (From Balch CM, Milton GW, Shaw HM, et al., eds. *Cutaneous Melanoma.* Lippincott; 1985, with permission.)

neurovascular bundles going to the sartorius muscle are divided to facilitate transposition, with care to preserve others to the maximal extent possible to ensure a vascularized pedicle. The rotated muscle is placed over the femoral vessels and tacked to the inguinal ligament, fascia of the adductor, and vastus muscle groups.

Wound Closure The skin edges are examined for viability and trimmed back to healthy skin, if necessary. Intravenous administration of fluorescein followed by examination using a Wood lamp may be used to identify poorly perfused skin edges. Two closed-suction drains are generally placed through separate small incisions superiorly. One is laid medially, and the other is laid laterally within the operative wound. The wound is closed with interrupted 3-0 undyed absorbable sutures in the dermis and followed by skin staples or a running 4-0 subcuticular suture. In some patients, interrupted nylon sutures are used overlying the area of skin crease.

Postoperative Management The patient begins ambulating the day following surgery; a custom-fit elastic stocking may be used during the day for 6 months. After this period, the stocking may be discontinued if no leg swelling occurs. Suction drainage is continued until output is less than 30 mL per day for 2 consecutive days. By approximately 4 weeks, the suction catheters are removed, regardless of the amount of drainage, to mitigate risk of infection.

Dissection of the Iliac and Obturator Nodes

General We generally perform a deep groin dissection—dissection of the iliac and obturator nodes—for the following indications: (a) known involvement of the nodes revealed by preoperative imaging studies, (b) more than three grossly positive nodes in the superficial lymph node dissection specimen, or (c) metastatic disease in Cloquet node, if performed.

Incision To gain access to the deep nodes, we extend the skin incision superiorly if performed concomitantly with a superficial groin dissection. If a deep groin dissection only is to be performed, we generally use a dedicated right lower quadrant incision.

Lymph Node Dissection The external oblique muscle is split from a point superomedial to the anterior superior iliac spine to the lateral border of the rectus sheath. The internal oblique and transversus abdominis muscles are divided, and the peritoneum is retracted superiorly. An alternative approach, sometimes used when extensive disease populates this region, is to split the inguinal ligament vertically, medial to the femoral vein. The ureter is exposed as it courses over the iliac artery. The inferior epigastric artery and vein are divided, if necessary. The bifurcation of the common iliac artery marks the cephalad extent of the dissection, and all nodes are taken along the external iliac artery to the inguinal ligament caudally. Nodes overlying the external iliac vein are dissected to the point at which the internal iliac vein courses under the internal iliac artery. The plane of the peritoneum is traced along the wall of the bladder, and the fatty tissues and lymph nodes are dissected off the perivesical fat starting at the internal iliac artery. Dissection is completed on the medial wall of the external iliac vein, and the nodal chain is further separated from the pelvic fascia until the obturator nerve is seen. Obturator nodes are located in the space between the external iliac vein and the obturator nerve (in an anteroposterior direction) and between the internal iliac artery and the obturator foramen (in a cephalad–caudad direction). The obturator artery and vein usually need not be disturbed.

Wound Closure The transversus abdominis, internal oblique, and external oblique muscles may be closed with running sutures. The inguinal ligament, if previously divided, is approximated with interrupted nonabsorbable sutures to Cooper ligament medially and to the iliac fascia lateral to the femoral vessels. A closed suction drain is placed in the deep pelvic space exiting through a separate small incision.

Postoperative Management Suction drainage is continued until output is less than 30 mL per day for 2 consecutive days. The pelvic drain is usually removed prior to hospital discharge. Ambulation is encouraged the day after surgery. Patients are hospitalized postoperatively for expectant management of potential ileus after deep pelvic surgery and for pain control, usually for a duration of 2 to 3 days.

Neck Dissection

Lymph node metastases from melanomas in the head and neck were previously believed to follow a predictable pattern. However, it is established that lymphatic drainage from melanomas of the head and neck can be multidirectional and unpredictable. SLNB may be misdirected in as many as 59% of patients if the operation is based on classic anatomical studies without preoperative lymphoscintigraphy. These findings strongly support the use of lymphoscintigraphy in patients with melanomas in the head and neck.

At MD Anderson, the approach for patients with melanoma in the head and neck region and clinically involved nodes is wide excision of the primary lesion with either modified radical neck dissection or selective neck dissection.

Melanomas arising on the scalp or face anterior to the pinna of the ear and superior to the commissure of the lip can metastasize to intraparotid lymph nodes because these nodes are contiguous with the cervical nodes. When intraparotid nodes are clinically involved, it is advisable to combine neck dissection with parotid lymph node dissection.

Morbidity of Lymph Node Surgery

Complications associated with SLNB for melanoma were evaluated in 2,120 patients in an analysis of data from the Sunbelt Melanoma Trial. Overall, 96 (4.6%) of the patients developed major or minor complications associated with SLNB, whereas 103 (23.3%) of 444 patients experienced complications associated with SLNB plus completion lymph node dissection. The authors concluded that SLNB alone is associated with significantly less morbidity compared to SLNB plus completion lymph node dissection. Similar to the Sunbelt Melanoma Trial, in MSLT-1, SLNB did not significantly add to the morbidity of melanoma surgery when compared to wide excision of the primary melanoma alone.

Formal lymphadenectomy is associated with higher complication rates than SLNB, and includes seroma, wound infection, cellulitis, lymphedema, and skin flap problems that may on occasion require surgical revision. Complication rates are higher in the inguinal region than in the axilla or neck. Cormier et al. prospectively followed 53 patients at MD Anderson who underwent inguinal lymphadenectomy for melanoma; using liberal objective criteria, investigators found the acute wound complication rate to be 77.4% with a wound infection rate of 54.7% and a wound dehiscence rate of 52.8%. In multivariate analysis, only body mass index was found to be associated with an increase in complications. The infection rate reported after lymphadenectomy in MSLT-1 was 12% and noted that lymphedema rates varied significantly depending on the lymph nodes basins that were dissected (i.e., 9.0% for axillary lymphadenectomy vs. 26.6% for inguinal lymphadenectomy).

Lymphedema is among the most serious long-term complications of formal lymphadenectomy. Inguinal lymphadenectomy–associated lymphedema was not altered significantly by the addition of a deep groin dissection. In addition, the number of lymph nodes removed did not appear to alter the lymphedema rate significantly. In the study by Cormier et al., the lymphedema rate at 3 months was 85% using qualitative measures and 45% by quantitative measures for patients who underwent inguinal lymphadenectomy. Lower extremity edema after groin dissection can be decreased by preventive measures, including perioperative antibiotics, elastic stockings, leg elevation exercises, and on occasion, diuretics. Even with preventive measures, patients should be counseled that lymphedema can still develop. Nonetheless, prophylactic measures are important because reversing the progression of lymphedema is difficult. The complication rate for axillary lymph node dissections is lower than that for inguinal dissection. The most frequent complication is wound seroma, varying from 3% to 23%. Other common complications include cellulitis and lymphedema (approximately 10%).

Special Clinical Situations
Metastatic Melanoma of Unknown Primary Site

Approximately 1% to 8% of patients with melanoma present with metastatic disease from melanoma of unknown primary (MUP) site. The most common presentation is in the axillary lymph node basin (>50%), followed by the cervical lymph node basin. Various reasons have been proposed for the phenomenon of MUP site. Anbari et al. suggested the following possibilities for primary lesions: an unrecognized melanoma, a treated melanoma that had been initially misdiagnosed, a spontaneously regressed melanoma, and malignant transformation of a melanocyte that had traveled to a metastatic location. For metastatic melanoma to be classified as MUP site, the histologic diagnosis must be confirmed, previous biopsies and/or excisions, if any, should be evaluated for a possible diagnosis of melanoma, and less common primary sites for melanoma should be thoroughly evaluated. A thorough history may also identify prior lesion that was excised or destroyed, but never pathologically examined. If the metastatic lesion is to a lymph node basin, the drainage areas of that basin should be rigorously examined. Furthermore, patients should undergo staging evaluation with CT of the chest, abdomen, and pelvis (also including neck CT if anatomically appropriate), and MRI of the brain. PET/CT can also be considered, particularly in the setting of extremity soft tissue metastasis associated with unknown primary.

Several studies have compared the survival of these patients to similar cohorts having equivalent nodal status and a known primary site. Although patients with unknown primary tumors were historically believed to have worse prognoses, recent studies have contradicted earlier findings by demonstrating that patients with MUP have a natural history that is similar to (if not better than) the survival of many patients with stage

III disease. Given their survival profile, such patients with nodal disease should be staged as stage III and treated like stage III patients with a known primary melanoma, including consideration for stage III clinical trials (Table 3.4, Fig. 3.1).

Management of Locoregional Non-Nodal Disease

Background

The presence of clinically or microscopically detectable locoregional non-nodal disease can be broadly categorized into three groups: satellites, in-transit metastasis, or microsatellite disease.

Satellite/in-transit patterns of recurrence are relatively unique to melanoma and occur in 3% to 10% of melanoma cases. Although the molecular determinants and pathophysiology of in-transit disease are not fully understood, they are likely an intralymphatic manifestation of melanoma metastases. Independent predictors of in-transit recurrence among patients who underwent sentinel node biopsy include age older than 50 years, a lower-extremity primary tumor, increasing tumor thickness, ulceration, and nodal involvement. Regional nodal metastases occur in about two-thirds of patients with in-transit disease and, if present, are associated with lower survival rates (Table 3.2, Fig. 3.3). Reported predictors of distant metastasis among patients with in-transit recurrence include positive SLN status, in-transit tumor size of at least 2 cm, and disease-free interval before in-transit recurrence of less than 12 months.

Approach to Treatment

The treatment landscape for patients with locoregional non-nodal disease continues to evolve and warrants a multidisciplinary team approach. Treatment options include surgery (particularly for patients with limited, resectable disease), regional approaches, intralesional therapy, and systemic therapy. If surgery is performed, it is recommended that clear histologic margins be obtained, as there is no clinical trial-informed data to support wider excision margins. In this era of more effective systemic therapy (see below), systemic treatment approaches have mostly supplanted regional-directed therapy for multifocal and/or unresectable disease. Patients with in-transit metastases confined to a limb that are not amenable to standard surgical measures (e.g., patients with recurrent and/or multiple in-transit metastases and patients with large-burden in-transit disease) and have failed or are not candidates for systemic therapy pose a unique treatment challenge. Importantly, amputation is rarely indicated.

Hyperthermic Isolated Limb Perfusion and Isolated Limb Infusion

Although infrequently employed as a component of the current melanoma treatment landscape, regional chemotherapy techniques such as isolated limb perfusion or hyperthermic isolated limb infusion (ILI) have been employed to treat in-transit metastases. Hyperthermic isolated limb perfusion (HILP) with melphalan was initially used to treat in-transit metastases of the extremities in the mid-1950s. With this procedure, a formal lymph node dissection is performed that provides exposure to the critical vessels of interest. Subsequently, cannulae are inserted and the extremity is placed on an extracorporeal (oxygenated) bypass circuit after a tourniquet is applied, effectively isolating the limb from systemic circulation. Melphalan has been the most employed agent for use in HILP. Overall response rates of 64% to 100% (median complete response rates of 58%) have been achieved, and the median response duration in patients with a complete response generally ranges from 9 to 19 months.

Although HILP was a rational treatment option for patents with in-transit metastases, the technique was also complex and invasive. To address these challenges, the technique of minimally invasive ILI was developed.

ILI is essentially a low-flow minimally invasive isolated limb perfusion performed via percutaneously inserted catheters, and without oxygenation of the circuit (Fig. 3.12). Using standard radiologic techniques, catheters are inserted percutaneously into the main artery and vein of the unaffected limb (or placed in the main artery and vein in the affected limb, i.e., brachial or popliteal artery and vein). Under general anesthesia, after a pneumatic tourniquet is inflated proximally, cytotoxic agents (generally melphalan and actinomycin-D) are infused through the arterial catheter and "hand-circulated" with a syringe technique for 20 to 30 minutes. Progressive hypoxia occurs because, in contrast to isolated limb perfusion, no oxygenator is used. The hypoxia and acidosis associated with ILI are therapeutically attractive because numerous cytotoxic agents, including melphalan, appear to damage tumor cells more effectively under hypoxic conditions; hypoxia and acidosis have been reported to increase the cytotoxic effects of melphalan in experimental models.

Although the limb tissues are exposed to the cytotoxic agent for only a short period (up to 30 minutes), the procedure has been shown to yield response rates roughly like those observed after conventional HILP; overall response rates of 85% (complete response rate, 41%; partial response rate, 44%) have been achieved in at least

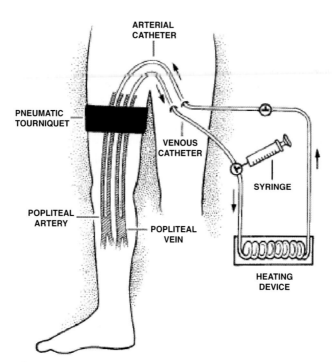

FIGURE 3.12 Schematic drawing depicting an isolated limb infusion. The catheters are typically placed percutaneously by an interventional radiologist via the contralateral extremity, with the catheter tips positioned in the tumor-bearing extremity just below the inguinal ligament in the superficial femoral artery and vein. After inflation of the tourniquet, chemotherapy is manually infused for 20 to 30 minutes, after which the limb is washed out with normal saline. (Reprinted by permission from Springer: Lindner P, Doubrovsky A, Kam PC, et al. Prognostic factors after isolated limb infusion with cytotoxic agents for melanoma. *Ann Surg Oncol.* 2002;9:127–136, with permission.)

one study. A multi-institutional study by Beasley et al. revealed a 31% complete response rate and a 33% partial response rate. Because of the relative simplicity of the isolated infusion technique, it became a more attractive option for patients with prohibitive comorbidities or the elderly, and in general became more widely used than HILP.

Toxicity and Morbidity of HILP and ILI
HILP and ILI can be associated with potentially significant regional adverse effects, including myonecrosis, nerve injury, compartment syndrome, and arterial thrombosis, sometimes necessitating fasciotomy or rarely amputation. Systemic leak of melphalan can result in additional toxicities. Following ILI, regional adverse events appear to be similar to those reported after conventional HILP, with 41% of patients experiencing grade II toxic effects and 53% experiencing grade III toxic effects. Both procedures require a high degree of technical expertise; if considered in the context of a multidisciplinary team-based approach, the procedure (almost exclusively ILI, as HILP is mostly of historical significance) should be performed only in centers that have experience with the technique. Moreover, in the era of modern targeted and immunotherapies, these techniques are rarely employed.

Intralesional Therapy
The concept of intralesional therapy for locoregional in-transit disease (or more broadly speaking for other accessible metastases) in melanoma is not new. A potential advantage of such a strategy is that a direct targeted approach may be associated with limited systemic toxicity while at the same time promoting a favorable local immune response and potentially direct cytotoxic activity. Historically, this approach has been considered for patients with unresectable, multiple, or locally advanced locoregional disease as well as patients with accessible M1a disease.

T-VEC (talimogene laherparepvec) is the only currently FDA-approved intralesional agent and leverages the role of granulocyte macrophage colony stimulating (GM-CSF) injection and its theoretical contribution to antitumor immunity. The agent is an attenuated oncolytic herpes simplex virus that has been modified to express the GM-CSF gene and is also capable of selective replication in tumor cells. The antitumor effect is thought to be due to a combination of a direct oncolysis from the viral infection and lytic replication, as well as the induction of a systemic immune response.

In a phase III trial reported by Andtbacka et al., 436 patients were enrolled and randomized to T-VEC or GM-CSF (control). All patients had unresectable, injectable stage III or IV melanoma with a limited visceral disease burden. T-VEC was administered by intralesional injections once every 2 weeks, while in the other arm GM-CSF was administered subcutaneously daily for 14 days in each 28-day cycle. The durable (defined as ≥6 months) response rate, the primary objective of the trial, was significantly increased in patients receiving T-VEC (16.3% vs. 2.1%), as was the overall response rate (26.4% vs. 5.7%). Some antitumor effects were observed in approximately one-third of uninjected lesions and in slightly more than 10% of visceral sites. OS was not significantly different among the arms of the trial; however, in subset analysis there appeared to be a survival advantage in patients with stage III or IV (M1a) disease (4-year OS 32% vs. 21%, HR 0.57, 95% CI 0.40 to 0.80). Treatment with T-VEC was well tolerated. Commonly reported adverse events included fatigue, chills, pyrexia, and other systemic flu-like symptoms. Based on these positive clinical results, in 2015, T-VEC became the first intralesional therapy approved by the FDA for the local treatment of unresectable cutaneous, subcutaneous, and nodal lesions in patients with melanoma recurrent after initial surgery.

Efforts have been made to build upon the success of ILI and intralesional therapy (T-VEC in particular). Ariyan et al. examined the safety and efficacy of combining ipilimumab with ILI in patients with in-transit disease. After administering combination therapy to 26 patients, they observed response rates of 85% at 3 months (62% CR) and progression-free survival (PFS) at 1 year of 57%. A recent positive phase II trial comparing T-VEC followed by surgery versus surgery alone in stage IIIB–IV(M1a) melanoma demonstrated an improvement in 2-year recurrence-free survival from 16.5% among 74 patients in the surgery alone arm to 29.5% in the 76 patients included in the T-VEC followed by surgery arm.

Management of Local Recurrence

True local recurrence is defined as recurrence at the site of the primary tumor, within or continuous with the scar, and is most likely the result of incomplete excision of the primary tumor; it represents a relatively rare pattern of recurrence. In many cases, such "local recurrences" may more appropriately be considered persistence of the primary tumor. A local recurrence consisting of a single lesion in a patient whose primary melanoma had favorable prognostic features may be appropriately treated with wide excision similar to a primary melanoma lesion. Patients with local recurrences consisting of multiple, small, and superficial lesions may be treated in a fashion similar to that used to treat patients with in-transit disease (see above).

Adjuvant Therapy

Systemic therapy options in melanoma have greatly increased in recent years, with a number of novel agents under active investigation. As these agents gain approval in the metastatic setting, many are considered and have demonstrated efficacy in the adjuvant arena. Currently approved adjuvant systemic treatment regimens are described below and summarized in Table 3.6.

Immune Checkpoint Blockade

Ipilimumab is a humanized monoclonal antibody that blocks CTLA-4, a key regulatory molecule of the immune system. The use of immune checkpoint blockade via monoclonal antibodies targeting anti-CTLA4 (ipilimumab; *Yervoy*) has been established as an effective treatment for stage IV disease since 2011.

Although approved in the metastatic setting for some time, the use of checkpoint blockade in the adjuvant setting has been more recently approved in stage III melanoma based on a number of randomized phase III trials. The randomized phase III clinical trial EORTC 18071 compared high-dose ipilimumab (10 mg/kg) to placebo, administered every 3 weeks for four doses, then every 3 months for 3 years unless toxicity or relapse prevented its continuation, and demonstrated both a decreased rate of recurrence and improved OS for patients in the ipilimumab arm, leading to the approval of adjuvant ipilimumab.

Despite the survival benefits noted in this adjuvant setting, opponents of this approach remark on the toxicity and paradoxical increased dosing seen in the adjuvant setting compared to metastatic disease (the latter of which employs a dose of 3 mg/kg every 3 weeks × four doses). The toxicity from ipilimumab in EORTC 18071 was significant; adverse events of any grade were noted in 98.7% of patients treated with ipilimumab, including 54.1% with grade 3 or 4 toxicity. The median number of ipilimumab doses was four. Furthermore, there were five treatment-related deaths in patients treated with ipilimumab (three due to colitis, one to myocarditis, and one to multiorgan failure associated with Guillain–Barré syndrome). While treatment-related

TABLE 3.6 FDA-Approved Therapies in the Adjuvant Setting and for Metastatic or Unresectable Melanoma

Adjuvant			
Agent	**Mechanism**	**Year Approved**	**Notes**
Interferon alfa	Indirect immune modulation	1995	No longer used
Ipilimumab	CTLA-4 inhibitor	2015	Current use as monotherapy very infrequent in adjuvant setting
Nivolumab	Anti-PD-1	2017	
Dabrafenib+trametinib	BRAFi/MEKi	2018	V600E or V600K mutations
Pembrolizumab	Anti-PD-1	2019	Recently also approved in adjuvant setting for Stage IIB and IIC
Metastatic or Unresectable Disease			
Dacarbazine	Alkylating agent	1795	Current use very infrequent
IL-2			Current use very infrequent
Ipilimumab	CTLA-4 inhibitor	2011	3 mg/kg dose; not generally first-line agent; often used in conjunction with nivolumab in metastatic setting; dosing may vary
Vemurafenib	BRAFi	2011	No longer used as monotherapy
Trametinib	MEKi	2013	No longer used as monotherapy
Dabrafenib+trametinib	BRAFi/MEKi	2014	V600E or V600K mutations
Pembrolizumab	Anti-PD-1	2014	
Nivolumab	Anti-PD-1	2014	
T-VEC	Oncolytic virus	2015	Administered via intratumoral injection
Vemurafenib+cobimetinib	BRAFi/MEKi	2015	V600E or V600K mutations only
Ipilumumab+nivolumab	CTLA-4 inhibitor/ anti-PD-1	2015	
Encorafenib+binimetinib	BRAFi/MEKi	2018	V600E or V600K mutations
Atezolizumab+vemurafenib+cobimetinib	Anti-PD-L1/ BRAFi/MEKi	2020	V600 positive mutations
Relatlimib+nivolumab	LAG-3 Inhibitor	2022	

Note–patients whose tumors contain other V600 mutations may sometimes also be offered BRAFi/MEKi-directed therapy.
BRAFi, BRAF inhibitor; MEKi, MEK inhibitor.

deaths may be encountered in any clinical trial, such events in the adjuvant setting raise caution; some argue whether the toxicity is worth the potential survival benefit. This is relevant since there is a fraction of patients who will never recur and therefore have no potential to benefit from any adjuvant therapy. Of course, the challenge is that it is currently not possible to know that information at the level of an individual patient. Therefore, the ability to prospectively identify *higher- and lower*-risk patients with biomarkers remains an area of intense clinical interest, as is interest on additional targets and combination therapies.

Following the success and approval of CTLA-4 inhibition, the study of programmed cell death protein-1 (PD-1) axis, which functions in the periphery to modulate T-cell responses, has produced success in a number of clinical trials. PD-1 interacts with two ligands, PD-L1 and PD-L2, to dampen T-cell responses, physiologically functioning to limit autoimmunity. The inhibitory effect of PD-1 is accomplished through a dual mechanism of promoting apoptosis in cytotoxic T-cells (programmed cell death, as the name implies) while simultaneously reducing apoptosis in regulatory T cells. PD-1 protein is upregulated on activated T cells, and blockade of this molecule upregulates the cellular immune system's antitumor activity.

The PD-1 axis of checkpoint blockade was explored in the adjuvant setting using the anti–PD-1 monoclonal antibody nivolumab. In a randomized, double-blind, phase III clinical trial (CheckMate 238) for patients with resected advanced melanoma, over 900 patients who underwent complete resection of stage IIIB, IIIC, or IV melanoma received either nivolumab (3 mg/kg every 2 weeks) or ipilimumab (10 mg/kg every 3 weeks × 4 doses and then every 12 weeks). Toxicity (grade 3 or 4 adverse events) was reported in 14.4% of the patients in the nivolumab group versus 45.9% of patients in the ipilimumab group; moreover, two deaths (0.4%) were reported and noted to be related to toxic effects in the ipilimumab group. Weber et al. concluded that nivolumab resulted in significantly longer RFS and a lower rate of grade 3 or 4 adverse events than adjuvant therapy with ipilimumab. Based upon the results of CheckMate 238, nivolumab was approved for adjuvant use by the FDA in 2017.

Another anti–PD-1 drug, pembrolizumab, was compared to placebo in the randomized, controlled, double-blind phase III EORTC 1325-MG/KEYNOTE-054 trial. AJCC 7th edition stage IIIA (if stage IIIA, SLN deposit had to be >1 mm metastasis), IIIB, and IIIC completely resected patients were included. RFS was 59.8% in the 514 patients receiving pembrolizumab versus 41.1% in the 505 patients on placebo after 42 months of follow-up (HR 0.59; 95% CI, 0.49 to 0.70) in the updated trial results published in 2021. Pembrolizumab was approved by the FDA for adjuvant use in stage III disease in 2019 after the initial trial results were released.

Building on the success of pembrolizumab in the stage III adjuvant setting, the phase III randomized clinical trial KEYNOTE-716 trial studied adjuvant pembrolizumab versus placebo in resected stage IIB or IIC melanoma patients, all of whom had a negative SLN biopsy. At the second interim analysis with a median follow-up of 18 months, this study demonstrated a significant reduction in relapse-free survival and distant metastasis among patients receiving pembrolizumab in an overall cohort of 1,182 patients. These findings led to the recently expanded indication for the use of pembrolizumab in the stage IIB and IIC setting.

As the indications continue to expand for the use of checkpoint blockade, their utilization in the meta-static, adjuvant, and neoadjuvant setting must be considered in view of their side effect profile. Adverse events are discussed below, but these become increasingly important to the surgical oncologist as immunotherapy is increasingly utilized in the adjuvant and neoadjuvant settings. Multidisciplinary care is ultimately crucial to these decisions in weighing the risks of a particular side effect profile, its potential downstream effects, and the potential benefit of these therapies.

Targeted Therapy

Targeted BRAF and MEK dual inhibition (BRAFi/MEKi) in BRAF V600 mutant melanoma has been associated with relatively rapid response, high disease control rates, and a survival benefit in stage IV melanoma. Unfortunately, this approach has also been associated with limited durability of response, leading some investigators to examine alternate stages of disease for this regimen. Long et al. investigated the efficacy of these agents in the adjuvant stage III setting in a randomized, double-blind, placebo-controlled, phase III trial (COMBI-AD), that randomly assigned patients with completely resected stage III melanoma and BRAF V600 mutations ($n = $ 870) to receive oral dabrafenib (150 mg BID) plus trametinib (2 mg once daily) versus placebo in a 1:1 fashion. At a median follow-up of 2.8 years, the estimated 3-year RFS was 58% in the combination-therapy group and 39% in the placebo group (HR for relapse or death, 0.47; 95% CI, 0.39 to 0.58; $P < .001$). In addition, the BRAFi/MEKi group had a significantly higher 3-year OS of 86% versus 77% in the placebo group (HR for death, 0.57; 95% CI, 0.42 to 0.79; $P = .0006$); authors noted that this level of improvement did not cross the prespecified interim analysis boundary of $P = .000019$. They concluded that combined dabrafenib plus trametinib in the adjuvant setting resulted in a significantly lower risk of recurrence in patients with stage III melanoma with BRAF V600 mutations and with an acceptable toxicity profile. This trial led to the 2018 FDA approval of dab-rafenib/trametinib for use in the adjuvant setting for those with stage III disease and BRAF V600E or V600K mutations.

Radiation Therapy

The role of radiation therapy in melanoma care continues to evolve, particularly in this emerging era of more effective systemic therapy. Overall, it is not as commonly utilized in contemporary practice compared to the era preceding the implementation of checkpoint blockade and targeted therapy. Radiation therapy is sometimes deployed in effort to enhance outcomes for melanoma patients. While local control is routinely achieved by primary tumor wide excision, adjuvant radiation therapy is sometimes used in the uncommon presentation of the potentially locally aggressive desmoplastic neurotropic melanoma subtype. The use of radiation in this setting is supported by various retrospective studies and the current national consensus guidelines. Radiation therapy is also sometimes used when surgery is not possible or feasible.

Although adjuvant radiation therapy has historically been offered to patients with multiple involved or matted regional nodes or with extracapsular extension of regional lymphatic metastases, its role in this context continues to rapidly evolve, and if considered, treatment plans should be developed in the context of the multidisciplinary care of the patient. Indeed, adjuvant radiation in the prevention of nodal relapse in high-risk populations was recently studied in the ANZMTG trial that randomized 250 patients with palpable regional nodal disease and high risk of nodal recurrence after lymphadenectomy to either adjuvant radiation therapy or observation. Although radiation therapy decreased nodal recurrence in the radiation arm (21% vs. 36%, $P = .02$), the additional therapy did not result in a significant difference in either overall or relapse-free survival.

The role of radiation therapy in the setting of progressively improving systemic treatment options remains an area of active clinical investigation. At MD Anderson, radiation therapy is sometimes used in the adjuvant setting to reduce in-basin failure in high-risk patients following lymphadenectomy. It is also used for the palliation of local symptoms and to reduce risk of local recurrence after failure of first-line therapy. More recently, radiation therapy has also been deployed in a clinical trial of nodal radiation therapy after SLN biopsy for patients with high-risk SLN-positive melanoma who are scheduled to have immunotherapy without completion lymph node dissection (i.e., undergoing nodal observation with active surveillance) (NCT04594187). Future research goals include clinical trials to further define the role of adjuvant radiation therapy alone or in combination with systemic therapies. Patients with multiple involved or matted regional nodes or with extracapsular extension of regional lymphatic metastases may be considered for adjuvant radiation therapy in the context of the multidisciplinary care of the patient with metastatic melanoma.

Neoadjuvant Therapy

Given the high risk of recurrence for patients with clinical regional lymphadenopathy or resectable distant metastasis and the effectiveness of systemic therapies, neoadjuvant therapy is being actively pursued in several clinical trials and is increasingly employed in the clinical setting for patients who present with clinical regional lymphadenopathy. Neoadjuvant therapy provides the opportunity to examine disease biology in response to therapy, reduce the morbidity of surgical resection, and potentially tailor the need for and approach to adjuvant therapy based on extent of response.

For BRAF V600 mutant patients, we completed a single-center, open-label phase II randomized neoadjuvant therapy trial with neoadjuvant BRAF/MEK combination inhibitor therapy dabrafenib + trametinib for 8 weeks followed by surgery versus surgery with adjuvant dabrafenib + trametinib (for patients in both study arms) in patients with resectable clinical stage IIIB/C or stage IV oligometastatic disease. The trial enrolled 14 patients to the neoadjuvant arm and 7 patients to the adjuvant arm. It was stopped early at a prespecified interim safety analysis after noting significantly longer event-free survival in the neoadjuvant arm (71% [10 of 14 patients] vs. 0% [0 of 7 patients]; median event-free survival 19.7 vs. 2.9 months; HR 0.016; 95% CI, 0.00012 to 0.14; $P < .0001$). There were no grade 4 adverse events in the neoadjuvant group, and importantly, we observed a pathologic complete response (pCR) in 58% of patients treated on the neoadjuvant arm. The trial was continued as a single-arm neoadjuvant study. The results were replicated in the phase II, single-arm NeoCombi study conducted in Australia, which found a 49% pCR in the cohort of 35 patients receiving neoadjuvant dabrafenib + trametinib.

Leveraging advances in the immunotherapy arena, several trials (OpACIN, OpACIN-Neo, Amaria et al., 2018) have investigated various regimens of nivolumab with or without ipilimumab, and one trial from the University of Pennsylvania investigated neoadjuvant single-dose pembrolizumab (Huang et al.). A recent meta-analysis of these four studies by Menzies et al. found that 38% ($n = 51$) of patients had a pCR, which correlated with improved RFS (100% vs. 72%, $P < .001$); no patients with a pCR had thus far died. In addition, in patients with pCR, near pCR, or partial pathologic response following neoadjuvant immunotherapy, the 2-year RFS was 96%, with very few relapses observed.

Of note, the optimal dose from OpACIN-Neo appeared to be ipilimumab 1 mg/kg and nivolumab 3 mg/kg, which was also better tolerated than the ipilimumab 3 mg/kg and nivolumab 1 mg/kg employed in the metastatic setting (see Adjuvant Therapy section for discussion of dosing). The ongoing PRADO trial (NCT02977052), based on an expansion cohort from OpACIN-Neo, is investigating whether CLND can be safely omitted in patients with a major pathologic response in the excised index lymph node after two cycles of neoadjuvant ipilimumab + nivolumab. The role of neoadjuvant therapy in patients with melanoma continues to rapidly evolve. When considered, this approach should be discussed in the context of a multidisciplinary care team, preferably in the context of a clinical trial.

Management of Distant Metastatic Disease

Common sites of distant metastasis in melanoma patients are, in order of decreasing frequency, skin and subcutaneous tissues (40%), lungs (12% to 36%), liver (15% to 20%), and brain (12% to 20%). Other sites include the gastrointestinal tract, bone, adrenal gland, distant skin, soft tissue, and/or lymph nodes, and less commonly, the spleen or pancreas. Historically, patients with systemic metastases have had a poor prognosis, with a median survival ranging from 6 to 12 months. Fortunately, a wave of effective systemic therapies have ushered in a new era of treatment options for patients with unresectable or distant metastatic disease (see Table 3.6

and sections on Immune Checkpoint Blockade and Targeted Therapy, below). Indeed, the approach to treatment for such patients is now associated with improved and sometimes durable long-term survival and continues to evolve. Contemporary systemic therapy represents the mainstay of treatment for most patients with distant metastatic disease, although surgery (curative or palliative) and other modalities (e.g., intralesional therapy) continue to play an evolving role in carefully selected patients as part of a multidisciplinary approach to the care of such patients. In view of continued advances in the clinical arena and the common need to often consider second- or subsequent line treatments, clinical trials represent an important and attractive option for many patients.

Surgery

The decision to perform surgery in patients with distant melanoma metastasis should be considered as part of a multidisciplinary approach to care. Overall, given the advances in systemic therapy, surgery as a sole component of the care of these patients is relatively uncommon, and the role of metastasectomy in this setting—whether curative or palliative in intent—continues to evolve. Indeed, most previous trials and retrospective series that have evaluated the role of surgery for patients with distant melanoma metastasis have mostly been conducted prior to this era of more effective systemic therapy. As such, if surgery is considered, the rationale, extent, timing, and decision to proceed should involve a multidisciplinary approach and thoughtful consideration of existing systemic treatment options. Common indications include palliation of symptoms (e.g., gastrointestinal obstruction or hemorrhage, difficulty in managing cutaneous metastases, intractable pain), isolated metastases not responding to otherwise successful systemic therapy, and isolated stable oligometastatic disease.

Complete metastasectomy may be considered in patients as part of a multidisciplinary approach to distant metastasis; indeed, in at least one legacy study, such as the Canvaxin phase III trial, patients underwent complete metastasectomy for stage IV melanoma as part of an adjuvant stage IV clinical trial; despite the overall negative trial results related to the Canvaxin vaccine, patients had a 40% 5-year survival, even though this trial was conducted prior to the era of contemporary systemic therapy. Other nonrandomized trials of highly selected patients demonstrated similar results after complete resection of distant metastases. Patient selection is critical for the strategy of complete surgical metastasectomy, whether for curative or palliative intent.

To aid in patient selection, a thorough imaging evaluation is indicated, including MRI of the brain and CT or PET/CT of the chest, abdomen, and pelvis to fully assess disease burden and the potential to offer either a complete or palliative resection.

Patient factors also play a role in patient selection. Patients should not have comorbidities that would preclude a possible full recovery from surgery within 4 to 8 weeks to allow for the initiation of adjuvant or systemic therapies. Moreover, the biology of the melanoma itself should be considered; patients whose distant metastasis developed following a longer disease-free interval or who present with isolated or oligometastatic disease are, in general, more likely to be considered for surgical resection. Lastly, the systemic options available and their demonstrated efficacy should be considered. This includes, but is not limited to, responsiveness and ability to tolerate immune checkpoint blockade, mutational status, and progression on other lines of therapy. Ultimately, these decisions should be made in collaboration with a multidisciplinary team.

Surgery may also offer effective palliation for isolated or oligometastatic accessible distant metastases. Examples of accessible lesions include isolated visceral metastases, isolated brain metastases, and occasionally isolated lung metastases. Palliative strategies may improve functional status and render patients more likely to tolerate systemic treatments. Importantly, surgery may also be considered to support consolidation of a mixed response to systemic therapy. Overall, the role of surgery in the context of the multidisciplinary management of the patient with distant metastases continues to evolve.

Brain Metastases

Melanoma ranks behind only small-cell carcinoma of the lung as the most common tumor that metastasizes to the brain. An unusual feature of brain metastases is their propensity for hemorrhage, which occurs much more frequently with melanoma than other primary tumors. Hemorrhage occurs in 33% to 50% of patients with brain metastases from melanoma. Prognosis worsens with an increasing number of lesions and the presence of neurologic symptoms; median survival has historically been reported to be 3 to 4 months.

With the description of combined immune checkpoint blockade for patients with brain metastasis by Tawbi et al., the prognosis for such patients has significantly improved. In this phase II study of 94 melanoma patients with nonirradiated measurable brain metastases, Tawbi et al. described a rate of radiologic clinical benefit of 57%

and complete response rate of 26%. As such, surgical resection is utilized less commonly than it has been historically. Currently, patients with brain metastases are generally treated with a combination of immune checkpoint
blockade and gamma knife radiation with the use of additional systemic or local therapies under the guidance of
a multidisciplinary treatment team. The role of targeted therapy remains unclear, although BRAF/MEK inhibition
appears to have superior control in extracranial rather than intracranial disease. Stereotactic radiosurgery is an
important option for patients with small to medium brain metastases who have a reasonable life expectancy and no
signs of increased intracranial pressure. Whole brain radiation therapy is not commonly utilized in contemporary
treatment strategies.

Targeted Therapy

Following an established track record set by other malignancies, such as breast cancer (trastuzumab) and
leukemia/GIST (imatinib), melanoma has undergone a paradigm change in cancer treatment. Of note, to
date, all targeted therapy agents used to treat melanoma have the advantage of oral administration. Given the
ease of administration and the often-profound disease control seen with these agents, it is our practice at MD
Anderson to routinely molecularly characterize tumors of patients with metastatic disease so that targeted
therapy treatment options can be integrated into an overall treatment strategy.

While the MAPK pathway is the most commonly targeted pathway in melanoma using BRAF/MEK inhibition
as detailed below, a number of other mutations have been targeted and described. These less common mutations
are of significant interest in a disease with an overall high prevalence. In the case of KIT mutations, several case
reports have demonstrated a benefit for individual patients with KIT mutations treated with a KIT inhibitor. In
a phase II study, 28 patients with unresectable metastatic KIT-mutated melanoma were treated with imatinib
mesylate. In this study, 16% of patients had durable responses that lasted more than a year. Continued work is
needed to identify and develop mechanisms to block additional known pathogenic mutations in melanoma.

BRAF Inhibitors

BRAF mutations have been found in approximately 50% of invasive cutaneous melanomas. The BRAF gene
encodes for production of B-RAF, a protein involved in cell signaling and growth. BRIM-3 was a randomized,
open-label, multicenter, phase III study that compared a BRAF inhibitor, PLX4032 (vemurafenib), to dacarbazine
for treatment of previously untreated, unresectable, stage IIIC or stage IV melanoma in patients harboring a BRAF
mutation. The inhibitor targets the common V600E BRAF mutation. Interim analysis of 675 patients revealed
superiority in OS and PFS for vemurafenib. The response rate of patients on vemurafenib was 48.4% compared to
5.5% for patients receiving dacarbazine. While such a response rate for single modality therapy was essentially
unprecedented in the treatment of metastatic melanoma, enthusiasm was tempered, at least to some extent, by
the observation that disease recurrence was observed in the majority of patients 6 to 8 months following initiation
of therapy. Also important was the observation that up to 25% of patients who received vemurafenib developed
squamous carcinoma of the skin, often in the form of keratoacanthomas. Dabrafenib, another agent targeting
BRAF V600 mutant melanoma, demonstrated similarly high OR rates in a phase III trial. Together, these findings
provided the basis for approval of each of these agents as monotherapy in 2011 and 2013, respectively.

MEK, a kinase downstream of RAF in the MAPK pathway, has been targeted in a similar fashion. MEK
inhibitors demonstrated benefit as monotherapy in patients with BRAF-mutant metastatic melanoma, leading to the FDA approval of trametinib in 2013. Of note, MEK inhibitors are rarely used as monotherapy for
patients with BRAF-mutant metastatic melanoma.

Numerous studies have elucidated acquired mechanisms of therapeutic resistance to BRAF-targeted therapy, and insights gained have led to treatment strategies to enhance responses to therapy. An outcome of this
is the use of combined BRAF and MEK inhibition—based on the observation that most BRAF-mutant melanomas demonstrate MAPK pathway reactivation at the time of therapeutic resistance. This combination was
tested in clinical trials in patients with BRAF-mutant melanoma, and results demonstrated that treatment
with combined BRAF and MEK inhibition (e.g., dabrafenib plus trametinib vs. dabrafenib monotherapy) was
associated with a higher overall response (76% vs. 54%), and with a longer PFS (9.4 months vs. 5.8 months)
than with BRAF inhibitor monotherapy. In January 2014, the FDA granted accelerated approval to combined
dabrafenib and trametinib for use in combination in patients with unresectable or metastatic BRAF-mutant
melanoma. The following year, the FDA also approved the BRAF/MEK inhibitor combination of vemurafenib
and cobimetinib (coBRIM study), and in 2018, encorafenib and binimetinib were added to the armamentarium (COLUMBUS trial). Importantly, neither BRAF inhibitor nor MEK inhibitor monotherapy is currently
deployed in the current melanoma treatment landscape. It should also be noted that BRAF inhibitors have
been shown to paradoxically stimulate growth in patients with wild-type BRAF status. The COMBI-MB clinical
trial enrolled patients with melanoma brain metastases to receive dabrafenib and trametinib. Across four

patient cohorts, intracranial response ranged from 44% to 59%, although duration of response was relatively short. As such, many medical oncologists prefer to use immunotherapy for brain metastases even in BRAF positive patients given the short duration of benefit with targeted therapy.

Immune Checkpoint Blockade

In a phase III, randomized prospective trial, Hodi et al. evaluated 676 patients who received ipilimumab, ipilimumab plus a peptide vaccine, or peptide vaccine alone. Overall response and disease control were highest in the ipilimumab alone cohort. Median OS was 10.1 months for this cohort and overall response was 10.9%. Disease control was 28.5%, with 60% of the ipilimumab cohort having a significant response at 2 years.

In March 2011, the FDA approved ipilimumab as a second-line treatment for metastatic melanoma. A subsequent study demonstrated the benefit of ipilimumab in the first-line setting. In a phase III, double-blind clinical trial of 502 metastatic melanoma patients randomized to ipilimumab plus dacarbazine versus placebo plus dacarbazine by Robert et al., the ipilimumab cohort was associated with a significantly higher OS (11.2 months vs. 9.2 months) and durable response (19.3 months vs. 8.3 months). As mentioned in the adjuvant section above, ipilimumab dosing has been studied at multiple levels and schedules. For patients with metastatic melanoma, the currently approved ipilimumab dose is 3 mg/kg by intravenous infusion given every 3 weeks for four doses.

The clinical use of PD-1 blocking antibodies has been tested in several clinical trials, including a phase I trial of 296 patients with either advanced melanoma or other solid tumors. Treatment with a monoclonal antibody targeting PD-1 (nivolumab) was associated with a 28% response rate in patients with metastatic melanoma, with long-term responses longer than 1 year in 50% of responders. Anti–PD-1-based therapy was associated with a lower rate of grade 3 or 4 adverse events compared to ipilimumab. Additional clinical trials have been performed (NCT01295827/NCT01704287), including a phase III trial with over 500 patients with metastatic melanoma whose disease was refractory to CTLA-4 blockade. In this trial (KEYNOTE-002), patients were randomized to pembrolizumab (2 mg/kg every 3 weeks), pembrolizumab (10 mg/kg every 3 weeks) or chemotherapy (carboplatin plus paclitaxel, paclitaxel alone, dacarbazine, or temozolomide per institutional standard). PFS was the primary endpoint and was significantly improved with both pembrolizumab arms compared to chemotherapy; 6-month PFS was 34%, 38%, and 16% for pembrolizumab 2 mg/kg, pembrolizumab 10 mg/kg, and chemotherapy, respectively.

Toxicity was limited in this trial; the most common adverse events included fatigue, pruritus, and rash. Grade 3 immune-related adverse events (IRAEs) were seen in two patients treated with pembrolizumab 2 mg/kg (hepatitis, hypophysitis) and in eight patients who received pembrolizumab 10 mg/kg (hepatitis, colitis, pneumonitis, and iritis/uveitis).

Cellular Therapies

Cellular therapy, also known as adoptive cell therapy (ACT), involves the in vitro expansion and activation, to supraphysiologic numbers ($10^{10\text{-}12}$), of highly specific cytotoxic T cells directed against a patient's own tumor and reinfusion after a lymphodepleting preparative regimen. These were originally procured by resection of a metastatic deposit and the growing of the so-called TILs. More recently, these cytotoxic lymphocytes have been created by gene modification of a patient's peripheral blood mononuclear cells (PBMCs) or the creation of chimeric antigen receptors (CARs) that further advance specificity and are not dependent upon a resectable lesion. At the National Cancer Institute (NCI), Rosenberg and others have reported their experiences with ACT using TILs that have principally been derived from metastatic tumors. An overall response rate as high as 72% was seen in patients with stage IV disease treated with ACT, with the addition of an extensive immune depletion preparative regimen (lymphodepleting chemotherapy + 12-Gy total-body irradiation [TBI]). A randomized, prospective study by the same group did not support the role of added TBI, but nonetheless reported an impressive overall response rate of 56%. Key steps affecting response include the effectiveness of lymphodepletion prior to T-cell transfer, extranodal source of TILs, short culture duration, short TIL doubling time, greater autologous tumor lysis by TIL, and TIL secretion of granulocyte–macrophage stimulating factor. Cellular therapies are becoming much more specific, with far less "off target" toxicity due to prior mentioned genetic modification. Recent evidence from the NCI suggests that neoantigens and their respective T-cell receptors (TCRs) can be identified in both tumors (including metastatic uveal) and in peripheral blood. Once procured, these can be massively expanded in vitro for subsequent infusion. Additional approaches employing in vitro pulsed dendritic cell infusion are also ongoing. Importantly, since these techniques require specialized expertise and an elaborate infrastructure, it is currently only being explored in select academic centers worldwide.

Interleukin-2 (IL-2) promotes the proliferation, differentiation, and recruitment of T, B, and NK cells and initiates cytolytic activity in a subset of lymphocytes. Although high-dose IL-2 has overall response rates of only 10% to 15% in appropriately selected patients, it is generally durable among the fraction of patients who have a complete response. Such durability of response was associated with approval by the U.S. FDA for metastatic melanoma in 1998. However, IL-2 administration is associated with multiple side effects, including, but not limited to the uncommon but potentially life-threatening "capillary leak syndrome." Therefore, it should be administered only by clinicians and teams experienced in the management of such therapies; in the context of the current metastatic melanoma treatment landscape, it is uncommonly used.

Combinatorial Strategies

Given the differential mechanisms of action of CTLA-4 blockade and PD-1 blockade, their use in combination has been explored. In the largest phase III clinical trial combining anti–PD-1 and anti–CTLA-4 checkpoint inhibition (CheckMate 067), over 900 treatment-naive patients were randomly assigned to nivolumab (1 mg/kg every 3 weeks) plus ipilimumab (3 mg/kg every 3 weeks) for four doses followed by nivolumab (3 mg/kg every 2 weeks), nivolumab alone (3 mg/kg every 2 weeks), or ipilimumab alone (3 mg/kg every 3 weeks for four doses). The primary endpoints of this trial were PFS and OS. At a median follow-up of 12 months, the median PFS for the combination arm or the nivolumab arm alone were superior to ipilimumab alone (11.5 months vs. 2.9 months and 6.9 months vs. 2.9 months, respectively). Not surprisingly, serious toxicities were more frequent with the combination than with either monotherapy arm alone. Despite the toxicity and based on survival data, the FDA granted accelerated approval in 2015 for the combination of ipilimumab and nivolumab for stage IV disease. Given the toxicities associated with this combination checkpoint inhibitor regimen, additional combinations are being explored, including combinations with other novel checkpoint inhibitors and other modalities such as targeted therapy. As an example, atezolumab + vemurafenib + cobimetinib—a combination of anti–PD-L1 and dual BRAF/MEK inhibitors—has been approved by the FDA based on results from the phase III randomized IMspire150 clinical trial. Recently, the RELATIVITY-047 trial demonstrated improved PFS when comparing the LAG-3 inhibitor (relatlimab) with nivolumab against nivolumab alone (10.1 months vs. 4.6 months, respectively). Importantly, grade 3 or 4 treatment-related adverse events (TRAEs) occurred in 18.9% of patients in the relatlimab–nivolumab group and in 9.7% of patients in the nivolumab group; the combination arm had fewer significant TRAEs than have been commonly observed for patients receiving standard dose ipilimumab and nivolumab combination checkpoint inhibitor therapy.

Lastly, with various systemic therapy options currently available, particularly for patients whose tumors have a BRAF mutation, the sequencing of agents has been suggested to play a potential role in clinical outcome. The recent results of the DREAMseq trial confirmed this hypothesis. Patients with *BRAF*-mutated melanoma were noted to have significantly improved 2-year OS when treated with immunotherapy followed by targeted BRAF/MEK inhibition, as compared to BRAF/MEK inhibition followed by immunotherapy (72% vs. 52%, $P = .0095$). As additional agents and avenues of treatment are described, it will become increasingly important for sequencing to be studied and optimized in preclinical models and translated to clinical trials to inform new standards in clinical care.

Tumor Vaccines

Tumor vaccines represent a longstanding area of exploration for the treatment of advanced melanoma and as adjuvant therapy for patients with high-risk melanoma. Such vaccines may contain: (1) irradiated tumor cells, usually obtained from the patient, (2) partially or completely purified melanoma antigens, or (3) tumor cell membranes from melanoma cells infected with virus (viral oncolysates). Synthetic vaccines containing genes that encode for tumor antigens and peptide antigens themselves are also being evaluated, as are vaccines containing genes encoding for immune costimulatory signal proteins.

Allogeneic tumor cell vaccines, generally prepared from cultured cell lines or lysates thereof, offer several potential important advantages over autologous tumor cell vaccines. Allogeneic vaccines are readily available and can be standardized, preserved, and distributed in a manner akin to other therapeutic agents. To date, most studies involving allogeneic tumor vaccines have been small, single-institution studies. None of these studies have demonstrated an unequivocal benefit for immunotherapy with allogeneic tumor cells administered in conjunction with BCG compared to no treatment or to treatment with BCG alone.

Additional vaccine strategies include administration of synthetic peptides based on known melanoma T-cell antigens, genetic vaccines, and combinations of vaccines with cytokines or costimulatory molecules. Morton et al. conducted nonrandomized studies of a polyvalent melanoma vaccine (Canvaxin) in patients with stage III or stage IV disease. Although matched-pair analyses of data from phase II trials demonstrated a consistent OS benefit for Canvaxin therapy in stage III or stage IV melanoma, two separate randomized phase III clinical trials of Canvaxin in patients with stage III or IV melanoma were discontinued due to lack of potential benefit based on interim analyses.

Follow-Up and Surveillance

Melanoma has a more variable and unpredictable clinical course than almost any other human cancer. At MD Anderson, the schedule of follow-up evaluations for patients with melanoma varies according to the risk of recurrence. In general, patients with early-stage invasive melanoma (e.g., ≤1-mm tumor thickness, nonulcerated, lymph-node negative) have follow-up visits every 6 months for 2 years and then annually. Patients with thicker or ulcerated melanomas and those with positive lymph nodes generally return for follow-up visits more frequently—every 3 to 4 months for 2 years, then every 6 months for 3 years, and annually thereafter. At each visit, the patient undergoes a physical examination concentrating on skin survey (to examine for additional primary melanomas, in-transit metastasis, satellite disease, and/or distant skin or soft tissue findings) and lymph node basin examination. Abnormal findings may prompt further workup. Extensive radiographic evaluation of asymptomatic patients with AJCC stage I or stage II melanoma who are clinically free of disease rarely reveals metastases, and thus is not routinely performed (although given the recognition that patients with stage AJCC 8th edition IIB and IIC disease have a risk profile that approaches that of AJCC 8th edition IIIB disease, and adjuvant anti–PD-1-based therapy has been approved, such patients often receive surveillance imaging). CT or PET/CT should be considered every 3 to 6 months (or according to clinical trial, if participating) to evaluate for progressive or new metastatic disease in patients with stage III or IV disease. MRI of the brain is also often performed for surveillance in patients who are stage III or IV, particularly in more advanced disease settings. Ultrasound surveillance of regional lymph node basins should be strongly encouraged for patients who have had a positive SLN as part of active surveillance in patients who have nodal observation and do not have CLND.

CASE SCENARIO

Case Scenario 1

Presentation

A 45-year-old female presents with a 2-year history of a changing pigmented lesion on her left shoulder that frequently becomes irritated and bleeds. She notes the lesion seems to crust over but never fully heals. She notes a history of frequent blistering sunburns in her youth and frequent use of tanning beds in her teens and twenties. Her past medical and family history are otherwise unremarkable.

Differential Diagnosis

Melanoma
Squamous cell carcinoma
Basal cell carcinoma
Merkel cell carcinoma
Atypical melanocytic lesion/dysplastic nevus
Irritated pigmented seborrheic keratosis

Confirmation of Diagnosis and Treatment

Performing a biopsy to obtain a histologic diagnosis is generally recommended when a patient notes a history of a changing skin lesion, particularly when there is asymmetry, border irregularity, variegation of color, a diameter greater than 6 mm, and/or an otherwise enlarging or evolving lesion. Most surgeons favor a punch or narrow margin excisional biopsy over a shave biopsy if melanoma is on the differential so that accurate depth of the lesion can be obtained. The clinical history should be available to the pathologist and the specimen is preferably reviewed by a dermatopathologist. If invasive melanoma is noted, melanoma tumor thickness, number of mitotic figures (measured using the hot spot approach as mitoses per mm^2), and presence or absence of ulceration should be recorded on the pathology report. In this case, a punch biopsy was performed which confirmed the diagnosis of a primary invasive melanoma with a tumor thickness of 2.4 mm that was ulcerated and had 4 mitotic figures per mm^2.

Surgical Approach—Key Steps

A ruler should be used to measure a 2-cm radial margin from any residual abnormal pigmentation or biopsy scar around the entire circumference of the lesion. If primary closure is planned, most surgeons generally extend the proposed resection to accommodate closure by marking out an ellipse around the area to be removed. The entire ellipse is then resected en bloc down to, but generally not including the underlying fascia. The specimen should be oriented for pathology so any involved margins can be identified postoperatively. In preparation for the SLNB, we recommend performing preoperative lympho scintigraphy in this case, as the shoulder region may drain to the axillary and/or cervical/periclavicular regions. Intradermal injection around the primary tumor with blue dye at the time of surgery should also be performed prior to SLNB as a dual tracer method is the most commonly employed approach to SLNB. If same-day lymphoscintigraphy is not performed, radiotracer is also intradermally injected at the same time as the blue dye. We generally harvest any lymph nodes that are stained blue and/or contain increased focal radiotracer uptake activity (the latter as detected by gamma probe scanning). Each SLN is sent for permanent histologic assessment with serial sectioning and immunohistochemical staining of the SLNs.

Postoperative Management

Patients who are otherwise healthy will usually be discharged home from the recovery area after the above procedure and follow-up in clinic in a few weeks, or sooner based on the specific reconstructive procedure performed. The patient returned to clinic for follow-up. Final pathology revealed the presence of metastatic melanoma in 3 of 3 axillary SLNs. The SLN tumor deposit location was subcapsular and the maximum SLN tumor diameter was 0.6 mm. Molecular analysis revealed no BRAF V600 mutation (i.e., it is BRAF wild type). After multidisciplinary tumor board the decision is made to initiate adjuvant checkpoint blockade.

Common Curve Balls

- Occult disease in SLNs on final pathology upstages the patient to stage III. It is appropriate to formally stage this patient with stage III disease via CT or PET/CT, often along with MRI brain, obtain molecular profiling of the tumor, and refer to medical oncology to participate in a multidisciplinary discussion of adjuvant therapy.
- Recurrence in the nodal basin after positive SLNB was as high as 33% at 3 years in MSLT-II; clinicians must remain vigilant during surveillance. Salvage lymph node dissection can be considered with isolated regional recurrence.
- The side effects of immunotherapy can develop during or following therapy and must be considered if a patient presents with any potential immune-related side effects.

Take Home Points

- It is important to consider both tumor thickness of the primary melanoma and its ulceration status, along with other clinicopathologic factors, when determining risk of SLN tumor involvement and recommendations for SLNB.
- Active nodal basin surveillance and omission of CLND after positive SLNB is supported by MSLT-II and the DeCOG-SLT trials.
- Checkpoint inhibitor immunotherapy is associated with many possible immune-related side effects, which in some cases can be severe and permanent.

Case Scenario 2

Presentation

A 59-year-old fair-skinned man presents after noticing a brown lesion on his right thigh that had been slowly growing over the past several years. A shave biopsy was performed by his dermatologist, and the final pathology revealed a melanoma that was recorded as 2.9 mm in tumor thickness with a positive (i.e., tumor involved) deep biopsy margin, 5 mitotic figures per mm^2, and no ulceration. He now presents to see you for an initial consultation. His past medical history is only notable for well-controlled HTN. He has no prior family or personal history of skin cancer. On examination, you notice residual pigmentation and a healing scab at the biopsy site, and an approximately 2-cm firm, palpable right inguinal lymph node. He also notes worsening headaches.

Differential Diagnosis
Inguinal Lymphadenopathy in the Setting of a Known Melanoma Primary

Metastatic melanoma
Reactive lymphadenopathy from the recent shave biopsy

| Lymphadenopathy from other infectious process in the right lower extremity |
| Concurrent lymphoma or other hematogenous disease |
| Metastatic disease from another solid tumor (rare) |

Confirmation of Diagnosis and Treatment

It is our practice at MD Anderson to have each patient's biopsy reviewed by our pathologists. Special attention should be paid to the primary tumor thickness, mitotic rate, presence of ulceration, lymphovascular and/or perineural invasion, and any positive biopsy margins. In the example above, the deep margin was positive so it can be inferred that the true depth of the lesion may be greater than 2.9 mm. This is particularly important to consider for lesions approaching 0.8 mm with a positive deep margin, as SLNB may be considered since the true depth of the lesion may be greater than what was noted on pathologic analysis.

You refer the patient for image-guided FNA of the right inguinal lymphadenopathy, which confirms metastatic melanoma on final pathology. Imaging shows inguinal adenopathy in the ipsilateral (right) inguinal nodal basin, which is also PET-avid, with no evidence of pelvic adenopathy or distant disease. No satellites or in-transit metastases are visualized or palpated on physical examination, nor are there any other FDG avid areas of uptake on PET/CT. The patient is referred to medical oncology for discussion of neoadjuvant therapy and participation in a clinical trial, the latter of which he is eager to enroll in. He is found to have a BRAF V600 mutation and is started on dual BRAF/MEK inhibitors. He receives 6 weeks of neoadjuvant therapy and is returns to your clinic for consideration of surgery.

Surgical Approach—Key Steps

For the primary lesion, a 2-cm margin wide excision is recommended. For a superficial groin lymph node dissection, key boundaries include the sartorius laterally, the adductor longus medially, approximately 5 cm above inguinal ligament superiorly, the apex of the femoral triangle inferiorly, and the femoral vessels deep to the dissection plane. All nodal tissue in the femoral triangle should be removed, as well as any nodal tissue that lies superficial to the external oblique above the inguinal ligament. A closed suction drain(s) should be placed prior to closure. There is generally no reason to resect the saphenous vein solely from an oncologic perspective. A Sartorius muscle transposition flap may be performed.

Postoperative Management

Our practice is to admit patients overnight after superficial groin dissection to ensure adequate pain control and mobility prior to discharge. Diet is advanced as tolerated, generally to clears on POD0 and regular on POD1. The patient is also instructed on drain care before discharge the following day. The drain generally remains in place until output is less than 30 cc for at least 2 consecutive days or until about 1 month after surgery if output remains high.

Common Curve Balls

- Development of postoperative seroma in the surgical bed. These can be observed if small and asymptomatic but may require drainage if there is concern for infected seroma or if causing symptoms.
- Postoperative cellulitis requiring at minimum oral antibiotics, but may require readmission and IV antibiotics if moderate or severe.
- Development of postoperative DVT necessitating therapeutic anticoagulation.

Take Home Points

- Full staging workup is required for stage III disease, and generally includes a brain MRI and either a PET/CT or CT chest, abdomen, and pelvis. PET/CT is often preferred as an initial staging approach for the patient with an extremity primary to include potential sites of satellite or in-transit metastases.
- FNA is the procedure of choice to confirm nodal disease.
- Neoadjuvant checkpoint inhibitor immunotherapy or targeted therapy (the latter only considered for patients with BRAF V600 tumor mutations) should be considered prior to surgery for those with clinically evident nodal disease at the time of diagnosis, ideally in the context of a clinical trial.

CASE SCENARIO REVIEW

Questions

1. What surgical procedure(s) would you propose for the patient in scenario 1's melanoma following their biopsy?

   A. Primary tumor wide excision with 0.5-cm margins only
   B. Primary tumor wide excision with 1-cm margins only
   C. Primary tumor wide excision with 0.5-cm margins and lymphatic mapping and sentinel lymph node biopsy
   D. Primary tumor wide excision with 2-cm margins and lymphatic mapping and sentinel lymph node biopsy

2. What is the next best step in the management of the above patient's melanoma after their initial operation?

   A. Nodal basin observation with active surveillance via serial ultrasound and physical examination; postoperative referral to medical oncology not recommended since primary tumor thickness less than 1 mm
   B. Nodal basin observation with active surveillance via serial ultrasound and physical examination; referral to medical oncology to discuss adjuvant PD-1 checkpoint inhibitor immunotherapy
   C. Axillary lymph node dissection; postoperative referral to medical oncology not recommended since primary tumor thickness less than 1 mm
   D. Axillary lymph node dissection; referral to medical oncology to discuss PD-1 adjuvant checkpoint inhibitor immunotherapy

3. The patient outlined in case 1 is offered adjuvant anti–PD-1 based immunotherapy to reduce her risk of recurrence. What are the possible immune side effect(s) of such therapy?

   A. Diabetes and other endocrinopathies
   B. Severe colitis and diarrhea
   C. Myocarditis
   D. All of the above

4. An otherwise healthy individual is diagnosed with a 2.9-mm melanoma of the right thigh with a positive deep margin and 5 mitoses per mm^2. On examination at the time of presentation he is noted to have right inguinal lymphadenopathy. FNA of his right inguinal lymph node confirms metastatic melanoma. After 6 weeks of neoadjuvant BRAF/MEK inhibition he presents to your surgical oncology clinic with a full staging workup (MRI brain and CT chest, abdomen, and pelvis) that does not reveal additional disease. What is the next best step in management for this patient following their neoadjuvant therapy?

   A. Proceed directly to the operating room for wide excision of the right thigh primary site and lymphatic mapping and sentinel lymph node biopsy
   B. Proceed directly to the operating room for open excisional biopsy of the suspicious nodes to assess for metastatic disease
   C. Proceed to the operating room for management of the primary site and nodal basin
   D. Obtain FNA biopsy of the palpable lymphadenopathy and if confirms metastatic melanoma

5. What surgical procedure(s) should you consent the above patient in question 4 for?

   A. Wide excision of the primary site only
   B. Wide excision of the primary site with SLNB
   C. Wide excision of the primary site and right superficial inguinal lymph node dissection
   D. Wide excision of the primary site with right superficial and deep inguinal lymph node dissection

Answers

1. **The correct answer is D.** *Rationale:* For an invasive melanoma whose tumor thickness is >2 mm, a 2-cm margin should be obtained. Lymphatic mapping and sentinel lymph node (SLN) biopsy (SLNB) should be considered for any primary lesions staged as T1b or higher, which includes melanomas with a tumor thickness at least 0.8 mm deep or those of any thickness with ulceration present.

2. **The correct answer is B.** *Rationale:* Results from the MSLT-II randomized clinical trial demonstrated no difference in survival for patients with a positive SLN who had completion lymph node dissection (CLND) compared to patients randomized to nodal basin observation with active surveillance. CLND (included in choices C and D) is therefore no longer recommended for most patients. Since she has stage III disease (more specifically, stage IIIC), referral to medical oncology is warranted to discuss the risks and benefits of immunotherapy. Indeed, for patients with stage AJCC 8th edition stage IIIA melanoma, the benefits may not outweigh the potential risks of therapy, and a multidisciplinary approach to decision-making, including active dialog with the patient, is important.

3. **The correct answer is D.** *Rationale:* Numerous immune-related side effects are possible with immunotherapy, including diabetes, hyperthyroidism, hypothyroidism, hypophysitis, pneumonitis, myocarditis, nephritis, colitis, and vitiligo. Many of these immune-related side effects are permanent even after stopping therapy. Side effects can sometimes be severe and may require hospitalization, IV steroids, IVIG, hormone replacement, and/or plasmapheresis in some cases. In general, adverse events are worse with ipilimumab (a CTLA-4 inhibitor) or combination anti-CTLA-4/anti–PD-1-based approach compared to anti-PD-1 alone, but may still occur with single-agent anti–PD-1 agents.

4. **The correct answer is C.** *Rationale:* Prior to the neoadjuvant therapy, this patient had clinically palpable biopsy-confirmed metastatic melanoma to the groin. Following neoadjuvant therapy, restaging of the patient is indicated to rule out additional regional and/or distant metastatic disease prior to proceeding with planned surgical treatment, as such findings would alter the treatment plan (excludes choices A and B). He also notes worsening headaches which should further prompt MRI brain to rule out brain metastases. Excisional biopsy is not indicated, as this is rarely indicated to confirm metastatic disease, and biopsy-proven metastatic melanoma to the inguinal basin was already confirmed prior to neoadjuvant therapy (excludes choice D).

5. **The correct answer is C.** *Rationale:* Based upon imaging, superficial lymph node dissection is all that is definitely indicated at this time. Iliac and obturator node dissection is indicated if staging reveals suspicious adenopathy and can be considered if Cloquet's node is biopsied and noted to be positive on frozen section analysis, although this latter approach has become uncommon. Of note, reports to date support that >50% of stage IIIB/IIIC patients treated with neoadjuvant BRAF/MEK inhibitors will have a pathologic complete response. Once lymph node metastasis is confirmed, there is no role for SLNB of the affected basin (choice B), and the current standard of care supports that lymph node dissection be performed for patients with stage III disease with regional lymph node metastasis who are medically fit to undergo the procedure (choice C). Deep groin nodal dissection can always be performed in the future if the patient develops resectable iliac or obturator disease without distant metastasis; there is no absolute indication for concomitant deep groin dissection in this scenario (choice D). Choice A does not consider surgical management of the known inguinal disease.

Recommended Readings

Aloia TA, Gershenwald JE. Utility of computed tomography and magnetic resonance imaging staging before completion lymphadenectomy in patients with sentinel lymph node-positive melanoma. *J Clin Oncol* 2006;24(28):2858–2865.

Amaria RN, Prieto PA, Tetzlaff MT, et al. Neoadjuvant plus adjuvant dabrafenib and trametinib versus standard of care in patients with high-risk, surgically resectable melanoma: a single-centre, open-label, randomized, phase 2 trial. *Lancet Oncol* 2018;19(2):181–193.

Amaria RN, Reddy SM, Tawbi HA, et al. Neoadjuvant immune checkpoint blockade in high-risk resectable melanoma. *Nat Med* 2018;24(11):1649–1654.

Andtbacka RH, Gershenwald JE. Role of sentinel lymph node biopsy in patients with thin melanoma. *J Natl Compr Canc Netw* 2009;7(3):308–317.

Andtbacka RH, Kaufman HL, Collichio F et al. Talimogene laherparepvec improves durable response rate in patients with advanced melanoma. *J Clin Oncol* 2015;33(25):2780.

Ariyan CE, Brady MS, Siegelbaum RH, et al. Robust antitumor responses result from local chemotherapy and CTLA-4 blockade. *Cancer Immunol Res* 2018;6(2):189–200.

Ascierto PA, Del Vecchio M, Mandalá M, et al. Adjuvant nivolumab versus ipilimumab in resected stage IIIB-C and stage IV melanoma (CheckMate 238): 4-year results from a multicentre, double-blind, randomised, controlled, phase 3 trial. *Lancet Oncol* 2020;21(11):1465–1477.

Atkins MB, Lee SJ, Chmielowski B, et al. DREAMseq: A phase III trial—ECOG-ACRIN EA6134. *ASCO Plenary Series*. Abstract 356154.

Balch CM, Soong SJ, Ross MI, et al. Long-term results of a multi-institutional randomized trial comparing prognostic factors and surgical results for intermediate thickness melanomas (1.0 to 4.0 mm). Intergroup Melanoma Surgical Trial. *Ann Surg Oncol* 2000;7:87–97.

Beasley GM, Caudle A, Peterson RP, et al. A multi-institutional experience of isolated limb perfusion: defining response and toxicity in the US. *J Am Coll Surg* 2009;208(5):706–715.

Blank CU, Rozeman EA, Fanchi LF, et al. Neoadjuvant versus adjuvant ipilimumab plus nivolumab in macroscopic stage III melanoma. *Nat Med* 2018;24:1655–1661.

Cancer Genome Atlas Network. Genomic classification of cutaneous melanoma. *Cell* 2015;161(7):1681–1696.

Chapman PB, Hauschild A, Robert C, et al. Improved survival with vemurafenib in melanoma with BRAF V600E mutation. *N Engl J Med*. 2011;364(26):2507–2516.

Cormier JN, Xing Y, Feng L, et al. Metastatic melanoma to lymph nodes in patients with unknown primary sites. *Cancer* 2006;106:2012–2020.

Curtin JA, Fridlyand J, Kageshita T, et al. Distinct sets of genetic alterations in melanoma. *N Engl J Med* 2005;353(20):2135–2147.

Davies H, Bignell GR, Cox C, et al. Mutations of the BRAF gene in human cancer. *Nature* 2002;417(6892):949–954.

Davies MA, Saiag P, Robert C, et al. Dabrafenib plus trametinib in patients with BRAFV600-mutant melanoma brain metastases (COMBI-MB): a multicenter, multicohort, open-label, phase 2 trial. *Lancet Oncol* 2017;18(7):863–873.

Dummer R, Gyorki DE, Hyngstrom J, et al. Neoadjuvant talimogene laherparepvec plus surgery versus surgery alone for resectable stage IIIB-IVM1a melanoma: a randomized, open-label, phase 2 trial. *Nat Med* 2021;27(10):1789–1796.

Eggermont AM, Blank CU, Mandala M, et al. Adjuvant pembrolizumab versus placebo in resected stage III melanoma (EORTC 1325-MG/KEYNOTE-054): distant metastasis-free survival results from a double-blind, randomised, controlled, phase 3 trial. *Lancet Oncol* 2021;22(5):643–654.

Eggermont AM, Chiarion-Sileni V, Grob JJ, et al. Adjuvant ipilimumab versus placebo after complete resection of high-risk stage III melanoma (EORTC 18071): a randomised, double-blind, phase 3 trial. *Lancet Oncol* 2015;16(5):522–530.

Eggermont AM, Chiarion-Sileni V, Grob JJ, et al. Prolonged survival in stage III melanoma with ipilimumab adjuvant therapy. *N Engl J Med* 2016;375(19):1845–1855.

Faries MB, Thompson JF, Cochran A, et al. The impact on morbidity and length of stay of early versus delayed complete lymphadenectomy in melanoma: results of the Multicenter Selective Lymphadenectomy Trial (I). *Ann Surg Oncol* 2010;17(12):3324–3329.

Faries MB, Thompson JF, Cochran AJ, et al. Completion dissection or observation for sentinel-node metastasis in melanoma. *N Engl J Med* 2017;376:2211–2222.

Flaherty KT, Infante JR, Daud A, et al. Combined BRAF and MEK inhibition in melanoma with BRAF V600 mutations. *N Engl J Med* 2012;367:1694–703.

Flaherty KT, Puzanov I, Kim KB, et al. Inhibition of mutated, activated BRAF in metastatic melanoma. *N Engl J Med* 2010;363(9):809–819.

Flaherty KT, Robert C, Hersey P, et al. Improved survival with MEK inhibition in BRAF-mutated melanoma. *N Engl J Med* 2012;367:107–114.

Gannon CJ, Rousseau DL Jr, Ross MI, et al. Accuracy of lymphatic mapping and sentinel lymph node biopsy after previous wide local excision in patients with primary melanoma. *Cancer* 2006;107(11):2647–2652.

Gershenwald JE, Andtbacka RH, Prieto VG, et al. Microscopic tumor burden in sentinel lymph nodes predicts synchronous nonsentinel lymph node involvement in patients with melanoma. *J Clin Oncol* 2008;26(26):4296–4303.

Gershenwald JE, Colome MI, Lee JE, et al. Patterns of recurrence following a negative sentinel lymph node biopsy in 243 patients with stage I or II melanoma. *J Clin Oncol* 1998;16:2253–2260.

Gershenwald JE, Ross MI. Sentinel-lymph-node biopsy for cutaneous melanoma. *N Engl J Med* 2011;364(18):1738–1745.

Gershenwald JE, Scolyer RA, Hess KR, et al. Melanoma Staging: Evidence-based Changes in the American Joint Committee on Cancer Eighth Edition Cancer Staging Manual. *CA Cancer J Clin.* 2017; 67(6): 472–492.

Gershenwald JE, Scolyer RA, Hess KR, et al. Melanoma of the skin. In: Amin MB, Edge SB, Greene FL, et al., eds. *AJCC Cancer Staging Manual.* 8th ed. Springer; 2017:563–585.

Gershenwald JE, Thompson W, Mansfield PF, et al. Multi-institutional melanoma lymphatic mapping experience: the prognostic value of sentinel lymph node status in 612 stage I or II melanoma patients. *J Clin Oncol* 1999;17:976–983.

Gershenwald JE, Tseng CH, Thompson W, et al. Improved sentinel lymph node localization in patients with primary melanoma with the use of radiolabeled colloid. *Surgery* 1998;124:203–210.

Hawkins WG, Busam KJ, Ben-Porat L, et al. Desmoplastic melanoma: a pathologically and clinically distinct form of cutaneous melanoma. *Ann Surg Oncol* 2005;12:207–213.

Hodi FS, Chesney J, Pavlick AC, et al. Combined nivolumab and ipilimumab versus ipilimumab alone in patients with advanced melanoma: 2-year overall survival outcomes in a multicentre, randomised, controlled, phase 2 trial. *Lancet Oncol* 2016;17(11):1558–1568.

Hodi FS, O'Day SJ, McDermott DF, et al. Improved survival with ipilimumab in patients with metastatic melanoma. *N Engl J Med* 2010;363(8):711–723. Erratum in: *N Engl J Med.* 2010;363(13):1290.

Huang AC, Orlowski RJ, Xu X, et al. A single dose of neoadjuvant PD-1 blockade predicts clinical outcomes in resectable melanoma. *Nat Med* 2019;25(3):454–461.

International Agency for Research on Cancer Working Group on Artificial Ultraviolet (UV) Light and Skin Cancer. The association of use of sunbeds with cutaneous malignant melanoma and other skin cancers: A systematic review. *Int J Cancer* 2007;120:1116–1122.

Keung EZ, Gershenwald JE. The eight edition American Joint Committee on Cancer (AJCC) melanoma staging system: implications for melanoma treatment and care. *Expert Rev Anticancer Ther* 2018;18(8):775–784.

Kroon HM, Moncrieff M, Kam PC, Thompson JF. Outcomes following isolated limb infusion for melanoma. A 14-year experience. *Ann Surg Oncol* 2008;15(11):3003–3013.

Larkin J, Ascierto PA, Dreno B, et al. Combined vemurafenib and cobimetinib in BRAF-mutated melanoma. *N Engl J Med* 2014;371:1867–1876.

Leiter U, Stadler R, Mauch C, et al. Complete lymph node dissection versus no dissection in patients with sentinel lymph node biopsy positive melanoma (DeCOG-SLT): a multicentre, randomised, phase 3 trial. *Lancet Oncol* 2016;17(6):757–767.

Leiter U, Stadler R, Mauch C, et al. Final analysis of DeCOG-SLT trial: no survival benefit for complete lymph node dissection in patients with melanoma with positive sentinel node. *J Clin Oncol* 2019;37(32):3000–3008.

Lo SN, Ma J, Scolyer RA, et al. Improved risk prediction calculator for sentinel node positivity in patients with melanoma: The Melanoma Institute Australia Nomogram. *J Clin Oncol* 2020;38(24):2719–2727.

Long GV, Atkinson V, Cebon JS, et al. Standard-dose pembrolizumab in combination with reduced-dose ipilimumab for patients with advanced melanoma (KEYNOTE-029): an open-label, phase 1b trial. *Lancet Oncol* 2017;18(9):1202–1210.

Long GV, Hauschild A, Santinami M, et al. Adjuvant dabrafenib plus trametinib in stage III BRAF-mutated melanoma. *N Engl J Med* 2017;377(19):1813–1823.

Long GV, Menzies AM, Nagrial AM, et al. Prognostic and clinicopathologic associations of oncogenic BRAF in metastatic melanoma. *J Clin Oncol* 2011;29(10):1239–1246.

Long GV, Saw RP, Lo S, et al. Neoadjuvant dabrafenib combined with trametinib for resectable, stage IIIB-C, BRAFV600 mutation-positive melanoma (NeoCombi): a single-arm, open-label, single-centre, phase 2 trial. *Lancet Oncol* 2019;20(7):961–971.

Marchetti MA, Coit DG, Dusza SW, et al. Performance of gene expression profile tests for prognosis in patients with localized cutaneous melanoma: a systematic review and meta-analysis. *JAMA Dermatol.* 2020;156(9):953–962.

Menzies AM, Amaria RN, Rozeman EA, et al. Pathological response and survival with neoadjuvant therapy in melanoma: a pooled analysis from the International Neoadjuvant Melanoma Consortium (INMC). *Nat Med* 2021;27(2):301–309.

Morton DL, Cochran AJ, Thompson JF, et al. Sentinel node biopsy for early-stage melanoma: accuracy and morbidity in MSLT-I, an international multicenter trial. *Ann Surg* 2005;242(3):302–311; discussion 311–313.

Morton DL, Thompson JF, Cochran AJ, et al. Final trial report of sentinel-node biopsy versus nodal observation in melanoma. *N Engl J Med* 2014;370(7):599.

Morton DL, Wen DR, Wong JH, et al. Technical details of intraoperative lymphatic mapping for early stage melanoma. *Arch Surg* 1992;127:392–399.

Murali R, Desilva C, Thompson JF, et al. Non-Sentinel Node Risk Score (N-SNORE): a scoring system for accurately stratifying risk of non-sentinel node positivity in patients with cutaneous melanoma with positive sentinel lymph nodes. *J Clin Oncol* 2010;28(29):4441–4449.

O'Meara AT, Cress R, Xing G, Danielsen B, Smith LH. Malignant melanoma in pregnancy. A population-based evaluation. *Cancer.* 2005;103:1217–1226.

Pawlik TM, Ross MI, Johnson MM, et al. Predictors and natural history of in-transit melanoma after sentinel lymphadenectomy. *Ann Surg Oncol* 2005;12:587–596.

Pawlik TM, Ross MI, Prieto VG, et al. Assessment of the role of sentinel lymph node biopsy for primary cutaneous desmoplastic melanoma. *Cancer* 2006;106(4):900–906.

Pawlik TM, Ross MI, Thompson JF, Eggermont AM, Gershenwald JE. The risk of in-transit melanoma metastasis depends on tumor biology and not the surgical approach to regional lymph nodes. *J Clin Oncol* 2005;23:4588–4590.

Pollock PM, Harper UL, Hansen KS, et al. High frequency of BRAF mutations in nevi. *Nat Genet* 2003;33(1):19–20.

Rosenberg SA, Yang JC, Sherry RM, et al. Durable complete responses in heavily pretreated patients with metastatic melanoma using T cell transfer immunotherapy. *Clin Cancer Res* 2011;17(13):4550–4557.

Rosenberg SA, Yannelli JR, Yang JC, et al. Treatment of patients with metastatic melanoma with autologous tumor-infiltrating lymphocytes and interleukin 2. *J Natl Cancer Inst* 1994;86:1159–1166.

Rozeman EA, Menzies AM, van Akkooi ACJ, et al. Identification of the optimal combination dosing schedule of neoadjuvant ipilimumab plus nivolumab in macroscopic stage III melanoma (OpACIN-neo): a multicentre, phase 2, randomised, controlled trial. *Lancet Oncol* 2019;20(7):948–960.

Scolyer RA, Prieto VG. Melanoma pathology: important issues for clinicians involved in the multidisciplinary care of melanoma patients. *Surg Oncol Clin N Am* 2011;20(1):19–37.

Scolyer RA, Thompson JF, McCarthy SW. Intraoperative frozen-section evaluation can reduce accuracy of pathologic assessment of sentinel nodes in melanoma patients. *J Am Coll Surg* 2005;201(5):821–823.

Tarhini AA, Lee SJ, Hodi FS, et al. Phase III study of adjuvant ipilimumab (3 or 10 mg/kg) versus high-dose interferon alfa-2b for resected high-risk melanoma: North American Intergroup E1609. *J Clin Oncol.* 2020;38(6):567–575.

Tawbi HA, Schadendorf D, Lipson EJ, et al. Relatlimab and Nivolumab versus Nivolumab in Untreated Advanced Melanoma. *N Engl J Med* 2022;386(1):24–34

Thompson JF, Soong SJ, Balch CM, et al. Prognostic significance of mitotic rate in localized primary cutaneous melanoma: an analysis of patients in the multi-institutional American Joint Committee on Cancer melanoma staging database. *J Clin Oncol* 2011;29(16):2199–2205.

Tripp MK, Watson M, Balk SJ, et al. State of the science on prevention and screening to reduce melanoma incidence and mortality: the time is now. *CA Cancer J Clin* 2016;66:460–480.

Uren RF. SPECT/CT lymphoscintigraphy to locate the sentinel lymph nodes in melanoma. *Ann Surg Oncol* 2009;16:1459–1460.

Weber J, Mandala M, Del Vecchio M, et al. Adjuvant nivolumab versus ipilimumab in resected stage III or IV melanoma. *NEJM.* 2017;377(19):1824–1835. doi:10.1056/NEJMoa1709030. Epub 2017 Sep 10.

Wolchok JD, Chiarion-Sileni V, Gonzalez R, et al. Overall survival with combined nivolumab in advanced melanoma. *N Engl J Med* 2017;377:1345–1356.

Wolchok JD, Neyns B, Linette G, et al. Ipilimumab monotherapy in patients with pretreated advanced melanoma: a randomised, double-blind, multicentre, phase 2, dose-ranging study. *Lancet Oncol* 2010;11(2):155.

4 Nonmelanoma Skin Cancers

Brandon M. Cope, Russell G. Witt, Rachel Feig, and Emily Z. Keung

Epidemiology

The term nonmelanoma skin cancers (NMSCs) encompasses a broad range of cutaneous neoplasms, including cutaneous lymphomas, Kaposi sarcoma, carcinosarcoma, and Merkel cell carcinomas (MCCs). However, the term is most commonly used to refer to the keratinocyte cancers, basal cell carcinomas (BCCs) and squamous cell carcinomas (SCCs). BCC and SCC together represent >95% of total malignant skin tumors. The incidence of both BCC and SCC continues to rise at nearly 10% per year with 2 to 3 million new cases diagnosed annually. Overall, BCC and SCC have a higher incidence in men and overall incidence increases with age.

Differential Diagnosis

The differential diagnosis for NMSC is extensive and consists of both benign and malignant processes. Recognition of the latter is important for both tumor surveillance and cancer prevention. Seborrheic keratoses, actinic keratosis (AK), melanoma, keratoacanthoma, cutaneous horns, and nevus sebaceous represent some of the entities on the differential diagnosis. Obtaining a biopsy of a suspicious lesion in order to reach a pathologic diagnosis is pivotal in determining appropriate management of the patient.

Seborrheic keratoses are benign proliferations of epidermis that can appear on any part of the skin, except mucous membranes, and usually appear after the age of 30 years. They are not related to sun exposure but are common on the face, neck, and trunk, often in large numbers. They initially appear as flat brown macules, eventually becoming larger, "stuck-on" brown plaques with dull crumbly surfaces (Fig. 4.1A). Seborrheic keratoses can sometimes be confused with skin cancer, and biopsy of these lesions is prudent if any sudden changes in size or color occur.

AKs are premalignant lesions with the potential to develop into SCCs. They are found mainly on sun-exposed areas. These lesions most commonly present as skin-colored, erythematous, or brown ill-defined patches with adherent scales (Fig. 4.1B). These lesions are extremely common on the face, scalp, ears, and lips and can often be better appreciated by palpation rather than by inspection with the naked eye.

Keratoacanthoma is a tumor that often occurs on older, sun-damaged skin and is most commonly found on the neck and face. These tumors originate in pilosebaceous glands and may grow rapidly as a red- or skin-colored dome-shaped nodule with a central crater. Maximum size may be attained at 6 to 8 weeks with slow regression over a period of months, leaving a residual scar. These tumors can be confused both clinically

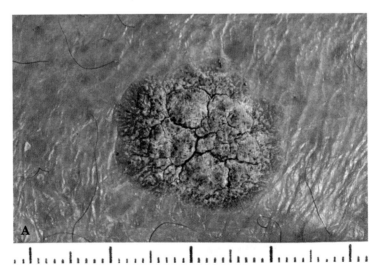

FIGURE 4.1 A: Seborrheic keratosis. (Reprinted with permission from Elder DE. *Lever's Dermatopathology: Histopathology of the Skin*. 12th ed. Wolters Kluwer; 2022. Figure 29.10.) *(continued)*

and histologically with SCC, and there are reports of progression of keratoacanthomas to invasive or meta-static carcinoma. Classification of these tumors as a well-differentiated variant of invasive SCC has been pro-posed. Surgical excision of keratoacanthomas with 3- to 5-mm margins is recommended, and Mohs surgery may be employed in cosmetically sensitive areas. These tumors are radiosensitive if surgery is not an option.

A cutaneous horn is the clinical description for a growth that appears as a dense cone of epithelium resem-bling a horn (Fig. 4.1C). They range in size from several millimeters to over a centimeter and are generally

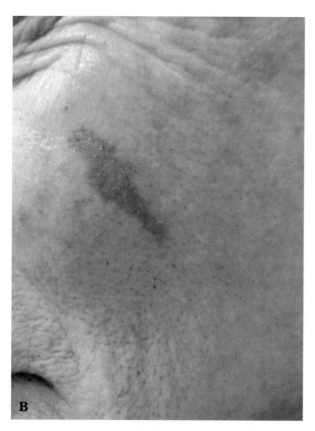

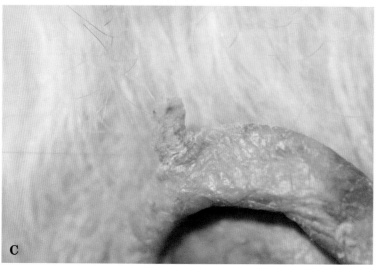

FIGURE 4.1 (Continued) B: Actinic keratosis. (Reprinted with permission from Rose M. Oncology in Primary Care. Philadelphia, PA: Wolters Kluwer; 2013. Figure 61.4.) **C:** Cutaneous horn. (Reprinted with permission from Elder DE. *Lever's Dermatopathology: Histopathology of the Skin*, 12th ed. Wolters Kluwer; 2023. Figure 29.54.)

white or yellowish in color; they also tend to appear on sun-exposed skin of older individuals. Histologically, cutaneous horns can develop from benign lesions such as warts or seborrheic keratoses, from premalignant lesions such as AKs and SCCs in situ or from malignant lesions such as SCCs. Up to 15% of cutaneous horns demonstrate invasive SCCs at the base, and excision of these tumors is always indicated.

Nevus sebaceous is a benign tumor of the scalp that appears at or soon after birth as a yellowish-orange, well-demarcated plaque. Initially, the surface has a smooth or waxy appearance that gradually becomes more warty or verrucous during puberty. In adulthood, approximately 10% of these lesions develop into BCC. It is therefore recommended that these lesions be excised or closely monitored for the life of the patient.

Basal Cell Carcinoma

BCC is the most common type of skin cancer and the most common cancer in the United States, affecting an estimated 2 million Americans annually. BCCs are believed to arise from hair follicle cells and are therefore found almost exclusively on hair-bearing skin. Most lesions are found on sun-exposed mask areas of the head and neck, but non–sun-exposed areas are also at risk. These tumors tend to grow slowly, but when untreated can lead to invasion of local structures including muscle, cartilage, and bone. Although metastasis is rare with a metastasis rate of <0.1%, local invasion can result in substantial local tissue destruction and disfiguration.

There are multiple histologic subtypes of BCC (Fig. 4.2), and subtype is predictive of its behavior. Less aggressive subtypes include nodular or superficial BCC while higher-risk subtypes include sclerosing, infiltrating, micronodular, morpheaform (or desmoplastic), and basosquamous carcinoma. The higher-risk subtypes tend to have subclinical extension exceeding the visible borders of the lesion, making treatment more difficult.

Nodular BCC is the classic lesion of this type of NMSC and occurs predominantly on the face (Fig. 4.2A). It appears as a pink translucent nodule with rolled edges and is often described as "pearly." In dark-skinned

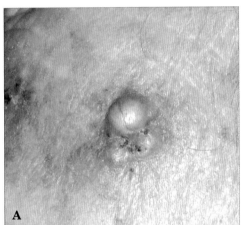
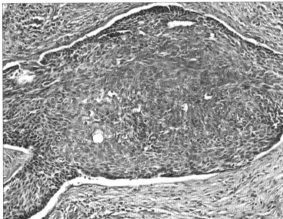
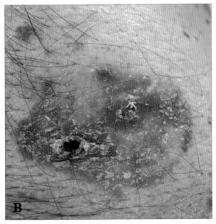
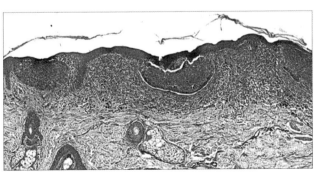

FIGURE 4.2 Basal cell carcinoma. **A:** Nodular type BCC. **B:** Superficial type BCC. (**A, B** from Dourmishev LA, Rusinova D, Botev I. Clinical variants, stages, and management of basal cell carcinoma. *Indian Dermatol Online J.* 2013;4(1):12–17.) *(continued)*

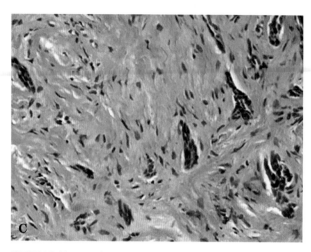

FIGURE 4.2 (Continued) C: Sclerosing type BCC. (Reprinted by permission from Springer: Crowson AN. Basal cell carcinoma: biology, morphology and clinical implications. *Mod Pathol.* 2006;19 Suppl 2:S127–S147.)

individuals, these tumors are often pigmented and can resemble melanoma. Overlying telangiectasias and ulceration are common.

Superficial BCC is a variant that is more common on the limbs and trunk, and on other areas with little or no sun exposure (Fig. 4.2B). It presents as a slow-growing, scaly pink plaque and can easily be confused with psoriasis, superficial SCC, or SCC in situ (Bowen disease). Gentle traction on the periphery of the lesion often demonstrates a shiny translucent surface characteristic of BCC which can assist with diagnosis.

The sclerosing or morpheaform type represents the rarest form of BCC and is often difficult to recognize (Fig. 4.2C). It presents as a poorly defined indurated or sclerotic plaque which can be mistaken for a scar. In addition, this type of BCC frequently is found to be larger histopathologically than is clinically evident. Therefore, both diagnosis and treatment remain a challenge.

Basosquamous carcinomas have histologic features of both BCC and SCC. Some of these lesions occur as a result of collision between adjacent BCC and SCC. These are aggressive tumors with potential to metastasize, with metastatic risk determined by the degree of squamous component present.

Squamous Cell Carcinoma

SCC is the second most common cutaneous carcinoma and is rapidly rising in incidence. SCC develops from keratinocytes of the epidermis and has many clinical variants. Due to the association with chronic sun exposure, SCC rates are higher in occupations involving outdoor work with higher incidences with increased age. Cutaneous SCC is also significantly associated with indoor tanning. SCC is most commonly found on sun-damaged skin, especially on the head, neck, or arms and is usually red, poorly defined plaques or nodules with an ulcerated friable surface (Fig. 4.3). Bowen disease, or SCC in situ, is characterized by a rapidly growing, well-demarcated ulcerating tumor in a pre-existing scaly, erythematous plaque. Up to 5% of Bowen disease may become invasive. SCC can arise from precursor lesions such as AKs or can develop at the base of a cutaneous horn (see "Differential Diagnosis"). Uncommonly, SCC presents de novo as a single lesion on otherwise normal-appearing skin.

Although distant metastasis due to NMSC is rare, SCC has higher metastatic potential than BCC, and is responsible for the majority of deaths from NMSC. SCC regional metastasis is associated with increased risk of recurrence and mortality and is associated with adverse pathologic features (lymphovascular invasion, poor differentiation, perineural invasion).

Risk Factors for NMSC

Development of NMSC is multifactorial and is related to various genotypic, phenotypic, and environmental risk factors. Ultraviolet (UV) solar radiation is considered to be the dominant risk factor for the development of both BCC and SCC, supported by the fact that most of these tumors tend to present on sun-exposed areas of the body. The development of BCC is thought to arise from intense intermittent sun exposure leading to burns, whereas SCC appears to be linked to the cumulative dose of UV solar radiation over time. Markers of

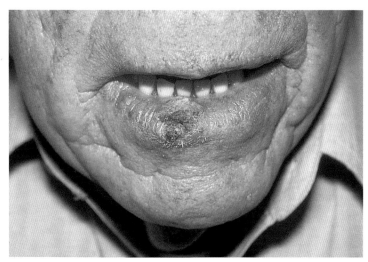

FIGURE 4.3 Squamous cell carcinoma. (From Goodheart HP, MD. *Goodheart's Photoguide of Common Skin Disorders*, 2nd ed. Lippincott Williams & Wilkins; 2003. Figure 8.18.)

UV sensitivity (e.g., fair skin, light eyes, blond or red hair) and intensity of exposure (i.e., increased incidence for individuals living in proximity to the equator) are associated with increased NMSC risk as is additional UV exposure from recreational tanning and UV light therapy. One case-controlled study demonstrated that the use of tanning devices was associated with an estimated twofold risk for both SCC (odds ratio = 2.5) and BCC (odds ratio = 1.5). Karagas et al. reported that treatment of psoriasis with oral psoralen in combination with light treatment resulted in an increased adjusted relative risk of 8.6 for SCC.

Another important risk factor for both BCC and SCC development is immunosuppression. Long-term immunosuppression therapy such as that used for solid organ transplant has been shown to increase the risk of BCC about 5- to 10-fold and SCC over 100-fold. SCC in immunosuppressed patients tends to behave more aggressively and is associated with greater depth, higher risk of recurrence, and perineural and/or lymphovascular invasion. BCC has not been found to be more aggressive in solid organ transplant recipients than the general population. Patients with acquired immunodeficiency syndrome also have an increased incidence of NMSC. This increased risk may result from decreased tumor surveillance by one's own immune system or may be attributed to immunosuppressive medications. Infection or reactivation of dormant human papillomavirus (HPV) in an immunosuppressed state is also believed to be a contributing factor. HPV has known carcinogenic effects in individuals infected with oncogenic virus subtypes, leading to SCC in mucosal and anogenital regions.

Prior receipt of ionizing radiation is associated with a threefold increased risk of NMSC and often presents decades after initial exposure. This risk has been shown to be dose dependent. Many other chemical exposures demonstrate a similar dose-dependent relationship; SCC has been associated with exposures to chemicals including arsenic, tar, soot, tobacco, and asphalt. SCC can also arise from areas of chronic inflammation and healing such as from scars, burn sites, or ulcers. This type of SCC is known as a Marjolin ulcer.

Patients with genetic syndromes including xeroderma pigmentosum, albinism, Muir–Torre syndrome, dystrophic epidermolysis bullosa, Fanconi anemia, Werner syndrome, nevoid basal cell syndrome, and Li–Fraumeni syndrome have an increased incidence of NMSC. Xeroderma pigmentosum is a rare autosomal recessive disease characterized by photophobia, severe sun sensitivity, and accelerated sun damage. Affected individuals have defective DNA excision repair, and when exposed to UV radiation, develop malignancies of the skin and eyes at a rate 1,000 times that of the general population. Aggressive sun protection in the form of full-body sun suits and regular skin examinations are critical for patients with xeroderma pigmentosum. Ideally, these patients should only go outside at night. Nevoid basal cell syndrome is an autosomal dominant disorder characterized by the development of multiple BCCs. BCCs in patients with nevoid basal cell syndrome are often quite small but can number in the hundreds on any given skin surface. The sonic hedgehog signaling pathway (PTCH1 gene, chromosome 9q) has been recognized as having a significant etiologic role in nevoid BCC syndrome, and is also present in 90% of sporadic BCC. These patients are exquisitely sensitive to radiation and should avoid excessive sun exposure and radiation therapy (RT). Regular follow-up is important, as such tumors are difficult to monitor and treat.

Workup and Biopsy Techniques

The initial evaluation of any suspected NMSC should include a thorough history, including reported duration, rate of growth, associated symptoms, previous treatment, and risk factors for NMSC and melanoma. Changes noted by the patient may be quite subtle and include itching, tenderness, bleeding, or changes in size, color, or texture. A detailed head-to-toe skin examination and lymph node examination should be performed; it is important to recognize that patients with suspected NMSC are at risk of additional NMSCs, melanoma, and premalignant lesions.

Any cutaneous lesion suspicious for malignancy should be biopsied for pathologic assessment. Punch or excisional biopsy of suspicious pigmented lesions is preferred. A punch biopsy usually ranges in size from 2 to 8 mm and involves removing a cylinder of tissue, ideally to the level of the subcutaneous fat. Often, entire lesions can be removed for pathologic examination; if not, the most suspicious aspect of the tumor may be sampled.

Excisional biopsy involves removal of the entire lesion with a margin of clinically clear tissue and is generally used for classic lesions such as superficial SCCs or nodular and superficial BCCs. Margins can be evaluated in the specimen, and further treatment is often unnecessary.

Shave biopsy may be considered for superficial lesions or nonpigmented lesions suspicious for BCC or SCC. It is also a good biopsy technique for cutaneous horns or keratoacanthomas, provided the base of the tumor is included in the specimen. A shave biopsy involves injecting local anesthesia into the epidermis and upper dermis and then performing a tangential incision at the base of the wheal. A sterile flexible razor blade or a 15-blade is recommended so that the mid-dermis is included in the biopsy specimen. If performed too superficially, invasion into the dermis cannot be evaluated and rebiopsy may be required.

A number of noninvasive diagnostic tools including dermoscopy, high-frequency ultrasound (HFUS), optical coherence tomography, and *in vivo* confocal microscopy/confocal laser scanning microscopy, and reflectance mode confocal microscopy (RCM) have been investigated for screening, diagnosis, and management of NMSC. The benefits of these modalities are that they allow the examination of large affected areas and monitoring and surveillance of selected skin sites for topical treatment modalities (e.g., patients with AK or BCC treated with imiquimod). However, any suspicious skin lesion still requires biopsy.

In general, radiologic studies are not necessary for the evaluation of patients with NMSC. However, if locally advanced/extensive disease (such as deep soft tissue involvement, perineural invasion, and/or bone involvement) and/or regional metastasis are of concern, staging imaging should be performed. A magnetic resonance imaging (MRI) study can be obtained to evaluate the extent of tumor involvement and ultrasound can be used for the evaluation of regional nodal basin(s). If there is concern for bone involvement, computed tomography (CT) with contrast is preferred unless contraindicated. Palpable or suspicious regional lymph nodes identified on physical examination or imaging should be biopsied by fine-needle aspiration or core needle biopsy. Patients with pathologically confirmed nodal disease should undergo either positron emission tomography (PET) with CT or chest/abdominal/pelvic CT with contrast to evaluate for distant metastatic disease.

Staging and Risk Assessment

The 8th edition of the American Joint Committee on Cancer (AJCC) *Cancer Staging Manual* states that there is no AJCC staging system for BCC outside the head and neck. The details of the head/neck staging are discussed further in Chapter 7, Cancer of the Head and Neck. However, although there is no AJCC staging system for BCC outside of the head and neck, there are well-described risk factors for BCC (Table 4.1) and SCC (Table 4.2) associated with recurrence and risk of metastasis and which guide management of these lesions.

Treatment of NMSC

The treatment of NMSC requires careful evaluation of tumor size, pathologic characteristics, anatomical location, age, overall health of the patient, cost to the patient, and cosmesis. Treatment modalities can be divided into surgical and nonsurgical therapies although surgical intervention is often the mainstay of treatment.

Surgical Techniques

Treatment of most NMSCs is primary surgical excision with a margin of clinically normal tissue to allow for subsequent evaluation of the entire specimen for clear margins. Complete excision with a margin of clinically normal tissue is associated with 5-year disease-free rates of over 98% for BCC and 92% for SCC. Predetermined margins of 4 to 10 mm should be performed with incisions made along Langer lines to achieve the best cosmetic result (Fig. 4.4).

Risk Stratification of Basal Cell Carcinomas (BCC)

	Low Risk	High Risk
Size <2 cm on the trunk/extremities	Yes	No
Location in "mask" areas of face[a]	No	Yes
Location on other high-risk areas[b]	No	Yes
Well-defined tumor borders	Yes	No
Primary BCC	Yes	No
Immunosuppressed patient	No	Yes
Site of prior radiation therapy	No	Yes
BCC subtype	Superficial, nodular	Aggressive growth pattern[c]
Perineural involvement present	No	Yes

[a]Central face, eyelids, eyebrows, periorbital, nose, lips, chin, mandible, preauricular, postauricular, temple, ear.
[b]Cheeks, forehead, scalp, neck, pretibial, genitalia, hands, feet.
[c]Having infiltrative, micronodular, morpheaform, basosquamous, sclerosing, or carcinosarcomatous differentiation features in any portion of the tumor.

For well-defined, low-risk lesions <2 cm, excision with a 4-mm margin around the tumor border is expected to definitively treat the tumor in 95% of cases. For high-risk tumors, a larger margin of at least 6 mm is indicated, and European guidelines suggest at least 10-mm margin should be used. Recurrent BCC is associated with a poor cure rate and a 10-mm excision margin is recommended. For incompletely excised lesions, re-excision is recommended if possible. Following excision of the lesion, appropriate reconstructive options include linear closure, skin grafting, or healing by secondary intention; if tissue rearrangement or skin grafting is required, intraoperative surgical margin assessment or temporary dressing placement with planned delayed reconstruction to allow for pathologic margin assessment should be considered.

Risk Stratification of Squamous Cell Carcinomas

	Low Risk	High Risk	Very High Risk
Location and size	Trunk/extremity location and <2 cm	Trunk/extremity location and between 2 and 4 cm or Head, neck, hands, feet, pretibial, anogenital location, any size	≥4 cm at any location
Borders	Well defined	Poorly defined	
Primary vs. recurrent	Primary	Recurrent	
Site of prior radiation therapy or chronic inflammation	No	Yes	
Immunosuppression	No	Yes	
Rapidly growing tumor	No	Yes	
Neurologic symptoms	No	Yes	
Degree of differentiation	Well or moderately differentiated		Poorly differentiated
Histologic features: acantholytic (adenoid), adenosquamous (mucin production), or metaplastic (carcinosarcomatous) subtypes	No	Yes	Desmoplastic SCC
Depth	≤6 mm without invasion beyond subcutaneous fat		>6 mm or invasion beyond subcutaneous fat
Perineural involvement	No	Yes	Tumor cells within nerve sheath of a nerve deeper than the dermis or measuring ≥0.1 mm
Lymphovascular involvement	No	No	Yes

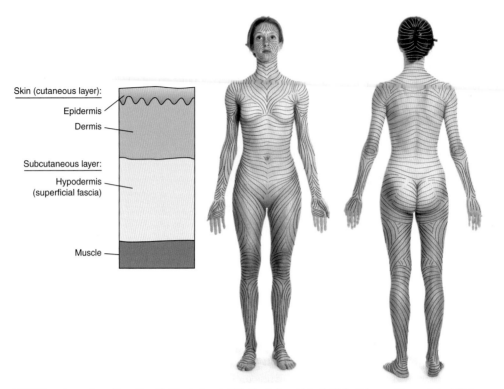

Skin (cutaneous layer):

Epidermis

Dermis

Subcutaneous layer:

Hypodermis
(superficial fascia)

Muscle

FIGURE 4.4 Langer lines. (From Clay JH, Allen L, Pounds DM. *Clay & Pounds' Basic Clinical Massage Therapy*, 3rd ed. Wolters Kluwer; 2015. Figure 1.4.)

Mohs micrographic surgery (MMS) involves removal of the clinical margins of the tumor under local anesthesia with immediate frozen section evaluation of the margins. Small incremental sections are removed until the margins are clear. This technique allows for the best cosmetic results by preserving normal tissue, while ensuring that larger lesions with subclinical extension are entirely removed. Two meta-analyses published in 1989 reported 5-year recurrence rate of 1% and 5.6% for primary and recurrent BCC, respectively, treated by MMS. MMS is a preferred surgical technique for high-risk SCC as it allows intraoperative analysis of the excision margin, with better 5-year local recurrence rate reported for both primary (3.1% vs. 8.1%) and recurrent (10% vs. 23%) lesions compared with surgical excision in one meta-analysis.

The reconstructive choices after Mohs surgery are similar to those available after traditional excision. Although MMS is time-consuming and requires skilled practitioners, the benefits of superior cosmesis and excellent cure rates make it the treatment of choice for many patients. However, MMS may not be appropriate for all cases and practitioners should carefully adhere to appropriate use criteria for MMS.

There has been considerable interest in performing sentinel lymph node (SLN) biopsy in selected patients with high-risk SCC in hopes that detection and treatment of subclinical nodal metastases will lead to improved outcomes for these patients. In a pooled evaluation of 83 high-risk SCC patients, all patients with a positive SLN had lesions >2 cm in diameter. Among patients with tumors <2 cm, 2.1 to 3 cm, and >3 cm in diameter, the proportions of patients with a positive SLN were 0%, 15.8%, and 30.4%, respectively. While the available data suggest SLN biopsy can accurately identify micrometastatic nodal disease in patients with SCC, studies to date are limited by small sample size, limited follow-up, and lack of uniform criteria. Additional studies will be needed before definitive guidelines can be established with respect to SLN biopsy.

When possible, NMSC nodal or distant metastases should be treated after discussion by a multidisciplinary tumor board. Regional lymph node dissection and adjuvant RT may be considered for selected patients.

Curettage and Electrodissection

Curettage and electrodissection (C&E) involves debulking the tumor under local anesthesia with a sharp curette until a firm layer of normal underlying dermis is reached and the base is then denatured by electrodessication. The process may be repeated up to three times in a session. The technique is based on the ability of the sharp curette to differentiate friable tumor tissue from normal dermis. If subcutaneous fat is reached during this technique, it is necessary to convert to surgical excision, as the curette will no longer be able to distinguish soft fat tissue from tumor. This technique does not allow for histologic margin assessment.

Data supporting use of C&E for localized BCC and SCC are based on older studies; national evidence-based review of the literature suggests that best results are obtained with surgery for patients with BCC. C&E should be reserved for small (<1 cm), low-risk, superficial primary BCCs tumors in non–hair-bearing areas. C&E may also be considered for low-risk local SCC in non–hair-bearing areas. C&E is not suitable for recurrent or ill-defined tumors.

Radiation Therapy

RT is often reserved for patients unable or unwilling to undergo surgical treatment of primary lesions or when clear margins cannot be obtained by Mohs or more extensive surgery. RT is also widely accepted as adjuvant treatment of recurrent or histologically aggressive tumors, particularly those with perineural invasion. For high-risk NMSC with perineural involvement or invasion into bone, RT is generally recommended in conjunction with surgical excision. RT can be further used as adjuvant or palliative treatment for lymph node metastases. Disadvantages of RT include acute and chronic radiation changes (dyspigmentation, telangiectasia, fibrosis), higher recurrence rates in BCC, lack of margin control, increased number of treatment sessions, and long-term complications such as nonhealing ulcers, tissue necrosis, and cataracts for lesions in the periorbital region. As RT can itself result in NMSC decades after exposure, it should be used cautiously in young patients. It is also contraindicated in nevoid BCC.

Superficial Therapies

Superficial therapies include topical treatment with 5-fluorouracil (5-FU) or imiquimod, photodynamic therapy (PDT), and cryotherapy and should be reserved for situations where surgery or radiation are contraindicated or impractical, as cure rates may be lower.

Topical therapies for superficial NMSC and AKs include 5-FU and imiquimod creams. 5-FU is an antineoplastic antimetabolite. Imiquimod is a synthetic immune response modifier that enhances cell-mediated immune response via the induction of proinflammatory cytokines. These topical therapies are most commonly used for AKs as well as for superficial BCCs and SCCs in situ when surgery or other treatment techniques are contraindicated or impractical. Topical 5-FU is not appropriate for nodular BCC and is not recommended for SCC due to high recurrence rates. Treatment regimens for AKs with 5-FU vary widely; in general, 5-FU is applied to the affected area once or twice daily for a period ranging from 2 to 6 weeks. Retreatment several months later, either with cryotherapy or other modalities, may be necessary. For the treatment of superficial BCC, 5-FU can be applied daily to the tumor and several millimeters of surrounding skin for a period of at least 4 weeks. After a 2- to 3-week respite, the area is then evaluated clinically for residual tumor. Biopsy is often indicated to ensure adequate therapy. Significant erythema, stinging, oozing, and crusting are often reported, especially with more aggressive treatment regimens. 5-FU can be applied to an entire region, such as the face, chest, arms, or hands.

Imiquimod therapy is approved for the treatment of AKs and superficial BCC but should not be used for SCC. In general, less local skin reaction is reported compared to 5-FU. For AKs, the cream is applied 2 nonconsecutive days a week for 16 weeks. For superficial BCC, the cream should be applied 5 nights a week for at least 6 weeks. After a 2- to 3-month respite, the lesion is evaluated either clinically or histologically (rebiopsy) to confirm adequate therapy. While imiquimod can also be used for nodular BCC, the treatment duration requires 12 weeks and the response is lower (76%) compared to a greater than 85% success rate for superficial BCC. Imiquimod is often well tolerated, causes minimal or no scarring, and is particularly useful for multiple lesions concentrated in one area.

PDT is another noninvasive method used for the treatment of AKs, superficial BCC and, at some institutions, SCC in situ. A photosensitizer (most commonly, aminolevulinic acid) is applied to the skin and activated with a light source. The tumor cells retain the photosensitizer for longer periods of time than normal cells, resulting in preferential killing. Cure rates for AKs are reported to be as high as 90%; however, recurrence rates at 5 years for superficial and nodular BCC have been reported to be as high as 14% to 22%, respectively. Side effects include burning or stinging pain during the treatment and posttreatment periods, erythema, swelling, and temporary hyper- or hypopigmentation, but overall the cosmetic results are superior in comparison to surgery or cryotherapy. Systemic PDT has also been tested as a treatment for BCC and may be appropriate for individuals presenting with multiple lesions or nevoid BCC syndrome.

Cryotherapy is a destructive method primarily reserved for the treatment of precancerous lesions such as AKs and occasionally for small, superficial, low-risk, primary BCCs or SCCs. Liquid nitrogen is either sprayed with a cryogen or is directly applied to the lesion with cotton-tipped applicators for a period of time such that the visible thawing of the lesions takes at least 15 seconds (30 seconds for superficial SCC or BCC). In prospective trials, cryotherapy for BCC and SCC results in recurrence rates ranging from 5% to 39% and 0% to 50%, respectively, and is associated with increased pain, longer time to complete healing, and poorer cosmetic outcomes compared with other treatment options.

Chemoprevention with low-dose oral retinoids and nicotinamide has shown some promise in the prevention of SCC for patients at high risk for AKs and SCCs, such as transplant recipients, those with xeroderma pigmentosa, psoriasis, and psoralen treatment with UV-A exposure. However, long-term therapy is needed as beneficial effects are often lost when these drugs are discontinued.

Systemic Therapies

Patients with advanced BCC who do not have local therapy options may be eligible for systemic treatment with one of two FDA-approved hedgehog pathway inhibitors (vismodegib, sonidegib). Unfortunately, advanced BCC can develop resistance to these agents, limiting the duration of response to treatment.

For patients with advanced BCC who do not have local therapy options, a first-in-class hedgehog pathway inhibitor, vismodegib, is a systemic therapy option. Vismodegib received Food and Drug Administration (FDA) approval based on a multicenter, single-arm, two-cohort, open-label, phase II trial (ERIVANCE) in which over 90% of patients were previously treated with surgery, RT, and/or systemic therapies. Objective response was 48% and 33% in patients with locally advanced and metastatic disease, respectively, with median duration of response of 9.5 and 7.6 months, respectively. Vismodegib can also be considered for BCC treatment and prophylaxis in patients with nevoid BCC syndrome.

Sonidegib is another hedgehog pathway inhibitor that has received FDA approval for the treatment of locally advanced BCC that has recurred after surgery or RT or in patients who are not candidates for surgery or RT. Sonidegib received FDA approval based on the phase II BOLT trial.

For patients with locally advanced or metastatic BCC previously treated with a hedgehog pathway inhibitor or who are not candidates for treatment with a hedgehog pathway inhibitor, cemiplimab-rwlc may be a systemic treatment option.

For patients with locally advanced, unresectable SCC and SCC with distant metastasis, there is limited evidence reporting response to systemic therapies. A number of small studies have reported responses to cytotoxic therapy (cisplatin alone or in combination with other agents), epidermal growth factor receptor (EGFR) inhibitors (cetuximab), and immune checkpoint inhibitors (anti–PD-1).

Surveillance, Screening, and Prevention

Patients with a previous diagnosis of NMSC are at increased risk of future NMSCs and melanoma; up to 35% and 50% of patients will develop another NMSC at 3 and 5 years, respectively. Thus, aggressive screening of patients at risk for skin cancer is essential to minimize the morbidity and mortality of NMSC. Patients at greatest risk include those with light skin types, immunosuppression, and a family or personal history of skin cancer. Exposure to UV radiation should be limited in children with regular use of broad-spectrum sunscreen from an early age. Appropriate Sun protection factor (SPF) level and application techniques should be emphasized for all patients, especially regarding applications to the face and neck.

Regular examination of the skin by a dermatologist is recommended for all patients at risk for skin cancer on at least a yearly basis. A complete skin examination includes examination of the entire skin surface, including the scalp, with particular attention to previous areas of skin cancer. For patients with a history of AKs or NMSCs, regular follow-up with a dermatologist is recommended. Patients with BCC should be followed with skin examinations every 6 to 12 months for 5 years, then annually for life. This schedule for follow-up highlights the fact that 30% to 50% of patients will develop another NMSC within 5 years and are at a 10-fold increase in risk compared to the general population. For patients with SCC, most recurrences or metastases will occur within 2 years of the initial therapy, and almost all recurrence will occur within 5 years. Therefore, close follow-up of these patients during this time period is critical. Patients should be monitored with regular physical examinations including complete skin and regional lymph node examination. For local SCC, monitoring during the first 2 years is the most critical, and examinations should occur at least every 3 to 12 months during this timeframe. If no further skin cancer develops in the first 2 years, then examinations every 6 to 12 months for another 3 years, then annually for life. For patients who had regional disease, a history and physical should be performed every 1 to 3 months for 1 year, then every 2 to 4 months for 1 year, then every 4 to 6 months for another 3 years, and then every 6 to 12 months for life. Surveillance using CT with contrast may be warranted to assess for regional or distant metastatic recurrence.

CASE SCENARIO

Case Scenario 1

Presentation

A 65-year-old male with a significant past medical history of a motor vehicle accident (MVA) 13 years ago, resulting in severe injuries to the left lower extremity requiring multiple operations and eventual skin grafting, now presents with an open wound at the site of the former skin graft. Despite aggressive local wound care, the wound has become larger and firmer during the past 6 months. Physical examination identifies an afebrile male in no acute distress with an open wound measuring 5.0 × 3.0 cm located anteriorly along the mid-tibia with crusting on the lateral margin. There is some mild surrounding erythema. The rest of the skin graft is well incorporated. There is also palpable lymphadenopathy in the left inguinal area. The patient reports no neurologic deficits which is confirmed on examination. The remaining skin and lymph node examination is otherwise negative for suspicious findings.

Differential Diagnosis

Marjolin ulcer/squamous cell carcinoma
Chronic nonhealing wound
Actinic keratosis
Allergic contact dermatitis
Atopic dermatitis
Basal cell carcinoma
Atypical fibroxanthoma
Bacterial cellulitis
Secondary malignancy with lymph node metastasis

Confirmation of Diagnosis and Treatment

Any suspicious nonhealing or ulcerative lesion that appears in a chronic scar should be biopsied to confirm the diagnosis. These should be taken from multiple locations of the ulcer including the edges of the wound to minimize false-negative results and determine the area of involved skin and guide extent of subsequent resection. In this case, multiple scouting punch biopsies revealed well-differentiated, invasive squamous cell carcinoma consistent with a Marjolin ulcer extending across most of the area of the patient's former split-thickness skin graft site.

Clinical evidence of lymphadenopathy warrants additional biopsy of the enlarged lymph nodes. Ultrasound-guided biopsy by a center or physician with expertise in fine-needle aspiration (FNA) is recommended. Core biopsy may be preferred over FNA in cases where primary tumor histology is uncertain or if a larger tissue sample is required for pathologic testing. In cases of positive lymph node biopsy, computed tomography (CT) with contrast of the nodal basin is performed to determine the size, number, and location of nodes. In addition, CT of the chest, abdomen, and pelvis with contrast or positron emission tomography (PET)/CT as clinically indicated. Histologically confirmed nodal disease without evidence of distant spread requires regional nodal basin lymphadenectomy with excision of the primary tumor. An MRI provides excellent soft tissue detail, such as tumor extent, depth, margins, underlying bone cortical or marrow involvement, or the involvement of adjacent neurovascular structures and can be employed prior to surgical excision to further evaluate the extent of primary disease.

Locally advanced resectable, inoperable, or incompletely resectable disease requires multidisciplinary consultation to discuss multimodal treatment options and consideration of systemic therapies (including in the neoadjuvant setting and clinical trials) and radiation therapy (RT) under the directive eye of multiple practitioners and sequencing of multimodal therapies.

Surgical Approach–Key Steps

The primary goals of treatment of squamous cell skin cancer (SCC) are the complete removal of the tumor and the maximal preservation of function and cosmesis. A common therapeutic option for SCC, including Marjolin ulcers, is standard surgical excision followed by postoperative pathologic evaluation of margins. Any peripheral rim of erythema around an SCC must be included in what is assumed to be the tumor. High-risk lesions such as Marjolin ulcers, poorly differentiated tumors, invasion of subcutaneous tissue, or large diameter (>2 cm) should require margins of at least 9 mm. If tissue rearrangement or skin graft placement is necessary to close the defect, permanent pathologic assessment of surgical margins is necessary before definitive closure. In many cases, this relies on the use of a temporary occlusive dressing or a vacuum dressing system in the interim. If margins are positive after excision, patients should undergo re-excision using standard margins. Split-thickness skin grafting or consideration of a free flap by plastic and reconstructive surgery may facilitate closure.

Postoperative Management

The value of adjuvant RT is widely debated due to lack of prospective randomized clinical trial data. For local SCC (i.e., without lymph node involvement), the national consensus guidelines recommend adjuvant RT for any SCC that shows evidence of extensive perineural or large nerve involvement. Adjuvant RT is also a recommended option in patients who are not candidates for surgical resection or if tissue margins are positive after definitive surgery without the option for re-excision. For those with regional or distant metastatic SCC, multidisciplinary consultation is recommended. A wide variety of cytotoxic therapies have been tested in these patients with clinical trials available to a subset of this population. The frequency of follow-up should be adjusted based on risk. For local SCC, monitoring during the first 2 years is the most critical, and examinations should occur at least every 3 to 12 months during this timeframe. If no further skin cancer develops in the first 2 years, then examinations every 6 to 12 months for another 3 years, then annually for life is recommended. For regional SCC, a history and physical should be performed every 1 to 3 months for 1 year, then every 2 to 4 months for 1 year, every 4 to 6 months for another 3 years, and then every 6 to 12 months for life. Surveillance CT with contrast may be warranted to screen for recurrence in the regional lymph node basin or distant metastatic disease.

Common Curve Balls

- A long latency period can exist between chronic wound, burn, or skin graft and development of Marjolin ulcer.
- An irregularly shaped, nonhealing ulcer resistant to healing despite best wound care should prompt biopsy.
- Enlarged lymph nodes require FNA biopsy and evaluation for regional and metastatic disease.
- Prior to definitive closure following wide local excision, margins must be assessed and clear of residual tumor. The use of a temporary or vacuum dressing is useful in these situations.

Take Home Points

- Marjolin ulcers are aggressive squamous cell cancers most commonly presenting in patients who have chronic wounds.
- Patients with suspicion for regional or distant metastasis should undergo staging imaging including CT scan of the chest, abdomen, and pelvis with contrast or PET/CT in addition to biopsy of nodal disease.
- Follow-up in the first 2 years should be in short intervals as recurrence is most common during this time period.

Case Scenario 2

A 61-year-old otherwise healthy female presents to your clinic with an enlarging right groin mass. She was seen prior to your visit by her primary care physician who obtained a CT scan with contrast of the abdomen and pelvis. The scan demonstrates isolated bulky nodal disease of the right inguinal pelvic regions with the largest node measuring 5.0 × 6.5 cm in the right pelvis. She mentions that about a year prior, she underwent a shave biopsy to remove what was thought to be another seborrheic keratosis on her right thigh, but no pathology report was obtained. The patient is up to date on all age-appropriate screening examinations including a colonoscopy, Pap smear, and urologic evaluation, all within the past 3 months and which were negative for disease.

*   On physical examination, she has a large, firm, fixed mass in the right inguinal region. She has no suspicious skin lesions on full-body examination. The patient is sent for biopsy that reveals metastatic squamous cell carcinoma.*

Differential Diagnosis

Firm, matted, nontender lymph nodes are concerning for malignancy. Malignancies to keep in mind, in this case, are those of the skin (including of the perineum), anorectal mucosa, and cervical mucosa that frequently drain to superficial inguinal lymph nodes. These tissues are typically of squamous cell origin and can present as squamous carcinoma in the inguinal lymph nodes. Pelvic nodal involvement could represent metastasis from the superficial nodes or, less commonly, could indicate a primary tumor residing in the rectum or in the genitourinary system. Consideration of infectious etiologies, specifically sexually transmitted infections, must remain in the differential diagnosis prior to biopsy and testing should be performed on a case-by-case basis. A thorough skin examination paying special attention to the lower extremities and perineal area may demonstrate wounds or skin lesions unbeknownst to the patient. Any lymphadenopathy could represent lymphoma or leukemia, particularly if the patient is experiencing fevers, night sweats, or unintentional weight loss.

Confirmation of Diagnosis and Treatment

The patient in question represents a case of inguinopelvic nodal SCC with an unknown primary at presentation. Examination of the anorectal region, a meticulous gynecologic examination, and cystoscopy are necessary investigations for these patients. It is possible that the previously presumed seborrheic keratosis removed on shave biopsy may have been an SCC and the primary lesion, highlighting the need for routine pathologic assessment of skin lesions. A PET/CT is invaluable to elicit total disease burden. Both distant metastatic disease and in cases where bulky nodal disease involves major blood vessels or neurologic structures, as in this case, require multidisciplinary consultation. A clinical trial or neoadjuvant systemic therapy should be considered in this patient with bulky lymphadenopathy and regionally advanced disease and who is at risk of both regional and distant recurrence following surgery.

Surgical Approach

Surgical intervention, likewise, may require the input of a multidisciplinary surgical team. Bulky nodal disease abutting major vessels may require the consultation of vascular surgeons. In this patient with isolated bulky metastases to the right superficial and deep pelvic lymph node basins, a right inguinofemoral and deep pelvic lymphadenectomy are performed.

Postoperative Management

The specimens taken during formal lymphadenectomy should be reassessed by the histopathologist. Evidence of extranodal extension and lymph node disease should be discussed with the multidisciplinary team. In such cases, a radiation oncologist should be evaluated for the potential utility of radiation therapy to the nodal basin due to high-risk features for regional recurrence. A detailed discussion of the rationale, logistics, and goals of radiation therapy should be undertaken with the patient and family. Additional adjuvant chemotherapy may be prescribed concurrently. Continued follow-up every 3 months with serial CT imaging as indicated is recommended. For regional recurrence or distant metastases, close involvement with a multidisciplinary team cannot be overemphasized.

Common Curve Balls

- Biopsies of skin lesions should be routinely assessed by a histopathologist.
- Neoadjuvant chemotherapy may be indicated given the degree of lymph node involvement or to help treat the tumor prior to safe resection.
- Lymph node dissection may require the specialized skills of several surgical teams for vascular reconstruction, ureteral stent placement, and reconstructive efforts in select cases of a reoperative field or advanced disease.
- Radiation and/or chemotherapy may be indicated postoperatively under the direction of multidisciplinary review.

Take Home Points

- Consideration should be given to performing FNA/CNB (core needle biopsy) of persistent lymphadenopathy.
- Lymph node dissection is indicated in patients with pathologically confirmed regionally metastatic SCC without distant sites of metastasis.
- RT to the lymph node basin may be considered for patients with extranodal extension or gross disease under the direction of a radiation oncologist.

CASE SCENARIO REVIEW

Questions

1. A 67 year-old male is referred to your clinic by their primary care physician following the development of a new, nonulcerated pearly lesion with rolled edges and subtle telangiectasia on the right cheek. Biopsy is performed which demonstrates a well-defined, low-risk basal cell carcinoma (BCC) approximately 1.5 cm in diameter. The patient would like surgical excision, what margin should be used?

   A. 2 mm
   B. 4 mm
   C. 7 mm
   D. 10 mm

2. A 43-year-old female reports a 6-month history of a briskly growing, 3.0-cm ulcerated lesion on her left leg. She was referred to your clinic where she underwent a punch biopsy, pathology results moderately differentiated squamous cell carcinoma (SCC). Comprehensive nodal examination is negative for lymphadenopathy. What is the next step in treatment?

   A. Curettage and Electrodissection (C&E)
   B. Radiation therapy
   C. Wide-local excision with sentinel lymph node biopsy (SLNB)
   D. Imiquimoid and photodynamic therapy

3. An 80-year-old male with nevoid basal cell syndrome whom you have followed for many years presents to your office with another lesion noted on his right thigh. He states that as with his previous lesions, he would like to proceed with curettage and electrodissection (C&E). After localizing the area with lidocaine, you proceed with the C&E. While curetting, you reach subcutaneous fat, what should be your next course of action?

   A. Suture the wound and follow-up in 2 weeks
   B. Apply topical imiquimod
   C. Consult photodynamic therapy
   D. Convert to open surgical resection

4. A 59-year-old male underwent resection of a right forearm lesion found to be basal cell carcinoma (BCC). Postoperative tissue defect after resection was 4.0 × 3.0 cm. Plastic and reconstructive surgery aided in the closure with a tissue advancement flap. Two weeks post operation, he presents to his follow-up appointment. Pathology demonstrates positive lateral margin. What is the next step in treatment?

   A. Re-excision, 1.0-cm lateral margin
   B. Re-excision, 2.0-cm lateral margin
   C. Observe
   D. Sonidegib

5. A 35-year-old male undergoes surgical excision for an ulcerated lesion he believed to be a nonhealing wound from a recent injury he sustained to his right forearm. Pathology reported poorly differentiated squamous cell carcinoma with negative margins but evidence of perineural involvement. Which of the following approaches should be taken?

   A. Observe
   B. CHOP chemotherapy
   C. Re-excision deep margin
   D. Adjuvant radiation

Answers

1. **The correct answer is B.** *Rationale:* A 4-mm margin around the tumor border is expected to definitively treat well-defined, low-risk BCC that are <2 cm in 95% of cases. Judicious margins that are maximally effective should be pursued to both limit recurrence and for improved cosmetic outcomes. Use of Mohs micrographic surgery should be considered here to limit the site of resection.

2. **The correct answer is C.** *Rationale:* Unlike basal cell carcinoma (BCC), SCC shows a greater propensity for nodal involvement. Nodal sampling is appropriate in patients with moderate- to high-risk SCC with positive sentinel lymph node (SLN) in lesions >2 cm. Among SCC tumors, those <2 cm, 2.1 to 3.0 cm, and >3 cm in diameter had positive SLN in 0%, 15.8%, and 30.4%, of cases.

3. **The correct answer is D.** *Rationale:* C&E refers to debulking the tumor with a sharp curette until a firm layer of normal healthy dermis is reached and then denaturing the area with an electrodessication technique. If subcutaneous fat is reached, the operator is no longer able to differentiate between friable tumor and normal tissue. The alternative techniques are available to use for varied nonmelanoma skin cancer (NMSC) and premalignant conditions, but classically, the removal of tumor, in this case, should be further explored with formal sharp excision.

4. **The correct answer is A.** *Rationale:* Recurrent BCC is associated with a poor cure rate and a 10-mm excision margin is recommended. For incompletely excised lesions, re-excision is recommended if possible. Observation is inappropriate as recurrent BCC must be dealt with surgically, particularly in young patients healthy enough for surgery. Sonidegib is a hedgehog pathway inhibitor that has received FDA approval for the treatment of locally advanced BCC that has recurred after surgery or RT or in patients who are not candidates for surgery or radiation therapy (RT). It would be inappropriate to begin systemic therapy when definitive curative resection is possible.

5. **The correct answer is D.** *Rationale:* National consensus guidelines recommend adjuvant RT for any SCC that shows evidence of extensive perineural or large nerve involvement. Observation would be against guidelines and would be a poor approach in a young patient with concern for local recurrence. CHOP chemotherapy is not used in cutaneous squamous cell carcinoma. Margins were noted to be negative.

Recommended Readings

American Academy of Dermatology, American College of Mohs Surgery, American Society for Dermatologic Surgery Association, Ad Hoc Task Force; Connolly SM, Baker DR, Coldiron BM, et al. AAD/ACMS/ASDSA/ASMS 2012 appropriate use criteria for mohs micrographic surgery: a report of the American Academy of Dermatology, American College of Mohs Surgery, American Society for Dermatologic Surgery Association, and the American Society for Mohs Surgery. *Dermatol Surg.* 2012;38:1582–1603.

Allen JE, Stolle LB. Utility of sentinel node biopsy in patients with high-risk cutaneous squamous cell carcinoma. *Eur J Surg Oncol.* 2015;41:197–200.

Arits AHMM, Mosterd K, Essers BA, et al. Photodynamic therapy versus topical imiquimod versus topical fluorouracil for treatment of superficial basal-cell carcinoma: a single blind, non-inferiority, randomised controlled trial. *Lancet Oncol.* 2013;14(7):647–654.

Bath-Hextall F, Ozolins M, Armstrong SJ, et al; Surgery versus Imiquimod for Nodular Superficial basal cell carcinoma (SINS) study group. Surgical excision versus imiquimod 5% cream for nodular and superficial basal-cell carcinoma (SINS): a multicentre, non-inferiority, randomised controlled trial. *Lancet Oncol.* 2014;15(1):96–105.

Brantsch KD, Meisner C, Schönfisch B, et al. Analysis of risk factors determining prognosis of cutaneous squamous-cell carcinoma: a prospective study. *Lancet Oncol.* 2008;9:713–720.

Chen AC, Martin AJ, Choy B, et al. A phase 3 randomized trial of nicotinamide for skin-cancer chemoprevention. *J Engl J Med.* 2015;373:1618–1626.

Chitwood K, Etzkorn J, Cohen G. Topical and intralesional treatment of nonmelanoma skin cancer: efficacy and cost comparisons. *Dermatol Surg.* 2013;39:1306–1316.

Chow LQM, Haddad R, Gupta S, et al. Antitumor activity of pembrolizumab in biomarker-unselected patients with recurrent and/or metastatic head and neck squamous cell carcinoma: results from the Phase Ib KEYNOTE-012 Expansion cohort. *J Clin Oncol.* 2016;34:3838–3845.

Flohil SC, van der Leest RJT, Arends LR, de Vries E, Nijsten T. Risk of subsequent cutaneous malignancy in patients with prior keratinocyte carcinoma: a systematic review and meta-analysis. *Eur J Cancer.* 2013;49(10):2365–2375.

Kadakia KC, Barton DL, Loprinzi CL, et al. Randomized controlled trial of acitretin versus placebo in patients at high-risk for basal cell or squamous cell carcinoma of the skin (North Central Cancer Treatment Group Study 969251). *Cancer.* 2012;118:2128–2137.

Karagas MR, McDonald JA, Greenberg ER, et al. Risk of basal cell and squamous cell skin cancers after ionizing radiation therapy. For The Skin Cancer Prevention Study Group. *J Natl Cancer Inst.* 1996;88(24):1848–1853.

Lansbury L, Bath-Hextall F, Perkins W, Stanton W, Leonardi-Bee J. Interventions for non-metastatic squamous cell carcinoma of the skin: systematic review and pooled analysis of observational studies. *BMJ.* 2013;347:f6153.

Lott DG, Manz R, Koch C, Lorenz RR. Aggressive behavior of nonmelanotic skin cancers in solid organ transplant recipients. *Transplantation.* 2010;90(6):683–687.

Maubec E, Petrow P, Scheer-Senyarich I, et al. Phase II study of cetuximab as first-line single-drug therapy in patients with unresectable squamous cell carcinoma of the skin. *J Clin Oncol.* 2011;29:3419–3426.

Mendenhall WM, Amdur RJ, Hinerman RW, Cognetta AB, Mendenhall NP. Radiotherapy for cutaneous squamous and basal cell carcinomas of the head and neck. *Laryngoscope.* 2009;119(10):1994–1999.

Migden MR, Guminski A, Gutzmer R, et al. Treatment with two different doses of sonidegib in patients with locally advanced or metastatic basal cell carcinoma (BOLT): a multicentre, randomised, double-blind phase 2 trial. *Lancet Oncol.* 2015;16(6):716–728.

Quirk C, Gebauer K, De'Ambrosis B, Slade HB, Meng TC. Sustained clearance of superficial basal cell carcinomas treated with imiquimod cream 5%: results of a prospective 5-year study. *Cutis.* 2010;85(6):318–324.

Reigneau M, Robert C, Routier E, et al. Efficacy of neoadjuvant cetuximab alone or with platinum salt for the treatment of unresectable advanced nonmetastatic cutaneous squamous cell carcinomas. *Br J Dermatol.* 2015;173:527–534.

Rhodes LE, de Rie MA, Leifsdottir R, et al. Five-year follow-up of a randomized, prospective trial of topical methyl aminolevulinate photodynamic therapy vs surgery for nodular basal cell carcinoma. *Arch Dermatol.* 2007;143(9):1131–1136.

Rogers HW, Weinstock MA, Feldman SR, Coldiron BM. Incidence estimate of nonmelanoma skin cancer (keratinocyte carcinomas) in the U.S. population, 2012. *JAMA Dermatol.* 2015;151(10):1081–1086.

Roozeboom MH, Arits AHHM, Nelemans PJ, Kelleners-Smeets NWJ. Overall treatment success after treatment of primary superficial basal cell carcinoma: a systematic review and meta-analysis of randomized and nonrandomized trials. *Br J Dermatol.* 2012;167(4):733–756.

Sekulic A, Migden MR, Oro AE, et al. Efficacy and safety of vismodegib in advanced basal-cell carcinoma. *N Engl J Med.* 2012;366(23):2171–2179.

Silverberg MJ, Leyden W, Warton EM, Quesenberry CP Jr, Engels EA, Asgari MM HIV infection status, immunodeficiency, and the incidence of non-melanoma skin cancer. *J Natl Cancer Inst.* 2013;105:350–360.

van Iersel CA, van de Velden HVN, Kusters CDJ, et al. Prognostic factors for a subsequent basal cell carcinoma: implications for follow-up. *Br J Dermatol.* 2005;153(5):1078–1080.

van Loo E, Mosterd K, Krekels GAM, et al. Surgical excision versus Mohs' micrographic surgery for basal cell carcinoma of the face: A randomised clinical trial with 10 year follow-up. *Eur J Cancer.* 2014;50(17):3011–3020.

Wehner MR, Shive ML, Chren MM, Han J, Qureshi AA, Linos E. Indoor tanning and non-melanoma skin cancer: systematic review and meta-analysis. *BMJ.* 2012;345:e5909.

5 Merkel Cell Carcinoma

Brandon M. Cope, Russell G. Witt, and Emily Z. Keung

Merkel cell carcinoma (MCC) is a rare but aggressive skin cancer with neuroendocrine features. The tumor was initially thought to arise from the Merkel cells of the epidermis, hair sheath, or sweat ducts, based on the dense core secretory granules seen in the cytoplasm of the tumor cells on electron microscopy, which are normally only seen in Merkel cells. However, more recent identification of neuroendocrine epithelial cells as well as sarcomatous elements within the tumors and the frequent identification of these tumors at noncutaneous sites, has led investigators to postulate the likelihood that these tumors may actually originate from a pluripotent stem cell. MCC appears to be rapidly increasing in incidence in the United States, from an age-adjusted incidence of 0.36/100,000 patient-years in the early 1990s, to greater than 0.7/100,000 patient-years by the early 2000s. MCC can grow rapidly and metastasize early with 26% to 36% of patients presenting with lymph node metastasis and 6% to 16% of patients presenting with distant metastasis at diagnosis. MCC is associated with a high mortality rate; an analysis of the Surveillance, Epidemiology, and End Results (SEER) database reported 5-year survival rates of 51%, 35%, and 14% for patients with localized, regional, and distant MCC disease, respectively.

Risk Factors

MCC typically affects older individuals with at least 90% of cases occurring in patients 50 years or older and greater than 76% of cases occurring in patients at least 65 years of age. In general, MCC is more likely to affect Caucasians, with a 1.4:1 male-to-female predominance.

Risk factors associated with MCC include sun exposure, with increased incidence in geographical regions with higher ultraviolet (UV) indices, on areas of skin exposed to the sun, and often in proximity to other UV-associated skin lesions. MCC also more commonly arises in individuals who are immunosuppressed, including those with organ transplants, lymphoproliferative disorders such as chronic lymphocytic leukemia, and human immunodeficiency virus (HIV). Merkel cell polyoma virus (MCPyV), a human polyoma virus, has been shown to be clonally integrated in 69% to 85% of MCC tumors. The role of MCPyV in MCC tumorigenesis is the subject of ongoing research in MCPyV-positive tumors but genetic analyses have found significantly higher tumor mutational burden with UV signature in MCPyV-negative tumors compared to MCPyV-positive tumors.

Clinical Presentation, Diagnosis, and Staging

MCC often presents as an asymptomatic lesion which can appear as a firm, well-defined nodule that is erythematous or violaceous without distinguishing features (Fig. 5.1A–D). The most frequent location of a primary MCC is the head and neck (48%), followed by the upper extremity (19%), lower extremity (16%), and trunk (11%). Patients often seek evaluation due to rapid growth over a period of weeks or months. Although MCC is often misdiagnosed and underrecognized at presentation, the mnemonic AEIOU may be helpful to recall relevant features of MCC: asymptomatic, expanding rapidly, immunosuppressed, older than 50 years, and UV exposure.

Initial evaluation of patients at presentation should include a thorough skin and nodal basin examination as it is common to find synchronous malignant and premalignant skin lesions. A biopsy of the suspicious lesion should then be performed; an incisional (i.e., punch) biopsy or excisional biopsy is preferred. Excisional biopsies should be oriented to facilitate a subsequent wide excision (e.g., axially on extremities) and minimize the need for skin graft for wound closure at the time of wide excision (Fig. 5.2D, E).

On hematoxylin and eosin (H&E) staining, MCC appears as round basophilic monomorphic cells with sparse cytoplasm, abundant mitoses, and dense granules in the cytoplasm (Fig. 5.2A, B). Histologically, MCC can appear similar to other small round blue cell tumors and immunohistochemistry is useful to distinguish MCC from other entities such as metastatic small cell lung cancer (SCLC). Cytokeratin 20 (CK20) is positive in 75% to 100% of primary MCC and rarely positive in SCLC while thyroid transcription factor-1 (TTF-1) should be negative in MCC tumors (Fig. 5.2C). Other neuroendocrine markers (chromogranin, synaptophysin, CD56, neuron-specific enolase) can also be expressed in, although are not specific for, MCC. An experienced dermatopathologist is an important member of the multidisciplinary team.

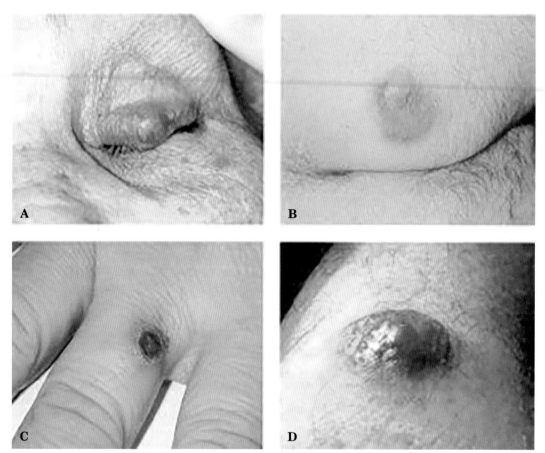

FIGURE 5.1 Clinical examples of primary Merkel cell carcinoma. **A:** Eyelid lesion thought to be rapidly growing chalazion. **B:** Nontender MCC that arose on buttock of patient with HIV. MCC diagnosis was markedly delayed because of history of multiple epidermoid cysts. **C:** Finger lesion that was clinically suggestive of pyogenic granuloma or amelanotic melanoma. **D:** MCC that arose on sun-exposed area of arm in man with fair skin. (Reprinted from Heath M, Jaimes N, Lemos B, et al. Clinical characteristics of Merkel cell carcinoma at diagnosis in 195 patients: the AEIOU features. *J Am Acad Dermatol.* 2008;58(3):375–381, with permission from Elsevier.)

MCC is staged clinically and pathologically according to the American Joint Committee on Cancer (AJCC) Eighth Edition staging system and is required to formulate management and treatment approaches as well as for prognostication. The Eighth Edition AJCC MCC staging system is based upon a National Cancer Database (NCDB) analysis of 9,387 patients with MCC treated between 1998 and 2012. The AJCC and the College of American Pathologists (CAP) strongly encourage synoptic reporting for MCC primary tumor specimens including, at a minimum, the parameters required to determine T stage (maximum tumor diameter, tumor extension), as well as other elements such as tumor site, peripheral and deep margin status, tumor thickness, lymphovascular invasion (LVI), mitotic rate, growth pattern, presence of infiltrating lymphocytes, and presence of additional malignancies.

After a diagnosis of primary MCC has been made by biopsy, clinical staging is required in order to develop the initial management and treatment approach. Patients with suspected regional nodal or distant metastasis on history and physical examination should undergo imaging to assess extent of disease. Biopsy of lesions concerning for regional or distant metastasis should be obtained to confirm the diagnosis. Brain magnetic resonance imaging (MRI) and whole-body fluorodeoxyglucose (FDG) positron emission tomography (PET) with fused axial computed tomography (CT) imaging should be considered in these cases. CT of the chest, abdomen, and pelvis with contrast, with CT of the head and neck in cases of primary MCC located in the head and neck region, may be used when whole-body FDG PET-CT is not available; however, there is some evidence to suggest that whole-body PET-CT may be more sensitive at detecting nodal and distant MCC compared with CT with contrast.

In patients without clinical evidence of regional or distant metastatic disease on history and physical at presentation, body imaging is not routinely indicated and should be selectively obtained only when clinically indicated. Detection of occult nodal disease is most reliably achieved by sentinel lymph node biopsy (SLNB) at

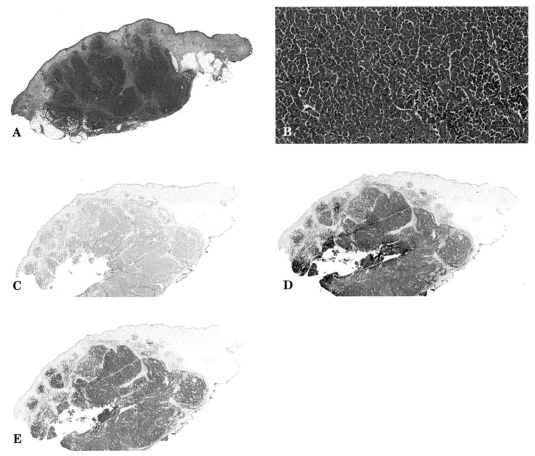

FIGURE 5.2 Histologic evaluation of Merkel cell carcinoma (MCC). **A:** Hematoxylin and eosin (H&E) stain of MCC. **B:** Magnification demonstrates blue rosettes of cells indicative of MCC. **C:** IHC staining for thyroid transcription factor type-1 (TTF-1) is negative. TTF-1 is rarely expressed in MCC. **D:** Immunohistochemical (IHC) staining for synaptophysin, a sensitive marker of neuroendocrine tumors. **E:** IHC staining for Merkel cell polyomavirus (MCPyV) stain, a specific marker of MCC. (Courtesy of Dr. Emily Keung, MD Anderson Cancer Center.)

the time of wide excision for primary MCC (see *Management of Regional Draining Nodal Basin* below) as MCC typically spreads to the regional lymph node basin prior to distant sites. Unlike melanoma, SLNB is warranted in all T stages for MCC. Standard pathologic SLNB reporting should include number of involved lymph nodes, size of largest metastatic deposit in millimeters (mm), and presence or absence of extracapsular extension (ECE) as retrospective studies suggest that MCC-associated survival is worse with increasing burden of nodal involvement and with the presence of ECE. Although the impact of SLNB on survival is unclear, SLN status is important for pathologic staging and to guide subsequent management of MCC.

Approximately 10% of patients will be diagnosed following biopsy of an enlarged lymph node where no primary cutaneous tumor is evident on physical examination. It is believed that the primary MCC may regress spontaneously in a subset of patients who may then have an overall improved prognosis compared to similarly staged patients with an identifiable primary tumor.

Management of Primary Disease

Patients without clinical evidence of regional or distant metastatic disease who are candidates for surgery are recommended to undergo wide excision of the primary MCC with SLNB in order to provide curative resection as well as definitive pathologic staging of the primary tumor and regional nodal basin. In general, SLNB should be performed prior to wide excision of the primary MCC so as to not disrupt the lymphatic drainage prior to retrieval of the lymph node. For MCCs of the head and neck region, lymphatic drainage patterns are often complex and special care should be taken in performing SLNB in these cases. At MD Anderson, preoperative lymphatic mapping by single-photon emission computed tomography imaging merged with CT (SPECT-CT) is often used to aid in identifying drainage pattern and localization of SLNs in the head and neck region.

Excision of primary MCC is typically performed with 1- to 2-cm margins with depth down to the investing fascia when feasible. There is insufficient evidence to support wider resection margins. The extent of planned surgical margins should also consider and be balanced against avoiding unnecessary delay of any planned adjuvant radiotherapy (RT) if possible. Adjuvant RT to the primary MCC site is typically recommended although observation may be considered for select patients who are immunocompetent with small (<1 cm) primary tumors without LVI and in whom widely negative margins of excision were attained.

For patients who are poor surgical candidates, definitive RT may be considered for treatment of primary and/or nodal MCC. In one study, 746 patients with MCC who received definitive RT and did not receive surgery, were found to have longer disease-specific survival (DSS) (5-year DSS 73% vs. 54% without definitive RT; $p < .0001$).

Management of Regional Draining Nodal Basin

Clinically Node-Negative Patients

Patients found to have occult regional nodal basin metastasis at the time of surgery (wide excision and SLNB) should then undergo systemic imaging, if not already performed preoperatively, to assess for other regional or distant metastases. Patients without distant metastatic disease identified on staging imaging may then undergo either completion lymphadenectomy (CLND) or RT to the nodal basin. In patients who undergo CLND, adjuvant RT should be considered only in those with multiple involved nodes or if ECE is present. Adjuvant RT also should be considered if SLNB was not performed or was unsuccessful.

Clinically Node-Positive Patients

Patients who present with clinically suspicious nodes should undergo baseline imaging to assess for regional and distant metastases. Fine-needle aspiration or core needle biopsy should be obtained for histologic confirmation of regional nodal metastasis. In patients without distant metastasis identified on staging imaging, either lymphadenectomy, definitive RT, or a clinical trial for neoadjuvant or adjuvant therapy could be considered. For patients who undergo lymphadenectomy, adjuvant RT may be considered particularly in patients with multiple involved nodes or if ECE is present.

Management of Local and/or Regional Recurrence

Treatment of local or regional MCC recurrence should be individualized and will depend on whether additional surgery or radiation is possible. Management approach should be based on input from a multidisciplinary team.

Management of Locally Advanced/Unresectable and Distant Metastatic Disease

The treatment of locally advanced/unresectable and distant metastatic disease requires multidisciplinary input, should be individualized for each patient, and may include a combination of systemic therapy, RT, and in highly selective circumstances, surgery. However, the mainstay of treatment for unresectable or metastatic MCC is systemic therapy and clinical trials should be considered if available.

Patients with MCC may respond to chemotherapy with reported response rates ranging as high as 70% in patients receiving first-line chemotherapy and 9% to 20% in those receiving subsequent lines of chemotherapy. Although MCC is chemosensitive, responses tend not to be durable with median progression-free survival (PFS) ranging from 3 to 5 months in the literature. A variety of chemotherapy regimens may be used to treat MCC, including platinum-based regimens in combination with etoposide and cyclophosphamide in combination with doxorubicin or epirubicin and vincristine.

The use of immune checkpoint blockade therapies has improved survival for many patients with advanced solid malignancies, and application of immunotherapy in MCC is an active area of investigation. In a phase II, single-arm multicenter trial (NCT02267603) of pembrolizumab (anti–PD-1) in patients with distant metastatic or unresectable locoregional disease, overall response rate was 56% although durability of response remains unknown. Preliminary results of the phase I/II Checkmate 358 trial suggest that patients with metastatic MCC may also respond to nivolumab (anti–PD-1). With median follow-up of 26 weeks (range 5 to 35 weeks), objective response rate was 68% among 22 evaluable patients with MCC (71% in patients without prior systemic treatment, 63% in patients who had one or two prior systemic therapies). The JAVELIN Merkel 2000 trial (NCT 02155647) was a multicenter trial which examined use of avelumab, an anti-PD-L1 antibody, in patients with distant metastatic MCC. In an interim analysis of patients for whom avelumab was their first line of systemic therapy and with a median follow-up of 5.1 months (range 0.3 to 11.3 months), the overall response rate was 62% for those with at least 3 months follow-up ($n = 29$) and 71% among those with at least 6 months follow-up ($n = 14$). The calculated PFS was 9.1 months. In the cohort of patients who failed prior lines of systemic therapy and with a median follow-up of 16.4 months, the overall response rate to avelumab was 33% for those with at least 12 months follow-up and median overall survival (OS) was estimated to be 12.9 months, compared to reported median OS of 4.4 to 5.7 months for patients with MCC treated with multiple lines of chemotherapy in retrospective series. Based on these data, avelumab received Federal Drug Administration (FDA) approval for treatment of metastatic MCC.

Although there are no trials comparing immune checkpoint therapy with chemotherapy for patients with metastatic MCC, immunotherapy appears to afford similar response rates and responses may be more durable. Thus, avelumab, nivolumab, and pembrolizumab should be considered as part of first-line treatment for patients presenting with metastatic or unresectable MCC. However, the side effects and toxicities of immune checkpoint blockade therapies differ from those of cytotoxic chemotherapies and for patients with contraindications to immunotherapy, cytotoxic systemic therapy regimens may be considered. Patients should be encouraged to participate in ongoing clinical trials evaluating the role of immunotherapy, chemotherapy, and the combination of those treatments, in order to help determine what is the best current treatment approach for patients with advanced MCC.

There are also several ongoing early-phase studies investigating the use of talimogene laherparepvec (TVEC) for the treatment of locally advanced or unresectable MCC either alone (NCT03458117) or in combination with RT (NCT02819843) or anti–PD-1 therapy (NCT02978625).

Follow-Up and Surveillance

Large retrospective series, meta-analyses, and more recent smaller studies have reported recurrence rates ranging 25% to 50%, with median time to recurrence of ~8 to 9 months and up to 90% of recurrence occurring within 24 months following completion of treatment. Patients who have had MCC are also at increased risk for additional primary malignancies, including another primary MCC and other cutaneous malignancies. Thus, close clinical follow-up is recommended for patients with MCC and, if clinically feasible, immunosuppressive treatments should be minimized with multidisciplinary input.

At MD Anderson, the schedule of follow-up evaluations for patients with MCC varies according to risk of recurrence. Physical examination should include a complete skin and lymph node examination every 3 to 6 months for the first 3 years, then every 6 to 12 months thereafter. Imaging studies should be performed as clinically indicated and should be considered in those who are immunosuppressed, with stage III disease, or who were MCPyV oncoprotein antibody seronegative at diagnosis as these individuals are at higher risk for recurrence. Surveillance imaging to monitor for recurrence/metastases may include brain MRI and whole-body FDG PET with fused axial CT imaging, which is especially useful to identify bone involvement. CT of the chest, abdomen and pelvis with contrast, with CT of the head and neck when appropriate, may be used when whole-body FDG PET-CT is not available. At MD Anderson, regional nodal basin ultrasonography is also used in the surveillance of select patients who are at risk of nodal relapse. Finally, rising titers may be an early indicator of recurrence in patients who were MCPyV oncoprotein antibody seropositive at diagnosis.

CASE SCENARIO

Case Scenario 1: Merkel Cell Carcinoma

Presentation

A 78-year-old male with an unremarkable past medical history presents with an erythematous nodule on the upper back. He first noted the lesion a month prior and noticed that it has become larger and more firm over the past month. He underwent shave biopsy and now presents to your surgical oncology office.

Differential Diagnosis

Melanoma
Squamous cell carcinoma
Basal cell carcinoma
Merkel cell carcinoma
Keratoacanthoma
Epidermal cyst
Kaposi sarcoma
Secondary malignancy

On physical examination, he has a healing biopsy incision site with surrounding erythema that is firm but without fluctuance or drainage. He has no palpable lymphadenopathy in the neck, bilateral axilla, or bilateral groin. Biopsy shows Merkel cell carcinoma, 3.8 × 0.8 mm (at least), tumor thickness 0.8 mm, mitotic count of 2 per mm², and carcinoma present at the deep tissue edge.

Confirmation of Diagnosis and Treatment

After confirmation of the Merkel cell carcinoma (MCC) diagnosis by an expert pathologist, the determination needs to be made whether staging imaging is indicated, particularly if there is clinical suspicion of regional or distant disease. Up to 25% of patients will have clinical evidence of regional lymphadenopathy, thus a careful and thorough history and physical examination is paramount to appropriate MCC management. In this scenario, as there is no clinical evidence of regional or distant disease, it is reasonable to proceed directly to wide local excision with sentinel lymph node biopsy (SLNB). Given the location on the upper back, we recommend performing preoperative lymphatic mapping to determine and localize the draining regional lymph node basin(s); this can be accomplished by either lymphoscintigraphy or single-photon emission computed tomography imaging merged with CT (SPECT-CT). It is also important to counsel the patient that adjuvant radiation may be recommended to both the primary and draining regional nodal basin based on pathologic findings following wide excision and SLNB.

Surgical Approach—Key Steps

The technical surgical approach is the same as that performed for melanoma (see Chapter 3 for the detailed description of the specific surgical approach to wide excision and SLNB). These principles are applied to the treatment of patients with Merkel cell carcinoma with the caveats that there is a more liberal use of SLNB, margins may be more difficult to assess intraoperatively and radiation therapy is used frequently and often not definitely recommended until the pathology is finalized. In view of these caveats, consideration should be given to delayed primary closure, especially if flap coverage might be required.

Postoperative Management

MCC is a radiosensitive tumor and adjuvant radiation therapy (RT) is often recommended/indicated in the multimodal care of these patients. For patients with positive margins or close margins, adjuvant RT should be given with consideration of adjuvant immune checkpoint blockade depending on sentinel node status. Patients who did not warrant preoperative staging imaging but who are found to have a positive sentinel node should undergo imaging assessment to evaluate for distant metastatic disease, consisting of brain MRI and whole-body fluorodeoxyglucose positron emission tomography (FDG PET) with fused axial CT imaging. If no distant metastatic disease is identified, patients with positive sentinel lymph nodes should be offered CLND and/or adjuvant radiation depending on the extent of nodal disease and ECE. In patients with significant comorbidities, definitive RT to the nodal basin can be considered.

Common Curve Balls

- Unable to identify a sentinel lymph node
- Positive margins
- Difficulty closing primary resection site

Take Home Points

- MCC is a highly aggressive skin malignancy with neuroendocrine features and high rates of regional and distant disease at diagnosis most commonly presenting in patients who are elderly or immunosuppressed.
- Patients with suspicion for regional or distant metastasis should undergo brain MRI and whole-body FDG PET with fused axial CT imaging (or CT if FDG PET-CT not available) prior to surgical resection.
- MCC is radiosensitive and RT is used commonly in the adjuvant setting or for definitive treatment.
- Patients without clinical evidence of regional disease undergoing wide local excision should undergo SLNB.
- Patients with positive SLNB should be offered either adjuvant RT to the nodal basin or completion lymph node dissection (CLND).
- Immunotherapy is a systemic treatment option in the metastatic setting with ongoing research assessing its role in the neoadjuvant setting.

Case Scenario 2: Merkel Cell Carcinoma

A 63-year-old male with a history of mantle cell lymphoma on immunosuppressive therapy following stem cell transplantation presents with a new skin lesion on his left thigh. A biopsy was performed which revealed Merkel cell carcinoma with positive margins. On examination, he is noted to have palpable lymphadenopathy in his left inguinal region; metastatic MCC was confirmed on core needle biopsy. Preoperative staging imaging revealed enlarged left inguinofemoral lymph nodes but no evidence of distant metastatic disease.

Confirmation of Diagnosis and Treatment

The patient has had early identification of regional metastatic disease at initial MCC presentation and diagnosis. Although regional MCC metastasis to the left inguinofemoral nodal basin was suspected due to the location of the primary MCC on the left thigh, biopsy is indicated to confirm clinical N1 disease in this immunosuppressed patient with a history of lymphoma. Multidisciplinary input should include discussion of the patient's multimodality treatment options, including systemic therapies, clinical trial options, RT, and surgery, as well as the sequencing of these potential treatments. The patient's performance status should also be evaluated at their initial presentation. This patient would require resection of the primary MCC as well as left inguinofemoral lymphadenectomy with possible consideration of neoadjuvant systemic therapy such as in clinical trial setting. Adjuvant radiation therapy would be recommended to the primary MCC site as well as potentially the regional nodal basin depending on the extent of regional lymph node involvement and presence of extracapsular extension (ECE).

Surgical Approach—Key Steps

Surgical management will require a wide excision of the primary MCC site of the left thigh as well as left inguinofemoral lymphadenectomy. At the time of surgery, the patient should be positioned, prepped, and draped with this in mind. For adequate exposure during the lymphadenectomy, the patient should be prepped with their leg flexed and externally rotated into a "frog-leg" position. If there is flap reconstruction planned, the type of flap coverage should be determined beforehand. In cases where the skin defect can be closed primarily, a Sartorius flap is often adequate for coverage of the femoral vessels. Although uncommonly required, the surgeon should be prepared for the possible need to perform en bloc vascular resection and reconstruction in cases where bulky nodal disease is inseparable from the adjacent/underlying vessels. The indication to perform a pelvic lymphadenectomy is controversial and needs to be individualized to the patient's risk of complication and the anticipated benefit provided. If performed, the technique of pelvic lymphadenectomy is the same as for melanoma (see Chapter 3, Melanoma) for specific surgical details.

Postoperative Management

The majority of patients undergoing lymphadenectomy without complications can be discharged from the hospital the following day. Patients should be fitted with compression stockings to limit their degree of lymphedema and their drain should be left in place until multiple days of low output. In this high-risk example, the patient would likely benefit from adjuvant RT to both the primary and regional nodal basin surgical sites after a period of healing has passed. Adjuvant systemic therapy could be considered on clinical trial basis. Patient must be educated to recognize and monitor for signs and symptoms of postoperative complications such as wound dehiscence, surgical site infections, seromas, deep venous thrombosis, as well as lymphedema and disease recurrence.

Common Curve Balls

- Complete gross resection of locally advanced and regional metastatic disease may be technically challenging.
- Surgery may not be the best first treatment modality for patients with resectable but bulky or borderline resectable regional disease. Such patients may benefit from participation in clinical trials of neoadjuvant therapy which may downstage and facilitate surgical resection.
- Postoperative wound complications.

Take Home Points

- Management of MCC with regional disease requires multidisciplinary input. Care should be tailored to the patient's individual risks.
- Patients with unresectable disease should be considered for definitive radiation and systemic therapy.
- Patient with regional disease without evidence of distant disease should be offered resection with lymphadenectomy if healthy enough for surgery. Clinical trials of neoadjuvant and adjuvant therapies should be considered if available.

CASE SCENARIO REVIEW

Questions

1. A 43-year-old female with a history of hypertension and polycystic kidney disease now 10 years post operation from a left renal transplant is referred to your Surgical Oncology clinic for a suspicious 2.0-centimeter (cm) lesion on the left upper chest. Outside biopsy was performed with findings consistent with Merkel cell carcinoma. Which of the following is a risk factor for the development of MCC?

   A. Female
   B. Immunosuppression
   C. Polycystic kidney disease
   D. Hypertension

2. An 80-year-old male is referred to your clinic by dermatology after discovery of a 0.25-cm Merkel cell carcinoma on the right forearm following shave biopsy. Margins are negative. Comprehensive history and physical examination reveal a 1-month history of a nodule to the right forearm without any other changes to his health. The surgical site is well healed without lymphadenopathy. Which is the best next step in management?

   A. Wide local excision with 1-cm margins and sentinel lymph node biopsy
   B. Wide local excision with 3-cm margins and sentinel lymph node biopsy
   C. Computed tomography of the chest, abdomen, pelvis, and brain
   D. PET/CT

3. A 65-year-old male is referred to your clinic by dermatology after discovery of a 3.0-cm Merkel cell carcinoma on the right forearm following shave biopsy. Margins are positive. The biopsy site is well healed and there is palpable right axillary lymphadenopathy on examination. What is the next best step in evaluation/management?

   A. Wide local excision with 2-cm margins and sentinel lymph node biopsy
   B. Neoadjuvant chemotherapy
   C. CT of chest, abdomen, and pelvis
   D. Biopsy of right axillary lymphadenopathy, PET/CT with brain MRI

4. The patient's (from Question 3) brain MRI was negative, however, PET/CT demonstrated FDG-avid nodules in the right axilla, three avid nodules in the liver, and an additional lesion in the lung. What is the next best course of treatment?

   A. Consult the liver transplant team, thoracic surgery, and begin neoadjuvant chemotherapy
   B. Complete lymph node dissection (CLND)
   C. Initiate multidisciplinary discussion
   D. Consult IR for liver, lung, and axillary biopsies

5. A 58-year-old female is 18 months postoperation for a 4-cm MCC to the back with advancement flap and adjuvant radiation. She presents as part of her regular scheduled surveillance. She reports that over the past 4 weeks, she has developed new nodularity at the superior margin of her incision. She otherwise is well and without complaint. Which of the following, in addition to imaging, could suggest recurrent disease?

   A. Chromogranin-A
   B. CEA
   C. MCPyV
   D. HPV

Answers

1. **The correct answer is B.** *Rationale:* Risk factors associated with MCC include sun exposure, with increased incidence in geographical regions with higher UV indices. MCC is also more common to arise in individuals who are immunosuppressed, including those with a history of organ transplantation and immunosuppressive medications, lymphoproliferative disorders such as chronic lymphocytic leukemia, and HIV. Male-to-female prevalence for MCC is 1.4:1. Neither polycystic kidney disease nor hypertension is risk factor for MCC.

2. **The correct answer is A**. *Rationale:* Patients without clinical evidence of regional or distant metastatic disease who are candidates for surgery are recommended to undergo wide excision of the primary MCC with SLNB in the same operative setting for the purpose of both curative resection and definitive pathologic staging of the primary tumor and regional nodal basin. SLNB should be performed prior to wide excision of the primary MCC. Excision of primary MCC is typically performed with 1- to 2-cm margins with depth down to the investing fascia when feasible. There is insufficient evidence to support wider resection margins. In patients without clinical evidence of regional or distant metastatic disease on history and physical at presentation, body imaging is not routinely indicated and should be selectively obtained only when clinically indicated.

3. **The correct answer is D**. *Rationale:* The patient in this question has palpable lymphadenopathy, highly concerning for clinically evident regional lymph node metastasis. Pathologic confirmation of lymph node metastasis by biopsy and staging imaging which should consist of PET-CT and brain MRI imaging should be performed prior to initiation of multimodal treatment. SLNB would be inappropriate in this patient with concern for node-positive disease and staging should be completed with the imaging. Neoadjuvant chemotherapy prior to staging or biopsy is inappropriate. PET/CT is preferred over CT alone.

4. **The correct answer is C**. *Rationale:* The patient has widely metastatic MCC and should be discussed at a multidisciplinary tumor board. MCC is radiosensitive and both the Checkmate and JAVELIN trials suggest promise for the use of immunotherapy treatments in this population of patients. Early multidisciplinary discussion should be sought. A liver transplant is not indicated in this patient with widely metastatic disease. Complete lymph node dissection would be inappropriate with evidence of widespread disease, although it could be considered in some instances for symptom control but not prior to multidisciplinary discussion. Consultation of interventional radiology (IR) for biopsy might be required for pathologic confirmation of metastatic disease, but biopsy of all three locations would be unnecessary, particularly if the patient had previous imaging for comparison.

5. **The correct answer is C**. *Rationale:* In addition to imaging and biopsy, a relative rise in MCPyV antibodies is associated with recurrence in Merkel cell carcinoma and can aid in postoperative surveillance. Patients must also be MCPyV seropositive prior to MCC treatment for this to be clinically relevant. Chromogranin-A is a marker of recurrence in neuroendocrine tumors. CEA is associated with colorectal tumor recurrence. HPV is the human papillomavirus and plays no role in surveillance postoperatively.

Recommended Readings

Albores-Saavedra J, Batich K, Chable-Montero F, Sagy N, Schwartz AM, Henson DE. Merkel cell carcinoma demographics, morphology, and survival based on 3870 cases: a population based study. *J Cutan Pathol.* 2010;37:20–27.

Cowey CL, Mahnke L, Espirito J, Helwig C, Oksen D, Bharmal M. Real-world treatment outcomes in patients with metastatic Merkel cell carcinoma treated with chemotherapy in the USA. *Future Oncol.* 2017;13:1699–1710.

D'Angelo SP, Russell J, Lebbé C, et al. Efficacy and safety of first-line avelumab treatment in patients with stage IV metastatic Merkel cell carcinoma: A preplanned interim analysis of a clinical trial. *JAMA Oncol.* 2018;4:e180077.

Fang LC, Lemos B, Douglas J, Iyer J, Nghiem P. Radiation monotherapy as regional treatment for lymph node-positive Merkel cell carcinoma. *Cancer.* 2010;116:1783–1790.

Feng H, Shuda M, Chang Y, Moore PS. Clonal integration of a polyomavirus in human Merkel cell carcinoma. *Science.* 2008;319:1096–1100.

Fields RC, Busam KJ, Chou JF, et al. Recurrence after complete resection and selective use of adjuvant therapy for stage I through III Merkel cell carcinoma. *Cancer.* 2012;118:3311–3320.

Frohm ML, Griffith KA, Harms KL, et al. Recurrence and survival in patients with Merkel cell carcinoma undergoing surgery without adjuvant radiation therapy to the primary site. *JAMA Dermatol.* 2016;152:1001–1007.

Harms KL, Healy MA, Nghiem P, et al. Analysis of prognostic factors from 9387 Merkel cell carcinoma cases forms the basis for the new 8th Edition AJCC Staging System. *Ann Surg Oncol.* 2016;23:3564–3571.

Hawryluk EB, O'Regan KN, Sheehy N, et al. Positron emission tomography/computed tomography imaging in Merkel cell carcinoma: a study of 270 scans in 97 patients at the Dana-Farber/Brigham and Women's Cancer Center. *J Am Acad Dermatol.* 2013;68:592–599.

Heath M, Jaimes N, Lemos B, et al. Clinical characteristics of Merkel cell carcinoma at diagnosis in 195 patients: the AEIOU features. *J Am Acad Dermatol.* 2008;58:375–381.

Jabbour J, Cumming R, Scolyer RA, Hruby G, Thompson JF, Lee S. Merkel cell carcinoma: assessing the effect of wide local excision, lymph node dissection, and radiotherapy on recurrence and survival in early-stage disease—results from a review of 82 consecutive cases diagnosed between 1992 and 2004. *Ann Surg Oncol.* 2007;14:1943–1952.

Kaae J, Hansen AV, Biggar RJ, et al. Merkel cell carcinoma: incidence, mortality, and risk of other cancers. *J Natl Cancer Inst.* 2010;102:793–801.

Kaufman HL, Russell JS, Hamid O, et al. Updated efficacy of avelumab in patients with previously treated metastatic Merkel cell carcinoma after ≥1 year of follow-up: JAVELIN Merkel 200, a phase 2 clinical trial. *J Immunother Cancer.* 2018;6:7.

Leech SN, Kolar AJ, Barrett PD, Sinclair SA, Leonard N. Merkel cell carcinoma can be distinguished from metastatic small cell carcinoma using antibodies to cytokeratin 20 and thyroid transcription factor 1. *J Clin Pathol.* 2001;54:727–729.

Lemos BD, Storer BE, Iyer JG, et al. Pathologic nodal evaluation improves prognostic accuracy in Merkel cell carcinoma: analysis of 5823 cases as the basis of the first consensus staging system. *J Am Acad Dermatol.* 2010;63:751–761.

Medina-Franco H, Urist MM, Fiveash J, Heslin MJ, Bland KI, Beenken SW. Multimodality treatment of Merkel cell carcinoma: case series and literature review of 1024 cases. *Ann Surg Oncol.* 2001;8:204–208.

Mojica P, Smith D, Ellenhorn JDI. Adjuvant radiation therapy is associated with improved survival in Merkel cell carcinoma of the skin. *J Clin Oncol.* 2007;25:1043–1047.

Nghiem P, Bhatia S, Lipson EJ, et al. Durable tumor regression and overall survival in patients with advanced Merkel cell carcinoma receiving pembrolizumab as first-line therapy. *J Clin Oncol.* 2019;37(9):693–702.

Paulson KG, Lewis CW, Redman MW, et al. Viral oncoprotein antibodies as a marker for recurrence of Merkel cell carcinoma: A prospective validation study. *Cancer.* 2017;123:1464–1474.

Paulson KG, Park SY, Vandeven NA, et al. Merkel cell carcinoma: current US incidence and projected increases based on changing demographics. *J Am Acad Dermatol.* 2018;78:457–463.

Satpute SR, Ammakkanavar NR, Einhorn LH. Role of platinum-based chemotherapy for Merkel cell tumor in adjuvant and metastatic settings. *J Clin Oncol.* 2014;32:9049–9049.

Servy A, Maubec E, Sugier PE, et al. Merkel cell carcinoma: value of sentinel lymph-node status and adjuvant radiation therapy. *Ann Oncol.* 2016;27:914–919.

Strom T, Carr M, Zager JS, et al. Radiation therapy is associated with improved outcomes in Merkel cell carcinoma. *Ann Surg Oncol.* 2016;23:3572–3578.

Tarantola TI, Vallow LA, Halyard MY, et al. Prognostic factors in Merkel cell carcinoma: analysis of 240 cases. *J Am Acad Dermatol.* 2013;68:425–432.

Topalian SL, Bhatia S, Hollebecque A, et al. Non-comparative, open-label, multiple cohort, phase 1/2 study to evaluate nivolumab (NIVO) in patients with virus-associated tumors (CheckMate 358): Efficacy and safety in Merkel cell carcinoma (MCC) [abstract]. Presented at the American Association for Cancer Research Annual Meeting; Abstract CT074.

Youlden DR, Youl PH, Peter Soyer H, Fritschi L, Baade PD. Multiple primary cancers associated with Merkel cell carcinoma in Queensland, Australia, 1982–2011. *J Invest Dermatol.* 2014;134:2883–2889.

6 Soft Tissue and Bone Sarcoma

Russell G. Witt and Christina L. Roland

Soft Tissue Sarcomas

Sarcomas are rare tumors; in 2021, the estimated number of new cases in the United States were 13,460 (0.7% of all new cancer cases), with an estimated number of deaths of 5,350 (0.8% of all cancer deaths), based on data from American Cancer Society. At the time of presentation, 60% to 80% of patients have localized disease, whereas 15% to 20% have metastatic disease. The overall 5-year survival rate for patients with all stages of soft tissue sarcoma is 50% to 60% but varies significantly by stage (approximately 80% in patients with localized disease and 20% in those with metastatic disease) and histologic subtype. Of the patients who die of sarcoma, most will succumb to metastatic disease, which 80% of the time occurs within 2 to 3 years of the initial diagnosis.

Soft tissue sarcomas arise predominantly from embryonic mesoderm but can also arise from the ectoderm. Mesodermal cells give rise to the connective tissues distributed throughout the body; therefore, soft tissue sarcomas can occur anywhere in the body. The majority of primary lesions originate in an extremity (45%), with the next most frequent anatomic site of origin being intra-abdominal (20%)/retroperitoneal (20%), followed by trunk (10%) and the head/neck region (5%) (Fig. 6.1). Sarcoma is a heterogeneous disease group that encompasses >100 histologic subtypes. Each subtype has its own unique behavior, different recurrence pattern, and distinct survival. Excluding gastrointestinal stromal tumors (GISTs), the most common histologic types of soft tissue sarcoma in adults are undifferentiated/unclassified sarcoma (with pleomorphic, round cell, and spindle cell variants), liposarcoma, leiomyosarcoma, synovial sarcoma, and malignant peripheral nerve sheath tumor (MPNST) (Fig. 6.2). Rhabdomyosarcoma is the most common soft tissue sarcoma of childhood.

For the past four decades, a multimodality approach has been utilized in the treatment of patients with soft tissue sarcomas, which has improved treatment outcomes and quality of life but recurrence rates and survival have made only incremental progress, highlighting the need for improved systemic therapy options.

Etiology

The vast majority of sarcomas are sporadic with unknown etiology, but a number of factors have been associated with increased risk of soft tissue sarcoma, including previous radiation exposure, chronic lymphedema,

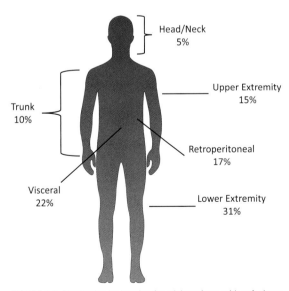

FIGURE 6.1 Distribution by location for adult patients with soft tissue sarcoma. (Data from DeVita VT Jr., Lawrence TS, Rosenberg SA, eds. *DeVita, Hellman, and Rosenberg's Cancer: Principles and Practice of Oncology.* 10th ed. Lippincott Williams & Wilkins; 2015:1253–1291.)

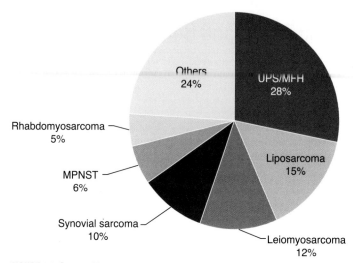

FIGURE 6.2 Common histologies of soft tissue sarcoma. (Data from Coindre JM, Terrier P, Guillou L, et al. Predictive value of grade for metastasis development in the main histologic types of adult soft tissue sarcomas a study of 1240 patients from the French Federation of Cancer Centers Sarcoma Group. *Cancer*. 2001;91:1914–1926.)

genetic predisposition, trauma, and occupational chemicals such as phenoxyacetic acids and wood preservatives containing chlorophenols.

Previous Radiation Exposure

External-beam radiation therapy is a rare but well-established cause of soft tissue sarcoma. An 8- to 50-fold increase in the incidence of sarcomas has been noted for patients treated with radiation therapy for cancers of the breast, cervix, ovary, testes, and lymphatic system. In addition, the risk of developing a sarcoma after radiation therapy increases in a dose dependent fashion. The median latency between irradiation and the development of a sarcoma is approximately 10 years but can range widely. The most common histologic types of radiation-associated sarcomas are osteogenic sarcoma, undifferentiated/unclassified sarcoma, angiosarcoma, and lymphangiosarcoma. Radiation-associated sarcomas are associated with a worse prognosis compared with non–radiation-associated sarcomas, even when matched for stage.

Chronic Lymphedema

In 1948, Stewart and Treves were the first to describe the association between chronic lymphedema following axillary dissection and subsequent lymphangiosarcoma. Lymphangiosarcoma has also been observed in patients after filarial infections and in the lower extremities of patients with congenital primary lymphedema.

Genetic Predisposition

Several well-described genetic predisposition syndromes have been associated with increased risk of certain subtypes of bone and soft tissue sarcomas. For example, patients with Gardner syndrome (familial adenomatous polyposis) have a higher-than-normal incidence of desmoid tumors; patients with germline mutations in the tumor suppressor gene *p53* (Li–Fraumeni syndrome) have a high incidence of various types of sarcomas; and patients with von Recklinghausen disease who have abnormalities in the neurofibromatosis type 1 gene have an increased risk of MPNST and GIST. Soft tissue sarcomas can also occur in patients with hereditary retinoblastoma (Rb) as a second primary malignancy.

Several oncogenes have been associated with the development of soft tissue sarcomas, including *MDM2*, *CDK4*, *N-myc*, *c-erbB2*, and members of the *ras* family. Amplifications of these oncogenes have been shown to correlate with an adverse outcome. Amplifications of MDM2 and CDK4 are frequently identified in well-differentiated or dedifferentiated liposarcomas and may be helpful in confirming histologic diagnoses as well as serving as potential treatment targets. Tumor suppressor genes, such as the Rb and the *p53* gene, also play a critical role in many cases of soft tissue sarcoma.

Histopathology

Histologic grade remains the most important prognostic factor for determining outcome for soft tissue sarcoma. However, emerging data suggest that pathologic classification may better determine outcomes when

TABLE 6.1	Breakdown of Common Sarcoma Histologic Type by Metastatic Potential

Low Metastatic Potential
Desmoid tumor
Atypical lipomatous tumor/well-differentiated liposarcoma
Dermatofibrosarcoma protuberans
Hemangiopericytoma

Intermediate Metastatic Potential
Myxoid liposarcoma
Myxofibrosarcoma (previous myxoid malignant fibrous histiocytoma)
Extraskeletal chondrosarcoma

High Metastatic Potential
Undifferentiated pleomorphic sarcoma (previously pleomorphic malignant fibrous histiocytoma)
Liposarcoma (dedifferentiated and pleomorphic)
Leiomyosarcoma
Angiosarcoma
Alveolar soft part sarcoma
Clear-cell sarcoma
Epithelioid sarcoma
Extraskeletal Ewing sarcoma
Extraskeletal osteosarcoma
Neurogenic sarcoma (malignant schwannoma)
Rhabdomyosarcoma
Synovial sarcoma

other pretreatment variables are considered. Tumor behavior varies significantly among histologic subtypes; for example, lymph node metastasis is rare in soft tissue sarcoma (<5%) except in a few histologic subtypes, such as epithelioid sarcoma, clear cell sarcoma, rhabdomyosarcoma, and angiosarcoma. However, at MD Anderson, routine lymphatic mapping is only performed on the two histologic subtypes that most frequently metastasize to LNs, epithelioid and clear cell sarcoma of the extremity. Chromosomal translocations have been found to be associated with specific histologic subtypes and can be used to help confirm the histologic diagnosis. Several variants of translocations between chromosomes 11 and 22 have been reported in Ewing sarcoma; similarly, a fusion of two novel genes (SYT at 18q11 and SSX at Xp11) has been identified as a causative translocation in most (perhaps all) synovial sarcomas. Other translocations or gene rearrangements are best characterized in myxoid liposarcoma (FUS-DDIT3), alveolar rhabdomyosarcoma (PAX3-FOXO1), and desmoplastic small round cell tumors (EWS-WT1). Table 6.1 shows a breakdown of the common histologic types of tumors according to their metastatic potential.

Grading of soft tissue sarcomas follows the French Federation of Cancer Centers (FNCLCC) grading system and is based on differentiation, mitotic count, and tumor necrosis. The scores for each factor are added to determine the grade (1 to 3) for the sarcoma. At MD Anderson Cancer Center (MDACC), the grading of soft tissue sarcoma uses histologic subtypes almost synonymously with the definition of grade in many cases. The following are high-grade by definition: undifferentiated pleomorphic sarcoma (UPS) (formerly malignant fibrous histiocytoma), synovial sarcoma, pleomorphic liposarcoma, dedifferentiated liposarcoma, MPNST, rhabdomyosarcoma, epithelioid sarcoma, clear-cell sarcoma, alveolar soft part sarcoma, Ewing sarcoma, primitive neuroectodermal tumor, osteosarcoma, and mesenchymal chondrosarcoma. Intermediate-grade soft tissue sarcomas include myxofibrosarcoma, myxoid liposarcoma, extraskeletal myxoid chondrosarcoma, and solitary fibrous tumor (hemangiopericytoma). Low-grade soft tissue sarcomas include well-differentiated liposarcoma. Grading for leiomyosarcoma, fibrosarcoma, and other unclassified sarcomas is determined individually by sarcoma pathologists on the basis of histologic morphology.

Important updates were made in 2020 in the fifth edition of the World Health Organization's *WHO Classification of Tumours of Soft Tissue and Bone*. The updated edition incorporated many changes in tumor classification and provided new genetic insight into the pathogenesis of many different tumor types. In the update, numerous classifications were added or changed as shown in Table 6.2.

Staging and Outcomes

The American Joint Committee on Cancer (AJCC) staging system includes the most widely accepted soft tissue sarcoma staging system in the world, and its eighth edition of *Cancer Staging Manual* was published

TABLE 6.2	Additions in 5th Edition of World Health Organization Classification of Soft Tissue Sarcoma and Bone

Adipocytic Tumors
Atypical spindle cell/pleomorphic lipomatous tumor
Myxoid pleomorphic liposarcoma
Epithelioid liposarcoma

Fibroblastic and Myofibroblastic Tumors
Angiofibroma of soft tissue
EWSR1-SMAD3-positive fibroblastic tumor
Superficial CD34-positibe fibroblastic tumor

Peripheral Nerve Sheath Tumors
Malignant melanotic nerve sheath tumor

Skeletal Muscle Tumors
Congenital spindle cell rhabdomyosarcoma with VGLL2/NCOA2/CITED2 rearrangement
MYOD1-mutant spindle cell/sclerosing rhabdomyosarcoma

Smooth Muscle Tumors
EBV-associated smooth muscle tumor
Inflammatory leiomyosarcoma

Vascular Tumors
Anastomosing hemangioma

Tumors of Uncertain Differentiation
NTRK-rearranged spindle cell neoplasm

in 2020. Staging of soft tissue sarcoma incorporates histopathologic grade (G), tumor size (T), nodal involvement (N), and distant metastases (M). There is a significant change from seventh edition, with one of the most notable changes dividing soft tissue sarcomas into the different staging systems by anatomic site: head and neck, extremity and trunk, abdomen/thoracic visceral organs, and retroperitoneum. In the eighth edition, T category criteria vary primarily by anatomic site, and the superficial versus deep distinction is eliminated. Prognostic stage grouping is also unique to each anatomic site category; however, the head/neck category and the abdomen/thoracic visceral organs category do not have stage grouping as insufficient data are available. Nodal involvement (N1 disease), which is rare but associated with poor survival in soft tissue sarcoma, is classified as stage IIIB in the retroperitoneal category, while it is classified as stage IV in the extremity/trunk category. Of note, desmoid tumors/deep fibromatosis and Kaposi sarcoma remained excluded from the sarcoma staging system while GISTs continue to have a unique staging system. Histologic grade (G1 to G3) continues to play an important role in soft tissue sarcoma staging utilizing the FNCLCC sarcoma grading system.

MDACC reported the results of a retrospective analysis of 1,225 patients with localized soft tissue sarcoma treated with surgical resection and radiation therapy. By multivariate analysis, high-grade histology was a risk factor for both local recurrence and distant metastases. The 5-year disease-specific survival rates were 96%, 87%, and 67% for low-, intermediate-, and high-grade tumors, respectively. The histologic subtypes rhabdomyosarcoma, epithelioid sarcoma, and clear-cell sarcoma were associated with shorter disease-specific survival (relative risk 1.6; 95% confidence interval [CI] 1.1 to 2.2; $P < .001$). Other risk factors for disease-specific survival included large tumor size (>5 cm), tumors located in the head/neck or deep trunk, age >64 years, and positive or uncertain margin status. Of note, rates of lymph node recurrence in this study were low (<3%) among all patients except for those with histologic subtypes of rhabdomyosarcoma (17% at 5 years), epithelioid sarcoma (18% at 5 years), and clear-cell sarcoma (15% at 5 years).

Multiple nomograms have been created to improve risk stratification of retroperitoneal sarcoma (RPS). MDACC published a postoperative nomogram for survival of patients with RPS, which was based on a retrospective analysis of 343 patients with RPS who underwent curative-intent surgery between 1996 and 2006. The nomogram incorporates the following factors: age (≥65 years), tumor size (≥15 cm), type of presentation (primary vs. recurrent), multifocality, completeness of resection, and histology. More recently, Gronchi et al. published a survival nomogram built on three cancer centers' data sets of RPS after primary resection and validated in 135 patients from a fourth institution. The analysis of 523 surgical patients with primary RPS revealed age, tumor size, grade, histologic subtype, multifocality, and extent of resection as prognostic factors for overall survival (OS).

Presentation and Diagnosis

Clinical presentation of soft tissue sarcoma depends on the anatomic site and depth of the tumor. Most extremity soft tissue sarcomas present as an asymptomatic mass. Although superficial tumors (e.g., back or hand tumors) become apparent early, a deeply located tumor (e.g., thigh tumors) can grow to 10 to 15 cm in diameter before it becomes apparent. RPSs generally present as a large mass (nearly 50% are larger than 20 cm when diagnosed) since they often do not produce symptoms until they are large enough to compress or invade adjacent organs. Occasionally, patients may present with neurologic symptoms resulting from lumbar or pelvic nerve compression, extremity edema/deep vein thrombosis from venous compression or obstructive gastrointestinal symptoms.

Radiographic Evaluation

The goals of pretreatment radiologic imaging are to accurately define the local extent of a tumor and to exclude metastatic disease. Magnetic resonance imaging (MRI) has supplanted computed tomography (CT) as the imaging technique of choice for soft tissue sarcomas of the extremities. MRI accurately delineates muscle groups and distinguishes between bone, vascular structures, neurologic structures, and tumor. In addition, sagittal and coronal views allow three-dimensional evaluation of anatomical compartments. A CT scan of the abdomen and pelvis and MRI of the spine should also be obtained in extremity myxoid liposarcomas because this disease is known to metastasize to the fatty tissue of the abdomen and retroperitoneum as well as to the axial skeleton.

For the vast majority of sarcomas, the predominant site of metastasis is the lung, and chest CT is used most often in patients with high-grade lesions to exclude metastatic disease. Specific radiologic evaluation of other areas can be indicated in certain histologies which have been shown to have unique patterns of metastatic spread. Examples of this include abdominal/retroperitoneal and bone imaging in patients with locally advanced extremity myxoid liposarcoma and brain imaging in patients with alveolar soft parts sarcoma. In other sarcoma histologies, searches for bone and brain metastases are rarely indicated unless a patient has associated symptoms. A retrospective study of 1,170 patients with extremity soft tissue sarcoma revealed that 10% had a distant metastasis at presentation, and 83% of these metastases were located in the lung. Among those patients with lung metastasis, 63% of metastases were detected by routine chest x-ray (CXR), whereas in 37%, the CXRs appeared to be normal. Higher risk of metastasis at presentation was observed in deep lesions (9% vs. 4%) and in high-grade tumors (11.8% vs. 7.0% in intermediate-grade and 1.2% in low-grade tumors). As for histologic subtypes, a higher risk of lung metastasis was observed in Ewing sarcoma (25%), MPNST (16%), extraskeletal chondrosarcoma (14%), and pleomorphic sarcoma (11%). The authors concluded that all patients with soft tissue sarcoma should have a CXR, with chest CT reserved for patients with a suspicious lesion on CXR or for patients with a high-risk tumor (large tumor size [>5 cm], deep tumor location, or intermediate/high-grade histology).

CT remains the imaging technique of choice for RPSs. In addition to giving invaluable information about anatomic considerations, radiologic subtleties between the various histologic types can be appreciated with CT. The role of positron emission tomography (PET) scan in patients with sarcoma has not been well defined. Many types of benign musculoskeletal tumors (e.g., Schwannoma) can show fluorodeoxyglucose F-18 (FDG) uptake in various degrees, making it difficult to establish the role of PET in the staging of patients with sarcoma.

Biopsy and Pathologic Evaluation

An accurate preoperative histologic diagnosis is critical in determining the primary treatment of a soft tissue sarcoma. The biopsy should yield enough tissue so that a pathologic diagnosis can be made without increasing the risk of complications. Core-needle biopsy has been demonstrated to be reliable for an accurate pathologic diagnosis, particularly when the pathologic findings correlate closely with clinical and imaging findings. Biopsy performed under ultrasound or CT guidance can improve the diagnostic accuracy. However, owing to heterogeneity within a tumor, sampling error can occur. Particularly in retroperitoneal liposarcomas, the failure to sample a nonlipogenic component of dedifferentiated liposarcoma can result in misdiagnosis. A retrospective study of 120 patients with retroperitoneal liposarcomas revealed that the overall subtype-specific diagnostic accuracy of percutaneous biopsy was 63%. The accuracy was especially lower in patients with dedifferentiated liposarcoma (36%), likely secondary to sampling error and to the morphologic variability of dedifferentiated liposarcoma. Incorporating radiographic information into histologic assessment is important to improve diagnostic accuracy in patients with deep extremity or RPSs. One potential application for PET scan is for biopsy guidance. Many RPSs are heterogeneous and PET scan *may* help to identify the presence of a highly active component within the heterogeneous tumor. When percutaneous image-guided biopsy is performed, the area identified as active on PET scan can be targeted.

Treatment Approach

The treatment of sarcomas requires a multidisciplinary approach, including discussion at multidisciplinary conferences that include radiologists, pathologists, surgical oncologists, medical oncologists, and radiation oncologists. Preoperative chemotherapy and/or radiation therapy are used frequently in selected patients. Treatment strategies should be discussed in individual cases and should be based on a number of factors, most notably on tumor location, size, and histologic grade/subtypes. Surgery for maximal locoregional control remains the mainstay of treatment, while the use of neoadjuvant and adjuvant chemotherapy and/or radiation are becoming increasingly individualized as our understanding of the disease improves.

Follow-Up

The rationale behind active follow-up strategies to detect recurrence in patients with soft tissue sarcomas is that early recognition and treatment of recurrent disease can prolong survival. Extremity sarcomas most frequently recur as pulmonary metastases, whereas retroperitoneal or intra-abdominal sarcomas more commonly recur locally. Recurrence patterns also vary depending on histologic subtypes. The majority of soft tissue sarcomas that recur do so within the first 2 years after the completion of therapy. Patients should therefore be examined every 3 months with chest imaging (as outlined previously) and primary site imaging during this high-risk period. Most experts recommend that the primary site be evaluated with either MRI for an extremity tumor or CT for intra-abdominal or retroperitoneal tumors. In some circumstances, ultrasonography can be used to look for local recurrence of an extremity tumor. Follow-up intervals may be lengthened to every 6 months, during years 2 through 5 after the completion of therapy. After 5 years, patients should be assessed annually, with chest and primary site imaging and physical examination.

Extremity Soft Tissue Sarcomas

More than 50% of soft tissue sarcomas originate in an extremity. The most common histologic subtypes include UPS, liposarcoma, synovial sarcoma, and fibrosarcoma, although various other histologic types are also seen in the extremities.

Surgery

The mainstay of treatment is margin-negative surgical resection. The extent of surgical resection is based on tumor location, tumor size, depth of invasion, involvement of nearby structures, and the patient's performance status. In the 1970s, 50% of patients with extremity sarcomas were treated with amputation. However, despite a local recurrence rate of less than 10% after amputation, many patients continued to die of metastatic disease. This realization led to the development of a consensus treatment algorithm consisting of limb-sparing surgical resection combined with postoperative radiation therapy. A landmark randomized trial from the National Cancer Institute by Rosenberg et al. in 1982 demonstrated no difference in survival among patients treated with limb-sparing surgery plus radiation therapy compared with patients treated with amputation. In 1985, on the basis of the limited data available, the National Institutes of Health developed a consensus statement recommending limb-sparing surgery for the majority of patients with high-grade extremity sarcomas. However, amputation remains the treatment of choice for patients whose tumor cannot be grossly resected with a limb-sparing procedure that preserves function (<5% of cases).

Radical, wide resection is the primary treatment of extremity sarcomas with ideally, a 2-cm margin, if possible. However, when this is not attainable (i.e., around neurovascular structures), surgeons should attempt to preserve major nerves since it is rare to have actual invasion into these structures. It is important to remember that there is generally a zone of compressed reactive tissue that forms a pseudocapsule around the tumors and that tumors may extend beyond this pseudocapsule. When possible, the biopsy site or tract should also be included en bloc with the resected specimen.

Before patients are referred to a specialized center, it is not uncommon for surgeons to perform a suboptimal resection due to inadequate surgical planning. For these patients, re-resection is preferred if it can be achieved without functional compromise, in conjunction with either pre- or postoperative radiation therapy. In cases where no radiologic or clinically evident tumor is apparent, in which re-resection would likely cause functional compromise, radiation therapy is an alternative option. At MDACC, among 666 patients who underwent apparent total tumor resection before presentation to MDACC without obvious macroscopic disease, 295 patients (44%) underwent re-resection. Among those who underwent re-resection, 136 (46%) patients had residual tumor. The 5-year local control rates were 85% in the re-resection group and 78% in the non–re-resection group ($P = .03$), even though the re-resection group had a higher proportion of positive margins at prereferral resection. Re-resection remained a significant predictor for improved survival after multivariate analysis.

Elective regional lymphadenectomy is rarely indicated in patients with soft tissue sarcomas. However, in patients with histologies that carry a high risk of lymph node metastasis (such as rhabdomyosarcoma, epithelioid sarcoma, clear-cell sarcoma, and UPS), fine-needle aspiration or core-needle biopsy should be performed of radiographically suspicious lymph nodes. In such cases, lymphadenectomy is recommended only if findings are positive. The role of sentinel lymph node biopsy in histologic subtypes susceptible to lymph node metastasis remains controversial. MDACC reported a retrospective study of 35 patients with synchronous (43%, $n = 15$) or metachronous (57%, $n = 20$) isolated nodal metastasis from extremity soft tissue sarcomas who underwent lymphadenectomy. Epithelioid sarcoma (23%), undifferentiated pleomorphic sarcoma (23%) and clear cell sarcoma (17%) were the most common histologic subtypes found to have undergone lymphadenectomy for lymph node metastases. The estimated 1-, 2-, and 5-year OS rates in patients with documented lymph node metastasis that underwent lymphadenectomy were 91%, 82%, and 60%, respectively. These outcomes more closely approximated the historical outcomes of patients with stage III disease (5-year OS 50%) compared to the 5-year OS of stage IV disease patients (25%), thus suggesting that aggressive surgical approaches, such as regional lymph node dissection in patients with confirmed lymph node metastasis, can have a positive impact on survival.

Multimodality Therapy

Radiation Therapy

The primary goal of radiation therapy is to optimize local tumor control. The evidence for adjunctive radiation therapy in patients eligible for limb-sparing surgical resection comes from two randomized trials and a number of single-institution reports. In the late 1990s, two index randomized controlled trials were published favoring postoperative radiation therapy for patients with extremity soft tissue sarcomas eligible for limb-sparing surgical resection. The study conducted at the National Cancer Institute randomized 91 patients with high-grade extremity tumors to limb-sparing surgery followed by chemotherapy alone or radiation therapy plus postoperative chemotherapy. A second group of 50 patients with low-grade tumors were treated with resection alone versus resection with radiation therapy. The overall 10-year local control rates were 98% with radiation therapy versus 70% without radiation therapy, and improved local control rates with radiation therapy were seen in both of the high- and low-grade tumor cohorts. However, quality-of-life analysis showed that radiation therapy resulted in worse limb strength, edema, and range of motion, although these adverse effects were often transient and had little effect on daily activities.

In a second randomized trial conducted at Memorial Sloan Kettering Cancer Center (MSKCC), 164 patients were randomized to observation or brachytherapy (42 to 45 Gy) following limb-sparing surgery for extremity or resection of superficial trunk soft tissue sarcomas. The 5-year local control rates were 82% in the brachytherapy group versus 69% in the no-brachytherapy group, respectively ($P = .04$). In subset analysis of the low-grade tumor cohort ($n = 45$), there was no benefit to brachytherapy in the local control ($P = .49$). There was no survival benefit observed in the radiation group in either study.

Brachytherapy

Brachytherapy, which involves the placement of multiple catheters in the tumor resection bed at the time of surgery, has been reported to achieve local control rates comparable to those achieved with external-beam radiation therapy. Guidelines have been established that recommend placing the afterloading catheters at 1-cm intervals with a 2-cm margin around the surgical bed. Usually, after the fifth postoperative day, the catheters are then loaded with radioactive wires (iridium-192) that deliver 42 to 45 Gy to the tumor bed over 4 to 6 days. The frequency of wound complications associated with brachytherapy is similar to that seen for postoperative radiation therapy (approximately 10%).

The primary benefit of brachytherapy is the shorter overall treatment time of 4 to 6 days, compared with the 4 to 6 weeks generally required by pre- or postoperative external-beam radiation therapy regimens. Brachytherapy also produces less radiation scatter in critical anatomical regions (e.g., gonads, joints), with improved function a potential clinical benefit. Cost-analysis comparisons of brachytherapy versus external-beam radiation therapy have further shown that the charges for postoperative irradiation with brachytherapy are lower than those for external-beam radiation therapy. However, with the increase in advanced radiation techniques (such as intensity-modulated radiation therapy [IMRT]), the utilization of brachytherapy has decreased over time.

On the basis of the evidence from these studies, radiation therapy in conjunction with margin-negative surgery is recommended for patients with intermediate- to high-grade tumors to improve local control. Because T1 tumors (<5 cm) are less frequently associated with local recurrences, radiation therapy can be omitted in cases with low risk of recurrence and wide margins (at least 1 cm). For low-grade tumors, radiation therapy can be considered in cases with positive or close margins (<1 cm).

Preoperative versus Postoperative Radiation Therapy

The optimal timing of radiation therapy for soft tissue sarcomas remains a focus of active investigation. There are potential advantages in both pre- and postoperative radiation approaches. In preoperative radiation therapy, the tumor itself displaces the normal structures and protects them from radiation exposure, which helps to limit the toxicity to surrounding normal structures. In addition, the potential exists for radiation therapy to reduce tumor burden and enable a more limited, conservative surgical resection. The postoperative approach allows better histologic examination of resected specimens without distortion from treatment effect and is associated with fewer acute wound complications.

A multicenter randomized trial comparing pre- and postoperative radiation therapy was conducted in Canada, which randomized 190 patients with primary (90%) or recurrent (10%), mostly intermediate- or high-grade (83%) extremity soft tissue sarcomas, to receive either 50 Gy of preoperative or 66 Gy of postoperative external-beam radiation therapy, in conjunction with limb-sparing surgical resection. Patients with positive margins in the preoperative group received a 16- to 20-Gy postoperative boost. This study was terminated at the interim analysis, due to a higher acute wound complication rate in the preoperative therapy group (35% vs. 17%, $P=.01$). In the update of this study with a median follow-up of 6.9 years, no significant differences were reported between the two groups in 5-year local control rates (93% in preoperative vs. 92% in postoperative therapy group) and 5-year OS rates (73% in preoperative vs. 67% in postoperative therapy group; $P=.48$). In regard to late toxicity, the study found a higher rate of grade 2 or greater fibrosis in the postoperative therapy group (48% vs. 32%; $P=.07$), which was associated with impaired function.

At MDACC, we favor the preoperative approach over the postoperative approach for most patients with extremity soft tissue sarcomas for several reasons. First, postoperative radiation therapy has a higher rate of late toxicity, which is usually irreversible (in contrast, acute wound complications are usually manageable and eventually heal). Second, lower doses and smaller field sizes can be used in the preoperative approach than in the postoperative approach. Third, rapidly improving radiation technologies, such as IMRT, are more effective in the preoperative setting, where the tumor can be precisely targeted and the radiation dose delivered to the surrounding structures can be minimized. This can be particularly important in preventing radiation damage to the joints. Finally, plastic surgery techniques that include advanced tissue transfer procedures are being used more frequently in patients with high-risk wounds, and this can achieve a high success rate (>90%) of healed wounds from a single-stage operation. The treatment strategy for extremity sarcomas treated at MDACC is summarized in Figure 6.3.

Certain histologic types of STS are more susceptible to radiation therapy, most notably myxoid liposarcoma. In the Dose Reduction of Preoperative Radiotherapy in Myxoid Liposarcoma (DOREMY) nonrandomized controlled trial, dose reduction of preoperative radiotherapy was attempted in myxoid liposarcoma given its known susceptibility to radiation. The objective was to determine if decreased overall radiation dosage resulted in decreased radiation toxicity without compromising oncologic outcomes. Seventy-nine patients were enrolled with 77 proceeding to surgical resection. They received a radiotherapy regimen of 36 Gy in once-daily 2-Gy fractions compared to the typical 50 Gy. Of the 77 who underwent surgical resection, extensive pathologic treatment response was seen in 70 patients (91%) with a local control rate of 100% and wound complication rate of 17% (compared to historical controls of 35%). This study demonstrated that reduction of radiation dosage was safe and remained oncologically effective for patients with myxoid liposarcoma of the extremity.

Chemotherapy

Despite improvements in local control, metastasis and death remain significant problems for patients with high-risk soft tissue sarcomas. This high-risk group includes localized sarcomas in nonextremity sites, tumors which show an intermediate- or high-grade histology, or large (T2) tumors. The treatment regimen for patients with high-risk localized disease, metastatic disease, or both, usually includes chemotherapy. Systemic chemotherapy is a particularly important component of treatment for several sarcomas that occur predominantly in children, such as rhabdomyosarcoma, Ewing sarcoma, and osteogenic sarcoma. It is also well recognized that myxoid liposarcoma and synovial sarcoma are chemosensitive soft tissue sarcomas.

Extremity Soft-Tissue Sarcoma Management

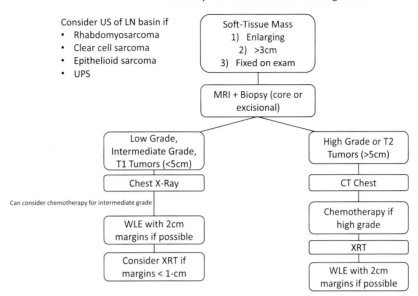

FIGURE 6.3 Treatment strategy for extremity soft tissue sarcomas. US, ultrasound; LN, lymph node; CT, computed tomography; MRI, magnetic resonance imaging; XRT, radiation therapy; UPS, unclassified pleomorphic sarcoma.

Only three drugs, doxorubicin, dacarbazine, and ifosfamide, have consistently achieved response rates of at least 20% as single-agent treatments in patients with advanced soft tissue sarcomas. The majority of active chemotherapeutic trials have included doxorubicin as part of the treatment regimen. The response rate to ifosfamide has been found to vary from 20% to 60% in single-institution series in which higher-dose regimens have been used or in which ifosfamide was given in combination with doxorubicin. Several newer agents have been FDA approved for patients with metastatic sarcoma including trabectedin, a DNA-binding agent is approved for patients with liposarcoma or leiomyosarcoma and eribulin, a microtubule-inhibiting agent approved in the treatment of liposarcoma. In 2015, trabectedin monotherapy after standard chemotherapy was compared to standard supportive care in patients with advanced, translocation-related sarcoma. Trabectedin significantly improved median progression-free survival (5.6 vs. 0.9 month, HR 0.07, 95% CI 0.03 to 0.16). Trabectedin was then studied in combination with doxorubicin versus doxorubicin alone as first-line therapy in patients with advanced soft tissue sarcomas. In this study, trabectedin plus doxorubicin did not show superiority over doxorubicin alone (median progression-free survival 5.5 vs. 5.7). A comparison between trabectedin at two different infusion rates versus doxorubicin was also performed and trabectedin was not found to be superior to doxorubicin in progression-free survival while having a higher rate of toxicity.

Eribulin was compared to dacarbazine in a phase III trial in patients with liposarcoma or leiomyosarcoma in 2016. Median OS was significantly improved in patients receiving eribulin compared to dacarbazine (median 13.5 months [95% CI 10.9 to 15.6] vs. 11.5 months [9.6 to 13.0]; HR 0.77 [95% CI 0.62 to 0.95]; $P = .0169$). Adverse events of grade 3 or higher were greater in the eribulin group (67%) than the dacarbazine group (56%). This study demonstrated the utility of this agent in those with refractory advanced liposarcoma and leiomyosarcoma.

Postoperative Chemotherapy

Individual randomized trials of postoperative chemotherapy have failed to demonstrate an improvement in disease-free survival or OS in patients with soft tissue sarcomas. However, there are several criticisms of these individual trials that may explain why they failed to demonstrate improvement in survival. First, the chemotherapy regimens used were suboptimal, in that single-agent drugs (most commonly doxorubicin) were studied and dosing schedules were less intensive. Second, the sample sizes in these trials were not large enough to allow the detection of clinically significant differences in survival. Third, the majority of patients who did not respond to the initial treatment regimen were started on other chemotherapeutic regimens that potentially affected disease-free and OS. Finally, most studies included patients at low risk for metastasis and death, that is, those with small (<5 cm) and low-grade tumors.

Hence, the role of postoperative chemotherapy in soft tissue sarcomas has been controversial. The first randomized trial of postoperative chemotherapy for soft tissue sarcomas was conducted at MDACC in 1973 and showed improved disease-free survival in the chemotherapy cohort. Since then, multiple randomized trials have been conducted with conflicting results, leading to a formal meta-analysis conducted by the Sarcoma Meta-Analysis Collaboration in 1997. This group analyzed data from 1,568 patients in 14 trials of doxorubicin-based postoperative chemotherapy to determine the effect of postoperative chemotherapy on localized, resectable soft tissue sarcomas. In this trial, with a median follow-up of 9.4 years, doxorubicin-based chemotherapy showed a trend toward improved OS in the postoperative therapy group (HR for death 0.89, 95% CI 0.76 to 1.03; $P = .12$). This led to a subsequent meta-analysis in 2008 of the randomized trials of doxorubicin-based postoperative chemotherapies in patients with resectable soft tissue sarcomas. The results from the analysis of data from 18 trials, which included 1,953 patients, demonstrated that the use of doxorubicin combined with ifosfamide was associated with improved OS (OR 0.56, 95% CI 0.36 to 0.85; $P = .01$), with absolute risk reduction of 11% (41% vs. 30%) (Table 6.3). Based on these analyses, a chemotherapy regimen including ifosfamide is generally recommended.

However, the use of postoperative chemotherapy for resectable soft tissue sarcomas remains controversial. The above-mentioned meta-analysis did not include the most recent two largest randomized trials conducted by the European Organisation for Research and Treatment of Cancer (EORTC). These studies tested doxorubicin/ifosfamide-containing regimens. The pooled analysis of a total of 819 patients from these two studies showed that postoperative chemotherapy was associated with improved recurrence-free survival (HR 0.74, 95% CI 0.60 to 0.92; $P = .006$), but not with OS.

Preoperative Chemotherapy

The potential advantages to preoperative chemotherapy over a postoperative approach include tumor reduction (which may enable more limited resection), early treatment of potential micrometastases, patient selection for surgery in cases with borderline resectable tumors or tumors with questionable metastases, and most importantly, in vivo evaluation of treatment effectiveness. Given that only 30% to 50% of patients respond to standard chemotherapeutic regimens, a preoperative approach enables the oncologist to identify patients who respond to specific regimens, as shown radiographically and pathologically. Treatment responders after four or six courses of chemotherapy subsequently undergo surgery, often after preoperative radiation therapy. After surgery, patients who did not respond to short courses of preoperative chemotherapy can be considered for either no postoperative chemotherapy or use of different chemotherapy agents.

Currently, there is no evidence available from phase III randomized controlled studies to define the role of preoperative chemotherapy in soft tissue sarcomas. A retrospective analysis of 356 patients with high-grade extremity soft tissue sarcomas conducted at MSKCC showed that preoperative chemotherapy (doxorubicin plus ifosfamide) improved disease-specific survival compared with survival in the surgery-alone cohort (HR 0.52, 95% CI 0.30 to 0.92; $P = .02$) after stratification by size, histology, and age. The authors concluded that preoperative chemotherapy is beneficial in patients with high-grade extremity soft tissue sarcomas >10 cm. The EORTC group conducted a phase II study that randomized 150 patients with high-risk soft tissue sarcomas (approximately 80% of which were located in extremities) to a preoperative chemotherapy (doxorubicin plus ifosfamide, three cycles) group versus a local treatment—only group. Postoperative radiation therapy was indicated based on margin status (<1 cm) irrespective of the study arm; 46% in the chemotherapy group and 54% in the local treatment—only group received radiation therapy. This study was closed before expansion into a phase III trial due to its slow accrual. Although the study was underpowered, precluding definitive

TABLE 6.3	Meta-Analysis of Adjuvant Chemotherapy for Soft Tissue Sarcoma				
Outcomes	No. of Trials	No. of Patients	Odds Ratio (95% CI)	P Value	Absolute Risk Reduction (%)
Local recurrence	17	1,700	0.73 (0.56–0.94)	0.02	3
Distant recurrence	18	1,747	0.69 (0.56–0.86)	0.001	9
Overall recurrence	18	1,747	0.67 (0.56–0.82)	0.0001	10
Overall survival (all regimens)	18	1,953	0.77 (0.64–0.93)	0.01	6
Overall survival (doxorubicin based + ifosfamide)	5	414	0.56 (0.36–0.85)	0.01	11

Data from Sarcoma Meta-Analysis Collaboration, 2008.

conclusions, it failed to show a survival benefit in those receiving preoperative chemotherapy; the 5-year OS rates were 64% in the local treatment—only group and 65% in the chemotherapy group ($P = .22$).

A cohort analysis of the combined databases from both MDACC and MSKCC was performed, evaluating the efficacy of chemotherapy in high-grade soft tissue sarcomas. The data on 674 patients with stage III extremity sarcoma who received either pre- or postoperative doxorubicin-based chemotherapy were reviewed to determine their outcomes (5-year disease-specific survival, as well as 5-year local and distant recurrence rates). The 5-year disease-specific survival rate was 61%, and the probability of local and distant recurrences at 5 years was 83% and 56%, respectively. An important conclusion from this study was that the clinical benefits of doxorubicin-based chemotherapy in patients with high-risk extremity sarcomas were not sustained beyond 1 year after therapy. The investigators then went on to compare their study with the Sarcoma Meta-Analysis Collaboration and made the following observations. First, the patient population of the Sarcoma Meta-Analysis Collaboration was more heterogeneous than that of the cohort study, in that it included patients with both primary and recurrent extremity and nonextremity sarcomas. Second, there were also fewer uncontrolled variables in the cohort study. On the basis of these findings, the authors urged caution when reviewing studies of chemotherapeutic regimens with a short-term follow-up and concluded that there remains no consensus regarding the role of chemotherapy in patients with localized high-risk soft tissue sarcomas.

As seen with outcomes, response rates to chemotherapy are likely related to histologic subtype. Certain subtypes of sarcoma have been shown to be more chemosensitive, such as synovial sarcoma. Eilber et al. reported a retrospective review of prospectively collected data of 101 patients with T2b extremity synovial sarcoma who underwent surgical resection. Sixty-seven percent of patients received ifosfamide-based therapy (85% preoperatively), which was associated with improved disease-specific survival (4 years, 88% vs. 67%; $P = .01$). The same group also reported a retrospective study of 245 patients with T2 high-grade extremity liposarcomas who underwent surgical resection. Approximately half (49%) of the patients had myxoid/round cell, 40% had pleomorphic, and 11% had dedifferentiated subtype of liposarcoma. Sixty percent of patients received pre- or postoperative chemotherapy (doxorubicin based [34%] or ifosfamide based [26%]). Ifosfamide-based chemotherapy was found to be associated with improved survival (5-year disease specific survival, 92% vs. 65%; $P < .001$), whereas doxorubicin-based chemotherapy was not.

In a phase III, randomized controlled, multicenter trial, Gronchi et al. evaluated histology-tailored neoadjuvant chemotherapy for patients with localized high-risk soft tissue sarcomas from five histologic subtypes: leiomyosarcoma, MPNST, myxoid liposarcoma, synovial sarcoma, and UPS. Patients were randomly assigned to receive epirubicin plus ifosfamide or a histology-tailored chemotherapy (gemcitabine and dacarbazine for leiomyosarcoma, etoposide and ifosfamide for MPNST, trabectedin for myxoid liposarcoma, ifosfamide for synovial sarcoma, and gemcitabine and docetaxel for UPS). No benefit was shown for histology-tailored chemotherapy over the standard chemotherapy regimen. In fact, there was a significant difference in the disease-free survival and OS at 3 years favoring the standard chemotherapy over the histology-tailored chemotherapy groups, demonstrating there is more work to be done for the optimal chemotherapy regimen for patients with localized disease.

At MDACC, we prefer the preoperative approach based on available data and the above-described theoretical advantages. Our standard treatment algorithm is described in Figure 6.3. We often use preoperative chemotherapy followed by radiation therapy in patients with large (T2) high-grade tumors. Future studies are warranted to determine the survival benefit of this approach and to define the most effective regimen.

Isolated Limb Perfusion Therapy

While limb salvage has become possible for the majority of patients with soft tissue sarcomas, it is not feasible in approximately 5% of patients. Regional therapy with isolated limb perfusion (ILP) or isolated limb infusion (ILI) has been evaluated in patients with advanced sarcoma for limb preservation. One of the largest series from the Netherlands used ILP with tumor necrosis factor-α (TNF-α) and melphalan in 217 patients with soft tissue sarcomas. The reported response rate was 75% and a limb salvage rate of 87%. ILI, as an alternative method of regional chemotherapy, seems equally as efficacious. The Sydney Melanoma Unit reported a response rate of 90% in 21 patients with sarcoma using ILI including 65% of patients with a complete response; however, the recurrence rate in this study, with a median follow-up of only 28 months, was 42%. It is important to note that these studies included infusion of TNF-α, which is not available in the United States. At MD Anderson, we have used ILP/ILI in patients with locally advanced extremity sarcomas who have amputation as their only treatment option. Although we have seen response rates similar to that seen in the studies noted above, these responses were not found to be durable with a significant early local recurrence rate. It is possible that the lack of availability of TNF-α contributed to this rapid recurrence rate; therefore, we have reserved offering this as a treatment option to patients until we have more active clinical agents available. As expected, it is difficult at this stage to interpret results for this technique since the data available represent a small population with heterogeneous histologies in which a variety of chemotherapeutic agents and indications have been used.

Management of Local Recurrence

Disease can recur in up to 20% of patients with extremity sarcoma, typically within 2 years after resection. Local recurrence is associated with shorter survival, although whether local recurrence is causative for shorter survival or is a marker of aggressive disease is controversial. Regardless, the adequacy of the surgical resection clearly plays a significant role in determining whether the disease recurs locally.

An isolated local recurrence should be treated aggressively by complete resection with a wide margin (10% to 20% of patients require amputation due to vital structure involvement) plus radiation therapy, commonly delivered preoperatively (for the reasons previously discussed) at MDACC. The use of pre- or postoperative chemotherapy is determined on a case-by-case basis. Several small studies have shown that patients with isolated local recurrences may be successfully retreated, with local recurrence-free survival rates approaching 72%. Treatment for patients who received previous irradiation can be complicated, since repeat irradiation increases complications such as impaired wound healing, osteonecrosis, and fibrosis, which can even result in future amputation due to these complications. However, simple wide resection harbors a high risk of local control failure, and amputation remains an option to provide adequate local control. Patients may be considered for brachytherapy or intraoperative radiation therapy. Use of plastic surgery techniques such as rotational tissue flaps is encouraged to enable more radical resection and improve wound healing.

We reported our experience in managing local recurrence in patients who had received previous irradiation at MDACC. Of 62 patients in this study, 25 had undergone resection alone, whereas 37 had received postoperative radiation therapy (33 receiving brachytherapy) after resection. Local control rate at 5 years was 51%. On multivariate analysis, positive margins were associated with higher risk of local failure. Postoperative radiation therapy did not improve the local control rate (5-year rates: 58% in the radiation group vs. 39% in the surgery-only group; $P = .4$) or disease-specific survival (5-year rates, 66% vs. 67%; $P = .8$). The wound complication rate was significantly higher in the irradiation group (80% vs. 17%, $P < .001$). Interpretation of these results is difficult because of selection bias; however, treating physicians need to be aware of the risk associated with re-irradiation in patients with recurrent soft tissue sarcoma.

Management of Distant Disease

Distant metastases occur in 40% to 50% of patients with intermediate- and high-grade extremity sarcomas. Most metastases to distant sites occur within 2 years of the initial diagnosis, and the predominant site of distant metastases from primary extremity sarcomas is the lung (>70%). The mainstay of treatment for metastatic disease is systemic chemotherapy, but metastasectomies can improve survival for selected patients.

Isolated lung metastases should be considered for resection if there are no extrapulmonary metastases, the patient is medically fit enough to withstand surgery, and the lesions are amenable to resection. While no randomized controlled trials have been performed evaluating pulmonary metastasectomy, multiple retrospective studies have demonstrated a survival benefit compared to best supportive care with reported 5-year survival rates ranging from 17% to 58% depending on the series. A disease-free interval of more than 12 months, the ability to resect all metastatic disease, age younger than 50 years, and the absence of preceding local recurrence were found to be independent prognostic factors in a multivariate analysis of patients who underwent resection of pulmonary metastases.

Extremity Sarcomas, General Recommendations (Fig. 6.3)

1. Soft tissue tumors that are enlarging, greater than 3 cm in diameter or fixed on physical examination should be evaluated with radiologic imaging (ultrasonography, CT, or MRI), and a tissue diagnosis made on the basis of core-needle biopsy findings.
2. Evaluation for metastatic disease once a sarcoma diagnosis is established: chest radiography for low- or intermediate-grade lesions and T1 tumors, and chest CT for high-grade or T2 tumors.
3. A wide local excision with 2-cm margins is adequate therapy for low-grade lesions and T1 tumors if they can be widely resected.
4. Radiation therapy plays a critical role in the management of intermediate- and high-grade tumors.

5. Patients with recurrent high-grade sarcomas or distant metastatic disease should be considered for chemotherapy.

6. An aggressive surgical approach should be taken in the treatment of patients with an isolated local recurrence or resectable distant metastases.

Retroperitoneal Sarcomas

Among soft tissue sarcomas in adults, 15% to 20% occur in the retroperitoneum. Most retroperitoneal tumors are malignant, and approximately one-third are soft tissue sarcomas. Benign entities include schwannoma and angiomyolipoma. The malignant differential diagnosis in a patient presenting with a retroperitoneal tumor includes lymphoma, germ cell tumors, and undifferentiated carcinomas. The most common RPSs are liposarcomas (50% to 65%, mainly well-differentiated or dedifferentiated liposarcomas), leiomyosarcomas (20% to 25%), and undifferentiated/unclassified sarcomas. Reported histologic frequencies in RPSs vary across studies; despite this, histology remains a key component to overall prognosis. Analysis of an MDACC database of 1,118 patients with RPSs revealed dramatic differences in behavior among the three subgroups of histologies (well-differentiated liposarcoma, other liposarcomas [mostly dedifferentiated liposarcoma], and other histologies [mainly leiomyosarcoma and undifferentiated/unclassified sarcomas]); 5-year OS rates were 95% in well-differentiated liposarcoma, 25% in other liposarcomas, and 43% in other histologies ($P < .001$). The importance of histologic subtypes in predicting tumor behavior and survival was also reported by two more recent large retrospective studies from MSKCC and the European Multi-Institutional Collaborative RPS Working Group. Based on these reports, liposarcoma has a high local recurrence rate (35% to 60%) and high metastasis rate if dedifferentiated (30%), whereas leiomyosarcoma has a higher distant metastasis rate (60%) and a low local recurrence rate (<20%). These two most common subtypes of RPS have characteristics distinct from each other. Treatment strategies should be individualized on the basis of tumor histology by dedicated multidisciplinary specialists in sarcoma.

Clinical Presentation

RPSs generally present as large masses; nearly 50% are larger than 20 cm at the time of diagnosis. They typically do not produce symptoms until they grow large enough to compress or invade contiguous structures. On occasion, patients may present with neurologic symptoms, resulting from the compression of lumbar or pelvic nerves, or obstructive gastrointestinal symptoms, resulting from the displacement or direct tumor involvement of an intestinal organ.

Evaluation

The workup of a patient with a retroperitoneal mass begins with an accurate history that should exclude signs and symptoms of lymphoma (e.g., fever, night sweats). A complete physical examination with particular attention to all nodal basins and a testicular examination in males is critically important. Laboratory assessment can be helpful; an increased lactate dehydrogenase level can be suggestive of lymphoma, whereas an increased β-human chorionic gonadotropin level, alpha-fetoprotein level, or both can indicate a germ cell tumor.

The radiologic assessment should include a CT scan of the abdomen and pelvis to define the extent of the tumor and its relationship to surrounding structures, particularly vascular structures. Imaging should include the liver in a search for metastases and discontinuous abdominal disease. The kidneys should also be evaluated to assess bilateral renal function. Thoracic CT is indicated to look for lung metastases in patients with high-grade tumors. A CT-guided core-needle biopsy is appropriate for obtaining a tissue diagnosis in patients who are potentially eligible for preoperative therapy.

Surgery

Complete surgical resection is the mainstay of treatment for primary RPSs. Wide, negative margins are frequently not possible due to anatomic constraints. In several retrospective assessments of patients with RPSs, complete surgical excision (R0 or R1) was achieved in only 40% to 60% of patients. Incomplete or debulking (R2) resection may improve local symptoms but does not improve survival.

The quality of surgical resection is important for outcomes. First, margin-positive resection increases the chance of local recurrence. This is vital since local recurrence is often the cause of mortality in RPS. Second, incomplete resection has also been associated with a risk of developing distant metastasis that is almost four times higher than in those who undergo complete resection. Finally, it has an important impact on survival. In an analysis of 500 patients with RPS treated at MSKCC, the median survival duration of patients who underwent complete resection was 103 months versus 18 months for patients who underwent incomplete resection, which was no different than the survival seen in patients treated with observation without resection, thus demonstrating that there is no survival benefit from debulking procedures.

Careful preoperative planning is of paramount importance when considering surgical resection. Multiorgan resection is often required to achieve complete resection. Multidisciplinary surgical teams are frequently necessary, such as vascular surgery when resection and/or reconstruction of great vessels are required.

How extensive the surgical resection should be is an area of active controversy. Extrapolating the treatment concept of "extended or compartmental resection" from the treatment algorithm for extremity sarcomas to the treatment of RPSs would potentially result in the resection of uninvolved adjacent organs. In a French retrospective study of 382 patients with RPSs reported by Bonvalot et al. in 2009, nephrectomy was performed in 42% and colectomy in 30% of patients. The local recurrence rate was 44%. The authors advocated for compartmental resection which was associated with improved local control (a 3.29 times lower rate of local recurrence than with simple complete resection). There was no improvement in OS in patients treated with such an approach. Moreover, a high surgical complication rate of 16% was reported; in half of these patients, further surgery was required to manage complications. Thirteen patients (3%) died perioperatively from surgical complications, and 3 (1%) died intraoperatively in this study.

Gronchi et al. from an Italian group evaluated the impact of compartmental resection compared to "standard" resection based on a change in institutional surgical "philosophy" over time. This study divided patients into two groups by time period, before and after the concept of extended resection was employed into practice. After such an approach was introduced, there was an associated improvement in the local recurrence rate from 48% to 28% ($P = .007$); however, the distant metastasis rate increased from 13% to 22% ($P = .013$), with no statistically significant change in OS (5-year rates, 51% vs. 60%; $P = .47$). Moreover, because of the nature of this design, patients in the extensive resection group had significantly shorter follow-ups (almost half), which may contribute to the differences in local recurrence.

Limitations of the extended or "compartmental resection" approach have hindered its adoption into clinical practice. RPSs are usually large, abutting multiple organs in all directions. Multivisceral resection, although often necessary, significantly increases the morbidity and mortality associated with resection, likely in an exponential fashion. This makes it difficult to justify the resection of uninvolved "adjacent" organs (e.g., kidney, pancreas, duodenum). Therefore, it is our practice to resect adjacent structures with evidence of invasion, either radiographically or at the time of surgical exploration. Structures that are clearly not invaded by the tumor are preserved (Fig. 6.4).

Multimodality Therapy
The high local and distant recurrence rates in RPS have resulted in a shift in treatment strategies for localized RPS toward multimodality therapy, such as perioperative use of chemotherapy.

Radiation Therapy
Although certain retrospective studies reported the benefits of postoperative radiation therapy, toxicity with postoperative radiation therapy can be significant and difficult to deliver. Radiation therapy to RPSs postoperatively, even with advanced techniques such as intensity-modulated radiation therapy is difficult due to the

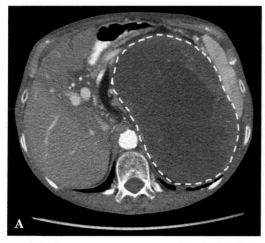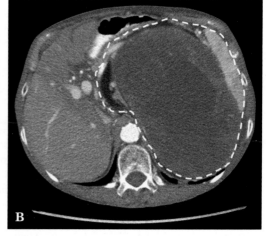

FIGURE 6.4 Cross-sectional imaging demonstrating the extent of resection by (**A**) a traditional organ-sparing resection as compared to (**B**) extended "compartmental" resection. Margin status of resection would be limited at the level of the aorta, the spine, and the body wall, regardless of extent of resection.

vicinity of bowel and other organs within the resected area. Therefore, postoperative radiation is generally not recommended.

The EORTC recently completed a prospective randomized phase III study (EORTC 62092, STRASS trial; NCT01344018) comparing preoperative radiation (50.4 Gy in 28 fractions) plus surgery to surgery alone for RPS. In the trial, 266 patients were enrolled with 133 being allotted to each treatment group. Median follow-up was 43.1 months. Of those within the surgery group, 126 (96%) made it to surgery and of those within the radiation group 119 (89%) underwent both surgery and radiation. Median recurrence-free survival in the radiation group was 4.5 years and 5.0 years in the surgery group ($P = .95$). Serious adverse events were reported in 30 (24%) of the patients in the radiation group and 13 (10%) within the surgery group. Based on these findings, preoperative radiation was not recommended for soft tissue sarcoma. Of groups treated, 75% were various liposarcoma subtypes (32% well-differentiated liposarcoma, 41% dedifferentiated liposarcoma, 3% other), 17% were leiomyosarcomas and 8% were other histologic types. Subgroup analysis showed that preoperative radiotherapy *may* improve outcomes in low-grade disease and liposarcoma but no benefit was seen in leiomyosarcoma and high-grade sarcomas. They were unable to draw any conclusions to the actual benefit in liposarcoma patients based on the low overall numbers.

The recently published American Society for Radiation Oncology guidelines for soft tissue sarcoma does not recommend the use of radiation therapy for RPS. If radiation therapy is to be considered, preoperative radiation therapy is recommended and postoperative radiation therapy is not recommended.

Postoperative brachytherapy has not been shown to be effective in combination with preoperative radiation therapy. Smith et al. reported the long-term follow-up of a phase II trial of 40 patients with RPS who had received preoperative radiation therapy with or without postoperative brachytherapy. The additional brachytherapy was associated with an unacceptable toxicity profile, typically associated with duodenitis/ duodenal stricture and death. Neither recurrence-free survival nor OS was improved in patients who received additional brachytherapy.

Chemotherapy

Data on post- or preoperative chemotherapy in RPS are very limited. Recently, a group from the Medical College of Wisconsin reported data from the National Cancer Database. Of 8,653 patients with surgically resected RPS, 1,525 (18%) received either preoperative (11%) or postoperative (7%) chemotherapy. Patients with tumors classified as intermediate/high-grade, leiomyosarcoma, or UPS histology and R2 resection status received chemotherapy more frequently. After propensity score matching, the median OS was shorter in patients who received chemotherapy (40 vs. 52 months; $P = .002$). Two other similar retrospective studies, reported by Singer et al. in 1995 and Bremjit et al. in 2014, showed adverse outcomes associated with postoperative or preoperative chemotherapy in RPS; however, because of innate selection bias associated with these retrospective studies, it is difficult to definitively assess the role of chemotherapy in RPS.

MDACC reported the safety of preoperative chemotherapy in a retrospective study of 309 patients with primary soft tissue sarcomas, including 108 located in retroperitoneum/viscera. Preoperative chemotherapy did not increase surgical complication rates in patients with RPS (29% vs. 34% in the upfront surgery group; $P = .66$). MDACC also evaluated the impact of radiographic response to preoperative chemotherapy on the extent of surgical resection. In this retrospective study of 65 patients with stage II or III sarcoma (23 retroperitoneal) who were treated with preoperative chemotherapy, the radiographic response was sufficient to decrease the extent of surgery in 13%. Patients with a radiographic response had a higher negative-margin resection rate, a better local recurrence-free survival rate, and a better OS rate than did nonresponders.

Traditional radiographic response criteria may not be the best indicator of response to therapy. MDACC reported on patients with retroperitoneal well-differentiated/dedifferentiated liposarcomas who underwent treatment with first-line chemotherapy. Eighty-two patients were included in the study, with 31 having received neoadjuvant chemotherapy and 51 having received definitive chemotherapy for unresectable recurrent or metastatic disease. Response Evaluation Criteria in Solid Tumors (RECIST) responses and analysis of their qualitative vascular responses (on contrast-enhanced CT) were performed. By RECIST criteria, 21% achieved partial response, 40% had stable disease and 39% had disease progression. All responses were seen in patients receiving chemotherapy. A qualitative vascular response was seen in 31% of patients. Clinical benefit (complete response, partial response, or stable disease greater than 6 months) was seen in 44% of patients. This study demonstrated that RECIST criteria did not adequately capture the response to therapy for large heterogeneous tumors and that other methods should be considered, such as qualitative vascular response.

Our practice is to determine treatment strategies for individual patients with RPS at a multidisciplinary sarcoma conference. We carefully use preoperative chemotherapy and/or radiation therapy, typically in patients with soft tissue sarcomas that are at high risk of distant metastasis, such as intermediate- or high-grade histology and large or recurrent tumors. Pretreatment biopsy and histologic confirmation are mandatory before initiating any preoperative therapy for RPS. The most commonly used regimen is doxorubicin plus ifosfamide, which is supported by data extrapolated from studies of extremity soft tissue sarcomas. The preoperative approach is preferred for several reasons, which were described in the previous section. In addition to the previous considerations, in patients with RPS that involve the kidney, preoperative multidisciplinary planning is critical as administration of ifosfamide requires two kidneys due to potential nephrotoxicity.

Targeted Therapy

Targeted therapy has been relatively unsuccessful for soft tissue sarcoma with most drugs achieving less than 10% overall response rates in trials (9.9% for trabectedin, 6.0% for pazopanib, and 4.0% for eribulin). Current studies are underway evaluating targeted therapy in combination with radiation therapy. A recent nonrandomized clinical trial by Martin-Broto et al. demonstrated that a combination of trabectedin with radiation therapy resulted in overall response rate of 60% in 25 patients with metastatic and unresectable STS. Dickson et al. published the results of a phase II trial of Palbociclib, a CDK4/6 inhibitor, administered to 60 patients with liposarcomas (47 dedifferentiated and 13 well differentiated). They reported one complete response lasting more than 2 years. The overall progression-free survival at 12 weeks was 57%. Early results are available from the TAPUR study, a phase II trial evaluating antitumor activity in patients with advanced tumors with genomic alterations, including 29 patients with STS. In subgroup analysis of patients with STS, monotherapy demonstrated antitumor activity in heavily pretreated STS patients with CDK4 amplification. Disease control rates (defined as partial responders, complete responders or stable disease at 16 weeks or greater) were 48%. MDM2 inhibitors for treatment of liposarcomas are also being investigated often in combination with other therapies. Further studies and further drugs are currently in development but there currently is no standardized targeted treatment available for patients with STS outside of clinical trials.

Treatment for Recurrent Disease

RPSs recur following complete surgical resection, in two-thirds of patients. In addition to recurring locally in the tumor bed and metastasizing to the lungs, retroperitoneal leiomyosarcomas frequently spread to the liver and soft tissues. RPSs can also recur diffusely throughout the peritoneal cavity (sarcomatosis). Not only does each local recurrence affect surgical therapy, it can also be associated with a change in the biology of the disease. For example, in as many as 25% of patients, well-differentiated liposarcoma may recur in a poorly differentiated form or develop areas of dedifferentiation. Dedifferentiated retroperitoneal liposarcoma is more aggressive with a greater propensity for distant metastasis than its well-differentiated precursor.

The approach to resectable recurrent disease after the treatment of an RPS is similar to the approach taken after the recurrence of an extremity sarcoma. However, the ability to adequately resect a recurrent RPS declines precipitously with each recurrence. A survival benefit of salvage surgery for recurrent RPS has been reported, but careful patient selection is critical.

Park et al. from MSKCC reported the results of a retrospective analysis of 105 patients with a first recurrent retroperitoneal liposarcoma, 61 of whom underwent salvage resection. The size and growth rate of the recurrent tumor were independently associated with the incidence of a second local recurrence. A recurrent tumor with a growth rate >0.9 cm/month was associated with a poorer outcome, and the authors concluded that patients with tumors such as these should be enrolled in clinical trials rather than undergo re-resection.

Keung et al. evaluated longer surveillance intervals for patients with retroperitoneal well-differentiated liposarcomas to determine if longer follow-up intervals would impact outcomes. While recurrence was common (60.2%, median time 27 months), it was determined that surveillance intervals of 4 and 6 months would not have impacted management of their recurrence. Timing of surgery is more often determined by symptoms or rate of disease progression rather than at time of initial recurrence. Resection of metastatic lesions also can be considered in selected patients. For example, patients with leiomyosarcoma have been reported to have a better survival after resection of distant metastasis as compared to other subtypes; therefore, patients with distantly recurred retroperitoneal leiomyosarcoma are occasionally considered for metastasectomies. A disease-free interval of >1 year from primary resection to recurrence was associated with improved outcomes after salvage surgery in our recent analysis at MDACC.

Gastrointestinal Stromal Tumors

GISTs constitute the majority of mesenchymal tumors involving the gastrointestinal tract, with an estimated 2,500 to 6,000 cases per year in the United States. Although the clinical presentation of these tumors varies depending on tumor size and anatomical location, most tumors are found incidentally at the time of endoscopy or radiologic imaging. GISTs arise most frequently in the stomach (60% to 70%), followed by the small intestine (20% to 25%), colon and rectum (5%), and esophagus (<5%). Most GISTs are sporadic and, in 95% of cases, solitary. Most patients with GISTs present in the fifth to seventh decades of life, and these tumors are equally distributed between the genders. Symptoms of these lesions include pain and gastrointestinal bleeding, with abdominal mass a frequent finding.

Since the late 1990s, GISTs have been recognized as having distinctive immunohistochemical and genetic features. GISTs originate from the intestinal pacemaker cells (the interstitial cells of Cajal), which express CD117, a transmembrane tyrosine kinase receptor that is the product of the c-KIT proto-oncogene. Expression of CD117, found in at least 95% of cases, has emerged as an important defining feature of GISTs. The pathogenesis of these tumors is related to mutations in the c-KIT gene. Exploitation of this genetic characteristic has led to significant inroads into the development of successful therapy for these tumors.

Treatment

GISTs are an example of success using targeted therapy in cancer therapeutics. In the past, surgical resection was the only curative treatment available for GISTs. Although surgery remains the standard treatment for resectable tumors, the addition of systemic therapy has markedly improved outcomes. The goal of surgery should be resection with a 1- to 2-cm margin if possible. For tumors located in the stomach, a wedge resection can often accomplish this goal. Minimally invasive techniques are commonly used in the management of GISTs. In cases with large tumors, preoperative therapy with a tyrosine kinase inhibitor (TKI) should be considered to decrease tumor size, which may downsize enough to change the extent of surgical resection. However, despite complete resection, recurrence is common in high-risk tumors. Factors such as large tumor size (>5 cm), tumor location in the duodenum or rectum, high mitotic count of >5 mitoses/50 high-power fields, and mutation status (such as deletion in KIT exon 9) are associated with increased risk of recurrence. In contrast, per national consensus guidelines, small GISTs (≤2 cm) with a low mitotic rate of ≤5 mitoses/50 high-power fields, located in the stomach are associated with low risk of further tumor progression and can be observed with serial endoscopic surveillance (6- to 12-month intervals).

The development of imatinib (Gleevec) has substantially increased the survival of patients with GISTs. Imatinib is a selective TKI of c-KIT and platelet-derived growth factor receptor alpha (PDGFR-α). Imatinib was approved in 2002 by the U.S. Food and Drug Administration after successful completion of trials that enrolled patients with metastatic and locally advanced disease (Table 6.4). Overall response rates were 48% to 71%, and median OS in patients with advanced GISTs who were treated with imatinib was 57 months compared with 9 months in historical controls. The genotype of the c-KIT mutation is important: patients with mutations in exon 11 had higher response rates than did those with exon 9 mutations, although both groups responded better than did those without a mutation (wild type).

The benefit of imatinib in the postoperative setting was shown in a randomized controlled trial (ACOSOG Z9001) that enrolled 713 patients with GIST and KIT mutations after complete surgical resection. Patients who received 1 year of daily 400-mg Gleevec had better relapse-free survival than a placebo group had (98% vs. 83%; $P < .001$). The optimal duration of postoperative therapy was investigated in another randomized trial of postoperative imatinib at 400 mg/day for 12 versus 36 months. The results showed superiority with use of long (36 months) postoperative imatinib therapy (5-year survival rate, 92% vs. 82%; $P = .02$).

TABLE 6.4	Summary of Clinical Trials of Imatinib Mesylate in Patients With Advanced Gastrointestinal Stromal Tumor						
Study, Year	Phase	No. of Patients	Overall Response	CR	PR	2-Yr Overall Survival	Progression-Free Survival
Van Oosterom et al., 2001	I	36	53%	0%	53%	—	—
Demetri et al., 2002	II	147	54%	0%	54%	—	—
Verwiej et al., 2003	II	27	71%	4%	67%	—	73% (1 yr)
Rankin et al., 2004	III	746					
– 400 mg daily			48%	3%	45%	78%	50% (2 yrs)
– 800 mg daily			48%	3%	45%	73%	53% (2 yrs)
Verweij et al., 2004	III	946					
– 400 mg daily			50%	5%	45%	69%	44% (2 yrs)
– 800 mg daily			54%	6%	48%	74%	55% (2 yrs)

CR, complete response; PR, partial response.

The PERSIST-5 Trial was a prospective, single-arm, phase II study which demonstrated that treatment with imatinib remains efficacious at 5 years. Ninety-one patients with resected primary GIST were enrolled. No patients with imatinib sensitive tumors had disease recurrence over the study period. Among those that recurred, recurrence was within 2 years of stopping imatinib therapy. Unfortunately, the rates of discontinuation of imatinib were relatively high, with approximately half stopping due to patient choice.

Because of the success of postoperative imatinib therapy for resectable disease and a reported high response rate to imatinib in advanced disease, imatinib has been used increasingly in a preoperative setting as well. The RTOG 0132/ACRIN 6665 phase II trial, which enrolled 63 patients with KIT-positive GIST, reported that 7% of patients had an objective response to preoperative imatinib (6 to 8 weeks), and stable disease was achieved in 83%. Whereas this study reported on the safety of preoperative imatinib therapy, Tirumani et al. reported that maximal tumor response is usually seen after 3 to 9 months, at which point surgery should be performed. However, even in patients who harbor the KIT mutation, 5% can still show primary resistance to imatinib and 14% will develop resistance at a later time. Sunitinib, another TKI with multiple targets including KIT, PDGFR, and VEGFR with different binding characteristics than those of imatinib, can be considered as second-line therapy in cases that do not respond or develop resistance to imatinib. Generally, in patients who undergo complete resection of their GIST but are at significant risk of recurrence due to tumor characteristics (>5 mitoses per 50 high power fields, tumor size greater than 5cm, non-gastric location). Adjuvant imatinib should be strongly considered In patients whom resection of their GIST will lead to significant morbidity. Appropriate neoadjuvant therapy should be considered based on molecular testing of a preoperative biopsy. Patients who receive neoadjuvant imatinib should be considered for continuation of imatinib adjuvantly. The lenght of time necessary to continue the adjuvant imatinib is still under active investigation; however, most studies suggest that patiemnts at high risk for recurrence should receive a minimum of 5 years of adjuvanmt treatment.

In patients with resectable disease that would carry significant morbidity, neoadjuvant targeted therapy should be considered prior to surgical resection. The use of adjuvant imatinib therapy should be considered in all patients with intermediate or high risk of recurrence, including those with tumor rupture during surgery. The optimal duration of adjuvant imatinib therapy is not known but it is generally accepted that treatment should be continued for a minimum of 3 years. As demonstrated in the PERSIST trial, 5 years of therapy remains efficacious and should be strongly considered in high-risk patients with imatinib-sensitive GIST.

Other Soft Tissue Sarcomas

Sarcoma of the Breast

Sarcomas of the breast are rare tumors, accounting for less than 1% of all breast malignancies and less than 5% of all soft tissue sarcomas. Various histologic subtypes occur within the breast, including angiosarcoma, stromal sarcoma, fibrosarcoma, and undifferentiated/unclassified sarcomas. Cystosarcoma phyllodes is generally considered to be a separate entity from other soft tissue sarcomas because these tumors are believed to originate from hormonally responsive stromal cells of the breast and the majority are benign.

Radiation-induced sarcomas of the breast are a separate sarcoma entity that arises after radiotherapy to the breast with histologic confirmation that it is a distinct malignancy from the patient's initial primary tumor. Radiation-induced sarcoma is quite rare and not limited to the breast but most often presents in the breast because of the widespread use of radiation therapy in breast cancer. Multiple different histologic subtypes can occur following radiation with angiosarcoma representing the most common. Reported 5-year survival rates range from 27% to 48%.

As with sarcomas at other anatomic sites, the histopathologic grade and size of the tumor are important prognostic factors. Complete resection with negative margins is the primary therapy. Total mastectomy carries no additional benefit if complete excision can be achieved by segmental mastectomy with 2-cm margins. Because of low rates of regional lymphatic spread, axillary nodal evaluation is not routinely indicated. Preoperative chemotherapy or radiation therapy may be considered for patients with large, high-risk tumors.

Desmoid Tumors

Desmoid tumors do not metastasize and are considered low-grade sarcomas. Approximately half of these tumors arise in the extremities, with the remaining ones originating in the trunk, abdominal wall, or abdomen/retroperitoneum (including the mesentery). Abdominal wall desmoids are frequently associated with pregnancy and are believed to arise as the result of hormonal influences. While patients with Gardner syndrome have a higher risk of mesenteric/retroperitoneal desmoid tumors than the normal population does, as an extracolonic manifestation. Although surgery was previously considered primary treatment of desmoid tumors, local recurrence was seen in up to one-third of patients that underwent margin-negative surgery, which has shifted primary treatment to nonsurgical therapies. Desmoids that are small, asymptomatic and in a favorable site (superficial), can be managed initially with active surveillance. For desmoids that are symptomatic or large, local therapy with definitive radiation therapy can control tumor growth for an extended time period and can be considered.

Significant advances have been made in the treatment of desmoid tumors with systemic therapy. A double-blind, placebo-controlled, randomized phase II study of sorafenib in patients with desmoid fibromatosis is notable for the response rate by RECIST in the sorafenib arm of 33% in contrast to 20% in the placebo arm, with a median time to response of 9.6 months versus 13.3 months with placebo, demonstrating that active surveillance is an increasingly appropriate strategy. Pazopanib is another multitargeted TKI with increasing evidence for its role in desmoid fibromatosis. Ongoing studies evaluating inhibition of β-catenin activity with Tegavivint and gamma-secretase/notch inhibitor Nirogacestat hold promise.

Doxorubicin-based chemotherapy can be considered for disease progression or recurrence. Progressive or recurrent desmoid tumors can be treated with systemic therapy, resection plus radiation therapy, or definitive radiation (if not previously irradiated). Routine follow-up with appropriate imaging every 3 to 6 months for 2 years and then annually is recommended to evaluate for recurrence.

Dermatofibrosarcoma Protuberans

Dermatofibrosarcoma protuberans is a neoplasm arising in the dermis that may occur anywhere in the body. Approximately 40% arise on the trunk, with most of the remaining tumors distributed between the head and neck and extremities. The lesion presents as a nodular, cutaneous mass that shows slow and persistent growth. Satellite lesions may be found in patients with larger tumors. Wide excision is recommended, ideally with 2-cm margins; recurrence rates can be as high as 50% with positive margins. Radiation therapy is recommended for positive margins if further re-resection is not able to be performed or for recurrent tumors. In genetic analysis, the COL1A1-PDGFB fusion gene/protein is often detected. This has clinical relevance in that some patients with metastatic dermatofibrosarcoma protuberans have responded to imatinib, a TKI of PDGFR. If fibrosarcomatous change is observed on pathologic review, tumors should be considered as high-grade soft tissue sarcomas and treated as such.

Bone Sarcomas

Osteosarcoma and Ewing sarcoma are the two most common malignant conditions of bone. Osteosarcoma has a peak frequency during adolescent growth, whereas Ewing sarcoma occurs most frequently in the second decade of life.

Presentation

The most common presentation of bone sarcomas (Ewing sarcoma or osteosarcoma) is pain or swelling in a bone or joint. As with soft tissue sarcomas in adults, often a traumatic event draws attention to the swelling and can delay the correct diagnosis. Osteosarcoma most commonly involves the metaphysis of long bones, especially the distal femur, proximal tibia, or humerus. Ewing sarcoma may involve flat bones or the diaphysis of tubular bones such as the femur, pelvis, tibia, and fibula. Ewing sarcoma may also occur in soft tissues. Chondrosarcoma occurs most commonly in the pelvis, proximal femur, and shoulder girdle.

Up to 25% of patients presenting with osteosarcoma or Ewing sarcoma have metastatic disease at presentation. The most frequent metastatic sites for osteosarcoma include the lung (>90%) and the bone (10%), whereas Ewing sarcoma metastases occur in the lung (50%), bone (25%), and bone marrow (25%).

Staging

As with soft tissue sarcomas, histopathologic grade is a crucial component of the staging of bone sarcomas. The surgical staging system for musculoskeletal sarcoma is based on the system by Enneking, which includes prognostic variables of histopathologic grade (G), the location of the tumor (T), and the presence of metastasis (M). The three stages are stage I (low grade), stage II (high grade), and stage III (metastatic). Stages I and II are then designated A (e.g., stage IA) if the lesion is confined within well-delineated surgical compartments and B if the lesion has extracompartmental invasion.

Diagnosis

The evaluation of patients with a suspected bone tumor should include a history and physical, plain radiographs, and MRI of the entire affected bone. Bone scanning and CT of the chest are also necessary. On plain radiographs, malignant bone tumors show irregular borders, and there is often evidence of bone destruction and a periosteal reaction. Soft tissue extension is also frequently seen.

A core-needle biopsy is the diagnostic procedure of choice when osteosarcoma is suspected. A core-needle biopsy performed under radiographic guidance should yield diagnostic findings in almost all cases of osteosarcoma.

Treatment
Effective multimodality therapy for childhood musculoskeletal tumors is critical to improve survival.

Surgery
Whenever feasible, limb salvage is the standard surgical approach to bone sarcomas. Successful limb-sparing surgery consists of three phases: tumor resection, bone reconstruction, and soft tissue coverage. Complete surgical extirpation of the primary tumor and any metastases is essential, particularly in osteosarcoma because it is relatively resistant to radiation therapy. It is also desirable to resect Ewing sarcoma. If surgical removal with a wide surgical margin can be achieved, the prognosis is favorable (12-year relapse-free survival rate of 60%). However, Ewing sarcoma most typically involves the pelvis with an extensive soft tissue mass that invades the pelvic cavity, which makes radical surgery difficult. Surgical resection is usually the only treatment indicated for the management of chondrosarcomas because this type of tumor is unresponsive to existing systemic therapies.

Chemotherapy
Chemotherapy has revolutionized the treatment of most bone sarcomas and is considered standard care for osteosarcoma and Ewing sarcoma. The bleak 15% to 20% survival rate with surgery alone during the 1960s has improved to 55% to 80% in more recent reports by the addition of chemotherapy to surgical resection. Preoperative chemotherapy is an attractive option because it can lead to the downstaging of tumors, which then enables the maximal application of limb-sparing surgery. In addition, tumor necrosis that occurs after preoperative chemotherapy has been shown to be the most important prognostic variable determining survival.

The optimal chemotherapy regimen for osteosarcoma has still not been established, but agents most commonly used include doxorubicin and cisplatin; a methotrexate-containing regimen is a reasonable alternative. Multiagent chemotherapy has also been shown to be effective in Ewing sarcoma. Standard multiagent regimens include doxorubicin plus cyclophosphamide and a combination of doxorubicin, vincristine, and cyclophosphamide with or without actinomycin D (VDCA or VDC).

Radiation Therapy
Because osteosarcomas are generally radiation resistant, radiation therapy is predominantly used for the palliation of large, unresectable tumors. In contrast, radiation therapy is the primary mode of treatment for most localized Ewing sarcomas. Preoperative irradiation may also be considered to reduce tumor volume before surgical resection is attempted.

Management of Recurrent Disease
Bone tumors disseminate through the bloodstream and commonly metastasize to the lungs and bony skeleton. In the past, only 10% to 30% of patients presenting with detectable metastatic osteosarcoma achieved long-term survival. More recent studies have shown that combined modality approaches consisting of surgical resection of the primary tumor and metastatic deposits in conjunction with multiagent chemotherapy can improve 5-year disease-free survival rates up to 47%.

Ewing sarcoma may recur in the form of distant disease as long as 15 years after the initial diagnosis. In a retrospective analysis of 241 patients with Ewing sarcoma of the pelvis, the major factors that influenced prognosis were tumor volume, responsiveness to chemotherapy, and adequate surgical margins.

Patients with suspected tumor recurrence should undergo a complete evaluation to determine the extent of disease. The resection of pulmonary metastases is the mainstay of treatment for patients with osteosarcoma. Prognosis can generally be determined by the response to previous therapy, duration of remission, and extent of metastases. Multimodality therapy, including chemotherapeutic agents not previously used, is the general recommendation for treatment.

Sacrococcygeal Chordoma
The notochord remnant is the site of origin of the rare sacrococcygeal chordoma tumor. Chordomas are locally aggressive tumors that have a high propensity to recur. Because symptoms can be vague, diagnosis can be delayed. Surgical resection should involve a multidisciplinary team that includes the surgical oncologist, neurosurgeon, and reconstructive plastic surgeon. A two-stage procedure is frequently used at MDACC. First, the blood supply to the tumor arising from the iliac vessels is controlled through an anterior approach. The following day, the tumor is resected via a posterior approach. Radiation therapy should be considered because of the high rates of local recurrence.

CASE SCENARIO

Case Scenario 1

Presentation

A 45-year-old male with an unremarkable past medical history presents with a mass in their left mid-thigh which has been slowly growing over the last year. He had a small lesion resected from that area 5 years ago that was diagnosed as a lipoma. Ultrasound performed showed a 7- × 4-cm mass within the quadriceps muscle. The ultrasound shows the mass is hypoechogenic, intermingled with anechoic areas and moderate vascularity.

Differential Diagnosis

Lipoma
Liposarcoma
Neurofibroma
Undifferentiated pleomorphic sarcoma
Epidermoid cyst
Synovial sarcoma
Lymphoma
Secondary malignancy
Hematoma or abscess
Other sarcoma or skin malignancy

On physical examination, he has a mass within the muscle with no evidence of palpable lymphadenopathy in the groin. Core-needle biopsy is performed which is read as myxoid liposarcoma.

Confirmation of Diagnosis and Treatment

Confirmation of the diagnosis should be made by an expert pathologist if possible as misdiagnosis is common. If need be, samples should be sent to a high-volume center for confirmation of diagnosis. After the diagnosis of myxoid liposarcoma has been made, further workup is warranted including an MRI of the affected extremity and a high-resolution CT scan of the chest to evaluate for pulmonary metastasis.

MRI imaging demonstrates the known mass within the quadriceps muscle, adjacent to the superficial femoral artery. CT imaging shows no pulmonary metastatic disease.

Management of the patient's soft tissue sarcoma is complicated and numerous factors must be considered including anticipated functional deficits after resection, histologic subtype, vicinity to other important structures, and the likelihood of R0 resection. The case should be discussed with a multidisciplinary team that includes the surgeon, radiologists, radiation oncologists, and medical oncologists. The patient's large tumor size and proximity to vascular structures indicate that they may benefit from multimodality therapy prior to surgical resection in order to increase the chance of R0 resection and decrease the amount of functional morbidity from the surgical resection. Preoperative chemotherapy can be considered based on the overall size of the tumor but it's use is subject to institutional preference due to the conflicting evidence on the efficacy as well as the question of what are the most appropriate chemotherapeutic regimens are to be used in patients with sarcomas. Radiation therapy is often advocated for improvement in local control of extremity sarcomas with the use of it in the neoadjuvant versus adjuvant setting being an active area of controversy. As discussed earlier in the chapter, at MDACC, we recommend the use of neoadjuvant radiation in most settings for soft tissue sarcomas. The patient's histology, myxoid liposarcoma, has been shown to be particularly radiosensitive. Lansu et al. demonstrated in a nonrandomized control trial that lower dose radiation therapy (36 Gy in daily 2 Gy fractions) was associated with lower morbidity and remained oncologically safe with those going on to receive surgery having a 100% local control rate. While this study demonstrated the utility in myxoid liposarcoma, at this time, 50.4 Gy remains the standard of care for radiation of extremity sarcomas.

The patient undergoes radiation to the left lower extremity prior to surgical resection.

Surgical Approach—Key Steps

It is important to assess the patient's planned surgical resection area and determine the appropriate flap coverage with a plastic surgeon, prior to presenting to the operating room. This will allow for appropriate positioning as well as appropriate counseling for postoperative expectations. In cases with close abutment of vascular structures, preparations should be made for a potential vascular resection with reconstruction as well. In the operating room, the preoperative MRI or CT should be reviewed, and patient positioned and draped appropriately to allow for vascular resection and reconstruction.

Margins should be marked out from the edges of the lesion and, ideally, a complete resection of the tumor performed en bloc with a margin of 2 cm. It is understandable that a 2-cm margin is not always achievable when attempting to preserve function postoperatively and therefore, it is up to the surgeon's discretion to balance the margin size with the proximity to important structures. Incisions should be oriented along the long axis of the extremity with inclusion of previous incisional biopsy scars. Fascial planes, when involved, should be included with the specimen. Areas of tumor that are close to the margins of the resected specimen can be sent for frozen section analysis, with the caveat that frozen section analysis can be difficult to interpret, particularly in patients who have received preoperative radiation therapy. If there is significant concern for a positive margin, however, further resection would significantly increase morbidity, a temporary closure can be performed using either a biologic matrix or vacuum-assisted device until permanent pathologic results return. This can then be followed by either further surgical resection or reconstruction.

After en bloc resection of the surgical specimen, the specimen should be oriented and taken to pathology directly by the surgeon to ensure that the specimen orientation and the true margins are accurately communicated to the pathologist. Clips should be placed along the edges of the surgical resection site for localization, if additional adjuvant radiation is needed and/or to help should additional surgical resection be needed. Surgical drains should be placed for areas at high risk for seroma and this should be discussed in conjunction with the reconstructive surgeon prior to placement.

The patient undergoes surgical resection with negative margins without the need for vascular or nerve resection. Complex rotational flap closure is performed.

The patients should be admitted to a floor based on the duration and complexity of their resection and reconstruction. This often warrants close monitoring of the flap used for soft tissue coverage. Physical therapy and occupational therapy should evaluate the patient and determine their outpatient needs prior to discharge. Diet can be advanced quickly in most cases and surgical drains can be removed when output is minimal for multiple days in a row, typically in outpatient follow-up. Further treatment should be dictated based on the margin status, histologic grade, and presence or absence of additional sites of disease. In cases where adjuvant radiation therapy is needed, this can usually be started 4 to 6 weeks following resection if no wound complications are present. Patients should follow up every 3 to 6 months for the first 2 to 3 years with a physical examination and depending on their risk of recurrence, repeat MRI and/or CT imaging of the chest. This should also be tailored based on their histologic type with certain histologic types potentially benefitting from regional nodal evaluation by MRI or ultrasound. If no evidence of disease after 2 to 3 years, follow-up can be spaced out to 6 months until 5 years when it can be changed to annually.

Common Curve Balls

- Difficult to assess intraoperative margin status
- Need for resection of vascular structures or major nerves
- Short interval local, regional or distant recurrence
- Myxoid liposarcoma is very responsive to RT

Take Home Points

- Preoperative imaging with MRI and or CT scan is essential for adequate surgical planning
- Management of STS is complex and warrants discussion at a multidisciplinary tumor board prior to resection
- Limb preservation with negative surgical margins and maximal preservation of function is the goal of surgical resection and can be facilitated with preoperative radiation
- High-grade STS should be evaluated for multimodality therapy as recurrence rates are high
- STS should be resected en bloc with a margin of uninvolved tissue when possible with care taken to preserve neurovascular structures when possible

Case Scenario 2

Presentation

A 52-year-old female with no significant past medical history presents with increasing abdominal distension and a mass felt. She has a firm mass felt in the right side of her abdomen, constipation, and early satiety. CT scan demonstrates a large retroperitoneal mass with displacement of her intra-abdominal organs to the left.

Differential Diagnosis

Liposarcoma
Dedifferentiated liposarcoma
Renal cell carcinoma
Germ cell tumor
Adrenal cortical carcinoma
Leiomyosarcoma
Primary liver malignancy
Lymphoma
Secondary malignancy
Retroperitoneal fibrosis
Other soft tissue sarcoma

Confirmation of Diagnosis and Treatment

Patients with retroperitoneal STS often present with nonspecific symptoms related to abdominal fullness or are found to have disease on incidental imaging for other causes. High-resolution CT imaging with IV and oral contrast are important for evaluation of the disease extent, determination of the tumor's relationship to vascular structures, adjacent organs, and the ureters, and can be helpful in narrowing down the differential diagnosis. Laboratory values can assist in narrowing the differential diagnosis by excluding functional adrenal cortical carcinoma (assessment of glucocorticoid excess and androgen excess) and germ cell tumor markers (alpha-fetoprotein and beta-human chorionic gonadotropin). Compression of the vascular structures can lead to development of lower extremity edema and possible deep vein thrombosis. Core-needle biopsy should be performed to confirm the diagnosis. Given the location, assessment of renal function should be performed as well with serum Cr and if the retroperitoneal mass appears to encase the kidney, consideration should be given to a renal mercaptoacetyltriglycine (MAG-3) scan to assess the involved kidney's function. MRI can be considered to further define the retroperitoneal mass but CT scan is often adequate.

Biopsy confirms the diagnosis of a dedifferentiated liposarcoma. No additional disease is noted on CT imaging of the chest.

Surgical Approach—Key Steps

Assessment should be made on the resectability of retroperitoneal mass which is often determined by the proximity to major vascular structures. If deemed resectable, a multidisciplinary tumor board should evaluate the case and determine the utility of multimodality treatment including chemotherapy and radiation therapy. While the guidelines for the use of radiation therapy are more established in extremity sarcoma, there are limitations to the use of RT in retroperitoneal sarcomas due to dose-related toxicity to adjacent organs and large treatment areas. Recent data from the STRASS trial (EORTC-62092) showed that preoperative radiation therapy did not provide a survival benefit but did result in an increase in adverse reactions. The conclusion from that trial was that preoperative radiation therapy should not be considered as the standard of care for retroperitoneal sarcomas but, based on subgroup analysis and analysis of the off-trial STREXIT cohort, can be considered in the care of well-differentiated liposarcomas and G1-G2 dedifferentiated liposarcomas. The evidence for the use of chemotherapy in the pre- and postoperative setting is limited and should be considered based on each individual patient's risk and potential benefit, particularly in patients in whom kidney resection is likely, particularly if chemotherapy is a consideration as ifosfamide, one of the commonly used chemotherapeutic agents is nephrotoxic and requires adequate renal function in order to be used).

Surgical resection should be performed with the goal of R0/R1 resection with as much organ preservation as feasible. The presence of peritoneal disease, involvement of the celiac artery or proximal SMA, or spinal cord involvement can preclude safe surgical resection, but are not absolute contraindications in centers of excellence that have significant operative experience in these areas. Debulking/R2 resection of large tumors is generally discouraged unless being done for palliative purposes. Patient positioning is dependent on tumor location, but most tumors can be adequately accessed and removed from the supine or "sloppy" lateral position with a large midline versus modified makuuchi incision. It is important when planning positioning and surgical resection, to make an incision large enough for safe exposure of all vital structures. Preoperative discussion with the anesthesia team for the appropriate epidural or regional block is important for early postoperative mobilization. Resection of the tumor should be performed en bloc with structures considered to be involved with the tumor; this can often include resection of a small bowel, colon, kidney, distal pancreas, adrenal glands, or portions of the IVC and aorta. In patients where kidney function is to be preserved, a renal capsulectomy can be considered if there is an adequate dissection plane between the tumor and the renal parenchyma.

After tumor resection, the edges of the surgical bed should be marked with metal clips for postoperative identification of the resection limits. Drain placement should be determined based on the surgical resection and are often not needed due to the intraperitoneal drainage of fluids. Drain placement should be considered when pancreatic resections are performed as they have a high postoperative leak rate in this setting.

Surgical resection of a 38- × 22- × 15-cm dedifferentiated liposarcoma is performed with en bloc resection of the right kidney due to significant ureteral involvement.

Postoperative management is determined primarily by the amount of manipulation of the intra-abdominal organs and if organ resection was required. In general, the longer the duration of the surgery and the more manipulation of the bowel, the longer the postoperative ileus. Patients who undergo extensive resections of retroperitoneal tissue frequently develop significant third-space fluid losses and, therefore, their intravenous fluid requirements will often be extremely high in the first 48 hours postoperatively. Patients should follow a similar surveillance pattern to extremity STS with physical examination and CT imaging every 3 to 6 months for the first 2 to 3 years followed by every 6 months until 5 years, then annually. Recurrence following resection of retroperitoneal sarcoma is very high and repeat surgical resection is common.

Common Curve Balls

- Postoperative wound complications
- Large retroperitoneal mass that is not a sarcoma
- Unresectable disease (critical vascular involvement, peritoneal disease) found during surgical exploration

Take Home Points

- Preoperative radiation therapy for retroperitoneal sarcoma is not the standard of care
- R0 resection with as much organ preservation as feasible is the goal of surgery
- Recurrence rates are very high following resection and surgical planning should take this into account when there is a high risk of surgical morbidity with extensive resection

CASE SCENARIO REVIEW

Questions

1. A 58-year-old male with a past medical history of hypertension presents with a 6-cm mass in his anterior thigh. On examination, the mass is firm and immobile with no associated neurovascular deficits or skin changes. What is the appropriate imaging choice for characterization of this mass?

    A. Plain radiographs of the femur
    B. Ultrasound
    C. CT with contrast
    D. PET/CT
    E. MRI with and without contrast

2. A 38-year-old female presents with an enlarging 3-cm mass in the posterior arm. Biopsy is performed which shows an undifferentiated pleomorphic sarcoma. Careful physical examination shows no other lesions. What imaging should be completed for adequate staging prior to treatment planning?

   A. CT Chest
   B. CT Chest/Abdomen Pelvis
   C. PET/CT
   D. No further imaging needed
   E. MRI of the head

3. Which of the following is associated with an increased risk of developing desmoid tumors?

   A. Neurofibromatosis type 1
   B. Familial adenomatous polyposis
   C. Anabolic steroids
   D. Lynch syndrome
   E. None of the above

4. A 63-year-old male presents with early satiety. Workup demonstrates a well-circumscribed 6-cm duodenal mass along the lateral aspect of the duodenum near the head of the pancreas. The patient is otherwise healthy and has no evidence of distant disease. Endoscopic biopsy is performed and confirms a gastrointestinal stromal tumor with a mitotic count of 6 and cKIT mutation in exon 11. What is the appropriate next step?

   A. Surgical resection
   B. Neoadjuvant radiation therapy
   C. Neoadjuvant imatinib
   D. Surgical bypass
   E. None of the above

5. Which of the following histologic subtypes of soft tissue sarcoma is high risk for metastasis to regional lymph nodes?

   A. Alveolar soft parts sarcoma
   B. Liposarcoma
   C. Leiomyosarcoma
   D. Epithelioid sarcoma
   E. Dermatofibromasarcoma protuberans

Answers

1. **The correct answer is E.** *Rationale:* MRI imaging is the preferred imaging modality for soft tissues as it allows better characterization of the mass compared to the other imaging choices. Plain radiographs will give an indication of the tumor's effect on the bone but will not provide information on the mass itself. Ultrasound is easy to perform but will provide little diagnostic information on the mass itself. CT of the extremity is a useful modality but is not as useful as MRI for determining soft tissue densities and the location of neural structures. PET imaging is not an appropriate first-line imaging and would provide limited information in characterization beyond a CT scan other than metabolic activity.

2. **The correct answer is A.** *Rationale:* Undifferentiated pleomorphic sarcomas are high-grade sarcomas with an increased risk of metastasis. The most common site of metastasis is the lung and these lesions can be identified with CT imaging of the chest. CT imaging of the abdomen and pelvis is not indicated at this time unless the patient has associated symptoms that would suggest metastatic disease in the abdomen or pelvis. PET/CT is also not indicated and would have little added value over CT imaging. MRI of the head is not indicated as these lesions very rarely metastasize to the brain.

3. **The correct answer is B.** *Rationale:* Gardner syndrome is a subset of familial adenomatous polyposis that has additional extracolonic manifestations of the disease. They have a higher risk of mesenteric/retroperitoneal desmoid tumors as well as osteomas of the skull, lipomas, neoplasms of the thyroid, adrenals, liver, and congenital hypertrophy of the retinal epithelium. Morbidity associated with mesenteric and retroperitoneal desmoid tumors is greater than their sporadic counterparts because of location.

4. **The correct answer is C.** *Rationale:* In cases with large tumors in difficult locations, preoperative therapy with a tyrosine kinase inhibitor (TKI) should be considered to decrease tumor size, which may downsize the tumor to allow for a smaller resection. In this case, the patient has multiple high-risk factors including a high mitotic rate, large tumor size, and duodenal primary. The patient's tumor location may require a Whipple procedure but if it is downsized, it may require a lateral duodenectomy which would be less long-term morbidity. Therefore, neoadjuvant imatinib is preferred in this situation.

5. **The correct answer is D.** *Rationale:* Epithelioid sarcoma, clear cell sarcoma, rhabdomyosarcoma, and undifferentiated pleomorphic sarcoma are higher risk for metastatic disease to the regional lymph nodes. The other listed histologies are lower risk for lymph node metastasis relative to these groups.

Recommended Readings

American Joint Committee on Cancer. *AJCC Cancer Staging Manual*. 8th ed. Lippincott-Raven; 2017.

Bonvalot S, Gronchi A, Le Péchoux C, et al. Preoperative radiotherapy plus surgery versus surgery alone for patients with primary retroperitoneal sarcoma (EORTC-62092: STRASS): a multicentre, open-label, randomised, phase 3 trial. *Lancet Oncol*. 2020;21(10):1366–1377.

Burgoyne, Adam M, et al. "Duodenal-jejunal flexure GI stromal tumor frequently heralds somatic NF1 and notch pathway mutations." *JCO precision oncology*. 2017;1:1–12.

Coindre JM, Terrier P, Guillou L, et al. Predictive value of grade for metastasis development in the main histologic types of adult soft tissue sarcomas: a study of 1240 patients from the French Federation of Cancer Centers Sarcoma Group. *Cancer*. 2001;91(10):1914–1926.

Demetri GD, von Mehren M, Blanke CD, et al. Efficacy and safety of imatinib mesulate in advanced gastrointestinal stromal tumors. *N Engl J Med*. 2002;347(7):472–480.

Dickson MA, Schwartz GK, Keohan ML, et al. Progression-free survival among patients with well-differentiated or dedifferentiated liposarcoma treated with CDK4 inhibitor palbociclib: a phase 2 clinical trial. *JAMA Oncol*. 2016;2:937–940.

Dineen SP, Roland CL, Feig R, et al. Radiation-associated undifferentiated pleomorphic sarcoma is associated with worse clinical outcomes than sporadic lesions. *Ann Surg Oncol*. 2015;22:3913–3920.

Eilber FC, Eilber FR, Eckardt J, et al. The impact of chemotherapy on the survival of patients with high-grade primary extremity liposarcoma. *Ann Surg*. 2004;240:686–695.

Eisenberg BL, Harris J, Blanke CD, et al. Phase II trial of neoadjuvant/adjuvant imatinib mesylate (IM) for advanced primary and metastatic/recurrent operable gastrointestinal stromal tumor (GIST): early results of RTOG 0132/ACRIN 6665. *J Surg Oncol*. 2009;99:42–47.

Gounder MM, Mahoney MR, Van Tine BA, et al. Sorafenib for advanced and refractory desmoid tumors. *N Engl J Med*. 2018;379(25):2417–2428.

Gronchi A, Ferrari S, Quagliuolo V, et al. Histotype-tailored neoadjuvant chemotherapy versus standard chemotherapy in patients with high-risk soft-tissue sarcomas (ISG-STS 1001): an international, open-label, randomised, controlled, phase 3, multicentre trial. *Lancet Oncol*. 2017;18(6):812–822.

Gronchi A, Palmerini E, Quagliuolo V, et al. Neoadjuvant chemotherapy in high-risk soft tissue sarcomas: final results of a randomized trial from Italian (ISG), Spanish (GEIS), French (FSG), and Polish (PSG) Sarcoma Groups. *J Clin Oncol*. 2020;38(19):2178–2186.

Gronchi A, Stacchiotti S, Verderio P, et al. Short, full-dose adjuvant chemotherapy (CT) in high-risk adult soft tissue sarcomas (STS): long-term follow-up of a randomized clinical trial from the Italian Sarcoma Group and the Spanish Sarcoma Group. *Ann Oncol*. 2016;27(12):2283–2288.

Grunhagen DJ, de Witt JHW, Graveland WJ, Verhoef C, van Geel AN, Eggermont AM. Outcome and prognostic factor analysis of 217 consecutive isolated limb perfusions with tumor necrosis factor-alpha and melphalan for limb-threatening soft tissue sarcoma. *Cancer*. 2006;106(8):1775–1784.

Guillou L, Coindre JM, Bonichon F, et al. Comparative study of the National Cancer Institute and French Federation of Cancer Centers Sarcoma Group grading systems in a population of 410 adult patients with soft tissue sarcoma. *J Clin Oncol*. 1997;15:350–362.

Issels RD, Lindner LH, Verweij J, et al; European Organisation for Research and Treatment of Cancer Soft Tissue and Bone Sarcoma Group (EORTC-STBSG). Neo-adjuvant chemotherapy alone or with regional hyperthermia for localised high-risk soft-tissue sarcoma: a randomised phase 3 multicentre study. *Lancet Oncol.* 2010;11:561–570.

Keung EZ, Rajkot N, Torres KE, et al. Evaluating the impact of surveillance follow-up intervals in patients following resection of primary well-differentiated liposarcoma of the retroperitoneum. *Ann Surg Oncol.* 2021;28(1):570–575.

Lansu J, Bovée JVMG, Braam P, et al. Dose reduction of preoperative radiotherapy in myxoid liposarcoma: a nonrandomized controlled trial. *JAMA Oncol.* 2021;7(1):e205865.

Le Cesne A, Ouali M, Leahy MG, et al. Doxorubicin-based adjuvant chemotherapy in soft tissue sarcoma: pooled analysis of two STBSG-EORTC phase III clinical trials. *Ann Oncol.* 2014;25:2425–2432.

Livingston JA, Bugano D, Barbo A, et al. Role of chemotherapy in dedifferentiated liposarcoma of the retroperitoneum: defining the benefit and challenges of the standard. *Sci Rep.* 2017;7(1):11836.

Martin-Broto J, Hindi N, Lopez-Pousa A, et al. Assessment of safety and efficacy of combined trabectedin and low-dose radiotherapy for patients with metastatic soft-tissue sarcomas: a nonrandomized phase 1/2 clinical trial. *JAMA Oncol.* 2020;6(4):535–541.

Nassbaum DP, Rushing CN, Lane WO, et al. Preoperative or postoperative radiotherapy versus surgery alone for retroperitoneal sarcoma: a case-control, propensity score-matched analysis of a nationwide clinical oncology database. *Lancet Oncol.* 2016;17:966–975.

Raut CP, Espat NJ, Maki RG, et al. Efficacy and tolerability of 5-year adjuvant imatinib treatment for patients with resected intermediate-or high-risk primary gastrointestinal stromal tumor: the PERSIST-5 clinical trial. *JAMA Oncol.* 2018;4(12):e184060–e184060.

Rosenberg SA, Tepper J, Glatstein E, et al. The treatment of soft tissue sarcomas of the extremities: prospective randomized evaluations of (1) limb-sparing surgery plus radiation therapy compared with amputation and (2) the role of adjuvant chemotherapy. *Ann Surg.* 1982;196:305–315.

Salerno KE, Alektiar KM, Baldini EH, et al. Radiation therapy for treatment of soft tissue sarcoma in adults: executive summary of an ASTRO clinical practice guideline. *Pract Radiat Oncol.* 2021;11(5):339–351.

Smith MJF, Ridgway PF, Catton CN, et al. Combined management of retroperitoneal sarcoma with dose intensification radiotherapy and resection: long-term results of a prospective trial. *Radiother Oncol.* 2014;110:165–171.

Stucky CCH, Wasif N, Ashman JB, Pockaj BA, Gunderson LL, Gray RJ. Excellent local control with preoperative radiation therapy, surgical resection, and intra-operative electron radiation therapy for retroperitoneal sarcoma. *J Surg Oncol.* 2014;109:798–803.

Tan MCB, Brennan MF, Kuk D, et al. Histology-based classification predicts pattern of recurrence and improves risk stratification in primary retroperitoneal sarcoma. *Ann Surg.* 2016;263:593–600.

Woll PJ, Reichardt P, Le Cesne A, et al. EORTC Soft Tissue and Bone Sarcoma Group and the NCIC Clinical Trials Group Sarcoma Disease Site Committee. Adjuvant chemotherapy with doxorubicin, ifosfamide, and lenograstim for resected soft-tissue sarcoma (EORTC 62931): a multicentre randomised controlled trial. *Lancet Oncol.* 2012;13:1045–1054.

Cancer of the Head and Neck

Yelda Jozaghi, Mark E. Zafereo, and Ryan P. Goepfert

INTRODUCTION

The head and neck is composed of many different anatomic sites with heterogeneous structures, functions, and cellular origins. Due to this diversity, cancers arising in each area often have distinct risk factors for carcinogenesis, different presenting signs and symptoms, and unique diagnostic considerations. A variety of treatment options and resultant outcomes are dependent upon the size and location of the tumor, histology and molecular profile, presence of regional and distant metastatic disease, specifics of prior treatment, comorbid disease status, and expected functional outcomes. This chapter will focus on cancers of the upper aerodigestive tract (divided into subsites), salivary gland, parapharyngeal space (PPS), sinonasal cavity, and temporal bone. Other cancers including melanoma, nonmelanoma skin cancer, carcinoma of the thyroid and parathyroid glands, sarcomas, and lymphomas are discussed separately in this handbook.

Epidemiology and Risk Factors

Cancers of the head and neck comprise 3% of all cancers in the United States, not including cancers of the skin and thyroid, and about 85% are squamous cell carcinomas (SCCs). Median age of diagnosis is in the early 60s. Men are disproportionately affected with an incidence ratio ranging from 2:1 to 4:1. Current global estimates project more than 500,000 new cases of head and neck cancer (HNC) annually with approximately 62,000 new cases and 13,000 deaths expected in the United States per year. Among aerodigestive sites, cancers of the oral cavity (OC), oropharynx (OP), and larynx are most common in the United States, though the latter is declining in incidence. Cancers of the nasopharynx (NP) are more common in Southeast Asia, while those of the OC are most common in the Indian subcontinent.

Risk factors for HNC are largely dependent upon anatomic location and differential exposures, explaining in part the geographic variations of the disease. Tobacco smoking is the most important carcinogen in HNC. Cigarette smokers have an estimated 5- to 25-fold increased risk, and cigar and pipe smokers also have an increased risk independent of cigarette smoking. The relative risk increases with duration of exposure but gradually declines after smoking cessation with no apparent excess risk by 20 years compared to nonsmokers. Long-term exposure to secondhand smoke also appears to be associated with increased risk of HNC. Alcohol is also an independent risk factor for cancers of the OC, pharynx, and larynx with consumption of 3.5 or more drinks per day increasing the risk of these cancers by two- or threefold. Chronic tobacco and alcohol use by the same patient substantially increases the risk. Betel quid chewing, a widespread practice in Southeast Asia and India, is associated with increased risk for OC carcinoma. Risk of cancer of the upper aerodigestive tract from smoking marijuana has not been established and is difficult to analyze given the high rates of concomitant tobacco and alcohol use.

Viral oncogenesis is a well-known mechanism of HNC development and has received a tremendous amount of attention in the last few decades. Human papilloma virus (HPV), particularly types 16 and 18, is recognized as the causative agent for greater than 70% of oropharyngeal carcinomas in the United States. Epstein–Barr virus (EBV) is the causative agent for most nasopharyngeal cancers, particularly in Southeastern China. Various occupational and/or environmental exposures have also been implicated in the development of HNC including asbestos, pesticides, wood, leather, cement dust, formaldehyde, and various petrochemical products. Studies of many of these exposures are limited by accurate quantification and potential misclassification, in addition to the possibility that hidden culprits in manufacturing processes may represent the actual causative factors. Though most important in thyroid cancers, prior irradiation is also a low but known risk factor for SCC, sarcomas, and salivary gland cancers. Finally, immunodeficiency such as that secondary to human immunodeficiency virus (HIV) or solid organ transplantation are associated with development of HNC (particularly nonmelanoma skin cancers), as are patients with congenital or acquired diseases such as Fanconi anemia, Li–Fraumeni syndrome, and Plummer–Vinson syndrome.

Initial Evaluation, Diagnosis, and Workup

The most important aspect of a HNC evaluation is an early diagnosis. Unfortunately, no population-level screening tests currently exist, though development of oral sampling tests analogous to the Papanicolaou smear used in cervical cancer represents a promising area of research. For patients already known to be at high risk for the disease, serial examination of high-risk areas such as the OC can be essential to identify early cancers or premalignant lesions. The initial evaluation of a patient with known or suspected cancer of the head and neck should involve comprehensive visual inspection and manual palpation (where possible) of the skin of the scalp, ears, face, and neck, and mucosal surfaces of the eyes, nose, mouth, and throat. Visualization of the pharynx and larynx is aided by transoral mirror examination or transnasal flexible endoscopy. Middle ear pathology may require otomicroscopy and intranasal pathology often requires rigid examination with specialized endoscopes. Palpation of the salivary glands, thyroid, and lateral neck to assess for masses and/or pathologic lymphadenopathy is essential. In cases when a palpable mass in the neck is the patient's reason for initial cancer evaluation, the location can help guide efforts to determine the location of the primary tumor. Finally, cranial nerve function should be carefully examined as both cancers and their subsequent treatments may result in nerve dysfunction.

Diagnostic imaging plays a central role in the evaluation and staging of HNC such that lack of need for cross-sectional imaging is rare in the workup of noncutaneous HNCs. Plain x-rays play a limited role in the modern evaluation of HNC with the exception of Panorex dental imaging and chest films for screening evaluation of primary thoracic malignancy or metastases. Computed tomography (CT) of the head and neck provides excellent delineation of bony anatomy and the addition of iodinated contrast can yield precise detail on the presence of metastatic lymphadenopathy and soft tissue invasion. Chest CT is also an important part of the initial evaluation since many patients may have concurrent lung pathology in addition to the fact that the lung is the most common site of distant metastases for cancers of the upper aerodigestive tract. Magnetic resonance imaging (MRI) is increasingly being used given its excellent soft tissue detail for tumors of mesenchymal or salivary origin, for identification of unknown primary tumors, and for identification of the presence or extent of perineural and/or dural invasion in the case of some cutaneous, salivary, paranasal sinus, and nasopharyngeal malignancies. Ultrasound is particularly sensitive in detecting cervical lymphadenopathy and has become the primary method for evaluation of thyroid and parathyroid pathology as well as regional lymphatic evaluation in many early-stage HNC patients. Positron emission tomography (PET) scans play a crucial role in the evaluation of distant metastases and may be used in the evaluation of unknown primary tumors or for initial posttreatment imaging to determine metabolic response to therapy.

Pathologic diagnosis of head and neck malignancy is made on the basis of histologic examination of primary tumor biopsies and/or cytopathologic examination of fine-needle aspiration (FNA) biopsy for regional lymphadenopathy. In many cases, in-office biopsy may be performed for lesions that are easily accessible. Alternatively, patients may require examination under anesthesia with biopsy in several scenarios: if the tumor is not easily accessible or there is concern for tumor bleeding; to determine the location of the primary tumor when unknown; to evaluate for synchronous malignant lesions of the upper aerodigestive tract; and to further delineate the specific extent of tumor prior to treatment planning. The latter scenario may be particularly important prior to surgical planning in certain oropharyngeal and laryngeal cancers. With modern ultrasound and cytopathology, the need for excisional biopsy of an undiagnosed neck mass should be rare and a last resort for establishing a diagnosis, as this may violate the principles of oncologic surgery, complicate further surgery, and necessitate more intense adjuvant therapy. Nevertheless, if a diagnosis cannot be made through location and/or biopsy of the primary tumor, if cytopathology with the aid of ultrasound or CT guidance cannot establish a diagnosis, or if tumor histology is needed in excess of that afforded by core biopsy, an excisional biopsy may be warranted. In some cases, surgical planning may be made based upon a patient's history, the tumor location, or specific imaging characteristics without having a preoperative pathologic diagnosis. With rare exception, a pathologic diagnosis should be considered a necessity prior to considering nonsurgical treatment with radiation and/or systemic therapy in HNCs. Benign tumors or lesions resulting from systemic inflammatory or infectious diseases may closely mimic malignant tumors of the upper aerodigestive tract such that pathologic diagnosis is critical, particularly when aspects of the history or examination are incongruous.

Staging and Treatment

Staging for HNC is based on the American Joint Committee on Cancer (AJCC) classification. The T stage defines the size and extent of the primary; the N stage defines the size, number, and location of nodal spread; and the M stage refers to the presence or absence of distant metastasis. Taken together, these form an overall TNM AJCC stage ranging from stage I to stage IV.

The mainstays of HNC treatment are surgery, radiation, and systemic therapy. In most cases, early cancers may be treated with a single modality, whereas advanced cancers require multimodality therapy. In some sites such as the OC, surgery represents the primary treatment modality largely due to the long-term morbidity of high-dose mandibular irradiation and the relative decreased sensitivity of these OC tumors to primary radiation therapy. In other areas such as the NP, radiation is preferred over surgery, given its high-degree effectiveness and relative surgical inaccessibility. Treatment of cancers of the larynx is largely dependent upon the size and location of the primary tumor and pretreatment function (i.e., respiratory, voice, and swallowing). In addition to these factors, extent of regional metastases, HPV status, and smoking history are also central to treatment decision making for oropharyngeal cancers. Overall, because of the many anatomic and histologic nuances of these cancers in addition to the functional impact of treatment, management of both early and advanced HNCs must be undertaken in a multidisciplinary setting and tailored to the patient. Providers routinely involved in these patients include radiation and medical oncologists, neuroradiologists, surgical and cytologic pathologists, dentists, speech–language pathologists, clinical dieticians, plastic and reconstructive surgeons, neurosurgeons, and thoracic surgeons.

Even though this text focuses on surgical oncology, a surgeon's understanding of head and neck radiation and medical oncology is indispensable when determining the role and extent of surgery in care of the HNC patient. Though surgical and nonsurgical treatment specifics will be discussed at length by anatomic site, there are a number of scenarios where nonsurgical therapy is preferred. When surgery is the preferred treatment modality, it is usually performed prior to administration of radiation and/or systemic therapy with few exceptions. For instance, certain diseases such as some sarcomas may be treated with preoperative chemotherapy and/or radiation, while systemic therapy may be given prior to determining whether a patient should have surgical or nonsurgical treatment of their laryngeal cancer. In any case, surgical management of primary tumors of the head and neck follows the principles of en bloc resection whenever possible. Clearing surgical margins without transection or spilling of tumor is considered a basic oncologic tenant with the exception of some endoscopic endonasal or transoral laser surgery where piecemeal resection has been shown to be oncologically equivalent. Specifics of resection are discussed in detail below. This chapter deals specifically with cancer of the head and neck, though many lesions in this area of the body may be benign. In these circumstances, recommendation for surgical excision must involve balancing the following considerations with the reasonable risks of the procedure: growth over time versus stability; risk of malignant transformation; challenge for surveillance or accurate sampling on biopsy; aggressive behavior with local destruction; cosmetically conspicuous; current or anticipated decrement in function (swallowing, breathing, nerve deficit); and patient concerns regarding surgery versus observation.

Radiation therapy is delivered through administration of ionizing radiation derived from either photons (e.g., x-rays and gamma rays) or particles (e.g., electrons, protons, neutrons, etc.) and can also be divided into external beam or brachytherapy. Photons are delivered by external beam and most commonly produced with a linear accelerator but can also be produced from a radioactive source (historically cobalt). Particles are also produced by a linear accelerator with the most common types being electron, often used in treatment of skin cancer since these particles do not penetrate deeply, and proton, which remains relatively uncommon but is increasing in use nationwide, including for certain HNCs. Brachytherapy refers to local deposition of a radioactive substance that releases radiation through decay. The most common substance used in treatment of HNC is iridium-192. Regardless of the type of radiation, all techniques are designed to deliver tumoricidal doses of radiation with minimization of treatment to normal tissues. Overall, external-beam photon treatment, delivered most commonly now through intensity-modulated radiation therapy (IMRT), represents the most common method for treatment of cancers of the upper aerodigestive tract. As far as dosing is concerned, primary treatment for cancers of the head and neck is typically administered between 66 and 70 Gy to the areas of known cancer (the primary and any positive nodes) and a slightly lesser dose to areas that may have cancer (the so-called elective treatment). When delivered after surgery (i.e., "postoperative" or "adjuvant" radiation), the dose is most commonly 60 Gy. Treatments are commonly given 5 days per week for 6 to 7 weeks. Dosing and algorithms for the treatment of other types of cancer such as melanoma, lymphoma, or sarcoma are different.

Systemic treatment in HNC most commonly refers to chemotherapy (i.e., cytotoxic drugs like cisplatin, 5-fluorouracil, or docetaxel), though also includes targeted treatments like monoclonal antibodies to EGFR (cetuximab) and checkpoint inhibitors to PD-1 (pembrolizumab, nivolumab). Systemic treatment can be given prior to surgery or radiation (i.e., "neoadjuvant" or "induction" therapy) in an effort to reduce the chance of distant spread of disease; as a type of "chemoselection" for patients whose cancers are particularly responsive to treatment; to reduce the size of large tumors prior to surgery or radiation; or prior to planned radiation in an effort to improve toxicity compared to concurrent treatment. When given together with radiation, chemotherapy acts as a radiation sensitizer, thereby producing greater treatment efficacy but also greater treatment side effects. Concurrent treatment is commonly used as a primary treatment for disease confined

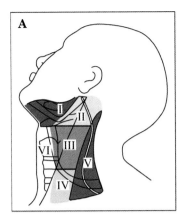
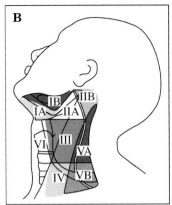
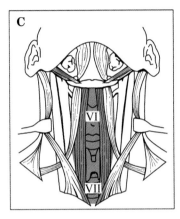

FIGURE 7.1 Anatomic lymph node levels. (Reprinted with permission from Fischer JE. *Fischer's Mastery of Surgery.* 7th ed. Wolters Kluwer; 2019. Figure 25.3.)

locoregionally as well as postoperatively in the setting of positive surgical margins or extracapsular extension in lymph node metastases. Cisplatin (either high dose or low dose) and cetuximab are the most commonly used systemic agents.

Nodal metastases to the parotid or neck may be treated effectively through surgery and/or radiation with decisions between them determined by tumor histology, location, and other specifics such as the number of positive nodes and the presence of extracapsular extension. Neck dissection refers to surgical removal of regional lymphatics from the cervical region and may be performed to remove known (macroscopic) sites of metastatic lymphadenopathy, or to provide prognostic information in the case of subclinical (i.e., microscopic) disease. Several variations of this procedure exist, all of which involve removing lymphatics from different anatomic levels of the neck (Fig. 7.1). *Radical neck dissection* (RND) refers to removal of lymphatics from levels I to V in addition to the sternocleidomastoid muscle (SCM), internal jugular vein (IJV), and spinal accessory nerve. Due to the morbidity of this procedure, it is rarely performed.

A *modified radical neck dissection* (MRND) reduces the morbidity of this procedure by preservation of one or more of these structures. Nevertheless, MRND is also often unnecessary since contemporary surgery seeks to confine dissection to levels which are at most risk for metastatic disease based upon location of the primary tumor. These surgeries are collectively referred to as *selective neck dissections* (SNDs) and can be subdivided into *supraomohyoid* (levels I to III), *lateral* (levels II to IV), and *posterolateral* (levels II to V). Indications for a specific type of SND are discussed by primary tumor site below. In cases where there is no evidence of nodal metastasis (stage N0), a neck dissection is called an *elective neck dissection* (END) and may be performed when the risk of regional metastasis exceeds a certain threshold. This threshold is generally recognized as 20% and is largely determined by known rates of microscopic nodal metastasis associated with a primary tumor of particular size and location. Finally, neck dissection may also be performed to remove persistent or recurrent cervical lymphadenopathy after nonsurgical treatment, with the specifics of these surgeries determined by the location of nodal disease, the extent of postradiation changes (i.e., fibrosis and/or inflammation), and need for or ability to receive additional radiation after surgery.

Prognosis and Functional Outcomes

As would be expected, prognosis for upper aerodigestive tract cancers is generally determined by the size of the primary, with bulkier disease being associated with a worse prognosis, in addition to the presence of regional and distant metastasis. Several other factors are also known to influence prognosis, typically through increased risk of regional and/or distant metastasis or local/regional recurrence. These include tumor grade, depth of tumor invasion, perineural and lymphovascular invasion by the primary tumor, close or positive margins, and the presence of extracapsular extension in lymph nodes. One advantage to surgical treatment is that pathologic determination of these factors is thus available (as opposed to that determined by clinical examination or imaging). Typically, presence of these factors often drives the decision for addition of adjuvant radiation or chemoradiation after surgery. Considering all sites and treatments, approximately 90% of patients achieve cure with stage I disease and roughly 70% with stage II. Survival continues to drop thereafter and the presence of nodal metastasis decreases survival by roughly 50%. This is largely associated with an increased risk of distant metastasis, which is estimated to occur in approximately 15% of all patients.

Similar to other disease sites, ongoing efforts to identify biologic and molecular markers that are either prognostic or targetable through systemic interventions represent the new frontier of personalized oncologic treatment. Though the field of investigative tumor biology in head and neck SCC is broad, the most well-recognized factors are disruptive TP53 mutations, epidermal growth factor receptor (EGFR) and tumor growth factor-alpha (TGF-α) overexpression, and p16 expression (often used as a marker for HPV-associated oropharyngeal tumors). Tumor expression of programmed death-ligand 1 (PD-L1) and cytotoxic T-lymphocyte–associated protein (CTLA-4) represents part of the evaluation of patients with recurrent or metastatic HNC during consideration of immunotherapy. Despite these advances, tailoring treatment on the basis of these molecular findings is often part of a clinical trial, particularly if those data are being used to reduce treatment intensity.

Apart from disease-specific outcomes, functional outcomes are also important considerations in the HNC population since both the tumor as well as treatment may have profound effects on normal function. Functional outcomes include both expected and unexpected sequelae of treatment and can also be divided into short- and long-term outcomes. In several areas of the head and neck, different types of treatment may achieve equal rates of cure, but one is often preferred based upon the anticipated functional outcome(s). For instance, in laryngeal cancer, a main goal of nonsurgical therapy is organ preservation through treatment of the cancer without removal of the larynx. In this scenario, the patient has the potential to retain their ability to speak, eat, and breathe through their native upper aerodigestive tract. Conversely, advanced laryngeal cancer may have already damaged normal laryngeal function. For this reason, surgery would be the preferred treatment modality, since this function will only be worsened through radiation-based treatment. Understanding these types of outcomes requires prospective gathering of data on baseline and/or longitudinal function since these may change over time. Clinical trials provide an ideal setting for gathering prospective data, and determination of functional outcomes is no exception. In part due to the fact that nonsurgical trials are historically much more common, comparatively robust data exist on the functional outcomes of patients treated with radiation with or without chemotherapy. Nevertheless, surgeons are becoming much more interested in prospectively tracking functional outcomes, particularly in treatment of cancers such as the OP and larynx where radiation is highly successful at treating the cancer but may have long-lasting side effects.

Similar to surgical risks and side effects, most radiation-associated side effects are predictable based upon the site(s) being treated. Indeed, many of the advances in radiation therapy delivery and technique have centered on maintaining treatment of the cancer while minimizing radiation to normal structures such as the salivary glands, muscles of deglutition and mastication, and the laryngeal framework (for nonlaryngeal cancers). These have resulted in improvements in xerostomia, dysphagia, aspiration, and trismus, though these remain among the most common long-term side effects. Other potential long-term risks include osteoradionecrosis (ORN) of the mandible and dental caries, thyroid dysfunction, sensorineural hearing loss, accelerated carotid atherosclerosis, and delayed cranial neuropathy. Given all of these considerations, functional outcome measures including patient-reported outcomes and clinician-determined metrics are essentially a mandatory component of both surgical and nonsurgical clinical trials and are increasingly becoming a common part of routine clinical care rather than reserved for patients with overt dysfunction.

Anatomic Sites

As previously discussed, the head and neck is composed of several different anatomic sites. Treatment of cancers in each area requires careful consideration of tumor histology and etiology, disease stage, location of surrounding structures, and preservation of function. The following sections will discuss HNC by these sites (and subsites), including relevant anatomy, common risk factors and cancer types, treatment considerations and rationale, and anticipated outcomes of therapy.

Oral Cavity

The OC refers to the region extending from the vermillion border of the lips to the circumvallate papillae of the tongue and junction between the hard and soft palate. Subsites include the lips, buccal mucosa, alveolar ridge, floor of the mouth, oral tongue, retromolar trigone, and hard palate. OC cancer is one of the most common cancers in the world, with an annual incidence of over 300,000 and nearly 150,000 deaths. Tracking incidence and mortality of this disease at a population level can be challenging though since skin cancers of the lips and cancers of the OP are often grouped together with it. Nevertheless, it is more common in men than women (~3–4 to 1) and occurs most commonly in the sixth and seventh decades. The majority of cancers in the OC are SCC, though cancers of the minor salivary glands also occur including mucoepidermoid carcinoma, adenoid cystic carcinoma, and adenocarcinoma.

Common risk factors for OC SCC include tobacco smoking and smokeless tobacco, alcohol, and betel quid chewing. HPV does not play a significant role in OC SCC carcinogenesis, although it is common for large tumors of the tonsil or base of tongue to extend secondarily to the OC. Although poor dental hygiene does appear to be an independent risk factor, chronic irritation from dentures or other oral appliances and use of mouthwash have not been supported as causative factors by further research. Finally, some patients have premalignant lesions including leukoplakia and erythroplakia. These lesions should be biopsied on initial evaluation and followed, if negative for malignancy, since they may transform into an invasive cancer. The risk of development of an invasive cancer for leukoplakia is estimated at between 1% and 18%, while erythroplakia is associated with a higher risk. In addition to detailed visual and manual physical examination, CT with contrast and/or MRI with gadolinium are very helpful for determining local extension of disease and presence of metastatic lymphadenopathy.

Surgery remains the treatment modality of choice for OC cancers in part due to the relative accessibility of these areas in addition to the long-term morbidity of high-dose OC radiation. OC cancers are also believed to be slightly less sensitive to ionizing radiation. Invasive cancers are typically removed with a 10- to 15-mm margin of normal-appearing tissue. Small excisions can be performed transorally and may be closed primarily, allowed to heal by secondary intention, or closed using a skin graft. Larger defects may necessitate a mandibulotomy or transcervical approach in addition to more complex reconstruction through local tissue rearrangement, regional flap reconstruction, or free tissue transfer. Lesions with periosteal involvement, extension into tooth roots, or frank invasion of the maxilla and/or mandible require bony resection to achieve negative margins.

The incidence of regional nodal metastasis correlates with the size, grade, and depth of invasion of the primary tumor. The primary nodal basins of the OC are levels I to III. Most data on the risk of occult metastases in clinically N0 patients derive from analysis of oral tongue carcinoma, where lesions with less than 2- to 4-mm depth of invasion have a low rate of regional metastasis. As such, lesions with greater than 4-mm depth of invasion typically are treated with wide local excision and simultaneous supraomohyoid neck dissection. Small lesions that are N0 with borderline thickness and/or those in the midline with the potential for bilateral lymph node metastasis may be amenable to sentinel lymph node biopsy and a recently initiated national trial promises to greatly expand our knowledge of early-stage OC cancer in general. In experienced hands, this procedure identifies sentinel nodes with a false-negative rate of less than 3%, which is comparable to that seen in melanoma. On the other hand, all patients with clinically evident or biopsy-proven nodal metastases from OC cancer should have a therapeutic neck dissection at the time of primary resection.

External-beam radiation or brachytherapy implants have been used extensively in the past for primary treatment of OC carcinoma. This is rarely performed contemporarily given high rates of radiation-associated toxicities and dismal rates of salvage in cases of radiation failure. Radiation therapy is commonly used in the adjuvant setting for patients at high risk of locoregional recurrence, including the pathologic risk factors described above (e.g., positive margins, perineural invasion, multiple metastatic lymph nodes, extranodal extension), as well as for patients with large primary tumors and/or need for extensive reconstruction, since margins may be more difficult to ascertain and monitoring for recurrence may be more challenging. Occasionally, if a patient is known preoperatively to have indications for radiation of the primary lesion but has no evidence of regional lymphadenopathy (N0), neck dissection may not be performed in favor of elective adjuvant nodal radiation. Use of concurrent chemotherapy is often recommended for positive margins or extracapsular extension. Treatment of early lesions of the OC (T1/T2) carries an 80% to 90% 5-year survival rate while more advanced lesions (T3/T4) have a 5-year survival of 30% to 60%, with decrements largely related to the presence of regional metastases.

Lips

Cancer of the mucosa (wet portion) of the lips is overwhelmingly SCC, with 90% being located on the lower lip, and largely results from smoking or chronic sun exposure. Cancers of the upper lip are much more commonly basal cell carcinomas and are typically classified as skin cancers. Lip cancer most commonly presents early as a nonhealing erythematous lesion with larger lesions causing pain or bleeding.

Lip cancers are almost always treated with primary surgery with the possible exception of lesions of the oral commissure, which present a challenge in reconstruction and may be better addressed with radiation. Beyond removal of the cancer, two primary goals of surgical management of lip cancer involve maintenance of oral competence and minimization of microstomia. Depending on the extent of resection, various types of closure or reconstruction may be needed ranging from wedge excision to local advancement or rotational flaps, to free tissue transfer such as the radial forearm free flap. Cancers of the lip uncommonly metastasize to regional lymph nodes, though elective dissection is recommended for tumors larger than 4 cm (T3/T4); those with perineural spread along the mental nerve; those with bony involvement; and for recurrent tumors. Use of adjuvant radiation or chemoradiation may then be recommended depending on final pathology.

Buccal Mucosa

Cancer of the buccal mucosa accounts for 5% to 10% of all OC cancers in the United States but upward of 40% in India. Smoking and concurrent alcohol use, smokeless tobacco, and betel quid chewing are the major risk factors. Pre-existing leukoplakia is more common for buccal mucosa cancer and patients also present with a nonhealing ulcer, pain, or cervical adenopathy. Induration of the cheek skin or facial paralysis indicates local invasion of tumor into adjacent structures, while trismus may be secondary to inflammation of the masseter or pterygoids or from frank pterygoid muscle invasion.

Early tumors (T1/T2) may be treated primarily with surgery or radiation, though the latter may result in high rates of xerostomia, trismus, and ORN. Surgery should consist of transoral excision at least down to the buccinator muscle, though this muscle is not considered an adequate anatomic barrier to spread into the buccal space and should be removed if invasion is suspected. Once the tumor extends to the buccal space, no anatomic barriers exist to contain its spread and tumor size is no longer predictive of prognosis. Small excisions may be reconstructed with split-thickness skin grafting, while larger defects necessitate regional or free tissue reconstruction to minimize trismus secondary to contracture as well as optimize wound healing in anticipation of need for adjuvant radiation. Transposition or ligation of the parotid duct may be required. Nodal metastasis is uncommon in early buccal cancers but patients with T3–T4, N0 tumors should have supraomohyoid neck dissection at the time of tumor resection. Moreover, given concerns for local recurrence, which has historically been higher in buccal cancers than many other sites, patients with T3/T4 disease and/ or extension into the buccal space should have adjuvant locoregional radiation regardless of nodal staging.

Alveolar Ridge

Alveolar ridge cancer is overwhelmingly SCC arising from the gingival mucosa if you exclude odontogenic tumors of the maxilla and mandible. Common risk factors include tobacco, alcohol, and possibly ill-fitting dentures. Patients usually present with a nonhealing ulcer, pain, bleeding, or loose teeth. Numbness of the teeth, lips, or chin, indicating invasion of the alveolar nerves (particularly the inferior branch) and extension onto the adjacent buccal mucosa, floor of mouth, or hard palate are also important considerations in the initial evaluation and treatment planning.

Due to the underlying bone in all of these cancers, surgery is the preferred treatment regardless of whether bone invasion actually exists, since primary radiation may result in exposed bone and predispose the patient to development of ORN. For inferior alveolar ridge (mandibular) lesions, marginal mandibulectomy is sufficient for early tumors with primary closure of mucosa or placement of a split-thickness skin graft. This should be done with caution in edentulous patients given the risks of subsequent fracture in an already atrophic mandible. Tumors with evidence of cortical bone invasion should be managed with segmental mandibulectomy and ideally should be reconstructed with osseous free tissue transfer such as a fibular free flap. Patients with comorbidities precluding extensive reconstruction may be allowed to "swing" without bony reconstruction. Titanium plating of the mandible without bony reconstruction has fallen into disfavor given short and long-term complications of chronic fistulization, plate exposure, hardware fracture, and infection. It is at times considered in the palliative setting for patients with poor surgical candidacy. For superior alveolar ridge (maxillary) lesions, inferior or infrastructure maxillectomy is typically required. The goal of reconstruction in these cases is to re-establish separation of the oral and sinonasal cavity which can be accomplished through placement of a prosthetic obturator or through free tissue reconstruction. Patients with T2–T4, N0 disease should have END with frequent use of adjuvant radiation for poor prognostic indicators on pathologic analysis of the primary tumor and lymph nodes.

Floor of the Mouth

Cancer of the floor of mouth accounts for approximately 10% to 15% of all OC cancers with the vast majority representing SCC. Patients may present with a nonhealing ulceration, obstruction of the submandibular duct, numbness of the tongue, or even dysarthria secondary to deep infiltration of the tongue or involvement of the hypoglossal nerve(s).

Surgery is the treatment of choice, though primary radiation may be used with similar efficacy with limitations and treatment sequelae similar to other OC sites. Transoral resection of the floor of mouth often involves removal of the submandibular duct orifice. This may require transposition of the duct posteriorly in the mouth if possible, or simply ligation as the submandibular gland should be removed during the level I neck dissection. Removal of early lesions may be reconstructed with split-thickness skin graft or allowed to heal by secondary intention. Larger tumors may require composite resection including partial glossectomy, or marginal versus segmental mandibulectomy. These cases require complex reconstruction for optimization of speech and eating, in addition to closure of the OC to prevent leakage of saliva into the neck.

Regional metastases are fairly common and may be bilateral. Patients with T2–T4, N0 cancer should have neck dissection(s) whereas those with T1 N0 disease lesions may be observed, subjected to sentinel node biopsy, or receive END. The use of adjuvant radiation or chemoradiation is then dictated by the pathologic details from surgical resection.

Oral Tongue

The oral tongue refers to the anterior two-thirds of the tongue in front of the circumvallate papilla. Cancer in this area is almost exclusively SCC with rare exception; represents the most common cancer of the OC; and most commonly occurs on the lateral surface of the tongue at the junction of the middle and posterior thirds. Tobacco use and alcohol are common risk factors, though an etiologic agent remains unidentified in a subset of patients younger than 40 years that may be increasing in incidence. Oral tongue cancer often presents as a painless mass, though larger tumors may cause local pain or numbness, bleeding, dysarthria, oral phase dysphagia, and referred otalgia.

Primary radiation (external beam and/or brachytherapy) can be effective for early tongue cancers but cannot provide pathologic information on the primary tumor or regional lymphatics, may require temporary tracheotomy placement, and patients are subject to the long-term sequelae of high-dose OC irradiation described above. As such, primary surgery is the treatment of choice and partial glossectomy is adequate for early tumors. Cancer can spread easily into the intrinsic and extrinsic tongue musculature, meaning that margins must be carefully assessed visually and by palpation during removal to ensure clear margins with the first specimen. Primary closure, healing by secondary intention, or split-thickness skin graft placement are appropriate for smaller defects. Larger defects should be reconstructed with regional or free tissue transfer as this results in improved speech and swallowing outcomes.

Occult regional metastases are common in oral tongue cancer and depth of invasion is the strongest predictor, such that all patients with tumors ≥4 mm should have END. Levels I to III should be dissected, though some also advocate inclusion of level IV for oral tongue cancers. Adjuvant radiation to both primary and regional lymphatics should be delivered for poor pathologic markers since locoregional recurrence is often unresectable and represents the most common cause of death.

Retromolar Trigone

The retromolar trigone refers to the mucosa posterior to the last molar overlying the ascending ramus of the mandible. Cancer of this region is rare though it is a common location of extension of tumors from other areas of the OC or OP. Patients often present with local pain, burning, and otalgia. Since the mandible is only covered by mucosa and periosteum in this area, tumors are often advanced at presentation with bone destruction. Trismus may indicate pterygoid involvement and numbness of the teeth and chin/lip may indicate mandibular invasion or direct spread along the inferior alveolar nerve. Surgery is the preferred treatment for all lesions and often requires at least marginal mandibulectomy. Primary radiation may be considered for early lesions though trismus, bone exposure, and local recurrence are significant risks. Transoral exposure frequently is assisted by a lip-splitting incision with a cheek flap or visor flap. Elective management of the neck through supraomohyoid neck dissection or radiation is recommended for T2–T4, N0 patients. Split-thickness skin grafting may be sufficient for small lesions but regional or free flap transfer for fasciocutaneous, myocutaneous, or osseocutaneous reconstruction is often required. Adjuvant radiation is frequently recommended for cancers with bone invasion and those with nodal metastases.

Hard Palate

Cancers of the hard palate are also rare, comprised equally of SCC and minor salivary gland cancers in the United States. Patients often present with a painless ulceration, although pain, bleeding, and ill-fitting dentures may also be seen at presentation. The palatal periosteum is a strong barrier to spread, although tumors may spread into the maxilla causing nasal symptoms and facial swelling or spread anteriorly/laterally to the alveolar ridge causing dental pain and loose teeth. Perineural spread can occur along the palatine branches of the maxillary nerve through the greater palatine foramen, into the pterygopalatine fossa, and into the cavernous sinus, particularly with adenoid cystic carcinoma. These patients may present with multiple cranial neuropathies including facial numbness and diplopia.

Surgery is the treatment of choice for cancers of the hard palate. Though preservation of bone may be possible in small lesions with wide local excision and healing by secondary intention or split-thickness skin graft placement, bone removal with partial palatectomy is the most oncologically sound approach. Larger tumors will require infrastructure maxillectomy or more extensive maxillectomy that may be aided by lip split with lateral rhinotomy or a facial degloving approach. Separation of the oral and sinonasal cavity may be accomplished by use of a prosthetic obturator or regional/free tissue reconstruction. END is controversial since occult nodal metastasis appears to be less common and patients often receive adjuvant radiation to the primary, thereby making elective nodal radiation a more common approach. Patients with extensive, unresectable perineural disease may be treated with primary radiation extending from the primary tumor following nerve branches to the skull base, though surgery may play a role for control of local disease and quality of life.

Nasopharynx

The NP refers to the region between the nasal cavity and OP, bounded anteriorly by the choanae, posteriorly by the posterior pharyngeal wall, superiorly by the body of the sphenoid, inferiorly by the soft palate, and laterally by the Eustachian tubes and superior pharyngeal constrictors. NP cancer is uncommon in most parts of the world with the exception of Southeastern China as well as areas of Southeast Asia and California that are home to Chinese immigrants. In these areas, the incidence is 10 to 20 times higher. It tends to affect patients at a younger age than many other cancers of the upper aerodigestive tract with a median age of approximately 50 years. SCC is by far the most common cancer but lymphomas, minor salivary gland cancers, melanomas, and sarcomas are also known to occur.

Carcinoma of the NP is traditionally classified according to histologic findings by the World Health Organization: Type 1, keratinizing SCC; type 2, nonkeratinizing SCC; and type 3, undifferentiated or poorly differentiated carcinoma (including "lymphoepithelioma"). Types 2 and 3, often combined together as nonkeratinizing types, are strongly associated with EBV. With regard to other risk factors, consumption of salted fish at an early age, which are high in nitrosamine compounds, also appears to play a role. Moreover, certain haplotypes and specific chromosomal alterations seem to be associated with increased risk and may explain why nasopharyngeal carcinoma is four times more common in first-degree relatives of patients with these tumors.

Carcinoma often arises in the lateral NP, particularly in the fossa of Rosenmüller, which is a recess posterior to the Eustachian tube orifice. Due to this location, patients may present with middle ear effusion, unilateral nasal obstruction, or bloody nasal secretions. As the tumor grows, it may cause complete nasal obstruction, hyponasal speech, and frank epistaxis in addition to localized pain, headaches, and trismus. However, a painless neck mass or bilateral neck masses are the most common presentation since the NP has rich lymphatic drainage. It may also invade superiorly into the cavernous sinus or laterally into the PPS causing both upper and lower cranial nerve deficits. Diagnosis is often made through FNA of cervical lymphadenopathy or endoscopic biopsy of the NP. In endemic areas, levels of immunoglobulin A against certain EBV-specific antigens have even been used as a screening tool for detection of early asymptomatic tumors.

Radiation therapy represents the mainstay of treatment for the primary tumor owing to the inherent radiosensitivity, its relative surgical inaccessibility, and its infiltrative nature. Radiation therapy alone is often reserved for T1N0 patients only. Chemotherapy is used in the treatment of all other stages, often delivered concurrently in the form of cisplatin and adjuvantly (after concurrent treatment) with cisplatin and 5-fluorouracil or neoadjuvantly with docetaxel, cisplatin, and 5-fluorouracil. Surgery, either through endoscopic or radical ("maxillary swing") procedures, remains a treatment that is almost entirely reserved for locally recurrent disease. However, reirradiation either through external beam or through brachytherapy is still the most common method for treatment of local recurrence. Persistent versus recurrent regional lymphadenopathy is addressed with neck dissection.

Survival is directly related to AJCC staging with approximately 90% 5-year overall survival for stage I dropping to less than 60% for stage IV. EBV-associated disease is generally accepted as a positive prognostic indicator compared to the keratinizing subtype. Moreover, posttreatment levels of EBV DNA in plasma appear to be a strong prognosticator for persistent disease and overall survival. Given reasonably high survival combined with disease occurring in younger patients, functional outcomes (particularly long-term radiation sequelae) are well known for survivors of nasopharyngeal carcinoma. Though improvements in imaging techniques to better delineate tumor location combined with advances in radiotherapy delivery have diminished some long-term effects, many remain including trismus, xerostomia, ORN of the facial bones and skull base, dysphagia, temporal lobe necrosis, and radiation-induced cranial neuropathies. Otologic complications are also common including chronic Eustachian tube dysfunction with serous effusions and sensorineural hearing loss, the latter of which may be exacerbated by concurrent treatment with cisplatin.

Oropharynx

The OP is composed of the soft palate, palatine tonsils, the base of the tongue, and the posterior and lateral pharyngeal walls from the soft palate to the pharyngoepiglottic fold. It is estimated that approximately 15,000 new cases of oropharyngeal cancer are diagnosed each year in the United States, which has been increasing steadily for almost four decades. The disease is more common in men than women with a ratio of 4:1. SCC is the most common type of cancer to arise in the OP but minor salivary gland tumors, lymphoma, and sarcoma can also occur.

SCC in the OP classically arises from chronic tobacco and alcohol use, though HPV-associated carcinogenesis has become the primary etiologic agent, such that at least 70% of oropharyngeal cancers are HPV-associated in the United States. HPV is a sexually transmitted infection, and although most sexually active people have been exposed to the virus, it remains unknown why a relatively small minority of the exposed population develops oropharyngeal malignancy, often many years following purported exposure. It appears that a long latency period exists and the risk for development of HPV-associated oropharyngeal cancer increases with the number of sexual partners, particularly related to oral sex. Compared to patients with non–HPV-associated disease, patients with HPV-associated oropharyngeal cancer on average are slightly younger and lack a history of heavy tobacco use.

Referred otalgia, dysphagia, bleeding, trismus, and halitosis are among the presenting signs and symptoms of oropharyngeal cancer patients, though by far the most common presentation is a painless neck mass. Indeed, cancers of the OP have a high likelihood for regional metastasis and have become increasingly common, such that physicians should have a high index of suspicion for this disease in an adult who presents with an asymptomatic neck mass. Small primary lesions and cystic regional lymphadenopathy are characteristic of HPV-associated oropharyngeal carcinoma, such that office-based pharyngoscopy may not reveal a primary lesion and FNA of the cystic fluid may fail to reveal malignant cells. In this circumstance, FNA should be repeated, ideally with ultrasound guidance, to sample the cyst wall. If this fails, one may consider examination under anesthesia with directed biopsies and excisional lymph node biopsy to establish a diagnosis. Alternatively, if the diagnosis is made on biopsy of a lymph node but no primary is identified on clinic examination or routine imaging (CT, MRI), a PET scan may be obtained to look for asymmetric uptake indicating a primary tumor, or examination under anesthesia performed with tonsillectomy and biopsies of the glossopharyngeal sulcus and tongue base.

Both surgery and radiation therapy are effective treatment modalities used in the primary treatment of oropharyngeal cancer and have been shown to have comparable oncologic outcomes. Treatment decisions are heavily based on the balance of expected oncologic and functional outcomes. Traditionally, surgery for oropharyngeal cancers consisted of transoral resection using self-retaining retractors and headlight-assisted, line-of-sight surgery; transcervical approach with suprahyoid or lateral pharyngotomy; or transmandibular approaches. Needless to say, strictly transoral resections were limited to small, accessible primaries. With the development of transoral surgical techniques using the CO_2 laser and transoral robotic surgery (TORS), these surgical approaches have been shown to have similar or improved oncologic outcomes with significantly lower complication rates as compared to open surgical approaches. In this context, surgery for oropharyngeal cancer has been given renewed consideration for the management of early-stage cancers in the past few decades. In general, primary surgery for OPC such as TORS is offered to T1, T2, and very select exophytic T3 tumors in which either single-modality treatment is likely, or the extent or adjuvant therapy can be tailored (ideally lessened) based on pathologic staging. This approach is supported by burgeoning data from multi-institutional trials largely demonstrating improved or equivalent disease and functional outcomes. Because of the high risk of nodal metastases, neck dissection should uniformly be performed in patients undergoing surgical resection of the primary tumor. Primary lymphatic drainage is to level II followed by levels III and IV. Retropharyngeal drainage also occurs and is of particular concern for lesions involving the soft palate.

Moreover, drainage can be bilateral for midline structures, particularly those of the base of the tongue. The decision for surgery must also consider the extent and location of the primary tumor, patient anatomy that allows for transoral access, and burden of nodal disease since the inability to achieve a margin-negative resection and/or pathologic nodal characteristics may trigger the recommendation for adjuvant radiation or even chemoradiation. Indeed, the prognostic value of various adverse features including the presence of extranodal extension, its extent, and the number of involved nodes in HPV-associated disease continues to be an area of active research.

An ever-growing body of evidence has shown that HPV-associated oropharyngeal cancers respond favorably to any treatment with over 80% 3-year overall survival compared to less than 60% with non–HPV-associated tumors. This, combined with the fact that these patients are often younger and healthier, has given rise to ongoing discussions about de-escalation of treatment through modern surgical techniques, lower radiation doses, and less toxic systemic agents or altered timing of administration. In fact, the most recent staging system unique to HPV-associated oropharyngeal carcinoma closely resembles that of nasopharyngeal carcinoma. Many treatment questions are under investigation through clinical trials that are planned, ongoing, or recently closed to accrual. Outside of a clinical trial, the current standard of care for treatment of early (T1 N0–1) to intermediate (T2N0–1) cancers is single-modality radiation therapy to 66 Gy or surgery alone in the absence of adverse features. Concurrent, cisplatin-based chemoradiation to 70 Gy for advanced disease (T1–2 N2+, T3 N+, and all T4). Induction chemotherapy using cisplatin and 5-fluorouracil or paclitaxel, ifosfamide, and cisplatin may also be considered for very bulky or low (level IV) nodal disease prior to definitive radiation or chemoradiation in an effort to improve regional and distant tumor control, though this approach has not been shown to improve local control or overall survival. Finally, functional outcomes, particularly long-term swallowing, have become a primary focus of oropharyngeal cancer treatment and prospective tracking of patient-reported and physician-determined functional outcomes has become paramount to allow for valid comparisons of treatment modalities beyond disease survival.

Hypopharynx

The hypopharynx (HP) is composed of the posterior pharyngeal wall (from the hyoid to esophageal inlet), the pyriform sinuses, and the postcricoid area. It's bounded laterally and posteriorly by the inferior constrictor and the most distal part of the middle constrictor. Upward of two-thirds of cancers in the United States are located in the pyriform sinus with another 20% arising from the posterior pharyngeal wall. Postcricoid tumors are quite rare. HP cancers are most closely linked to chronic tobacco and alcohol use with SCC being the predominant histologic type. Rarely, cancers of the minor salivary gland, neuroendocrine tumors, or lymphomas can also arise. Patients commonly present with dysphagia, sore throat, referred otalgia, dysphonia from vocal cord paralysis, and weight loss. Neck masses are also common owing to the rich, bilateral lymphatic drainage of the HP. On initial examination, patients should undergo fiberoptic examination of the pharynx and larynx to assess tumor location and extent in addition to evaluation of vocal cord mobility. Imaging is often obtained using CT scan with improved visualization of the HP through dynamic maneuvers such as Valsalva.

Cancers of the HP can be treated with either surgery or radiation as the primary modality. Numerous partial open pharyngectomy procedures can be found in head and neck surgical textbooks along with descriptions of transoral techniques. Overall, laryngeal-preserving surgery for management of HP cancer is not common since this requires lesions to be small and not involve the pyriform apex. Treatment of at least the unilateral nodal basin is mandatory either through neck dissection or postoperative radiation, though bilateral nodal treatment is typically necessary owning to the bilateral lymphatic drainage of the HP. As a result, most patients with early and advanced disease are treated nonsurgically with either radiation alone or concurrent chemoradiation with high-dose cisplatin. Unfortunately, trials examining both surgical and nonsurgical treatment often group sites of disease within the pharynx and larynx such that HP cancer represents a minority of cases. This makes extrapolation of findings more challenging. For the most advanced cancers (mostly T4) causing vocal cord paralysis, laryngeal cartilage destruction, and/or pretreatment evidence of aspiration, surgery consisting of total laryngectomy with partial or total pharyngectomy is the treatment of choice and is often followed by adjuvant radiation or chemoradiation. For recurrent cancers after nonsurgical treatment, total laryngectomy is arguably the only option though partial laryngectomy procedures may be considered in highly select cases. Despite advances in treatment intensification, survival remains poor for patients with HP cancer due to the rarity of patients presenting at an early stage, the aggressiveness of the disease with propensity for locoregional recurrence and distant metastases, and the numerous comorbidities that patients often have. Considered as a group, 5-year survival is less than 50% with most patients dying from a second primary tumor, from recurrent disease, or from distant metastases.

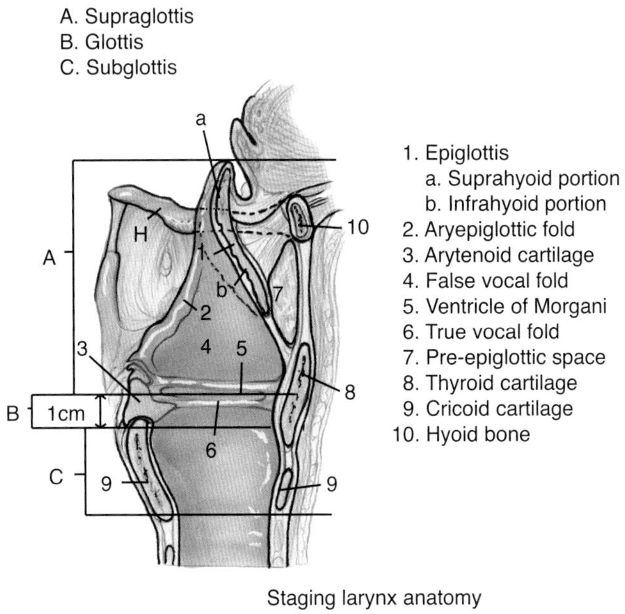

A. Supraglottis
B. Glottis
C. Subglottis

1. Epiglottis
   a. Suprahyoid portion
   b. Infrahyoid portion
2. Aryepiglottic fold
3. Arytenoid cartilage
4. False vocal fold
5. Ventricle of Morgani
6. True vocal fold
7. Pre-epiglottic space
8. Thyroid cartilage
9. Cricoid cartilage
10. Hyoid bone

Staging larynx anatomy

FIGURE 7.2 Laryngeal anatomy. (Reprinted with permission from Johnson J. *Bailey's Head and Neck Surgery.* 5th ed. Wolters Kluwer; 2013. Figure 124.2)

Larynx

The larynx consists of three main subsites, the supraglottis, glottis, and subglottis, each with its own distinct anatomic features and embryologic origins (Fig. 7.2). These in turn explain differences in the clinical behavior of cancers that can occur in each subsite. The supraglottis is composed of the epiglottis, aryepiglottic folds, arytenoid cartilage, false vocal cords, and the upper half of the laryngeal ventricle. The supraglottis has rich lymphatic drainage, which in part explains the more aggressive behavior of cancers in this area, particularly those arising in the "marginal zone" (the suprahyoid epiglottis and aryepiglottic folds). The glottis includes the lower half of the ventricle, the vocal cords including the anterior and posterior commissure, and the area extending 1 cm below the apex of the ventricle. The vocal cords (or folds) are comprised of several layers: epithelium, a gelatinous superficial layer, and more dense intermediate and deep layers (called the vocal ligament). The conus elasticus extends from the superior edge of the cricoid cartilage to the inferior surface of the vocal cord to merge with the vocal ligament. This structure is a strong barrier to lateral extension of cancer from the glottis and subglottis and also accounts for the relative paucity of lymphatic drainage in the area. Finally, the subglottis extends from the inferior margin of the glottis to the inferior border of the cricoid.

SCC is the most common histology encountered in laryngeal cancer, though tumors can also originate from the minor salivary glands, cartilage, and neuroendocrine cells. Over 13,000 new cases are currently diagnosed annually in the United States, with approximately 60% starting in the glottis and 35% to 40% in the supraglottis. Tumors originating in the subglottis are very rare. Men are much more likely to develop both glottic and supraglottic cancer than women though the ratios are gradually declining. Overall, the incidence of laryngeal cancer is falling by 2% to 3% per year, in large part due to fewer smokers, which is the predominant risk factor and is dose-dependent. Alcohol has a synergistic effect with tobacco, particularly for cancers of the supraglottis. Certain occupational exposures are also known to be risk factors including wood and cement dust, asbestos, and certain fuels or industrial solvents. Secondhand smoke and HPV have much less commonly been implicated in laryngeal carcinogenesis.

The initial presentation of patients with laryngeal cancer depends in part on the anatomic location, though common symptoms include dysphagia or odynophagia, dysphonia, otalgia, weight loss, hemoptysis, and local pain. Patients with glottic cancer more often present with early-stage disease, since lesions cause a change in voice, while patients with supraglottic cancer may be asymptomatic and present at a later stage. Evaluation of these patients should include laryngoscopy, ideally guided by a flexible or rigid laryngoscope, to precisely determine the location and size of the lesion in addition to the mobility of the vocal cords. Advanced lesions also require evaluation of swallowing function to determine the presence of clinical or subclinical aspiration prior to treatment. Patients require cross-sectional imaging of the neck and larynx for locoregional staging as well as imaging of the chest to assess for metastasis or secondary malignancies. Finally, patients may require examination under anesthesia to establish a diagnosis or to assist with accurate delineation of tumor anatomy. In cases where airway compromise is impending or represents a significant risk, tracheotomy may be necessary.

As would be anticipated, either surgery or radiation can be reasonable primary treatment of laryngeal cancer, depending on multiple factors including the location and stage of the cancer, its etiology and the presence of comorbidities, and the patient's pretreatment swallowing and respiratory status. Early cancers may be amenable to excision via transoral or open techniques or by radiation alone. Endoscopic and partial open laryngectomies are technically challenging procedures that demand specific discussion outside the limits of this chapter. Lesions of the supraglottis may extend into the pre-epiglottic or paraglottic spaces and also have bilateral lymphatic drainage. For these reasons, surgical resection of early lesions must be carefully selected. Otherwise, radiation therapy is preferred. Early glottic lesions are approached similarly with regard to surgical resectability, though regional lymphatics are not a concern with smaller glottic tumors. Narrow-field radiation fields are used in these tumors, which spares some of the chronic sequelae of radiation. Treatment of T1a lesions may have better voice results with radiation alone, though it may prohibit use of radiation for future malignancy in high-risk patients. It is debatable whether lesions involving the anterior commissure have a higher propensity for recurrence given spread through Broyles ligament, though these are more challenging to resect and functional outcomes may be inferior to radiation.

Over the last several decades, treatment of advanced laryngeal cancer has undergone major changes, largely in the form of nonsurgical intensification aiming at laryngeal preservation without decrement in survival outcomes. Several large studies in the United States and Europe have demonstrated the feasibility of two nonsurgical approaches, namely induction chemotherapy followed by radiation, or concurrent chemoradiation. Specific results from these trials and the implications of their results can be found in the recommended readings. The goal of therapy for most patients with T1–T3 cancers is tumor eradication with preservation of laryngeal function. Total laryngectomy is often recommended for patients who have poor function, those with T4 cancers (usually from laryngeal cartilage destruction), and others who would not be able to tolerate nonsurgical treatment. Functional outcomes including speaking (or voice rehabilitation) and swallowing are a primary concern for laryngeal cancer survivors.

Salivary Glands

Tumors of the salivary glands can arise in any of the paired major salivary glands, the parotid, submandibular, or sublingual glands, or the minor salivary glands found throughout the mucosa of the upper aerodigestive tract. Cancer of the salivary glands is rare and is comprised of a heterogeneous group of malignancies with different biologic behavior. Upward of 70% of salivary gland tumors are found in the parotid gland, the majority of which are benign compared to the minor salivary glands, which are mostly malignant. Of note, the parotid gland is divided into two lobes, superficial and deep, by the course of the facial nerve. The superficial lobe contains lymph nodes that serve as the primary echelon of nodal drainage for anterolateral scalp, lateral face, and auricular cutaneous malignancies, meaning that a superficial parotidectomy should be included in surgical treatment of these malignancies when there is evidence of regional metastasis.

Parotid and submandibular tumors most commonly present as a painless mass. Pain, facial nerve weakness (parotid), weakness or numbness of the tongue (submandibular or sublingual), or hypomobility of the mass are indicators of possible malignancy. Tumors of the minor salivary glands often present with symptoms similar to SCC of the same areas though lesions are typically submucosal. Certain histologies may have a predilection for perineural spread such that numbness in the distribution of trigeminal nerve branches may be the only symptom. Risk factors include prior radiation exposure and smoking (for Warthin tumors) though most salivary gland neoplasms have no known environmental etiology. Lesions are typically evaluated with FNA for the major salivary glands or directed biopsy for the minor glands. FNA in this circumstance is most useful for providing a determination of the mass as salivary gland in origin, malignant versus benign, and possibly tumor grade (low vs. high). At times, a specific tumor type may be identified on cytopathology. Imaging may not be necessary for small, mobile lesions in the superficial parotid gland though both CT and MRI play an important role in clarification of the extent of all other lesions.

Among benign tumors, pleomorphic adenoma (also known as benign mixed tumor) is the most common, though Warthin tumors and monomorphic adenomas can also occur. Malignant tumors include mucoepidermoid carcinoma, adenoid cystic carcinoma, acinic cell carcinoma, salivary duct carcinoma, adenocarcinoma, SCC, lymphoma, and carcinoma ex pleomorphic adenoma, which arises from a pre-existing benign mixed tumor. In the case of a benign mixed tumor, there is approximately a 10% risk of malignant transformation over a 15-year period. Even though each of these malignant tumors has different defining characteristics with regard to propensity for locoregional recurrence or distant metastasis, surgery represents the mainstay of primary therapy in virtually all locoregional cases amenable to resection. Tumors of the superficial lobe of the parotid gland are addressed with superficial parotidectomy while total parotidectomy is reserved for lesions involving the deep lobe and/or those requiring facial nerve sacrifice. In general, all attempts are made to preserve the facial nerve in cases where it is functioning properly prior to surgery. For extensive tumors, this may require identification of the facial nerve within the temporal bone through mastoidectomy. Similarly, submandibular gland tumors require excision of the entire gland at a minimum but extension of tumor into the surrounding tissues may require en bloc resection including surrounding soft tissue and potentially the hypoglossal, lingual, or marginal mandibular nerves if there is preoperative evidence of dysfunction or histologic involvement with tumor at the time of surgery. Surgery for tumors of the minor salivary gland tumors is also performed in en bloc fashion (with the possible exception of endoscopic endonasal resection).

Tumor grade is often important for treatment planning including need for neck dissection and use of adjuvant radiation therapy. Recommendations for END vary in the literature though it is generally performed for high-grade lesions, when there is evidence of major nerve invasion, or in the presence of intraparotid lymph node metastases. Radiation therapy is often recommended in an adjuvant setting for high-grade cancers as well as in those with advanced locoregional disease and with adverse features on pathologic review of the resected specimen. Moreover, radiation including proton and neutron therapy is sometimes used for control of disease in inoperable tumors though this broader application is based on results from small, published case series and is therefore challenging to interpret. Use of chemotherapy in salivary gland tumors is not common though high-grade tumors may respond favorably. Close follow-up surveillance is very important for higher-grade malignancies as they have a high rate of locoregional recurrence and distant metastasis.

Parapharyngeal Space

The PPS represents an anatomically complex potential space between investing layers of the deep cervical fascia where tumors can either arise primarily or spread from adjacent sites. Most often described as an inverted pyramid starting at the skull base and extending down to the greater cornu of the hyoid bone, the PPS is bounded medially by the constrictor muscles, laterally by the deep lobe of parotid and ramus of the mandible, posteriorly by the prevertebral musculature, and anteriorly by the pterygoid muscles. The carotid sheath is the most important group of structures located in this space, containing the carotid artery, IJV, and vagus nerve but cranial nerves XI and XII also exit the skull base through the jugular foramen and the cervical sympathetic chain runs just posterior to the carotid sheath.

Tumors arising in the PPS are uncommon and approximately 80% benign. Deep lobe parotid tumors extending into the PPS are the most common lesions (specifically pleomorphic adenomas) followed by paragangliomas, schwannomas, and neurofibromas. Numerous other tumors including sarcomas, meningiomas, and lymphomas can also rarely occur. Patients most often present with an asymptomatic neck mass causing blunting of the mandibular angle or inferior displacement of the submandibular gland. Alternatively, tumors may present with fullness of the soft palate or lateral pharyngeal wall and/or medial displacement of the palatine tonsil. This can mistakenly lead to the impression of tonsillar asymmetry and even a diagnosis of tonsil cancer. Lesions arising from nerves may present with corresponding deficits but the presence of pain, multiple cranial neuropathies, or trismus should raise clinical suspicion for a malignant process. Examination should include a complete cranial nerve assessment and palpation of the OP, parotid, and neck. Imaging prior to biopsy or other intervention is critical. Both CT and MRI are appropriate for evaluation of the PPS though MRI is often preferred for soft tissue detail. Diagnosis is often able to be made on radiographic appearance of the lesion and the pattern of displacement of neurovascular structures. At times, angiography may be beneficial to evaluate the blood supply of the tumor and even for embolization to minimize blood loss if surgery is planned. FNA may be beneficial, particularly to evaluate for a suspected malignant tumor, as these lesions require more extensive treatment and counseling of patients is accordingly more important. Finally, syndromes involving hereditary or multiple paragangliomas require special consideration as tumors of the head and neck may by bilateral, may be associated with tumors in other areas of the body, and may rarely possess catecholamine secretory function.

Treatment of tumors of the PPS depends largely on the type of lesion, the presence of functional deficits, the tumor's natural history, and the patient's overall health status. A period of observation of benign tumors is common to establish the rate of change, which is indolent for many PPS tumors. Benign tumors without significant and rapid growth may be monitored indefinitely, as sometimes the morbidity of surgery may exceed the potential benefit. When treatment is indicated, surgery is the mainstay of therapy for most lesions, with the goal being simultaneous tumor removal and preservation of neurovascular structures. Surgery is accomplished transorally in a minority of cases. More commonly, a transcervical or transparotid approach is used. For lesions requiring high exposure of the skull base, sometimes an anterior mandibulotomy is performed, although nasal intubation with anterior subluxation of the mandibular condyle is often sufficient to allow transcervical removal, especially for benign tumors. Suspected or known malignant tumors are treated with radical surgery and adjuvant radiation. Radiation has been advocated for local control of growth in patients who were unfit or declined surgical intervention. This approach is not widely performed since lesions often have a very slow growth rate and the long-term side effects of carotid sheath radiation are significant.

Nasal Cavity and Paranasal Sinuses

The nasal cavity extends in a dorsoventral dimension from the external nasal dorsum and pyriform aperture to the choanae and in a craniocaudal dimension from the nasal roof (frontal, ethmoid, and sphenoid bones or anterior skull base) to the nasal floor (maxilla and palatine bones). The nasal septum, which is composed of cartilage anteriorly and the vomer and perpendicular plate of the ethmoid bones posteriorly, divides the nasal cavity in half in the sagittal plane. There are four paired paranasal sinuses, maxillary, frontal, ethmoid, and sphenoid, each of which communicates with the nasal cavity through their respective ostia. The nasolacrimal duct also drains into the nasal cavity. Finally, three turbinates are found in each side of the nasal cavity (inferior, middle, and superior) that serve to warm and humidify air during nasal respiration.

The nasal cavity and paranasal sinuses are lined by mucosa derived from ectoderm as opposed to endoderm like the rest of the upper aerodigestive tract. The mucosa is pseudostratified ciliated columnar epithelium containing mucinous and minor salivary glands, except at the nasal vestibule, which is lined by keratinizing squamous epithelium, and the superior septum/ethmoid roof, which is olfactory neuroepithelium. The sensory innervation to the nasal and paranasal mucosa is from branches of the trigeminal nerve (V1 and V2). The blood supply is from the external carotid (superior labial, angular, and internal maxillary arteries) and internal carotid (anterior and posterior ethmoidal arteries) arteries. Lymphatic drainage of the paranasal sinuses occurs via the retropharyngeal, parapharyngeal, and upper cervical lymph nodes.

Benign tumors of the sinonasal cavity are reasonably common and include antrochoanal polyp, squamous papilloma, schneiderian papilloma, angiofibroma, osteoma, fibrous dysplasia, hemangioma, schwannoma, and benign minor salivary gland tumors. Nasal papillomas may result from HPV virus with squamous variants typically arising in the nasal vestibule. Schneiderian papillomas most often arise on the nasal septum or lateral nasal wall, can be locally destructive, and have a 5% to 15% risk of harboring carcinoma. Angiofibromas (also called juvenile nasopharyngeal angiofibromas) are benign, locally destructive, fibrovascular tumors occurring almost exclusively in adolescent males. Other benign tumors also have more common locations of origin, appearance on endoscopy, and imaging characteristics that aid in their diagnosis.

Sinonasal malignancies are rare, accounting for less than 5% of head and neck malignancies. The differential diagnosis for sinonasal malignancy is broad, including SCC, sinonasal undifferentiated carcinoma (SNUC), small-cell neuroendocrine carcinoma, mucosal melanoma, several types of sarcoma, non-Hodgkin lymphoma, esthesioneuroblastoma (also called olfactory neuroblastoma), adenocarcinoma, and adenoid cystic carcinoma. SCC is the most common type, occurring predominantly in males in the sixth to eighth decades. Mucosal melanomas are rare (1% to 2% of all melanomas), with a fairly equal male-to-female ratio. Up to one-third may be amelanotic, and immunohistochemical analysis is important to establish the diagnosis. Risk factors for sinonasal malignancy are often thought to occur through occupational exposure. These include metals such as nickel, aluminum, and chromium for SCC, and wood and leather dust for adenocarcinoma. Smoking also plays an etiologic role in development of SCC and some evidence suggests outdoor air pollution is also correlated.

The most common presenting symptoms for sinonasal tumors are unilateral nasal obstruction, facial pressure, pain, or numbness, rhinorrhea, anosmia, and epistaxis. Patients may also present with unilateral serous otitis media (due to obstruction of the Eustachian tube orifice), epiphora (due to obstruction of the nasolacrimal duct), or diplopia (from extension into the orbit or cavernous sinus). Nodal metastases are uncommon in sinonasal malignancies. Evaluation of the nose and paranasal sinuses includes external and endoscopic inspection. Unilateral masses are more common to be neoplastic rather than inflammatory (i.e., polyps). Imaging (both CT scan and MRI scan) is important to determine the anatomic extent of the disease and can even provide the likely diagnosis in some cases. Imaging should often be obtained prior to biopsy since biopsy could potentially cause extensive bleeding or even cerebrospinal fluid leak.

As would be expected from such a broad group of tumors, treatment largely depends on the nature of the lesion. The development of endoscopic endonasal surgery has provided a natural orifice surgical option that appears to have similar oncologic outcomes and lower relative morbidity in the hands of high-volume surgeons in comparison to traditional transfacial and craniofacial resections. Surgery is the treatment of choice in almost all circumstances for benign lesions and most commonly is the primary treatment for malignancies as well. Exceptions to this include certain sarcomas treated with neoadjuvant radiation, lymphomas treated entirely by local radiation and chemotherapy, and certain biologically aggressive or initially unresectable lesions such as SCC, SNUC, small-cell neuroendocrine carcinoma, olfactory neuroblastoma, or salivary gland carcinoma that may be treated with neoadjuvant chemotherapy or chemoradiation. For instance, in the context of SNUC, induction chemotherapy seems to biologically select patients with the greatest chance of improved survival. In those who demonstrate a favorable response to induction chemotherapy, definitive chemoradiation has led to improved survival as compared to definitive surgery. However, those without at least partial response to induction chemotherapy had significantly compromised survival outcomes. Nevertheless, they achieved slightly improved survival with surgery, when feasible, followed by chemoradiation. For advanced lesions invading the orbit, surrounding bony structures, or skin of the face, surgery may entail a partial or total rhinectomy, partial or total maxillectomy and adjacent sinuses (ethmoid and frontal), and orbital exenteration. Lesions involving the skull base with or without intracranial extension require collaboration with neurosurgery through endoscopic or craniofacial resection. Prognosis largely depends on the type and stage of the cancer, with most experts agreeing that survival is improved with multimodal therapy including surgery, radiation, and sometimes chemotherapy. Five-year overall survival approaches 60% for all types, is best for olfactory neuroblastoma (>70%), and worst for undifferentiated carcinoma (20% to 40%) and mucosal melanoma (10% to 30%).

Ear and Temporal Bone
The ear is composed of the external ear (pinna, auricle, and external canal), the middle ear, and the inner ear. The epithelium over the external ear is squamous with adjacent adnexal and glandular (sebaceous) structures while ciliated epithelium and glands line the middle ear. The framework of the auricle and outer third of the external canal is comprised of elastic cartilage, while the inner third of the external canal, the middle ear, the mastoid, and the inner ear are part of the temporal bone.

Although cutaneous malignancies of the pinna and auricle are common, cancers of the temporal bone are rare and account for less than 1% of all HNCs. The majority of tumors of the ear involve the auricle (>80%), followed by the ear canal, middle ear, and mastoid. Males are more commonly affected, and sun exposure is a major risk factor. SCC is the most common histologic cancer of the outer ear, followed by basal cell carcinomas. Paragangliomas, rhabdomyosarcomas, and adenocarcinomas can occur in the middle ear. More commonly, the temporal bone and ear are involved with cancer by extension from tumors or lymph node metastases of the parotid, temporomandibular joint, infratemporal fossa, or periauricular skin. Pain, aural fullness, conductive hearing loss, ulceration, and chronic otorrhea are common presenting symptoms. Deep extension may be associated with cranial neuropathies such as facial paralysis, vestibular symptoms, or sensorineural hearing loss.

Surgery is often the preferred therapy for SCC and basal cell carcinoma, although radiation therapy may play a role in highly selected cases. Small lesions of the outer ear are treated effectively by wide local excision, but partial or total auriculectomy may be required for larger lesions. Early external canal lesions can be effectively treated by sleeve resection. Lateral temporal bone resection is necessary for large tumors with medial extension or bony erosion, and subtotal temporal bone resections may be required for the most extensive tumors, though this treatment should be carefully considered in a multidisciplinary setting as prognosis remains poor. Extensive paragangliomas or sarcomas may be treated with primary radiation. Lesions arising elsewhere and invading the ear and/or temporal bone may require auriculectomy and/or lateral temporal bone resection. Adjuvant radiation therapy is commonly recommended. Survival for cancers of the outer ear is greater than 90% for cancers confined to the auricle, with worsening prognosis for those with medial extension into the ear canal, and middle ear extension with less than 30% long-term survival. Temporal bone malignancies have an overall survival rate of 20% to 30% at 5 years.

CASE SCENARIO

Case Scenario 1
Presentation
A 53-year-old male is referred to a head and neck cancer center by his dentist after noting a left floor of mouth ulcer present over the past 3 months.

He has smoked one pack of cigarettes per day for 30 years and consumes alcohol only on social occasions. The clinical examination denotes a left floor of mouth ulcerated lesion measuring 1.5 cm which extends to the inner mandibular gingiva. The lesion feels mobile with respect to the mandible (no obvious fixation to the mandible). There is no palpable cervical lymphadenopathy, though some fullness of the left submandibular area is noted. A biopsy demonstrates a well-differentiated squamous cell carcinoma (SCC).

A CT neck with contrast demonstrates a left floor of mouth lesion which abuts the inner cortex of the mandible, without evidence of erosion. Two enlarged lymph nodes are noted adjacent to the left submandibular gland. A CT chest shows areas of ground glass opacification, but no focal lesions. He is clinically staged as cT1 N2b M0.

The patient is taken to the operating room where he undergoes dental extractions, floor of mouth resection with a composite marginal resection of the mandibular inner cortex, and level Ia, Ib, IIa, III, and supraomohyoid level IV neck dissection. A radial forearm free flap reconstruction is performed. A tracheostomy is also performed, given anticipated postoperative oral edema.

The final pathology shows a 1.8-cm well-differentiated SCC with 0.6-cm depth of invasion and 1.0 cm closest mucosal margin. It abuts the mandibular cortex but does not invade it. There is no perineural invasion. Three level Ib nodes have metastatic SCC. One of these is notable for ENE extending into the submandibular gland. The pathologic staging is established as pT2N3bM0. Following a multidisciplinary review of surgical pathology, he undergoes adjuvant radiation with concurrent cisplatin chemotherapy within 6 weeks of his surgery.

Take Home Points

- The AJCC 8th edition has made significant changes to the N classification as it pertains to extra-nodal extension (ENE). A single, ipsilateral involved node of ≤3 cm with ENE is classified as N2a. All other scenarios of ENE are classified as N3b.
- Depth of invasion, not tumor thickness, contributes to the T classification of oral cavity SCC. The depth of invasion is defined as the distance between the level of the basement membrane of the closest adjacent normal mucosa down to the deepest point of tumor invasion. The perpendicular line measuring the depth of invasion is referred to as the "plumb line."
- When an oral cavity tumor abuts the mandible without radiographic evidence of invasion, a marginal mandibulectomy is recommended to provide adequate oncologic clearance of the surgical margin. These patients are often best reconstructed with a soft tissue free flap such as a radial forearm free flap.
- General indications for postoperative radiation in head and neck SCC include large/invasive primary tumor, perineural invasion, multiple metastatic lymph nodes, extranodal disease extension, and positive/close surgical margin. Indications for postoperative concurrent chemoradiation therapy include extranodal disease extension and positive surgical margins.

Case Scenario 2

Presentation

A 46-year-old male presents with a left neck mass which he noted while shaving 2 months ago.

He is otherwise well and asymptomatic. He does not smoke and rarely consumes alcohol. A physical examination demonstrates an approximate 3-cm mobile, nontender, left mid (level 3) neck mass. An oral examination demonstrates fullness of the left tonsil which is comparatively firm to palpation. A CT neck with contrast demonstrates a single 3-cm cystic left level 3 lymph node and an enhancing 1.5-cm left tonsillar mass confined to the tonsil. CT chest demonstrates no pulmonary disease. He is clinically staged as cT1N1M0.

Following multidisciplinary assessment, he is offered a surgical approach versus ipsilateral radiation alone. The patient decides to go forward with surgery. TORS (transoral robotic surgery) left tonsillectomy with lateral pharyngectomy, and left level IIa, III, and IV neck dissection with lingual artery ligation are performed. Following the lateral pharyngectomy, the specimen is sent for margin assessment by frozen section. The assessment indicates a 1-mm margin at the glossotonsilar sulcus. This margin is revised and a subsequent adjacent specimen is sent for assessment, with a negative margin.

The final pathology shows a 2-cm tonsillar SCC with a clear revised margin. Of the 24 nodes in the specimen, a single 3-cm node is involved without evidence of ENE. Following a multidisciplinary review, no further adjuvant treatment is recommended.

Take Home Points

- The recommendation for surgery in patients with T1-2 oropharyngeal cancer should be limited to patients for whom adjuvant radiation therapy is unlikely. The potential short and long-term functional gains associated with TORS (vs. radiation alone) are diminished with the addition of adjuvant treatment. When possible, single-modality therapy (i.e., surgery alone or radiation alone) is preferred over multimodality therapy (i.e., surgery plus radiation).

■ Intraoperative margin analysis by frozen section is an invaluable tool in the operative management and clearance of margins for patients with oropharyngeal carcinoma in whom single-modality treatment is targeted.

CASE SCENARIO REVIEW

Questions

1. A 1-cm gingival SCC with superficial erosion of the mandibular cortex is classified as T4a.
   A. True
   B. False

2. A patient presents with a 2-cm cutenous SCC of the skin of the right temple anterior to the plane of the ear, with an ipsilateral level 1B and an ipsilateral level 2 metastatic lymph node, both approximately 1 cm. In addition to wide excision of the primary tumor, what is the most appropriate treatment recommendation for this patient?
   A. Radiation therapy to the primary site, parotid, and ipsilateral neck with concurrent chemotherapy
   B. Ipsilateral level I to IV neck dissection with postoperative radiation therapy
   C. Superficial parotidectomy, ipsilateral level I to IV neck dissection, and postoperative radiation therapy
   D. Superficial parotidectomy and ipsilateral level I to IV neck dissection

3. Which of these oral cavity lesions has the highest risk of malignant transformation?
   A. Leukoplakia
   B. Lichen planus
   C. Erythroplakia
   D. Aphthous ulcer

4. Per national consensus guidelines, a patient with p16+ 1.5-cm left tonsillar SCC confined to the tonsil and a single 3-cm ipsilateral cystic lymph node without radiographically apparent extranodal extension can be treated by which of the following approaches?
   A. TORS lateral oropharyngectomy and ipsilateral neck dissection
   B. Primary radiation
   C. Concurrent systemic therapy and radiation
   D. All of the above

5. Nonoropharyngeal p16+ head and neck cancers are consistently associated with better prognosis as compared to their p16– counterparts.
   A. True
   B. False

Answers

1. **The correct answer is B.** *Rationale:* Under the AJCC 8th edition staging, superficial erosion of bone or tooth socket alone by a gingival primary is not sufficient to classify a tumor as T4. This tumor would be classified as T1. Nevertheless, a marginal mandibulectomy would be recommended.

2. **The correct answer is C.** *Rationale:* Patients with upper facial and scalp skin cancers anterior to the ear generally require superficial parotidectomy with level I to IV neck dissection, while cancers of the scalp posterior to the ear generally are recommended for posterolateral (level I to IV, including postauricular lymph nodes) neck dissection. Postoperative radiation therapy would be recommended on account of multiple metastatic lymph nodes.

3. **The correct answer is C.** *Rationale:* Over 50% of erythroplakic lesions will demonstrate invasive SCC upon biopsy. Nearly 90% will demonstrate at least carcinoma in situ.

4. **The correct answer is D**. *Rationale:* In the context of the p16+ T0-2 N1 (single node ≤3-cm) oropharyngeal SCC, at this time the national consensus guidelines provide the following four treatment options:
   1. Resection of primary +/− ipsilateral or bilateral neck dissection
   2. Definitive radiation
   3. Concurrent systemic therapy and radiation
   4. Clinical trial
   However, most centers will recommend single-modality treatment for such patients.

5. **The correct answer is B**. False. *Rationale:* At this time, various analyses of nonoropharyngeal head and neck SCC have continued to demonstrate mixed results, which is supported by national consensus guidelines in 2021. This continues to be an area of active research. On the other hand, p16+ oropharynx cancers have consistently demonstrated improved prognosis compared to p16− oropharynx cancers.

Recommended Readings

Agrawal A, Civantos FJ, Brumund KT, et al. [(99m)Tc]Tilmanocept accurately detects sentinel lymph nodes and predicts node pathology status in patients with oral squamous cell carcinoma of the head and neck: results of a phase III multi-institutional trial. *Ann Surg Oncol.* 2015;22(11):3708–3715.

Al-Sarraf M, LeBlanc M, Giri PG, et al. Chemoradiotherapy versus radiotherapy in patients with advanced nasopharyngeal cancer: phase III randomized Intergroup study 0099. *J Clin Oncol.* 1998;16(4):1310–1317.

Amin MB, Edge SB, Greene FL, et al. *AJCC Cancer Staging Manual.* 8th ed. Springer Science+Business Media; 2016.

Amit M, Abdelmeguid AS, Watcherporn T, et al. Induction chemotherapy response as a guide for treatment optimization in sinonasal undifferentiated carcinoma. *J Clin Oncol.* 2019;37(6):504–512.

Ang KK, Berkey BA, Tu X, et al. Impact of epidermal growth factor receptor expression on survival and pattern of relapse in patients with advanced head and neck carcinoma. *Cancer Res.* 2002;62(24):7350–7356.

Ang KK, Harris J, Wheeler R, et al. Human papillomavirus and survival of patients with oropharyngeal cancer. *N Engl J Med.* 2010;363(1):24–35.

Ang KK, Jiang GL, Frankenthaler RA, et al. Carcinomas of the nasal cavity. *Radiother Oncol.* 1992;24(3):163–168.

Ang KK, Trotti A, Brown BW, et al. Randomized trial addressing risk features and time factors of surgery plus radiotherapy in advanced head-and-neck cancer. *Int J Radiat Oncol Biol Phys.* 2001;51(3):571–578.

Arriaga M, Curtin H, Takahashi H, Hirsch BE, Kamerer DB. Staging proposal for external auditory meatus carcinoma based on preoperative clinical examination and computed tomography findings. *Ann Otol Rhinol Laryngol.* 1990;99(9 Pt 1):714–721.

Baan R, Straif K, Grosse Y, et al; WHO International Agency for Research on Cancer Monograph Working Group. Carcinogenicity of alcoholic beverages. *Lancet Oncol.* 2007;8(4):292–293.

Bäckström A, Jakobsson PA, Nathanson A, Wersäll J. Prognosis of squamous-cell carcinoma of the gums with cytologically verified cervical lymph node metastases. *J Laryngol Otol.* 1975;89(4):391–396.

Bae WK, Hwang JE, Shim HJ, et al. Phase II study of docetaxel, cisplatin, and 5-FU induction chemotherapy followed by chemoradiotherapy in locoregionally advanced nasopharyngeal cancer. *Cancer Chemother Pharmacol.* 2010;65(3):589–595.

Byers RM, Clayman GL, McGill D, et al. Selective neck dissections for squamous carcinoma of the upper aerodigestive tract: patterns of regional failure. *Head Neck.* 1999;21(6):499–505.

Byers RM, Newman R, Russell N, Yue A. Results of treatment for squamous carcinoma of the lower gum. *Cancer.* 1981;47(9):2236–2238.

Byers RM, Wolf PF, Ballantyne AJ. Rationale for elective modified neck dissection. *Head Neck Surg.* 1988;10(3):160–167.

Chan ATC, Lo YMD, Zee B, et al. Plasma Epstein-Barr virus DNA and residual disease after radiotherapy for undifferentiated nasopharyngeal carcinoma. *J Natl Cancer Inst.* 2002;94(21):1614–1619.

Chaturvedi AK, Engels EA, Pfeiffer RM, et al. Human papillomavirus and rising oropharyngeal cancer incidence in the United States. *J Clin Oncol.* 2011;29(32):4294–4301.

Department of Veterans Affairs Laryngeal Cancer Study Group; Wolf GT, Fisher SG, Hong WK, et al. Induction chemotherapy plus radiation compared with surgery plus radiation in patients with advanced laryngeal cancer. *N Engl J Med*. 1991;324(24):1685–1690.

Diaz EM Jr, Holsinger FC, Zuniga ER, Roberts DB, Sorensen DM. Squamous cell carcinoma of the buccal mucosa: one institution's experience with 119 previously untreated patients. *Head Neck*. 2003;25(4):267–273.

Dietz A, Ramroth H, Urban T, Ahrens W, Becher H. Exposure to cement dust, related occupational groups and laryngeal cancer risk: results of a population based case-control study. *Int J Cancer*. 2004;108(6):907–911.

Eden BV, Debo RF, Larner JM, et al. Esthesioneuroblastoma. Long-term outcome and patterns of failure—the University of Virginia experience. *Cancer*. 1994;73(10):2556–2562.

Evans JF, Shah JP. Epidermoid carcinoma of the palate. *Am J Surg*. 1981;142(4):451–455.

Fang Y, Guan X, Guo Y, et al. Analysis of genetic alterations in primary nasopharyngeal carcinoma by comparative genomic hybridization. *Genes Chromosomes Cancer*. 2001;30(3):254–260.

Fee WE Jr, Roberson JB Jr, Goffinet DR. Long-term survival after surgical resection for recurrent nasopharyngeal cancer after radiotherapy failure. *Arch Otolaryngol Head Neck Surg*. 1991;117(11):1233–1236.

Forastiere AA, Goepfert H, Maor M, et al. Concurrent chemotherapy and radiotherapy for organ preservation in advanced laryngeal cancer. *N Engl J Med*. 2003;349(22):2091–2098.

Forastiere AA, Zhang Q, Weber RS, et al. Long-term results of RTOG 91-11: a comparison of three nonsurgical treatment strategies to preserve the larynx in patients with locally advanced larynx cancer. *J Clin Oncol*. 2013;31(7):845–852.

Fordice J, Kershaw C, El-Naggar A, Goepfert H. Adenoid cystic carcinoma of the head and neck: predictors of morbidity and mortality. *Arch Otolaryngol Head Neck Surg*. 1999;125(2):149–152.

Fukano H, Matsuura H, Hasegawa Y, Nakamura S. Depth of invasion as a predictive factor for cervical lymph node metastasis in tongue carcinoma. *Head Neck*. 1997;19(3):205–210.

Garden AS, Morrison WH, Clayman GL, Ang KK, Peters LJ. Early squamous cell carcinoma of the hypopharynx: outcomes of treatment with radiation alone to the primary disease. *Head Neck*. 1996;18(4):317–322.

Garden AS, Weber RS, Ang KK, Morrison WH, Matre J, Peters LJ. Postoperative radiation therapy for malignant tumors of minor salivary glands. Outcome and patterns of failure. *Cancer*. 1994;73(10):2563–2569.

Gidley PW, Roberts DB, Sturgis EM. Squamous cell carcinoma of the temporal bone. *Laryngoscope*. 2010;120(6):1144–1151.

Gidley PW, Thompson CR, Roberts DB, Weber RS. The results of temporal bone surgery for advanced or recurrent tumors of the parotid gland. *Laryngoscope*. 2011;121(8):1702–1707.

Ginsberg LE, DeMonte F. Imaging of perineural tumor spread from palatal carcinoma. *AJNR Am J Neuroradiol*. 1998;19(8):1417–1422.

Goepfert H, Dichtel WJ, Medina JE, Lindberg RD, Luna MD. Perineural invasion in squamous cell skin carcinoma of the head and neck. *Am J Surg*. 1984;148(4):542–547.

Goepfert RP, Hutcheson KA, Lewin JS, et al. Complications, hospital length of stay, and readmission after total laryngectomy. *Cancer*. 2017;123(10):1760–1767.

Gordon I, Boffetta P, Demers PA. A case study comparing a meta-analysis and a pooled analysis of studies of sinonasal cancer among wood workers. *Epidemiology*. 1998;9(5):518–524.

Grandis JR, Melhem MF, Gooding WE, et al. Levels of TGF-alpha and EGFR protein in head and neck squamous cell carcinoma and patient survival. *J Natl Cancer Inst*. 1998;90(11):824–832.

Greenberg JS, Fowler R, Gomez J, et al. Extent of extracapsular spread: a critical prognosticator in oral tongue cancer. *Cancer*. 2003;97(6):1464–1470.

Hanna E, Sherman A, Cash D, et al. Quality of life for patients following total laryngectomy vs chemoradiation for laryngeal preservation. *Arch Otolaryngol Head Neck Surg*. 2004;130(7):875–879.

Herbst RS, Soria JC, Kowanetz M, et al. Predictive correlates of response to the anti-PD-L1 antibody MPDL3280A in cancer patients. *Nature*. 2014;515(7528):563–567.

Huang CJ, Chao KS, Tsai J, et al. Cancer of retromolar trigone: long-term radiation therapy outcome. *Head Neck*. 2001;23(9):758–763.

Hutcheson KA, Lewin JS. Functional outcomes after chemoradiotherapy of laryngeal and pharyngeal cancers. *Curr Oncol Rep*. 2012;14(2):158–165.

Johnson JT, Barnes E, Myers EN, Schramm VL Jr, Borochovitz D, Sigler BA. The extracapsular spread of tumors in cervical node metastasis. *Arch Otolaryngol*. 1981;107(12):725–729.

Johnson JT, Myers EN, Hao SP, Wagner RL. Outcome of open surgical therapy for glottic carcinoma. *Ann Otol Rhinol Laryngol.* 1993;102(10):752–755.

Jorgensen K, Elbrond O, Andersen AP. Carcinoma of the lip. A series of 869 cases. *Acta Radiol Ther Phys Biol.* 1973;12(3):177–190.

Jungehulsing M, Scheidhauer K, Damm M, et al. 2[F]-fluoro-2-deoxy-D-glucose positron emission tomography is a sensitive tool for the detection of occult primary cancer (carcinoma of unknown primary syndrome) with head and neck lymph node manifestation. *Otolaryngol Head Neck Surg.* 2000;123(3):294–301.

Kakarala K, Bhattacharyya N. Survival in oral cavity minor salivary gland carcinoma. *Otolaryngol Head Neck Surg.* 2010;143(1):122–126.

Kandoth C, McLellan MD, Vandin F, et al. Mutational landscape and significance across 12 major cancer types. *Nature.* 2013;502(7471):333–339.

Kowalski LP, Hashimoto I, Magrin J. End results of 114 extended "commando" operations for retromolar trigone carcinoma. *Am J Surg.* 1993;166(4):374–379.

Kraus DH, Zelefsky MJ, Brock HA, Huo J, Harrison LB, Shah JP. Combined surgery and radiation therapy for squamous cell carcinoma of the hypopharynx. *Otolaryngol Head Neck Surg.* 1997;116(6 Pt 1):637–641.

Laccourreye H, Laccourreye O, Weinstein G, Menard M, Brasnu D. Supracricoid laryngectomy with cricohyoidoepiglottopexy: a partial laryngeal procedure for glottic carcinoma. *Ann Otol Rhinol Laryngol.* 1990;99(6 Pt 1):421–426.

Laccourreye H, Laccourreye O, Weinstein G, Menard M, Brasnu D. Supracricoid laryngectomy with cricohyoidopexy: a partial laryngeal procedure for selected supraglottic and transglottic carcinomas. *Laryngoscope.* 1990;100(7):735–741.

Langevin SM, McClean MD, Michaud DS, Eliot M, Nelson HH, Kelsey KT. Occupational dust exposure and head and neck squamous cell carcinoma risk in a population-based case-control study conducted in the greater Boston area. *Cancer Med.* 2013;2(6):978–986.

Lee AWM, Sze WM, Au JSK, et al. Treatment results for nasopharyngeal carcinoma in the modern era: the Hong Kong experience. *Int J Radiat Oncol Biol Phys.* 2005;61(4):1107–1116.

Lewin F, Norell SE, Johansson H, et al. Smoking tobacco, oral snuff, and alcohol in the etiology of squamous cell carcinoma of the head and neck: a population-based case-referent study in Sweden. *Cancer.* 1998;82(7):1367–1375.

Maier H, De Vries N, Snow GB. Occupational factors in the aetiology of head and neck cancer. *Clin Otolaryngol Allied Sci.* 1991;16(4):406–412.

McGuirt WF Jr, Johnson JT, Myers EN, Rothfield R, Wagner R. Floor of mouth carcinoma. The management of the clinically negative neck. *Arch Otolaryngol Head Neck Surg.* 1995;121(3):278–282.

Mendenhall WM, Parsons JT, Stringer SP, Cassisi NJ. Management of Tis, T1, and T2 squamous cell carcinoma of the glottic larynx. *Am J Otolaryngol.* 1994;15(4):250–257.

Morita A, Ebersold MJ, Olsen KD, Foote RL, Lewis JE, Quast LM. Esthesioneuroblastoma: prognosis and management. *Neurosurgery.* 1993;32(5):706–714; discussion 714–715.

Myers JN, Hanna EYN, Myers EN. *Cancer of the Head and Neck.* 5th ed. Wolters Kluwer; 2017.

Nair MK, Sankaranarayanan R, Padmanabhan TK. Evaluation of the role of radiotherapy in the management of carcinoma of the buccal mucosa. *Cancer.* 1988;61(7):1326–1331.

Narasimhan K, Kucuk O, Lin HS, et al. Sinonasal mucosal melanoma: a 13-year experience at a single institution. *Skull Base.* 2009;19(4):255–262.

Nason RW, Sako K, Beecroft WA, Razack MS, Bakamjian VY, Bakamjian VY. Surgical management of squamous cell carcinoma of the floor of the mouth. *Am J Surg.* 1989;158(4):292–296.

Nicholson RI, Gee JM, Harper ME. EGFR and cancer prognosis. *Eur J Cancer.* 2001;37(suppl 4):S9–S15.

Pan JJ, Ng WT, Zong JF, et al. Proposal for the 8th edition of the AJCC/UICC staging system for nasopharyngeal cancer in the era of intensity-modulated radiotherapy. *Cancer.* 2016;122(4):546–558.

Poeta ML, Manola J, Goldwasser MA, et al. TP53 mutations and survival in squamous-cell carcinoma of the head and neck. *N Engl J Med.* 2007;357(25):2552–2561.

Pop LA, Eijkenboom WM, de Boer MF, et al. Evaluation of treatment results of squamous cell carcinoma of the buccal mucosa. *Int J Radiat Oncol Biol Phys.* 1989;16(2):483–487.

Reibel J. Prognosis of oral pre-malignant lesions: significance of clinical, histopathological, and molecular biological characteristics. *Crit Rev Oral Biol Med.* 2003;14(1):47–62.

Sale KA, Wallace DI, Girod DA, Tsue TT. Radiation-induced malignancy of the head and neck. *Otolaryngol Head Neck Surg*. 2004;131(5):643–645.

Sandulache VC, Vandelaar LJ, Skinner HD, et al. Salvage total laryngectomy after external-beam radiotherapy: a 20-year experience. *Head Neck*. 2016;38(suppl 1):E1962–E1968.

Sankaranarayanan R, Masuyer E, Swaminathan R, Ferlay J, Whelan S. Head and neck cancer: a global perspective on epidemiology and prognosis. *Anticancer Res*. 1998;18(6B):4779–4786.

Siegel RL, Miller KD, Jemal A. Cancer statistics, 2016. *CA Cancer J Clin*. 2016;66(1):7–30.

Simons MJ, Wee GB, Chan SH, Shanmugaratnam K. Probable identification of an HL-A second-locus antigen associated with a high risk of nasopharyngeal carcinoma. *Lancet*. 1975;1(7899):142–143.

Spiro RH. Salivary neoplasms: overview of a 35-year experience with 2,807 patients. *Head Neck Surg*. 1986;8(3):177–184.

Spiro RH, Huvos AG, Wong GY, Spiro JD, Gnecco CA, Strong EW. Predictive value of tumor thickness in squamous carcinoma confined to the tongue and floor of the mouth. *Am J Surg*. 1986;152(4):345–350.

Steiner W. Results of curative laser microsurgery of laryngeal carcinomas. *Am J Otolaryngol*. 1993;14(2):116–121.

Stern SJ, Goepfert H, Clayman G, et al. Squamous cell carcinoma of the maxillary sinus. *Arch Otolaryngol Head Neck Surg*. 1993;119(9):964–969.

Tan EH, Adelstein DJ, Droughton ML, Van Kirk MA, Lavertu P. Squamous cell head and neck cancer in nonsmokers. *Am J Clin Oncol*. 1997;20(2):146–150.

Turner JH, Reh DD. Incidence and survival in patients with sinonasal cancer: a historical analysis of population-based data. *Head Neck*. 2012;34(6):877–885.

Weber RS, Berkey BA, Forastiere A, et al. Outcome of salvage total laryngectomy following organ preservation therapy: the Radiation Therapy Oncology Group trial 91-11. *Arch Otolaryngol Head Neck Surg*. 2003;129(1):44–49.

Wei WI, Sham JST. Nasopharyngeal carcinoma. *Lancet*. 2005;365(9476):2041–2054.

Wyss A, Hashibe M, Chuang SC, et al. Cigarette, cigar, and pipe smoking and the risk of head and neck cancers: pooled analysis in the International Head and Neck Cancer Epidemiology Consortium. *Am J Epidemiol*. 2013;178(5):679–690.

Yu MC, Yuan JM. Epidemiology of nasopharyngeal carcinoma. *Semin Cancer Biol*. 2002;12(6):421–429.

Zafereo ME, Hanasono MM, Rosenthal DI, et al. The role of salvage surgery in patients with recurrent squamous cell carcinoma of the oropharynx. *Cancer*. 2009;115(24):5723–5733.

Zafereo ME, Xu L, Dahlstrom KR, et al. Squamous cell carcinoma of the oral cavity often overexpresses p16 but is rarely driven by human papillomavirus. *Oral Oncol*. 2016;56:47–53.

Zitsch RP 3rd, Lee BW, Smith RB. Cervical lymph node metastases and squamous cell carcinoma of the lip. *Head Neck*. 1999;21(5):447–453.

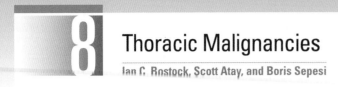

8 Thoracic Malignancies

Ian C. Bostock, Scott Atay, and Boris Sepesi

Primary Neoplasms of the Lung

In 2020, lung cancer accounted for an estimated 135,720 deaths and 228,000 new cases of cancer in the United States. With approximately 25% of all cancer deaths attributable to lung cancer, it is the most common cause of cancer-related death in both men and women, killing more people than the next three most common cancers combined (breast, prostate, and colon). Fortunately, the overall age-adjusted death rates for lung cancer have been decreasing since 2015. This trend has been attributed to an overall decrease in the number of males who smoke and to no further increases in the number of women who smoke. Unfortunately, this good news is countered by a disturbing increase in smoking among certain minority and adolescent age groups. The overall 5-year survival rate for lung cancer is only 25%, primarily because the disease is usually advanced at presentation; if the disease is diagnosed and treated at an early stage, however, the 5-year survival rate approaches 60%.

Epidemiology

Smoking is the primary cause of more than 80% of lung cancers. The second most common cause of lung cancer is radon exposure. The third most common cause is secondhand smoke, which increases the risk of lung cancer by 30%. Despite the strong association between lung cancer and smoking, lung cancers develop in only 15% of heavy smokers. Giant bullous emphysema and airway obstructive disease can act synergistically with smoking to induce lung cancer, perhaps because of poor clearance and trapping of carcinogens. In addition, exposure to industrial and environmental carcinogens, including asbestos, uranium, cadmium, arsenic, and terpenes, have been implicated. The risk of cancer associated with smoking emerging nontobacco products such as e-cigarettes/e-liquids is unknown. Importantly, the incidence of lung cancer in nonsmokers and women has been increasing in the past decade.

Pathology

Lung cancer can be broadly separated into two groups: non–small cell lung carcinoma (NSCLC) and small cell lung carcinoma (SCLC). This is a popular division because, for the most part, localized NSCLC is often managed with surgery, whereas SCLC is almost always managed with chemotherapy with or without radiation therapy. The three major types of NSCLC are adenocarcinoma, squamous cell carcinoma, and large cell carcinoma (Table 8.1). Significant advances in molecular profiling have extended the classification of lung cancer and influenced the prognosis, treatment strategies offered, and the expected response to different treatments.

Non–Small Cell Lung Carcinoma

Adenocarcinoma is the most common type of NSCLC and accounts for more than 40% of cases. It is the most common lung cancer found in nonsmokers and women. The lesions tend to be located in the periphery of the

TABLE 8.1	Frequency of Histologic Subtypes of Primary Lung Cancer
Cell Type	**Estimated Frequency (%)**
Non–Small Cell Lung Cancer	
Adenocarcinoma	40
Bronchoalveolar	2
Squamous cell carcinoma	25
Large cell carcinoma	7
Small Cell Lung Cancer	
Small cell carcinoma	20
Neuroendocrine, well differentiated	1
Carcinoids	5

lung and are more likely to develop systemic metastases, even in the face of small primary tumors. Obtaining tumor molecular profiling during the staging process has become standard of care, particularly in the setting of advanced disease.

Bronchoalveolar cell carcinoma/adenocarcinoma with lepidic growth is a subset of adenocarcinoma. The incidence of this tumor appears to be increasing. It occurs more frequently in women and nonsmokers and can present as a single mass, ground-glass opacity, multiple nodules, or an infiltrate. The clinical course can vary from indolent progression to rapid diffuse dissemination. This carcinoma, defined by tumor cells proliferating along the surface of intact alveolar walls without stromal or vascular invasion, is now referred to as adenocarcinoma with *lepidic* growth.

Squamous cell carcinoma accounts for approximately 25% of all lung cancers. Most (66%) present as central lesions, and cavitation is found in 7% to 10% of cases. Unlike adenocarcinoma, the tumor often remains localized, tending to spread within the pulmonary lobe or to regional lymph nodes rather than systemically; invasion of the chest wall, mediastinum, or other intrathoracic organs is also known to occur. In addition, squamous cell carcinoma tends to show a better response to novel immunotherapy agents, particularly if programmed death ligand-1 (PDL-1) receptors are highly expressed within the tumor.

Large cell carcinoma accounts for approximately 7% to 10% of all lung cancers. Clinically, large cell carcinomas behave aggressively, with early metastases to the regional nodes in the mediastinum and distant sites such as the brain.

Small Cell Lung Carcinoma

Small cell carcinoma is associated with neuroendocrine carcinoma due to the ultrastructural and immunohistochemical similarities. Small cell carcinomas are believed to represent a spectrum of disease beginning with the well-differentiated, benign/typical carcinoid tumor, moving to the intermediate less differentiated atypical carcinoids or neuroendocrine carcinomas, and ending with the undifferentiated malignant small cell carcinomas. Small cell carcinomas, which tend to grow fast and present with metastatic and regional spread, are usually treated with chemotherapy with or without radiation therapy. In addition, novel immunotherapy agents have shown promise in small cell carcinoma. Even with seemingly low intrathoracic disease volume, brain metastases may occur. Therefore, close follow-up with brain MRIs is warranted. Multiple studies have evaluated prophylactic whole-brain irradiation but this strategy is currently only offered in selective cases.

Carcinoids tend to arise from major bronchi and as such are frequently central tumors that often present with cough or hemoptysis. Metastases are rare, and surgery is frequently curative. Immunohistochemically, carcinoids express neuron-specific enolase, chromogranin, and synaptophysin virtually without exception. They generally demonstrate fewer than two mitotic figures per high power field under the microscope.

Neuroendocrine carcinomas or *atypical carcinoid*s occur more peripherally than typical carcinoids and have a more aggressive course, although surgery should still be considered according to clinical stage. Without appropriate immunostaining, they may be classified inadvertently as large cell carcinomas. They are diagnosed by more than two mitotic figures per high power field and Ki67 staining is used to estimate the aggressiveness of their behavior, and guide the decisions for systemic therapy.

Diagnosis

Signs and symptoms of lung carcinoma depend on the tumor size and location within the thorax. Some tumors may cause cough, hemoptysis, dyspnea, wheezing, and fever (often due to infection from proximal bronchial tumor obstruction). Regional spread of the tumor within the thorax can lead to pleural effusions or chest wall pain. Less common but worrisome symptoms are superior vena cava syndrome (dyspnea, upper extremity and face swelling, distended neck veins, and/or cough), Pancoast syndrome (shoulder and arm pain, Horner syndrome [miosis, ptosis, anhidrosis], and weakness or atrophy of the hand muscles), and symptoms secondary to involvement of the recurrent laryngeal nerve, the phrenic nerve, the vagus nerve, or the esophagus. Paraneoplastic syndromes are found in 10% of patients with lung cancer, most commonly in those with SCLC. These syndromes are numerous and can affect endocrine, neurologic, skeletal, hematologic, and cutaneous systems. With the frequent use of computed tomography (CT), as high as 40% of tumors are discovered incidentally in otherwise asymptomatic patients.

A standard chest radiograph (CXR) is the initial diagnostic study for the evaluation of suspected lung carcinoma, but contrast CT is mandatory. CT should include imaging of the liver and adrenal glands to rule out two common sites for intra-abdominal metastases. CT with intravenous contrast helps assess local extension to other thoracic structures and the presence of mediastinal adenopathy. At present, magnetic resonance imaging (MRI) adds little to the information gained by CT imaging, although it is indicated when evaluating superior sulcus tumors with concern for neurovascular or spine involvement. Positron emission tomography

(PET), especially integrated PET-CT, is another standard of care radiologic examination. Although the accuracy of PET scanning in evaluating a pulmonary nodule can exceed 90% in some studies, clinicians should be aware that false-negative PET scans occur in patients with neoplasms having low metabolic activity (carcinoids and lepidic growth adenocarcinomas). Even with advances in imaging, histologic confirmation is always required to distinguish benign from malignant disease and to determine the histologic type of cancer and obtain tissue for molecular profiling. For a small solitary lesion with a high index of suspicion (using Fleischner criteria based on size, growth, and risk category of the patient), histologic confirmation can be obtained at the time of surgery (thoracotomy or video-assisted thoracic surgery [VATS]) by using frozen sectioning of a wedge resection or a needle biopsy. If immediate surgery is not appropriate, then tissue from the tumor can be obtained by sputum cytology, bronchoscopy, or biopsy for central lesions; by electromagnetic/robotic bronchial navigation–guided biopsy or fine-needle aspiration (FNA) for more peripheral lesions; or by CT-guided core-needle biopsy or FNA. Patients with benign lesions should be monitored for interval growth with cross-sectional imaging performed every 6 months for at least 2 years to ensure stability.

Staging

The primary goal of pretreatment staging is to determine the extent of disease so that prognosis and treatment can be determined. In SCLC, most patients present with metastatic or advanced locoregional disease. A simple two-stage system classifies the SCLC as limited or extensive disease. Limited disease is confined to one hemithorax, ipsilateral or contralateral hilar or mediastinal nodes, and ipsilateral supraclavicular lymph nodes. Extensive disease has spread to the contralateral supraclavicular nodes or distant sites such as the contralateral lung, liver, brain, or bone marrow. Staging for SCLC requires a whole-body PET-CT scan and brain MRI.

The staging system for NSCLC—the International Lung Cancer Staging System or International Staging System (ISS)—was initially proposed in 1985. This system is based on tumor, node, and metastasis (TNM) classifications. Survival rates for patients with NSCLC by stage of disease are shown in Figure 8.1. Because of

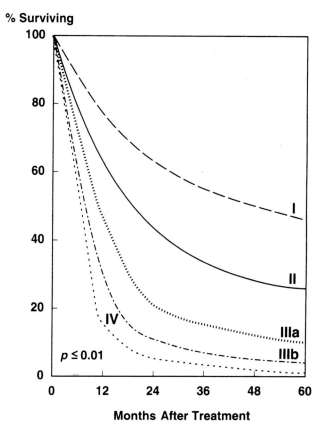

FIGURE 8.1 Cumulative survival according to clinical stage of non–small cell lung cancer.

heterogeneity within groups, the staging system has been continuously refined, with the most recent *AJCC Cancer Staging Manual*, eighth edition, staging classification released in late 2016. This edition has further refinement of T-status, as well as additional subgroupings for metastatic disease, which are beyond the scope of this chapter. The new staging schema will likely account for molecular profiling of lung cancer and its prognostic value.

Staging of NSCLC involves a thorough medical history and physical examination, CXR, CT scanning of the chest and upper abdomen, and PET-CT scanning to look for occult metastases. Unfortunately, CT cannot definitively predict mediastinal nodal involvement because not all malignant lymph nodes are enlarged, and many enlarged nodes are simply larger because of previous infection. Lymph nodes larger than 1 cm on the short axis have a 30% chance of being benign, whereas lymph nodes smaller than 1 cm still have a 15% chance of containing tumor. PET-CT has a higher negative predictive value in the evaluation of mediastinal N2 disease (96%), although false positives can occur in patients with granulomatous disease, inflammatory processes, and rheumatoid nodules. Patients with subtle signs of possible distant metastases need to be examined more carefully, and PET scan represents an ideal test in this situation. A solitary site of possible metastasis by PET requires a biopsy of the site in question. Patients with discrete nodal enlargement on CT should undergo tissue confirmation of these nodes regardless of PET findings. Multiple medical societies recommend tissue confirmation of PET-positive mediastinal lymph nodes. Conversely, most investigators also agree that patients with early-stage (T1N0) lung cancer who have a PET-CT–negative mediastinum do not necessarily need invasive mediastinal staging to prove that the mediastinum is free of disease, since the addition of mediastinoscopy achieves only a <10% positive detection of N2 nodes in such a circumstance. With respect to the method of mediastinal sampling, both cervical mediastinoscopy and endobronchial ultrasound (EBUS) with biopsy are appropriate; lymphatic tissue harvest must be documented to ensure quality of nodal sampling. Brain MRI is indicated in larger or central tumors or clinical stage II disease. National consensus guidelines can be consulted for further recommendations regarding staging and treatment algorithms.

Treatment
Pretreatment Assessment

Once a patient has been staged clinically with noninvasive tests, a physiologic assessment should be performed to determine the patient's ability to tolerate various therapeutic modalities. In addition to a general evaluation of the patient's overall medical status, specific attention should be paid to the cardiovascular and respiratory systems. Cardiovascular screening should include a history and physical examination, as well as a CXR and electrocardiography. Patients with signs and symptoms of significant cardiac disease should undergo further noninvasive testing, including either exercise testing, echocardiography, or nuclear perfusion scans. Significant reversible cardiac problems should be addressed before therapy (i.e., chemotherapy, radiation therapy, or surgery) has begun.

The pulmonary reserve of patients with lung cancer is commonly diminished as a result of tobacco abuse. Simple spirometry is an excellent initial screening test to quantify a patient's pulmonary reserve and ability to tolerate surgical resection. A predicted postoperative forced expiratory volume in 1 second (FEV_1) of less than 40% of predicted or less than 0.8 L is associated with an increased risk of perioperative complications, respiratory insufficiency, and death. The predicted postoperative FEV_1 is estimated by subtracting the contribution of the lung to be resected from the preoperative FEV_1. In certain instances, the lung to be resected does not contribute much to the preoperative FEV_1 because of tumor, atelectasis, or pneumonitis. Thus, more accurate determination of predicted postoperative FEV_1 can be obtained by performing a ventilation–perfusion scan and subtracting the exact contribution of the lung to be resected. In good-performance patients with borderline spirometry criteria, oxygen consumption studies can be obtained that measure both respiratory and cardiac capacity. A maximum oxygen consumption (VO_2 max) of greater than 15 mL/min/kg indicates low risk, whereas a VO_2 max of less than 10 mL/min/kg is associated with high risk (a mortality rate of more than 30% in some series). Additional risk factors for complications with lung resection include a predicted postoperative diffusing capacity or maximum voluntary ventilation of less than 40% and hypercarbia (>45 mm CO_2) or hypoxemia (<60 mm O_2) on preoperative arterial blood gases. For a summary of risk classification, refer to Table 8.2. In conjunction with clinical assessment (6-minute walk and number of flights of stairs climbed), these tests can help identify those patients at high risk of complications during and after surgical resection.

Preoperative training with an incentive spirometer, initiation of bronchodilators, weight reduction, good nutrition, physical "prehabilitation," and cessation of smoking for at least 2 weeks before surgery can help minimize complications and improve performance on spirometry for patients with marginal pulmonary reserve.

TABLE 8.2	Pulmonary Assessment and Risk for Thoracic Resection		
Average Risk		**High Risk**	**Prohibitive Risk**
ppoFEV$_1$% >40		ppoFEV$_1$% 20–40	ppoFEV$_1$% <20
ppoDLCO% >40		ppoDLCO% 20–40	ppoDLCO% <20
pO$_2$ >60		pO$_2$ 45–60	pO$_2$ <45
pCO$_2$ <45		pCO$_2$ 45–60	pCO$_2$ >60
VO$_2$ max >15		VO$_2$ max 10–15	VO$_2$ max <10

FEV1- Forced Expiratory Volume; DLCO-Diffusion lung capacity.

Treatment of Non–Small Cell Lung Carcinoma

Surgery is a critical part of treatment in early-stage NSCLC, however, further investigation of novel clinical trials of perioperative systemic immunotherapy or targeted therapy are underway to decrease the moderate recurrence rates observed following surgical resection. Unfortunately, more than 50% to 70% of NSCLC patients present with advanced disease and require careful multidisciplinary evaluation and therapy. An algorithm for treatment based on clinical stage is presented in Figure 8.2. Physiologically fit patients with stage I disease are treated with surgery alone or possibly stereotactic body radiation therapy (SBRT). Stage II patients are treated with surgery, systemic chemotherapy, and possibly targeted therapy if their tumors harbor an actionable epidermal growth factor receptor (EGFR) mutation. A lesser resection (such as segmentectomy or wedge resection) or nonsurgical treatment (such as stereotactic radiation therapy) is indicated if lobectomy cannot be tolerated and in otherwise poor operative candidates. Chest wall involvement without nodal spread (T3N0) is ideally treated with surgical resection coupled with adjuvant systemic therapy or chemoradiation.

The remainder of patients with stage III A/B disease (N2 disease or chest wall with nodal involvement) require multidisciplinary evaluation and multimodality therapy. Patients with this stage of disease display a very heterogenous spectrum of biology and depending on the circumstance and surgical operability patients can be treated with induction systemic therapy on or off a clinical trial followed by surgical resection, and adjuvant therapy based on pathologic response rates. Unresectable stage III A/B patients are generally treated with chemoradiation followed by 1 year of immunotherapy.

The standard treatment for stage IV disease has evolved rapidly over the last 5 years. Chemotherapy alone is rarely used now. Depending on the molecular profiling, and PD-L1 tumor expression, patients can be treated with either targeted therapy alone, immunotherapy alone, or concomitant chemotherapy and

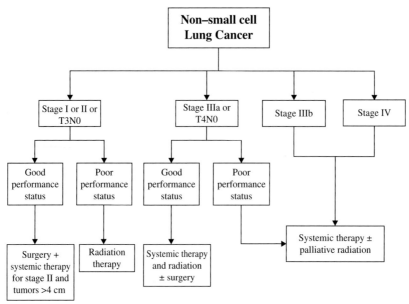

FIGURE 8.2 Algorithm for treatment of non–small cell lung cancer.

immunotherapy. With these regimens and current understanding of the lung cancer biology, the median survival of metastatic NSCLC has increased from 12 months to 4 years.

Metastatic disease is treated surgically or with radiation for local disease control only in the unusual circumstance of a solitary brain or adrenal metastasis with a node-negative lung primary. In a phase II randomized oligometastatic trial, improved progression-free survival (PFS) and overall survival (OS) rates were demonstrated after locoregional disease control with either surgery or radiation therapy for up to three metastatic sites, compared with survival rates with chemotherapy alone. The benefit of early locoregional disease control in stage IV NSCLC is now well recognized as it improves both PFS and OS as well the time to the appearance of new metastases.

Surgery

Pneumonectomy

The removal of the whole lung was historically the most commonly performed operation for NSCLC; it now accounts for less than 10% of all resections. It is associated with a higher mortality (4% to 10%) and morbidity than anatomical lobectomy. Advances in bronchoplastic and vascular reconstruction techniques, and also in induction therapies, have further obviated the need for pneumonectomy, even when faced with central tumors or those involving the lobar bronchi or pulmonary artery.

Lobectomy

Lobectomy remains the "workhorse" of lung cancer surgery. It is the most common procedure performed for lung cancer, with a perioperative mortality rate of approximately 2%, depending on the risk stratification. From an oncologic standpoint, lobectomy usually achieves complete tumor removal along with the resection of intralobar lymph nodes and the lymphatic pathway; it is the procedure against which all the other procedures and treatment modalities for local lung cancer are measured.

Lesser Resections

Segmentectomies and nonanatomical wedge resections may be employed, or even preferable, for tumors smaller than 2 cm in size, although they are associated with increased local recurrence when compared with lobectomy. The advent of CT screening for lung cancer has led to increased identification of early-stage primary lung cancers and premalignant lesions such as adenocarcinoma in situ or atypical adenomatous hyperplasia. In a phase III randomized controlled trial, perioperative mortality and morbidity did not seem to differ between lobar and sublobar resection in physically and functionally fit patients with clinical T1aN0 non–small cell lung cancer.

Minimally Invasive Thoracic Surgery

Minimally invasive thoracic surgery, defined as VATS or robotic-assisted thoracic surgery (RATS) has emerged as the preferred technique for many primary thoracic malignancies, with thoracotomy being reserved for more advanced disease or complex resections. A growing body of literature suggests that minimally invasive techniques are oncologically equivalent to open resection and may be associated with an improved perioperative morbidity profile. There are few, if any, absolute contraindications to a VATS or RATS. Although the degree of difficulty is increased with chest wall involvement, central tumors, significant hilar adenopathy, or calcified hilar lymph nodes, patients with these conditions can often be safely treated via minimally invasive techniques. VATS following prior thoracotomy is possible, as the degree of adhesions and the ability to mobilize the lung adequately varies among patients. The degree of emphysema, comorbidities, and age are not contraindications, and patients so affected are not treated differently from patients undergoing standard thoracotomy.

Extended Operations

Improvements in neoadjuvant strategies, surgery, and critical care have allowed some previously unresectable tumors to be removed with acceptable morbidity and mortality. Carinal resections, sleeve resections, and extended resections for superior sulcus tumors with hemivertebrectomy and instrumentation of the spine can now be performed in a small subset of patients. These procedures are preferably limited to patients without mediastinal nodal involvement although this is slowly changing with increasingly effective systemic therapy options. Experienced multidisciplinary care is critical when addressing such advanced disease.

Mediastinal Lymph Node Dissection   Complete mediastinal lymph node dissection improves the accuracy of lung cancer staging, improves indications for subsequent adjuvant therapy, and may decrease locoregional recurrence, but improvement in overall survival has not been conclusively demonstrated. In experienced hands, the morbidity rate associated with the addition of complete nodal dissection is not increased compared to that associated with nodal sampling (removal of one or two nodes only from each accessible nodal station).

Radiofrequency Ablation and Targeted Radiation Therapy   Interest in nonsurgical local ablative therapies has increased in recent years in an effort to provide curative intent therapies to patients with early-stage lung cancer who are either unwilling or unfit to undergo operative pulmonary resection. With the advent of SBRT also known as stereotactic ablative body radiation (SABR) and encouraging short-term results in nonoperable patients, the use of SBRT as the first-line therapy for patients with resectable NSCLC and adequate pulmonary reserve has been gaining momentum among radiation oncologists. Two phase III randomized controlled trials (ROSEL and STARS) sought to answer the question of equivalency of SBRT to surgical resection; unfortunately, neither was able to accrue sufficient numbers of patients (only 3% of expected accrual). In a controversial publication, data from the two trials were pooled into an analysis of 58 patients, and the authors concluded that SBRT is at least equivalent to lobectomy for early-stage NSCLC. In contrast, a review of the National Cancer Database suggested that SBRT was far inferior to surgical lobectomy with respect to overall survival at 5 years (29% vs. 59%). Given the lack of level I evidence and the uncertainty with respect to long-term outcomes, the role of SBRT/SABR for early-stage lung cancer is best reserved for patients with comorbidities precluding surgical resection, although even operable patients warrant a multidisciplinary discussion of their treatment options.

Chemotherapy

The addition of chemotherapy remains the standard of care for surgically resected patients with stage II and III NSCLC. The benefit of chemotherapy appears to be the same whether given in the neoadjuvant or adjuvant setting. At the time of this writing, numerous phase II and one phase III trial demonstrated superior results with combined chemoimmunotherapy as compared to chemotherapy in terms of short-term outcomes, such as major or complete pathologic response rates. It is anticipated that chemoimmunotherapy will become a part of standard of care in the future in selected operable patients. In the adjuvant setting, patients with resected stage IB–III disease and targetable EGFR should be treated with 3 years of targeted therapy to decrease disease recurrence. Likewise, the same patient group with higher PD-L1 expression could be treated with adjuvant immunotherapy after chemotherapy to decrease recurrence although this regimen is not yet fully approved.

As mentioned before, chemotherapy was the only type of treatment for stage IV lung cancer for decades. Molecular tumor profiling has quickly become the standard of care, and there are at least 11 detectable targets for which novel targeted therapies are available. Response rates to these drugs are superior to those of standard chemotherapy. For a more complete list of biologic or genetic markers and their prognostic value, see Table 8.3. Depending on the biomarkers, immunotherapy has also become the standard of care in the metastatic setting in patients without targetable mutations.

TABLE 8.3	Biologic or Genetic Markers and Their Prognostic Value	
Biologic Variable	**Prognostic Factor**	**Reference**
bcl-2	Favorable	Martin et al., 2003
TTF1	Adverse	Berghmans et al., 2006
Cox2	Adverse	Mascaux et al., 2006
EGFR overexpression	Adverse	Nakamura et al., 2006 Meert et al., 2002
Ras	Adverse	Mascaux et al., 2006 Hunckarek et al., 1999
Ki67	Adverse	Martin et al., 2004
HER2	Adverse	Meert et al., 2004 Nakamura et al., 2005
VEGF	Adverse	Delmotte et al., 2002
Microvascular density	Adverse	Meert et al., 2002
p53	Adverse	Steels et al., 2001 Mitsudomi et al., 2000 Huncharek et al., 2000
Aneuploidy	Adverse	Choma et al., 2001

bcl-2 = B-cell lymphoma 2.

Immunotherapy

Immune modulation as a potential therapeutic strategy for the treatment of advanced NSCLC was established with the Food and Drug Administration (FDA's) approval (2015) of nivolumab, a human monoclonal antibody that targets the programmed death-1 (PD-1) cell surface membrane receptor. This checkpoint inhibitor disrupts the binding of PD-1 to its ligand (PD-L1) and allows the release of cytotoxic T cells to attack tumor cells. As a result, PD-L1 has become one of the most studied biomarkers to predict the response to immunotherapy. Studies evaluating the prognostic role of PD-L1 in NSCLC demonstrated that high PD-L1 expression correlated with diminished overall survival and poor tumor differentiation in immunotherapy-naive patients; however, high expression of PD-L1 was associated with a good response to immunotherapy suggesting value of PD-L1 as a predictive biomarker.

There are currently five immunotherapy drugs approved for metastatic lung cancer, two anti–PD-1, two anti–PD-L1, and one anti–CTLA-4 inhibitor. The choices and decisions for therapy are complex and are beyond the scope of this chapter, but recommendations can be reviewed in national consensus guidelines.

Surveillance

Historically, the limited treatment options for tumor recurrence in NSCLC limited the cost-effectiveness of aggressive radiologic surveillance after surgical resection. This has changed with the availability of novel treatments. Accordingly, guidelines for surveillance depend on the disease stage, treatment type, treatment responses, and toxicities. There is an increased incidence of second primary lung cancers (2% per year), and annual or semiannual cross-sectional imaging may help detect these lesions, in addition to possible recurrences. Patients who experience symptoms in the interim should be aggressively evaluated for recurrence or a new primary. The lung, brain, bone, adrenals, and liver are the most common sites of metastases.

Small Cell Lung Carcinoma

Unlike NSCLC, SCLC tends to be disseminated at presentation and is therefore rarely amenable to curative surgery or thoracic radiation therapy alone. Without treatment, the disease is rapidly fatal, with few patients surviving more than 6 months. Fortunately, SCLC is very sensitive to chemotherapy, and more than two-thirds of patients achieve a partial response after systemic therapy with multidrug regimens. Treatment of SCLC, therefore, focuses on systemic chemotherapy and immunotherapy. A treatment algorithm based on the extent of disease is presented in Figure 8.3. Complete response is seen in as many as 20% to 50% of patients with limited disease. Unfortunately, these responses are rarely durable, and the 5-year survival rate is still less than 10%.

Chemotherapeutic regimens for SCLC most commonly include combinations of cyclophosphamide, cisplatin, etoposide, doxorubicin, and vincristine. Immunotherapy has now been added to this regimen. Thoracic radiation therapy has been shown to improve local control of the primary tumor and is often included as part of the treatment for limited SCLC. In addition, although brain metastases occur in 80% of patients with SCLC

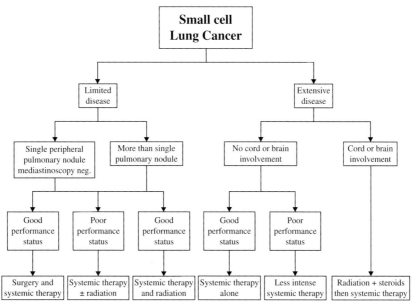

FIGURE 8.3 Algorithm for treatment of small cell lung cancer.

during the course of their disease, prophylactic whole-brain cranial irradiation has become controversial due to the development of cognitive side effects. Decisions for whole-brain radiation should be individualized and MRI surveillance should be considered.

An infrequent, but beneficial, role for surgical resection of SCLC does exist. Solitary peripheral pulmonary nodules with no evidence of metastatic disease after evaluation with CT of the abdomen and chest, MRI of the brain, PET-CT, and EBUS/mediastinoscopy can be treated with lobectomy, postoperative chemotherapy, and prophylactic brain irradiation. In these selected patients, a 5-year survival rate of 50% has been achieved for peripheral T1N0 and T2N0 staged disease.

Metastatic Neoplasms to the Lung

Pathology

The biology of the underlying primary malignancy determines the behavior of its metastases. Metastases may occur via any route, including direct extension to the chest.

Diagnosis

Because of their often peripheral localization, most pulmonary metastases remain asymptomatic, with fewer than 5% showing symptoms at presentation. Diagnosis is commonly made during radiographic follow-up after treatment of the primary malignancy. Planning of surgical interventions should be based on CT findings, even though CT scanning may still miss some small nodules found at surgery. As the resolution of CT scanning continues to improve, the number of missed nodules will likely decrease, whereas the number of subcentimeter, clinically insignificant nodules will rise.

When multiple new pulmonary nodules are present in patients with a known previous malignancy, the likelihood of metastatic disease approaches 100%. New solitary lesions, however, can represent new primary lung cancers as many of the risk factors are similar.

Staging

No valid staging system exists for pulmonary metastases. The International Registry of Lung Metastases has identified three parameters of prognostic significance: resectability, disease-free interval, and number of metastases. The criteria for offering patients resection of metastases include technical feasibility to achieve complete resection of all metastases, adequate predicted postoperative pulmonary reserve, plan to control the primary tumor, and plan to control any extrathoracic metastasis with other local therapies. This final criterion should be viewed as only a relative contraindication, since patients with liver and lungs metastases from colorectal primaries have achieved durable results with complete resection. Patients who meet these criteria could be offered metastasectomy. Favorable histologies for long-term survival after resection include sarcoma, breast, colon, and genitourinary metastases. Unfavorable histologies include melanoma, esophageal, pancreatic, and gastric cancers. It should be mentioned, however, that the landscape of systemic treatment options for various malignancies is rapidly evolving with the availability of novel chemotherapy, hormonal therapy, targeted therapy, and immunotherapy that patient selection of pulmonary metastasectomy should be based on the latest knowledge and treatment options for that particular disease process.

Treatment

Surgery

Preoperative evaluation for resection of pulmonary metastases is similar to that of any other pulmonary resection. Because of the increased risk of recurrent metastases and the need for future thoracotomies, parenchyma-conserving procedures (wedge resection, laser, or cautery excision) are performed whenever possible. A variety of surgical approaches can be used.

Median sternotomy allows bilateral exploration with one incision. Lesions located near the posterior hilum can be difficult to reach, and exposure of the left lower lobe is poor, especially in patients with obesity, cardiomegaly, or an elevated left hemidiaphragm.

Bilateral anterothoracosternotomy (clamshell procedure) allows excellent exposure of both hemithoraces, including the left lower lobe, although some surgeons think that this incision is unnecessarily morbid due to severe postoperative pain.

Posterolateral thoracotomy allows excellent visualization of one hemithorax. However, this approach necessitates a second-stage operation when treating bilateral metastases, usually performed about 2 to 4 weeks after the first surgery.

VATS resection offers a well-tolerated and effective approach for limited-volume and relatively superficial lesions. Pleural-based lesions are therefore easily visualized and excised. Unfortunately, the ability to carefully evaluate the parenchyma for deeper or smaller nonvisualized lesions is poor, and some reports suggest an increased risk of local recurrence with thoracoscopy, likely due to intraoperative tumor rupture, especially in sarcomas.

At surgery, wedge resections with a 1- to 2-cm margin depending on the tumor size are preferred. Using staplers that allow the specimen side to be staple-free enhances the pathologist's ability to adequately examine the true parenchymal margin. If multiple nodules residing within one segment, lobe, or lung preclude resection with multiple wedges, then laser or cautery resections ("lumpectomy") can be performed. Anatomical resection can be used when central lesions are resected but should be performed carefully since the likelihood of recurrence is high; every effort should be made to preserve lung parenchyma.

Chemotherapy and Radiation as Adjuvant Treatment for Pulmonary Metastases

The role of radiation therapy for pulmonary metastases is limited to the palliation of symptoms of advanced lesions with extensive pleural, bony, or neural involvement, although SBRT has gained significant traction in the management of pulmonary metastases from colon cancer. The value of chemotherapy preoperatively or postoperatively in metastatic clinical situations is dependent on the specific disease process and its biology. Systemic therapy is generally indicated in the metastatic setting to treat any potential microscopic disease deposits and determine the biology of the disease. Disease progression on chemotherapy is usually associated with a poor outcome, even after local control of metastases.

Surveillance

The frequency and intensity of follow-up after resection are determined by the primary tumor but usually involve CT scans.

Neoplasms of the Mediastinum

The mediastinal compartment can harbor numerous lesions of congenital, infectious, developmental, traumatic, or neoplastic origin. While advances in CT and MRI allow intricate characterization of these masses, biopsy should be performed on all but selected smaller mediastinal masses, which may be completely resected without prior biopsy. Surgical resection is a feasible first step for small (<4 cm) tumors that have characteristics of a thymoma on imaging and when a surgeon believes that complete R0 resection can be readily achieved. Otherwise, histologic diagnosis is beneficial before initiation of treatment to avoid incomplete surgical resections of tumors such as thymoma, thymic carcinoma, germ cell tumors, or lymphoma. With the utilization of VATS and RATS, many mediastinal masses can be resected without need for a sternotomy. Skill and patient selection are both important factors in the success of these procedures.

Pathology

A study combining nine previous series was performed to better approximate the true incidence of mediastinal lesions (Table 8.4). In adults, neurogenic and thymic tumors contribute 23% and 19%, respectively, to the overall incidence, whereas in children they contribute 39% and 3%, respectively. This section does not attempt to describe the myriad cystic and other rare miscellaneous lesions but instead concentrates on the more common diagnoses.

Diagnosis

Mediastinal lesions are most commonly asymptomatic. When symptoms do occur, they result from compression of adjacent structures or systemic endocrine or autoimmune effects of the tumors. Children, with their

TABLE 8.4	Overall Incidence of Mediastinal Tumors
Thymic	19 (3)[a]
Neurogenic	23 (39)[a]
Lymphoma	12
Germ cell	12
Cysts	18
Mesenchymal	8
Miscellaneous	8

[a]Numbers in parentheses represent incidence in children.

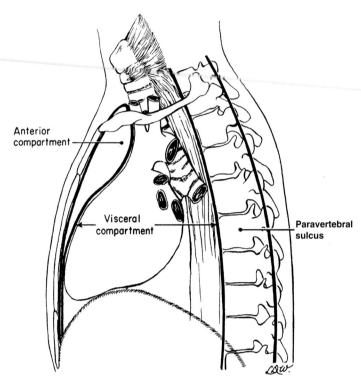

FIGURE 8.4 Anatomical boundaries of mediastinal masses according to one commonly used classification.

smaller chest cavities, tend to have symptoms at presentation (two-thirds of children vs. only one-third of adults) and more commonly have malignant lesions (greater than 50%). Symptoms can include cough, stridor, and dyspnea (more common in children), as well as symptoms of local invasion such as chest pain, pleural effusion, hoarseness, Horner syndrome, upper-extremity and back pain, paraplegia, and diaphragmatic paralysis. Most symptoms are nonspecific with regard to the tumor histology with the exception of myasthenia gravis, which is strongly suggestive of thymoma.

Fifty percent of lesions are diagnosed by CXR. The position of the tumor within the mediastinum on lateral projection can help tailor the differential diagnosis (Fig. 8.4, Table 8.5). The standard for further assessment of the lesion is contrast CT. Certain tumors and benign conditions can be diagnosed or strongly suggested by their appearance on CT scans. Angiography or MRI may be required if a major procedure is planned and vascular or cardiac involvement is suspected. Nuclear imaging such as thyroid and parathyroid scanning,

TABLE 8.5	Usual Location of Common Primary Tumors and Cysts of Mediastinum	
Anterior Compartment	**Visceral Compartment**	**Paravertebral Sulci**
Thymoma	Enterogenous cyst	Neurilemmoma (schwannoma)
Germ cell tumors	Lymphoma	Neurofibroma
Lymphoma	Pleuropericardial cyst	Malignant schwannoma
Lymphangioma	Mediastinal granuloma	Ganglioneuroma
Hemangioma	Lymphoid hamartoma	Ganglioneuroblastoma
Lipoma	Mesothelial cyst	Neuroblastoma
Fibroma	Neuroenteric cyst	Paraganglioma
Fibrosarcoma	Paraganglioma	Pheochromocytoma
Thymic cyst	Pheochromocytoma	Fibrosarcoma
Parathyroid adenoma	Thoracic duct cyst	Lymphoma
Aberrant thyroid		

Cell Type	Estimated Frequency (%)	Standard Therapy
Chondrosarcoma	35	Surgical resection
Plasmacytoma	25	Radiation + chemotherapy
Ewing sarcoma	15	Surgery + chemotherapy
Osteosarcoma	15	Surgery + chemotherapy
Lymphoma	10	Chemotherapy ± radiation

gallium scanning for lymphoma, and metaiodobenzylguanidine scanning for pheochromocytomas may also be indicated. The use of serum markers is essential in the diagnosis of germ cell and some rare neuroendocrine tumors.

FNA and a transthoracic core needle biopsy should be performed for most tumors, although the diagnosis of lymphoma may require larger amounts of tissue for tumor typing. Extended mediastinoscopy, VATS, or the Chamberlain procedure may aid in the diagnostic process. Use of a sternotomy or thoracotomy should be exceedingly rare for a tissue diagnosis.

Tumor Types and Their Treatment

Therapy, like staging, is determined by the type of tumor and its histologic characteristics (Table 8.6).

Neurogenic tumors include schwannoma, neurofibroma, ganglioneuroblastoma, neuroblastoma, pheochromocytoma, and paraganglioma. They are the most common tumors arising in the posterior compartment. Complete surgical resection is generally curative, except in highly malignant tumor subtypes, which may require additional therapy depending on specific histologic findings.

Thymoma arises from thymic epithelium, although its microscopic appearance is a mixture of lymphocytes and epithelial cells. Thymomas are classified as lymphocytic (30% of cases), epithelial (16%), mixed (30%), or spindle cell (24%). Histologic evidence of malignancy is difficult to obtain because benign and malignant lesions can have similar histologic and cytologic features. Surgical evidence of invasion at the time of resection is the most reliable method of differentiating between malignant and benign thymomas. Completeness of resection is the best predictor of survival. Adjuvant radiation can be employed in the unresectable or incompletely resected disease.

Lymphomas make up approximately 50% of childhood and 20% of adult anterior mediastinal malignancies. They are generally treated nonsurgically but may require surgical biopsy to establish the diagnosis.

Germ cell tumors comprise teratomas, seminomas, and nonseminomatous germ cell tumors. Teratomas, the most common type, are typically benign and are treated with surgical resection. Malignant teratomas are very rare and are often widely metastatic at diagnosis. Seminomas progress in a locally aggressive fashion and are both chemosensitive and radiosensitive. Nonseminomatous malignant tumors include embryonal carcinoma and choriocarcinoma, both of which carry a poor prognosis, and the more favorable endodermal sinus tumor. Chemotherapy is the first-line and second-line option for nonseminomatous germ cell tumors, with the endpoint goal being the normalization of tumor markers. Surgical resection is indicated for any residual mass, which is usually comprised of the remaining teratoma component of the tumor.

Miscellaneous cysts and mesenchymal tumors include thyroid goiters, thyroid malignancies, mediastinal parathyroid adenomas, bronchogenic cysts, pericardial cysts, duplications, diverticula, and aneurysms. Surgical resection is often employed for these tumors.

Surveillance

The frequency and intensity of follow-up after resection are determined by the primary tumor. CXR remains the mainstay of surveillance, with CT scanning reserved for the evaluation of subsequent abnormal CXR findings.

Neoplasms of the Chest Wall

Primary chest wall malignancies account for less than 1% of all tumors and include a wide variety of bone and soft tissue lesions. The absence of a large series evaluating the behavior of these tumors makes it difficult to come up with a definitive treatment algorithm. As more patients with these tumors are treated at large referral institutions, the initiation of multi-institutional databases may help settle some of the more controversial aspects of therapy; conduction of clinical trials will likely not be feasible.

Pathology

Primary chest wall tumors include chondrosarcoma (20%), Ewing sarcoma (8% to 22%), osteosarcoma (10%), plasmacytoma (10% to 30%), and, infrequently, soft tissue sarcoma. Chondrosarcomas arise from the ribs in 80% of cases and from the sternum in the remaining 20%. They are related to prior chest wall trauma in 12.5% of cases and are very resistant to radiation and chemotherapeutic agents. Ewing sarcoma is part of a spectrum of disease having primitive neuroectodermal tumors at one end and Ewing sarcoma at the other. Multimodality therapy, including both radiation therapy and chemotherapy, has been shown to be beneficial for this tumor. Osteosarcomas are best treated with neoadjuvant therapy, with prognosis being predicted by the tumor's size, grade, response to chemotherapy, and completeness of resection. Solitary plasmacytoma confined to the chest must be confirmed by evaluating the remaining skeletal system. Surgery can then be used to confirm the diagnosis. If radiation therapy is unable to achieve local control, then resection may be indicated. Soft tissue sarcomas are rare and are primarily resected. Adjuvant therapy is based on specific histologic findings.

Diagnosis

Chest wall tumors are asymptomatic in 20% of patients, whereas the remaining 80% present with an enlarging mass. A total of 50% to 60% of these patients will have associated pain. Radiographic assessment usually includes CXR and CT; however, MRI is being used instead of CT with increasing frequency because of its ability to image in multiple planes with superior anatomical distinction. Pathologic diagnosis is made by FNA (64% accuracy) or core biopsy (96% accuracy). Incisional biopsies, if necessary, should be carefully planned to allow complete excision of the scar and the tumor during the definitive procedure.

Staging

Chest wall lesions are staged according to the primary tumor identified. Sarcomas are staged based on tumor size and grade.

Treatment

As outlined previously, the treatment of chest wall lesions is determined by the diagnosis. Most, with few exceptions, require resection as part of the treatment. Posterior lesions covered by the scapula or that require resection of less than two ribs do not require reconstruction of the chest wall. However, all other, mainly anterior, defects require some form of stable reconstructive technique. A simple mesh closure using Marlex, Prolene, Gore-Tex, or Biologic mesh is acceptable as long as the material is secured in position under tension. A more rigid prosthesis is methyl methacrylate sandwiched between two layers of Marlex mesh. Sternal- and rib-plating systems exist to enhance stabilization of a rigid repair. Our study comparing pulmonary and infectious outcomes after chest wall reconstruction with flexible or rigid prosthesis did not identify significant differences between these two techniques. The pulmonary complication rate increased with the number of resected ribs, and there is a bias toward more rigid prosthesis use with larger defects.

If the chest wall lesion involves the overlying muscle or the skin, a large defect may be present after resection. This may require a muscle or myocutaneous flap, especially if the field was or will be irradiated.

Surveillance

Once treated and in remission, chest wall tumors tend to recur either locally or with pulmonary or hepatic metastases. Regular follow-up with careful examination and CT scanning should suffice to monitor all significant sites of recurrence.

Neoplasms of the Pleura

There are two main types of pleural neoplasms. The first, malignant pleural mesothelioma, remains an uncommon and highly lethal tumor with no adequate method of treatment. It behaves as a locally aggressive tumor in half of the patients and the other half develops distant metastatic disease. Its relationship with asbestos exposure was suggested in the 1940s and 1950s and clearly established in 1960. The second, a more localized pleural tumor known as solitary fibrous tumor (SFP) is generally benign; however, malignant variants exist. Complete resection is usually curative, although malignant SFP is known to recur. Prolonged survival with disease is at times possible due to the lesser tumor aggressiveness compared with mesothelioma.

Pathology

Localized mesotheliomas and malignant SFPs of the pleura are very rare. There is some controversy as to whether these lesions are even mesothelial at all because no epithelial component may be identifiable. More commonly, a benign SFP of the pleura is found. However, diffuse pleural mesothelioma is always a malignant process. There are decades of latency before the development of this disease after exposure to asbestos. The incidence of this disease reflects the widespread use of asbestos in the 1940s and 1950s, and the presence of mesothelioma will still continue because mechanisms for limiting occupational asbestos exposure were not instituted until the 1970s. Mesothelioma commonly presents as an epithelial histology and less commonly as a very aggressive sarcomatoid or mixed histology. It can be hard to differentiate this lesion from metastatic adenocarcinoma to the pleura. Immunohistochemical analysis, electron microscopy, and calretinin staining have aided pathologic diagnosis.

Diagnosis

The presentation of mesothelioma is often vague and nonspecific, with dyspnea and pain common in 90% of patients. Radiographic diagnosis in the early stage is often difficult, with the findings limited to a pleural effusion in many cases. Even CT may fail to identify any other abnormalities at this stage. The classic finding of a thick, restrictive pleural rind is a late finding. Thoracentesis is diagnostic in 50% of patients and pleural biopsy is positive in 33%. If the diagnosis remains elusive, thoracoscopy is diagnostic in 80% of patients.

Staging

A staging system for diffuse malignant pleural mesothelioma was initially proposed by Rusch and the International Mesothelioma Interest Group (IMIG). The most recent staging system can be found in the *AJCC Cancer Staging Manual*, eighth edition.

Treatment

The treatment of mesothelioma continues to evolve. Attempts at radical resections, such as extrapleural pneumonectomy or pleurectomy and decortication, have led to some improvements in local control, but have had only a limited impact on survival at the cost of a significantly increased operative risk. There is no level I evidence that has established surgical therapy as an effective treatment for mesothelioma, and patients should continue to be treated on protocols and clinical trials. The addition of adjuvant radiation therapy has increased local control. Although the removal of the entire lung facilitates radiation delivery, intensity-modulated radiation therapy (IMRT) techniques have allowed for adjuvant radiation even after pleurectomy and decortication. The only therapy that has been demonstrated to improve survival in patients with mesothelioma in a randomized trial, albeit for 3 additional months, has been chemotherapy consisting of cisplatin and pemetrexed. In addition, a recent trial demonstrated the benefit of immunotherapy over chemotherapy, especially in patients with biphasic and sarcomatoid histology. The median survival from the time of diagnosis in untreated patients ranges between 6 and 9 months. With trimodality therapy, the median survival has been extended to 17 to 20 and in one trial to 35 months; however, this has been at the cost of multiple cycles of chemotherapy, gruesome surgery, and 5 to 6 weeks of adjuvant radiation therapy totaling approximately 6 months of intensive treatment. Survival with immunotherapy in nonoperable patients was 18 months, which is the current benchmark to which all other treatment modalities are compared.

Surveillance

CT scans every 3 months are required to detect recurrences or monitor residual disease. Unfortunately, treatment options are limited, although some phase I trials are demonstrating encouraging results in anecdotal cases.

CASE SCENARIO

Case Scenario 1: Lung Cancer

Presentation

A 63-year-old male with a past medical history of hypertension, diabetes, and chronic smoking with a 50 pack per year history, underwent a lung cancer screening Computed Tomography (CT) chest that was notable for a 4-cm mass to his right upper lobe. The patient was subsequently referred for a Positron Emission Tomography-Computed Tomography (PET-CT), which showed that the lesion in the right upper lobe was PET-avid with an Standard Uptake Value (SUV) of 6, without associated subcarinal lymphadenopathy or PET-avidity. The patient appears fit for his age. Reports that he routinely performs his own yard work and appears to have a performance status of Eastern Coopertive Oncology Group (ECOG) 0. He reports a dry cough for the past 6 months but denies any chest pain, shortness of breath, hemoptysis, or weight loss. His pulmonary reserve is assessed with pulmonary function testing, which reveals a predicted Forced Expiratory Volume (FEV1) of 83% and a predicted Diffusion Lung Capacity (DLCO) of 86%.

Lung cancer
Metastastatic lesion
Inflammatory or inflammatory etiologies

Subsequently, he underwent a CT-guided biopsy, which showed findings consistent with lung adeno-carcinoma. Tumor markers were sent and his PDL-1 levels were >80%. He now arrives at the Thoracic Surgery clinic for further evaluation. After evaluating the imaging and pulmonary function tests, you determine that he is a good candidate for a minimally invasive right upper lobectomy with medias-tinal lymph node dissection. The 4-cm right upper lobe mass meets criteria for mediastinal staging and you perform a mediastinoscopy with endobronchial ultrasound. Sampled lymph node stations include 4R, 4L, and 7. Review of his pathology shows no evidence of metastatic disease, giving a stage of T2aN0M0, or stage IB. He is discussed at multidisciplinary tumor board with agreement to offer surgical resection and adjuvant chemotherapy given the size of the mass. Furthermore, the use of immunotherapy is discussed as a potential adjuvant option given his Programmed death-ligand 1 (PDL-1) levels, but with the understanding that this is not yet standard of care.

He is consented for a video-assisted thoracic surgery (VATS). During the operation, the patient is noted to have a significant amount of scar tissue and adhesion at the apex of the lung making exposure and definition of the anatomy quite difficult. As such, the operation is converted to an open lobectomy and complete without any further difficulty. He recovers well, utilizing specific enhanced recovery protocols proven to make the postoperative recovery after open surgery equivalent to a minimally invasive opera-tion without compromising oncologic principles.

- Different pathology on biopsy
- Poor functional status or pulmonary function tests limit resection
- More advanced stage requiring additional therapy modalities, change in sequencing
- Difficult dissection forcing conversion to open

- Understand staging and preoperative evaluation for lung cancer
- Ealy lung adenocarcinoma can be treated with upfront surgical resection
- Understand the role of chemotherapy and immunotherapy in the treatment of lung cancer

Case Scenario 2: Mediastinal Mass
An 18-year-old male with no remarkable past medical history presents to his primary care physician with complaints of mild shortness of breath, intermittent chest pain, and palpitations. His physician orders a CT chest with findings concerning for a 6- × 4-cm anterior mediastinal mass. He arrives at the Thoracic Surgery clinic to discuss these findings, with the conversation focusing on a differential diagnosis.

Lymphoma
Thymoma
Germ cell tumors

He is sent for a CT-guided biopsy. Pathology is consistent with a germ cell tumor. These tumors are broadly categorized as seminomas and nonseminomas. Serum biomarkers are sent to differentiate between a seminoma and nonseminomatous germ cell tumor. High levels of lactate dehydrogenase suggest a diagnosis of seminoma. High levels of beta-HCG (Human Chorionic Gonadotrophin) (>5,000 U) are usually indicative of a nonseminomatous germ cell tumor. Furthermore, seminomas do not secrete alpha-fetoprotein, hence its presence suggests a nonseminomatous germ cell tumor. After investigating these biomarkers, the patient was found to have high levels of beta-HCG and Alpha feto protein (AFP) in his serum making the diagnosis of a nonseminomatous germ cell tumor.

His case is discussed at multidisciplinary tumor board. He is referred to medical oncology as non-seminomatous germ cell tumors are typically responsive to chemotherapy. His management plan is for upfront chemotherapy with interval evaluation of serum biomarkers. On review of his imaging, the patient is noted to have a persistent mediastinal mass, now measuring 4 cm × 3 cm but his biomarkers are now within normal limits.

Surgical Approach—Key Steps

With this persistent disease in the setting of normalized biomarkers after chemotherapy, he is now appropriate for surgical resection. In many instances, these lesions are found to be teratomas with a benign biology; nonetheless, resection is recommended based on the high risk of malignant transformation.

Common Curve Balls

- Different pathology on biopsy
- Different biochemical markers confirming alternative diagnosis
- Tumor unresponsive to initial therapies

Take Home Points

- Understand mediastinal mass differential diagnosis for mediastinal masses
- Understand biochemical evaluation for chest tumors

CASE SCENARIO REVIEW

Questions

1. What is the best method to assess a patient's fitness to undergo a pulmonary resection?
   - **A.** 6-minute walk test
   - **B.** Physical examination
   - **C.** Pulmonary function testing
   - **D.** Ventilation perfusion scan

2. A 59-year-old patient presents with an isolated positron emission tomography (PET) avid 4-cm right upper lobe mass, percutaneously biopsied as adenocarcinoma. What other preoperative staging is necessary?
   - **A.** None, proceed directly to the operating room
   - **B.** Mediastinoscopy/endobronchial ultrasound
   - **C.** CT-guided biopsy of the subcarinal lymph node
   - **D.** CT angiography of the chest

3. A 21-year-old nonsmoking male presents with a 9-cm mediastinal mass. Biopsy reveals a germ cell tumor. Which of the following laboratory markers if extremely elevated would suggest this to a non-seminomatous subtype?
   - **A.** LDH
   - **B.** Beta-HCG
   - **C.** Alpha-fetoprotein
   - **D.** B and C

4. A patient is 2 days postop following resection of a posterior mediastinal mass and develops new hypoxia. Chest X-ray shows an elevated hemidiaphragm. What surgical complication should be included in the differential diagnosis?
   - **A.** Large volume ascites
   - **B.** Diaphragm herniation

     C. Phrenic nerve injury

     D. Tension pneumothorax

5. A 70-year-old woman has a newly diagnosed T2N0M0 right upper lobe adenocarcinoma. Staging examinations are complete and the patient has an ECOG of 0 with good pulmonary testing. What is the most appropriate next step in management?

     A. Proceed with surgical resection, mediastinal lymphadenectomy, and adjuvant chemotherapy

     B. Referral to medical oncology for consideration of definitive chemotherapy

     C. Referral to medical oncology for consideration of definitive immunotherapy

     D. Referral to radiation oncology and medical oncology for definitive chemoradiation

Answers

1. **The correct answer is C.** *Rationale:* The simplest way to determine if the patient's pulmonary function is adequate is to perform pulmonary function tests.

2. **The correct answer is B.** *Rationale:* The patient was found to have a 4-cm right upper lobe mass which meets criteria for mediastinal staging.

3. **The correct answer is D.** *Rationale:* Serum biomarkers are extremely helpful when dealing with a differential diagnosis of germ cell tumors. High levels of lactacte dehydrogenase suggest a diagnosis of seminoma. High levels of beta-HCG (>5,000 U) are usually indicative of a nonseminomatous germ cell tumor. Seminomas do not secrete alpha-fetoprotein.

4. **The correct answer is C.** *Rationale:* Injury to the phrenic nerve from traction or cautery is frequently observed after resection of a large mediastinal mass and should be high on the differential diagnosis in a patient with respiratory dysfunction and an elevated diaphragm on chest x-ray.

5. **The correct answer is A.** *Rationale:* The patient is stage IB. She should be considered for upfront surgical resection and likely adjuvant chemotherapy given the size of the mass. Furthermore, there is data to support the use of immunotherapy in an adjuvant setting particularly with high PDL-1 levels, but this is not yet standard of care.

Recommended Readings

Detterbeck FC, Vansteenkiste JF, Morris DE, Dooms CA, Khandani AH, Socinski MA. Seeking a home for a PET, part 3: emerging applications of positron emission tomography imaging in the management of patients with lung cancer. *Chest.* 2004;126(5):1656–1666.

Erasmus JJ, Connolly JE, McAdams HP, Roggli VL. Solitary pulmonary nodules: part I. Morphologic evaluation for differentiation of benign and malignant lesions. *Radiographics.* 2000;20(1):43–58.

Erasmus JJ, McAdams HP, Connolly JE. Solitary pulmonary nodules: part II. Evaluation of the indeterminate nodule. *Radiographics.* 2000;20(1):59–66.

Gonzalez-Stawinski GV, Lemaire A, Merchant F, et al. A comparative analysis of positron emission tomography and mediastinoscopy in staging non-small cell lung cancer. *J Thorac Cardiovasc Surg.* 2003;126(6):1900–1905.

Reed CE, Harpole DH, Posther KE, et al; American College of Surgeons Oncology Group Z0050 trial. Results of the American College of Surgeons Oncology Group Z0050 trial: the utility of positron emission tomography in staging potentially operable non-small cell lung cancer. *J Thorac Cardiovasc Surg.* 2003;126(6):1943–1951.

Adjuvant Chemotherapy for Early-Stage Lung Cancer

Pignon JP, Tribodet H, Scagliotti GV, et al; LACE Collaborative Group. Lung adjuvant cisplatin evaluation: a pooled analysis by the LACE Collaborative Group. J Clin Oncol. 2008;26(21):3552–3559.

Additional References

Altorki NK, Wang X, Wigle D, et al. Perioperative mortality and morbidity after sublobar versus lobar resection for early-stage non-small-cell lung cancer: post-hoc analysis of an international, randomised, phase 3 trial (CALGB/Alliance 140503). *Lancet Respir Med.* 2018;6(12):915–924.

American Joint Committee on Cancer (AJCC). *AJCC Cancer Staging Manual.* 8th ed. Springer International Publishing AG Switzerland; 2017.

Borghaei H, Paz-Ares L, Horn L, et al. Nivolumab versus docetaxel in advanced nonsquamous non-small-cell lung cancer. *N Engl J Med.* 2015;373(17):1627–1639.

Bracken-Clarke D, Kapoor D, Baird AM, et al. Vaping and lung cancer—A review of current data and recommendations. *Lung Cancer.* 2021;153:11–20.

Brahmer J, Reckamp KL, Baas P, et al. Nivolumab versus docetaxel in advanced squamous-cell non-small-cell lung cancer. *N Engl J Med.* 2015;373(2):123–135

Chance WW, Rice DC, Allen PK, et al. Hemithoracic intensity modulated radiation therapy after pleurectomy/decortication for malignant pleural mesothelioma: toxicity, patterns of failure, and a matched survival analysis. *Int J Radiat Oncol Biol Phys.* 2015;;91(1):149–156.

Ferguson MK, ed. *Difficult Decisions in Thoracic Surgery: An Evidenced-Based Approach.* Springer; 2007.

Ginsberg RJ, Rubinstein L. The comparison of limited resection to lobectomy for T1N0 non-small cell lung cancer. LCSG 821. *Chest.* 1994;106(suppl 6):318S–319S.

Goldstraw P, Chansky K, Crowley J, Rami-Porta R, Asamura H, Eberhardt WE, Nicholson AG, Groome P, Mitchell A, Bolejack V; International Association for the Study of Lung Cancer Staging and Prognostic Factors Committee, Advisory Boards, and Participating Institutions; International Association for the Study of Lung Cancer Staging and Prognostic Factors Committee Advisory Boards and Participating Institutions. The IASLC Lung Cancer Staging Project: Proposals for Revision of the TNM Stage Groupings in the Forthcoming (Eighth) Edition of the TNM Classification for Lung Cancer. *J Thorac Oncol.* 2016;11(1):39–51. doi: 10.1016/j.jtho.2015.09.009.

Halmos B, Burke T, Kalyvas C, et al. A Matching-Adjusted Indirect Comparison of Pembrolizumab + Chemotherapy vs. Nivolumab + Ipilimumab as First-Line Therapies in Patients with PD-L1 TPS ≥1% Metastatic NSCLC. *Cancers (Basel).* 2020;12(12):3648.

Hellmann MD, Chaft JE, William WN Jr, et al; University of Texas MD Anderson Lung Cancer Collaborative Group. Pathological response after neoadjuvant chemotherapy in resectable non-small-cell lung cancers: proposal for the use of major pathological response as a surrogate endpoint. *Lancet Oncol.* 2014;15(1):e42–e50.

MacMahon H, Austin JHM, Gamsu G, et al. Guidelines for the management of small pulmonary nodules detected on CT scans: a statement from the Fleischner Society. *Radiology.* 2005;237:395–400.

Rusch VW. A proposed new international TNM staging system for malignant pleural mesothelioma. From the International Mesothelioma Interest Group. *Chest.* 1995;108(4):1122–1128.

Sculier JP, Chansky K, Crowley JJ, et al. The IASLC lung cancer staging project. *J Thor Oncol.* 2008;3(5):457–466.

9 Esophageal Carcinoma

Bradford J. Kim and Wayne L. Hofstetter

INTRODUCTION

In the United States and other western societies, cancer of the esophagus is relatively uncommon, representing only a small percentage of newly diagnosed invasive malignancies. However, it is the eighth most common malignancy worldwide comprising approximately 4% of the newly diagnosed tumors per year. The yearly incidence of esophageal cancer is comparable to its yearly total of cancer-related deaths. Treatment paradigms are individualized and are primarily related to clinical stage at presentation. Although surgical resection has traditionally been the mainstay of therapy, most newly diagnosed cancers present at a late stage and are therefore precluded from curative resection. Symptoms such as dysphagia, weight loss, regurgitation, or back pain are alarming as they potentially herald advancing disease. Those patients who have been fortunate to have their disease discovered at a very early stage may be candidates for esophageal sparing mucosal resections or esophagectomy. Patients with locally advanced tumors will typically undergo multimodality approaches that combine concurrent chemoradiation followed by reevaluation for surgery. These approaches have resulted in 5-year survival rates of 40% to 75% in the subset of patients who have a complete or near complete pathologic response after preoperative therapy. Finally, patients who present with advanced disease are treated with palliative measures, which include chemotherapy, radiation, mechanical devices such as stents and/or feeding tubes, and supportive care.

Epidemiology

According to the National Cancer Institute database for 2016, there will be an estimated 16,910 new cases of esophageal cancer diagnosed in the United States, and 15,690 will die of the disease. Data provided on the SEER website indicate an 18.6% 5-year overall survival and relatively consistent incidence of events and mortality since data began being tracked from 1991 to 2016. In the past, squamous cell carcinomas (SCCs) accounted for more than 95% of cases, but in recent years, adenocarcinoma arising in the background of Barrett esophagus has become increasingly more common, and it now accounts for more than 75% of the esophageal cancers at most major American centers. Esophageal carcinoma, particularly SCC, has substantial geographic variation, from 1.5 to 7 cases per 100,000 people in most parts of the world, including the United States, to 100 to 500 per 100,000 people in its endemic areas such as northern China, South Africa, Iran, Russia, and India. Males have a 2- to 3-fold higher overall risk than females, and a 7- to 10-fold higher risk for the development of adenocarcinoma. Furthermore, in the United States, SCC is approximately five times more common among African Americans than it is among Whites, whereas adenocarcinoma occurs approximately three to four times more often in Whites, particularly in men. Thankfully, SCC among African American males has been on a sharp decline in the past two decades. Both major histologic types are rare in patients younger than 40 years, but the incidence increases thereafter.

Etiology and Risk Factors

Several different environmental and genetic risk factors have been identified as potential causes of esophageal cancers, particularly SCC. A well-established risk factor is the combination of smoking and alcohol consumption which has a synergistic effect on the development of esophageal SCC, increasing the risk by as much as 44 times. Other risk factors or associations for esophageal SCC include SCC of the head and neck (presumably because of the risk associated with alcohol and smoking), achalasia (as high as 30 times increased risk), strictures resulting from ingestion of caustic agents such as lye, Zenker diverticulum, esophageal webs in Plummer–Vinson syndrome, prior radiation, and familial connective tissue disorders such as tylosis (50% have cancer by 45 years). In geographic areas where esophageal SCC reaches epidemic levels, such as in China, definitive risk factors other than the typical causative agents listed above, are currently unknown. Some risk factors may include diets that are deficient in vitamins A, C, riboflavin, and protein, and have excessive nitrates and nitrosamines. Fungal contamination of foodstuffs with the associated aflatoxin production may be another important risk factor outside of Western societies.

For adenocarcinoma, the typical patient is a middle-class, overweight male in his 60s or 70s. The primary etiologic factors are obesity and Barrett esophagus, with an estimated annual incidence of malignant transformation of approximately 0.5% per year, representing 125 times greater risk than that in the general population. This risk seems to be mediated through reflux disease. Esophageal adenocarcinomas are known to progress through a metaplasia–dysplasia–cancer sequence, similar to colon cancers. Gastroesophageal reflux disease results in the overexposure of the esophageal mucosa to acid and bile. Specifically, the conjugated bile salts (secondary bile acids) are believed to synergistically damage the mucosa, leading to increased DNA methylation and variations in ploidy (as well as other genetic and molecular changes) and the formation of intestinal metaplasia (Barrett mucosa) or cardiac metaplasia. Both are recognized as precursor lesions to esophageal/gastroesophageal junction cancers. Tobacco use and the eradication of *Helicobacter pylori* are also linked to the increased incidence of esophageal adenocarcinoma in the United States.

Pathology

Esophageal cancer consists of two main histologic types: SCC and adenocarcinoma. In the United States, approximately 20% of cases of SCC involve the upper third of the esophagus, 50% involve the middle third, and the remaining 30% extend from the distal part of the esophagus to the gastroesophageal junction. SCC rarely invades the stomach, and there is usually a discrete segment of normal mucosa between the cancer and the gastric cardia. In contrast, nearly 97% of adenocarcinomas develop in the middle and distal esophagus, and many extend into the stomach if they are centered near the gastroesophageal junction. Cancers arising in a Barrett esophagus are believed to comprise upward of 50% to 70% of all adenocarcinomas involving the distal esophagus and gastroesophageal junction. They can vary in length and range in contour from flat, infiltrative lesions to fungating, polypoid masses. Ulceration is often present and may even be deep enough to cause perforation. Because symptoms appear late in the progress of the disease, the typical esophageal carcinoma is a circumferential, exophytic, fungating mass that is nearly or completely transmural. Early access to the submucosal lymphatics allows tumors to spread freely along a submucosal plane and present with very long tumors or multiple mucosal lesions. Similarly, early metastases to lymph nodes or distant sites are common. This is because there is a rich submucosal lymphatic system that tumors may infiltrate at a very early period of growth. This lymphatic system leads directly to the bloodstream by way of the thoracic duct, facilitating early dissemination of disease. Microscopically, adenocarcinomas can resemble cells of the gastric cardia or colon, and most are well or moderately differentiated. Signet ring differentiation may signify a gastric cardia origin, but this is not an absolute rule.

Other less common primary malignant neoplasms of the esophagus include neuroendocrine tumors, gastrointestinal stromal tumors, variants of SCC or adenocarcinomas (e.g., adenosquamous), melanomas, sarcomas, and lymphomas.

Clinical Features

Clinical presentation is generally insidious, and typical symptoms occur late in the course of the disease, usually precluding an easy cure. Most patients experience symptoms for 2 to 6 months before they seek medical attention. The most common symptom is progressive dysphagia, which occurs in as many as 80% to 90% of patients. This is usually a late sign because the esophageal lumen must be reduced to 50% to 75% of its original size before patients experience this symptom. Typically, malignant dysphagia will begin when the esophageal functional diameter approaches 12 to 13 mm. Weight loss is also common, with an estimated mean weight loss of 10 kg from the onset of symptoms. This sign is also an independent predictor of poor outcome, as is presentation with advanced stage. Other symptoms include varying degrees of odynophagia (in approximately 50%), as well as emesis, cough, regurgitation, anemia, hematemesis, and aspiration pneumonia. Hoarseness can be due to invasion of the recurrent laryngeal nerve, and Horner syndrome indicates invasion of the sympathetic trunk. Hematemesis and melena usually indicate friability of the tumor or its invasion into major vessels. Bleeding from the tumor mass occurs in 4% to 7% of patients and may cause considerable difficulty with treatment.

Diagnostic Evaluation

Results of the physical examination may depend in large part on the degree of weight loss and cachexia. Enlarged cervical or supraclavicular lymph nodes can be biopsied with fine-needle aspiration (FNA) and are indicative of advanced disease. In the past, there was significance placed on plain CXR, barium swallow studies, and bone scans. However, these have been replaced by modern imaging. Computed tomography (CT) scans of the chest and abdomen should be obtained to assess the degree of any local invasion of mediastinal structures, adenopathy, or for evidence of dissemination/distant metastasis, especially in the lungs.

In addition to a high-resolution CT scan, integrated positron emission tomography (PET) is being used in the diagnostic staging algorithm. It has been shown to alter the treatment course in approximately 15% of patients with locally advanced tumors, which in and of itself has rendered it cost efficient. This modality is helpful in determining the significance of nonregional adenopathy or distant lesions and may carry prognostic information in terms of the level of initial nucleotide uptake and midterm response to preoperative treatment. It is also very efficient at detecting bone-related metastases and has primarily replaced the use of bone scans. As PET–CT is not sensitive for brain evaluation, any neurologic signs or complaints (e.g., headaches, visual disturbances, and new-onset weakness) should be assessed with magnetic resonance (MR) imaging (preferred) or CT scan of the brain.

Upper endoscopy is currently the most widely used technique for the diagnosis and staging of esophageal cancer. Flexible endoscopy allows magnified visual observation and histologic sampling of the esophagus, as well as visualization of the stomach. A detailed description of tumor location within the esophagus and stomach is critical to surgical and radiation treatment planning. Biopsy and brush cytology can produce diagnostic accuracy of nearly 100% with adequate sampling, and gentle endoscopic dilation of tight strictures can be performed by experienced endoscopists to allow passage of the endoscope beyond the tumor. The addition of endoscopic ultrasound (EUS) should be used to assess the T and N status of the lesion. EUS is most accurate in predicting the depth of invasion of the primary lesion, and this can provide very good insight into the potential of surrounding organ or lymph node involvement. Regional lymph nodes in the mediastinal, paraesophageal, paragastric, porta hepatis, and celiac areas are routinely identified and can be biopsied via transesophageal or bronchoscopic ultrasound-guided aspiration (FNA) for diagnosis. Tumors that involve the upper or middle third of the esophagus should be evaluated by flexible and/or rigid bronchoscopy to rule out tracheobronchial involvement.

Staging

The staging system of the American Joint Committee on Cancer (AJCC) uses the TNM classification and is the most commonly used system in the United States. Although CT scanning is probably the most widely used noninvasive staging modality worldwide, its accuracy is quite limited. Overall accuracy in determining resectability and T status has been estimated at 60% to 70%, whereas accuracy in determining N status is generally less than 60%. Accuracy in the detection of metastatic disease is somewhat better, estimated at 70% to 90% for lesions larger than 1 cm. The use of combined imaging with PET–CT has improved the accuracy of both tests. The ability to combine anatomical irregularity to areas of abnormal fluorodeoxy glucose uptake on a superimposed CT image increases the predictive value over PET alone or CT alone. Studies with this technique have reported overall accuracy levels of nearly 60% and 90% in the ability to detect both locoregional nodal metastases and distant diseases, respectively.

Currently, EUS is likely to be the most accurate means available for determining T and N status. Reported overall accuracy for depth of invasion is 76% to 90%; overall accuracy in predicting resectability is approximately 90% to 100% for adenocarcinoma but decreases to 75% to 80% for SCC. Studies comparing EUS and CT scanning generally agree that EUS is superior in determination of overall T status and assessment of regional lymph nodes (70% to 86% accuracy). The precise differentiation between benign and malignant nodes occasionally remains problematic, however, due to micrometastases that are undetectable by EUS and enlarged inflammatory lymph nodes that are incorrectly classified as metastatic. FNA can be helpful in making this determination. Minimally invasive techniques such as thoracoscopy and laparoscopy may also be utilized in the staging of esophageal cancer. Thoracoscopy allows visualization of the entire thoracic esophagus and the periesophageal nodes, when performed through the right hemithorax, or the aortopulmonary and periesophageal nodes and the lower esophagus, when performed through the left chest. Lymph nodes can be sampled for histologic evaluation, the pleura can be examined, and adjacent organ invasion (T4) can be confirmed. The overall accuracy for detecting lymph node involvement has been reported to be as high as 81% to 95%. Laparoscopy and laparoscopic ultrasonography are useful in evaluating the peritoneum, liver, gastrohepatic ligament, gastric wall, diaphragm, and the perigastric and celiac lymph nodes. Biopsies and peritoneal washings can be performed to confirm nodal or metastatic disease. These modalities are especially useful in patients with gastroesophageal junction or proximal gastric tumors. In addition, a feeding jejunostomy can be placed for nutritional support before treatment begins. Studies have suggested that the overall accuracy of laparoscopy in staging and determination of resectability in esophageal cancer is as high as 90% to 100% and that invasive staging procedures may prevent unnecessary surgical resection in as many as 20% of patients.

Prospective comparisons with CT and EUS have suggested that laparoscopy and laparoscopic ultrasonography have superior overall accuracy in staging, particularly for lymph nodes and metastatic diseases. Mediastinoscopy can also prove helpful in assessing regional lymph nodes at the right and left paratracheal lymph node stations, along the mainstem bronchi, in the aortopulmonary window, or in the subcarinal area.

Treatment

Treatment options vary according to presenting stage, patient performance status, and local expertise.

Stage 0 to I

Patients with in situ carcinoma (high-grade dysplasia, HGD) or tumors that are limited to the mucosa (stages 0 and I) may be candidates for esophageal-preserving techniques of endoscopic resection and ablation. This modality is typically limited to patients with smaller lesions (~2 cm) located within the mucosa generally penetrating no deeper than the muscularis mucosae. Favorable factors include the ability to completely resect the mass, well–moderate differentiation, and no evidence of lymphovascular invasion (LVI). Patients with disease beyond the very superficial submucosa, or those with endoscopically unresectable lesions, or with evidence of poor differentiation and LVI should be considered for formal surgical resection if medically fit. Because accurate clinical staging of early-stage disease is difficult, patients in whom there is a question of depth of mucosal invasion should be considered for a diagnostic endoscopic mucosal resection (EMR) at a center of expertise with high volume. Confirmation of very early stage may result in a therapeutic organ-preserving endoscopic resection. Tumors found to be more deeply invasive (stages I, T1b) may not be amenable to definitive EMR but have a lower risk of metastatic lymphadenopathy and should be considered for curative resection. EMR helps to differentiate watershed staging overlaps that will significantly alter the therapeutic recommendations. For example, T1a versus T1b can be difficult to differentiate on EUS, and similarly, the treatment paradigm between T1 and T2 would be very different.

Stage II to III

Tumors that invade more deeply harbor a higher probability of regional lymph node involvement. In fact, there is a direct correlation of depth of invasion to lymph node involvement, where deep submucosal lesions have approximately a 30% risk of regional lymphadenopathy and transmural tumors carry risk of 80% to 100%. Because results with surgery alone in patients with regional lymph node metastasis are relatively poor, clinical studies began to focus on including multimodality treatment in conjunction with surgery. Recent randomized trials with locally advanced disease have shown a survival advantage in groups treated with neoadjuvant chemoradiation followed by surgery compared to those treated with surgery alone. However, debate continues regarding the most appropriate treatment of a clinically staged T2N0 patient. Many argue for surgery followed by selective chemoradiation based on surgical pathology. This approach is supported by both retrospective and some prospective data. However, an equally compelling argument stands with the same level of evidence that preoperative staging is inaccurate in many patients, resulting in upstaging in approximately 40% of operated patients from N0 to N+ status. These data prompt some groups to advocate for neoadjuvant treatment at centers of excellence, where therapy including surgery can be given with very low (2% to 3%) 30-day mortality and good overall survival.

There is little debate that locally advanced adenocarcinoma, stage IIb and III diseases, should be treated with concurrent neoadjuvant chemoradiation followed by restaging and consideration for surgical resection. Squamous cancers are increasingly being treated with definitive chemotherapy and radiation, especially those located in the cervical and very proximal esophagus. Treatment for SCC tumors located in the mid-distal esophagus is often individualized. Two European trials (Bedenne, 2007); (Stahl, 2005) have shown statistical survival equipoise in groups treated with definitive chemoradiation versus chemoradiation plus surgery if they responded to therapy. However, both of these trials suffered from excessive mortality in the surgical arm, and disease-free survival (DFS) was significantly favored in the surgical arm of one trial. Nonetheless, in patients with SCC of the esophagus who have had a clinical complete response to therapy there are advocates for observation rather than surgical resection; a decision our group makes on a case-by-case basis. Nonresponding patients and those with tumor behind the airway should be considered for resection, based on presence of disease remaining after systemic treatment and for disease located in high-risk recurrence areas.

Stage IV

Patients who present with nonregional lymph node involvement or other distant metastatic disease are candidates for palliative chemotherapy. On occasion, patients with stage IV disease whose tumor burden is systemically controlled become candidates for consolidative local regional therapy (chemoradiation). As there is a significant morbidity and mortality associated with palliative surgical resections, this procedure is generally not recommended unless a patient has uncontrolled bleeding or perforation and would otherwise be expected to have a significant life span despite metastatic or advanced esophageal cancer. Given this, there are also nonoperative methods of controlling these complications such as mechanical stents for perforation or trachea–esophageal fistula and radiation for local control of bleeding. The concept of incorporating surgery in the treatment algorithm for oligometastatic disease, that is well controlled over a period of time, is gaining some traction.

Operative Approaches

There are many available techniques for performing esophageal resection, and most often this choice is based on surgeon preferences and/or tumor location. Esophageal tumors located distally or at the gastroesophageal junction can be managed by subtotal esophagectomy, esophagogastrectomy, or segmental esophagectomy with bowel interposition. The extent of gastric and esophageal involvement, as well as the stage of the primary tumor, should guide the surgeon to an appropriate approach. A subtotal esophagectomy through a right thoracotomy and laparotomy (Ivor Lewis or Tanner–Lewis esophagectomy) allows for generous resection of the stomach because the esophageal reconstruction takes place in the chest at or above the level of the azygos vein. Locally advanced tumors with involvement of the distal esophagus and proximal stomach lend themselves to this approach because a lymphadenectomy is easily performed in two fields and negative margins can be obtained on the stomach with less concern for gastric necrosis. However, tumors with extensive involvement of the stomach and esophagus may require an esophagogastrectomy, with interposition of small or large bowel for reconstruction. Early distal tumors or short-segment Barrett esophagus with HGD should be treated endoscopically, though a rare patient may not have a salvageable esophagus due to extent of disease. These can be treated with standard esophagectomy, segmental esophagectomy with small bowel interposition (Merendino procedure), or vagal-sparing esophagectomy with gastric or bowel interposition.

Proximally located (e.g., upper and midesophageal) tumors often require a total esophagectomy because it is difficult to achieve negative margins with segmental or subtotal resections (e.g., Ivor Lewis esophagectomy). Given the propensity for esophageal cancers to spread to the submucosal lymphatic system, it is recommended that a minimum of a 5-cm margin, and preferably a 10-cm margin, be taken on the esophagus. This is a critical decision-making factor when formulating a treatment algorithm for an individual patient. The two most popular methods to achieve a total or near-total esophagectomy differ according to whether thoracotomy is used for esophageal mobilization. The esophagus can be mobilized using a right thoracotomy with the conduit brought either through the posterior mediastinum (preferred) or substernally to the neck for anastomosis (McKeown or three-field approach). Alternatively, a transhiatal esophagectomy can be performed with mobilization of the intrathoracic esophagus from the esophageal hiatus to the thoracic inlet without the need for thoracotomy. The advantage of the transhiatal technique is that it avoids thoracotomy while achieving a complete removal of the esophagus. The potential disadvantages of this technique include a limited periesophageal and mediastinal lymphadenectomy, the risk of causing tracheobronchial or vascular injury during blunt dissection of the esophagus, and significantly higher locoregional recurrence rates. In addition, the use of a cervical anastomosis is associated with a higher rate of anastomotic leakage than an intrathoracic anastomosis (12% vs. 5%, respectively) although the morbidity may be less with a cervical leak than it is with a thoracic leak. Other potential downsides to a cervical anastomosis include pharyngeal reflux, nocturnal aspiration, prolonged swallowing dysfunction after surgery, and an increased incidence of recurrent laryngeal nerve palsy. This last complication is underestimated in its importance; a patient with an intrathoracic stomach and limited ability to protect their airway is at great danger in the immediate postoperative period and is also in chronic danger of aspiration. On the other hand, intrathoracic anastomoses are hampered by a higher reoperation incidence when there is a postoperative anastomotic leak (approximately 4% to 10%).

Patients who present with cervical esophageal carcinomas have several treatment options. Advances in chemoradiotherapy have relegated resection of most localized cervical lesions to salvage procedures. Patients who have persistent locoregional, limited disease after definitive medical therapy are candidates for segmental resections with immediate or delayed reconstruction. Small bowel, neck, or musculocutaneous free flaps are well suited to esophageal reconstructions in the cervical area, with or without pharyngolaryngectomy. An alternative option for patients with early-stage disease is immediate resection and reconstruction. At the other end of the spectrum, lengthy lesions with involvement into the thoracic esophagus may require a complete esophagectomy via a three-field approach.

Extent of Resection/Lymphadenectomy

Although it is generally agreed that surgical resection has a therapeutic role in the treatment of local and locoregional disease, great controversy remains over the extent of the resection necessary and over the value and extent of lymphadenectomy. There is one group of thought that lymph node metastases are markers for systemic disease and that removal of involved nodes in most cases offers no survival benefit. This is very likely to be true when more than six lymph nodes are involved with cancer on the surgical specimen. However, many well-respected and experienced surgeons believe that some patients with affected lymph nodes can be successfully cured with an aggressive surgical approach that focuses on wide peritumoral excision and extended lymphadenectomy using a transthoracic/thoracoabdominal and cervical approach (en bloc or radical esophagectomy). There is currently no definitive evidence to support the superiority of either philosophy; however, many collaborative, multi-institutional reports that have focused on specific subsets of patients in stages IIb to III have shown that patients who have undergone complete lymphadenectomy have improved survival and can still look forward to excellent locoregional control. Proponents of radical resection have reported increased survival rates with more extensive surgical procedures and excellent locoregional control, but most of these comparisons have been retrospective. Furthermore, it is unclear whether more extensive dissection actually leads to improved survival or whether these superior results are a function of more accurate staging (stage migration effect). Nonetheless, several recent studies have shown a positive association between the number of lymph nodes resected and overall survival. The question of optimal number of nodes examined in a specimen can be a moving target based on the pTNM stage of an individual patient and a function of whether or not preoperative chemoradiation was administered. Retrieval goals of 18 to 30 nodes per patient, regardless of treatment seem to be reasonable. To summarize the controversy, a good lymphadenectomy either improves overall survival or it improves the pathologic staging of the patient. It also happens to be a marker of surgical (and pathology) quality. In any case, so long as it does not increase the risk of the operation, performing regional lymphadenectomy including all of the at-risk nodal basins should be considered an essential part of the resection.

Regarding the technique of resection, prospective randomized studies in the United States and Western Europe have failed to show any significant difference in morbidity, mortality, recurrence, or overall survival rate when comparing transhiatal esophagectomy with transthoracic or total thoracic esophagectomy. However, there is a survival trend favoring more radical transthoracic resections over a transhiatal approach, and local regional recurrence is known to be substantially higher after a transhiatal resection. In fact, subset analyses have shown that tumors located in the thoracic esophagus and cancers with positive but limited lymph node involvement benefit from a complete (at least two-field, including a thoracic dissection) esophagectomy compared to a transhiatal resection. The choice among surgical resection techniques should be individualized to the particular characteristics of the patient. The salient points that emerge from historical comparisons of these procedures are that a transhiatal resection has a tendency toward higher locoregional recurrence, but perhaps a lower respiratory complication incidence as it does not require thoracotomy to complete. We personally reserve a transhiatal approach for extremes in age and stage, or for patients at high risk for thoracotomy.

Minimally invasive esophagectomy (MIE) is offered in many centers around the world. Patients with appropriate lesions have the option of undergoing esophageal resection with combined thoracoscopic and laparoscopic resection followed by a small neck incision with an esophagogastric anastomosis performed in the neck, or a minimally invasive Ivor Lewis resection. Complete laparoscopic (transhiatal) resections can also be accomplished, but again, this approach makes extensive en bloc resection of mediastinal lymph nodes difficult. Results on several hundred patients resected in this manner show no difference in survival, and a benefit in less blood loss, earlier return of bowel function, and a slightly shortened hospital stay. Disadvantages of this modality include a fairly steep learning curve, especially for surgeons with limited laparoscopic esophageal experience and prolonged anesthetic times (although very experienced surgeons can effectively resect the esophagus in a similar amount of time as open procedures). The key point in the discussion of MIE versus open resection is that MIE should not compromise the surgical/oncologic principles. If these goals can be maintained, then a less invasive option may be very attractive.

Reconstruction After Resection

The stomach, colon, and jejunum have all been successfully used as replacement conduits after esophagectomy. The stomach is used far more frequently because of the ease of mobilization, a hearty and redundant blood supply, limited perioperative morbidity, and the need to perform only one anastomosis.

The colon is a commonly used alternative replacement conduit. However, some surgeons prefer this conduit over the stomach in younger patients who are expected to have a prolonged survival because it provides a barrier between the stomach remnant and the residual esophagus, and this may prevent significant pharyngeal reflux and future esophageal metaplasia or dysplasia within the esophageal remnant. Either the right colon or the left colon can be used, but the segment of left and transverse colon that is supplied by the ascending branch of the left colic artery, arc of Riolan, and the marginal artery is generally a better size match to the esophagus and has more reliable arterial arcades. The colonic arterial anatomy should be evaluated preoperatively by arteriography in any patient who is expected to have extensive limiting atherosclerosis or is suspected to have had a previous bowel resection. Otherwise, in patients with a naive abdomen, evaluation of the vasculature can take place in the operating theater. Another alternative is CT or MR angiography. Colonoscopy is necessary to rule out pathologic conditions preoperatively, such as telangiectasia, polyposis, synchronous neoplasm, or extensive diverticulosis, which would preclude the use of the colon.

Jejunal reconstruction can be performed for lesions anywhere in the esophagus. Segmental free flaps transferred to the neck have been used successfully after resection of hypopharyngeal or upper cervical esophageal tumors. In this case, the mesenteric vessels are typically anastomosed to the external carotid artery and the internal jugular vein. Pedicled grafts are being used when segmental distal esophageal resection is performed for benign lesions requiring resection or confirmed short segment Barrett esophagus with HGD that is recalcitrant to efforts at endoscopic ablation. Pedicled jejunal flaps with proximal microvascular augmentation (long-segment supercharged jejunum) will allow for total esophageal replacement with the small bowel. This has some advantages over the colon in that small bowel has a good size match to the esophagus, is relatively free of intrinsic disease, and does not require preparation before transfer.

Finally, musculocutaneous flaps are also frequently used for segmental cervical reconstruction and can be harvested from any of multiple areas with minimal physiologic or aesthetic effect.

Few prospective studies have been performed to evaluate the use of different replacement conduits, but evidence from several nonrandomized and small, randomized trials supports that overall survival is unchanged regardless of the technique used. A review performed by Urschel (2001) was unable to reach definitive results that would cause one technique to be favored over another. The basic principles are that the stomach has the most reliable blood supply and is associated with the lowest immediate postoperative morbidity. Cervical leaks from a colon interposition tend to be well tolerated and stricture rarely occurs. If strictures do occur, they are more easily dilated than those that occur with esophagogastric anastomoses. Graft loss can occur with any conduit in any position, cervical or intrathoracic. Pyloroplasty or pyloromyotomy may be required to avoid gastric stasis secondary to the division of the vagus nerves during esophagectomy; however, with a trend toward using narrower conduits rather than whole stomach, this step remains somewhat controversial and several centers are reporting the omission of gastric drainage procedures without significant change in outcomes.

Results of Surgical Therapy

Perioperative mortality rates for transhiatal or transthoracic esophagectomies are now less than 3%, and realistic morbidity rates range from 35% to 65%. Overall survival rates after surgical resection correspond to the stage of the disease and vary drastically. The 5-year survival rates have been reported to be 60% to 95% for stage I, 30% to 60% for stage II, 5% to 30% for stage III, and 0% to 20% for stage IV (Fig. 9.1). Unfortunately, the vast majority (70%) of patients present with advanced stage III or IV disease at diagnosis.

When examining the patterns of failure after surgical resection, one finds that most patients experience either distant metastasis or both locoregional and distant recurrence, while a small percentage experience solely a recurrence of localized disease. Novel treatment modalities focusing on these patterns of failure have been explored to improve on the relatively poor prognosis afforded by surgery alone in most patients with esophageal carcinoma.

Adjuvant Therapy

Results of several randomized prospective trials on the use of adjuvant radiation therapy (45 to 56 Gy) after resection have been published. Traditionally clinicians would consider radiation therapy in patients with unexpected locally advanced disease, positive margins, or an R2 resection, although there is no scientific proof of benefit. Treatment-related toxicity can be severe. Overall, although reductions in local recurrences have been noted and specific subsets may benefit, no significant survival advantage has been found using adjuvant radiotherapy alone for esophageal carcinoma.

According to the results of prospective randomized trials, postoperative combination chemotherapy with various agents, including 5-fluorouracil (5-FU), cisplatin, mitomycin C, vindesine, and paclitaxel, have also not been proven to have a role in the treatment of completely resected lesions. Furthermore, adjuvant

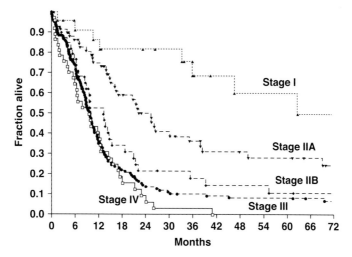

FIGURE 9.1 Survival curves for patients with esophageal cancer.

chemotherapy is generally poorly tolerated, and many patients fail to complete their treatment regimen. This treatment modality, therefore, is not recommended outside clinical trial settings.

Adjuvant chemoradiotherapy may benefit patients with esophageal carcinoma. This modality has the advantage of better patient selection because the pathologic stage will guide the decision to proceed to therapy. Patients with a high risk of recurrence (stage IIb and above) should be considered to selectively undergo treatment. In theory, chemoradiotherapy may increase survival by decreasing both distant and local disease. There is phase III evidence that has shown favorable results in a select group of patients with gastroesophageal junction adenocarcinomas treated with adjuvant chemoradiation, but compliance with treatment was not ideal. Most recently, the CheckMate 577 trial, a global, randomized double-blind, placebo-controlled phase III trial evaluated checkpoint inhibitor (nivolumab) as adjuvant therapy to resection. This trial was in patients with resected (R0) stage II or III esophageal or gastroesophageal junction cancer who had received neoadjuvant chemoradiotherapy and residual pathologic disease. This study demonstrated significantly improved median DFS in the intervention nivolumab arm (22.4 months) compared to the control arm (11.0 months). Data on patients with squamous cancers, on the other hand, has been mixed. Most studies have not shown benefit from adjuvant chemoradiation after complete resection.

Neoadjuvant Therapy

Largely because of the difficulty administering adjuvant therapy to postesophagectomy patients and the disappointing results of trials with adjuvant chemotherapy or radiation monotherapy, researchers turned their attention toward the use of preoperative or neoadjuvant therapy. Preoperative radiation therapy has been investigated in several prospective randomized trials, and the results have been subjected to meta-analysis. Despite some initial responses, the results of these trials have shown marginal benefit in terms of overall survival rate. Preoperative radiation therapy alone is, therefore, not generally recommended, even in the setting of a clinical trial.

Results of phase II studies of induction chemotherapy were promising, but many small subsequent prospective randomized trials using multiple different drug combinations failed to show any advantage in overall or progression-free survival. This is despite the observation that neoadjuvant chemotherapy was capable of significant tumor response in the majority of patients. However, the net gain in survival was not significantly different from controls. Conjecture on the reasons for this is that toxicity and failure to receive all of the therapy, including an issue that the overall resection rate was lower in patients undergoing neoadjuvant therapy, abolished any potential therapy benefit. In contrast, the largest trial on induction chemotherapy involving more than 800 patients with esophageal carcinoma (squamous and adenocarcinoma) performed in Europe (MRC Trial, 2002) did show a significant survival advantage over surgery alone. Furthermore, the long-term follow-up of the MRC trial continued to show a survival advantage in the treatment arm. Because complete response is a relatively rare event with preoperative chemotherapy, and tumor viability is a surrogate endpoint to survival, interest in chemotherapy as a neoadjuvant monotherapy has been mostly diverted to combined chemoradiotherapy.

Neoadjuvant chemoradiation therapy (CXRT) for esophageal carcinoma has been shown to be feasible and effective. Radiation to 50.4 Gy is given concurrently with a doublet of chemotherapy (fluorouracil and a platinum combination is currently the most common regimen) which is well tolerated without significantly increasing perioperative mortality (in experienced centers). Phase II trials reported excellent overall response rates (complete responses in 25% to 35%) and relatively decent compliance with therapy. Survival compared favorably to historical controls. The following decade of multiple small, prospective randomized trials lead to confusion over the potential benefit of preoperative CXRT. Some trials showed benefit while others did not. Complicating the issue was the fact that the studies showing benefit had significant study design flaws. At this point, three randomized trials comparing preoperative CXRT to surgery alone have observed survival benefit with therapy. The Walsh trial, conducted at the University of Dublin with 113 patients with adenocarcinoma, evaluated neoadjuvant cisplatin plus 5-FU and 40 Gy of radiation with surgery alone. The investigators reported a 25% complete pathologic response rate, as well as a significant increase in median survival (16 vs. 11 months) and 3-year survival rate (32% vs. 6%) for the patients receiving the neoadjuvant treatment. Much of the debate over this study has focused on the poor survival in the surgery-only arm of 6% at 3 years, erratic preoperative clinical staging, and questions of miscalculations within the statistics. The CALGB trial (Tepper et al.) also showed a significant survival advantage with CXRT but the trial reached only 10% of its accrual goals and had a very poor outcome in the surgical arm, similar to the Walsh trial. Finally, the CROSS trial published in 2012 showed a significant improvement in survival with doublet chemotherapy cocktail given concurrently with 41 Gy of radiation. A positive finding in this study was that patients in the surgery-alone arm fared reasonably well, but not as well as with CXRT. In addition, the R0 resection rate was better after preoperative therapy. There was limited toxicity in the trial, with similar perioperative morbidity and mortality in both arms of the trial. On the critical side, the study combined SCC and adenocarcinoma. The differential hazard ratios indicate that the following variables: male sex, N0, SCC, and good performance status really pushed the trial to significant differences in outcome. Subsequent long-term results of the CROSS trial were reported confirming the overall survival benefits of neoadjuvant chemoradiotherapy in patients who underwent resection of esophageal or gastroesophageal junction cancers (median overall survival: 48.6 months) compared to surgery alone (median overall survival: 24.0 months). Despite the controversy in this randomized data, three separate meta-analyses have been published comparing neoadjuvant therapy to a surgery-alone arm. All favored the treatment arm, although squamous cancers and the Walsh trial may be adding a significant amount of weight to the calculated hazard ratios.

Definitive Chemoradiation Therapy

Although surgical resection remains the preferred therapy for esophageal cancer, definitive radiation therapy and CXRT have been used in patients who opt out of, or who are not candidates for, surgical resection. Local control rates ranged between 40% and 75%, and median and 2-year survival rates ranged from 9 to 24 months and from 18% to 38%, respectively. Several prospective randomized trials have shown that definitive CXRT is superior to radiation therapy alone in the treatment of esophageal cancer. A trial published by Stahl et al. (2005) from Germany sought to evaluate the additional benefit of surgery in patients with SCC after neoadjuvant chemoradiotherapy. The trial showed significantly improved locoregional control in the surgery arm compared with chemoradiotherapy alone and greater freedom from the use of palliative procedures after surgery. However, despite a local–regional recurrence rate approaching 60% in both the German and the French definitive chemoradiation trials (FFCD, Bedenne et al., 2007), neither trial was able to demonstrate a statistically significant difference in overall survival after surgery, largely due to the fact that these multicenter trials had a high perioperative mortality incidence, and both modalities failed to prevent death from distant disease.

Other Therapeutic Modalities

In certain parts of the world, particularly in areas where esophageal cancer is endemic, mass screening and advances in diagnostic techniques have led to the detection of increased numbers of superficial esophageal cancers. Studies from Japan and the United States have suggested that for lesions confined to the epithelium and lamina propria, lymphatic spread is rare. In some of these patients, EMR is a feasible option, although experience with this technique is still limited. Endoscopic ablative therapy using radiofrequency ablation, cryotherapy, and photodynamic therapy can be used for palliating large otherwise untreatable tumors, but in patients with superficial cancers and carcinoma in situ, these methods can also be curative. Although experience with these techniques is limited, investigators have reported tumor-free survival for several months after therapy, although recurrence rates after 1 year can be significant. Similarly, photodynamic therapy has been used in nonsurgical candidates, and results of preliminary studies in patients with early-stage tumors have suggested that tumor-free survival can last several months and that complete remission is possible in some patients (at 2-year follow-up). However, long-term studies are still needed.

Palliation for Unresectable Tumors

Common indications for palliation in patients with advanced disease include dysphagia, presence of esophagorespiratory fistula, recurrent bleeding, and prolongation of survival. Tumor debulking surgery has been performed, and although survival duration seems somewhat improved relative to that in patients who did not undergo resection, few randomized trials have been performed, and morbidity can be significant. Other options for palliation include (a) dilation, which is a safe and effective method to relieve dysphagia, although it usually requires multiple procedures; (b) stents, both rigid and expandable, which have become very popular in recent years for relieving dysphagia and for treating fistulas and bleeding; (c) laser therapy, which has been effective in relieving dysphagia from shorter strictures and those with intraluminal rather than infiltrative growth; (d) photodynamic therapy, which results in fewer perforations than do dilations or laser therapy and is tolerated better but requires more frequent sessions; (e) bipolar electrocautery and coagulation with tumor probes that use heat to destroy tumor cells and cause circumferential injury; and (f) brachytherapy, which delivers radioactive seeds intraluminally.

All of these techniques have advantages and disadvantages, and short-term success rates of 80% to 100% have been reported. If these treatment options fail, an endoscopic prosthesis can often be placed with good results. These techniques are not without complications, however, and ulceration, obstruction, dislocation, and aspiration have all been reported. Recently, improvements in definitive radiation therapy and chemotherapy have also provided excellent means for short-term palliation. With nonoperative treatment, however, long-term local control is still poor (40% locoregional failure). Which method to use therefore depends on the experience of the physician and the particular needs and condition of the patient.

Surveillance

A barium swallow study should be obtained in the first postoperative month as a baseline study. Asymptomatic patients can be assessed with yearly physical examinations and chest radiography. Any symptoms (e.g., pain, dysphagia, and weight loss) should be evaluated aggressively with CT scanning, barium studies, or endoscopy. Benign strictures at the anastomosis should be treated with dilation. Unfortunately, treatment options are limited for locoregional or distant recurrences. If radiation therapy was not given preoperatively or postoperatively, it can be used along with the previously mentioned nonoperative methods of palliation (i.e., dilation, stenting, laser, photodynamic, or thermal resection).

CASE SCENARIO

Case Scenario 1

Presentation

A 65-year-old female presents to the surgical oncology clinic with a 2-month history of dysphagia and unintentional weight loss of 15 lb. The dysphagia started with solids and progressively worsened with liquids. On review of systems, she reports increasing fatigue. She walks 2 miles per day and her ECOG performance status is 1. Past medical history is significant for gastroesophageal reflux disease and hypertension. She does not report any past surgical history. She drinks a glass of wine per day and has a 10-pack year smoking history (quit 10 years ago). There is no family history for malignancy. She lives with her retired husband. On physical examination, she does not have cervical, axillary, supraclavicular, or inguinal lymphadenopathy. Her abdominal examination is normal without tenderness.

Esophagogastroduodenoscopy identifies a tumor in the lower third of the esophagus 3 cm away from the gastroesophageal junction.

Differential Diagnosis

Adenocarcinoma
Squamous Cell Carcinoma
Gastrointestinal Stromal Tumor
Neuroendocrine tumor
Leiomyoma

A biopsy of this tumor is determined by pathologic evaluation to be adenocarcinoma. She undergoes staging with a CT of the chest, abdomen, and pelvis with no evidence of metastatic disease on computed tomography. Endoscopic ultrasound identifies the tumor to be invading the muscularis propria. The patient's case is discussed at multidisciplinary tumor board and given the clinical staging of cT2N0M0, and the patient is recommended for neoadjuvant therapy. Following completion of neoadjuvant therapy, the patient undergoes repeat staging which determines no evidence of metastases. The esophagectomy is performed without complication. The pathology evaluation demonstrates a poorly differentiated T3N0M0 adenocarcinoma with negative margins. After recovery from surgery, they are started on adjuvant nivolumab as supported by the CheckMate 577 trail.

Common Curveballs

- Different location of the tumor along the esophagus
- Involvement or invasion of aorta, bronchial tree, or peritoneal structures
- Endoscopic treatment of very early–stage esophageal cancer
- Difference in surgical approach and management of related postoperative complications

Take Home Points

- Stage and location of esophageal cancer will dictate treatment approach
- Neoadjuvant chemoradiation should be considered in stage II and III patients

CASE SCENARIO REVIEW

Questions

1. What is the next best step in the management of a patient who presents with a newly diagnosed Siewert I adenocarcinoma?

    A. Neoadjuvant chemoradiation
    B. Upfront esophagectomy
    C. Definitive radiation alone
    D. CT chest, abdomen, and pelvis
    E. Diagnostic laparoscopy

2. What is the most appropriate treatment for the management of a patient with esophageal adenocarcinoma with invasion into the muscularis propria without evidence of nodal or distant metastatic disease?

    A. Endomucosal resection (EMR)
    B. EMR followed by radiation therapy
    C. Neoadjuvant chemoradiation
    D. Definitive radiation therapy
    E. Esophagectomy

3. A 57-year-old man with pT3N1M0 esophageal carcinoma has completed neoadjuvant chemoradiation and underwent Ivor Lewis esophagectomy. Final pathology confirmed an R0 resection with a modest but incomplete pathologic response. What is the most appropriate next step in his management?

    A. Repeat local radiation therapy
    B. Repeat surgical resection
    C. Chemotherapy alone
    D. Chemoradiation
    E. Checkpoint blockade therapy

Answers

1. **The correct answer is D.** *Rationale:* Before any therapy is decided upon, the patient must be adequately staged with a CT of the chest, abdomen, and pelvis to evaluate for evidence of metastatic disease. This should also be supplemented with an endoscopic ultrasonography to provide the most accurate tumor depth information. If there is suspicion for aortic invasion, magnetic resonance imaging may be considered. For occult metastatic disease, positron emission tomography can also be

utilized. Finally, diagnostic laparoscopy is not considered in patients for distal tumors not involving the gastroesophageal junction unless there are signs suspicious for carcinomatosis. High-risk Siewart type II and all Siewert type III should be considered for diagnostic laparoscopy.

2. **The correct answer is C.** According to the 8th edition of the American Joint Committee on Cancer Staging Criteria for Esophageal Cancer, the tumor is identified to be a T2 tumor. EMR should only be considered for superficial tumors that appear to be ≤T1. Although there is no evidence of metastatic disease, neoadjuvant therapy should be considered before esophagectomy. Definitive

3. **The correct answer is E.** *Rationale:* The CheckMate 577 trial was a global randomized double-blind, placebo-controlled phase III trial that evaluated the use of nivolumab as adjuvant therapy in R0 resected patients with stage II or III esophageal or gastroesophageal junction cancer that underwent neoadjuvant chemoradiotherapy and had residual pathologic disease after esophagectomy. The trial demonstrated a 22.4-month versus 11.0-month disease-free survival benefit in the nivolumab arm compared to control.

Recommended Readings

Ajani JA. Current status of new drugs and multidisciplinary approaches in patients with carcinoma of the esophagus. *Chest.* 1998;113(suppl 1):112S–119S.

Akiyama H, Tsurumaru M, Udagawa H, Kajiyama Y. Esophageal cancer. *Curr Probl Surg.* 1997;34:767–834.

Bedenne L, Michel P, Bouché O, et al. Chemoradiation followed by surgery compared with chemoradiation alone in squamous cancer of the esophagus: FFCD 9102. *J Clin Oncol.* 2007;25(10):1160–1168.

Bedenne L, Micherl P, Boiuché O, et al. Chemoradiation followed by surgery compared with chemoradiation alone in squamous cancer of the esophagus: FFCD 9102. *J Clin Oncol.* 2007;25(10):1160–1168. DOI: 10.1200/JCO.20056.04.7118.

Bosset JF, Gignoux M, Triboulet JP, et al. Chemoradiotherapy followed by surgery compared with surgery alone in squamous-cell cancer of the esophagus. *N Engl J Med.* 1997;337:161–167.

Goldminc M, Maddern G, LePrise E, Meunier B, Campion JP, Launois B. Oesophagectomy by transhiatal approach or thoracotomy: a prospective randomized controlled trial. *Br J Surg.* 1993;80:367–370.

Gore RM. Esophageal cancer: clinical and pathologic features. *Radiol Clin North Am.* 1997;35:243–263.

Herskovic A, Martz K, al-Sarraf M, et al. Combined chemotherapy and radiotherapy compared with radiotherapy alone in patients with cancer of the esophagus. *N Engl J Med.* 1992;326:1593–1598.

Kelly RJ, Ajani JA, Kuzdzal J, et al; CheckMate 577 Investigators. Adjuvant nivolumab in resected esophageal or gastroesophageal junction cancer. *N Engl J Med.* 2021;384(13):1191–1203.

Kelsen DP, Ginsberg R, Pajak TF, et al. Chemotherapy followed by surgery compared with surgery alone for localized esophageal cancer. *N Engl J Med.* 1998;339:1979–1984.

Knyrim K, Wagner HJ, Bethge N, Keymling M, Vakil N. A controlled trial of an expansile metal stent for palliation of esophageal obstruction due to inoperable cancer. *N Engl J Med.* 1993;329:1302–1307.

Kolh P, Honore P, Degauque C, Gielen J, Gerard P, Jacquet N. Early stage results after oesophageal resection for malignancy-colon interposition versus gastric pull-up. *Eur J Cardiothorac Surg.* 2000;18:293–300.

Medical Research Council Oesophageal Cancer Working Group. Surgical resection with or without preoperative chemotherapy in oesophageal cancer: a randomised controlled trial. *Lancet.* 2002;359:1727–1733.

Omloo JM, Lagarde SM, Hulscher JB, et al. Extended transthoracic resection compared with limited transhiatal resection for adenocarcinoma of the mid/distal esophagus: five-year survival of a randomized clinical trial. *Ann Surg.* 2007;246(6):992–1000.

Orringer MB, Marshall B, Iannettoni MD. Transhiatal esophagectomy: clinical experience and refinements. *Ann Surg.* 1999;230:392.

Pech O, Behrens A, May A, et al. Long-term results and risk factor analysis for recurrence after curative endoscopic therapy in 349 patients with high-grade intraepithelial neoplasia and mucosal adenocarcinoma in Barrett's oesophagus. *Gut.* 2008;57(9):1200–1206.

Rizk NP, Ishwaran H, Rice TW, et al. Optimum lymphadenectomy for esophageal cancer. *Ann Surg.* 2010;251(1):46–50.

Roth JA, Pass HI, Flanagan MM, Graeber GM, Rosenberg JC, Steinberg S. Randomized clinical trial of preoperative and postoperative adjuvant chemotherapy with cisplatin, vindesine and bleomycin for carcinoma of the esophagus. *J Thorac Cardiovasc Surg.* 1988;96:242–248.

Shapiro J, van Lanschot JB, Hulshof MCCM, et al; CROSS study group. Neoadjuvant chemoradiotherapy plus surgery versus surgery alone for oesophageal or junctional cancer (CROSS): long-term results of a randomized controlled trial. *Lancet Oncol.* 2015;16(9):1090–1098.

Stahl M, Stuschke M, Lehmann N, et al. Chemoradiation with and without surgery in patients with locally advanced squamous cell carcinoma of the esophagus. *J Clin Oncol.* 2005;23(10):2310–2317. Erratum in: *J Clin Oncol.* 2006;24(3):531.

Tepper J, Krasna MJ, Niedzwiecki D, et al. Phase III trial of trimodality therapy with cisplatin, fluorouracil, radiotherapy, and surgery compared with surgery alone for esophageal cancer: CALGB 9781. *J Clin Oncol.* 2008;26(7):1086–1092.

Urba SG, Orringer MB, Turrisi A, Iannettoni M, Forastiere A, Strawderman M. Randomized trial of preoperative chemoradiation versus surgery alone in patients with locoregional esophageal carcinoma. *J Clin Oncol.* 2001;19:305–313.

Urschel JD. Does the interponat affect outcome after esophagectomy for cancer? *Dis Esophagus.* 2001;14(2):124–130.

Walsh TN, Noonan N, Hollywood D, Kelly A, Keeling N, Hennessy TP. A comparison of multimodal therapy and surgery for esophageal adenocarcinoma. *N Engl J Med.* 1996;335:462–467.

Primary Gastric Malignancies

Derek J. Erstad, Seth J. Concors, Naruhiko Ikoma, and Brian D. Badgwell

INTRODUCTION

Gastric cancer is a common solid organ malignancy and a leading cause of cancer-related death worldwide. The treatment of gastric cancer is evolving rapidly, including advances in our understanding of the molecular underpinnings of this disease, development of robotic minimally invasive surgical techniques, and optimization of chemotherapy and chemoradiation systemic treatments. Gastric cancer is a malignancy that truly demands multidisciplinary collaboration between medical, radiation, and surgical oncologists. Additional expertise in nutritional assessment and endoscopy are also critical components to achieving successful outcomes in centers treating gastric cancer. The timing and interplay between systemic chemotherapy, operative resection, and radiation therapy are areas of intense study in an effort to improve survival outcomes. While peritoneal metastases have historically been a contraindication to operative treatment for gastric cancer, there are many recent and ongoing studies evaluating the utility of regional therapy in improving the extremely low reported median survival rates for patients with carcinomatosis. The treatment of advanced, incurable disease is particularly challenging and requires thoughtful consideration of the patient's needs and goals. This chapter will cover these topics, mostly as they relate to gastric adenocarcinoma. Brief mention will be made of the treatment of other gastric malignancies, including gastric lymphoma and gastric neuroendocrine tumors (NETs). Gastrointestinal stromal tumors (GISTs) are discussed in Chapter 6, Soft-Tissue and Bone Sarcoma.

Epidemiology, Risk Factors, and Genetics

Epidemiology

The incidence and public health burden of gastric adenocarcinoma varies greatly worldwide. The incidence in the United States has declined steadily over the last century. Whereas it was a leading cause of cancer-related deaths in the first half of the 20th century, responsible for 20% to 30% of all cancer-related deaths in the United States in the 1930s, currently it accounts for only about 2% of cancer-related deaths. Approximately 26,000 new cases of gastric adenocarcinoma and nearly 11,000 deaths are expected in the United States in 2021. Globally, gastric adenocarcinoma remains a significant public health burden, although the incidence has been steadily declining over the last several decades. It is the fifth most common malignancy worldwide and the third leading cause of cancer death. The incidence tends to be higher in developing countries compared to industrialized countries.

In the United States, incidences and death rates vary by race, gender, and ethnicity. Incidence rates are approximately twofold higher in non-Hispanic Blacks and Asian/Pacific Islanders compared to non-Hispanic Whites. Mortality rates are also approximately twice as high in non-Hispanic Blacks and Asian/Pacific Islanders compared to non-Hispanic Whites. Across all races and ethnicities, incidence and death rates are approximately twice as high in males compared to females.

Risk Factors

There is a complex interaction between environment and ethnicity contributing to differences in incidence rates of gastric cancer. The highest rates are seen in Japan and other eastern Asian countries, including China and Korea. Ethnicity may play some role in variable global rates of gastric cancer, though local environment appears to be a more impactful factor. For example, epidemiologic studies have provided evidence that first-generation migrants who move from high-incidence to low-incidence countries have the same risk of gastric cancer as that of their native country. However, subsequent generations acquire the risk rate of their new environment, indicating that the local environment is a dominant factor over long periods of time.

Atrophic gastritis, intestinal metaplasia, dysplasia, and infection with *Helicobacter pylori* have been identified as important steps in the pathogenesis of gastric cancer. *H. pylori* plays a critical role in the development of gastric cancer. *H. pylori* is common in patients with distal (noncardia) cancer but not in patients with proximal cancer. A falling incidence of both *H. pylori* infection and distal gastric cancers in developed countries coincides with rising rates of cardia and gastroesophageal junction (GEJ) tumors, which are often associated with obesity, reflux, and a Western lifestyle. *H. pylori* infection is more prevalent in the populations of developing nations than in industrialized nations. *H. pylori* infection is disproportionately associated with intestinal-type gastric cancer, in which the incidence of *H. pylori* infection is almost 90%, compared to 32% in diffuse type. The risk of adenocarcinoma is increased in patients with evidence of *H. pylori* antibodies and in patients with prolonged (>10 years) infection.

Diet is believed to play a major role in the pathogenesis of gastric adenocarcinoma and is likely an important factor in the geographic differences in gastric cancer incidence. Diets rich in salt, smoked or poorly preserved foods, nitrates, nitrites, and secondary amines are associated with an increase in gastric cancer. Prolonged exposure to this type of diet results in alterations in the gastric environment with the generation of carcinogenic *N*-nitroso compounds. Diets high in raw vegetables, fresh fruits, vitamin C, vitamin A, calcium, and antioxidants are associated with a decreased risk of gastric cancer.

Lifestyle factors are associated with an increased risk of gastric cancer in the United States. Occupational-associated increased risk may exist for metal workers, miners, and rubber workers, as well as for workers exposed to wood or asbestos dust. Obesity is associated with proximal gastric cancers. Cigarette smokers have a two to three times increased risk of proximal gastric cancer. Alcohol consumption has not been correlated with the development of gastric cancer.

Unlike colorectal adenocarcinoma, polyps are rarely precursor lesions of gastric adenocarcinoma. Hyperplastic polyps are the most common type of polyps found in the stomach. In general, they are not associated with increased risk of malignancy when there is no dysplasia present. However, dysplasia can be present in some hyperplastic polyps and these lesions have an increased risk of subsequent malignancy. Risk factors for malignancy in hyperplastic polyps include size >1 cm and a pedunculated shape. Villous adenomas, though rare, are associated with increased risk of invasive cancer, both in the polyp itself and elsewhere in the stomach. Chronic atrophic gastritis and intestinal metaplasia are known precursor lesions for gastric adenocarcinoma. *H. pylori* is the most important risk factor for these precursor lesions, and the eradication of *H. pylori* is recommended when these lesions are discovered. The role of acid reduction by H_2 blockade or with proton pump inhibitors in order to reduce the risk of invasive malignancy when these precursor lesions are found is unclear.

Pernicious anemia is a risk factor for multiple types of gastric cancer. The presence of pernicious anemia in US elderly population was associated with a 2-fold increased risk of noncardia gastric adenocarcinoma and an 11-fold increased risk of gastric NETs. A history of surgery for benign peptic ulcers is associated with an increased risk of gastric cancer. Adenocarcinoma in the gastric remnant may appear several decades after the index peptic ulcer operation and appears to increase over time. Chronic, nonhealing gastric ulcers must be carefully evaluated endoscopically with multiple biopsies to determine if an underlying invasive malignant component is present. Epstein–Barr virus (EBV) infection is associated with a specific phenotype of gastric adenocarcinoma. It is more prevalent in Hispanics and non-Hispanic Whites compared to Asians, more often in the cardia and body, and more often diffuse type. Each of the above risk factors contributes a marginal increase to the lifetime risk of gastric cancer, meaning that even in the presence of these risk factors, the absolute lifetime risk may still be small.

Genetics

Most gastric carcinomas occur sporadically, however, 1% to 3% have an inherited familial component. Patients with germline mutations in p53 (Li–Fraumeni syndrome) and BRCA2 are at increased risk for developing gastric cancer and should be followed under close endoscopic surveillance. Gastric cancer can also develop as part of the hereditary nonpolyposis colon cancer syndrome (HNPCC), as well as part of the gastrointestinal polyposis syndromes, including familial adenomatous polyposis (FAP), MUTYH-associated adenomatous polyposis, juvenile polyposis syndrome, PTEN-associated hamartoma tumor syndrome (Cowden syndrome), and Peutz–Jeghers syndrome.

Germline mutations in the gene *CDH1* encoding the cell adhesion protein E-cadherin result in an autosomal-dominant predisposition to gastric adenocarcinoma, known as hereditary diffuse gastric cancer. The cumulative risk of invasive gastric cancer in patients with the *CDH1* mutation is 70% in men and 56% in women. Endoscopic surveillance is not a reliable strategy to prevent invasive malignancy in these patients. The lesions are diffuse type and difficult to identify endoscopically. Prophylactic gastrectomy should be offered to carriers of this mutation, ideally when the patient is young (in their 20s), but no later than 10 years prior to the earliest age of gastric cancer diagnosed in their family. Virtually all carriers of this mutation have multiple foci of intramucosal adenocarcinoma in the resected specimen.

Pathology

The vast majority of gastric cancers are adenocarcinomas that arise almost exclusively from the mucus-producing rather than the acid-producing cells of the gastric mucosa. The remaining types of gastric cancer include lymphoma, neuroendocrine, leiomyosarcoma, adenosquamous and squamous cell carcinoma, and GISTs. Gastric tumors are classified according to their site in the proximal (cardia) and distal (noncardia) stomach. The Siewert classification system was proposed in the 1908s as a way to categorize tumors based on proximity to the GEJ and direct management differently for these groups. This system is still found to be therapeutically relevant, and proximal tumors in the cardia (Siewert II) are staged as esophageal tumors in the latest edition of the *AJCC Staging Manual*. Although the incidence of distal gastric cancer is decreasing in the United States, the incidence of proximal gastric tumors continues to increase. Cancers of the gastric cardia currently account for nearly 50% of all cases of gastric adenocarcinoma. Gastric cardia tumors are five times more common in men than in women, whereas noncardia gastric tumors are only twice as common in men than in women. Nine percent of patients have tumor that involves the entire stomach. This is known as linitis plastica or "leather bottle" stomach, and the prognosis for these patients is dismal. In general, gastric tumors are more common on the lesser curve of the stomach than on the greater curve. In the United States, the incidence of synchronous gastric lesions is 2.2%, compared to an incidence of up to 10% in Japanese patients with pernicious anemia.

The most common histologic classification scheme is a two-category system called the Lauren classification, delineating intestinal versus diffuse types. The intestinal type is found in geographic regions where there is a high incidence of gastric cancer and is characterized pathologically by the tendency of malignant cells to form glands. These tumors are usually well to moderately differentiated and associated with metaplasia or chronic gastritis. They occur more commonly in males and older patients. These tumors tend to spread through both lymphatics and hematogenously to distant organs, most often the liver. Conversely, the diffuse type typically lacks organized gland formation, is poorly differentiated, and has many signet ring cells. If more than 50% of the tumor cells contain intracytoplasmic mucin, then it is designated as signet ring subtype. Diffuse-type tumors are more common in younger patients with no history of gastritis and spread transmurally and by lymphatic invasion. Diffuse-type tumors appear to be associated with obesity. Although the incidence of these tumors varies little from country to country, their overall incidence appears to be increasing worldwide. It is difficult to apply the Lauren classification in patients who have had a significant response to preoperative therapy and in those who have limited volume endoscopic tissue samples to evaluate. An alternative classification scheme is recognized by the World Health Organization, classifying gastric adenocarcinomas according to their histologic appearance: tubular, mucinous, papillary, and signet ring cell types.

Recently, advances in next-generation sequencing (NGS) and molecular phenotyping have led to new insights regarding the biologic underpinnings of gastric cancer pathogenesis. A comprehensive, genome-wide analysis of DNA, RNA, and protein from 295 primary gastric adenocarcinomas was recently performed by The Cancer Genome Atlas (TCGA) research network. In this study, the authors proposed a new molecular classification for gastric adenocarcinoma with four distinct subtypes: EBV positive, microsatellite unstable, genomically stable, and chromosomal instability (CIN). EBV tumors are associated with recurrent PI3K mutations, DNA hypermethylation, JAK2 amplification, and expression of programmed death ligands PD-L1 and PD-L2, which are activating ligands for the T-cell PD-1 receptor. Microsatellite unstable tumors exhibit elevated tumor mutational burden, including targetable driver genes. Genomically stable tumors are associated with few targetable mutations, a diffuse gastric cancer histologic phenotype, and RHO-family GTPase mutations. Finally, CIN lesions have frequent aneuploidy and receptor tyrosine kinase (RTK) amplifications. The translation of this type of molecular phenotyping into more effective therapies and personalized treatment is still in its infancy. Nonetheless, molecular phenotyping has been helpful in identifying gastric cancer patients who may have favorable responses to immunotherapy (EBV and microsatellite instability [MSI] tumors). Going forward, this type of tumor analysis will likely become foundational to deciding on individual treatment approaches for gastric cancer patients, particularly as immune and targeted therapies continue to diversify and improve.

Clinical Presentation

Gastric adenocarcinoma is insidious in onset, lacking outward signs of early disease. Patients and physicians often ignore the vague epigastric discomfort that in hindsight was present for months prior to diagnosis. The most frequent presenting symptoms are weight loss, pain, vomiting, and anorexia. Physical examination will reveal a palpable mass in up to 30% of patients. Chronic anemia is a common laboratory finding that prompts endoscopic evaluation which reveals an otherwise occult gastric cancer. Dysphagia is more commonly associated with tumors of the cardia or GEJ. Tumors in the antrum may cause symptoms of gastric outlet obstruction, which is an ominous sign of advanced disease. Although rare, large tumors that directly invade the transverse colon may present with colonic obstruction.

Approximately 40% of patients in the National Cancer Database with gastric adenocarcinoma have stage IV metastatic disease at the time of presentation. As with incidence, stage at presentation varies with race and ethnicity. Physical examination findings that suggest metastatic disease include a palpable left supraclavicular lymph node (Virchow node), a palpable mass on rectal examination (Blumer shelf), a palpable periumbilical mass (Sister Mary Joseph node), the presence of ascites, and jaundice. Intestinal-type gastric cancer most commonly metastasizes to the liver and diffuse type routinely metastasizes to the peritoneum.

Assessment

National consensus guidelines have been developed for the clinical evaluation and staging of patients suspected of having gastric adenocarcinoma. The recommended initial evaluation requires complete history and physical examination and laboratory studies including complete blood count, chemistry panels, and carcinoma embryonic antigen (CEA) levels. CEA may only be elevated in approximately 30% of patients with gastric carcinoma, but in those patients with CEA elevation, it is a useful marker to trend for treatment response and to monitor for recurrence. Nutrition labs may be helpful to identify subclinical malnutrition, evidenced by an albumin level less than 3.5 g/dL, and to guide decision making regarding operative timing.

Chest, abdominal, and pelvic computed tomography (CT) scans should be performed early to assess the overall staging of patients with newly diagnosed gastric cancer. This allows expeditious identification of solid organ metastases, malignant ascites, or large peritoneal metastases. The major limitations of CT as a staging tool are in the evaluation of early gastric tumors and small (<5 mm) metastases on peritoneal surfaces or in the liver. The use of fluorodeoxyglucose (2-deoxy-2-[^{18}F]fluoro-D-glucose) positron emission tomography (FDG-PET) may improve the detection of otherwise occult metastases in patients with locally advanced (T3, T4, or node positive) disease and can be considered as part of the staging workup. Esophagogastroduodenoscopy, an essential part of the staging evaluation, allows for direct anatomic localization of the tumor and sampling of tissue for diagnostic purposes. Endoscopic ultrasound (EUS) is a useful tool to predict the tumor (T) classification of the tumor and identify suspicious perigastric lymphadenopathy. An added benefit of EUS is the ability to perform fine-needle aspiration biopsy of suspicious lymph nodes to confirm node-positive disease. The addition of EUS to cross-sectional CT imaging greatly improves the accuracy of both T and nodal (N) classification.

For newly diagnosed patients, national consensus guidelines recommend universal testing for MSI by polymerase chain reaction (PCR) and for mismatch repair (MMR) defects by immunohistochemistry (IHC). For patients found to have metastatic disease at diagnosis, additional testing for HER2 and PD-L1 expression by IHC is also recommended. If sufficient tissue is present from the biopsy sample, NGS may be considered.

Staging laparoscopy is a critical part of the initial assessment and staging of patients with newly diagnosed gastric adenocarcinoma for lesions designated cT1b or higher. This minimally invasive procedure serves two purposes: (1) to identify small (<5-mm) peritoneal metastases often undetected on CT imaging, and (2) to obtain peritoneal washings for cytology to identify microscopic peritoneal metastatic disease. Our preference is to perform this procedure as an outpatient surgery as part of the initial staging workup, rather than immediately preceding a definitive resection. The intent is identification of metastatic peritoneal disease; intraoperatively interpreted cytology studies are often not as accurate as those collected and processed during separate staging laparoscopy. In our experience at MD Anderson, routine laparoscopy performed in patients with gastroesophageal or gastric adenocarcinoma identified radiographically occult macroscopic peritoneal metastases in 21% of patients, positive cytology in lavage specimens in another 13% of patients, and unexpected clinically relevant findings (such as liver metastases or cirrhosis) in another 6% of patients. The total yield of diagnostic laparoscopy in these patients was 36%. Patients with microscopically positive peritoneal cytology findings have a prognosis similar to that of patients with macroscopic visceral or peritoneal disease. A repeat diagnostic laparoscopy prior to planned resection in patients with locally advanced disease after neoadjuvant treatment can also be considered and may identify radiographically occult metastatic disease in a minority of patients.

Staging

The American Joint Committee on Cancer (AJCC) staging guidelines, based on the tumor (T), node (N), and metastasis (M) classification is the most commonly used system to stage gastric adenocarcinoma. The Japanese classification historically refers to the extent of lymph node dissection by D classification. The Japanese classification is harmonized with the AJCC TNM system, but contains more detail regarding the preoperative macroscopic appearance of the lesions and the designation of the nodal stations involved.

American Joint Committee on Cancer Staging System

The eighth edition of the *AJCC Staging Manual* published in 2016 preserved most of the significant changes found in the seventh edition in 2010, while updating the distinction between gastric and esophageal adenocarcinoma of the GEJ. Tumors at the GEJ with the epicenter of the tumor greater than 2 cm into the proximal stomach are staged as gastric cancer; those with an epicenter less than 2 cm into the proximal stomach are staged as esophageal cancers and will be discussed in a separate chapter. The staging system relies on the TNM classification. The updated eighth edition defines clinical, pathologic, and postneoadjuvant therapy stage groupings. The system is designed to stratify patients according to their overall survival. Stages are grouped to identify survival differences, thus there is a mix of T and N classifications in each stage designation (Table 10.1).

When comparing studies from different time periods, care must be paid to changes in staging definitions. The T classification regarding depth of invasion was aligned with other gastrointestinal tract malignancies, such as the esophagus and small and large bowel. The modification of T stage in the seventh edition from previous editions include: tumor penetrates subserosal tissue (previously T2b, currently T3), serosa (previously T3, currently T4a), and adjacent structures (previously T4, currently T4b). These modifications are preserved in the eighth edition.

The nodal classification in the eighth edition is the same as the seventh edition. The evaluation of the lymph nodes and the extent of lymph node resection have always been contentious issues in gastric cancer. The AJCC staging guidelines make no recommendations as far as extent of lymph node dissection required for accurate staging, only suggesting that at least 16 regional lymph nodes be removed and assessed pathologically. Under the AJCC eighth edition, 16 or more positive lymph nodes correspond to an N-category of 3b, and therefore a minimum of 16 nodes is necessary for adequate staging. A pN0 designation can be assigned based on the actual number of lymph nodes evaluated microscopically.

The presence of metastatic disease is simply designated M1 without subclassification. Metastases to nonregional lymph node groups, including the retropancreatic, para-aortic, portal, retroperitoneal, or mesenteric groups is considered M1 disease. Both microscopically positive peritoneal cytology and macroscopic peritoneal disease are also considered M1 disease.

Japanese Classification

Since 1962, when the first version of the Japanese Classification of Gastric Cancer was published, frequent modifications have been applied up to the current 14th version. The Japanese Classification not only defines pathologic staging, but also describes all aspects of preoperative staging, intraoperative findings, how to handle resected specimens, rules of treatment effect on pathology, and detailed histologic classifications. There are also a series of Japanese Treatment Guidelines of Gastric Cancer, which summarize current consensus of stage-specific treatment strategies, currently in its fifth edition. The greatest advantage of the detailed Japanese Classification is the standardization of the description of specific tumor status, which creates a standard format used by Japanese surgeons in each case. The disadvantages include its complexity which limits its broader acceptance and the frequent updates which make it difficult to compare results to historical literature. Efforts have been made to correlate the Japanese Classification to the AJCC staging system. The pathologic staging and grouping are now essentially identical to those of AJCC in the current version. N stage was previously defined by location of involved lymph nodes (stations) but is now defined by the number of involved lymph nodes in accordance with AJCC convention. However, GEJ tumors in the Japanese Classification are not staged as esophageal cancers, thus Siewert type II tumors are classified as gastric. The current interest in Japan is to create a new classification for Siewert type II tumors, and a prospective study is underway to define the optimal surgical approach (right thoracotomy vs. transhiatal approach and examining the extent of lymph node dissection) for these tumors.

Operative Treatment

Operative resection offers the only significant potential for cure of gastric cancer. Preoperative staging should demonstrate the extent of disease, define the patient's prognosis, and permit treatment planning. The type of surgery is then dependent upon tumor depth, growth pattern, and tumor location. Early gastric cancer confined to the mucosa (Tis or T1a) can be treated endoscopically with endoscopic mucosal resection (EMR). All other surgical resections are based on the location of the tumor and potential lymph node metastases, with the intent of microscopically negative surgical margins and clearance of the at-risk lymph node groups.

Endoscopic Mucosal Resection

Gastric adenocarcinoma confined to the mucosa (T1a lesions) has a very low rate of lymph node metastases (~2% to 6% for T1a disease). As such, if complete resection of these lesions is possible via an endoscopic

TABLE 10.1	TNM Classification of Carcinoma of the Stomach

Definition of Primary Tumor (T)

T Category	Criteria
Tx	Primary tumor cannot be assessed
T0	No evidence of primary tumor
Tis	Carcinoma in situ: intraepithelial tumor without invasion of the lamina propria, high-grade dysplasia
T1	Tumor invades the lamina propria, muscularis mucosae or submucosa
T1a	Tumor invades the lamina propria or muscularis mucosae
T1b	Tumor invades the submucosa
T2	Tumor invades muscularis propria[a]
T3	Tumor penetrates the subserosal connective tissue without invasion of the visceral peritoneum or adjacent structures[b,c]
T4	Tumor invades the serosa (visceral peritoneum) or adjacent structures[b,c]
T4a	Tumor invades the serosa (visceral peritoneum)
T4b	Tumor invades adjacent structures/organs

Definition of Regional Lymph Node (N)

N Category	Criteria
Nx	Regional lymph node(s) cannot be assessed
N0	No regional lymph node metastasis
N1	Metastasis in 1 or 2 regional lymph nodes
N2	Metastasis in 3–6 lymph nodes
N3	Metastasis in 7 or more regional lymph nodes
N3a	Metastasis in 7–15 regional lymph nodes
N3b	Metastasis in 16 or more regional lymph nodes

Definition of Distant Metastasis (M)

M Category	Criteria
M0	No distant metastasis
M1	Distant metastasis

Clinical (cTNM)

When T is...	And N is...	And M is...	Then the Stage Group is...
Tis	N0	M0	0
T1	N0	M0	I
T2	N0	M0	I
T1	N1, N2, or N3	M0	IIA
T2	N1, N2, or N3	M0	IIA
T3	N0	M0	IIB
T4a	N0	M0	IIB
T3	N1, N2, or N3	M0	III
T4a	N1, N2, or N3	M0	III
T4b	Any N	M0	IVA
Any T	Any N	M1	IVB

Pathologic (pTNM)

When T is...	And N is...	And M is...	Then the Stage Group is...
Tis	N0	M0	0
T1	N0	M0	IA
T1	N1	M0	IB
T2	N0	M0	IB
T1	N2	M0	IIA
T2	N1	M0	IIA
T3	N0	M0	IIA
T1	N3a	M0	IIB
T2	N2	M0	IIB

TABLE 10.1   TNM Classification of Carcinoma of the Stomach (Continued)

When T is...	And N is...	And M is...	Then the Stage Group is...
T3	N1	M0	IIB
T4a	N0	M0	IIB
T2	N3a	M0	IIIA
T3	N2	M0	IIIA
T4a	N1	M0	IIIA
T4a	N2	M0	IIIA
T4b	N0	M0	IIIA
T1	N3b	M0	IIIB
T2	N3b	M0	IIIB
T3	N3a	M0	IIIB
T4a	N3a	M0	IIIB
T4b	N1	M0	IIIB
T4b	N2	M0	IIIB
T3	N3b	M0	IIIC
T4a	N3b	M0	IIIC
T4b	N3a	M0	IIIC
T4b	N3b	M0	IIIC
Any T	Any N	M1	IV

Postneoadjuvant Therapy (ypTNM)

When T is...	And N is...	And M is...	Then the Stage Group is...
T1	N0	M0	I
T2	N0	M0	I
T1	N1	M0	I
T3	N0	M0	II
T2	N1	M0	II
T1	N2	M0	II
T4a	N0	M0	II
T3	N1	M0	II
T2	N2	M0	II
T1	N3	M0	II
T4a	N1	M0	III
T3	N2	M0	III
T2	N3	M0	III
T4b	N0	M0	III
T4b	N1	M0	III
T4a	N2	M0	III
T3	N3	M0	III

Postneoadjuvant Therapy (ypTNM)

When T is...	And N is...	And M is...	Then the Stage Group is...
T4b	N2	M0	III
T4b	N3	M0	III
T4a	N3	M0	III
Any T	Any N	M1	IV

[a]A tumor may penetrate the muscularis propria with extension into the gastrocolic or gastrohepatic ligaments, or into the greater or lesser omentum, without perforation of the visceral peritoneum covering these structures. In this case, the tumor is classified T3. If there is perforation of the visceral peritoneum covering the gastric ligaments or the omentum, the tumor should be classified as T4.
[b]The adjacent structures of the stomach include the spleen, transverse colon, liver, diaphragm, pancreas, abdominal wall, adrenal gland, kidney, small intestine, and retroperitoneum.
[c]Intramural extension to the duodenum or esophagus is not considered invasion of an adjacent structure, but is classified using the depth of the greatest invasion in any of these sites.
Note: A designation of pN0 should be used if all examined lymph nodes are negative, regardless of the total number removed and examined.
Adapted from Stomach. In: Amin MB, Edge SB, Greene FL, et al., eds. *AJCC Cancer Staging Manual*. 8th ed. Springer; 2017.
Used with permission of the American Joint Committee on Cancer (AJCC). The Original Source for This Material is the *AJCC Cancer Staging Manual*. 8th ed. Springer Science and Business Media LLC; 2017. www.springer.com

approach, acceptable locoregional disease control can be achieved with minimal morbidity. EMR, generally performed with a snare-based technique, has very well-defined indications proposed by the Japanese Gastroenterological Endoscopy Society and the Japanese Gastric Cancer Association. The standard indication for EMR is a well-differentiated tumor less than 2 cm in diameter confined to the mucosa without ulceration (T1a lesion). The expanded indications include nonulcerated, well-differentiated lesions greater than 2 cm in diameter; ulcerated, well-differentiated lesions less than 2 cm in diameter; and undifferentiated, nonulcerated T1a lesions less than 2 cm in diameter. When EMR is performed for lesions meeting the strict criteria of well-differentiated tumors without ulceration less than 2 cm in size confined to the mucosa, survival outcomes are excellent, similar to operative resection, on the order of 95% 5-year overall survival. Local recurrence rates are notably higher (approximately 6% vs. 1%) with EMR compared to standard surgical resection.

An alternative technique is endoscopic submucosal dissection (ESD), which was developed in Japan in the 1990s. In this approach, the submucosal tissue plane is identified and dissected en bloc from the muscular wall. A common approach involves injecting fluid into the luminal wall to separate out the layered tissue planes, followed by resection with an endoscopic knife or energy device. Indications for ESD include nonulcerated, differentiated T1a carcinomas greater than 2 cm in length; ulcerated, differentiated T1a carcinomas less than 3 cm in length; and nonulcerated, undifferentiated T1a carcinomas less than 2 cm in length. Local recurrence rates after ESD for appropriately selected patients is less than 1%, similar to surgical resection. In a recent meta-analysis comparing ESD to EMR, ESD was associated with higher rates of en bloc tumor resection (vs. piecemeal), higher rates of histologically complete resection, and a lower local recurrence rate. However, ESD is more costly, time-intensive, and is associated with a higher rate of gastric perforation.

While the advantages and outcomes of EMR and ESD for early T1a gastric cancer are attractive, they must be considered only in the appropriate clinical context. The reported experience is mostly from eastern Asia, where intense surveillance programs are in place and the incidence of early T1a gastric cancer is high. As such, experience with this complicated endoscopic technique is very robust in these countries. Gastric cancer is rarely diagnosed at such an early stage in Western countries lacking dedicated surveillance programs. The approach remains an option for treatment in very early-stage gastric cancer, but the appropriate endoscopic expertise and commitment to long-term follow-up are necessary.

Extent of Resection

Tumors involving the GEJ with the tumor epicenter no more than 2 cm into the proximal stomach are staged as esophageal cancers (Siewert type II). A margin-negative resection is the goal for treatment of these tumors. The operation to achieve complete resection may require an esophagogastrectomy, subtotal esophagectomy with resection of the proximal stomach, or total gastrectomy with resection of the distal esophagus, further described below. The approach can be abdominal, abdominothoracic, transhiatal, or transthoracic, via either an open or minimally invasive technique. Tumors at the GEJ and proximal stomach are treated via a multiteam approach at the MD Anderson Cancer Center. Siewert type I lesions that are associated with Barrett's esophagus or that are true esophageal cancers descending into the GEJ are typically treated with an esophagectomy. Siewert type II lesions lying within 2 cm of the squamocolumnar junction at the level of the cardia or type III lesions in the subcardia region of the stomach are usually treated with a total gastrectomy, with resection of the distal esophagus only to the extent needed to achieve negative margins. This is performed with input from both the thoracic and surgical oncology teams, usually via an open transabdominal approach. We favor this approach so that a D2 lymph node dissection including the greater curvature lymph nodes can be performed. We reported that extended (D1+D2) lymph node dissection, including celiac and hepatic artery lymph nodes, was associated with improved survival in patients with GEJ tumors who underwent resection after neoadjuvant treatment.

Tumors located in the body and antrum make up the remaining 65% to 70% of gastric cancers. The surgeon must decide whether to perform a distal, subtotal, or total gastrectomy in these patients on a case-by-case basis. As long as a margin-negative resection is performed, survival is equivalent among these operations. Quality of life and long-term nutrition status appears to be better in subtotal versus total gastrectomy. In candidates for subtotal gastrectomy, we favor whatever extent of resection is needed to achieve a gross 5-cm margin. An adequate remnant proximal gastric pouch needs to be present to consider a subtotal gastrectomy. We do not generally perform proximal subtotal gastrectomies with an esophagogastrostomy in more proximal body tumors in order to avoid postoperative alkaline reflux esophagitis.

Lymphadenectomy

The extent of lymphadenectomy has been a much debated topic in gastric cancer treatment over the last several decades. Japanese surgeons have espoused radical lymphadenectomy and meticulous pathologic analysis, with low perioperative morbidity and mortality. Western studies attempting to replicate these findings initially demonstrated alarmingly high rates of perioperative morbidity and mortality without survival benefit in extended lymphadenectomy. More recent data have supported more extensive lymphadenectomy for advanced disease, as long as it can be performed by experienced surgeons with good outcomes.

The Japanese definition of D1 or D2 lymph node dissection is complicated even after recent simplification. The extent of D1/D2 lymph node dissection changes based on the extent of gastrectomy, and D3 is no longer defined. An important update of the D1/D2 classification in the current Japanese Classification is that the left gastric artery lymph nodes (station 7) should be included in a D1 lymph node dissection in addition to perigastric lymph nodes, regardless of the procedure type or tumor location. The right paracardial lymph nodes (station 1) are also included in a D1 lymph node dissection in any tumor location or procedure type, whereas the left paracardial lymph nodes (station 2) and splenic hilar nodes (station 10) are not included in either a D1 or D2 dissection for distal tumors in the antrum or body that can be treated with distal subtotal gastrectomy. The description in national consensus guidelines defining D1/D2 lymph nodes is simple: D1 lymph nodes are defined as the perigastric lymph nodes in stations 1, 3, 5 (lesser curvature) and stations 2, 4, 6 (greater curvature), and D2 lymph nodes are defined as left gastric (station 7), common hepatic artery (station 8), celiac artery (station 9), splenic artery (station 11), and splenic hilar lymph nodes (station 10) (Fig. 10.1). A lymph node dissection is classified as D0, D1, or D2. D0 refers to an incomplete sampling of nodal stations. The extended D3 lymph node dissection, while it is no longer entitled as such, included further extent of lymphadenectomy such as resection of para-aortic (station 16) and retropancreatic (station 13) nodes.

The relevant clinical trials examining D1, D2, and D3 lymphadenectomies are summarized in Table 10.2. The Dutch and UK trials initially reported high perioperative morbidity, high pancreatectomy and splenectomy rates, and high perioperative mortality, without any survival benefit for D2 versus D1 lymphadenectomy. Long-term follow-up in the Dutch trial reported a statistically significant difference in overall survival, favoring D2 (15-year survival 29% vs. 21%). The Italian study, with strict quality control measures regarding definition of D1 and D2 dissections and the experience level of the participating surgeons, reported much lower perioperative morbidity and mortality rates, reassuring the medical community that experienced surgeons could perform extended lymphadenectomy for gastric cancer safely. The Italian data also suggested a survival

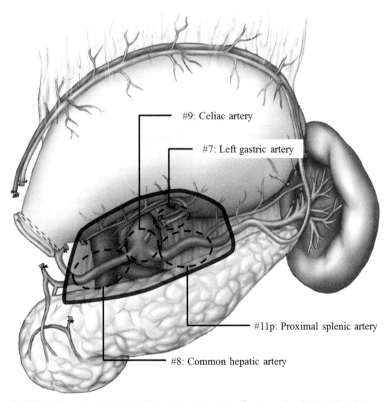

FIGURE 10.1 Lymph node stations for D2 lymph node dissection. (Courtesy of Paul F. Mansfield, MD.)

		Table 10.2 Summary of Clinical Trials Comparing Extent of Lymph Node Dissection in Gastric Cancer				

Author, Trial Name, Journal, Year	Comparison	Perioperative Mortality	Morbidity	5-yr Survival	Comments
Cuschieri, MRC Trial, Br J Cancer, 1999	D1 vs. D2	6.5% vs. 13%	28% vs. 46%	35% vs. 33%	Very high perioperative mortality, high rates of pancreatectomy and splenectomy in D2 group associated with morbidity and mortality
Bonenkamp, Dutch Trial, NEJM, 1999 (*Songun, Lancet Oncol, 2010)	D1 vs. D2	4% vs. 10%	25% vs. 43%	45% vs. 47% *15-yr survival showed difference (21% vs. 29%)	Incomplete lymph node dissection in 50% of D2 group, high rate of splenectomy and pancreatectomy
Sano, JCOG 9501, J Clin Oncol, 2004	D2 vs. D3	0.8% vs. 0.8%	21% vs. 28%	69% vs. 70%	D3—para-aortic lymph node dissection established that D2 could be performed with acceptable mortality/ morbidity
Wu, Taipei trial, Br J Surg, 2004	D1 vs. D2 + retropan-creas LN	Not reported	Not reported	61% vs. 54%	D3: D2 + retropancreatic lymph nodes.
Degiuli, Italian Gastric Cancer Study Group trial, Eur J of Surg Onc, 2004 (*Degliuli, BJS, 2015)	D1 vs. D2	3.0% vs. 2.2%	12% vs. 18%	67% vs. 64%	Survival benefit for D2 in patients with T2–4 and N+ disease (59% vs. 38%)

benefit in subgroups with advanced disease (T2–4 tumors with positive lymph nodes). The Japanese Clinical Oncology Group Study 9501 reported excellent perioperative outcomes for D2 and D3 lymphadenectomies, without long-term survival benefit from the addition of a D3 dissection of the para-aortic lymph nodes.

The interpretation and implementation of these trial findings can be complicated. A limited D1 lymphadenectomy may be sufficient for early-stage gastric cancer, particularly in low-volume centers that may have higher complication rates. A more extensive D2 lymphadenectomy may be performed in the hands of experienced gastric surgeons who can do so with limited morbidity and mortality. The additional resection of para-aortic lymph nodes is not necessary to improve locoregional disease control or survival. At MD Anderson Cancer Center, our standard approach is a D2 lymphadenectomy with emphasis on splenic preservation.

Splenectomy and En Bloc Multivisceral Resection

Splenectomy was once considered a part of D2 lymph node dissection in proximal gastric adenocarcinoma, however, it is associated with increased morbidity and mortality. It is of paramount importance not to perform splenectomy with a distal gastrectomy, as the loss of the short gastric vessels can make the remnant stomach ischemic and increase the risks of complications. The Japanese JCOG 0110 trial failed to a show survival benefit with splenectomy (and associated lymph node dissection of station 10) in patients with proximal gastric adenocarcinoma not invading the greater curvature. It is still controversial whether a splenectomy should be performed (or station 10 lymphadenectomy) in tumors located at the proximal greater curvature, but based on currently available evidence, the spleen should be preserved unless directly involved. At MD Anderson, splenectomy is not performed unless the tumor adheres to or invades the spleen or its vascular supply.

Locally advanced tumors which invade adjacent structures are classified as T4b lesions. Resection of the involved organs in an effort to achieve negative R0 margins is acceptable if the patient can tolerate such an extensive operation. Lymph node metastases are common with locally invasive disease; they are present on the order of 60% to 90%. Perioperative morbidity increases with the extent of resection, with the highest complications being associated with concomitant pancreatectomy, although perioperative mortality is similar in patients who do and do not undergo multivisceral resections. If the patient is physically fit to undergo an extensive operation, has no evidence of metastatic disease, and an R0 resection is expected, we perform a multivisceral resection in locally advanced disease.

Operative Technique

Staging Laparoscopy and Enteral Access

Diagnostic laparoscopy is performed in newly diagnosed patients without radiographic evidence of systemic or peritoneal metastases. The procedure is usually performed as an outpatient and a vascular port is also placed in anticipation of systemic chemotherapy. Either a closed optical trocar or open technique can be used to obtain laparoscopic access. The stomach, peritoneal lining, and the rest of the visceral organs are visually inspected in a systematic fashion. Any suspicious lesions are biopsied and sent for permanent pathologic analysis. One liter of normal saline is instilled into the right and left upper quadrants, then evacuated and collected for cytologic analysis.

If the patient has evidence of malnutrition, based on nutrition labs or precipitous weight loss, a poor performance status that is expected to decline during systemic chemotherapy treatments, or evidence of near complete or complete gastric outlet obstruction prohibiting adequate oral intake, a jejunostomy feeding tube is placed at the time of staging laparoscopy. A location at least 20 cm past the ligament of Treitz is chosen at a point that easily reaches the abdominal wall. When a feeding tube is placed, the patient is admitted to the hospital while tube feeds are initiated, and patient education is performed.

Total Gastrectomy

Our approach for a total gastrectomy begins with an upper midline incision that extends to or below the umbilicus (Fig. 10.2). The greater omentum is separated from the transverse colon up to and including the short gastric vessels (Fig. 10.3). While the perigastric lymph nodes in the greater omentum are resected en bloc, the more inferior portion of the omentum is preserved to form an omental pedicle flap. Dissection around the GEJ is performed, starting at the right crus and then progressing over to the left crus anterior to the esophagus. The GEJ is encircled with a Penrose drain, mobilizing 7 to 8 cm of the distal esophagus to ensure an adequate proximal margin. The vagus nerves may be divided to provide additional mobilization. The right gastroepiploic vessels are ligated at their origin, and the subpyloric nodes are resected with the specimen. The first portion of the duodenum is mobilized and divided 2 cm distal to the pylorus with a stapling device (Fig. 10.4). The gastrohepatic ligament is opened, and the left gastric artery is ligated at its origin. A replaced or accessory left hepatic artery may originate from the left gastric artery and reside in the gastrohepatic ligament and should be preserved. A

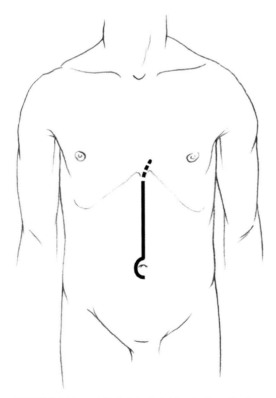

FIGURE 10.2 Upper midline incision for total gastrectomy. (Courtesy of Paul F. Mansfield, MD.)

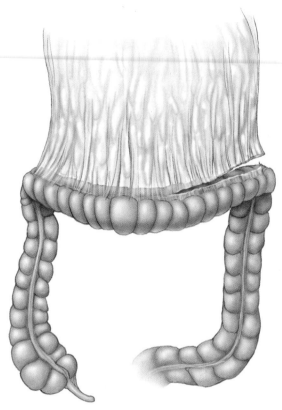

FIGURE 10.3 Mobilization of the omentum off of the transverse colon. (Courtesy of Paul F. Mansfield, MD.)

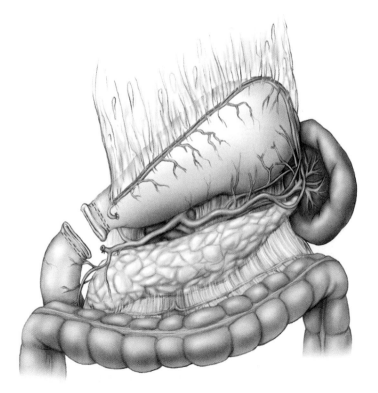

FIGURE 10.4 Division of the duodenum for total gastrectomy, 2 cm distal to the pylorus. (Courtesy of Paul F. Mansfield, MD.)

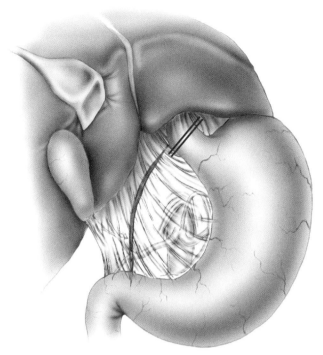

FIGURE 10.5 Division of the esophagus for total gastrectomy, 2 to 3 cm proximal to the gastroesophageal junction. (Courtesy of Paul F. Mansfield, MD.)

vascular clamp is placed across the esophagus, then the esophagus is divided either sharply or with cautery 2 to 3 cm proximal to the GEJ, and the specimen is passed off the field for frozen section evaluation of the margins (Fig. 10.5). Full-thickness stay sutures are placed to prevent the esophageal mucosa from retracting proximally. The hepatic, celiac, and splenic lymph node packets are then dissected and passed off separately to complete the D2 lymphadenectomy. If the tumor adheres to the spleen, pancreas, liver, diaphragm, colon, or mesocolon, the involved organ or organs are removed en bloc.

The most frequent reconstruction used is a Roux-en-Y anastomosis (Fig. 10.6). If a significant portion of the distal esophagus is resected, a left thoracoabdominal or right thoracotomy incision (Ivor Lewis approach) may be necessary. A 60-cm Roux limb is created and passed in a retrocolic fashion. The enteroenterostomy is performed. A hand-sewn single-layer esophagojejunostomy is performed with interrupted sutures. The previously preserved omentum is wrapped around the anastomosis. If available, a falciform patch is placed over the transected duodenal stump. No drain is placed. A feeding jejunostomy tube is placed 10 to 20 cm distal to the jejunojenal for postoperative nutritional support.

Subtotal Gastrectomy

The mobilization for subtotal gastrectomy is identical to that for total gastrectomy described in the preceding section, except that the short gastric vessels are preserved and only approximately 75% to 80% of the distal stomach is resected. A gross 5-cm margin is obtained proximal to the tumor. The small pouch of stomach that remains is supplied by the remaining short gastric vessels and the posterior gastric artery arising from the splenic artery. We often use Roux-en-Y reconstruction after subtotal gastrectomy, although a loop gastrojejunostomy (Billroth II) or less frequently a gastroduodenostomy (Billroth I) may be employed.

Laparoscopic Resection

Data continue to emerge that laparoscopic resection for gastric cancer is safe and oncologically sound. The technique was first attempted in distal gastrectomies for early gastric cancer, with promising results regarding patient-reported outcomes. The KLASS-01 trial randomized 1,416 patients with clinical stage I (T1N0, T1N1, or T2aN0) gastric adenocarcinoma to either laparoscopic-assisted or open distal gastrectomy. Long-term results demonstrated no significant difference in perioperative morbidity and mortality (5-year cancer-specific survival 97% for both groups, $P = .91$).

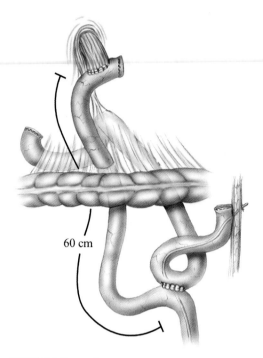

FIGURE 10.6 Roux-en-Y reconstruction for total gastrectomy, with jejunostomy feeding tube. (Courtesy of Paul F. Mansfield, MD.)

Now data are accumulating regarding the safety of minimally invasive approaches in advanced gastric cancers. Several meta-analyses have reported short-term outcomes that favor laparoscopic over open approaches in advanced gastric cancer. Long-term results from the KLASS-02 trial, a trial examining laparoscopic versus open distal gastrectomy with D2 lymphadenectomy for patients with advanced (T2–4aN0–3) gastric adenocarcinoma, report no differences in 3-year relapse-free survival (81% for open surgery, 80% for laparoscopy, $P=.726$). However, open surgery was associated with a significantly higher rate of short- and long-term complications.

Some additional randomized trials have been performed. The STOMACH trial was a European study of 13 hospitals that randomized patients with gastric cancer to minimally invasive versus open total gastrectomy. Median number of retrieved nodes was 43 and 41 for open and minimally invasive surgery, respectively ($P=.617$). One-year survival was 90% for open surgery and 85% for minimally invasive surgery ($P=.701$). The authors concluded that minimally invasive surgery was not inferior to standard open total gastrectomy. The LOGICA study similarly evaluated laparoscopic versus open gastrectomy

As experience with the technique grows and the technical aspects of the procedure are refined, laparoscopic resection for gastric cancer is being performed more frequently in both the East and West. Nonetheless, optimization of the minimally invasive approach remains under investigation. In particular, while circular stapling and flexible stapling devices may make this operation technically feasible, there is some controversy over the safety of the esophagojejunostomy when laparoscopic total gastrectomies are performed. The use of this technique is dependent on the surgeon's minimally invasive skills. Longer-term oncologic outcomes evaluating locoregional disease control and survival will have to be assessed before laparoscopic resection becomes more widely utilized.

Robotic Resection

There has been a trend toward the use of minimally invasive techniques for gastrointestinal surgery over the last three decades, primarily the use of laparoscopy. However, robotic technology for surgical applications has drastically improved over the last two decades, and this has been associated with wider adoption and expanded surgical indications, often replacing conventional laparoscopy. Much of the early adaptation for robotic surgery occurred with gynecologic and urologic procedures focused in the pelvis, a challenging location where structures can be difficult to visualize and manipulate due to limited operative angles. Robotic platforms are particularly useful in this context due to enhanced camera visualization and increased dexterity with jointed instruments.

Like the pelvis, the foregut is another location, particularly near the esophageal hiatus, where visualization and tissue manipulation can be challenging and lends itself to the advantages of a robotic platform. Robotic gastrectomy is a new technique performed primarily at tertiary centers within the last 10 years. The largest trial evaluating robotic gastrectomy to date was performed by Kim et al. in South Korea. They recently completed a prospective, multicenter study comparing laparoscopic versus robotic total gastrectomy in which 223 and 211 patients underwent robotic and laparoscopic gastrectomy, respectively. There was no difference in complication rates (11.9% robotic, 10.3% laparoscopic), though operative time was significantly longer and costs higher in the robotic group. Survival data has not yet been reported.

Although there is limited supporting data, robotic gastrectomy is likely to become a commonly used technique for the surgical management of gastric adenocarcinoma, and further studies are necessary to evaluate its safety and long-term survival outcome measures compared to laparoscopic and open techniques.

Surgical Outcomes

Complications

Complications from gastric cancer resection are similar to other major abdominal operations and include bleeding, infection, cardiac and pulmonary issues, and venous thromboembolism. The rates of major and minor complications are approximately 20% to 30% and 40% to 45% in our most recent series. One of the most potentially devastating complications is an anastomotic leak, which occurs in 2% to 15% of patients. Leaks can occur late in the postoperative course, including after the patient has been discharged home and is presumably doing well; therefore, continued vigilance is necessary. Endoscopic techniques, such as the use of covered stents over anastomotic leaks, have been described to manage leaks with good outcomes. Our approach to anastomotic leaks is to attempt to manage conservatively with adequate drainage using percutaneous drains, endoscopic stenting, and nutritional support with jejunostomy feedings. Complications may have long-term effects on oncologic outcomes, thus further emphasizing the need for high-quality, comprehensive care of these patients in experienced centers. With improved anesthesia, preoperative risk stratification, perioperative care, and early recognition and rescue of complications, perioperative mortality has improved after gastrectomy. In the most recent MD Anderson experience, the 90-day perioperative mortality was 3%.

Oral feeding is typically started 4 to 7 days postoperatively, often after return of bowel function. Supplemental jejunostomy feedings are started the day after surgery and continued until oral intake is adequate, which usually occurs after discharge. Upper gastrointestinal tract contrast studies are performed on the basis of clinical indications only (e.g., fever, tachycardia, and tachypnea). A total gastrectomy drastically changes the patient's eating habits. A significant proportion of patients will eventually eat regular meals plus snacks, but this will take time. Patients are counseled preoperatively that their eating habits will never return completely back to their preoperative baseline. Within several months, most patients are able to increase their oral intake capacity and eat larger meals less frequently (three or four meals per day). We utilize nutritional support from registered dieticians heavily in both the immediate postoperative course and in the long-term follow-up for these patients. About 10% of patients will develop clinically significant dumping syndrome. Early dumping typically occurs 15 to 30 minutes after a meal; signs and symptoms include diaphoresis, abdominal cramps, palpitations, and watery diarrhea. Late dumping is usually associated with hypoglycemia and hyperinsulinemia. The medical management for dumping symptoms should include dietary modification (increased fiber diet, avoidance of concentrated sweets, and avoidance of hyperosmolar liquids) and, if refractory, a somatostatin analog.

Survival

Overall 5-year survival in patients with gastric cancer in most Western series, including the most recent AJCC staging report, is approximately 30%. The survival rates clearly change for patients with localized versus nodal or metastatic disease. Five-year survival for patients with gastric cancer localized to the stomach is approximately 70%, while patients with nodal disease only have an approximately 32% 5-year survival. Survival in reports from Japan and Asia is usually higher, thought to be related to differences in stage, epidemiologic factors, tumor biology, and medical comorbidities.

The differences in outcomes in Eastern and Western series have been studied extensively to discern to what extent patient factors, treatment factors, and early-screening factors play a role in the different outcomes. In a direct comparison of two series from US and Korea, Strong et al. found significant differences in age, BMI, site of tumor (more proximal in the United States), early-stage tumors (more common in Korea), and higher number of lymph nodes identified in Korean patients. After multivariable analysis, the disease-specific survival was still significantly better in Korean patients. The authors noted that it was likely that lower node positivity and early-stage tumors accounted for the differences in disease-specific survival. Outcomes in patients of Asian descent treated in US were compared to Caucasians in a recent SEER analysis, which also found that after controlling for relevant risk factors and treatment differences, survival remained higher for patients of Asian descent compared to Caucasian patients.

Locoregional recurrence rates after R0 resection for gastric adenocarcinoma remain high. Recurrence patterns are complex and often involve multiple regions, typically classified as locoregional, distant, or peritoneal. Recurrence patterns may be affected by treatment strategy, such as use of preoperative therapies. Data from MD Anderson demonstrated that in patients treated with neoadjuvant therapy, the most common recurrence sites after potentially curative gastrectomy are peritoneal, followed by locoregional, and liver metastases. Most (~80%) recurrences will occur within 2 years after resection. Median survival after recurrence is a dismal 6 months.

Adjuvant Therapy

Patients with localized node-negative gastric cancer have excellent outcomes in both Western and Eastern series with a favorable chance at durable cure. Lymph node involvement decreases 5-year survival rates by as much as 10% to 30%. Unfortunately, recurrence develops in most patients who undergo potentially curative resection for gastric cancer. Recurrence patterns are variable (as discussed above), but often involve nonlocoregional failure, for which the only reasonable strategy would be systemic chemotherapy. Adjuvant therapy after potentially curative R0 resection has been studied in numerous patients, with particular interest in improving outcomes for high-risk node-positive patients.

Adjuvant Chemotherapy

Randomized trials investigating the effects of adjuvant chemotherapy alone on survival after complete resection of gastric adenocarcinoma have produced inconsistent results. Some of the more recent trials are summarized in Table 10.3. The JCOG 8801 trial of adjuvant 5-FU–based chemotherapy showed no survival benefit in early-stage (T1 and T2) gastric cancers. The ACTS-GC trial from Sakuramoto et al. later demonstrated a survival benefit with an adjuvant oral fluoropyrimidine-based therapy in stage II or III gastric cancer after D2 lymphadenectomy. The CLASSIC study from South Korea, China, and Taiwan compared D2 gastrectomy alone to D2 gastrectomy plus adjuvant capecitabine/oxaliplatin and reported a modest improvement in overall and disease-free survival. In the CLASSIC trial, subgroup analysis showed that the survival benefit was limited to node-positive patients. Meta-analyses of the available adjuvant trials have demonstrated a modest benefit to adjuvant chemotherapy when compared to surgery alone.

Adjuvant Chemoradiation Therapy

Radiation treatment is added to adjuvant therapy regimens in an effort to improve locoregional disease control. Radiation therapy is usually combined with a sensitizing chemotherapy agent such as 5-FU. Radiation alone without any chemotherapy, sensitizing, or otherwise, is rarely used outside of the palliative setting. The Southwest Oncology Group national intergroup trial (INT-0116) established the data supporting adjuvant chemoradiation after resection for GEJ or gastric adenocarcinoma. Median overall survival was improved from 27 to 36 months compared to surgery alone. Criticisms of the trial raised concern that most patients underwent what would be considered an inadequate lymph node dissection and perhaps the radiation therapy was simply making up for inadequate surgery; 54% underwent a "D0" dissection. Subsequent reports with longer follow-up continue to support the long-term survival benefit of adjuvant chemoradiation versus surgery alone in the trial.

The ARTIST trial from Korea improved upon the INT-0116 trial in two important areas: (1) operative quality was controlled, with all patients undergoing standard D2 lymphadenectomy and (2) the control arm was treated with systemic cisplatin-based chemotherapy. The initial report and subsequent follow-up report found no difference in disease-free or overall survival between adjuvant chemo alone and adjuvant chemoradiation. However, subgroup analysis found that patients with node-positive disease and intestinal-type pathology had improved disease-free survival with the addition of adjuvant radiation therapy. These findings formed the basis for the next ARTIST trial, which is essentially a repeat of the original ARTIST trial, but limited to node-positive patients.

The CRITICS trial took a combined perioperative approach to treatment. All patients received neoadjuvant chemotherapy and gastric resection. Postoperatively, patients received either chemotherapy alone or chemoradiation. The initial report shows no difference in 5-year overall survival between the two groups (41.3% vs. 40.9%). However, postoperative treatment in this study was significantly limited by substantial patient drop out. Adjuvant therapy was hampered by unresectability at the time of surgery (~18% of all patients

TABLE 10.3	Randomized Controlled Trials of Perioperative Treatment of Gastric Cancer

Author, Trial Name, Journal, Year	Country	Treatment	Survival Difference	Indication	Tumor location: % Esophageal % EGJ	% of D2 LND % of R0	% of pT1 Patients	% of pN0 Patients
Al-Batran, FLOT4, Lancet 2019	Germany	Pre + postop ECF/ECX (3 cycles) vs. Pre + postop FLOT (4 cycles)	5-yr OS 36% vs. 45%	c-Stage T2 or higher, cN+ or higher, M0	Eso: 0% EGJ: 56%	53%/57% (ECF/ECX vs. FLOT) 78%/85% (ECF/ECX vs. FLOT)	15% vs. 25% (ECF/ECX vs. FLOT)	41% vs. 49% (ECF/ECX vs. FLOT)
Cunningham, MAGIC, NEJM 2006	UK	Pre + postop CTx vs. surgery only	5-yr OS 38% vs. 11%	c-Stage II/III excluding cT1	Eso: 15% EGJ: 12%	41% 66%[b] (surgery) 60%[b] (chemo)	8% (surgery) 16% (chemo)	27% (surgery) 31% (chemo)
Ychou, FNCLCC/FCD, JCO 2011	France	Pre + postop CTx vs. surgery only	5-yr OS 38% vs. 24%	All curatively resectable pts	Eso: 11% EGJ: 64%	NA (D2 rec'd) 74% (surgery) 84% (chemo)	[c]32% (surgery) 42% (chemo)	20% (surgery) 33% (chemo)
Macdonald, INT-0116, NEJM 2001	USA	Postop CRTx vs. surgery only	3-yr OS 50% vs. 41%	Stage IB/II/III	Eso: 0% EGJ: 20%	10% (54% D0) 100%	NA (pT1–3 31%)	15%
Bang, CLASSIC, Lancet 2012	Korea China Taiwan	Postop CTx vs. surgery only	3-yr OS 83% vs. 78%	Stage II/III	Eso: 0% EGJ: 2%	100% 100%	1%	10%
[a]Lee, ARTIST, JCO 2012	Korea	Postop CTx vs. CRTx	3-yr DFS[a] 74% vs.78%	Stage IB/II/III excluding T2N0	Eso: 0% EGJ: NA	100% 100%	22%	31%
Sakuramoto, ACTS-GC, NEJM 2007	Japan	Postop CTx vs. surgery only	3-yr OS 80% vs. 70%	Stage II/III excluding T1	Eso: 0% EGJ: NA	100% 100%	0%	11%
[a]Nakajima, JCOG 8801 Lancet 1999	Japan	Postop CTx vs. surgery only	5-yr OS[a] 86% vs. 83%	c-Stage IB/II/III	Eso: 0% EGJ: NA	NA 100%[b]	33%	53%

[a]No difference in survival.
[b]Curative surgery rate.
[c]Rate of pT0-2, NA: not documented.
Stage is adjusted to AJCC 8th definition. Stage IB: T1N1, T2N0, Stage II: T1N2, T2N1, T3N0.

underwent a palliative gastrectomy at time of planned resection), early postoperative progression, worsening of overall health (~20%), and approximately 20% of patients who refused additional therapy. Further, the doses of adjuvant chemotherapy were decreased to below 80% to 90% of recommended doses. Per-protocol post hoc analysis demonstrated higher 5-year survival with adjuvant chemotherapy over chemoradiotherapy (57.9% vs. 45.5%). More studies are needed to define the patient population that might benefit from adjuvant chemoradiation therapy.

Neoadjuvant Therapy

The use of neoadjuvant chemotherapy in the treatment of gastric cancer evolved from preoperative treatment strategies used for esophageal and rectal cancers. There are several potential advantages of neoadjuvant therapy for gastric cancer. These include theoretical biologic advantages (decreased tumor seeding at surgery) and the opportunity to assess in vivo tumor sensitivity to a particular chemotherapeutic regimen. If the tumor responds to the neoadjuvant therapy, the same treatment can be continued postoperatively. Another theoretical advantage is an improved R0 resection rate due to tumor consolidation and decrease in size. By giving chemotherapy upfront before an operation, oncologists can avoid issues with patients' inability to tolerate timely chemotherapy due to deconditioning, malnutrition, or other postoperative complications after operative resection. Micrometastatic disease, which is ultimately the cause of death from gastric cancer, is addressed early, prior to development of macroscopic disease spread. Finally, the interval required for neoadjuvant therapy provides a time in which progression of disease can be evaluated to identify patients with aggressive disease who would not benefit from operative resection, thus sparing them the morbidity of surgical resection when no benefit in quality of life or life prolongation would be provided by surgery. An advantage specific to preoperative radiation therapy is a smaller treatment area and displacement of uninvolved contiguous structures by the intact tumor, both leading to reduced radiation therapy toxicity.

There are potential disadvantages to a neoadjuvant treatment strategy. One potential is that patients with initially resectable primary tumors may progress during therapy rendering them unresectable. Whether this is simply a reflection of extremely aggressive disease as most believe or an actual loss of window of opportunity is impossible to discern. It is also possible that the toxicity from preoperative treatment may delay operative intervention or increase surgical morbidity. Finally, there is a risk of overtreating patients with early-stage disease, although improved pretreatment staging with EUS minimizes this risk.

Neoadjuvant Chemotherapy

Various combinations of etoposide, cisplatin, 5-FU (ECF), and doxorubicin as neoadjuvant treatment for gastric cancer have been evaluated in several trials. Clinical response rates have ranged from 21% to 31%, with complete pathologic response rates ranging from 0% to 15%. Multivariable analysis of three phase II trials of neoadjuvant therapy at MD Anderson identified response to neoadjuvant chemotherapy as the single most important predictor of overall survival after treatment for gastric cancer.

Survival results of the UK Medical Research Council Adjuvant Gastric Infusion Chemotherapy (MAGIC) trial were reported in 2006. In this multi-institutional, prospective, randomized trial, 503 patients with stage II or higher gastric cancer were randomized to receive perioperative chemotherapy (preoperative chemotherapy followed by surgery followed by additional postoperative chemotherapy) or to undergo surgery alone. Those randomized to the perioperative treatment arm received three cycles of ECF, followed by surgery and then three additional postoperative cycles of ECF. While completion of the preoperative therapy was a respectable 88%, only 42% of patients completed the postoperative portion of treatment even though they were allowed up to 12 weeks after surgery to begin. Both progression-free survival and overall survival were improved in the treatment arm; 5-year survival was 36% in the treatment plus surgery group and 23% in the surgery-only group. Despite these promising results, the MAGIC trial is not without some criticism. First, the trial included patients with distal esophageal cancers, which may affect the external validity when applied to pure gastric cancer. Second, the staging in this trial may have been suboptimal due to lack of EUS or staging laparoscopy. Finally, only 40% of patients had a D2 lymph node resection. The findings of the French FNCLCC/FFCD trial were similar. In this trial, patients with GEJ or gastric adenocarcinoma were randomized to two or three preoperative cycles of 5-FU and cisplatin, followed by surgery and three to four postoperative cycles, or surgery alone. Five-year overall survival favored the chemotherapy and surgery group compared to surgery alone (38% vs. 24%). This trial was confounded by a high number of GEJ and esophageal tumors (~75% of the study), so the generalizability of its findings to purely gastric adenocarcinoma is unclear.

Of course, the preceding studies did not address whether chemotherapy given in a strictly neoadjuvant setting improves survival, as the treatments were considered perioperative therapy with cycles given both before and after operative resection. The EORTC 40954 trial attempted to address that question, comparing neoadjuvant 5-FU/cisplatin and surgery to surgery alone in locally advanced gastric and GEJ adenocarcinoma. The trial was stopped early for poor accrual; no survival difference was demonstrated in the limited results. Interesting findings from the trial include increased R0 rates in the neoadjuvant group (82% vs. 67%), more lymph node metastases identified in the surgery alone group (77% vs. 61%), and a nonsignificant trend toward greater postoperative morbidity in the neoadjuvant group (27% vs. 16%).

In the German FLOT4 trial, patients with T2 category or higher or node-positive gastric or GEJ adenocarcinoma were randomized to perioperative treatment with ECF/ECX (etoposide, cisplatin, and capecitabine) or FLOT (fluorouracil, leucovorin, oxaliplatin, and docetaxel). The ECF/ECX arm received six cycles of chemotherapy (three preoperative and three postoperative), whereas the FLOT arm received four preoperative and four postoperative cycles. Overall, survival was significantly higher in the FLOT group, with a median overall survival of 50 months in the FLOT group compared to 35 months in the ECF/ECX group. Notably, FLOT was also associated with a significantly improved margin-negative resection rate (85% vs. 78%).

Neoadjuvant Chemoradiation

Radiation alone is rarely given in the neoadjuvant setting. Most studies report experience with the combination of chemotherapy and radiation therapy in the neoadjuvant setting. The general approach to gastric adenocarcinoma at MD Anderson includes neoadjuvant chemoradiation therapy except in select patients with early-stage, localized cancers. This approach has been built on the basis of our early experiences with 5-FU–based chemoradiation therapy published in the 2000s.

In 2004, Ajani et al. demonstrated that with a three-step multimodal approach consisting of induction chemotherapy (5-FU, leucovorin and cisplatin) followed by chemoradiation therapy (45 Gy plus concurrent 5-FU) then gastrectomy, a complete pathologic response can be achieved in 30% of cases. The R0 resection rate in the series was 70%. At a median follow-up of 50 months, the median survival was 33.7 months, and 2-year survival rate was 54%.

Ajani et al. then reported a prospective, nonrandomized study of preoperative paclitaxel-based chemo-radiation therapy. The neoadjuvant regimen was two cycles of 5-FU, cisplatin, and paclitaxel for 28 days, followed by chemoradiation therapy. All patients underwent gastrectomy with spleen preserving D2 lymph-adenectomy after radiographic and endoscopic restaging. At the time of analysis, 78% of patients had under-gone an R0 resection, 20% had a complete pathologic response, and 15% had a partial pathologic response. In this study, R0 resection, pathologic complete response, pathologic partial response, and postsurgical T and N status were factors associated with overall survival. This was followed by a second multi-institutional study evaluating two cycles of 5-FU, leucovorin, and cisplatin followed by concurrent radiation and chemotherapy (infusional 5-FU and weekly paclitaxel). The pathologic complete response rate was 26% with an R0 resection rate of 77%. Pathologic response was a major determinant of outcome.

In a recent experience at MD Anderson with neoadjuvant chemoradiation therapy for gastric cancer, we reported a series of 195 patients receiving either induction chemotherapy followed by chemoradiation (79%) or chemoradiation alone (21%) followed by gastrectomy with curative intent. An R0 resection was achieved in 93% of patients, and a complete pathologic response was demonstrated in 20% of patients. Median overall survival was 5.8 years. Nodal status was the most important independent predictor of overall survival. This strategy of preoperative chemotherapy or chemoradiation therapy followed by resection is effective and well tolerated by patients. Concerns about increased postoperative morbidity or failure to continue on to resec-tion are not apparent in our results. The rates of 90-day major and minor complications and mortality are no different in patients undergoing upfront surgery, neoadjuvant chemotherapy, or neoadjuvant chemoradiation therapy. Preoperative therapy is completed by 81% of patients undergoing chemotherapy alone and 93% of patients undergoing chemoradiation. Toxicities from chemotherapy (2%) and chemoradiation (6%) rarely result in the inability to undergo operative resection. In approximately 25% of patients, progressive, unre-sectable, or metastatic disease is identified during preoperative therapy—this is a subset of patients that was spared the morbidity of a noncurative operation.

In a more recent analysis that combined patients treated at MD Anderson with those at H. Lee Moffitt Can-cer Center, patients undergoing neoadjuvant chemotherapy were compared to neoadjuvant chemotherapy plus chemoradiation. Comparison of 113 propensity-matched patients demonstrated higher rates of complete pathologic response to therapy (15% vs. 4%) with the addition of chemoradiation, as well as longer disease-free survival (45 months with chemotherapy vs. 113 months with the addition of chemoradiation). Overall survival was 130 months with chemotherapy plus chemoradiation, versus 53 months with chemotherapy alone.

Metastatic Disease

Up to 40% of patients will have metastatic disease at the time of their initial presentation, and an additional subset will be deemed unresectable based on local tumor advancement or patient comorbidities. These patients are thus treated not with curative intent but with the goal of symptom relief and palliation to improve not only the duration of their remaining life but the quality as well. Furthermore, a sizable number of patients will recur after definitive surgical resection with metastatic disease and are thus incurable. Palliation is an essential set of skills that must be mastered by physicians regularly treating gastric cancer. Optimal palliation relieves symptoms while causing minimal morbidity and improving the patient's quality of life. Prolonged survival is generally not a goal of palliative treatment, but palliation may relieve debilitating and potentially life-threatening problems, such as gastrointestinal bleeding or gastric outlet obstruction, which may impact short-term survival.

Nonoperative Palliation

Systemic chemotherapy can be offered with palliative intent in patients with metastatic or recurrent gastric cancer. Chemotherapy is associated with prolonged survival, with more benefit from combination therapy compared to single-agent 5-FU. Aggressive palliative chemotherapy regimens must be balanced with patient expectations, side effects, and expected improvements in quality of life. For example, radiation therapy can be used to reduce bleeding from unresectable, advanced gastric cancer. Malignant ascites are often a source of patient discomfort and distress in advanced gastric cancer. Repeat therapeutic paracenteses can be performed, possibly with the aid of an indwelling catheter, in certain clinical scenarios to give the patient control of managing these symptoms.

Operative Palliation

Operative palliation for advanced gastric cancer may involve minimally invasive endoscopic approaches to provide symptomatic decompression or to relieve obstruction. Operative palliative resection, including palliative total or subtotal gastrectomy, may have a role in carefully selected patients. A thorough understanding of the patient's symptoms, goals, expectations, and systemic therapy options is necessary to decide on the most appropriate approach to operative palliation.

Palliation with endoscopic techniques may be appropriate for patients with peritoneal disease, hepatic metastases, extensive nodal metastases, or ascites and for patients with problems that include bleeding or gastric obstruction. Both morbidity and mortality from these seemingly minimal risk procedures are relatively high in these patients and must be discussed carefully. Laser recanalization or simple dilatation with or without stent placement can be used to treat gastric outlet obstruction. Repeat endoscopy may be required at periodic intervals. Stenting may be used at the GEJ or in distal tumors. Operative gastrojejunostomy is sometimes necessary to adequately address the obstruction and provide symptom relief. A venting gastrostomy tube, placed by either interventional radiology or endoscopy, may be useful for distal gastric outlet obstructions. Laparoscopic hyperthermic intraperitoneal chemotherapy (HIPEC) may be considered to palliate debilitating malignant ascites.

The selection of patients for palliative gastrectomy is complex. In patients with an excellent performance status, experienced surgeons can perform palliative distal gastrectomy with minimal morbidity and acceptable mortality rates. Palliative total gastrectomy and esophagogastrectomy, however, should be approached with great caution because the morbidity from these procedures is higher. Median survival is less than 1 year in most studies examining palliative gastric resection. Symptom resolution may be achieved in less than 50% of patients undergoing palliative gastrectomy and additional procedures are often necessary to control evolving symptoms.

Hyperthermic Intraperitoneal Chemotherapy

Due to the tendency of gastric cancer to form peritoneal metastases, local therapy with HIPEC with or without cytoreduction has been attempted to either prevent or treat this unique, somewhat localized form of metastatic disease. The technique can be applied to two clinical situations with different treatment goals: (1) a combined cytoreductive surgery (CRS) with HIPEC can be performed at the time of gastrectomy to render a patient with existing macroscopic peritoneal metastases disease free, or (2) HIPEC can be performed at the time of gastrectomy in an adjuvant setting to reduce the risk of peritoneal recurrence in situations in which there is no macroscopic or microscopic evidence of peritoneal metastases, but the primary tumor penetrates the serosa and is considered high risk.

CRS-HIPEC for Metastatic Disease

CRS-HIPEC in combination with gastrectomy for M1 disease localized to the peritoneum should only be considered in carefully selected patients with low-volume peritoneal disease. Peritonectomy is associated with high rates of postoperative morbidity and mortality, so the risk and benefits of aggressive cytoreduction must be weighed carefully. A complete cytoreduction is associated with improved survival over an incomplete one, thus the procedure should only be undertaken in patients with a low peritoneal cancer index (PCI). Mitomycin C or oxaliplatin-based regimens have been described. The addition of HIPEC to a cytoreduction alone does appear to improve overall survival in patients with peritoneal metastases without an increase in postoperative morbidity according to a randomized clinical trial reported by Yang et al. Reported 5-year survival rates in most series are still relatively low, in the range of 10% to 30%. However, theses survival rates must be considered in the context of other patients with M1, stage IV gastric cancer.

One of the initial concerns regarding CRS-HIPEC in combination with gastrectomy was the potential for procedural morbidity and mortality, given the severity of intervention. This led to trialing techniques that space out procedures, one approach being neoadjuvant laparoscopic HIPEC (LS-HIPEC) to potentially reduce the volume of peritoneal disease. At MD Anderson, we have performed several studies to better clarify the role of LS-HIPEC for carefully selected patients. In a phase II trial, we performed neoadjuvant LS-HIPEC in 19 patients with peritoneal disease (6 with positive cytology only). Patients who experienced resolution of their peritoneal disease were then treated with gastrectomy. LS-HIPEC was associated with complications in 11% of patients, 0% mortality, while median overall survival was 20 months, and 3-year overall survival was 44%.

In a follow-up retrospective analysis, 25 patients were treated with LS-HIPEC and compared to 27 patients treated with standard of care systemic therapy. Gastrectomy was performed in 28% of LS-HIPEC patients after clearance of peritoneal disease, while no patients in the standard of care group progressed to resection of the primary. Median overall survival for LS-HIPEC was 24.7 months compared to 21.3 months for chemotherapy alone ($P = .08$). Among patients treated with LS-HIPEC and gastrectomy, median overall survival was improved to 25.3 months ($P = .05$ compared to standard of care chemotherapy).

More recently, the Japanese Intraperitoneal Chemotherapy Study Group performed a trial of intraperitoneal paclitaxel administered via an abdominal port combined with intravenous paclitaxel (PHOENIX-GC Trial). 114 patients received intravenous paclitaxel plus tegafur/gimeracil/oteracil (S1) and intraperitoneal paclitaxel compared to 50 patients receiving intravenous paclitaxel or S1 plus cisplatin. The primary endpoint was overall survival, and follow-up analysis demonstrated a 3-year overall survival of 22% in the intraperitoneal group versus 6% in the systemic only group.

Taken together, it remains inconclusive whether intraperitoneal chemotherapy modalities add additional therapeutic value beyond standard of care systemic chemotherapy for patients with peritoneal metastatic disease. While there are some promising trends based on preliminary studies, further multi-institutional studies with larger patient volumes are necessary to better clarify the clinical value of neoadjuvant LS-HIPEC. There is newfound interest in pressurized intraperitoneal aerosol chemotherapy (PIPAC), performed every 3 to 4 weeks. Retrospective studies of this technique showed median overall survival of 19.1 months in 42 patients, however, comparative randomized trials are lacking.

General Approach and Follow-Up

The practice algorithm for the treatment of gastric cancer at MD Anderson can be found online in a continually updated format on the MD Anderson website. A comprehensive initial evaluation is performed to assign a clinical stage, which is the basis on which further workup or treatment is recommended. Early T1a lesions are considered for EMR. Upfront gastrectomy without neoadjuvant therapy is usually only considered in select cases with T1b or T2 disease without any evidence of nodal disease. Otherwise, most patients are evaluated for neoadjuvant chemotherapy or chemoradiation therapy. Restaging is preferred with cross-sectional imaging after the completion of neoadjuvant therapy prior to resection. After gastrectomy, node-negative patients may be simply observed or recommended for adjuvant chemotherapy. T3 or greater patients, or those with positive nodes, usually receive adjuvant chemoradiation or chemotherapy depending on their neoadjuvant regimen. All patients are evaluated for inclusion in relevant, appropriate clinical trials.

Patients are typically seen every 3 months for the first 2 years following resection. A careful history and physical examination are performed, along with laboratory studies (complete blood cell count, liver function tests, chemistries, prealbumin, vitamin B12, and vitamin D levels). Chest, abdominal, and pelvic CT is performed every 6 months after surgery for 2 years and then yearly thereafter. It is important to balance the intensity of follow-up with the likely ability to benefit a patient who does have a recurrence. In patients who have undergone a subtotal gastrectomy, endoscopy should be considered at the end of the first postsurgical year, again the following year, and finally once more 5 years after surgery. Patients who receive protocol-based therapy often have more frequent staging studies, but this has never been shown to impact patient survival. The most important reasons to follow patients closely are to recognize and address any postgastrectomy sequelae and to acquire accurate recurrence and survival data on patients in clinical trials.

Other Gastric Malignancies

Gastric Lymphoma

The gastrointestinal tract is the most common site of extranodal non-Hodgkin lymphoma (NHL). Two-thirds of gastrointestinal lymphomas occur in the stomach, while less than 5% of gastric neoplasms are lymphoma. The two primary histologic types are low-grade marginal zone B-cell lymphomas of the mucosa-associated lymphoid tissue (MALT) type and high-grade diffuse large B-cell lymphoma (DLBCL); the latter contains a low-grade MALT component in approximately one-third of cases. Whether high-grade lymphomas derive from MALT lymphomas remains unresolved, however, the pathogenesis for both is frequently attributed to chronic gastritis and infection with *H. pylori*. The initial symptomatology of gastric lymphoma is often nonspecific and delay in diagnosis is common. The most frequent symptoms at the time of presentation are pain (88%), loss of appetite (47%), weight loss (25%), bleeding (19%), and vomiting (18%). Obstruction and perforation are possible, but uncommon, presenting symptoms.

Diagnosis is established with upper endoscopic evaluation and biopsy. Multiple biopsies should be taken in each region of the stomach, duodenum, and GEJ. All suspicious lesions should be sampled, as well as normal-appearing mucosa. Deeper biopsies, including possible EMR, may be necessary to establish the diagnosis. The presence of *H. pylori* must be determined through histopathology, urease enzyme levels (breath test), and serology. Testing for the t(11;18) translocation should be performed in cases of MALT lymphoma, as its presence is associated with resistance to certain treatments, including *H. pylori* eradication. Laboratory evaluation includes lactate dehydrogenase and beta-2-microglobulin levels as well as bone marrow aspiration and biopsy. The extent of disease is assessed with cross-sectional imaging of the chest, abdomen, and pelvis.

The general trend over the last several decades has been away for surgical treatment for gastric lymphoma and toward nonsurgical therapy. Initial therapy for early-stage, low-grade MALT lymphoma consists of regimens of antibiotics and proton pump inhibitors for the eradication of *H. pylori* and results in long-term remission in a majority of patients. Assessment of failure of MALT lymphoma to resolve with *H. pylori* eradication can only be made after several years, as the median time to tumor remission is 15 months. Serial endoscopic evaluation is used to assess response. There is evidence that patients with limited residual disease may either be safely observed or treated with an alternative *H. pylori*-directed therapy. Patients with the t(11;18) translocation are often resistant to *H. pylori* eradication and may need to be treated with multimodal therapy.

For patients with persistent MALT lymphoma after *H. pylori* therapy or those without evidence of *H. pylori* infection, external beam radiation therapy has a 90% to 100% rate of complete response and results in durable remission in a majority of patients. Alternatively, single-agent chemotherapy or rituximab (anti-CD20 monoclonal antibody) may be administered if radiation is contraindicated or may be preferential to receiving radiotherapy to minimize impact on future treatment options should a patient subsequently develop a gastric or GEJ adenocarcinoma (which we have seen on several occasions). Combination chemotherapy, often combined with rituximab, is reserved for patients with GI bleeding, bulky local disease, or progressive systemic disease. Close monitoring without treatment is also an option in asymptomatic patients with medical comorbidities that preclude aggressive radiation or systemic therapy.

DLBCL is the most common type of gastric lymphoma. Treatment varies but typically consists of aggressive anthracycline-based combination chemotherapy, including CHOP (cyclophosphamide, doxorubicin, vincristine, and prednisone) and R-CHOP (with rituximab). The addition of operative resection to systemic chemotherapy does not improve survival. In patients with gastric DLBCL containing a low-grade MALT component, *H. pylori* eradication can result in complete response and sustained remission. The role of consolidation radiotherapy remains unclear. Retrospective studies suggest that patients with localized disease (stages I and II) may have lower local relapse rates with the addition of consolidation radiotherapy. The development of these regimens has resulted in a significant improvement in overall survival rates. Patients who relapse are treated with high-dose chemotherapy followed by autologous stem-cell transplantation. CD19 T-cell (CAR-T) immunotherapy in relapsed or recurrent DLBCL is a promising therapy for these patients, however, the sequence of utilization of this therapy remains ill-defined, given a known risk of perforation during therapy.

Currently, the most common indications for surgical intervention in gastric lymphoma include bleeding, perforation, obstruction, and the rare finding of localized residual disease after primary therapy. While operative resection historically has demonstrated excellent outcomes for gastric lymphoma, it has largely been abandoned in favor of chemotherapy and radiation regimens with comparable oncologic outcomes and superior quality of life results. Complications requiring operative intervention during treatment for gastric lymphoma are rare (~5%). Patients with large, bulky, transmural tumors are those at greatest risk of treatment-related complications such as perforation. In these patients, a dose reduction for the first cycle of chemotherapy may be used as a precaution while the patient is carefully observed.

Neuroendocrine Tumors

Gastric NETs constitute less than 10% of all NETs, but the incidence is increasing in the United States. Whether this is due to the increased use of endoscopy and subsequent increased number of asymptomatic tumors being diagnosed or an actual increase in the incidence of these tumors is unclear. Four distinct types of gastric NETs have been described with variable clinical courses and prognosis. Gastric NETs are also graded by WHO criteria into three classifications: well-differentiated (carcinoid), well-differentiated neuroendocrine carcinoma (malignant carcinoid), and poorly differentiated neuroendocrine carcinoma.

Type 1 gastric NETs are the most frequent, accounting for 70% to 80% of all cases. Typically, these are asymptomatic, small (usually <1 cm), well differentiated, and multifocal. The majority of patients are women (70% to 80%) and the condition develops in the setting of chronic atrophic gastritis and enterochromaffin-like (ECL) cell hyperplasia. These patients have elevated plasma gastrin levels and low gastric acid production.

Regional lymph node metastases are rare and usually occur only in larger tumors that penetrate the muscularis propria. Endoscopic resection is the treatment of choice for small tumors (<2 cm). Surgical excision or resection is considered for larger or more invasive tumors. Endoscopic surveillance alone is also an option in small, asymptomatic tumors. Type 1 tumors have a tendency to recur, and larger, more advanced tumors may be associated with concomitant adenocarcinoma. Careful, long-term endoscopic surveillance is required. These patients have an excellent prognosis with 5- and 10-year survivals that are comparable to the general population.

Type 2 gastric NETs are associated with multiple endocrine neoplasia type 1 (MEN-1)–associated Zollinger–Ellison syndrome (ZES). They account for 5% to 6% of NETs. These tumors rarely develop in sporadic ZES patients (<0.1%), however, they are relatively common in MEN-1/ZES patients (15% to 30%). The disease tends to develop late in the course of MEN-1/ZES disease (15 to 20 years). The tumors are typically well differentiated, multifocal, small (<1.5 cm), and limited to the mucosa/submucosa. ECL hyperplasia is common. These patients have elevated plasma gastrin levels and high gastric acid production. In tumors larger than 2 cm or with invasion of the muscularis propria, there is up to a 30% incidence of regional lymph node spread or metastatic disease. Therapy is directed toward localizing and removing the source of hypergastrinemia; most commonly this requires local excision of the gastrin-producing gastrinoma. Somatostatin analogs are used to inhibit tumor growth, particularly in patients in whom hypergastrinemia cannot be surgically corrected. Resection of type 2 NETs is reserved for tumors with suspicious or proven signs of malignancy. Type 2 gastric NET patients have 5-year survival rates of 60% to 75%.

Between 14% and 25% of gastric NETs are type 3. These are more aggressive sporadic neoplasms not associated with ECL hyperplasia, hypergastrinemia, or any other diseases of the stomach. They are more common in males. The tumors tend to be solitary, large (3 to 5 cm), and are well differentiated. Plasma gastrin levels and gastric acid production are usually within normal limits (though the use of proton pump inhibitors may impact this and should be accounted for during evaluation). Penetration of the muscularis propria is common and invasion of all layers of the gastric wall is seen in approximately 50% of patients. Metastases are present in greater than 50% of patients with larger lesions. Treatment is similar to gastric adenocarcinoma and consists of operative resection to achieve negative margins, lymph node dissection, and consideration of systemic chemotherapy. Because of the generally favorable biology of these tumors, aggressive surgical or ablative therapies should be considered, as reasonably prolonged overall survival is reported, even in patients with metastatic disease.

Type 4 gastric NET is the newest classification and accounts for 6% to 8% of gastric NETs. These tumors occur more frequently in men and consist of highly malignant, poorly differentiated (small cell) neuroendocrine carcinoma. Patients commonly present at an advanced stage with large (>5 cm), often ulcerated primary masses exhibiting local invasion and often have metastases. As such, surgical intervention is rarely appropriate for these patients, but may be considered in the rare event of localized disease.

Systemic chemotherapy has limited efficacy in metastatic gastric NETs. Most studies have evaluated treatments for metastatic NETs from multiple primary sites. Somatostatin analogs have been evaluated in metastatic settings with some improvement in time to tumor progression. Everolimus has an impact on the survival of patients with pancreatic NETs, but there are limited data reporting its efficacy in gastric NETs.

Our general approach to gastric NETs at MD Anderson considers the type of NET, WHO grade, and patient comorbidities. Regardless of type, both tumor size and grade predict recurrence and survival. For type 1 and 2 gastric NETs, operative resection is recommended for NETs greater than 2 to 3 cm in diameter. Because of the indolent nature of type 1 and type 2 gastric NETs, nonsurgical management may be preferable in older patients or those with significant comorbidities. Somatostatin analogs can promote the regression of small (<1 cm) gastric NETs and may also prevent recurrence after resection. When complete R0 resection is achievable, aggressive surgical and/or ablative therapy may be considered in carefully selected type 1, 2, and 3 patients with metastatic disease.

Conclusion

Gastric cancer demands a thoughtful, multidisciplinary approach in order to achieve successful long-term outcomes. Durable cure may only be possible in a minority of patients in whom early gastric cancer is identified. However, all patients with gastric cancer can benefit from evaluation by an experienced surgeon in conjunction with a multidisciplinary team to formulate a comprehensive treatment plan that meets each patient's needs and goals. New therapies, including the promise of immunotherapy, continue to be evaluated in gastric cancer. The surgeon will always play an essential role in the diagnosis, staging, and treatment of this disease.

CASE SCENARIO

Case Scenario 1

A 65-year-old male with hypertension, type 2 diabetes, and a history of reflux underwent an elective esophago-gastroduodenoscopy (EGD) for epigastric pain. A 1-cm ulcer located in the antrum of the stomach along the greater curvature was biopsied. The pathology was notable for the presence of well-differentiated adenocarcinoma involving the mucosa only. Antral biopsy was also notable for the presence of H. pylori. The patient was started on antibiotics by his primary care provider (PCP) and was referred to your clinic for further management.

Case Discussion

Based on the preliminary studies, the patient has a T1a gastric adenocarcinoma, which is isolated to the gastric mucosa. Deep to the mucosa lies the submucosa, and this tissue layer contains dense lymphatic and vascular channels that are a common source of regional and distant metastatic spread. Very early lesions isolated to the mucosa are associated with a low risk of local, regional, or distant spread. For this reason, T1a lesions are potentially amenable to endoscopic mucosal resection (EMR) or endoscopic submucosal dissection (ESD) techniques. EMR generally involves a snare-based resection technique. The Japanese Gastroenterological Endoscopy Society and the Japanese Gastric Cancer Association have very well–delineated indications for EMR, which involves well-differentiated tumors less than 2 cm in diameter confined to the mucosa without ulceration. Expanded criteria include the presence of ulceration, as is the case with our patient who has a 1-cm well-differentiated adenocarcinoma confined to the mucosa. Long-term overall survival is equivalent to surgical resection, approximately 95% at 5 years, however, there is a higher risk of local recurrence (6% vs. 1%). This increased risk of local recurrence should be discussed with the patient when considering available treatment options. ESD is a more technically challenging endoscopic procedure in which the operator dissects down to the level of the submucosa and then lifts the overlying tissue for an en bloc resection. This technique is frequently performed with a thermal knife or hydrodissection. Indications for ESD include lesions greater than 2 cm that are limited to the mucosal layer or ulcerated lesions.

According to national consensus guidelines, all gastric cancer patients should undergo a formal diagnostic and staging workup before proceeding with any treatment. This includes a complete history and physical examination, EGD with biopsy to confirm the diagnosis, and staging CT chest, abdomen, and pelvis with oral and intravenous contrast. For early-stage disease, endoscopic ultrasound is the most sensitive technique to determine the depth of invasion. It would be reasonable to confirm the depth of invasion in this patient by repeating the EGD and performing an Endoscopic ultrasound (EUS). However, endoscopic resection techniques are both diagnostic and therapeutic, and in the absence of distant spread, the surgeon could also directly proceed with endoscopic mucosal resection or dissection to remove the lesion. Pathology would need to be followed up to confirm that the lesion is limited to the mucosa, in which case no further treatment is necessary if negative margins were obtained. National consensus guidelines note that EMR or ESD can be considered adequate therapy when the mass is ≤2 cm, well or moderately differentiated, limited to the superficial submucosa, without lymphovascular invasion, and with clearly negative deep and lateral margins. However, if the lesion is found to have invasion into deeper tissue layers of the gastric wall, the patient will be upstaged and will require further workup and treatment.

If the lesion is found to invade into the submucosa after EMR, the patient should undergo diagnostic laparoscopy and multidisciplinary evaluation. If the staging CT is negative and the diagnostic laparoscopy is negative for peritoneal metastatic spread, the patient should be considered for upfront surgical resection, perioperative chemotherapy, or neoadjuvant chemoradiation.

CASE SCENARIO REVIEW

Case Scenario 1 Questions

1. A patient is referred to your clinic with a "T1" gastric cancer. A repeat EUS ordered by you reveals invasion into the muscularis propria. What is the appropriate next step in management?

   A. Watch and wait approach with repeat EGD in 3 months

   B. Resection of the ulcer bed with endoscopic submucosal dissection

   C. Proceed to the distal gastrectomy

   D. Proceed with multidisciplinary evaluation for additional staging and treatment

2. After undergoing preoperative therapy for a cT2 antral adenocarcinoma, the patient is taken to the operating room for a distal gastrectomy with D2 lymphadenectomy. What are the appropriate nodal stations to sample for a D2 lymphadenectomy?

   A. Perigastric lymph nodes
   B. Perigastric lymph nodes and left gastric artery nodal packet
   C. Perigastric lymph nodes and nodes along left gastric artery, common hepatic artery, celiac axis, and proximal splenic artery
   D. Perigastric lymph nodes, nodes along left gastric artery, common and proper hepatic artery, celiac axis, and splenic artery

3. You are seeing a patient in clinic with cN+ gastric adenocarcinoma of the body of the stomach to discuss their upcoming operation. You plan to perform a subtotal gastrectomy. The patient reports that she has read the literature extensively and wants to know how many lymph nodes you plan to retrieve. What is your answer?

   A. 15 nodes
   B. 16 nodes
   C. 30 nodes
   D. Number of nodes does not matter as long as all stations for a D2 lymphadenectomy are sampled

Case Scenario 1 Answers

1. **The correct answer is D.** *Rationale:* The patient was presumed to have T1 disease, potentially amenable to EMR. Unfortunately, in this case, the tumor has invaded into the muscularis propria, and is therefore at increased risk for local regional and distant spread (cT2). Multidisciplinary evaluation and consideration of upfront surgery, perioperative chemotherapy, or preoperative radiation would be appropriate next steps. Of note, in situations in which a patient is treated with EMR and has a positive deep margin, it might be difficult to distinguish T1b from T2+ disease, and as such, these tumors should be managed as a T2 or higher lesion. According to national consensus guidelines, the next step for the above patient would be multidisciplinary evaluation for additional staging and treatment considerations.

2. **The correct answer is D.** *Rationale:* Answers A, B, C, and D correlate to the 0, D1, D1+, and D2 lymphadenectomy for gastric cancer. A formal D2 lymphadenectomy includes all lymph node stations along the lesser and greater curvature of the stomach, lymph nodes lining the common hepatic artery, and more distally beyond the gastroduodenal artery takeoff to include the proper hepatic artery lymph nodes. It also includes nodal dissection along the celiac axis including the left gastric artery and the entire length of the splenic artery to the splenic hilum.

3. **The correct answer is C.** *Rationale:* The most recent AJCC staging guidelines (8th edition) recommend a minimum of 16 nodes to be sampled, whereas this number was previously 15. The rationale for 16 relates to appropriate staging. In the current staging system, N3 nodal disease is subcategorized into N3a (6 to 15 positive nodes) and N3b (16 or greater positive nodes). Therefore, 16 is necessary at minimum to distinguish N3a from N3b disease in patients with a high positive nodal burden. However, there is a second question of theoretical oncologic value by retrieving more nodes. Several single and multi-institutional studies have been published investigating the optimal number of nodes resected in association with outcome measures such as recurrence and survival using institutional and national registry data found in SEER and the NCDB. Based on the currently available data, retrieval of 30 nodes appears to be optimally associated with outcome measures and also addresses issues related to stage migration.

CASE SCENARIO

Case Scenario 2

A 70-year-old female with a history of GERD and hypertension presents to her primary care doctor with several weeks of fatigue. A complete blood count identifies a hemoglobin of 6.5 g/dL, and a fecal occult blood test was positive. An upper endoscopy was performed, and a large fungating mass was identified in the antrum of the stomach. Biopsy of the mass confirmed adenocarcinoma. On endoscopic ultrasound, the mass penetrated the muscular layer of the gastric wall. CT of the chest, abdomen, and pelvis with IV and oral contrast was notable for enlarged perigastric lymph nodes along the gastroepiploic and left gastric arteries without evidence of distant disease.

Case Discussion

Based on these staging studies, the patient has clinical T3N1M0 disease at minimum. Based on the American Joint Committee on Cancer (AJCC) staging guidelines, the patient is clinical stage III. National consensus guidelines recommend additional tumor testing for microsatellite instability and mismatch repair defects, as well as for HER2 and PD-L1 expression if metastatic disease is suspected. In addition to transfusion and stabilization, staging should be completed with a diagnostic laparoscopy with peritoneal cytology. Based on our experience at MD Anderson, approximately 21% of patients are found to have macroscopically positive peritoneal metastases, and positive cytology with malignant cells is observed in an additional 13% of patients. In instances where peritoneal cytology is positive, outcomes are similar to those with macroscopically positive peritoneal disease.

After completion of the clinical staging evaluation, the patient should be discussed in a multidisciplinary setting. For stage 3 disease, neoadjuvant therapy with chemotherapy or chemotherapy plus chemoradiotherapy should be considered. The current standard of care for systemic therapy is based on the FLOT4 clinical trial, which is predicated on a perioperative regimen of fluorouracil, leucovorin, oxaliplatin, and docetaxel. Patients are treated with four cycles of neoadjuvant chemotherapy followed by an additional four cycles after successful recovery from surgery.

After completion of preoperative therapy, patients should be restaged before proceeding to the operating room for surgical resection. Regarding the type of resection, tumor location and size determine the extent of gastric resection, and in this case, an antral tumor may safely be treated with a subtotal gastrectomy. With a 5-cm margin negative resection, there is equivalent survival between total and subtotal gastrectomy, with the latter having improved quality of life and long-term nutritional parameters. Gastric resection should be accompanied by D2 lymphadenectomy.

CASE SCENARIO REVIEW

Case Scenario 2 Question

1. After completion of preoperative therapy, the surgeon is contemplating a minimally invasive approach to gastric resection. Which of the following is true regarding published data for minimally invasive gastrectomy for gastric cancer?

   A. Data strongly favors laparoscopic or robotic resection
   B. In some meta-analyses, minimally invasive resection is associated with poorer lymph node yields
   C. Most studies have shown no difference in long-term survival or oncologic outcomes with minimally invasive approaches
   D. Robotic resection is considered superior to laparoscopic resection in terms of short-term complications and cost

Case Scenario 2 Answer

1. The correct answer is **C**. *Rationale:* Available data has demonstrated no significant differences in long-term survival or oncologic outcomes after minimally invasive gastrectomy compared to open surgery. The KLASS-01 trial demonstrated no significant difference in perioperative morbidity or mortality, with similar 5-year cancer-specific outcomes between laparoscopic-assisted and open gastrectomy. Similarly, the STOMACH trial showed no significant difference in 1-year survival for open and minimally invasive surgery. The LOGICA trial, which compared laparoscopic and open gastrectomy, similarly showed no difference in outcome measures. Limited prospective trials exist for robotic resection, however, when comparing laparoscopic versus robotic resection in South Korea, there were no differences in short-term complication rates.

CASE SCENARIO

Case Scenario 3

A 55-year-old male with a history of hyperlipidemia and 30 pack-year of smoking tobacco presents to his primary care physician complaining of 3 weeks of progressive abdominal bloating, crampy abdominal pain, low-grade fevers, and nausea. A CT scan is performed and identifies a thickened stomach, without evidence of distant disease. Upper endoscopy identifies a raised lesion in the prepyloric region. Biopsies are taken at the lesion, as well as the gastroesophageal junction, cardia, and antrum. Biopsies of this mass are significant for a diagnosis of mucosa-associated lymphoid tissue (MALT) lymphoma. Subsequent testing for H. pylori *with urease breath test and serology are positive.*

Case Discussion

The stomach is the most common site of gastrointestinal lymphoma and may be either high-grade diffuse B-Cell or MALT subtype. Classic symptoms include pain, early satiety, weight loss, and gastrointestinal bleeding. After gastric biopsy and diagnosis, staging CT scans should be performed as well as bone marrow biopsy and *H. pylori* testing.

Eradication of *H. pylori* with antibiotics and proton pump therapy is the initial preferred treatment for MALT lymphoma and induces tumor regression in an average of 15 months. Certain genetic subtypes, specifically t(11;18) translocation, are resistant to *H. pylori* eradication, and may require multimodal therapy. Remission of disease is evaluated with serial endoscopy. If triple therapy does not induce remission, external beam radiation or single-agent chemotherapy with anti-CD20 monoclonal antibiotics are acceptable treatment strategies. Surgical therapy for gastric lymphoma is typically reserved for cases of perforation, bleeding, or obstruction.

CASE SCENARIO REVIEW

Case Scenario 3 Question

1. The patient in the above scenario underwent gastric biopsy and was found to have high-grade diffuse large B-cell lymphoma. Which of the following is true of this malignancy?

   A. Surgical resection is a mainstay of treatment

   B. Anthracycline-based chemotherapy is the preferred systemic treatment

   C. Radiation has a clear role in the treatment paradigm

   D. *H. pylori* implicated in pathogenesis and eradication is vital to treatment

Case Scenario 3 Answer

1. **The correct answer is B.** *Rationale:* Diffuse large B-cell lymphoma is an aggressive form of gastric lymphoma, and is primarily treated with cyclophosphamide, doxorubicin, vincristine, and prednisone with or without rituximab. Radiation may have utility in persistent disease, and stem cell transplant and CAR-T immunotherapy have emerging roles in advanced disease. Some patients with diffuse large B-cell lymphoma may have a MALT component, necessitating *H. pylori* eradication, though this is not universal.

Recommended Readings

Ajani JA, Mansfield PF, Crane CH, et al. Paclitaxel-based chemoradiotherapy in localized gastric carcinoma: degree of pathologic response and not clinical parameters dictated patient outcome. *J Clin Oncol.* 2005;23(6):1237–1244.

Al-Batran, SE, Homann N, Pauligk C et al; FLOT4-AIO Investigators. Perioperative chemotherapy with fluorouracil plus leucovorin, oxaliplatin, and docetaxel versus fluorouracil or capecitabine plus cisplatin and epirubicin for locally advanced, resectable gastric or gastro-oesophageal junction adenocarcinoma (FLOT4): a randomised, phase 2/3 trial. *Lancet.* 2019;393:1948–1957. https://doi.org/10.1016/S0140-6736(18)32557-1

Al-Refaie WB, Tseng JF, Gay G, et al. The impact of ethnicity on the presentation and prognosis of patients with gastric adenocarcinoma. Results from the National Cancer Data Base. *Cancer.* 2008;113(3):461–469.

Badgwell B, Blum M, Elimova E, et al. Frequency of resection after preoperative chemotherapy or chemoradiotherapy for gastric adenocarcinoma. *Ann Surg Oncol.* 2016;23(6):1948–1955.

Badgwell B, Blum M, Estrella J, et al. Predictors of survival in patients with resectable gastric cancer treated with preoperative chemoradiation therapy and gastrectomy. *J Am Coll Surg.* 2015;221(1):83–90.

Badgwell B, Ikoma N, Murphy MB, et al. A phase II trial of cytoreduction, gastrectomy, and hyperthermic intraperitoneal perfusion with chemotherapy for patients with gastric cancer and carcinomatosis or positive cytology. *Ann Surg Oncol.* 2021;28(1):258–264.

Bajetta E, Catena L, Fazio N, et al. Everolimus in combination with octreotide long-acting repeatable in a first line setting for patients with neuroendocrine tumors: an ITMO group study. *Cancer.* 2014;120(16):2457–2463.

Bang YJ, Kim YW, Yang HK, et al; CLASSIC trial investigators. Adjuvant capecitabine and oxaliplatin for gastric cancer after D2 gastrectomy (CLASSIC): a phase 3 open-label, randomised controlled trial. *Lancet.* 2012;379(9813):315–321.

Cardona K, Zhou Q, Gönen M, et al. Role of repeat staging laparoscopy in locoregionally advanced gastric or gastroesophageal cancer after neoadjuvant therapy. *Ann Surg Oncol.* 2013;20(2):548–554.

Chicago Consensus Working Group. The Chicago Consensus on peritoneal surface malignancies: management of gastric metastases. *Cancer.* 2020;126(11):2541–2546.

Choi IJ, Lee JH, Kim YI, et al. Long-term outcome comparison of endoscopic resection and surgery in early gastric cancer meeting the absolute indication for endoscopic resection. *Gastrointest Endosc.* 2015;81(2):333–341.

Csendes A, Burdiles P, Rojas J, Braghetto I, Diaz JC, Maluenda F. A prospective randomized study comparing D2 total gastrectomy versus D2 total gastrectomy plus splenectomy in 187 patients with gastric carcinoma. *Surgery.* 2002;131(4):401–407.

Degiuli M, Sasako M, Ponti A, et al; Italian Gastric Cancer Study Group. Randomized clinical trial comparing survival after D1 or D2 gastrectomy for gastric cancer. *Br J Surg.* 2014;101(2):23–31.

Eveno C, Jouvin I, Pocard M. PIPAC EstoK 01: pressurized intraperitoneal aerosol chemotherapy with cisplatin and doxorubicin (PIPAC C/D) in gastric peritoneal metastasis: a randomized and multicenter phase II study. *Pleura Peritoneum.* 2018;3(2):20180116.

Facchiano E, Scaringi S, Kianmanesh R, et al. Laparoscopic hyperthermic intraperitoneal chemotherapy (HIPEC) for the treatment of malignant ascites secondary to unresectable peritoneal carcinomatosis from advanced gastric cancer. *Eur J Surg Oncol.* 2008;34(2):154–158.

Glehen O, Gilly FN, Arvieux C, et al; Association Française de Chirurgie. Peritoneal carcinomatosis from gastric cancer: a multi-institutional study of 159 patients treated by cytoreductive surgery combined with perioperative intraperitoneal chemotherapy. *Ann Surg Oncol.* 2010;17(9):2370–2377.

GASTRIC (Global Advanced/Adjuvant Stomach Tumor Research International Collaboration) Group; Paoletti X, Oba K, Burzykowski T, et al. Benefit of adjuvant chemotherapy for resectable gastric cancer: a meta-analysis. *JAMA.* 2010;303(17):1729–1737.

Hanna A, Kim-Kiselak C, Tang R, et al. Gastric neuroendocrine tumors: reappraisal of type in predicting outcome. *Ann Surg Oncol.* 2021;28:8838–8846. https://doi.org/10.1245/s10434-021-10293-7

Honda M, Hiki N, Kinoshita T, et al. Long-term outcomes of laparoscopic versus open surgery for clinical stage I gastric cancer: the LOC-1 study. *Ann Surg.* 2016;264(2):214–222.

Hyung WJ, Yang HK, Park YK et al; Korean Laparoendoscopic Gastrointestinal Surgery Study Group. Long-term outcomes of laparoscopic distal gastrectomy for locally advanced gastric cancer: the KLASS-02-RCT randomized clinical trial. *J Clin Oncol.* 2020;38(28):3304–3313.

Ikoma N, Blum M, Chiang YJ, et al. Yield of staging laparoscopy and lavage cytology for radiologically occult peritoneal carcinomatosis of gastric cancer. *Ann Surg Oncol.* 2016;23(13):4332–4337.

Kim BS, Park YS, Yook JH, Oh ST, Kim BS. Differing clinical courses and prognoses in patients with gastric neuroendocrine tumors based on the 2010-WHO classification scheme. *Medicine (Baltimore).* 2015;94(44):e1748.

Kim HH, Han SU, Kim MC, et al; Korean Laparoendoscopic Gastrointestinal Surgery Study (KLASS) Group. Effect of laparoscopic distal gastrectomy vs open distal gastrectomy on long-term survival among patients with stage I gastric cancer: the KLASS-01 randomized clinical trial. *JAMA Oncol.* 2019;5(4):506–513.

Kim MS, Kim WJ, Hyung WJ, et al. Comprehensive learning curve of robotic surgery: discovery from a multi-center prospective trial of robotic gastrectomy. *Ann Surg.* 2021;273(5):949–956.

Kondoh C, Shitara K, Nomura M, et al. Efficacy of palliative radiotherapy for gastric bleeding in patients with unresectable advanced gastric cancer: a retrospective cohort study. *BMC Palliat Care.* 2015; 14:37.

Lee J, Lim DH, Kim S, et al. Phase III trial comparing capecitabine plus cisplatin versus capecitabine plus cisplatin with concurrent capecitabine radiotherapy in completely resected gastric cancer with D2 lymph node dissection: the ARTIST trial. *J Clin Oncol.* 2012;30(3):268–273.

Lee JH, Kim SH, Han SH, An JS, Lee ES, Kim YS. Clinicopathological and molecular characteristics of Epstein-Barr virus-associated gastric carcinoma: a meta-analysis. *J Gastroenterol Hepatol.* 2009;24(3):354–365.

Li TT, Qiu F, Qian ZR, Wan J, Qi XK, Wu BY. Classification, clinicopathologic features and treatment of gastric neuroendocrine tumors. *World J Gastroenterol.* 2014;20(1):118–125.

Lian J, Chen S, Zhang Y, Qiu F. A meta-analysis of endoscopic submucosal dissection and EMR for early gastric cancer. *Gastrointest Endosc.* 2012;76(4):763–770.

Macdonald JS, Smalley SR, Benedetti J, et al. Chemoradiotherapy after surgery compared with surgery alone for adenocarcinoma of the stomach or gastroesophageal junction. *N Engl J Med.* 2001;345(10):725–730.

Mezhir JJ, Shah MA, Jacks LM, Brennan MF, Coit DG, Strong VE. Positive peritoneal cytology in patients with gastric cancer: natural history and outcome of 291 patients. *Ann Surg Oncol.* 2010;17(12):3173–3180.

Newhook TE, Agnes A, Blum M, et al. Laparoscopic hyperthermic intraperitoneal chemotherapy is safe for patients with peritoneal metastases from gastric cancer and may lead to gastrectomy. *Ann Surg Oncol.* 2019;26(5):1394-1400.

Pacelli F, Cusumano G, Rosa F, et al; Italian Research Group for Gastric Cancer. Multivisceral resection for locally advanced gastric cancer: an Italian multicenter observational study. *JAMA Surg.* 2013;148(4):353–360.

Park SH, Sohn TS, Lee J, et al. Phase III trial to compare adjuvant chemotherapy with capecitabine and cisplatin versus concurrent chemoradiotherapy in gastric cancer: final report of the adjuvant chemoradiotherapy in stomach tumors trial, including survival and subset analyses. *J Clin Oncol.* 2015;33(28):3130–3136.

Pyo JH, Lee H, Min BH, et al. Long-term outcome of endoscopic resection vs. surgery for early gastric cancer: a non-inferiority-matched cohort study. *Am J Gastroenterol.* 2016;111(2):240–249.

Ramos RF, Scalon FM, Scalon MM, Dias DI. Staging laparoscopy in gastric cancer to detect peritoneal metastases: a systematic review and meta-analysis. *Eur J Surg Oncol.* 2016;42(9):1315–1321.

Sano T, Sasako M, Mizusawa J, et al; Stomach Cancer Study Group of the Japan Clinical Oncology Group. Randomized controlled trial to evaluate splenectomy in total gastrectomy for proximal gastric carcinoma. *Ann Surg.* 2017;265(2):277–283.

Sano T, Sasako M, Yamamoto S, et al. Gastric cancer surgery: morbidity and mortality results from a prospective randomized controlled trial comparing D2 and extended para-aortic lymphadenectomy—Japan Clinical Oncology Group study 9501. *J Clin Oncol.* 2004;22(14):2767–2773.

Sasako M, Sano T, Yamamoto S, et al; Japan Clinical Oncology Group. D2 lymphadenectomy alone or with para-aortic nodal dissection for gastric cancer. *N Engl J Med.* 2008;359(5):453–462.

Schuhmacher C, Gretschel S, Lordick F, et al. Neoadjuvant chemotherapy compared with surgery alone for locally advanced cancer of the stomach and cardia: European Organisation for Research and Treatment of Cancer randomized trial 40954. *J Clin Oncol.* 2010;28(35):5210–5218.

Song H, Zhu J, Lu D. Long-term proton pump inhibitor (PPI) use and the development of gastric pre-malignant lesions. *Cochrane Database Syst Rev.* 2014(12):CD010623.

Songun I, Putter H, Kranenbarg EMK, Sasako M, van de Velde CJH. Surgical treatment of gastric cancer: 15-year follow-up results of the randomised nationwide Dutch D1D2 trial. *Lancet Oncol.* 2010;11(5):439–449.

Strong VE, Song KY, Park CH, et al. Comparison of gastric cancer survival following R0 resection in the United States and Korea using an internationally validated nomogram. *Ann Surg.* 2010;251(4):640–646.

Sun J, Song Y, Wang Z, et al. Benefits of hyperthermic intraperitoneal chemotherapy for patients with serosal invasion in gastric cancer: a meta-analysis of the randomized controlled trials. *BMC Cancer.* 2012; 12:526.

Tanabe S, Ishido K, Higuchi K, et al. Long-term outcomes of endoscopic submucosal dissection for early gastric cancer: a retrospective comparison with conventional endoscopic resection in a single center. *Gastric Cancer.* 2014;17(1):130–136.

van der Post RS, Vogelaar IP, Carneiro F, et al. Hereditary diffuse gastric cancer: updated clinical guidelines with an emphasis on germline CDH1 mutation carriers. *J Med Genet.* 2015;52(6):361–374.

Verheij M, Jansen EP, Cats A, et al. A multicenter randomized phase III trial of neo-adjuvant chemotherapy followed by surgery and chemotherapy or by surgery and chemoradiotherapy in resectable gastric cancer: First results from the CRITICS study. *ASCO Meeting Abstracts.* 2016;34(suppl 15):4000.

Yonemura Y, Ishibashi H, Hirano M, et al. Effects of neoadjuvant laparoscopic hyperthermic intraperitoneal chemotherapy and neoadjuvant intraperitoneal/systemic chemotherapy on peritoneal metastases from gastric cancer. *Ann Surg Oncol.* 2017;24(2):478–485.

Yonemura Y, Kawamura T, Bandou E, Takahashi S, Sawa T, Matsuki N. Treatment of peritoneal dissemination from gastric cancer by peritonectomy and chemohyperthermic peritoneal perfusion. *Br J Surg.* 2005;92(3):370–375.

11 Small Bowel Malignancies

Meredith C. Mason and Abhineet Uppal

INTRODUCTION

Small bowel malignancies are rare. Fewer than 12,000 patients are diagnosed annually in the United States (US) and an estimated 2,000 die per year from these cancers. There are multiple histologic types of primary small bowel malignancies, the most common include adenocarcinoma, carcinoid or neuroendocrine, sarcoma, and lymphoma. Metastases from other tumor types such as melanoma, lung, colon, and ovarian cancers should also be included in the differential diagnosis of small bowel masses. This chapter will focus on the most common primary small bowel malignancies (adenocarcinoma, carcinoid/neuroendocrine, lymphoma, and sarcoma).

Epidemiology

The incidence of small bowel malignancies rose from 11.8 cases per million in 1973 to 22.7 cases per million in 2004. Since 2012, incidence has been stable at this rate. African Americans in US have the highest age-adjusted incidence of small bowel cancers in the world.

Neuroendocrine tumors (NETs) and adenocarcinomas are the most common primary malignancies of the small bowel. A study by Bilimoria et al. using the National Cancer Data Base and the Surveillance Epidemiology and End Results database found that of the 67,843 patients identified with small bowel masses, 37.4% had NETs, 36.9% adenocarcinoma, 17.3% lymphoma, and 8.4% stromal tumors. The rise in the incidence of NETs of the small intestine in US was from 2.1 per million in 1973 to 9.3 per million in 2004, representing a 340% increase. The reason for the rising incidence is unclear but may be related to increased detection rate.

NETs are more common in the ileum while adenocarcinomas are more common in the duodenum, followed by the jejunum and least commonly, the ileum. Stromal tumors and lymphomas are most commonly seen in the distal small bowel but can be found throughout.

Risk Factors

Despite the small intestine accounting for 75% of the length of the gastrointestinal (GI) tract, small bowel malignancies comprise <5% of all GI cancers. Protective factors released by the small intestine, lower bacterial load, and lower levels of carcinogenic factors may explain this discrepancy. Another factor thought to contribute to the relatively low incidence is secretion of immunoglobulin A by the small intestine, which serves an integral role in mucosal immunity.

Familial inherited syndromes are also associated with small bowel cancers. These include familial adenomatous polyposis (FAP), Peutz–Jeghers, Lynch syndrome, Cowden syndrome, and von Recklinghausen neurofibromatosis. Autoimmune bowel diseases are also associated with increased risk of small bowel malignancies, particularly Crohn disease and celiac disease.

Clinical Presentation

Patients with small intestine malignancies are more likely to present with GI complaints compared to patients with benign lesions. Common presenting symptoms include abdominal pain (75%), weight loss (28%), bowel obstruction (25%), and bleeding (24%). Duodenal tumors can also present with jaundice if the ampulla is involved. Diagnosis of small bowel tumors is often delayed unless the presentation involves acute symptoms such as obstruction, bleeding, or perforation. Bowel perforation is the presenting symptom in 10% of patients and is more often seen with lymphoma or gastrointestinal stromal tumors (GISTs).

Diagnostic Workup

Initial workup consists of performing a comprehensive history and exam including history of familial syndromes, personal history of malignancy or inflammatory bowel diseases, as well as a complete physical examination. Laboratory tests should include a complete blood count, serum electrolytes, liver enzymes, and 5-hydroxyindoleacetic acid (5-HIAA) if there is clinical suspicion for a NET. Additionally, tumor markers including carcinoembryonic antigen (CEA) and carbohydrate antigen 19-9 (CA 19-9) should be included in initial workup.

These tumor markers may be normal in up to half of patients with masses. If the initial presenting symptom is obstruction, cross-sectional imaging may identify the location and characterize the cause of obstruction. Computed tomography (CT) imaging carries a sensitivity of 80% for small bowel lesions and increases to 85% to 95% with CT or MR enterography. For NETs, radio-labeled somatostatin analog [^{111}In-DTPA^0] octreotide scintigraphy (OctreoScan) can be used as an adjunct for identification of the primary and extra-abdominal lesions, with a sensitivity of 88% and specificity of 97%. 68Ga-DOTATATE PET/CT offers 95% sensitivity and 98% specificity but may not be available at all institutions.

Endoscopy allows for the detection and biopsy of proximal small bowel malignancies in the duodenum, however, evaluation of lesions in the more distal small bowel are challenging. Single and double balloon enteroscopy allow for examination of the mucosa beyond the ligament of Treitz but do not allow for visualization for the entire small bowel. Takano et al. compared single to double balloon enteroscopy and found higher completion rates with double balloon (0% vs. 57%, $p = .002$) but no difference in therapeutic outcomes (single balloon 28% vs. double balloon 35%, $p = .63$). Use of single or double balloon enteroscopy is still dependent on physician preference and availability.

Video capsule endoscopy (VCE) is another modality that is increasingly used to evaluate the small intestine. A pill-shaped camera is ingested and transmits images of the entire small intestine. A pooled meta-analysis by Lewis et al. found a lower rate of missed pathology compared to enteroscopy with equivalent completion rate. VCE has poor diagnostic yield when used in patients with delayed gastric emptying, previous abdominal operations, and poor bowel preparation. Risks with VCE include retention of capsule requiring either repeat endoscopy or surgical retrieval in 1% of patients.

Despite the multiple diagnostic tools available, an accurate preoperative diagnosis of small intestinal malignancy remains difficult and is only made in approximately half of cases. When no diagnosis has been made but clinical suspicion is high with symptoms of GI bleeding or obstruction, exploratory surgery should be performed. Intraoperative endoscopy can be done with surgeon assistance to allow for complete visualization of the small intestine mucosa.

Specific Types of Small Bowel Malignancies

Adenocarcinoma

Pathology

Small bowel adenocarcinomas (SBAs) historically accounted for 50% of all small bowel malignancies but contemporary studies have found rates of 36.9%. Over half of these lesions arise in the duodenum, followed by the jejunum and ileum. Much like colorectal adenocarcinoma, these tumors invade into the bowel wall and can involve adjacent structures, and generally metastasize early to locoregional lymph nodes. Tumor enlargement can cause obstructive symptoms. Violation of the mucosal layer can lead to GI bleeding and acute or chronic anemia.

Genetic analyses reveal mutations in several key genes. The adenomatous polyposis coli (*APC*) gene is mutated in 10% to 18% of SBA compared to 80% of sporadic colorectal cancers (CRCs). This suggests the pathways to adenocarcinoma may differ between small and large bowel adenocarcinomas.

Germline mutations in the *APC* gene are found in FAP. Patients with FAP develop duodenal adenomas in 80% of cases and 4% develop adenocarcinoma. Due to the risk of malignant transformation, endoscopic surveillance with a side-view scope to evaluate the ampulla is recommended. Frequency of surveillance is determined by the number and size of polyps present in the individual patient (Spiegelman score).

Lynch syndrome is associated with germline inactivation in one or more of the mismatch repair (MMR) genes (*MLH1*, *MSH2*, *MSH6*, and *PMS2*), leading to microsatellite instability. This inactivation is found in over 90% of Lynch syndrome patients. Sporadic mutations, particularly in *MLH1*, can also occur with resulting inactivation of the MMR system occurring in 15% of CRC. SBAs have a sporadic deficiency in MMR (dMMR) in up to 35% of cases, much higher than that in CRC, once again suggesting the molecular mechanisms behind the development of SBA are different from large bowel adenocarcinomas. SBA in patients with dMMR is more often located in the proximal small intestine rather than the ileum.

Additional important proteins frequently mutated in SBA are *KRAS*, p53, and SMAD4, with mutation rates as high as 53%, 52%, and 47% respectively. Crohn's disease is also associated with SBA, with a standardized incidence ratio of 18 to 46 compared to the non-IBD population. Patients with a long disease duration and stricture-forming disease are at increased risk.

Clinical Course

The clinical symptoms of SBA are often nonspecific, therefore more than half of patients present with stage III or IV disease. Prognosis is based on the stage of disease, with 5-year disease-specific survival rates of 90% for stage I, 78% for stage II, 64% to 73% for stage III and 43% to 47% for stage IV disease. Five-year overall survival rates are significantly lower, reflecting the older age of diagnosis for many patients (61%, 46%, 32%, and 8% for stages I to IV, respectively). Compared to other small bowel malignancies such as neuroendocrine, lymphoma, and stromal tumors, SBAs have a worse prognosis.

Lymph node metastases are present in approximately 24% of patients at the time of diagnosis and 32% will have distant disease, usually in the liver. A SEER database study by Overman et al. examining the prognostic value of lymph nodes in SBA found that there was a survival benefit with a greater total number of lymph nodes examined in patients with stage I to III disease. Furthermore, in patients with stage III disease, there was a worse 5-year disease-specific survival when ≥3 positive lymph nodes were found compared to <3 (37% vs. 58%).

CEA and CA 19-9 are elevated in 30% and 40% patients, respectively. These markers can be used as prognostic factors for progression-free and overall survival and in surveillance for disease recurrence.

Surgical Treatment
The primary treatment for SBA involves wide segmental resection with locoregional lymphadenectomy. Patients with unresectable disease have a 5-year overall survival of 0% compared to 54% for resectable disease.

Proximal duodenal lesions in the first and second portions of the duodenum are typically managed with pancreaticoduodenectomy with locoregional lymphadenectomy. For distal duodenal lesions, wide excision with lymphadenectomy may be appropriate as long as negative margins are obtained and there is no ampullary involvement. Jejunal and ileal lesions are treated with wide segmental resection and regional lymph node dissection. For ileal lesions close to the cecum, a right colectomy or ileocecectomy may be required in order to obtain negative margins and appropriate lymphadenectomy.

Adjuvant Therapy
Recurrence after resection for SBA can be as high as 39% lending credence to the argument for adjuvant therapy. Of those with recurrences, 56% are distant, 19% are carcinomatosis, and 17% are local. Prospective randomized data examining the optimal adjuvant regimen for SBA is lacking, with current recommendations guided primarily by retrospective data as well as extrapolation from colon cancer data. Despite the paucity of high-quality data, a National Cancer Database study found the rate of adjuvant chemotherapy use has increased from 8% in 1985 to 22% in 2005 ($p < .0001$). Based on the data that is available, 5–fluorouracil–based chemotherapy with oxaliplatin is the standard for patients with high-risk SBA (+ lymph nodes). Capecitabine with oxaliplatin is also an acceptable regimen. Currently, neoadjuvant therapy is not routinely employed in the treatment of SBA.

To address this paucity of data for adjuvant therapy, the International Rare Cancers Initiative (IRCI) was created. This is a joint initiative between Cancer Research UK (CRUK), the National Institute of Health Research Clinical Research Network: Cancer (NIHR CRN: Cancer), the National Cancer Institute (NCI), the European Organization for Research and Treatment of Cancer (EORTC), the Institut National Du Cancer (INCa), and the National Cancer Institute of Canada Clinical Trials Group (NCIC CTG), whose aim is to "facilitate the development of international clinical trials for patients with rare cancers in order to boost the progress of new treatments for these patients." For SBA, the BALLARD study is a large, prospective, randomized trial specifically evaluating the impact of adjuvant chemotherapy for small intestinal adenocarcinomas. It began accruing in 2017 and 5-year survival data is anticipated in the near future.

Hyperthermic Intraperitoneal Chemotherapy
Hyperthermic intraperitoneal chemotherapy (HIPEC) with cytoreductive surgery (CRS) is the standard of care for pseudomyxoma peritonei, peritoneal mesothelioma, and CRC with isolated peritoneal metastases, but is emerging as a potential therapy for highly selected patients with SBA. This technique involves removing all visible peritoneal disease and perfusing the abdominal cavity with heated chemotherapy. In a study examining prognostic factors for SBA from MDACC, 25% of patients with stage IV disease were found to have peritoneal carcinomatosis. For this highly selective group of patients, HIPEC/CRS has a potential role in treatment. In a multi-institutional study from the Netherlands by van Oudheusden et al. examining HIPEC/CRS for SBA, complete resection was obtained in 93.8% with median overall survival of 30.8 months versus 7.1 months in patients not undergoing resection.

At MDACC, the treatment algorithm for patients with metastatic SBA with isolated peritoneal disease (i.e., absence of liver, lung, or other distant metastasis) includes case discussion at a multidisciplinary tumor board with evaluation of the extent of disease and initiation of systemic chemotherapy with serial evaluation for progression via cross-sectional imaging and/or diagnostic laparoscopy. If there is no progression and the limited disease is amenable to complete resection, HIPEC with CRS is offered in appropriate surgical candidates.

Metastatic Disease

Systemic chemotherapy is the primary treatment for patients with metastatic SBA. Data from retrospective studies have found improved overall survival with systemic chemotherapy, 13 months versus 4 months (p = .02). These studies used a wide variety of agents, but standard therapy should entail use of bevacizumab with CAPOX (capecitabine and oxaliplatin), FOLFOX (5-fluorouracil, leucovorin, and oxaliplatin), or FOLFOXIRI (5-fluorouracil, leucovorin, oxaliplatin, and irinotecan), depending on the patients' performance status. Second-line therapy for mismatch-repair deficient (dMMR) tumors includes checkpoint blockade with anti–PD-1 or anti-CTLA4 monoclonal antibodies, extrapolating from data from dMMR CRC. For mismatch-repair proficient tumors, taxane-based regimens are recommended as second-line based on small retrospective studies. Ongoing clinical trials are currently investigating use of targeted therapies to help determine optimal regimens for metastatic SBA.

Neuroendocrine Tumors

Epidemiology

NETs, formerly referred to as carcinoid tumors, are a diverse group of tumors that arise from enterochromaffin cells found throughout the body. They can arise from the foregut, midgut, or hindgut and have the ability to secrete various hormones and peptides leading to functional syndromes.

The peak incidence of NETs is in the seventh to eighth decades. For jejunal/ileal NETs, higher rates occur in males compared to females (0.8 vs. 0.57/100,000). Small bowel tumors account for 42% of NETs of the GI tract and most commonly arise from the terminal ileum. Overall, the incidence of small bowel NETs is increasing, with a sixfold rise from 1973 to 2012 based on SEER data. Small bowel NETs have overtaken SBA as the most common primary tumor of the small intestine.

Risk factors for the development of small bowel NETs include a family history of prostate or CRC among first-degree relatives, tongue or mouth cancer in siblings, and endometrial, kidney, skin, or non-Hodgkin lymphoma in parents.

Environmental risk factors for development of NETs are unclear. Cigarette smoking was found to increase the risk of developing small bowel NETs in a European population-based case-control study, but not in a US-based case-control study, while alcohol consumption did not increase the risk in either study.

Pathology

Multiple nomenclature systems exist to describe NETs, adding to the confusion and limiting applicability of data when different systems are used.

In an effort to standardize terminology, the European Neuroendocrine Tumor Society (ENETS) and World Health Organization established criteria to ensure clinicians are referring to the same tumor subtype. Based on these criteria, small bowel NETs are differentiated into three grades based on the number of mitoses and Ki-67 proliferative index (Table 11.1). The term "Carcinoid tumor," refers to low/intermediate-grade tumors, well-differentiated tumors, or NET grades 1 and 2 (also rare well-differentiated grade 3 tumors).

TABLE 11.1	Neuroendocrine Tumor of Midgut Grading System			
Grade	Differentiation	Traditional	ENETs, WHO	Criteria
Low grade	Well differentiated	Carcinoid tumor	Neuroendocrine tumor grade 1 (G1)	<2 Mitoses/10 high-power fields, and <3% Ki-67 index
Intermediate grade	Well differentiated	Carcinoid tumor	Neuroendocrine tumor grade 2 (G2)	2–20 Mitoses/10 high-power fields, or 3–20% Ki-67 index
High grade	Poorly differentiated	Small cell carcinoma Large cell neuroendocrine carcinoma	Neuroendocrine carcinoma grade 3 (G3), small cell carcinoma Neuroendocrine carcinoma grade 3 (G3), large cell carcinoma	>20 Mitoses/10 high-power fields or >20% Ki-67 index

ENET, European Neuroendocrine Tumour Society; WHO, World Health Organization.
Adapted from Boudreaux JP, Klimstra DS, Hassan MM, et al. The NANETS consensus guideline for the diagnosis and management of neuroendocrine tumors: well-differentiated neuroendocrine tumors of the jejunum, ileum, appendix, and cecum. *Pancreas.* 2010;39(6):753–766.

Small bowel NETs are often multiple, appear as tan or brown intramural or submucosal nodules, and are capable of releasing biologically active substances such as serotonin, amines, and prostaglandins. Because multiple tumors are often found, careful evaluation of the entire small bowel is needed during the time of operation. The liver should also be carefully examined for metastatic disease. As a whole, at the time of presentation, regional lymph node involvement is seen in 70% of patients and liver metastasis in over half.

Clinical Presentation

NETs of the small bowel are typically indolent. This can lead to a delay in diagnosis, with many patients having symptoms for an average of 5 years before a diagnosis is made. As with SBA, the majority of these patients present with nonspecific chronic abdominal pain and/or obstruction.

Twenty to 30% of patients present with carcinoid syndrome. Carcinoid syndrome symptoms include flushing (94%), watery diarrhea (80%), wheezing, abdominal pain, and pellagra related to niacin deficiency. Flushing can be triggered by the consumption of alcohol, blue cheese, chocolate, or red wine. Long-term carcinoid syndrome can ultimately lead to development of right-sided heart failure (carcinoid heart disease). Preoperative echocardiogram should be considered to evaluate for carcinoid heart disease and any valvular disease in high-risk patients.

The most extreme manifestation of carcinoid syndrome is a carcinoid crisis. Symptoms include hemodynamic instability, shock nonresponsive to vasopressors, hyperthermia, arrhythmia, and/or bronchoconstriction. Those individuals at greatest risk of developing carcinoid crisis are patients with flushing and large bulky tumors. Carcinoid crisis can be triggered by surgery and therefore all patients with NETs should be given octreotide preoperatively.

Diagnosis

The diagnosis of small bowel NETs is made by the clinical picture, biochemical testing, and imaging. Chromogranin A (CgA) is a polypeptide present in the secretory granules of neuroendocrine cells. CgA is elevated in 60% to 100% of patients with functional or nonfunctional NETs and have sensitivity and specificities of 70% and 100%, respectively. False elevations in CgA can be seen with renal and liver failure, chronic gastritis, and in patients taking proton pump inhibitors (PPIs). PPIs should be stopped 2 weeks before CgA evaluation.

One of the major hormones released by NETs is serotonin, which is metabolized by the liver into 5-hydroxyindoleacetic acid (5-HIAA) and then excreted into the urine. Direct measurement of serum serotonin levels can be inaccurate as there is significant daily variation based on stress and activity level. A 24-hour urinary 5-HIAA level provides a more accurate measurement of global serum serotonin activity. Elevations are found in over half of patients and carry specificity as high as 88% for NET tumors. However, like CgA, 5-HIAA can be falsely elevated, with incorrect results seen after recent consumption of alcohol, nuts, tomatoes, and over-the-counter cold/cough medications.

Because CgA and 5-HIAA levels can be reflective of overall tumor burden, they are most useful in evaluating tumor response in the treatment of metastatic disease. These studies can also be followed to detect tumor recurrence after initial resection.

In situations where 5-HIAA is not elevated, additional testing should consist of measurements of urinary 5-hydroxytryptamine (5-HT, serotonin) and 5-hydroxytryptophan (5-HPT), plasma 5-HPT, platelet 5-HT, and serum levels of CgA, neuron-specific enolase (NSE), substance P, and neuropeptide K.

With any imaging modality used, at least 25% of patients will have underestimation of the extent of disease. Cross-sectional imaging with CT or MRI can identify small bowel NETs with 77% to 80% sensitivity. NETs are hypervascular lesions and CT imaging should be done with thin slices with an arterial and late venous phase in order to identify arterial enhancement and venous washout. This technique is particularly helpful in cases of liver metastases. On MRI, NETs can have a variable appearance on T1-weighted images, being hypointense or isointense, while appearing bright on T2-weighted images.

OctreoScan can be used as an adjunct to CT or MRI in the identification of locoregional or distant disease. It carries sensitivity as high as 90% and unlike localized cross-sectional imaging, it examines the entire body for occult lesions. OctreoScan identifies somatostatin receptors 2 and 5 in tumors. In some cases, patients with poorly differentiated NETs have lost these receptors and these lesions cannot be detected with OctreoScan.

68Ga-DOTATATE PET/CT has been approved for detection of small bowel NETs, with a 96% sensitivity and 93% specificity. This modality combines cross-sectional imaging with whole-body evaluation for metastatic disease but is not available at all centers.

Treatment of Localized Disease

Complete resection of the primary tumor with regional lymphadenectomy is standard therapy for nonmetastatic disease. Prior to any surgery, patients with symptoms of carcinoid syndrome should be pretreated with

It should be noted that melanoma metastases to the small bowel that are treated with systemic immunotherapy are at risk for involution and subsequent perforation. These patients may require urgent or delayed resection, even in the setting of complete response, for management of the perforation itself. Delay to surgery may be appropriate for patients with very recent exposure to chemotherapy to avoid unnecessary morbidity, to be decided on a case-by-case basis. For metastases from other primaries, resection of the lesion is sufficient for palliation without needing to perform a regional lymphadenectomy.

Palliation

Metastatic lesions to the small bowel are often bulky and not amendable to resection. In addition, multipoint obstructions are common due to disseminated carcinomatosis. Most patients have multiple sites of partial obstruction and are best palliated with decompressive gastrostomy tube placement. Palliative care consultation is recommended, as life expectancy is limited after development of unresectable small bowel metastases. Palliative surgery may have a role in patients with indolent disease biology and focal points of obstruction amenable to resection or enteric bypass. In situations of GI bleeding, angiography with selective embolization can be considered. However, one major complication of embolization is delayed bowel ischemia, and patients should be closely monitored. Both surgical and angiographic procedures have high morbidity, are temporizing, and rarely lead to resumption of systemic therapy or prolonged overall survival. In addition, patients often have poor performance status due to effects of systemic therapy and malnutrition. The morbidity of interventions and limited life expectancy must be carefully balanced through shared decision-making between the patient and medical team.

CASE SCENARIO

Case Scenario 1

Presentation

A 67-year-old male presents to clinic with a several month history of vague abdominal pain, bloating, melena, and a 10-lb unintentional weight loss. His only relevant history is celiac disease, which was diagnosed 20 years ago, and his physical exam is unremarkable. Initial workup includes a CBC, electrolyte panel, liver panel, and tumor markers including CEA and CA 19-9. Laboratory studies are significant for mild anemia and CEA 3× the upper limit of normal. He is sent for CT abdomen and pelvis which reveals prominent lymphadenopathy in the small bowel mesentery, but no discrete mass. He is then sent for EGD and colonoscopy, which are unremarkable. Because there is high suspicion for a small bowel mass, he is sent for push enteroscopy, which reveals a 3-cm mass in the proximal jejunum that is biopsied.

Differential Diagnosis

Benign small bowel pathology	Malignant small bowel pathology
Focal bowel ischemia	Adenocarcinoma
Inflammatory bowel disease	Neuroendocrine tumor
Infection	Lymphoma
Adenoma	Gastrointestinal stromal tumor (GIST)
Leiomyoma	Metastasis to small bowel
Lipoma	

The biopsy confirms moderately differentiated adenocarcinoma of the jejunum. The patient's metastatic workup including CT chest/abdomen/pelvis is negative for evidence of metastatic disease. Because his tumor is resectable and he has no evidence of metastases, the patient is scheduled for upfront wide segmental resection with regional mesenteric lymphadenectomy.

Surgical Approach—Key Steps

Wide segmental resection with associated mesentery/regional lymph nodes can be undertaken minimally invasively (laparoscopically/robotically) or open. The procedure should begin with thorough exploration to ensure no evidence of intra-abdominal metastatic disease, taking special care to evaluate the liver and peritoneal surfaces. The small bowel should be visually and manually (if possible) evaluated in its entirety. After exploration, wide segmental resection should be performed with a 5-cm margin proximally and distally. Reanastomosis in a side-to-side fashion can be performed either by hand-sewing or with a surgical stapler.

Postoperative Management

Postsurgical care after small bowel resection should be focused on pain control, early ambulation, and return of bowel function. This patient underwent laparoscopic wide segmental resection of a mid-jejunal adenocarcinoma with negative margins and 3/20 positive lymph nodes on final pathologic evaluation. He was then recommended to undergo adjuvant FOLFOX and is followed in clinic every 4 months with tumor markers and cross-sectional imaging for 2 years, followed by annually thereafter.

Case Scenario 2

Presentation

A 48-year-old female presents to clinic with vague abdominal pain over the previous 12 months. She is otherwise asymptomatic but has a family history of a sister with a colorectal cancer. She has had multiple previous abdominal operations including an open cholecystectomy, appendectomy, and ventral hernia repair. Her physical exam is unremarkable. She is sent for a CT abdomen/pelvis with contrast that reveals a distal ileal mesenteric mass without evidence of other intra-abdominal disease. Her laboratory studies are significant for elevated chromogranin A and urinary 5-HIAA levels. Her EGD and colonoscopy are unremarkable.

An ileal neuroendocrine tumor is suspected based on preoperative workup. Due to the patient's previous surgical history, she is planned for an exploratory laparotomy and open wide segmental ileal resection with regional mesenteric lymphadenectomy.

Surgical Approach—Key Steps

Wide segmental resection with associated mesentery/regional lymph nodes can be undertaken minimally invasively (laparoscopically/robotically) or open as in this case. The procedure should begin with thorough exploration, either laparoscopically or open, to ensure no evidence of intra-abdominal metastatic disease, taking special care to evaluate the liver. The small bowel should be visually and manually evaluated in its entirety, as NETs may present as multiple primary lesions that are relatively small and challenging to visualize on cross-sectional imaging. After exploration, wide segmental resection should be performed with a 5-cm margin proximally and distally. Reanastomosis in a side-to-side fashion can be performed either by hand-sewing or with a surgical stapler.

Postoperative Management

Postsurgical care after small bowel resection should be focused on pain control, early ambulation, and return of bowel function. This patient underwent exploratory laparotomy and open wide segmental resection of two small (<2 cm) distal well-differentiated ileal neuroendocrine primary tumors with negative margins and 2/16 positive lymph nodes on final pathologic evaluation. She recovered well after surgery and is followed in clinic every 3 months for biochemical testing and cross-sectional imaging for 1 year, followed by every 6 to 12 months thereafter for at least 10 years.

CASE SCENARIO REVIEW

Questions

1. A 54-year-old female with a history of FAP who had undergone total proctocolectomy with ileal pouch–anal anastomosis presented for her routine screening EGD and was found to have a large polyp in the second portion of her duodenum. She was asymptomatic. The polyp was biopsied but was not able to be snared due to close proximity to the ampulla. The pathology was consistent with high-grade dysplasia. What is the next best step in the management of this patient?

    A. Continue endoscopic surveillance
    B. Repeat endoscopy with additional attempt to endoscopically remove the polyp
    C. Initial systemic chemotherapy
    D. Pancreaticoduodenectomy
    E. Segmental duodenectomy

2. A 64-year-old woman presents with a 14-month history of weight loss, bloating, and recent episode of bilious emesis. She underwent upper endoscopy and enteroscopy, which revealed a near-obstructing mid-jejunal mass, which was biopsied and consistent with moderately differentiated adenocarcinoma. CT scan of the chest, abdomen, and pelvis were negative for metastatic disease. The patient

was taken to the OR for a laparoscopic small bowel resection and lymphadenectomy. However, during diagnostic laparoscopy, two subcentimeter peritoneal masses were encountered. A frozen biopsy of each lesion was consistent with adenocarcinoma. What is the next step in management?

A. Perform surgical bypass, then close and refer to GI medical oncology for chemotherapy

B. Convert to open and perform wide segmental jejunal resection with resection of peritoneal lesions

C. Close without any resection and refer to GI medical oncology for chemotherapy

D. Perform laparoscopic wide segmental jejunal resection without resection of peritoneal lesions and refer to GI medical oncology for chemotherapy

E. Close and call palliative care for goals of care discussion

3. A 72-year-old man presented to the emergency center with bright red hematemesis. He is hemodynamically stable. Upper endoscopy reveals a 4-cm friable mass along the posterior wall of the first portion of the duodenum with evidence of ulceration but no identified source of bleeding. Biopsy is consistent with duodenal adenocarcinoma. What is the next best step in management?

A. IR embolization of GDA

B. CT of the chest, abdomen, and pelvis

C. Pancreaticoduodenectomy

D. Referral to GI medical oncology for chemotherapy

E. Radiation therapy

4. An 83-year-old woman with multiple medial comorbidities with a history of small bowel neuroendocrine tumor and diffuse liver metastases presents for follow up with wheezing, palpitations, flushing, and diarrhea. Due to her age, she has been under close observation for several years, with stable liver metastases on surveillance CT scans. What is the next best step in her management?

A. Obtain DOTATE scan to identify additional sites of metastases

B. Refer to GI medical oncology for initiation of systemic chemotherapy

C. Proceed to the operating room for liver debulking given symptoms of carcinoid syndrome

D. Continue observation

E. Initiate octreotide therapy to help control her symptoms

5. A 50-year-old woman presents after being diagnosed with a 5-cm right lower quadrant mesenteric mass that was found on CT abdomen/pelvis obtained during an evaluation for vague abdominal pain. The patient denies weight loss and fatigue. Her first colonoscopy was 3 months ago, during which two benign polyps were removed from within the descending colon. Laboratory testing revealed an elevated chromogranin A and 24-hour urine 5-HIAA. What is the next step in management?

A. EGD

B. Proceed to the OR for wide segmental resection of the mass

C. DOTATATE PET/CT

D. IR-guided biopsy of the mass

E. Initiate octreotide therapy

Answers

1. **The correct answer is D.** *Rationale:* Polyps with high-grade dysplasia should be surgically resected due to increased risk of associated adenocarcinoma. For a polyp near the ampulla, a pancreaticoduodenectomy is the appropriate surgical procedure rather than a segmental resection that has the potential to compromise the ampulla or narrow the proximal duodenum. Systemic therapy is not appropriate without a diagnosis of cancer, and generally not recommended in the neoadjuvant setting for SBA. Surveillance is also not appropriate with high-grade dysplasia.

2. **The correct answer is A.** *Rationale:* In cases when unexpected metastatic disease is encountered, formal resection should not be performed, and the patient should be referred for systemic chemotherapy. However, in this case, the patient has a near-obstructing tumor and surgical bypass should be done at the time of the operation to prevent complete obstruction in the near future.

3. **The correct answer is B.** *Rationale:* The patient should be staged fully before surgical resection is undertaken. If metastatic disease is found, patient should be referred for systemic therapy and should not undergo resection. The lesion is no longer bleeding, and the patient is stable, so GDA embolization is not appropriate. Radiation is not generally considered for small bowel adenocarcinoma unless patient is palliative and cannot tolerate surgery and/or chemotherapy.

4. The correct answer is E. *Rationale:* This patient is symptomatic from carcinoid syndrome and should be started on a somatostatin analog. She is elderly and has multiple comorbid conditions and should not undergo surgery. If the patient were fit for surgery, a debulking procedure resecting 90% of the liver disease would be recommended to decrease symptoms. Continued observation is not appropriate, as she is symptomatic. Obtaining further imaging will not change management.

5. The correct answer is C. *Rationale:* This patient likely has a small bowel neuroendocrine tumor based on imaging and laboratory studies, but imaging should be completed with DOTATATE to ensure no additional metastatic disease are present. Proceeding straight to the OR is inappropriate before staging workup is complete. Biopsy carries significant risk and will not change management, and octreotide therapy before final diagnosis and complete workup is also not appropriate.

Recommended Readings

Annesse V. Small bowel adenocarcinoma in Crohn's disease: an underestimated risk? *J Crohn's and Colitis.* 2020;14(3):285–286.

Aparicio T, Svrcek M, Zaanan A, et al. Small bowel adenocarcinoma phenotyping, a clinicobiological prognostic study. *Br J Cancer.* 2013;109(12):3057–3066.

Aparicio T, Zaanan A, Mary F, Afchain P, Manfredi S, Evans TR. Small bowel adenocarcinoma. *Gastroenterol Clin N Am.* 2016;45(3):447–457.

Arai M, Shimizu S, Imai Y, et al. Mutations of the Ki-ras, p53 and APC genes in adenocarcinomas of the human small intestine. *Int J Cancer.* 1997;70(4):390–395.

Benson A, Venook AP, Al-Hawary MM, et al. Small bowel adenocarcinoma NCCN clinical practice guidelines in oncology version 1.2020. *J Natl Compr Canc Netw.* 2019;17(9):1109–1133.

Bilimoria KY, Bentrem DJ, Wayne JD, Ko CY, Bennett CL, Talamonti MS. Small bowel cancer in the United States: changes in epidemiology, treatment, and survival over the last 20 years. *Ann Surg.* 2009;249(1):63–71.

Boudreaux JP, Klimstra DS, Hassan MM, et al. The NANETS consensus guideline for the diagnosis and management of neuroendocrine tumors: well-differentiated neuroendocrine tumors of the jejunum, ileum, appendix, and cecum. *Pancreas.* 2010;39(6):753–766.

Cerutti A, Rescigno M. The biology of intestinal immunoglobulin A responses. *Immunity.* 2008;28(6):740–750.

Chambers AP, Pasieka JL, Dixon E. The role of imaging studies in the staging of midgut neuroendocrine tumors. *J Am Coll Surg.* 2008;207(3):s18.

Czaykowski P, Hui D. Chemotherapy in small bowel adenocarcinoma: 10–year experience of the British Columbia Cancer Agency. *Clin Oncol (R Coll Radiol).* 2007;19(2):143–149.

Dabaja BS, Suki D, Pro B, Bonnen M, Ajani J. Adenocarcinoma of the small bowel: presentation, prognostic factors, and outcome of 217 patients. *Cancer.* 2004;101(3):518–526.

Haselkorn T, Whittemore AS, Lilienfeld DE. Incidence of small bowel cancer in the United States and worldwide: geographic, temporal and racial differences. *Cancer Causes Control.* 2005;16(7):781–787.

Howe JR, Karnell LH, Scott-Conner C. Small bowel sarcoma: analysis of survival from the National Cancer Data Base. *Ann Surg Oncol.* 2001;8(6):496–508.

Keat N, Law K, Seymour M, et al. International rare cancers initiative. *Lancet Oncol.* 2013;14(2):109–110.

Kim MK, Warner RRP, Roayale S, et al. Revised staging classification improves outcome prediction for small intestinal neuroendocrine tumors. *J Clin Oncol.* 2013;31:3776–3781.

Kvols LK, Martin JK, Marsh HM, Moertel CG. Rapid reversal of carcinoid crisis with a somatostatin analogue. *N Engl J Med.* 1985;313(19):1229–1230.

Lewis BS, Eisen GM, Friedman S. A pooled analysis to evaluate results of capsule endoscopy trials. *Endoscopy.* 2005;37(10):960–965.

Modlin IM, Pavel M, Kidd M, Gustafsson BI. Review article: somatostatin analogues in the treatment of gastroenteropancreatic neuroendocrine (carcinoid) tumors. *Aliment Pharmacol Ther.* 2010;31(2):169–188.

Nakamura S, Matsumoto T, Iida M, Yao T, Tsuneyoshi M. Primary gastrointestinal lymphoma in Japan: a clinicopathologic analysis of 455 patients with special reference to its time trends. *Cancer.* 2003;97(10):2462–2473.

Overman MJ, Hu CY, Wolff RA, Chang GJ. Prognostic value of lymph node evaluation in small bowel adenocarcinoma: analysis of the surveillance, epidemiology, and end results database. *Cancer.* 2010;116(23):5374–5382.

Overman MJ, Pozadzides J, Kopetz S, et al. Immunophenotype and molecular characterisation of adenocarcinoma of the small intestine. *Br J Cancer*. 2010;102(1):144–150.

Overman MJ, Varadhachary GR, Kopetz S, et al. Phase II study of capecitabine and oxaliplatin for advanced adenocarcinoma of the small bowel and ampulla of Vater. *J Clin Oncol*. 2009;27(16):2598–2603.

Pape UF, Perren A, Niederle B, et al. ENETS Consensus Guidelines for the management of patients with neuroendocrine neoplasms from the jejuno-ileum and the appendix including goblet cell carcinomas. *Neuroendocrinology*. 2012;95(2):135–156.

Pappalardo G, Gualdi G, Nunziale A, Masselli G, Floriani I, Casciani E. Impact of magnetic resonance in the preoperative staging and the surgical planning for treating small bowel neoplasms. *Surg Today*. 2013;43(6):613–619.

Parris WC, Oates JA, Kambam J, Shmerling R, Sawyers JF. Pre-treatment with somatostatin in the anaesthetic management of a patient with carcinoid syndrome. *Can J Anaesth*. 1988;35(4):413–416.

Pavel ME, Hainsworth JD, Baudin E, et al. Everolimus plus octreotide long-acting repeatable for the treatment of advanced neuroendocrine tumours associated with carcinoid syndrome (RADIANT-2): a randomised, placebo-controlled, phase 3 study. *Lancet*. 2011;378(9808):2005–2012.

Pilleul F, Penigaud M, Milot L, Saurin J-C, Chayvialle J-A, Valette P-J. Possible small-bowel neoplasms: contrast-enhanced and water-enhanced multidetector CT enteroclysis. *Radiology*. 2006;241(3):796–801.

Raghav K, Overman MJ. Small bowel adenocarcinomas—existing evidence and evolving paradigms. *Nat Rev Clin Oncol*. 2013;10(9):534–544.

Rinke A, Muller HH, Schade-Brittinger C, et al. Placebo-controlled, double-blind, prospective, randomized study on the effect of octreotide LAR in the control of tumor growth in patients with metastatic neuroendocrine midgut tumors: a report from the PROMID Study Group. *J Clin Oncol*. 2009;27(28):4656–4663.

Shenoy S. Primary small-bowel malignancy: update in tumor biology, markers, and management strategies. *J Gastrointest Cancer*. 2014;45(4):421–430.

Shenoy S. Small bowel sarcoma: tumor biology and advances in therapeutics. *Surg Oncol*. 2015;24(3):136–144.

Takano N, Yamada A, Watabe H, et al. Single-balloon versus double-balloon endoscopy for achieving total enteroscopy: a randomized, controlled trial. *Gastrointest Endosc*. 2011;73(4):734–739.

van Oudheusden TR, Lemmens VE, Braam HJ, et al. Peritoneal metastases from small bowel cancer: results of cytoreductive surgery and hyperthermic intraperitoneal chemotherapy in the Netherlands. *Surgery*. 2015;157(6):1023–1027.

Wheeler JM, Warren BF, Mortensen NJ, et al. An insight into the genetic pathway of adenocarcinoma of the small intestine. *Gut*. 2002;50(2):218–223.

Yantiss RK, Odze RD, Farraye FA, Rosenberg AE. Solitary versus multiple carcinoid tumors of the ileum: a clinical and pathologic review of 68 cases. *Am J Surg Pathol*. 2003;27:811–817.

Yao JC, Hassan M, Phan A, et al. One hundred years after "carcinoid": epidemiology of and prognostic factors for neuroendocrine tumors in 35,825 cases in the United States. *J Clin Oncol*. 2008;26(18):3063–3072.

12 Peritoneal Malignancies

Michael G. White and Keith F. Fournier

INTRODUCTION

Peritoneal carcinomatosis was historically considered a terminal disease regardless of the site of origin. Left untreated, patients with carcinomatosis experience significant abdominal pain, bloating, bowel obstruction, and eventual death with a median overall survival from the time of diagnosis of 6 months. Palliative chemotherapy increased the median overall survival duration to only 12 months. While surgery was typically reserved for emergency situations and palliation of other symptoms, the last two decades have seen a rapid increase in data supporting cytoreductive surgery (CRS) as a potential viable treatment option. This new data demonstrates marked improvement in survival in many patients and potentially offers a cure to select patients.

The advent of CRS can be traced to the early 1980s, when a small number of surgeons evaluated the feasibility of complete resection of all disease for patients with peritoneal malignancies. Fernandez and Daly initially reported on 38 patients with pseudomyxoma peritonei (PMP) treated at MD Anderson and concluded that the initial treatment for these individuals should be surgical cytoreduction, including omentectomy, appendectomy, and, in female patients, bilateral oophorectomy. That same year, Spratt reported on the successful use of extensive abdominal resection with the addition of intraoperative, intraperitoneal hyperthermic chemotherapy in a patient with the clinical syndrome of PMP. A few years later, Sugarbaker would begin what has become one of the largest series of patients undergoing CRS and intraperitoneal chemotherapy (IPEC) for peritoneal surface malignancies.

Concurrently, surgical resection for oligometastatic disease was refined for a variety of histologies including melanoma, colorectal cancer, and sarcoma. Not until recently, however, have peritoneal malignancies been approached as a type of regional failure rather than distant metastasis. The observation that many malignancies, such as appendiceal adenocarcinoma, colorectal adenocarcinoma, and peritoneal mesothelioma, remain confined to the peritoneal cavity without extra-abdominal spread led to the investigation of CRS as the preferred treatment modality for peritoneal surface malignancies. The goal of CRS is to systematically evaluate all visceral and parietal peritoneal surfaces and remove all visible disease. The concern that cytoreduction alone may miss microscopic cells leading to early recurrence propelled the study and use of IPEC to eradicate microscopic residual disease that may be present at the conclusion of CRS.

The efficacy of IPEC depends on several pharmacologic principles, including molecular size, affinity to lipids, first-pass clearance from the plasma by the liver, and the permeability of the peritoneal-plasma barrier. Optimization of these variables allows for a 10- to 100-fold increased concentration of chemotherapy drug in the peritoneal cavity. High drug concentration within the peritoneal cavity is important, but the drugs must also penetrate tissue to reach invasive cancers growing into the subperitoneal surface. The estimated penetration depth of IPEC is only 1 to 3 mm maximum. The addition of hyperthermia (41 °C to 42 °C) to intraperitoneal chemotherapy (HIPEC), quickly gained favor given hyperthermia's direct cytotoxic effects and synergism with chemotherapy, resulting in increased drug penetration of tissue and inhibition of DNA repair mechanisms. Administering HIPEC at the time of surgery rather than in the early postoperative period allows for the safe use of hyperthermia and assures better distribution of chemotherapy prior to the early adhesion formation that limits diffusion throughout the abdomen.

HIPEC does, however, come with some distinct disadvantages. The addition of HIPEC at the time of surgical resection may double the rate of anastomotic leak and increases the risk of bone marrow suppression, intra-abdominal abscess, and fever. Patients receiving HIPEC at the time of surgery have a prolonged hospital stay of on average 10 days, a 10% readmission rate, an overall morbidity rate of 40%, and a mortality rate of 2% in historic series. Recent results of a randomized control trial of CRS versus CRS + HIPEC demonstrated that the addition of HIPEC increased 60-day morbidity from 13.6% to 24.1% and increased length of stay from 14 to 18 days. Single institutions with high case volumes have reported lower morbidity and mortality rates, suggesting that experience can mitigate some of the adverse events associated with surgery for peritoneal surface malignancies. However, these institutions with high case volumes still report significant morbidity and measurable mortality rates. Both the individual and institutional learning curves are steep, with studies reporting that 33 to 70 cases are needed to decrease morbidity rates and 140 to 220 cases are needed to improve the completeness of cytoreduction (CCR).

In order to obtain a complete cytoreduction, all visible disease must be removed, at times requiring multiple organ resections, leading to significant morbidity and decreased quality of life (QOL). The most common postoperative complications after CRS and HIPEC are delayed gastric emptying, extended postoperative ileus, intra-abdominal abscess, gastric or small intestinal perforation, anastomotic leak, postoperative bleeding, fistula, sepsis, respiratory distress, hematologic toxicity, and urinary disturbances. The most common causes of death include anastomotic leakage, sepsis, and postoperative hemorrhage. Improvements in these outcomes have correlated with improving surgical technique, standardization of care at high volume centers, and implementation of enhanced recovery pathways.

There are several unique toxicities specific to each IPEC agent. Bone marrow toxicity occurs in 40% of patients receiving intraperitoneal mitomycin C (dosage: 20 mg/m^2 in patients who received previous systemic chemotherapy and 25 mg/m^2 for chemo-naïve patients); nadirs in absolute neutrophil count typically occur around postoperative day 7 to 9 and last for 2 days. Importantly, this is not associated with increased mortality, infection, or length of hospital stay. Cisplatin (dosage: 200 mg/m^2) is associated with renal toxicity, and renal protective measures are employed when the drug is used (discussed later). Finally, oxaliplatin (dosage: 200 mg/m^2) has historically been used for carcinomatosis of colorectal origin. Oxaliplatin has been associated with unexplained hemoperitoneum and hepatic dysfunction in phase 1 trials. Moreover, oxaliplatin was felt to be unstable in chloride-containing carrier solutions, necessitating the use of 5% dextrose/water carrier solutions. The use of this solution often resulted in severe intraoperative hyperglycemia, electrolyte abnormalities, and even led to the death of several patients secondary to cerebral edema. More recent work has suggested that more balanced carriers can be effectively used while avoiding the above noted issues.

QOL is dramatically reduced postoperatively in patients undergoing CRS and HIPEC, with a return to baseline functioning taking 6 to 12 months. Therefore, care must be taken in selecting patients for CRS and HIPEC. It is imperative to exclude patients at the highest risk for significant morbidity or early recurrence, given that these individuals are unlikely to benefit from these treatments and yet incur a significant decline in QOL. Clinical factors such as advanced age, history of extensive and current tobacco use, extensive prior surgery, low albumin level, and poor performance status have all been associated with increased rates of morbidity, readmission, reoperation, and mortality. Although multiple factors have been evaluated in an attempt to identify patients at the highest risk for early recurrence, the ability to achieve a complete cytoreduction remains the most important predictor of outcome. Studies have reported clinical and radiographic scoring systems that can predict the ability to achieve complete cytoreduction and will be discussed later in this chapter.

Appendiceal Neoplasms

Epidemiology

Appendiceal adenocarcinoma is a unique entity with a broad spectrum of behavior. Although rare, its incidence has increased from 0.6 cases per 1,000,000 people in 1973 to 2.8 cases per 1,000,000 people in 2011. While this increased incidence is at least partially due to improvements in detection and recognition of the disease, there has been a disproportionate increase in incidence in younger patients (age <50 years). This observation parallels the rising incidence of early-onset colorectal cancer in the United States during the same time period. Obesity, physical inactivity, and the Western-style diet are commonly cited as potential contributing factors for early-onset colorectal cancer, although these observations remain purely correlative. Given the increased frequency with which colorectal polyps and cancers are diagnosed in patients with appendiceal neoplasms, it is possible that the risk factors for these diseases also influence the incidence of appendiceal neoplasms in young adults.

Clinical Presentation

Male patients are most commonly diagnosed with an appendiceal neoplasm at the time of appendectomy for presumed appendicitis (34%) or when mucin is identified in an inguinal hernia sack at the time of hernia repair (25%). In female patients, the disease is most often discovered during resection of a presumed ovarian cancer. As many as 5% of all patients with an appendiceal neoplasm are completely asymptomatic and are diagnosed incidentally after undergoing surgery or radiographic imaging for an unrelated cause. Approximately one-third of all patients with an appendiceal neoplasm present with PMP; a clinical condition characterized by abdominal distension, mucinous ascites, and nausea/vomiting from extensive carcinomatosis.

Appendiceal neoplasms are unique in that they metastasize predominately through peritoneal seeding after serosal invasion or appendix perforation. A distinctive feature of mucinous neoplasms is the redistribution phenomenon that follows the physiologic flow of peritoneal fluid. This distributes malignant cells in a clock-wise manner within the peritoneal cavity to sites of fluid absorption through lymphatic lacunae and lymphoid aggregates. Consequently, the tumor tends to spare mobile loops of small intestine early in the disease process and first accumulates in other sites such as the pelvis, paracolic gutters, omentum, liver capsule, and right hemidiaphragm. Bulky accumulations can develop as mucin is absorbed at the lymphatic lacunae. Epithelial cells are then "filtered out" and concentrated into sheets of tumor. Only late in the disease process do mucinous implants develop on the bowel, eventually leading to obstruction. Malignant bowel obstructions from appen-diceal neoplasms are therefore a late and ominous finding associated with a decreased probability of complete cytoreduction and subsequent survival. Occasionally, mucinous neoplasms from other sites of origin, including the ovary, colon, urachus, and pancreas, may also present with the clinical appearance of classic PMP. As such, the term PMP should be used only to describe the clinical condition of mucinous ascites and does not refer to any specific histology.

Pathology

Appendiceal neoplasms are also unique in that they are the only malignancies classified according to the histologic features of the metastatic deposits rather than the primary tumor. The complexities of this classi-fication system reflect the heterogeneity of disease phenotypes observed clinically. A retrospective review by Ronnett proposed three prognostic groups based on histologic findings: disseminated peritoneal adenomuci-nosis (low grade), peritoneal mucinous carcinomatosis (high grade), and peritoneal mucinous carcinomatosis intermediate (intermediate grade). Subsequent single-institution studies validated the prognostic distinc-tion of this three-tiered staging system. Others, however, including the seventh edition of the American Joint Committee on Cancer (AJCC) *Cancer Staging Manual* have suggested a two-tier system combining interme-diate- and high-grade groups, because of the expected similar outcomes for these two groups. Large popula-tion-based analysis of the National Cancer Database contradicts these observations and noted significantly different survival outcomes between patients with intermediate- and high-grade classifications. Similarly, a review of 265 consecutive patients with mucinous appendiceal adenocarcinoma treated with CRS and HIPEC at MD Anderson also noted significantly different disease-free and overall survival rates among patients with well-differentiated, moderately differentiated, and poorly differentiated appendiceal adenocarcinoma. The eighth edition of the AJCC has since adopted a three tiered staging.

An expert panel at the 2012 World Congress of the Peritoneal Surface Oncology Group published original guidelines that were later updated in 2016 and concluded that a two-tier staging system was best and indi-cated that the terms "low-grade mucinous adenocarcinoma" or "disseminated peritoneal adenomucinosis" were to be used for appendiceal tumors with low-grade histologic features, and the terms "high-grade muci-nous adenocarcinoma" or "peritoneal mucinous carcinomatosis" were to be used for appendiceal tumors with high-grade histologic features. A tumor with >50% signet ring cells would be classified as having signet ring cell histology. Appendiceal tumors without infiltrative invasion and bland cytologic architecture would be classified as low-grade appendiceal mucinous neoplasms (LAMNs); those with more high-grade cytology are called high-grade appendiceal mucinous neoplasms (HAMNs). If no epithelial cells are identified in deposits outside the appendix, then the designation of "acellular mucin" is used.

Another important prognostic variable in appendiceal neoplasm is the identification of mucinous his-tologic features. Tumors with mucinous histology (>50%) tend to be well differentiated with scant cellular-ity, minimal cellular atypia, and are accompanied by slow, progressive accumulation of mucinous ascites, resulting in the clinical condition of PMP. Patients with mucinous tumors have an excellent median survival duration of 109 months. In contrast, patients with nonmucinous tumors, which are often moderately or poorly differentiated, are characterized by solid peritoneal metastases and associated with surrounding desmopla-sia/invasion have a median survival duration of only 35 months.

The presence of signet ring cells is a poor prognostic factor for moderately and poorly differentiated tumors. Shetty et al. proposed a classification system that categorized appendiceal adenocarcinoma by grade as low-grade tumors, high-grade tumors without signet ring cells, or high-grade tumors with signet ring cells, with the last group having the poorest prognosis. A review of cases from MD Anderson confirmed that the presence of signet ring cells was an independent predictor of poor survival. Signet ring cells stratified outcome within each histologic grade and therefore represented a complimentary, rather than redundant, prognostic variable.

The final subtype of appendiceal neoplasm that deserves mention is the goblet cell adenocarcinoma. This tumor type was previously termed goblet cell carcinoid tumor. The decision to change the name is related to the term "carcinoid tumor," which historically has suggested a less aggressive tumor biology. The change in the name better reflects this tumor's biology which demonstrates a propensity for perineural and lymphatic spread and for peritoneal dissemination. Although various classification systems exist, these tumors should be managed similar to a high-grade adenocarcinoma of the appendix.

Staging

In 2010, the AJCC released the seventh edition of its Cancer Staging Manual, which for the first time distinguished appendiceal adenocarcinoma from colorectal adenocarcinoma. In the most recent, eighth edition, M1a disease is now defined as intraperitoneal mucin without identifiable tumor cells, while M1b includes any intraperitoneal metastasis and M1c includes patients with extraperitoneal metastasis. Stage IV is further classified into IVA, IVB, and IVC, depending on histologic grade and presence of extraperitoneal metastasis. Stage IVA includes patients with intraperitoneal mucin and negative lymph nodes, along with well-differentiated mucinous adenocarcinoma (grade 1) with any lymph node status, whereas stage IVB includes both moderately and poorly differentiated (grade 2 and 3) mucinous tumors, irrespective of lymph node status. Stage IVC is any patient with metastases outside the peritoneum. The AJCC staging system has been infrequently applied in published studies that estimate prognosis; many centers instead report the prognostic significance of mucinous or nonmucinous histologic features, grade of the tumor, lymph node status, and signet ring cell histologic features. Moreover, the most important independent predictors of outcome for patients with appendiceal neoplasms remain factors that can be assessed only at/after surgery, such as the extent of tumor burden (peritoneal carcinomatosis index [PCI]) and the ability to remove all visible disease (complete cytoreduction).

The Lyon prognostic index, described by Gilly for peritoneal carcinomatosis from gastrointestinal malignancies, accounts for the size of metastatic implants and whether or not the disease is diffuse or localized to one region. This staging system was designed to be applied at the time of cytoreduction as well as after cytoreduction and HIPEC. The extent of remaining disease is recorded as the downstaging index resulting from the cytoreduction. The stages are as follows: stage 0, no macroscopic disease; stage 1, tumor <5 mm localized to one part of abdomen; stage 2, tumor <5 mm and diffused to whole abdomen; stage 3, tumor ≥5 mm but ≤2 cm; and stage 4, tumor >2 cm. This staging system is often used by medical oncologists because of its simplicity and reproducibility. It has been used in numerous clinical trials, including EVOCAPE-1, which demonstrated a median survival duration of 6 months for patients with stage 1 or 2 disease compared with a median survival of 3 months for patients with stage 3 or 4 disease.

The PCI scoring system created by Sugarbaker documents the volume and distribution of mucinous implants throughout the abdomen (Fig. 12.1) as determined at the time of operative exploration. After lysis of adhesions and inspection of the entire parietal and visceral peritoneum, the abdomen is divided into 13 regions. Implants within each region are scored as lesion size (LS) 0 through 3. LS-0 means no implants are present throughout the region, LS-1 means implants of up to 0.5 cm are present, LS-2 means implants greater than 0.5 cm and up to 5 cm are present, and LS-3 means that there are

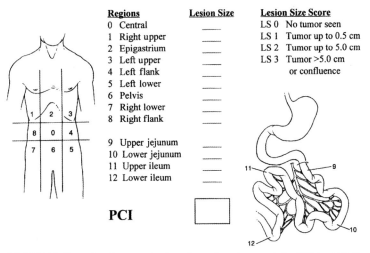

FIGURE 12.1 Illustration demonstrating how the peritoneal cancer index (PCI) is obtained. (Reprinted by permission from Springer: Carmignani CP, Esquivel J, Sugarbaker PH. Cytoreductive surgery and intraperitoneal chemotherapy for the treatment of peritoneal surface malignancy. *Clin Transl Oncol.* 2003;5:192–198.)

CC-0   CC-1   CC-2   CC-3

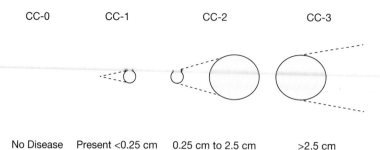

No Disease   Present <0.25 cm   0.25 cm to 2.5 cm   >2.5 cm

FIGURE 12.2 Illustration of the completeness of cytoreduction (CCR) score that is calculated after completing cytoreduction. (Reprinted by permission from Springer: Sugarbaker P. Management of peritoneal surface malignancy: a short history. In: González-Moreno S, ed. *Advances in Peritoneal Surface Oncology. Resent Results in Cancer Research.* Vol. 169. Springer; 2007:1–9.)

implants 5 cm or greater in diameter or that there is a tumor confluence (the rule of 5's). The PCI is the most commonly reported prognostic scoring system for appendiceal neoplasms and has been well correlated with survival in numerous studies. Despite its widespread use, several limitations exist. First, the PCI requires the surgeon to divide the abdomen into 13 compartments with no sharp anatomic boundaries. In response to this complexity, the Dutch have reported a simplified peritoneal carcinomatosis assessment score in which disease volume is graded as large (>5 cm), moderate (1 to 5 cm), small (<1 cm), or absent in seven abdominal areas: the left and right subdiaphragmatic areas, subhepatic area, omentum/transverse colon, small intestine/mesentery, ileocecal area, and pelvic area. Second, the PCI can be determined only at the time of surgery, limiting its prognostic utility. Determining the PCI based on preoperative imaging is difficult and inaccurate because the extent of disease is often underestimated. A small series from the Mayo Clinic comparing radiographic and clinical PCI at the time of CRS reported a correlation of 0.59 for appendiceal and 0.62 for colon adenocarcinoma. Furthermore, 46% of patients with a radiologic PCI score ≥20 were able to undergo adequate cytoreduction and would have been turned away if a radiographic PCI of 20 was used as a strict criterion for CRS and HIPEC. More recently, MRI has demonstrated improved correlation with surgical PCI scoring with correlation nearing 0.80. Further study and optimization of such protocols are needed before they are adopted into clinical pathways. Therefore, radiographic PCI is helpful in evaluating the volume and distribution of disease, but it offers no definite cut-off values for appendiceal neoplasms that are sensitive/specific enough to warrant patient inclusion/exclusion from CRS and HIPEC.

Sugarbaker also developed a CCR score describing the amount of disease remaining at the completion of the cytoreduction (Fig. 12.2). The scores are as follows: CCR-0, no visible tumor nodules remaining; CCR-1, persistence of tumor nodules <2.5 mm; CCR-2, tumor nodules ≥2.5 mm but ≤2.5 cm; and CCR-3, tumor nodules >2.5 cm (rule of 2.5). Because hyperthermic IPEC is thought to penetrate to a depth of 3 mm, scores of CCR-0 or CCR-1 are considered a complete cytoreduction, while scores of CCR-2 and CCR-3 indicate incomplete cytoreduction. This scoring system has been consistently demonstrated to be the most important prognostic factor for patients with carcinomatosis of appendiceal origin who undergo CRS and HIPEC.

Given the importance of a complete cytoreduction to long-term survival, various scoring systems have been proposed that predict the likelihood of accomplishing complete cytoreduction. One such scoring system for patients with well-differentiated appendiceal adenocarcinoma is the Simplified Preoperative Assessment for Appendix Tumor (SPAAT) scoring system, developed at MD Anderson. SPAAT utilizes preoperative computed tomography (CT) studies to grade the volume of disease in five anatomic locations. The presence of scalloping or indentation of the liver, spleen, pancreas, or portal vein from mucinous implants is assessed, and one point is given for each location where scalloping or indentation is present. The bowel is also assessed for involvement, and if the small bowel appears to float to the abdominal wall without evidence of mesenteric foreshortening, it is scored as a 0. Patients with mesenteric foreshortening, which causes the small bowel to appear tethered or cocoon-like on CT images (a condition termed "cauliflowering" of the bowel), are given a score of 3. SPAAT scores range from 0 to 7, and a score of ≥3 has 100% sensitivity and 93% specificity with 95% positive predictive value for identifying patients in whom a complete cytoreduction will not be obtainable. These patients are not offered CRS and HIPEC for cure because of reduced overall survival. The exception to this recommendation is the symptomatic patient with minimal comorbidities and preserved nutritional and functional status. In these patients, we offer an organ-sparing, tumor debulking. Omentectomy is performed and potential sources of GI tract obstruction are addressed at this time. The patients also receive HIPEC for ascites control. A small study from MD Anderson evaluated the outcomes of 28 patients who were taken to the operating room for CRS and HIPEC with a palliative intent. In this palliative group median overall survival was 79 months and ascites well controlled over the long term with only one patient requiring a single paracentesis post operatively for ascites control.

Diagnostic Workup

Appendiceal neoplasms are most often found incidentally at appendectomy or at the time of an unrelated surgical procedure. The pathology should be reviewed by an experienced gastrointestinal pathologist at a center familiar with peritoneal surface malignancies. The operative report for the index operation should be carefully reviewed for details regarding the extent and location of disease. If an appendiceal neoplasm is encountered unexpectedly at the time of an unrelated operation, the recommendation is to perform limited resection to confirm the histologic diagnosis and document the extent of disease without performing an unnecessary dissection. The rationale for this approach can be found in the prior surgical score (PSS). The PSS takes into account the extent of any surgeries prior to definitive CRS and HIPEC. The more extensive the previous surgery, the more morbidity is expected, and the lower the likelihood of obtaining a complete cytoreduction. PSS scores are as follows: PSS-0, no previous surgery or biopsy only; PSS-1, previous surgery involving only one region; PSS-2, two to five regions previously dissected; and PSS-3, previous attempt at CRS and HIPEC. Patients scoring PSS-2 or PSS-3 are less likely to undergo complete cytoreduction because the previous extensive dissection entraps residual tumor cells in scar tissue. Dense adhesions not only increase the morbidity of subsequent operations but also makes it difficult to distinguish between tumor implants and normal tissue. In addition, local growth factors associated with an extensive operation may promote the growth of residual neoplastic cells. Therefore, partial debulking surgery at the time of incidental diagnosis is strongly discouraged as it offers no benefit to patients, delays definitive treatment, and hinders the chances of a complete cytoreduction in the future. Data from our institution has confirmed these findings in patients with appendiceal neoplasms. We have found that the patient who is most likely to have recurrent disease after definitive CRS and HIPEC is the female patient who had extensive TAH/BSO and debulking at the time of their index operation for what was inaccurately presumed to be ovarian cancer.

If no histologic diagnosis has been obtained and the patient is found to have an incidentally identified appendiceal mass, some imaging characteristics may suggest a diagnosis. A review of 332 cases of appendiceal neoplasms and 136 control cases at MD Anderson found mural calcifications in the appendix to be associated with a mucinous neoplasm with a specificity of 99%. An appendix with a diameter >15 mm and a soft-tissue mass/wall thickening, or a finding of mucin outside of the appendix, is also highly suspicious for an appendiceal malignancy. A percutaneous biopsy of the area of most dense nodularity should be performed in an effort to obtain cellular material. Difficulty aspirating fluid during paracentesis is also suggestive of the thick mucin associated with mucinous appendiceal malignancies.

Once a histologic diagnosis has been confirmed, the extent of disease must be assessed by high-quality imaging of the abdomen and pelvis in the form of multidetector CT with enteric and parenteral contrast reconstructed to <2.5 mm axial, sagittal, and coronal planes or magnetic resonance imaging (MRI) with diffusion-weighted imaging and intravenous gadolinium contrast. CT studies are the most commonly used cross-sectional imaging. They are routinely available and are the imaging modality of choice at MD Anderson. Because CT does not detect disease < ~3 mm, systematic underestimation of the PCI is possible, particularly with higher-grade malignancies. Other institutions have reported that preoperative PCI scores established through gadolinium-enhanced MRI correlate better with surgically determined PCI than CT. Some studies have also suggested that gadolinium-enhanced MRI offers notable improvements in the detection of small bowel nodules compared with CT. Regardless of the imaging modality, having the patient's cross-sectional imaging interpreted by an experienced radiologist/surgeon is critical because imaging of peritoneal disease is often subtle and requires a high index of suspicion.

A preoperative colonoscopy is highly recommended because there is a higher incidence of colonic polyps and invasive adenocarcinoma in patients with appendiceal neoplasms. Synchronous colon polyps have been reported in 42% of patients and metachronous colonic cancers in 5% to 21%. The use of colonoscopy for the diagnosis of appendiceal adenocarcinoma is of low yield as only 10% of patients in a large colonoscopy series was able to identify the appendix as the site of tumor origin.

Preoperative evaluation of the patient's candidacy for CRS and HIPEC includes a complete history and a physical examination detailing comorbidities and functional status. Obtaining a social history is also important because smoking is a significant independent predictor of morbidity. Smoking cessation should be highly encouraged. Patients must have preserved renal, hepatic, and cardiac functions to tolerate the effects of a long operation that includes significant fluid shifts. Medications must be reviewed to ensure cessation of any anticoagulants prior to surgery. Nutritional status can be assessed with body mass index, recent weight changes, body habitus, and albumin and prealbumin levels. At MD Anderson, the patients considered to be the best candidates for CRS and HIPEC are <70 years old, do not smoke, have an Eastern Cooperative Oncology Group (ECOG) functional status of 0 or 1, and have maintained their nutritional reserves (albumin >3.5 g/dL).

The tumor marker, CEA, is elevated in 56% of patients with appendiceal adenocarcinoma and CA 125 and CA 19-9 is elevated in ~65% of patients. However, serum CEA, CA-125, and CA 19-9 levels are not useful for definitive diagnosis of appendiceal adenocarcinoma as they lack sensitivity and specificity. Although the absolute level of a tumor marker does not correlate with prognosis, a normal value for each of the tumor markers is associated with improved survival. Furthermore, elevated preoperative levels of CEA or CA 19-9 should return to baseline within 7 days after complete resection, and residual disease should be suspected if these levels do not return to baseline. Caution needs to be maintained, however, as extensive residual inflammation may falsely elevate tumor markers. We suggest obtaining serum CEA, CA 19-9, and CA 125 levels prior to surgery and at each follow-up visit for at least the first 5 years after CRS and HIPEC, even if preoperative levels were normal. Carmignani reported elevated serum CEA levels in 35% of 110 patients determined to have recurrent disease during surveillance. In addition, CA 19-9 was elevated in 63% of patients, and at least one of the tumor markers was elevated in 68% of patients. An elevated CEA level at the time of recurrence indicates a poorer prognosis. Studies in colorectal cancer suggest that elevation of tumor markers precedes findings on imaging by 1.5 to 6 months. Utility of circulating tumoral DNA has been demonstrated in localized colorectal cancers but studies utilizing contemporary assays are ongoing to characterize its utility in other metastatic GI malignancies including appendiceal adenocarcinoma.

Operative Steps

Dissemination of disease for patients with peritoneal metastases is unique to each patient. Of primary importance is that these procedures be performed at a high-volume center by a surgical oncologist familiar with this treatment modality. As with other complex oncologic procedures, there is a significant institute and surgeon learning curve and the surgical treatment of these patients should be a part of a comprehensive peritoneal surface malignancy program. Experience performing CRS and the longitudinal follow-up of these patients have exposed common sites of unnoticed disease and underlines the importance of a thorough, meticulous survey of the abdomen and all peritoneal surfaces. Diagnostic laparoscopy and biopsy should be utilized prior to any consideration of CRS/HIPEC in patient with high-grade appendiceal adenocarcinoma and liberally in other grades.

At the initiation of surgery, all mucinous ascites should be removed. Complete lysis of all adhesions should follow. Once this is completed, a formal exploration of the entire peritoneal cavity ensues and the surgeon should pause and record the PCI score and determine if a complete cytoreduction is possible. Once the decision has been made that a complete cytoreduction is possible, a systemic approach to extirpate all tumor should be followed for every procedure. Although the exact sequence of the operation differs between surgeons and centers, it is imperative that each individual surgeon has a standard, thorough approach to each procedure.

The falciform ligament should be taken down and the round ligament identified and followed into the umbilical fissure of the liver. If there is no disease, the ligament can be suture ligated and passed off the table. If disease if present, the ligament is left in situ and will be addressed further with the porta-hepatis dissection.

In general, a complete omentectomy should be performed early to allow full exposure to the peritoneal cavity, as a bulky omental cake impairs visualization. During this process, the left lobe of the liver should be mobilized, giving full exposure to the upper stomach, left upper quadrant, and spleen. Once the omentum has been full mobilized from the right side of the abdomen to the left, the spleen and left upper quadrant are now well exposed. If there is disease in the left upper quadrant or on the spleen, a left upper quadrant peritonectomy, splenectomy, and completion omentectomy can be performed with one procedure. If the spleen is not involved, routine resection is to be avoided and omentectomy is completed in the splenic hilum.

The dissection now turns to the right upper quadrant and the surgery proceeds in a clockwise manner. It is important to fully mobilize the liver to the bare area to avoid missed disease that is often hidden in the fold created by the ligament and the bare area. Once the liver is fully mobilized, a fixed retractor can be placed giving excellent exposure of the entire right upper quadrant. If indicated, a complete right upper quadrant peritonectomy is then started near the costal margin, to include the peritoneum of the hepatorenal recess and the peritoneum overlying the vena cava. Care is taken medially to avoid the hepatic veins superiorly and the adrenal gland inferiorly.

The surface of the liver is next inspected and resection of tumor on the capsule of the liver can now proceed. It is recommended to do this after the right upper quadrant peritonectomy as injury to the liver or removal of the capsule of the liver makes the liver vulnerable to fracture.

The gallbladder is inspected. If there is tumor present, cholecystectomy is performed. If there is tumor present in the porta hepatis, utilization of the gallbladder and identification of the cystic duct can assist with getting in the proper plane in order to help avoid injury of the portal structures.

Once within the port-hepatis, the previously mobilized round ligament is identified. The pont hepatique should be opened and the peritonectomy can be carried into the porta hepatis and lesser omentum. Lesser omentectomy should be performed if disease is present, with attempts made to preserve the right gastric vascular pedicle.

It is important to evaluate the space posterior to the porta hepatis. If disease is visualized or palpable, Kocherization of the duodenum can allow excellent exposure to this area. Tumor is removed from the right side toward the caudate lobe of the liver. The dissection can be completed from the lesser sac. The caudate lobe and peritoneum over the crus of the diaphragm should be inspected and tumor removed at this time.

The lesser sac is now well visualized. Peritonectomy of the lesser sac is now performed if disease is present. Unless a gastrectomy is planned, it is important to identify and protect the left gastric vascular pedicle from injury. The subpyloric space is a common site of missed disease and this area should be opened and inspected. If high volume disease is present in this area, distal gastrectomy may be indicated.

The upper abdomen has now been cleared of all disease, and the mid abdomen is approached by identifying the ligament of Treitz. There are a number of fossa is this area, each of these needs to be carefully inspected as they are common sites of missed disease if they are not intentionally evaluated.

The small bowel is now meticulously evaluated with disease being resected with electrocautery and sharp dissection as needed. Resection of small bowel is done only when absolutely necessary in an effort to preserve as much intestinal function as possible.

Upon reaching the terminal ileum, the decision to perform an appendectomy versus formal right colectomy is dictated by disease burden and grade of the tumor. High-grade tumors require formal right colectomy, whereas low-grade tumors require a margin-negative appendectomy only. The right lower quadrant and right paracolic gutter peritonectomies are performed at this time.

Evaluation of the transverse colon and transverse mesocolon is now performed and all disease not previously removed with the omentectomy is removed with peritonectomy as indicated. The descending colon is inspected as is the left paracolic gutter, if there is tumor present, peritonectomy is performed. If colon resection is needed, the colon is freed along Toldt line at this time. The decision to divide the colon is made only after evaluation of the pelvis.

If there is extensive disease in the pelvis, complete extraperitoneal resection is indicated. The peritoneum is scored circumferentially beginning at the distal extent of the previous left paracolic dissection. This is continued anteriorly over the bladder over to the right side of the abdomen and ends at the previous right lower quadrant/paracolic gutter peritonectomy site.

The peritonectomy is then carried circumferentially toward the rectum. Care is taken to avoid injury to the bladder. The dissection ends at the cervix in females or the seminal vesicles in males. The bilateral ovarian pedicels (if present) are identified and doubly tied, suture ligated, and divided. It is crucial to identify the ureters at this stage to avoid injury. Preoperative ureteral stent placement can make this easier. If present, the round ligaments are divided distally. The circumferential extra peritoneal dissection continues centripetally inferiorly. The uterus is usually divided above the cervix if there is no disease present. This provides a muscular barrier to tumor invasion into the vagina in the future. The rectosigmoid dissection is completed at the appropriate level based on disease. If necessary, the rectum is then divided distally with a green contour stapler—although this is generally able to be avoided. The proximal colon is divided with a blue load GIA stapler.

Anterior abdominal wall peritonectomy should be performed with full thickness excision of any port sites and careful examination for any umbilical hernia and associated hernia sac. Visceral resection should only be performed when absolutely necessary, as more extensive, prophylactic resections can increase morbidity without improvement in long-term outcome

Once all visible disease is excised, the perfusion inflow and outflow cannulas can be placed and the abdomen temporarily closed. The patient is cooled and HIPEC is initiated. Inflow temperatures are kept between 41 °C to 42 °C. We like to maintain a flow rate of 1 to 1.5 L/min. The chemotherapy is removed at the completion of HIPEC and the abdomen irrigated with sterile water. We attempt to achieve patient core temperature between 38 and 38.5 degrees celsius for at least 30 minutes.

Agent	Duration	Penetration	Indication	Hyperthermia
Mitomycin C	90–120 min	2 mm	Appendiceal Colorectal Gastric Ovarian	HIPEC
Oxaliplatin	30 min	1–2 mm	Appendiceal Colorectal Ovarian	HIPEC
Cisplatin	30–90 min	1–3 mm	Ovarian Colorectal Gastric Mesothelioma	HIPEC
Doxorubicin	60–90 min	4–6 cell layers	Ovarian Colorectal	HIPEC
Carboplatin	90 min	1 mm	Ovarian	HIPEC
5-Fluorouracil		0.2 mm	Colorectal	EPIC
Taxane		>80 cell layers	Colorectal Gastric Ovarian	EPIC

It is our practice to perform any enteric anastomoses after resection, although this point is debated among high-volume surgeons. Finally, the choice of agent and duration is variable between practices. Common regimens and their indications are summarized in Table 12.1.

Well-Differentiated Mucinous Appendiceal Neoplasms (Low Grade)

Our algorithm for treating LAMN, HAMN, and well-differentiated mucinous appendiceal adenocarcinoma is shown in Figure 12.3. Patients with localized disease have most often had a previous laparoscopic appendectomy prior to referral to MD Anderson (see case 1). Postoperatively, if imaging shows no evidence of residual disease, tumor markers are normal, the margins on the appendiceal base are negative, and the colonoscopy is normal, then we would not recommend performing a right hemicolectomy because the incidence of nodal metastasis for low-grade appendiceal neoplasms is <5%. Instead, we recommend surveillance every 6 months with a history and physical examination, CT imaging, and determination of tumor marker levels for the first 2 years and then annually thereafter. Any change on imaging or tumor markers would warrant consideration of a diagnostic laparoscopy.

If a patient has residual disease on baseline imaging, we recommend determining the patient's SPAAT score to determine whether complete cytoreduction is possible. If a patient's medical comorbidities, nutritional status, and functional status permit, we then offer potentially curative CRS and HIPEC to a patient with a SPAAT score <3. We typically wait 1 to 2 months from the last operation to allow inflammation to resolve. An ileocecectomy is recommended for patients with low-grade tumors only when there is a positive appendiceal margin or visible serosal disease. For patients with a SPAAT score ≥3 who are symptomatic but have manageable comorbidities and preserved functional and nutritional status, we offer palliative, organ-preserving debulking and HIPEC. This approach attempts to balance morbidity and the benefits of tumor debulking. For patients with unresectable low-grade appendiceal neoplasms, we do not recommend palliative chemotherapy because there has been no demonstrable benefit to systemic chemotherapy in these patients. These individuals are best managed with supportive care or one of the clinical trials ongoing at MD Anderson.

Low-grade appendiceal neoplasms generally have a more indolent course. In those patients with recurrent disease after surgery, the mean time to identification is 18 months. We therefore recommend surveillance consisting of a history and physical examination, serial tumor markers (CEA, CA 19-9, and CA 125), and serial imaging of the abdomen and pelvis every 6 months for 2 years and then annually thereafter. Given that there is no clear time interval where risk of recurrence is zero, we follow patients until they feel comfortable following up with their primary care physicians for a history and physical examination alone. Our longest interval recurrence for well-differentiated tumors was 100 months. Also, given the slow progression of the disease, new findings on imaging can be followed for clinical behavior to help distinguish recurrent tumors from residual acellular mucin or scars.

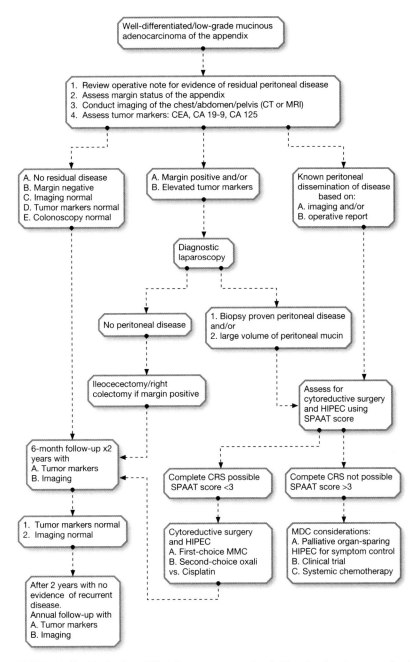

FIGURE 12.3 Algorithm for the multidisciplinary management of well-differentiated mucinous appendiceal adenocarcinoma.

Moderately and Poorly Differentiated Appendiceal Adenocarcinoma (High Grade)

Our algorithm for treating moderately and poorly differentiated appendiceal adenocarcinoma is shown in Figure 12.4. Briefly, patients with localized disease often have had a previous laparoscopic appendectomy at an outside institution prior to referral to MD Anderson. If no evidence of residual disease is seen on postoperative imaging and tumor markers are not elevated, we recommend performing a diagnostic laparoscopy; and if no peritoneal disease is present, then we would proceed with a formal right hemicolectomy to assess lymph node metastasis as the risk of lymph node involvement approaches 40% in this cohort. If the ileocolic lymph nodes are positive, we recommend adjuvant systemic chemotherapy as lymph node metastases are associated with poor 5-year overall survival rates (33% compared with 74% for patients without lymph node involvement). If no peritoneal disease is evident on laparoscopic exploration, and the ileocolic lymph nodes are negative,

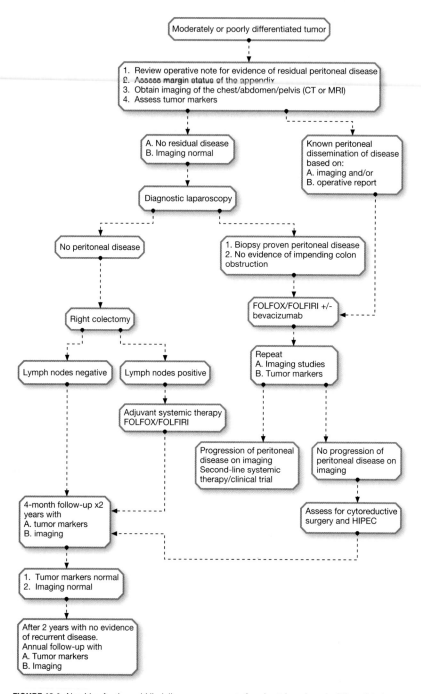

FIGURE 12.4 Algorithm for the multidisciplinary management of moderately and poorly differentiated appendiceal adenocarcinoma.

we recommend surveillance follow-up only. Follow-up should include a history and physical examination; CT imaging of the chest, abdomen, and pelvis; and testing of tumor markers every 3 to 4 months for the first 2 years. Follow-up can then be done every 6 months until the 5-year mark is reached and can thereafter be done annually.

If the patient has radiographic evidence of peritoneal disease, we recommend careful evaluation of the CT scan for evidence of small bowel mesenteric involvement (cauliflowering of the bowel) or porta-hepatis involvement; these are the two most difficult areas from which to surgically clear disease. In general, a PCI score <20 is considered more favorable for a complete cytoreduction and improved overall survival. We do not, however, use this as an absolute cut-off as select patients with a PCI score ≥20 may have meaningful long-term survival. We recommend all patients receive neoadjuvant systemic chemotherapy, preferably folinic acid, fluorouracil, and oxaliplatin (FOLFOX) or folinic acid, fluorouracil, and irinotecan hydrochloride (FOLFIRI) with bevacizumab, for six to 12 cycles. Potential benefits of the neoadjuvant approach include better tolerance of chemotherapy and, as a result, an increased likelihood of completing the intended therapy. Preoperative therapy also facilitates the assessment of tumor biology and chemosensitivity. Modern chemotherapy regimens with FOLFOX or FOLFIRI and bevacizumab have radiographic response rates of 38% to 50%, which corresponds to an improved median disease-free survival duration of 27 months and median overall survival duration of 48 months. Patients who are not candidates for surgical resection also have improved rates of progression-free and overall survival when receiving this type of chemotherapy regimen. A lack of response to systemic therapy may indicate that the patient is unlikely to benefit from CRS and HIPEC, as patients who do not respond to FOLFOX or FOLFIRI and bevacizumab have a median disease-free survival duration of only 14 months and a median overall survival duration of 22 months. A lack of response may also indicate a need to change the chemotherapy regimen to one that potentially will induce more of a clinical, biochemical, or radiographic response. We have demonstrated that neoadjuvant systemic chemotherapy had no detrimental effects on blood loss, operative time, hospital length of stay, or morbidity in this population, provided the bevacizumab is completed 8 weeks prior to CRS and HIPEC.

After patients recover from neoadjuvant chemotherapy, we offer them a diagnostic laparoscopy, to determine if the extent and volume of disease is amenable to complete cytoreduction, given that CT studies consistently underestimate PCI. Diagnostic laparoscopy has been demonstrated to be a safe and feasible adjunct to preoperative imaging in the vast majority of patients. We have found it to be particularly useful in identifying small bowel and mesenteric metastases, which are often missed on imaging and can greatly impact the ability to obtain a complete cytoreduction. The current literature suggests a high percentage (20% to 44%) of patients undergo incomplete cytoreduction in the absence of preoperative laparoscopy. In one study, the use of diagnostic laparoscopy spared half of patients a nontherapeutic laparotomy and its associated morbidity. With the judicious use of diagnostic laparoscopy, we have been able to reduce our rate of incomplete cytoreduction to <10% for high-grade adenocarcinoma.

Moderately and poorly differentiated tumors usually follow an aggressive course and can recur rapidly (median time to recurrence: <16 months). We therefore recommend close surveillance for affected patients. Surveillance consists of a history and physical examination, an assessment of serial tumor markers (CEA, CA 19-9, and CA 125), and imaging of the chest, abdomen, and pelvis every 3 to 4 months for 2 years. Patients then receive surveillance every 6 months until the 5-year mark and annually thereafter. Our longest interval to recurrence was 74 months for a moderately differentiated tumor.

Outcomes

An improvement in survival for patients with appendiceal neoplasms was observed from 1973 to 2006 mainly owing to better survival in patients with advanced disease. Major advances in the management of advanced appendiceal neoplasms during this period led to the recognition of the benefit of complete surgical cytoreduction and the introduction of HIPEC described previously.

A review of 265 patients with mucinous appendiceal adenocarcinoma treated with CRS and HIPEC at MD Anderson demonstrated 5-year overall survival rates of 94% for patients with well-differentiated tumors, 71% for moderately differentiated tumors, and 30% for patients with poorly differentiated/signet ring cell tumors. The corresponding 5-year disease-free survival rates were 66%, 21%, and 0%. If acellular mucin alone was found outside the appendix at the time of CRS and HIPEC in a patient with well-differentiated appendiceal adenocarcinoma, then the prognosis was excellent; all such patients remained alive without evidence of disease after a median follow-up of 54 months. Other independent predictors of improved survival included mucinous histology, lower histologic grade, lower PCI score, and the ability to obtain a complete cytoreduction. Patients with mucinous tumors had a median overall survival duration of 109 months. Those with non-mucinous tumors did significantly worse with a median overall survival duration of only 36 months.

Approximately 40% of patients with appendiceal neoplasms develop a recurrence after complete CRS and HIPEC. More than half of these patients are candidates for repeat CRS and HIPEC, and a second complete cytoreduction is achieved in most of them. Patients who undergo a repeat CRS with or without HIPEC have improved survival outcomes compared with those who do not undergo repeat CRS and HIPEC, and this is true even after controlling for clinical and pathologic factors. Patients are carefully selected for repeat CRS and HIPEC. The morbidity (37%) and mortality (0%) rates for repeat cytoreduction and HIPEC are similar to those for primary CRS and HIPEC (55% and 0.8%, respectively). Some clinicians have found that early recurrence within 12 months of a complete cytoreduction is an indicator of a poor prognosis, associated with a median overall survival duration of 38 months. In contrast, patients who remain disease-free for more than 12 months have a more favorable prognosis and are the best candidates for repeat CRS and HIPEC with a median overall survival duration of 97 months. Data from MD Anderson have shown that patients with preserved functional status, absence of signet ring cells, absence of distant metastasis, low PCI, and those able to undergo complete cytoreduction may have the most pronounced benefit from repeat CRS ± HIPEC.

Peritoneal Carcinomatosis in Patients With Colorectal Cancer

Incidence and Risk Factors

A Swedish population study demonstrated that approximately 8.3% of patients with colorectal cancer will also have synchronous or metachronous peritoneal carcinomatosis. Peritoneal carcinomatosis was the first and only type of metastasis in 4.8% of these patients. The prevalence of synchronous peritoneal carcinomatosis was 4.3%, and the cumulative incidence of metachronous peritoneal carcinomatosis was 4.2%. Each year, there are an estimated 104,610 new patients with colon cancer and 43,340 new patients with rectal cancer in the United States. Of these, approximately 7,100 patients have or will develop peritoneal carcinomatosis and might be candidates for CRS and HIPEC.

Independent predictors of metachronous peritoneal carcinomatosis are right-sided colon cancer, primary stage T4 tumors, advanced nodal status, emergency surgery, perforated primary tumor, and nonradical resection of the primary tumor. Patients older than 70 years have a decreased risk of metachronous peritoneal carcinomatosis.

Staging

The colorectal cancer section in the eighth edition of the AJCC Cancer Staging Manual classifies any metastasis to the peritoneal surface as stage IVC. However, distinct survival differences between stage IVA (metastasis to a single organ, excluding the peritoneum), stage IVB (metastasis to multiple organs, excluding the peritoneum), and stage IVC (peritoneal surface metastases), have not been published. As is the case with appendiceal adenocarcinoma, the Lyon and PCI staging systems are important for staging peritoneal carcinomatosis of colorectal origin. The SPAAT score was intended for low-grade appendiceal adenocarcinoma and has not been evaluated for peritoneal carcinomatosis from colorectal cancer. Instead, the Peritoneal Surface Disease Severity Score (PSDSS) was introduced as a means of categorizing patients with colorectal peritoneal carcinomatosis into prognostic groups to improve patient selection. The PSDSS accounts for symptoms, the extent of carcinomatosis, and primary tumor histologic features to assign a score between 2 and 22 points. Stage I is defined as <4 points, stage II as 4 to 7 points, stage III as 8 to 10 points, and stage IV as >10 points. In a validation cohort of 1,013 patients with peritoneal carcinomatosis of colorectal origin, the median overall survival duration was 86 months for stage I, 43 months for stage II, 29 months for stage III, and 28 months for stage IV. Several studies have demonstrated that the PSDSS is an independent prognostic factor, and it has proven to be better than the PCI in stratifying overall survival and progression-free survival. Another group externally validated the PSDSS but suggested modifying the nomogram to include four important prognostic factors; age, PCI score, locoregional lymph node status, and signet ring cell histologic features. The resultant precytoreduction nomogram, which has been termed the colorectal peritoneal metastases prognostic surgical score (COMPASS), is more accurate than the PSDSS in predicting overall survival of patients undergoing CRS with HIPEC. Therefore, the PCI and PSDSS remain the most commonly used staging/scoring systems for peritoneal carcinomatosis of colorectal origin.

Treatment

National consensus guidelines recommend complete cytoreduction and/or IPEC at experienced centers for select patients with limited peritoneal metastasis and for whom an R0 resection can be achieved. Long-term outcomes after CRS and HIPEC for colorectal peritoneal carcinomatosis depend on the volume and distribution of peritoneal spread as measured by the PCI. Therefore, to improve the probability of a complete cytoreduction and long-term survival, it is important to diagnose and treat peritoneal recurrences early. Population-based studies suggest that patients with T4a primary tumors, N1 or N2 node status, mucinous histologic features, and a history of incomplete or emergency resection are at the highest risk of peritoneal relapse. Between 18% and 50% of patients with a T4 primary tumor develop peritoneal carcinomatosis as a result of the intra-abdominal exfoliation of cancer cells. Our experience at MD Anderson has demonstrated that 21% of T4 tumors will develop a peritoneal recurrence with a median time to recurrence of 12 months and 42% of these relapses will be isolated peritoneal recurrences.

Because diagnostic imaging is insufficient for the identification of early peritoneal disease. Other approaches have been attempted. Two recent studies have addressed potential treatment algorithms for these patients at high risk for peritoneal recurrence. Both were, unfortunately, negative studies but provide important information.

The PROPHYLOCHIP trial randomized patients to standard care surveillance versus second look laparoscopy with oxaliplatin-HIPEC at 6 months postoperatively. Disease-free survival was equivalent between the groups. In the second look arm, 52% of patients were diagnosed with recurrent peritoneal disease while only 33% developed clinically evident peritoneal disease in the surveillance arm. Similarly, the COLOPEC trial randomized T4 or perforated colorectal cancer patients to adjuvant HIPEC at 8 weeks postoperatively along with systemic chemotherapy versus surveillance and systemic chemotherapy and demonstrated no difference in disease-free survival. Therefore, second-look surgery and/or prophylactic HIPEC cannot be recommended outside of a clinical trial.

Our algorithm for treating peritoneal metastasis from colorectal cancer is similar to the algorithm for moderately and poorly differentiated appendiceal adenocarcinoma shown in Figure 12.4. Patients with synchronous or metachronous peritoneal carcinomatosis from colorectal cancer undergo a detailed history and physical examination recording comorbidities and functional and nutritional status. If a colonoscopy had not been done recently, one is performed to evaluate for synchronous colon cancers or polyps. High-quality imaging of the chest, abdomen, and pelvis is performed to exclude other sites of metastatic disease and to determine the radiographic PCI score. A PCI score of >17 is considered a relative contraindication to CRS and HIPEC; Gore demonstrated that patients with peritoneal carcinomatosis of colorectal origin and a PCI score >17 who undergo CRS and HIPEC have a similar survival rate to those patients who undergo palliative operations only. Our long-standing algorithm is similar to the 2018 Chicago Consensus Guidelines in that we routinely recommend neoadjuvant systemic chemotherapy with bevacizumab in all patients with colorectal peritoneal carcinomatosis. We recommend that all patients undergo neoadjuvant systemic chemotherapy with FOLOFOX or FOLFIRI with bevacizumab for four to six cycles and then are reassessed for response. We then recommend further systemic therapy or diagnostic laparoscopy for all patients who have stable or responsive disease according to the restaging imaging studies. The intent of the diagnostic laparoscopy is to get a more accurate PCI score and to evaluate the involvement of the bowel and portal structures and to assess for the ability to obtain a complete cytoreduction.

Recently, the utility of HIPEC in conjunction with CRS has been called into question. The PRODIGE-7 trial randomized patients with peritoneal colorectal cancer to CRS and bidirectional oxaliplatin (systemic and peritoneal administration) versus CRS and systemic oxaliplatin alone. The study did demonstrate a rather unexpectedly high OS in the group of patients undergoing CRS alone (42 months); however, the study failed to demonstrate a difference in survival between the two arms. It did demonstrate, however, a significant drop in QOL in the patients undergoing HIPEC. Criticisms of this study include a short duration of HIPEC (30 minutes), inclusion of patients with a PCI of up to 25 and a potentially underpowered study given the surprising OS of 42 months in the CRS only group.

For patients at MD Anderson, we currently offer cytoreduction alone for patients with peritoneal dissemination of their colorectal cancer. We generally limit this to patients with a PCI <20, evidence of disease control on systemic chemotherapy for at least 6 months, and no evidence of retroperitoneal or extra-abdominal metastasis. Patients with concomitant liver metastases not necessitating an extended liver resection are also candidates for CRS. HIPEC is considered for patients who present with ascites or have a mucinous histology. Our overall survival from surgery for this group of patients is >60 months.

Outcomes

A study in the Netherlands by Verwaal et al. randomized 105 patients to receive either (1) standard treatment consisting of systemic chemotherapy (5-fluorouracil and leucovorin) with or without palliative surgery, or (2) cytoreduction with HIPEC, followed by the same systemic chemotherapy regimen. The trial demonstrated a near twofold increase in median overall survival for patients who received CRS and HIPEC compared with those who received systemic chemotherapy only (22 months compared with 12 months). Furthermore, patients who had a complete cytoreduction achieved a 5-year overall survival rate of 45%. Critics of this study cite the use of 5-fluorouracil and leucovorin as an inadequate and rarely used single chemotherapy regimen and suggest that median overall survival is improved with the use of newer chemotherapy regimens with oxaliplatin, irinotecan, and bevacizumab. However, a pooled analysis of 2,095 patients enrolled in two prospective randomized trials of oxaliplatin and irinotecan demonstrated that peritoneal carcinomatosis from colorectal cancer is associated with a significantly shorter median overall survival (duration of 12 months) and progression-free survival (duration of 6 months) compared to patients with other sites of metastatic colorectal cancer (liver and lung). Subsequent single-institution studies have demonstrated that overall survival following CRS and HIPEC in patients with peritoneal carcinomatosis from colorectal cancer is similar to that of patients undergoing hepatic resection for colorectal liver metastasis. Some centers have reported 5-year overall survival rates exceeding 50%.

A consensus statement published in 2020 recommended the use of CRS and HIPEC for carefully selected patients with peritoneal carcinomatosis of colorectal origin. The ability to obtain a complete cytoreduction is the most predictive factor of long-term survival in these individuals. Variables associated with a complete cytoreduction include:

1. Preserved ECOG performance status (≤2)
2. No evidence of extra-abdominal disease
3. No more than three small, resectable hepatic metastases
4. No evidence of biliary obstruction
5. No evidence of ureteral obstruction
6. No evidence of intestinal obstruction at more than one site
7. Small bowel involvement: no gross small bowel mesenteric involvement causing segmental partial bowel obstruction
8. Small-volume disease in the gastrohepatic ligament

Median overall survival for select patients with colorectal cancer metastasis undergoing CRS with or without HIPEC ranges from 32 to 62 months. Unfortunately, disease recurrence occurs in 50% to 70% of patients at a median interval of 12 months. Between 30% and 60% of these patients will present with isolated peritoneal recurrence. Several retrospective studies suggest that 10% to 40% of patients with peritoneal recurrences may be candidates for repeat CRS ± HIPEC. Again, these patients must be carefully selected; CCR and a low tumor burden are the predominant predictors of improved survival. Morbidity and mortality for repeat CRS and HIPEC has been demonstrated to be similar to the first CRS and HIPEC. Given the importance of obtaining a complete cytoreduction on the second CRS and HIPEC and the potential for significant morbidity, we strongly caution against repeat CRS and HIPEC in patients with diffuse intra-abdominal recurrence because these patients have much poorer long-term survival.

Malignant Peritoneal Mesothelioma

Epidemiology

Mesothelioma is a rare malignancy affecting the cuboidal cells lining the pleura (75% of cases), peritoneum (20%), pericardium (5%), or tunica vaginalis (<1%). The disease is regarded as universally fatal and remains poorly understood. Exposure to asbestos increases the risk of mesothelioma after a latency period of 20 to 40 years. Although asbestos is the environmental factor most commonly associated with mesothelioma, it does not transform human mesothelial cells in tissue culture. This indicates a potentially complex and multifactorial carcinogenic process that potentially involves additional carcinogens to induce mesothelial carcinogenesis. Recent evidence suggests that simian virus 40, a polyomavirus that can transform hamster mesothelial cells, acts with asbestos to produce mesothelioma in several independent animal models and human cell lines. Compared with other cell types, human mesothelial cells are unusually susceptible to simian virus 40-induced malignant transformations; 50% to 60% of human mesotheliomas contain and express simian virus 40's DNA and proteins. The presence of simian virus 40 in mesothelioma has been associated with activation of specific oncogenic pathways, direct induction of telomerase activity, and downregulation of the tumor suppressor p53.

Approximately 250 to 400 cases of malignant peritoneal mesothelioma (MPM) are diagnosed annually in the United States. However, the association between asbestos exposure and MPM is weaker than that between asbestos exposure and other types of mesothelioma; only 29% to 58% of males and 2% to 23% of female patients with MPM report known asbestos exposure. Other environmental exposures associated with an elevated risk of developing MPM include thorium, talc, erionite, and mica.

Recently, germline mutations in BRCA-1 associated protein (BAP-1) have been found in a growing number of families. BAP-1 is inherited in an autosomal dominant manner with incomplete penetrance. "BAP-1 cancer syndrome" is associated with increased susceptibility to uveal and cutaneous melanoma, basal cell and squamous cell carcinoma, renal cell cancer, cholangiocarcinoma, and peritoneal mesothelioma. Early identification of this mutation has important implications for cancer screening, potential preventative measures, and for improving overall outcomes for all the associated malignancies.

Clinical Presentation

Patients with MPM present with nonspecific signs and symptoms, including abdominal pain, swelling, anorexia, weight loss, and ascites. A characteristic paraneoplastic syndrome associated with MPM may include thrombocytosis, hypoglycemia, venous thrombosis, hepatopathy, wasting syndrome, fevers, and night sweats. In half of patients, MPM spreads in confluent sheets over the parietal and visceral peritoneum, encasing abdominal organs and creating a dominant, solid, heterogeneous, enhancing, soft-tissue peritoneal mass with little to no ascites, creating a "dry" appearance on CT studies. This presentation is commonly associated with abdominal pain. In contrast to the masses seen in pleural mesothelioma, the masses seen in MPM are not usually calcified. In the other half of patients presenting with MPM, significant abdominal distension occurs; patients have mild to moderate volume of ascites on CT studies and widespread peritoneal nodules without a predominant mass, a so-called "wet" presentation. In MPM, presentation type does not correlate with histologic subtype or prognosis, and a precise diagnosis based on imaging findings alone is not possible.

Diagnosis

Given its nonspecific symptoms, MPM is not easy to diagnose early; the mean time between the presentation of symptoms and diagnosis is 122 days. The cytology of the ascites in "wet" MPM rarely leads to a definitive diagnosis; therefore, a diagnostic laparoscopy is often necessary because there are few or no peritoneal tumor nodules available for image-guided biopsy. Because port-site recurrence is commonly observed at trocar sites, we recommend placing trocars along the linea alba, when possible, to facilitate resection of the port sites at the time of CRS and HIPEC. For "dry" MPM, an image-guided biopsy of the dominant mass is usually successful. Even when tissue is obtained, establishing a histologic diagnosis of MPM often requires the use of several immunohistochemical stains; no marker by itself is diagnostic. It is also important when obtaining biopsies to include some normal surrounding tissue. One of the hallmarks of MPM is invasion into underlying fat. MPM is characterized by positive staining for EMA, calretinin, WT1, cytokeratin 5/6, antimesothelial cell antibody-1, and mesothelin. Cytokeratins can help to confirm invasion and distinguish mesothelioma from sarcoma and melanoma. Serum markers may also be elevated in MPM. These include mesothelin-related protein (elevated in 84% of cases), CA 125 (elevated in 58%), CA 15-3 (elevated in 50%), and CA 19-9 (elevated in 2.3%). Because of their low sensitivity and specificity, these tumor markers are best used for surveillance rather than diagnostic purposes.

Pathology

Epithelioid is the most common histologic subtype of MPM (60% of cases), followed by sarcomatoid (20%) and biphasic (20%). Epithelioid mesothelioma can grow in four different morphologic patterns: tubular, papillary, diffuse, and deciduoid. These morphologic patterns have no influence on prognosis. Epithelioid mesothelioma, which typically is confined to the peritoneal cavity, is locally expansive without invading solid organs, and not prone to hematogenous or lymphatic metastasis, and is commonly associated with a better prognosis than the other subtypes. Therefore, when possible, treatment with CRS and HIPEC is recommended. In contrast, sarcomatoid mesothelioma, named after its sarcoma-like proliferation of spindle cells seen at magnification, is more commonly associated with asbestos exposure and is more likely to have calcified plaques. The prognosis for patients with this type of mesothelioma is dismal with a median overall survival duration of 5 months, regardless of treatment modality. Biphasic mesothelioma demonstrates both epithelioid and sarcomatoid features within the tumor. Its natural history tends to mimic that of sarcomatoid mesothelioma, that is, it often leads to locally aggressive and bulky disease that may invade solid organs. It is unclear whether the poor prognoses of biphasic and sarcomatoid mesothelioma are attributable to aggressive growth patterns, frequent chemoresistance of mixed/sarcomatoid tumors, or other biologic factors. These patients are far less likely to benefit from surgical resection and caution is recommended.

Finally, there are other rare forms of mesothelioma with borderline malignant potential including well-differentiated/papillary and multicystic mesothelioma. These unique forms of MPM typically occur in women who have not been exposed to asbestos. The multicystic variant has the appearance of thin walled, cystic structures scattered throughout the peritoneal cavity and are often easily seen on imaging. The well differentiated/papillary variants are often not well visualized and found incidentally at the time of operation for an unrelated issue. Unfortunately, these tumors are not well understood but can cause considerable pain and impairment in QOL long term. Although they are not invasive, these forms have a tendency toward local recurrence, and malignant transformation has been described. We therefore recommend CRS and HIPEC for multifocal or recurrent disease. Although patient cohorts are small, results of CRS and HIPEC appear to reduce incidence of recurrence compared with CRS alone.

Staging

There is no universally accepted system for staging MPM, as the eighth edition of the AJCC *Cancer Staging Manual* does not specifically address peritoneal mesothelioma. However, eight international institutions have proposed a tumor-node-metastasis–based staging system that resulted in significant stratification of survival by stage. The proposed staging system replaces the traditional T classification with the PCI: T1 corresponds to PCI 1 to 10, T2 corresponds to PCI 11 to 20, T3 corresponds to PCI 21 to 30, and T4 corresponds to PCI 30 to 39. Any positive lymph nodes are classified as N1 and any extra-abdominal metastases are classified as M1. Overall survival for stage I patients with T1 PCI 1 to 10 N0 M0 is significantly superior to the overall survival durations in patients in the other groups. Overall survival in patients with T2 PCI 11 to 20 and T3 PCI 21 to 30, in the absence of N1 or M1 disease, is similar, and therefore individuals meeting these criteria are categorized as stage II. Overall survival in patients with T4 PCI 30 to 39, N1, and/or M1 is also similar and is poor, and individuals in this group are therefore categorized as stage III. The 5-year overall survival rates are 87% for stage I, 53% for stage II, and 29% for stage III disease. The proposed staging system was found to be an independent predictor of survival but has not been subsequently validated. Important prognostic factors to consider in determining which MPM patients should undergo CRS and HIPEC include epithelioid histology, low disease burden (PCI <20), the likelihood of achieving complete cytoreduction, patient age is <60 years, whether the duration of environmental asbestos exposure was <20 years, and whether the patient's ECOG performance status is <2. A nomogram that includes histologic subtype, pre-CRS PCI, and preoperative serum CA 125 has been developed and demonstrated to correlate with overall survival, but it has not been subsequently validated and therefore is not largely used. Recently, Ki-67 has been demonstrated to be a powerful independent prognosticator that, along with the PCI score and histologic subtype, predicts overall survival in patients with MPM. One particular study found that patients with a Ki-67 >9% and a PCI score >17 are less likely to benefit from CRS and HIPEC.

Treatment

Our treatment algorithm for peritoneal mesothelioma is shown in Figure 12.5. Briefly, patients are evaluated with a history, physical examination, assessment of CA 125, and high-quality imaging (CT or MRI). Pathologic results are carefully reviewed, and the patient's case is discussed during a multidisciplinary conference. For patients with epithelioid MPM, the CT imaging is reviewed. If the estimated PCI is <20, the ECOG status <2, there are limited comorbidities without renal insufficiency, no bicavitary disease, or significant lymph node involvement, then the patient is offered a diagnostic laparoscopy. If the PCI at that time is less than or equal to 10, the patient is offered CRS and HIPEC with cisplatin (200 mg/m²) for 60 minutes. We utilize a renal protective strategy that includes perioperative fluid hydration, avoidance of perioperative CT imaging with contrast, avoidance of nephrotoxic medications, and the use of sodium thiosulfate at the time of HIPEC and

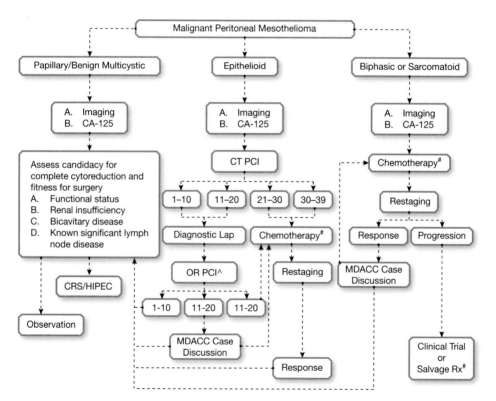

^PCI: Peritoneal Cancer Index (CT – Imaging; OP – Operative)
#Chemotherapy: ECOG Performance Status = 0–2; Cisplatin/Carboplatin + Pemetrexed ± Avastin (Typical Course: 3 cycles q3wks); Salvage Rx (Gemcitabine + Docetaxel, Vinorelbine, Gemcitabine).

FIGURE 12.5 Algorithm for the multidisciplinary management of malignant peritoneal mesothelioma.

during the subsequent 12 hours. Implementation of this strategy has greatly reduced cisplatin-related nephrotoxicity in our experience.

If the estimated CT PCI is 11 to 20, the patient is discussed at a multidisciplinary tumor board to decide upon neoadjuvant systemic therapy or upfront CRS/HIPEC. Patients with an estimated CT PCI >20 or a PCI >20 identified at diagnostic laparoscopy are offered neoadjuvant systemic therapy with cisplatin or carboplatin and pemetrexed. If there is no disease progression on systemic therapy and a complete cytoreduction is believed to be possible, we offer CRS and HIPEC with Cisplatin.

All patients with biphasic MPM are offered neoadjuvant systemic chemotherapy with cisplatin and pemetrexed to evaluate tumor biology. CRS and HIPEC are offered after careful multidisciplinary discussion. Patients with sarcomatoid variant are generally not considered candidates for CRS and HIPEC because of the aggressive nature of these tumors.

Immune checkpoint blockade regimens are currently being studied here at MD Anderson and show promising early results with response rates of ~20% even among patients who progressed on first-line cisplatin/carboplatin therapy. Further study is needed before these agents are incorporated into treatment algorithms.

Surveillance for all surgically resected patients consists of a history, physical examination, assessment of CA 125, and CT imaging every 4 months for the first 2 years. Thereafter, they are monitored every 6 months until the 5-year mark is reached, after which annual surveillance is continued.

Outcomes

Systemic chemotherapy is associated with relatively low response rates (0% to 35%) and significant toxicity (24% to 60% grade III/IV toxicity) in patients with MPM (Table 12.2), but the adoption of CRS and HIPEC has resulted in improved outcomes for these individuals. Multiple single-institution series of patients with MPM treated with CRS and HIPEC have reported median overall survival durations of 30 to 92 months; this compares favorably to the results of systemic chemotherapy trials for MPM, which have reported median overall survival durations of 6 to 15 months (Table 12.3). Although a randomized, controlled trial comparing systemic chemotherapy and CRS and HIPEC has not yet been done, a recent systematic review and meta-analysis of 1,047 patients concluded that patients treated with intraperitoneal cisplatin had an improved 5-year overall survival rate.

Despite these encouraging survival results, approximately 40% to 60% of patients developed disease progression at a median of 11 to 28 months following comprehensive treatment. The majority of these patients (82%) experience peritoneal-only recurrence; involvement of the pleura, liver, and/or lymph nodes is rare. Unfortunately, the small bowel is frequently involved (up to 70% of patients) at times limiting the utility of repeat CRS and HIPEC (only 8% of patients with recurrent disease underwent repeat CRS and HIPEC at the National Cancer Institute of Milan).

The primary predictor of disease progression is an incomplete (>2.5 mm) cytoreduction. Recurrent disease is most commonly treated with systemic chemotherapy; however, repeat CRS and HIPEC may be associated with improved survival and similar morbidity to the first CRS and HIPEC in highly selected patients. Independent predictors of reduced survival following surgery include a time-to-progression <9 months, poor performance status, and a need for supportive care.

TABLE 12.2   Clinical Trials of Systemic Chemotherapy for Malignant Peritoneal Mesothelioma

Study	Median OS	Response Rate (%)	Grade III/IV Complications
Ifosfamide/mesna	6.9	3	50%
Doxorubicin/ifosfamide	7	32	36%
Cisplatin/MMC	7.7	26	40%
Raltitrexed/cisplatin	7.7	20	30% stopped treatment due to toxicity
Cisplatin/doxorubicin	8.8	14	40%
Irinotecan	9.3	0	43%
Sorafenib	9.7	6	24%
Tremelimumab	10.7	7	14%
Cisplatin/IFN α2a	12	38	70%
Gemcitabine/cisplatin/bevacizumab	15.6	24	42%
Gemcitabine/pemetrexed	26.8	15	60%

Median overall survival (OS), response rate, and grade III/IV complications are reported.

TABLE 12.3 Clinical Studies of Cytoreduction and Intraperitoneal-Heated Chemotherapy for Malignant Peritoneal Mesothelioma

Study	n	Median OS (Months)	Survival	
			3 yrs (%)	5 yrs (%)
Blackham (2010)	38	41	56	17
Brigand (2006)	15	36	43	29
Baratti (2010)	83	44	–	50
Feldman (2003)	49	92	59	59
Yan (2006)	100	52	55	46
Kluger (2010)	47	55	62	49
Tudor (2010)	20	30	46	–
Yan (2009)	401	53	60	47

Median overall survival (OS), and 3- and 5-year survivals are reported.

CASE SCENARIO

Case Scenario 1

Presentation

A 34-year-old female presents to her outside gynecologist with a several-month history of lower abdominal pain. The gynecologist obtains an U/S in the office which notes an abnormal mass in the right lower quadrant. Given her age she was taken to the operating room for a laparoscopic appendectomy. At the time of appendectomy, however, the referring surgeon encounters mucin throughout the pelvis and diffuse white peritoneal plaques. These lesions and their locations were well photographed and biopsies were obtained. The appendix was inflamed and at the tip, a mass lesion was identified. The base of the appendix appeared normal. An appendectomy was performed. No further procedures were performed. The patient recovered well and presented to your surgical oncology office.

Differential Diagnosis

Appendiceal Tumor	Secondary Malignancy
Low-grade appendiceal mucinous neoplasm (LAMN)	Colorectal adenocarcinoma
High-grade appendiceal mucinous neoplasm (HAMN)	Ovarian
Appendiceal adenocarcinoma (AA)	Pancreatic adenocarcinoma
Goblet cell adenocarcinoma (GCA)	Gastric adenocarcinoma
	Cholangiocarcinoma
	Peritoneal mesothelioma
	Primary peritoneal malignancy

Confirmation of Diagnosis and Treatment

Tissue diagnosis and review by an expert pathologist is of paramount importance in these patients. Primary appendiceal malignancies are rare and subtle pathologic differences can have a major impact on treatment and outcome. Once an appendiceal primary is confirmed, the decision to initiate systemic neoadjuvant treatment is made. While high-grade (moderate/poorly differentiated/signet ring cell) adenocarcinomas and GCA with peritoneal dissemination of disease may benefit from neoadjuvant cytotoxic therapy; LAMN, HAMN, well-differentiated adenocarcinoma, and neuroendocrine disease are treated primarily with cytoreductive surgery with hyperthermic intraperitoneal chemotherapy.

In this case, the patient was diagnosed with a high-grade AA. She was started on a course of neoadjuvant FOLFOX prior to planned definitive surgical therapy. She had stability of disease and underwent subsequent diagnostic laparoscopy with the finding of a PCI of 17. She was offered an accepted CRS and HIPEC.

Surgical Approach—Key Steps

The patient underwent a full cytoreduction to CC-0 following the operative steps as described in the main text. Perfusion was completed with a core body temperature >38 °C being obtained during the perfusion.

Postoperative Management

In the immediate postoperative period, close attention should be given to patient's urine output given the cytotoxic nature of most chemotherapy agents. Postoperative ileus is common in these patients, therefore routine nasogastric tube placement has been adopted as part of our practice. Routine use of G tubes and J tubes is discouraged.

Various enhanced recovery pathways have been studied. In general, progression to safe discharge and expeditious return to intended oncologic therapy should be one's primary outcome of interest. Similarly, long-term physical and emotional sequalae of the procedure should be frankly discussed preoperatively and be managed by the operative surgeon given their experience with this unique and oftentimes extended recovery.

This patient had a complete cytoreduction and was placed on surveillance with tumor markers and imaging as outlined in the text.

Common Curve Balls

- Perfusion/pump problems
- Postoperative neutropenia/AKI/bleeding secondary to perfusate
- Unexpected PCI or histology
- Unable to obtain CCR = 0/1 resection
  - Porta-hepatitis infiltrative disease
  - Extensive vascular resection
  - Extensive bowel serosa/mesentery involvement
  - Ureteral involvement
- Postoperative change in histology

Take Home Points

- Histology is a strong predictor of outcome and determines the need for neoadjuvant therapy.
- Patients should be treated at high-volume cytoreductive centers with established cytoreduction and HIPEC protocols.
- A low threshold should exist for diagnostic laparoscopy/documentation of extent and location of disease/biopsy if it may assist in diagnostic confirmation or operative planning but extensive surgery prior to CRS and HIPEC is highly discouraged.
- Full cytoreduction should be followed by hyperthermic intraperitoneal chemotherapy, the exact regimen and agents continue to be refined based on patient histology.
- Surveillance program is needed for all patients with peritoneal surface malignancy including low-grade malignancies.

Case Scenario 2

Presentation

A 74-year-old gentleman is noted to have a rising CEA and a new mass in the right pelvis on surveillance CT scan. He notably has a history of a microsatellite stable T4 N0 M0 moderately differentiated colonic adenocarcinoma who underwent a right hemicolectomy followed by adjuvant FOLFOX 3 years prior. He had previously shown no evidence of disease recurrence during screening.

Differential Diagnosis

Recurrent colorectal cancer
Peritoneal metastasis from a new primary
Colorectal—second primary
Gastric adenocarcinoma
Cholangiocarcinoma
Pancreatic adenocarcinoma
Small Bowel adenocarcinoma

Confirmation of Diagnosis and Treatment

In cases such as this, a tissue diagnosis can typically be obtained by IR biopsy and should be compared against slides obtained from the patient's initial resection. Additionally, full staging scans should be completed if not already obtained during surveillance imaging to evaluate for pulmonary, hepatic, or bone metastases. Appropriate stains should be used to confirm a lower gastrointestinal origin and a colonoscopy should rule out an occult second primary. While still in its nascency, quantifying circulating tumoral DNA can be useful in measuring response to therapy and in confirmation of minimal residual disease following any eventual resection. After confirmation of a peritoneal recurrence of this colorectal cancer, the next step would be presentation at a multidisciplinary tumor board and initiation of neoadjuvant chemotherapy.

Cross-sectional imaging should be carefully evaluated pre and post treatment by a surgeon and radiologist well versed in peritoneal disease. Specifically, signs of advanced and likely unresectable disease should be confirmed to be absent, such as cauliflowering of the small bowel or porta-hepatis disease, and a SPAAT score calculated.

Surgical Approach—Key Steps

When technically feasible, a diagnostic laparoscopy should be the first operative procedure to confirm extent of disease and determine if a complete cytoreduction is possible. Even in the presence of an extensive surgical history, we will attempt an open entry and evaluation with laparoscopy. This can be completed with very low morbidity. Once the disease has been deemed resectable, a midline laparotomy incision is made and the abdomen is thoroughly inspected again, including evaluation of all peritoneal surfaces. Once again, it is important to ensure that all visible disease can and will be removed with surgery.

Surgical resection should be undertaken with basic tenets of cytoreductive surgery (described in main chapter text) ensuring clear margins and striving for an R0 resection. Complete omentectomy is always performed. Involved organs should be removed en bloc when feasible and weighed against their associated morbidity. In female patients who are postmenopausal, consideration to of bilateral oophorectomy should be strongly considered.

In this case, the patient was able to undergo an RLQ peritonectomy to completely excise this peritoneal recurrence. Following our current practice and guidance from recent randomized control trials, we currently perform cytoreduction without HIPEC.

Postoperative Management

In the absence of a peritoneal perfusion, patients' fluid balance and hematologic parameters do not experience the same derangements as they have following CRS and HIPEC. Postoperative cytoreductive patients can be excellent candidates for ERAS protocols and fluid restrictive postoperative resuscitation when appropriate. This patient was able to advance to a CLD on postoperative day 2 and a regular diet the following day being discharged home on day 4 post surgery.

Common Curve Balls

- Peritoneal disease from a new primary
- Discussing the role of surveillance laparoscopy in resected high-risk colorectal cancers
- "Fitness" for surgical resection-Physiologic age versus chronologic age.
- Whether or not/when to perform HIPEC and with what agent
- Unexpected PCI or histology
- Disease identified outside the peritoneum (liver metastasis identified at the time of exploration)
- Timing of surgery when the patient is unable to tolerate neoadjuvant cytotoxic therapy

Take Home Points

- Diagnostic laparoscopy prior to laparotomy for cytoreduction can decrease rates of aborted explorative laparotomy-allowing patients with unresectable disease to return to systemic therapy in a more expedited fashion.
- In colorectal cancer, a more targeted cytoreduction can be performed for single sites of metastasis and a formal peritoneal quadrantectomy for diffuse or miliary disease.
- Current evidence suggests minimal benefit to HIPEC in colorectal adenocarcinoma. Our current practice is to perform cytoreduction alone in these patients. Patients who present with ascites or mucinous histology are considered for HIPEC on a case by case basis.
- Patients with gastric or ovarian primaries, however, may benefit from HIPEC in select cases.

CASE SCENARIO REVIEW

Questions

1. Which of the following histologic subtypes of malignant peritoneal mesothelioma are not currently offered cytoreduction and HIPEC?

   A. Biphasic
   B. Well-differentiated
   C. Sarcomatoid
   D. Epithelioid
   E. Multicystic

2. In which of the following patients would a right hemicolectomy be indicated after the following incidental finding on pathologic review of an appendectomy specimen?

   A. 1.5-cm moderately differentiated appendiceal adenocarcinoma
   B. 0.8-cm well-differentiated neuroendocrine tumor with no tumor at the cut margin
   C. 4.2-cm well-differentiated mucinous appendiceal adenocarcinoma with clear margins and no serosal disease
   D. 2.3-cm low-grade mucinous neoplasm with clear margins undergoing cytoreduction and HIPEC for disseminated disease along the right diaphragm and omentum
   E. None of the above

3. Which of the following represents a contraindication to cytoreduction of peritoneal spread of colorectal adenocarcinoma?

   A. Primary tumor in place
   B. Inability to tolerate neoadjuvant chemotherapy
   C. A single peripheral liver metastasis
   D. Peritoneal carcinomatosis index (PCI) score of 16
   E. Splenic capsular involvement

4. What is the best initial treatment for a female patient who is taken to the operating room for presumed ovarian cancer and is instead found to have an appendiceal mass with widespread mucinous-appearing peritoneal deposits.

   A. Appendectomy/TAH/BSO and debulk disease to <1 cm in size
   B. Call in the perfusionist and proceed with CRS/HIPEC immediately
   C. Perform an appendectomy/document extent of disease/biopsy representative lesions and stop the operation
   D. Call in a general surgeon to perform a formal right colectomy
   E. Appendectomy/TAH/BSO/attempt complete debulking

5. Which of the following correlates least well with predicting overall long-term survival after CRS and HIPEC for appendiceal malignancies:

   A. The ability to obtain a complete cytoreduction
   B. The grade of peritoneal deposits
   C. The peritoneal carcinomatosis index
   D. CA 19-9 of 200 (normal value is 35) but a normal CEA
   E. CA 19-9 of 50 (normal is 35) and a CEA of 10 (normal is 3.8)

Answers

1. **The correct answer is C.** *Rationale:* Sarcomatoid mesothelioma is a particularly aggressive mesothelioma histology with a median survival of 5 months. As such, there is not a role for cytoreduction for these patients outside of a clinical trial. CRS and HIPEC should be considered for the other listed histologies in the appropriate clinical setting. Notably, biphasic peritoneal mesothelioma would require neoadjuvant therapy.

2. **The correct answer is A.** *Rationale:* Given the rarity of lymph node disease in mucinous neoplasms of the appendix or well-differentiated neuroendocrine tumors less than 2 cm, margin-negative

appendectomy is the appropriate definitive management for these patients. In the case of appendiceal adenocarcinoma, rates of positive lymph nodes in moderate (17%) and poorly (72%) differentiated adenocarcinoma justify the need for a completion right hemicolectomy.

3. **The correct answer is B.** *Rationale:* Neoadjuvant and adjuvant chemotherapies are key components in the management of patients with carcinomatosis of colorectal origin. Inability to tolerate cytotoxic chemotherapy should be considered a contraindication for cytoreduction. Various PCI score cutoffs have been used in carcinomatosis of colorectal origin, but 16 is classically below all of them. None of the other choices are associated with prohibitive operative risk. This includes concurrent resection of colorectal liver metastasis at the time of CRS-HIPEC. Multiple case series have demonstrated safety and equivalent outcomes to isolated peritoneal disease.

4. **The correct answer is C.** *Rationale:* A less is more approach is optimal for patients in whom an unexpected appendiceal adenocarcinoma with peritoneal disease is encountered. The more extensive a procedure is undertaken at this stage, the less likely a complete cytoreduction will be able to be accomplished when a definitive procedure is undertaken.

5. **The correct answer is D.** *Rationale:* CA 19-9 is elevated in 67.1% of appendiceal cancers while CEA is elevated in 56% of these patients. At the time of recurrence an elevated CEA was associated with a worse prognosis, while CA 19-9 levels did not correlate with prognosis. The other factors (completeness of cytoreduction, grade of disease, and PCI) all strongly correlate with long-term survival in patients undergoing CRS and HIPEC for appendiceal malignancies.

Recommended Readings

Addiss DG, Shaffer N, Fowler BS, Tauxe RV. The epidemiology of appendicitis and appendectomy in the United States. *Am J Epidemiol.* 1990;132(5):910–925.

Amin MB, Greene FL, Edge SB, et al. American Joint Committee on Cancer. *AJCC Cancer Staging Manual.* 8th ed. Springer; 2017.

Andreasson H, Lorant T, Påhlman L, Graf W, Mahteme H. Cytoreductive surgery plus perioperative intraperitoneal chemotherapy in pseudomyxoma peritonei: aspects of the learning curve. *Eur J Surg Oncol.* 2014;40(8):930–936.

Bailey CE, Hu CY, You YN, et al. Increasing disparities in the age-related incidences of colon and rectal cancers in the United States, 1975–2010. *JAMA Surg.* 2015;150(1):17–22.

Blackham AU, Russell GB, Stewart JH 4th, Votanopoulos K, Levine EA, Shen P. Metastatic colorectal cancer: survival comparison of hepatic resection versus cytoreductive surgery and hyperthermic intraperitoneal chemotherapy. *Ann Surg Oncol.* 2014;21(8):2667–2674.

Blair NP, Bugis SP, Turner LJ, MacLeod MM. Review of the pathologic diagnoses of 2,216 appendectomy specimens. *Am J Surg.* 1993;165(5):618–620.

Bradley RF, Stewart JH 4th, Russell GB, Levine EA, Geisinger KR. Pseudomyxoma peritonei of appendiceal origin: a clinicopathologic analysis of 101 patients uniformly treated at a single institution, with literature review. *Am J Surg Pathol.* 2006;30(5):551–559.

Carbone M, Pass HI, Miele L, Bocchetta M. New developments about the association of SV40 with human mesothelioma. *Oncogene.* 2003;22(33):5173–5580.

Carmignani CP, Hampton R, Sugarbaker CE, Chang D, Sugarbaker PH. Utility of CEA and CA 19-9 tumor markers in diagnosis and prognostic assessment of mucinous epithelial cancers of the appendix. *J Surg Oncol.* 2004;87(4):162–166.

Cashin PH, Graf W, Nygren P, Mahteme H. Cytoreductive surgery and intraperitoneal chemotherapy for colorectal peritoneal carcinomatosis: prognosis and treatment of recurrences in a cohort study. *Eur J Surg Oncol.* 2012;38(6):509–515.

Ceelen W, Van Nieuwenhove Y, Putte DV, Pattyn P. Neoadjuvant chemotherapy with bevacizumab may improve outcome after cytoreduction and hyperthermic intraperitoneal chemoperfusion (HIPEC) for colorectal carcinomatosis. *Ann Surg Oncol.* 2014;21(9):3023–3028.

Chua TC, Liauw W, Morris DL. Early recurrence of pseudomyxoma peritonei following treatment failure of cytoreductive surgery and perioperative intraperitoneal chemotherapy is indicative of a poor survival outcome. *Int J Colorectal Dis.* 2012;27(3):381–389.

Collins DC. 71, 000 human appendix specimens. A final report, summarizing forty years' study. *Am J Proctol.* 1963;14:265–281.

Connor SJ, Hanna GB, Frizelle FA. Appendiceal tumors: retrospective clinicopathologic analysis of appendiceal tumors from 7,970 appendectomies. *Dis Colon Rectum.* 1998;41(1):75–80.

Deraco M, Baratti D, Cabras AD, et al. Experience with peritoneal mesothelioma at the Milan National Cancer Institute. *World J Gastrointest Oncol.* 2010;2(2):76–84.

Di Fabio F, Aston W, Mohamed F, Chandrakumaran K, Cecil T, Moran B. Elevated tumour markers are normalized in most patients with pseudomyxoma peritonei 7 days after complete tumour removal. *Colorectal Dis.* 2015;17(8):698–703.

Dineen SP, Royal RE, Hughes MS, et al. A simplified preoperative assessment predicts complete cytoreduction and outcomes in patients with low-grade mucinous adenocarcinoma of the appendix. *Ann Surg Oncol.* 2015;22(11):3640–3646.

Elias D, Goéré D, Di Pietrantonio D, et al. Results of systematic second-look surgery in patients at high risk of developing colorectal peritoneal carcinomatosis. *Ann Surg.* 2008;247(3):445–450.

Elias D, Lefevre JH, Chevalier J, et al. Complete cytoreductive surgery plus intraperitoneal chemohyperthermia with oxaliplatin for peritoneal carcinomatosis of colorectal origin. *J Clin Oncol.* 2009;27(5):681–685.

Esquivel J, Sticca R, Sugarbaker P, et al. Cytoreductive surgery and hyperthermic intraperitoneal chemotherapy in the management of peritoneal surface malignancies of colonic origin: a consensus statement. Society of Surgical Oncology. *Ann Surg Oncol.* 2007;14(1):128–133.

Esquivel J, Sugarbaker PH. Clinical presentation of the pseudomyxoma peritonei syndrome. *Br J Surg.* 2000;87(10):1414–1418.

Esquivel J, Sugarbaker PH. Second-look surgery in patients with peritoneal dissemination from appendiceal malignancy: analysis of prognostic factors in 98 patients. *Ann Surg.* 2001;234(2):198–205.

Franko J, Shi Q, Goldman CD, et al. Treatment of colorectal peritoneal carcinomatosis with systemic chemotherapy: a pooled analysis of north central cancer treatment group phase III trials N9741 and N9841. *J Clin Oncol.* 2012;30(3):263–267.

Glockzin G, Gerken M, Lang SA, Klinkhammer-Schalke M, Piso P, Schlitt HJ. Oxaliplatin-based versus irinotecan-based hyperthermic intraperitoneal chemotherapy (HIPEC) in patients with peritoneal metastasis from appendiceal and colorectal cancer: a retrospective analysis. *BMC Cancer.* 2014;14:807.

Goere D, Glehen O, Quenet F, et al. Second-look surgery plus hyperthermic intraperitoneal chemotherapy versus surveillance in patients at high risk of developing colorectal peritoneal metastases (PROPHYLO-CHIP-PRODIGE 15): a randomised, phase 3 study. *Lancet Oncol.* 2020;21(9):1147–1154.

Goere D, Souadka A, Faron M, et al. Extent of colorectal peritoneal carcinomatosis: attempt to define a threshold above which HIPEC does not offer survival benefit: a comparative study. *Ann Surg Oncol.* 2015;22(9):2958–2964.

Hill AR, McQuellon RP, Russell GB, Shen P, Stewart JH 4th, Levine EA. Survival and quality of life following cytoreductive surgery plus hyperthermic intraperitoneal chemotherapy for peritoneal carcinomatosis of colonic origin. *Ann Surg Oncol.* 2011;18(13):3673–3679.

Jafari MD, Halabi WJ, Stamos MJ, et al. Surgical outcomes of hyperthermic intraperitoneal chemotherapy: analysis of the American College of Surgeons National Surgical Quality Improvement Program. *JAMA Surg.* 2014;149(2):170–1755.

Jayne DG, Fook S, Loi C, et al. Peritoneal carcinomatosis from colorectal cancer. *Br J Surg.* 2002;89(12):1545–1550.

Kepenekian V, Elias D, Passot G, et al. Diffuse malignant peritoneal mesothelioma: evaluation of systemic chemotherapy with comprehensive treatment through the RENAPE Database: multi-institutional retrospective study. *Eur J Cancer.* 2016;65:69–79.

Klaver CEL, Wisselink DD, et al. Adjuvant hyperthermic intraperitoneal chemotherapy in patients with locally advanced colon cancer (COLOPEC): a multicentre, open-label, randomised trial. *Lancet Gastroenterol Hepatol.* 2019;4(10):761–770.

Konigsrainer I, Horvath P, Struller F, Forkl V, Königsrainer A, Beckert S. Risk factors for recurrence following complete cytoreductive surgery and HIPEC in colorectal cancer-derived peritoneal surface malignancies. *Langenbecks Arch Surg.* 2013;398(5):745–749.

Kusamura S, Baratti D, Virzì S, et al. Learning curve for cytoreductive surgery and hyperthermic intraperitoneal chemotherapy in peritoneal surface malignancies: analysis of two centres. *J Surg Oncol.* 2013;107(4):312–319.

Kusamura S, Torres Mesa PA, Cabras A, Baratti D, Deraco M. The role of Ki-67 and pre-cytoreduction parameters in selecting diffuse malignant peritoneal mesothelioma (DMPM) patients for cytoreductive surgery (CRS) and hyperthermic intraperitoneal chemotherapy (HIPEC). *Ann Surg Oncol.* 2016;23(5):1468–1473.

Lambert LA, Armstrong TS, Lee JJ, et al. Incidence, risk factors, and impact of severe neutropenia after hyperthermic intraperitoneal mitomycin C. *Ann Surg Oncol.* 2009;16(8):2181–2187.

Leung V, Huo YR, Liauw W, Morris DL. Oxaliplatin versus mitomycin C for HIPEC in colorectal cancer peritoneal carcinomatosis. *Eur J Surg Oncol.* 2017;43(1):144–149.

Levine EA, Stewart JH 4th, Shen P, et al. Intraperitoneal chemotherapy for peritoneal surface malignancy: experience with 1,000 patients. *J Am Coll Surg.* 2014;218(4):573–585.

Lord AC, Shihab O, Chandrakumaran K, Mohamed F, Cecil TD, Moran BJ. Recurrence and outcome after complete tumour removal and hyperthermic intraperitoneal chemotherapy in 512 patients with pseudomyxoma peritonei from perforated appendiceal mucinous tumours. *Eur J Surg Oncol.* 2015;41(3):396–369.

Marmor S, Portschy PR, Tuttle TM, Virnig BA. The rise in appendiceal cancer incidence: 2000–2009. *J Gastrointest Surg.* 2015;19(4):743–750.

Marudanayagam R, Williams GT, Rees BI. Review of the pathological results of 2660 appendicectomy specimens. *J Gastroenterol.* 2006;41(8):745–749.

McCall JL, Black RB, Rich CA, et al. The value of serum carcinoembryonic antigen in predicting recurrent disease following curative resection of colorectal cancer. *Dis Colon Rectum.* 1994;37(9):875–881.

Milovanov V, Sardi A, Studeman K, Nieroda C, Sittig M, Gushchin V. The 7th edition of the AJCC staging classification correlates with biologic behavior of mucinous appendiceal tumor with peritoneal metastases treated with cytoreductive surgery and hyperthermic intraperitoneal chemotherapy (CRS/HIPEC). *Ann Surg Oncol.* 2016;23(6):1928–1933.

Moran B, Baratti D, Yan TD, Kusamura S, Deraco M. Consensus statement on the loco-regional treatment of appendiceal mucinous neoplasms with peritoneal dissemination (pseudomyxoma peritonei). *J Surg Oncol.* 2008;98(4):277–282.

Passot G, Vaudoyer D, Cotte E, et al. Progression following neoadjuvant systemic chemotherapy may not be a contraindication to a curative approach for colorectal carcinomatosis. *Ann Surg.* 2012;256(1):125–129.

Polanco PM, Ding Y, Knox JM, et al. Institutional learning curve of cytoreductive surgery and hyperthermic intraperitoneal chemoperfusion for peritoneal malignancies. *Ann Surg Oncol.* 2015;22(5):1673–1679.

Quenet F, Elias D, Roca L, et al. Cytoreductive surgery plus hyperthermic intraperitoneal chemotherapy versus cytoreductive surgery alone for colorectal peritoneal metastases (PRODIGE 7): a multicentre, randomised, open-label, phase 3 trial. *Lancet Oncol.* 2021;22(2):256–266.

Reuter NP, Macgregor JM, Woodall CE, et al. Preoperative performance status predicts outcome following heated intraperitoneal chemotherapy. *Am J Surg.* 2008;196(6):909–913; discussion 913–914.

Ripley RT, Davis JL, Kemp CD, Steinberg SM, Toomey MA, Avital I. Prospective randomized trial evaluating mandatory second look surgery with HIPEC and CRS vs. standard of care in patients at high risk of developing colorectal peritoneal metastases. *Trials.* 2010;11:62.

Sadeghi B, Arvieux C, Glehen O, et al. Peritoneal carcinomatosis from non-gynecologic malignancies: results of the EVOCAPE 1 multicentric prospective study. *Cancer.* 2000;88(2):358–363.

Segelman J, Granath F, Holm T, Machado M, Mahteme H, Martling A. Incidence, prevalence and risk factors for peritoneal carcinomatosis from colorectal cancer. *Br J Surg.* 2012;99(5):699–705.

Shaib WL, Goodman M, Chen Z, et al. Incidence and survival of appendiceal mucinous neoplasms: a SEER analysis. *Am J Clin Oncol.* 2017;40(6):569–573.

Shetty S, Natarajan B, Thomas P, Govindarajan V, Sharma P, Loggie B. Proposed classification of pseudomyxoma peritonei: influence of signet ring cells on survival. *Am Surg.* 2013;79(11):1171–1176.

Simkens GA, van Oudheusden TR, Luyer MD, et al. Predictors of severe morbidity after cytoreductive surgery and hyperthermic intraperitoneal chemotherapy for patients with colorectal peritoneal carcinomatosis. *Ann Surg Oncol.* 2016;23(3):833–841.

Smeenk RM, Verwaal VJ, Zoetmulder FA. Learning curve of combined modality treatment in peritoneal surface disease. *Br J Surg.* 2007;94(11):1408–1014.

Sugarbaker PH. Pseudomyxoma peritonei. A cancer whose biology is characterized by a redistribution phenomenon. *Ann Surg.* 1994;219(2):109–111.

Sugarbaker PH, Acherman YI, Gonzalez-Moreno S, et al. Diagnosis and treatment of peritoneal mesothelioma: the Washington Cancer Institute experience. *Semin Oncol.* 2002;29(1):51–61.

Tarraga Lopez PJ, Albero JS, Rodriguez-Montes JA. Primary and secondary prevention of colorectal cancer. *Clin Med Insights Gastroenterol.* 2014;7:33–46.

Verwaal VJ, Boot H, Aleman BM, van Tinteren H, Zoetmulder FA. Recurrences after peritoneal carcinomatosis of colorectal origin treated by cytoreduction and hyperthermic intraperitoneal chemotherapy: location, treatment, and outcome. *Ann Surg Oncol.* 2004;11(4):375–379.

Verwaal VJ, van Ruth S, de Bree E, et al. Randomized trial of cytoreduction and hyperthermic intraperitoneal chemotherapy versus systemic chemotherapy and palliative surgery in patients with peritoneal carcinomatosis of colorectal cancer. *J Clin Oncol.* 2003;21(20):3737–3743.

Votanopoulos KI, Russell G, Randle RW, Shen P, Stewart JH, Levine EA. Peritoneal surface disease (PSD) from appendiceal cancer treated with cytoreductive surgery (CRS) and hyperthermic intraperitoneal chemotherapy (HIPEC): overview of 481 cases. *Ann Surg Oncol.* 2015;22(4):1274–1279.

Wagner PL, Austin F, Zenati M, et al. Oncologic risk stratification following cytoreductive surgery and hyperthermic intraperitoneal chemotherapy for appendiceal carcinomatosis. *Ann Surg Oncol.* 2016;23(5):1587–1593.

Yan TD, Deraco M, Elias D, et al. A novel tumor-node-metastasis (TNM) staging system of diffuse malignant peritoneal mesothelioma using outcome analysis of a multi-institutional database*. *Cancer.* 2011;117(9):1855–1863.

Cancer of the Colon, Rectum, and Anus

Naveen V. Manisundaram, Neal Bhutiani, and Y. Nancy You

Epidemiology

Colorectal cancer (CRC) is a major cause of cancer-related morbidity and mortality. It is the third most commonly diagnosed cancer in men and in women and is the third leading cause of cancer deaths in the United States. There are approximately 149,000 new cases of CRC diagnosed annually including 104,270 colon cancers and 45,230 rectal cancers. Efforts aimed at prevention, early detection, and screening have resulted in a significant decrease in CRC incidence of about 2% to 3% per year over the past 15 years. Despite these improvements, CRC still accounts for just over 53,000 deaths per year in the United States as well as for 8.7% of overall cancer deaths.

In the United States, the lifetime risk of developing CRC is about 1 in 23 (4.3%) in men, and 1 in 25 (4%) in women. Age is a major risk factor in the development of sporadic CRC. Approximately 90% of all CRCs are diagnosed in patients aged 50 or greater. While population-based CRC screening beginning at age 50 has been a standard recommendation since the late 1980s, adoption rates have remained imperfect. At the time of diagnosis, 37% of patients will have localized disease, 36% will have regional spread, and 22% will have distant metastasis. The overall survival (OS) rates for CRC are highly dependent on disease stage at diagnosis, with 5-year OS for local, regional, and metastatic disease being approximately 91%, 72%, and 15%, respectively.

However, CRC incidence is increasing in the segment of the population younger than age 50. These young patients tend to present with more left-sided and rectal cancers when compared to the overall CRC patient population. These patients also tend to present at more advanced stages and many are symptomatic at diagnosis. Indeed, the American Cancer Society in 2018 and the US Preventive Services Task Force (USPSTF) in 2021 lowered the age to commence average-risk CRC screening from 50 to 45 years old, in response to the increasing incidence rates in the younger populations.

Risk Factors

Age

Advanced age predisposes to CRC development. CRC incidence increases progressively after age 40 and rises exponentially after age 50. More than 80% of new CRC cases and 90% of CRC deaths occur in patients over age 50 years. The incidence of CRC in patients aged >60 years is approximately 30-fold higher than patients <40 years.

Race

In the United States, CRC incidence and mortality are highest among African Americans when compared to all other ethnic/racial groups. African American men and women have a 14% higher CRC incidence and 30% higher CRC mortality when compared to their White counterparts. CRC incidence and mortality among Hispanic and Asian/Pacific Islander ethnic groups are lower than those seen in Whites. Over the past 10 years, American Indian/Alaskan Native ethnic groups now have higher CRC incidence and mortality rates compared to their White counterparts.

Although there has been a national decline in CRC rates in the last decade, this decline has been disproportionate within demographic subpopulations. The disparity is likely linked to variations in access to screening and advanced treatment modalities, as well as multifactorial reasons. For example, African Americans in general are less likely than Whites to receive the most appropriate surgery, chemotherapy, and radiation treatments after a cancer diagnosis; however, in some clinical trial settings, where treatment variation is eliminated, these racial differences in survival disappear. Socioeconomic status is a major confounder. Using the type of insurance as a surrogate for economic status, studies have shown that the 5-year survival for CRC is 30% higher among African American patients who are privately insured when compared to those without health insurance.

Diet

Many dietary factors have been studied regarding their effect on CRC. Consumption of red meat, processed meat, and animal fat, as well as the presence of high fecal levels of cholesterol, correlate with an increased risk of CRC. In 2015, the World Health Organization declared red meat and processed meat as probable carcinogens. Some studies suggest that people who eat a diet high in natural fiber or whole grains have a lower risk of CRC. Additionally, people whose diet is low in fruits and vegetables have a higher risk of CRC. Differences in dietary fiber intake have been hypothesized to contribute significantly to geographic differences in CRC incidence globally. Additionally, an increased risk of CRC development has also been linked to moderate (30 g or approximately 2 drinks/day) and heavy alcohol consumption (greater than 3 drinks/day). Conversely, folate supplements have been shown to be protective against CRC. Calcium supplements have been shown to decrease the formation of new adenomas in patients with a history of adenomas as well as reduce the risk of CRC. Vitamins with antioxidant properties including beta-carotene, vitamins A, C, E, and selenium have been studied, and at present there are no prospective data that demonstrate a protective effect when these vitamins are derived from food sources, but a daily multivitamin supplement showed a relative risk reduction for CRC with its use. Currently, there is ongoing research focusing on the role of the microbiome in CRC tumorigenesis. Some studies have found a higher abundance of pro-carcinogenic microbial species—including *Fusobacterium nucleatum*, *Escherichia coli*, and *Bacteroides fragilis*—in CRC tumor tissue and stool, but the role these microorganisms play in the initiation or progression of CRC has not been fully elucidated. Given the potential role of the microbiome in tumorigenesis, there has been interest in the use of gut microbial modulation in decreasing the risk of CRC development. The use of gut microbial markers has also been postulated to augment CRC screening algorithms. Currently, causal mechanisms linking gut or tumoral microbes to CRC growth have been demonstrated in preclinical models through potential roles in inducing antiproliferative and apoptotic responses or altering intestinal mucosal barriers or local immune responses.

Physical Activity and Obesity

Physical inactivity and obesity are two modifiable lifestyle-related risk factors linked to the development of CRC. Regular physical activity has been shown to decrease the risk of CRC with the strongest evidence noted in colon cancer. Obesity in particular has been shown to have differences in the risk incurred between men and women, with obese men having a higher risk of both colon (50%) and rectal cancer (25%) compared to men of normal weight. While the biologic mechanisms are still being elucidated, the metabolic effect of activity on insulin resistance and gut motility have been implicated. Obesity, specifically excess central adiposity, has been shown to correlate with increased circulating insulin and decreased insulin sensitivity, both of which are believed to increase cancer risk.

Cigarette Smoking

Cigarette smoking contributes to the development of adenomatous polyps, particularly more aggressive adenoma precursor lesions for CRC. Some studies have shown that long-term smoking increases the risk of developing CRC, particularly rectal cancer, and demonstrate an earlier average age of onset of CRC in cigarette smokers. Furthermore, smoking is associated with lower CRC-specific survival.

Medications

Several medications have demonstrated protective effects for CRC. Hormone replacement therapy has been shown to significantly decrease mortality from CRC in women. Aspirin and other nonsteroidal anti-inflammatory drugs have also demonstrated protective effects. In an international double-blind randomized trial featuring Lynch syndrome, patients received either 600-mg aspirin daily or placebo. The aspirin group had a significantly reduced hazard ratio of 0.65 in development of CRC compared to the placebo group after long-term follow-up. There were no significant differences in adverse events between the two groups. Recent studies with sulindac and the selective cyclooxygenase-2 inhibitor celecoxib demonstrated the ability of these agents to cause regression of colon polyps in patients with FAP. However, the cyclooxygenase-2 inhibitors have been associated with an increased risk for cardiovascular complications; therefore, their role in chemoprevention remains unclear.

Colorectal Tumorigenesis

The majority of CRCs arise as sporadic cancers in patients without a significant family history of CRC (Fig. 13.1). An additional 10% to 20% are associated with a familial predisposition with no identifiable hereditary mutation. An estimated 3% to 5% of CRC can be directly attributed to known inheritable genetic syndromes. Hereditary CRC syndromes arise from inheritable germline mutations and are typically associated with well-characterized clinical presentations. Lynch syndrome (LS, also termed hereditary non-polyposis CRC, HNPCC) and familial adenomatous polyposis (FAP) are the most common hereditary CRC syndromes. Other rarer syndromes that predispose to CRC and are outlined in Table 13.1 and are briefly discussed below.

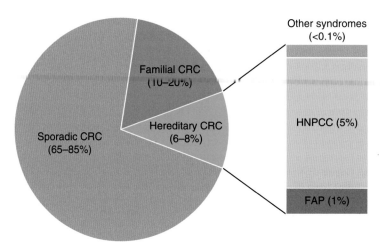

FIGURE 13.1 Pie chart showing proportion of CRC cases believed to be sporadic, familial or due to hereditary cancer syndromes. HNPCC, hereditary nonpolyposis colon cancer; FAP, familial adenomatous polyposis.

Genetic Syndromes With an Inherited Predisposition to Development of CRCs

Syndrome	Mutations	Life Time CRC Risk	Age at Dx	Phenotype
Nonpolyposis Syndromes				
Hereditary nonpolyposis colorectal cancer (HNPCC)/Lynch syndrome Autosomal dominant inheritance	MLH1 (30–40%) MSH2 (50%) MSH6 (7–10%) PMS2 (5%) EPCAM (1–3%)	50–80%	40–60 yrs	Synchronous tumors Microsatellite unstable tumors (MSI-H) Other associated cancers: Endometrial, ovarian, stomach
Adenomatous Polyposis Syndromes				
Familial adenomatous polyposis (FAP) Autosomal dominant inheritance	APC	≈100%	30–40 yrs	100–1,000s adenomatous polyps, duodenal and gastric polyps (fundus) Congenital hypertrophy of retinal pigment epithelium
Gardner syndrome Autosomal dominant inheritance	APC	≈100%	30–40 yrs	Same as FAP—simply a phenotypic variant Additionally associated with desmoid tumors (15%), osteomas of the skull and thyroid cancer
Turcot syndrome Autosomal dominant inheritance	APC (60–70%) MLH1, PMS (30%)	50–100%	20–40 yrs	Same as FAP—colon polyps, CRC and CNS tumors primarily medulloblastoma Lynch type—no polyps, CRC and CNS tumors primarily glioblastoma multiforme
Attenuated familial adenomatous polyposis coli Autosomal dominant inheritance	APC	Unknown	50 yrs	<100 polyps Right-sided tumors and polyps with rectal sparing
MYH-associated polyposis Autosomal recessive inheritance	MYH	80%	50 yrs	10–100s adenomatous polyps Somatic KRAS mutation (G12C) Microsatellite stable tumors (MSS)
Hamartomatous Polyposis Syndromes				
Juvenilepolyposis Autosomal dominant inheritance	SMAD4/DPC4 BMPR1a	60–70%	60 yrs	Hamartoma of colon and stomach, GI bleed, children <10 yrs Associated with facial abnormalities including cleft lip or palate and macrocephaly
Peutz–Jeghers Autosomal dominant inheritance	LKB1 STK11	85%	50 yrs	Hamartomatous GI polyps, hyperpigmented macules on the lips and oral mucosa, breast caner
Cowden Autosomal dominant inheritance	PTEN	16%	50–60 yrs	Hamartomas of skin, mucous membranes, thyroid, breast

Hereditary CRC Syndromes

Lynch Syndrome

LS is the most commonly inherited CRC syndrome (Fig. 13.1). This autosomal dominant syndrome results from germline mutations in DNA mismatch match repair (MMR) genes leading to accumulation of mutations predisposing to the development of colorectal, endometrial, ovarian, gastric, and hepatobiliary malignancies. A molecular signature of MMR mutations is the finding of microsatellite instability in the tumor. Microsatellites are short, repetitive DNA sequences typically consisting of one to five base pairs. Impaired DNA repair results in microsatellite repeat replication errors that go unchecked inactivating tumor suppressor genes and leading to genetic instability. These resulting cancers are characterized by a high level of microsatellite instability (MSI-H). Consequently, microsatellite instability occurs in nearly all malignancies associated with LS. In general, these cancers afford a better overall prognosis when compared to microsatellite stable tumors.

Mutations in *MLH1* and *MSH2* account for the majority of all LS patients, with mutations in *MSH6, PMS2,* and *EPCAM* accounting for the remainder of cases. Patients typically inherit one germline MMR gene mutation and subsequently acquire an inactivating mutation in the remaining allele. For this reason, penetrance varies widely within families ranging from 30% to 70%. The risk of developing a CRC by the fourth and fifth decades of life approaches 80% depending on the specific gene mutated. At the time of diagnosis, up to 20% of patients may have synchronous tumors, so careful evaluation of the entire colon and rectum prior to surgical intervention must be performed in patients with LS presenting with a cancer. About 20% to 60% of patients may develop a metachronous CRC after the index cancer. Therefore, when planning surgical resection, consideration should be given to extending the resection beyond a segmental colectomy with the intent of preventing future CRCs. Furthermore, the time it takes for an adenoma to progress to malignancy is shorter in LS than the time frame seen in sporadic CRC. Therefore, the development of adenomatous polyps at an early age may be a clinical clue to LS, and endoscopic clearance of all synchronous adenomas is extremely important in patients with LS.

When compared to sporadic CRC, CRCs associated with LS are more likely to arise proximal to the splenic flexure (60% to 70%), at a younger age (≈45 years of age), at a less advanced stage at diagnosis, and have an increased rate of metachronous and synchronous tumors (20%).

A major challenge in the management of patients with LS is the identification of those individuals who should be tested. A detailed family history should be obtained in all patients with CRC and may identify high-risk conditions where the patients would benefit from genetic counseling. Potentially affected individuals may also be identified by screening using Amsterdam criteria or Bethesda guidelines (Table 13.2). Although

TABLE 13.2   Amsterdam Criteria and Bethesda Guidelines

Amsterdam I

At least three relatives must have histologically verified colorectal cancer	1. One must be a first-degree relative of the other two 2. At least two successive generations must be affected 3. At least one of the relatives must have received the diagnosis before age 50

Amsterdam II

Similar to Amsterdam I, but may include any combination of cancers associated with HNPCC (e.g., colorectal, endometrial, gastric, ovarian, ureter or renal pelvis, brain, small bowel, hepatobiliary tract, sebaceous gland adenomas, keratoacanthomas)

Bethesda Guidelines

1. Amsterdam criteria are met
2. Two colorectal or HNPCC-related cancers, including synchronous and metachronous presentation
3. Colorectal cancer and a first-degree relative with colorectal and/or an HNPCC-related cancer and/or a colonic adenoma; one of the cancers must be diagnosed before age 45 and the adenoma diagnosed before age 40
4. Colorectal or endometrial cancer diagnosed before age 45
5. Right-sided colorectal cancer with an undifferentiated pattern (solid/cribriform) on histopathology, diagnosed before age 45
6. Signet ring cell–type colorectal cancer diagnosed before age 45 (>50% signet ring cells)
7. Colorectal adenomas diagnosed before age 40

Revised Bethesda Guidelines

1. Early-onset colorectal cancer (before age 50)
2. Synchronous, metachronous, or other HNPCC-associated tumors, regardless of age
3. Colorectal cancer with high microsatellite instability diagnosed before age 60
4. Colorectal cancer diagnosed in one or more first-degree relatives with an HNPCC-related tumor, with one of the cancers being diagnosed before age 50
5. Colorectal cancer diagnosed in two or more first- or second-degree relatives with HNPCC-related tumors, regardless of age

lacking in specificity, the use of these criteria and guidelines is associated with 60% to 94% sensitivity for identifying individuals with LS. At the MD Anderson Cancer Center (MDACC), we advocate for universal screening with testing for MMR gene protein expression in all colorectal tumors. If loss of protein expression is noted, genetic counseling and confirmatory germline testing should be performed. Probands with confirmed pathogenic mutation in MMR genes should be enrolled in specialized lifelong screening and surveillance programs. Screening colonoscopy in affected individuals should begin by 20 to 25 years of age and should be repeated every 1 to 2 years. Surgical treatment of patients with LS and confirmed colon cancer should favor subtotal colectomy with ileorectal anastomosis (IRA). Annual surveillance of the remnant rectum is indicated thereafter. Prophylactic hysterectomy and bilateral salpingo-oophorectomy should be discussed as an option in women after the completion of childbearing.

Familial Adenomatous Polyposis

FAP is the second most commonly inherited CRC syndrome accounting for about 1% of all CRCs. It is an autosomal dominant genetic disorder that results from a germline mutation in *APC*. Classic FAP manifests with hundreds to thousands of colorectal adenomas beginning in adolescence that develop into CRCs almost universally by the fourth decade of life. Most patients will present with a strong history of early colon cancers in first- and second-degree relatives, though about 25% of patients will present as the proband due to "de novo" APC gene mutations. The lifetime incidence of CRC in patients with FAP approaches 100%.

Prophylactic surgery is essential, especially in patients with classic FAP, to decrease mortality related to CRC. Preventative surgery should be considered when the polyp burden exceeds the ability for endoscopic clearance or surveillance, when there is evidence of dysplasia, and by patient preference, which often occurs by the fourth decade. Prophylactic surgery should comprise either total proctocolectomy with ileoanal pouch anastomosis or total abdominal colectomy with IRA and must balance the polyp and disease burden in the rectum, the extent of surgery, with long-term quality of life. Prophylactic colorectal resection must be followed up by frequent surveillance of the remaining GI tract to identify and remove other adenomas. Although as many as 90% of patients can develop polyps in the upper GI tract, particularly the duodenum, only about 5% of duodenal polyps progress to invasive carcinomas. Duodenal adenocarcinoma is the most common cause of death in FAP patients who have had prophylactic colorectal surgery.

Variants of classic FAP, arising also from *APC* gene mutations, have been described, and similarly predispose to development of CRC (Table 13.1). There are genotype–phenotype correlations between the severity of disease and the nature of the APC mutations. Attenuated adenomatous polyposis coli (aFAP) is often described as a less aggressive variant of FAP. These patients develop fewer polyps, typically confined to the proximal colon and rarely affect the rectum. CRCs can manifest later, in the fifth decade of life.

Other Inherited CRC Syndromes

Table 13.1 summarizes other hereditary syndromes that predispose to the development of CRC. MYH-associated polyposis is an autosomal recessive disorder that results from biallelic germline mutations in *MYH*, a base excision repair gene. For this reason, patients typically will not have a generational family history of cancers but most will develop CRC before age 60 years. Other syndromes result in hamartomas of the colon and rectum with varying lifetime risk of development of CRC. *SMAD4, PTEN,* and *STK11* are several of the genes implicated in the development of these tumors.

Sporadic CRC

Advances in molecular biology have increased our knowledge of the genetic and epigenetic events that drive CRC tumorigenesis. The Cancer Genome Atlas Network (TCGA) in their recent comprehensive molecular analysis of CRC demonstrated that colon and rectal cancers can be molecularly distinguished into hypermutated versus nonhypermutated subcategories. These and other investigations have led to the identification of multiple pathways that lead to the development of CRC (Fig. 13.2). The classic adenoma-to-carcinoma pathway was initially described by Vogelstein and colleagues. Approximately 70% of sporadic CRC arise via this adenoma-to-carcinoma progression, driven by loss of APC and/or p53 tumor suppressor genes with accumulation of chromosomal instability over time. A second pathway involves the loss of DNA mismatch repair and is exemplified by the germline mutations seen in LS or by acquired MLH1 gene promoter hypermethylation. BRAF mutated cancers appear to act via a third pathway; the serrated/methylator pathway in which tumors are characterized by the methylation of CpG islands that cause the silencing of critical tumor suppressor genes resulting in CpG island methylator phenotype (CIMP) tumors. The CRC Subtyping Consortium (CRCSC) has worked to further characterize the genetic and epigenetic features of CRC by integrating tumor mutation status, DNA copy number variations, gene methylation, microRNA, and protein expression. This effort

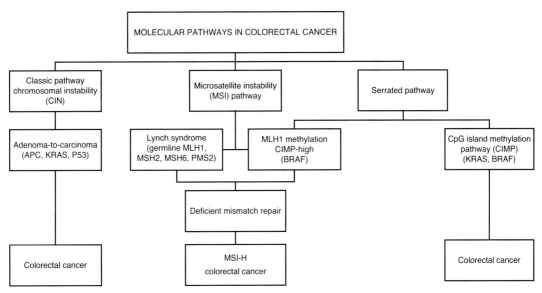

FIGURE 13.2 CRCs develop via three distinct molecular pathways. The classic or chromosomal instability (CIN) pathway accounts for 30% to 70% of CRCs resulting from adenoma progressing to carcinoma. Germline mismatch repair mutations lead to Lynch syndrome, which accounts for approximately one-quarter of all MSI CRCs. The Serrated/Methylated pathway is driven by hypermethylation.

has better elucidated CRC tumor heterogeneity and may have direct implications on patient prognosis and response to therapies. They describe four distinct consensus molecular subtypes (CMS) with unique molecular characteristics, tumor phenotype, and prognosis (Table 13.3). CMS1 CRCs are predominantly MSI—high tumors and tend to be hypermutated, methylated, and/or enriched for *BRAF* mutations. CMS2 and CMS4 are driven by chromosomal instability typically resulting in microsatellite stable tumors arising from high copy number alterations. CMS4 tumors display proangiogenic properties driven by multiple pathways including vascular endothelial growth factor (VEGF) signaling. For this reason, these tumors are associated with a poor prognosis manifest as early relapse and distant failure. CMS3 tumors are driven by metabolic reprogramming, exhibiting fewer copy number alterations and enriching for mutations known to affect metabolic adaptation such as *KRAS* and *PIK3CA* mutations.

TABLE 13.3   Consensus Molecular Subtype (CMS) Classification of CRC

Consortium Subtype	Molecular Features	Clinical Characteristic	Incidence (%)
CMS1 MSI Immune	Hypermutated MSI—high CIMP—high BRAF mutated Immune activation/expression	Right-sided tumors Older age at diagnosis Females Intermediate survival Worse survival after relapse	14
CMS2 Canonical	High CIN MSS WNT/MYC pathway activation TP53 mutated EGFR amplification/overexpression	Left-sided tumors Better survival	37
CMS3 Metabolic	CIN-low Mixed MSI and MSS tumors Metabolic derangement KRAS mutated PIK3CA mutated IGFBP2 overexpression	Intermediate survival	13
CMS4 Mesenchymal	CIN-high MSS TGF-beta activation NOTCH3/VEGFR2 overexpression	Stromal infiltration Younger age at diagnosis Worse relapse-free and overall survival	23

While the efforts of the TCGA, CRCSC, and others have significantly improved our understanding of CRC carcinogenesis, the mutational landscape of CRC continues to evolve. There remains a need to identify and validate novel translational paradigms to accurately subtype CRC to allow for a truly personalized approach to treatment.

Genetic Testing

Germline genetic testing is the method by which inherited mutations responsible for hereditary CRC predisposition syndromes can be detected. When patients present with classic phenotypic features highly suggestive of a particular syndrome, targeted testing focused on the gene or genes corresponding to the syndrome is sensible. However, because phenotypes can be overlapping and/or ambiguous, multi-gene panel testing has emerged as an efficient approach to genetic testing. This multi-gene panel approach ensures clinically significant and actionable genes are not overlooked as they may be in a targeted gene approach. Patients who may benefit the most from multi-gene panel testing include CRC patients diagnosed under the age of 50 (regardless of MSI status), patients with >cumulative 10 adenomatous polyps or >3 cumulative hamartomatous polyps, and CRC patients diagnosed greater than the age of 50 with one first-degree relative with CRC or endometrial cancer as well as patients with any synchronous LS-associated cancers.

CRC Screening

Screening Guidelines and Methods

The overall incidence of CRC is decreasing in the United States; this has been largely attributed to improved population-based screening for CRC, which allows for detection and removal of potentially precancerous lesions. As previously discussed, the majority of CRCs arise via the classic adenoma-to-carcinoma pathway so that the identification and timely removal of premalignant lesions can prevent progression to carcinoma. Current guidelines for CRC screening and surveillance as recommended by the US Multi-Society Preventive Task Force are outlined in Table 13.4. Recently, several societies have issued qualified recommendations to commence average-risk screening at age 45 instead of 50. African Americans are more likely to be develop CRC than other populations and tend to present at a younger age. For this reason, many experts advocate initiating screening at age 45 years in this population. The goals of screening are detection of early cancers and prevention of cancer by finding and removing adenomas. It is important to realize that patients with predisposing conditions are considered at high risk for CRC, and specific guidelines for these patients should be followed (summarized in Table 13.4). Common known conditions that increase CRC risk include a personal history of polyps, personal history of CRC, or family history of CRC or polyps, a known or suspected diagnosis of hereditary CRC syndrome, and longstanding inflammatory bowel disease (IBD).

Stool-Based Screening Tests

Multiple methods of CRC screening are currently employed in average-risk patients with demonstrated efficacy and sensitivity. Blood in the stool is a nonspecific finding but can point to large adenomas or occult tumors. Fecal tests for blood are either guaiac-based (gFOBT) or immunohistochemical-based (FIT). Guaiac-based tests rely on pseudoperoxidase-mediated oxidation which is catalyzed in the presence of heme or hemoglobin. FIT utilizes antibodies to detect human globulin. Most recently however, FOBT has largely been replaced with FIT. Prospective randomized trials have shown that FOBT screening followed by colonoscopy detects cancers at an earlier stage when compared to patients that are not screened. The Minnesota Colon Cancer Control Study demonstrated a relative reduction of 32% in CRC cancer-related mortality but no impact on all-cause mortality. A meta-analysis of FOBT randomized trials indicates that hemoccult testing is associated with a 15% to 43% reduction in the mortality rate from CRC. However, the sensitivity of these tests is highly variable and two to three samples are often needed to complete the test with acceptable sensitivity.

FIT screening has been compared to endoscopic screening methods in recently published trials. In one randomized controlled trial, asymptomatic adults ages 50 to 69 received screening by either one-time colonoscopy or FIT every 2 years. The study found that those in the FIT group were more likely to participate than those in the colonoscopy group (34.2% vs. 24.6%). The number of trial subjects in whom CRC was detected was found to be similar between the two groups. In a separate trial, asymptomatic individuals aged 50 to 74 were randomized to either one-time flexible sigmoidoscopy (FSIG) or FIT screening every 2 years. Detection in the FIT group after multiple rounds of screening was higher than that of the FSIG group.

Both FIT and FOBT can be utilized in screening asymptomatic patients; symptomatic patients require diagnostic rather than screening tests as detailed below. Similarly, if FOBT or FIT is positive, a complete colonoscopy should be performed.

| TABLE 3.4 | US Multi-Society Task Force on CRC Guidelines for Colonoscopy Screening and Surveillance |

Patients With Average Risk

Screening beginning at age 50 yrs (consider screening at age 45 yrs for African Americans) with one of the following:
- Colonoscopy every 5–10 yrs
- Flexible sigmoidoscopy (FSIG) every 5 yrs
- Computed tomography colonography (CTC) every 5 yrs
- Fecal occult blood test (FOBT) annually
- Fecal immunochemical testing (FIT) annually

Patients at Increased Risk due to Personal History of Polyps

Risk Category	Recommendation
Small rectal hyperplastic polyps	Same as average risk
1–2 small (<1 cm) tubular adenomas with low-grade dysplasia	Colonoscopy 5–10 yrs after polypectomy
3–10 small adenomas Any adenoma >1 cm Any adenoma with high-grade dysplasia Any adenoma with villous features	Colonoscopy 3 yrs after complete polypectomy
>10 adenoma on a single examination	Colonoscopy <3 yrs after polypectomy
Sessile adenomas removed in pieces	Colonoscopy 2–6 months to verify complete excision

Patients at Increase Risk due to Personal History of Sporadic CRC

Risk Category	Recommendation
At time of CRC diagnosis	• Colonoscopy aimed at evaluating the entire colon preoperatively to rule out synchronous cancer and remove premalignant polyps • If unable to traverse the tumor due to obstruction colonoscopy within a 3–6 month interval after surgery
Surveillance after curative CRC resection	• Colonoscopy 1 year after surgery or 1 year after clearing perioperative colonoscopy • Next colonoscopy after a 3-year interval (4 yrs after surgery) • Subsequent colonoscopies every 5 yrs * If polyps are found the recommended interval for polyp surveillance above should be performed

Patients at Increased Risk due to Family History of CRC

Risk Category	Recommendation
CRC or adenomatous polyp in first-degree relative <60 yrs CRC or adenomatous polyp in 2 or more first-degree relatives any age	Screening colonoscopy beginning at age 40 yrs or 10 yrs prior to age of youngest affected immediate family member and every 5 yrs there after
CRC or adenomatous polyp in first-degree relative ≥60 yrs CRC or adenomatous polyp in 2 or more second-degree relatives any age	Screening colonoscopy beginning at age 40 yrs and every 10 yrs there after

Patients at High Risk

Risk Category	Recommendation
Familial adenomatous polyposis (FAP) confirmed or suspected	• Screening beginning at ages 10–12 yrs with annual FSIG • Genetic testing and counseling • Early prophylactic colectomy
Lynch syndrome (HNPCC) confirmed or suspected Known family history of HNPCC	• Screening colonoscopy beginning at ages 20–25 yrs and every 1–2 yrs there after • Genetic testing and counseling to patient and all first-degree relative s if HNPCC confirmed
Inflammatory bowel disease (IBD) *Crohn colitis and ulcerative colitis*	• Consider referral to tertiary center with IBD expertise • Screen prior to 8 yrs after onset of pancolitis or prior to 12–15 yrs after onset of left-sided colitis with colonoscopy and biopsy to assess for dysplasia

Direct Visualization Endoscopic Screening Tests

Endoscopic screening tools are the most frequently utilized as they offer diagnostic and therapeutic options. FSIG allows for endoscopic examination of the distal colon and rectum. Case-control studies have demonstrated a 60% to 80% reduction in CRC mortality with routine FSIG screening over nonscreened counterparts. Additionally, recent data from randomized clinical trials have shown that FSIG is associated with a 25% reduction in CRC incidence and a 30% reduction in CRC mortality. This is because most sporadic CRCs arise in the left colon or rectum. However, FSIG is only effective for the area inspected and should be performed with insertion of the endoscopy to at least 40 cm or to the splenic flexure to be considered adequate. FSIG as a screening tool has found favor because it can be easily performed. The procedure is often done in the office without sedation and patients must only undergo bowel preparation in the form of enemas. As a screening test, FSIG, when normal, should be repeated every 5 years. Because of its limited evaluation of the colon, FSIG is often used in conjunction with radiographic evaluation of the more proximal colon or annual fecal occult blood testing. If polyps are found on FSIG, a full colonoscopy is warranted.

Colonoscopy is one of the most frequently performed procedures in the United States and is considered the gold-standard CRC screening tool. Colonoscopy involves inspection of the entire rectum and colon to the ileocecal valve. Given that up to 40% of colon cancers arise proximal to the splenic flexure, colonoscopy offers added sensitivity of CRC detection over FSIG. In 2015, the American Society of Gastrointestinal Endoscopy (ASGE)/American College of Gastroenterology (ACG) Task Force on Quality in Endoscopy recommended a benchmark ADR of ≥25% for an average-risk population. Of note, each 1% increase in a physician's ADR is associated with a 3% decrease in the risk of CRC-related deaths. Observational studies have shown that colonoscopy has been associated with a reduction in the incidence of proximal colon cancers, not accessible by FSIG. Limitations of colonoscopy include the need for prolonged bowel preparation and dietary restrictions, the need for sedation and monitoring and wide variation in operator-skill. Cost is also an important consideration; however, studies have shown screening colonoscopy to be cost-effective if a 10-year interval is used and if the colon is appropriately cleared of polyps. Despite these limitations, colonoscopy remains the gold-standard for examination of the colon and rectum. All positive findings found with other screening modalities require a colonoscopy to definitively assess and/or clear the colon.

Additional Screening Modalities

Computed tomography (CT) colonography (virtual colonoscopy) has emerged as a technique for the diagnosis of colonic polyps of 10 mm or more in the screening population using three-dimensional reconstruction of the air-distended colon. At the National Naval Medical Center, in 1,223 average-risk adults who subsequently underwent conventional (optical) colonoscopy, virtual colonoscopy was as good or better at detecting relevant lesions. A more recent multi-institutional study looking at 2,600 asymptomatic patients 50 years of age or older found that CT colonography identified 90% of patients with adenomas or cancers measuring 10 mm or more in diameter and further strengthened published data on the role of CT colonography in screening patients with an average risk of CRC. A recent meta-analysis that included 4,086 patients estimated that CT colonography had a specificity of 98.7% for polys >10 mm and 97.6% for adenomas >10 mm. However, some of the major limitations included the need for full bowel preparation and follow-up colonoscopy for diagnostic and therapeutic intervention on the radiographic abnormalities. Because virtual colonoscopy is considerably time and labor intensive from the standpoint of the radiologist, active investigations into methods of automating the evaluation process are ongoing. Current American Cancer Society screening recommendations are for virtual colonoscopy every 5 years with subsequent colonoscopy if a lesion is found. There has been significant interest in identifying circulating blood biomarkers as a screening tool for CRC. Examples have included carcinoembryonic antigen (CEA), carbohydrate antigen (CA 19.9), tissue polypeptide-specific antigen (TPS), tumor-associated glycoprotein-72 (TAG-72), hematopoietic growth factors, macrophage-colony stimulating factor (M-CSF) and granulocyte-macrophage-colony stimulating factor (GM-CSF), interleukin-3, or interleukin-6. Emerging techniques such as circulating cancer cells (CTCs) and circulating tumor (ctDNA) have also been investigated. An analysis of SEPT9 hypermethylation and associated methylation markers has shown the most accuracy. At present, however, none of these blood tests have demonstrated sufficient diagnostic accuracy to be performed as a stand-alone screening test for CRC.

CEA is the most commonly tested biomarker for CRC. It is a glycoprotein found in the cell membranes of many tissues, including CRC. Some of the antigen enters the circulation and is detected by radioimmunoassay of serum; although CEA is also detectable in various other body fluids. Elevated serum CEA is not specifically associated with CRC; abnormally high levels are also found in sera of patients with malignancies of the pancreas, breast, ovary, prostate gland, head and neck, bladder, and kidney. CEA levels are high in approximately

30% to 80% of patients with cancer of the colon, but less than half of patients with localized disease are CEA positive. False-positive results occur in benign disease (lung, liver, and bowel). The CEA level is also increased in smokers. Overall, 60% of tumors will be missed by CEA screening alone. Therefore, CEA has no role in screening for primary lesions. The role of CEA in surveillance following treatment and resection of CRC is discussed in a subsequent section of this chapter.

Indications for Endoscopic Intervention on Screening

Polyps

Polyps represent the most frequent indication for endoscopic intervention during colonoscopy. As previously mentioned, CRCs often arise from polyps, however polyps differ and carry varying risks of malignant progression. Colorectal polyps are classified histologically as either neoplastic (which may be benign or malignant), adenomatous polyps (including serrated adenomatous) or nonneoplastic polyps (including hyperplastic, mucosal, inflammatory, and hamartomatous). Adenomatous polyps are found in approximately 33% of the general population by age 50 and in approximately 50% of the general population by age 70. Most lesions are less than 1 cm in size, with 60% of people having a single adenoma and 40% having multiple lesions. Sixty percent of lesions will be located distal to the splenic flexure. These polyps have the potential to progress to CRC via the classic or serrated molecular pathways previously discussed.

The National Polyp Study showed that colonoscopic removal of adenomatous polyps significantly reduced the risk of developing CRC. Polyps coexist with CRC in 60% of patients and are associated with an increased incidence of synchronous and metachronous colonic neoplasms. Patients with a primary cancer and a solitary associated polyp have a lower incidence of synchronous and metachronous lesions when compared to patients with multiple polyps. The natural history of polyps supports their timely removal as invasive cancer will develop in 24% of patients with untreated polyps at the site of that polyp within 20 years.

The risk of associated malignancy varies with polyp histology and size. There are three main histologic variants of adenomatous polyps (Table 13.5). Tubular adenomas are found with equal distribution throughout the colon and carry the lowest risk of associated malignancy. Villous adenomas have a predilection for the rectum and are much less common but carry a 35% to 40% risk of harboring an underlying malignancy. Polyps may be pedunculated (usually tubular or tubulovillous), sessile (usually tubulovillous or villous), or nonpolypoid (flat or depressed). Nonpolypoid neoplasms are more difficult to detect because of subtle similarities to normal mucosa. Depressed nonpolypoid lesions have been shown to carry a high risk of cancer at the time of diagnosis. Polyp size and the degree of dysplasia also correlate with malignant potential. Small adenomas (<1 cm) are associated with malignancy in only 1.3% of cases while adenomas >2 cm harbor malignancy 46% of the time. Similarly, a higher degree of dysplasia is associated with increasing risk of malignancy; adenomatous polyps with mild, moderate, and severe dysplasia are found to have malignant cells on complete excision of the polyp in 5.7%, 18%, and 34.5% of the time, respectively.

High-grade dysplasia characterizes severely dysplastic adenomas where malignant transformation has not invaded through the muscularis mucosa. When this is the finding on a biopsy report, one should be alerted to the possibility for a risk of deeper invasion or nodal dissemination on final pathology. Approximately 5% to 7% of adenomatous polyps contain high-grade dysplasia and 3% to 5% harbor invasive carcinoma at the time of diagnosis. Increasing dysplasia and malignant potential correlate with increasing size, villous component, and patient age. If a polyp containing high-grade dysplasia is completely excised endoscopically, the patient may be considered cured.

Overall, 8.5% to 25% of polyps harboring invasive carcinoma will metastasize to regional lymph nodes. Unfavorable pathologic features increase the probability that regional lymph nodes will be involved and include (a) poor differentiation, (b) vascular and/or lymphatic invasion, (c) invasion below the submucosa, and (d) positive resection margin as defined by the presence of tumor within 1 to 2 mm from the transected margin and/or the presence of tumor cells within the diathermy of the transected margin. Approximately 4%

TABLE 13.5 Neoplastic Polyps and Risk of Malignancy

Histologic Subtype	Incidence (%)	Risk of Malignancy (%)
Tubular adenoma	75–85	<5
Tubulovillous adenoma	8–15	20–25
Villous adenoma	5–10	35–40

TABLE 13.6	Haggitt Classification for Colorectal Carcinomas Arising in Adenomas

Classification	Depth of Invasion
0	Carcinoma confined to the mucosa
1	Head of polyp
2	Neck of polyp
3	Stalk of polyp
4	Submucosa of the underlying colonic wall

to 8% of malignant polyps are poorly differentiated. Poorly differentiated lesions (grade 3) are associated with a higher incidence of lymphovascular involvement when compared with well- and moderately differentiated lesions (grades 1 and 2, respectively). The presence of one or more of these adverse features should prompt evaluation for surgical resection.

Depth of invasion is another important prognostic factor for nodal involvement. In 1985, Haggitt et al. classified the level of invasion from the head of the polyp to the submucosa of the underlying colonic wall (Table 13.6). In a multivariable analysis, only invasion into the submucosa of the underlying bowel wall (level 4) was a significant prognostic factor. This is in keeping with previous pathologic studies that have shown that the lymphatic channels do not penetrate above the muscularis mucosa. Although these findings have been confirmed by other studies, there are frequently multiple adverse prognostic factors seen in patients with higher levels of invasion (i.e., levels 3 and 4), which makes it difficult to assign depth as the single factor. Later in 1995, Kikuchi et al. created a separate classification system to describe sessile and flat malignant colorectal polyps into the submucosa (Table 13.7). Using this system, a lower third (Sm3) lesion was associated with an increased risk of lymphatic spread up to 23%. However, the main challenge in using this classification system is that pathologists require a significant portion of the submucosa and sometimes up to the muscularis propria to provide the proper designation for the examined polyp.

A negative resection margin has consistently been shown to be associated with a decreased risk for adverse outcomes (i.e., recurrence, residual carcinoma, lymph node metastases, and decreased survival). Twenty-seven percent of patients with positive or indeterminate tumor margins will have adverse outcomes, compared with 18% with negative margins and poor prognostic features and 0.8% with negative margins and no other poor prognostic features. Therefore, multiple risk factors should be assessed together.

Colonoscopic polypectomy is safe and effective for excision of nearly all pedunculated polyps. For polyps not amenable to polypectomy, endoscopic mucosal resection (EMR) may be utilized and is particularly advantageous in the removal of small (not >1 cm), flat or depressed lesions. EMR results in the en-bloc removal of the lesion and the deep submucosal layer, providing additional pathologic information. Furthermore, EMR alone may be sufficient treatment for early cancers without aggressive features. For larger lesions, endoscopic submucosal dissection (ESD) is a technique in which saline is injected into the submucosa to lift the lesion of interest, thus facilitating dissection of the submucosa using an electrosurgical endoscopic knife. ESD is more technically challenging for the endoscopist, and the risks for bleeding and perforation complications that require surgical intervention may be higher when compared to EMR (3% vs. 0.4%). For lesions approaching 20 mm in size, ESD is difficult to be achieved in a nonpiecemeal fashion, raising concerns for potentially higher risk of recurrence at the polypectomy site and the need for surveillance colonoscopy at a shorter interval. A more recent approach for large or difficult to resect polyps is Endoscopic Full Thickness Resection (EFTR), a technique in which all layers of the colon wall are removed. This maneuver is ideal for nonlifting lesions; however, similar to ESD, it requires technical expertise by the endoscopist and can be associated with increased risk for complications.

TABLE 13.7	Kikuchi Classification for Colorectal Carcinomas Arising in Sessile and Flat Polyps

Classification	Depth of Invasion
Sm1	Invasion into upper 1/3 of submucosa
Sm2	Invasion into middle 1/3 of submucosa
Sm3	Invasion into lower 1/3 of submucosa close to muscularis propria

Surgical resection is recommended for lesions that are large with high-risk for malignancy, particularly those that are considered endoscopically unresectable. Fungating, ulcerated, or distorted lesions destroying the surrounding bowel wall indicate the presence of invasive cancer and are contraindications to polypectomy. Additionally, any lesions previously removed by optimal endoscopic polypectomy and found to have positive margins likely require surgical resection. Surgical resection is also indicated for patients with residual invasive carcinoma and for those at high risk for lymph node metastases despite complete endoscopic polypectomy. Management of high-risk polyps should be done in conjunction with the endoscopist. Marking of the polyp or polypectomy site, usually in the form of tattooing, should be performed at the time of colonoscopy or within 2 weeks of the initial endoscopy to improve accuracy of identifying the target lesion at the time of surgical resection.

Polyps with the high-risk pathologic features previously described (margin ≤2 mm, poor differentiation, Haggitt level 4, and vascular and/or lymphatic invasion) confer an increased risk of lymph node metastasis. In a review of 17 studies to evaluate the frequency of lymph node metastases or residual carcinoma in low-risk patients with pedunculated polyps, only a 1% incidence was found. In sessile polyps with low-risk features, the incidence was increased to 4.1%. Surgical polypectomy should thus be considered in these high-risk polyps to limit the potential for lymph node metastasis and distant spread.

Stalk invasion in pedunculated polyps is not considered an adverse histologic feature, and treatment of polyps with stalk invasion is the same as that of polyps without stalk invasion (based on risk stratification). Large villous adenomas of the rectum may be amenable to transanal local excision. This provides a complete diagnostic evaluation for malignancy, and if excised with negative margins (with other favorable prognostic features), it may be the only therapeutic procedure needed.

Inflammatory Bowel Disease
Ulcerative Colitis
Chronic ulcerative colitis carries a risk for CRC that is 30 times greater than that of the general population. A recent population-based cohort study analyzing patients in Denmark and Sweden from 1969 to 2017 found that individuals with ulcerative colitis were at increased risk of developing CRC, were diagnosed with less advanced stages of CRC, and had increased mortality compared to individuals without ulcerative colitis. The cancer risk in IBD increases significantly 8 years after the onset of pancolitis and 12 to 15 years after left-sided colitis. This risk continues to increase by 0.5% to 1% per year after 10 years and is 18% to 35% at 30 years. The severity, extent, and duration of inflammation, as well as family history of CRC and history of primary sclerosing cholangitis, are risk factors for the development of cancer. In contrast to sporadic CRCs, these cancers are more often multiple, broadly infiltrating, and poorly differentiated. They can be extremely difficult to identify due to chronic inflammation and scarring, as well as the fact that many of them arise from dysplasia-associated lesions or masses (DALMs) which are often flat lesions easily missed during endoscopy. Initiation of surveillance colonoscopy is recommended 8 to 10 years from the start of IBD symptoms, with a frequency of every 1 to 2 years with random 4-quadrant biopsies every 10 cm throughout the affected area. A minimum of 33 biopsies is recommended for patients with extensive disease. In patients with ulcerative colitis, consideration should be given to taking biopsies every 5 cm in the distal sigmoid and rectum where their cancer risk is highest. Findings of CRC, a nonadenoma dysplasia-associated lesion or mass (DALM), or high-grade dysplasia are accepted indications for total proctocolectomy, with or without IPAA. Studies have found these findings are associated with 43% to 50% risk of a concomitant malignancy discovered at the time of the colectomy. Adenoma DALM, on the other hand, can sometimes be managed via endoscopic polypectomy. However, as discussed previously, large or high-risk DALMs require a collaborative approach involving the endoscopist and the surgeon, with surgery often being the preferred option for ensuring en-bloc resection of the lesion. The management of low-grade dysplasia in UC patients remains controversial. Studies have shown progression rates to high-grade dysplasia as high as 53% and the risk of cancer upward of 20%. Continued close surveillance endoscopy versus proctocolectomy can be considered on a case-by-case basis.

Crohn's Disease
Longstanding Crohn's colitis is associated with significantly higher CRC risk. Surveillance colonoscopy for individuals with Crohn's disease is endorsed by multiple medical societies; however, there is controversy regarding the frequency of these examinations. Similar to patients with UC, patients with Crohn's disease should undergo initial screening colonoscopy within 8 years of the onset of their symptoms. Screening typically requires random 4-quadrant biopsies at 10-cm intervals (total of >32 biopsies) with white-light colonoscopy or targeted biopsies via chromoendoscopy. There is currently no consensus on the recommended

interval between future screenings. The American Society for Gastrointestinal Endoscopy recommends that patients with active inflammation, history of CRC or dysplasia in a first-degree relative, or anatomic abnormalities such as strictures receive annual screening. Average-risk patients can receive surveillance every 1 to 3 years, and this time interval can be extended beyond 3 years after 2 consecutive colonoscopies without any abnormal endoscopic or histologic findings.

Visible dysplasia found in Crohn's patients should be completely excised endoscopically if possible; these patients should continue endoscopic surveillance following complete resection. In patients with lesions not amenable to endoscopic resection, with multifocal dysplasia, or with colorectal adenocarcinoma, total colectomy or proctocolectomy rather than segmental colonic resection is favored, because studies have shown that 14% to 40% of patients with Crohn's colitis who underwent segmental CRC resection developed metachronous CRC. Individuals with invisible low- or high-grade dysplasia should be referred to an experienced endoscopist for high-definition colonoscopy with chromoendoscopy for repeat random biopsies within 3 to 6 months. If patients are found to have these same pathologies on repeat biopsies, they should undergo total colectomy or proctocolectomy.

Diagnosing CRC

Clinical Presentation

Patients with CRC can be asymptomatic (cancers found on screening colonoscopy) or present with symptoms such as rectal bleeding, unexplained anemia, fatigue, shortness of breath, abdominal pain, change in bowel habits, anorexia, weight loss, nausea, and/or vomiting. Pelvic pain or tenesmus may point to rectal cancer. Metastatic disease may present as abdominal pain, fevers, hepatomegaly, ascites, effusions, and supraclavicular adenopathy. Central nervous system and bone metastases are seen in less than 10% of autopsy cases and are rare in the absence of advanced liver or lung disease. The routine use of CT for *diagnosis* of CRC is discouraged because cross-sectional imaging can easily miss mural disease in the hollow viscus. Endoscopy with biopsy is recommended for histologic diagnosis. Subsequent cross-sectional imaging of the abdomen and pelvis should be used for clinical staging and for assessing complications such as obstruction or perforation which may warrant urgent or emergent intervention. For patients that present with impending or complete mechanical obstruction, the most common symptoms and physical signs are the absence of passage of flatus or stool and abdominal distention. The incidence of complete obstruction at the time of presentation is 5% to 15%. In a large study from the United Kingdom, 49% of obstructions occurred at the splenic flexure, 23% occurred in the left colon, 23% occurred in the right colon, and 7% occurred in the rectum. Obstruction increases the risk of death from CRC 1.4-fold and is an independent covariate on multivariable analyses. Perforation occurs in 3% to 12% of colorectal carcinoma cases, commonly at the location of the primary tumor due to tissue necrosis and friability but also at other site due to increased pressure at colonic wall. Perforation increases the risk of death from cancer 3.4-fold, with some studies reporting the mortality from peritonitis secondary to a perforation being as high has 30% to 50%.

Pathology

Endoscopy with biopsy is often the most efficient method of acquiring tissue for diagnosis. More than 90% of colon cancers are adenocarcinomas. On gross appearance, there are four morphologic variants of adenocarcinoma, including ulcerative (most commonly found distal to the splenic flexure), exophytic (also known as polypoid or fungating, most commonly found in the proximal colon), annular (scirrhous, associated with the classic apple core appearance), and rarely, a submucosal infiltrative pattern similar to linitis plastica seen with gastric adenocarcinoma. Other epithelial histologic variants of colon cancer that are occasionally seen include mucinous (colloid) carcinoma, signet-ring cell carcinoma, adenosquamous and squamous cell carcinoma (SCC), and undifferentiated carcinoma. Other rare colorectal histologies include carcinoids, leiomyosarcomas, and lymphoma.

Staging

Clinical Staging

A thorough history including family history and physical examination focusing on abdominal, digital rectal, and lymph node examinations should be performed. Complete evaluation of the lower GI tract with colonoscopy should be performed prior to treatment whenever feasible. CT colonography can be considered if tumor-related obstruction prevents endoscopic evaluation of the colon proximal to the tumor. National consensus guidelines recommend a CT scan of the chest, abdomen and pelvis, complete blood cell count, CEA and chemistry profile for workup, and clinical staging of colon cancer. For rectal cancer, national consensus guidelines recommend the addition of endoscopic rectal ultrasound (ERUS) and/or pelvic magnetic resonance imaging (MRI). In the modern era, high-quality pelvic MRI is generally preferred to ERUS. Additionally, we recommend that the operative surgeon performs a proctoscopy him- or herself to accurately determine the distance of the most distal border of the tumor from the anal verge for more accurate preoperative planning. When neoadjuvant therapy is being considered, tattooing the distal edge of the tumor prior to therapy is prudent because a proportion of the patients may experience significant tumor regression or even complete clinical response. Transaminases and tests assessing synthetic function of the liver (e.g., PT/INR) are not as useful for determining liver metastasis. Abnormal tests are present in only approximately 15% of patients with liver metastases and may be elevated without liver metastases in up to 40%. Preoperative CEA level can reflect the extent of the disease and prognosis: CEA levels surpassing 10 to 20 ng/mL are associated with increased chances of treatment failure for both node-negative and node-positive patients. Approximately 18% to 25% of patients will present with stage IV disease at diagnosis. Patient's should be asked about their baseline bowel, urinary, and sexual function. Patients who present with urinary symptoms should undergo evaluation of their urinary tract with CT urogram, and/or cystoscopy as appropriate.

Positron emission tomography (PET) is not routinely indicated in the clinical staging of CRC. Although potentially useful in patients presenting with locally recurrent or metastatic disease, it has not been helpful in the primary evaluation of patients with colon cancer due to poor sensitivity, false positives, and high costs.

The clinical staging of rectal cancer warrants more discussion as it has significant therapeutic implications. The decision to proceed with surgery or preoperative multimodality therapy as the first step in treatment of rectal cancer and is based on clinical stage. It is also extremely important to accurately assess the local spread of disease, including the potential involvement of the levator muscles and other pelvic structures. ERUS is an accurate tool in determining tumor (T) stage. Performed using rigid or flexible probes, the layers of the rectal wall can be identified with 67% to 93% accuracy. The ERUS characteristics of T1 and T3 tumors make them relatively easy to differentiate. However, the distinction between T2 and T3 tumors is more difficult. One recent systematic review found that for identifying T2 disease, the sensitivity was 81%, and the specificity was 96%; whereas for T3 disease, the sensitivity was 96% and the specificity was 91%. ERUS is highly operator-dependent, and it can be difficult to differentiate lymph nodes from blood vessels and other structures or peritumoral edema from tumor. Furthermore, ERUS is limited in its ability to evaluate tumors that are pedunculated, bulky, or obstructing. An additional limitation is that ERUS cannot adequately assess the distance to the CRM. As a result of these factors, overstaging occurs in approximately 20% of cases and understaging in approximately 10% to 20%. Stenotic lesions may make ERUS impossible secondary to the inability to pass the probe. ERUS evaluation of T stage is superior to that of CT scanning (52% to 83% accuracy) and to rectal MRI (59% to 95% accuracy). Pelvic MRI can additionally delineate the relationship of the tumor to the mesorectal fascia, surrounding viscera, and pelvic structures as well as predict risk for involvement of circumferential margins. The MERCURY Study Group (2006) found that MRI accurately predicted whether surgical margins would be clear or affected by tumor. The relative accuracy of ERUS versus MRI for rectal cancer staging can be operator and institution dependent. At MDACC, pelvic MRI is the preferred modality for clinical staging in rectal cancers, and ERUS is utilized to clarify any potential discrepancies in early T-staging. Lymph node staging in rectal cancer has proven more difficult than primary tumor staging, with ERUS accuracies of 62% to 83%, CT accuracies of 35% to 73%, and MRI accuracies of 39% to 84% reported. Despite descriptions of methods to radiologically predict metastases in lymph nodes, only nodal enlargements can be detected with most current technologies. Approximately, 50% to 75% of positive lymph nodes in rectal cancer may be normal in size, thereby limiting accurate evaluation. Similarly, lymph nodes may be enlarged from inflammation, giving false-positive results. Combining size and radiographic characteristics can increase accuracy. For ERUS, lymph nodes that are greater than 3 mm and hypoechoic are more likely to contain metastatic deposits. In addition, it is possible to perform fine-needle aspiration of suspicious lymph nodes under ERUS guidance. While ERUS or MRI can evaluate lymph node status in patients prior to preoperative therapy, assessment of response to neoadjuvant therapy can be difficult due to the obliteration of tissue planes by edema and fibrosis secondary to the treatment.

The staging of patients presenting with locally recurrent rectal cancer is complicated by radiation and posttreatment changes that are often difficult to distinguish from tumor. CT is useful to assess the extent of the disease and adjacent organ involvement. In cases where recurrence is unknown but suspected, comparison to prior CT is helpful. Pelvic MRI, rather than ERUS, is the imaging modality of choice. It provides detailed anatomic delineation of the extent of the tumor and its relationship to critical pelvic structures, thereby enabling an accurate assessment of resectability. PET has been shown to be up to 95% sensitive, 98% specific, and 96% accurate in the detection of cancer recurrence particularly when the other imaging modalities fail to localize the disease. When used appropriately, it can help distinguish patients who would benefit from surgery for recurrent cancer from those who have unresectable disease, and it is most useful when images are correlated with those from the MRI. Currently at MDACC, we obtain CT scan of the chest, abdomen and pelvis, MRI of the pelvis, and PET for patients who present with locally recurrent rectal cancer. We believe these studies are complimentary to provide accurate clinical staging, to rule out distant metastatic disease, and to assess local resectability.

Pathologic Staging

British Pathologist Cuthbert Dukes proposed a classification system for colon cancer in 1932 to develop a uniform language that could reliably estimate disease burden and portend patient prognosis. The American Joint Committee on Cancer (AJCC) Staging System is currently used to stage CRC. The AJCC published its 8th edition TNM Classification of Colon and Rectum Cancer in 2018. This system uses a standardized pathologic assessment of depth of tumor penetration (T), extent of regional nodal involvement (N), and the presence absence of metastatic disease (M). A prefix of "c" denotes a clinical classification (cTNM), "p" denotes the pathologic classification (pTNM), and "y" for tumors classified after neoadjuvant therapy (ypTNM). The current AJCC Staging is outlined in Table 13.8. The Astler-Coller Modified Duke staging is sometimes utilized internationally and in the setting of clinical trials. It is detailed in Table 13.9.

Surgical Management of Colon Cancer

The goal of primary surgical treatment of colon carcinoma is to eradicate disease in the colon, the draining nodal basins, and contiguous involved organs. Careful surgical planning is essential to achieve this goal. The stage of disease, presence of synchronous colonic lesions or pathology, and the presence of underlying CRC syndromes are significant factors in determining the optimal surgical approach. The patient's general medical condition is also important because most perioperative mortality can be related to cardiovascular or pulmonary comorbidities.

Anatomy

Thorough knowledge of the arterial, venous and lymphatic anatomy of the colon and rectum is essential for appropriate surgical management (Fig. 13.3). The cecum, ascending and proximal transverse colons are embryologically derived from the midgut and receive their arterial blood supply from the superior mesenteric artery via the ileocolic, right, and middle colic arteries. The distal transverse, descending, and sigmoid colon are hindgut derivatives whose arterial blood supply arises from the inferior mesenteric artery (IMA) through the left colic and sigmoid arteries. The rectum, also a hindgut derivative, receives its blood supply to the upper third from the IMA via the superior hemorrhoidal artery. The middle and lower thirds of the rectum are supplied by the middle and inferior hemorrhoidal arteries, which are branches of the hypogastric artery. Collateral blood supply for the colon is provided through the marginal artery of Drummond and the arc of Riolan. The venous drainage of the colon and rectum parallels the arterial supply, with the majority draining directly into the portal venous system. This provides a direct route for metastatic spread of tumor to the liver. The only minor anatomical variation in the venous drainage compared with the arterial supply is that the inferior mesenteric vein (IMV) joins the splenic vein before emptying into the portal system. The rectum has dual venous drainage; the upper rectum drains into the portal system, and the distal one-third of the rectum drains into the inferior vena cava via the middle and inferior hemorrhoidal veins, providing a direct route for hematogenous spread outside the abdomen.

The lymphatic drainage of the bowel is more complex than the vascular supply. Lymphatics begin in the bowel wall as a plexus beneath the lamina propria and drain into the submucosal and intramuscular lymphatics. The epicolic lymph nodes drain the subserosa and are located close to the colon wall. This nodal group runs along the inner bowel margin between the intestinal wall and the arterial arcades. These nodes drain into the paracolic nodes, which follow the routes of the marginal arteries. The epicolic and paracolic nodes represent the majority of the colonic lymph nodes and are the most likely sites of regional metastatic disease. The paracolic nodes drain into the intermediate nodes, which follow the main colic vessels. Finally, the intermediate nodes drain into the principal nodes, which begin at the origins of the superior and inferior mesenteric arteries and are contiguous with the para-aortic chain.

The route of lymphatic flow parallels the arterial and venous distribution of the colon. The right colon will drain to the superior mesenteric nodes through the intermediate nodes or to the portal system via the lymphatics of the superior mesenteric vein. The left colon's lymphatic drainage follows the marginal artery to the left colic intermediate nodes and finally to the inferior mesenteric nodes. The lymphatic drainage of the upper third of the rectum follows the IMV, whereas the lower two-thirds drain into the hypogastric nodes, which, in

TABLE 3.8 TNM Staging Classification of CRC

Primary Tumor (T)

TX	Primary tumor cannot be assessed
T0	No evidence of primary tumor
Tis	Carcinoma in situ, intramucosal carcinoma
T1	Tumor invades submucosa
T2	Tumor invades muscularis propria
T3	Tumor invades through the muscularis propria into pericolorectal tissues
T4a	Tumor invades through the visceral peritoneum
T4b	Tumor directly invades or is adherent to other organs or structures

Regional Lymph Nodes (N)

NX	Regional lymph nodes cannot be assessed
N0	No regional lymph node metastasis
N1	One to three regional lymph nodes are positive, or any number of tumor deposits are present and all identifiable lymph nodes are negative
N1a	One regional lymph node is positive
N1b	Two or three regional lymph nodes are positive
N1c	No regional lymph nodes are positive but there are tumor deposit(s) in the subserosa, mesentery, or nonperitonealized pericolic or perirectal tissues
N2	Four or more regional lymph nodes are positive
N2a	Four to six regional lymph nodes are positive
N2b	Seven or more regional lymph nodes are positive

Distant Metastases (M)

M0	No distant metastasis by imaging
M1	Metastasis to one or more distant sites or organs or peritoneal metastasis
M1a	Metastasis confined to one organ or site without peritoneal metastasis
M1b	Metastases to two or more sites or organs without peritoneal metastasis
M1c	Metastasis to the peritoneal surface alone or with other site or organ metastases

Stage	T	N	M	MAC[a]
0	Tis	N0	M0	—
I	T1	N0	M0	A
	T2	N0	M0	B1
IIA	T3	N0	M0	B2
IIB	T4a	N0	M0	B2
IIC	T4b	N0	M0	B3
IIIA	T1–T2	N1/N1c	M0	C1
	T1	N2a	M0	C1
IIIB	T3–T4a	N1/N1c	M0	C2
	T2–T3	N2a	M0	C1/2
	T1–T2	N2b	M0	C1
IIIC	T4a	N2a	M0	C2
	T3–T4a	N2b	M0	C2
	T4b	N1–N2	M0	C3
IVA	Any T	Any N	M1a	—
IVB	Any T	Any N	M1b	—
IVC	Any T	Any N	M1c	—

[a]MAC—Modified Astler-Coller Classification.

Stage	Description
A	Lesion not penetrating submucosa
B1	Lesion invades but not through the muscularis propria
B2	Lesion through intestinal wall, no adjacent organ involvement
B3	Lesion involves adjacent organs
C1	Lesion B1 invasion depth; regional lymph node metastasis
C2	Lesion B2 invasion depth; regional lymph node metastasis
C3	Lesion B3 invasion depth; regional lymph node metastasis
D	Distant metastatic disease

TABLE 13.9 Modified Astler–Coller Classification of the Dukes Staging System for CRC

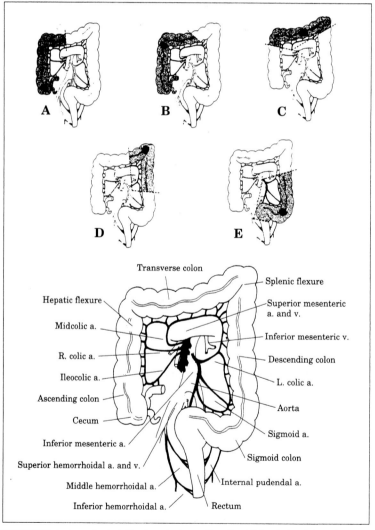

FIGURE 13.3 Anatomy of colonic blood supply along with a pictorial description of the various anatomical resections used for colon carcinoma. **A:** Right hemicolectomy. **B:** Extended right hemicolectomy. **C:** Transverse colectomy. **D:** Left hemicolectomy. **E:** Low anterior resection. (From Sugarbaker PH, MacDonald J, Gunderson L. CRC. In: DeVita VT, Hellman S, Rosenberg SA, eds. *Cancer: Principles and Practice of Oncology*. 3rd ed. Lippincott; 1984, with permission.)

turn, drain into the para-aortic nodes. The lower third of the rectum can also drain along the pudendal vessels to the inguinal nodes.

Surgical Options

Curative-intent surgical resection should be conducted anatomically based on the location of the tumor and the corresponding arterial supply and lymphatic drainage. At resection, the primary tumor and its lymphatic, venous, and arterial supply are extirpated taking care to perform a high ligation of appropriate vessels. In parallel with the concept of the total mesorectal excision (TME) for rectal cancers, complete mesorectal excision (CME) with central vascular ligation (CVL) has emerged as the new standard for the management of colon cancer. In CME, the surgeon dissects in the embryologically defined mesocolic planes, creating a distinct separation between the visceral and retroperitoneal planes. This technique allows for complete mobilization of the entire mesocolon with a surrounding mesocolic fascial envelope, and it ensures safe exposure and ligation of the supplying colonic arteries at their origin. Additionally, incorporating CVL allows removal of any possible metastatic lymph nodes. A retrospective study with data collected from the Danish Colorectal Cancer Group compared patients with stage I–III colon adenocarcinoma who underwent CME versus those who received conventional colon resections. The study found that the CME group had a significant improvement in 4-year disease-free survival (DFS) (85.8%) compared to the non-CME group (75.9%). After propensity-score matching, CME surgery was found to be highly prognostic of DFS regardless of stage. If there is contiguous organ involvement, those organs are removed en bloc with the tumor, aiming for microscopically negative margins (R0). Circumferential resection margin (CRM) status, previously been found to be one of the most important prognostic factors in the management of rectal cancer, has also been found to have significant prognostic value in predicting local control of colon cancer. A recent retrospective study investigating patients in the National Cancer Database who underwent colon resections from 2010 to 2015 found the CRM positivity to be 11.6%.

Right Hemicolectomy

This operation involves removal of a portion of the distal ileum, appendix, right colon, hepatic flexure, and portion of the transverse colon, typically to the right of the main middle colic artery. The ileocolic, right colic, and right branch of the middle colic vessels are ligated at their takeoffs from the central mesenteric vessels, typically superior mesenteric artery and vein. This procedure is indicated for right colon lesions. Operative morbidities can include ureteral injury, duodenal injury, and rarely bile acid deficiency. Anastomotic dehiscence is a risk with all bowel resections that include reconstruction.

Extended Right Hemicolectomy

This procedure includes resection of an extended portion of the transverse colon (typically including ligation of the entire middle colic artery at its origin) in addition to the structures removed in the right hemicolectomy. It generally requires mobilization of the splenic flexure to allow a tension-free anastomosis. Indications for the procedure are hepatic flexure or transverse colon lesions. Morbidities include splenic injury in addition to those associated with right hemicolectomy. Ninety percent of the fecal water is absorbed in the proximal colon; therefore, extended resections are associated with the potential for diarrhea.

Transverse Colectomy

This procedure involves the segmental resection of the transverse colon. Transverse colectomy for mid transverse colon cancer should only be performed in selected patients who are elderly, infirm, or in whom there is risk for debilitating postoperative diarrhea. The oncologically appropriate operation for transverse colon cancer in most patients is an extended right or extended left hemicolectomy. To prevent anastomotic dehiscence, a well-vascularized and tension-free anastomosis is mandated and mobilization of both the right and the left colons and both hepatic and splenic flexures is needed.

Left Hemicolectomy

This resection involves the removal of the transverse colon distal to the right branch of the middle colic artery and the left colon up to, but not including, the rectum. The left branch of the middle colic, and either the IMA or its branches, are ligated. This operation may be tailored to the location of the lesion. Indications for the procedure are left colon and splenic flexure lesions. Morbidities include splenic and ureteral injury.

Low Anterior Resection

When performed for lesions of the distal sigmoid colon or proximal rectum, this procedure includes removal of the sigmoid colon and a portion of the rectum. The arterial ligation should be performed at the highest level on the superior rectal artery as a minimum, when no clinically suspicious nodes are present above this level. Ligation should occur at the level of the proximal IMA for central lymphadenectomy and when necessary to achieve a tension-free anastomosis. The splenic flexure is routinely mobilized, and the reconstruction is performed using the descending colon. The use of the sigmoid colon is discouraged, especially for distal reconstruction as the thickened and hypertrophic muscle of the sigmoid is less compliant and less well vascularized than the descending colon. The IMV can be ligated at the inferior border of the pancreas to gain additional length in order to ensure a tension-free anastomosis. For lesions involving the rectum, the mesorectum should be divided at least 5 cm distal to the distal aspect of the tumor. A 2-cm distal margin is acceptable only for rectal cancers arising from within 5 cm of the anal verge. Morbidities include anastomotic dehiscence, which is higher with more distal reconstruction and approaches 10%, and bowel ischemia (secondary to inadequate flow through the marginal artery of Drummond). For routine low anterior resections (LARs) for sigmoid or upper rectal lesions without radiation, a defunctioning ileostomy is not typically necessary.

Low anterior resection syndrome (LARS) describes a constellation of symptoms that can be experienced in up to 80% of the patients after a low anterior resection. The most commonly reported symptoms include fecal incontinence, stool frequency, urgency, evacuatory dysfunction, and poor gas-stool discrimination. One commonly used tool to measure this negative functional outcome for patients is the LARS score, which ultimately stratifies patients into "No LARS," "Minor LARS," and "Major LARS" based on their reported symptoms on a patient-completed survey.

Total Abdominal Colectomy

This resection involves the removal of the entire colon to the rectum with an IRA. Subtotal colectomy refers to removal of nearly the entire colon with an anastomosis above the rectum. These procedures are typically indicated for multiple synchronous colonic pathologies arising in different anatomic regions, for selected patients with FAP with rectal sparing, and for selected patients with colon cancer in the setting of HNPCC. Most patients experience frequent loose bowel movements and they should be counseled regarding the need for a bowel regimen and perianal care. The risk for anastomotic leak after IRA is approximately 5% or less.

The surgical treatment of the familial polyposis syndromes must be individualized to the polyp burden, the feasibility of endoscopic clearance, as well as the preferences and priorities of the patient. Surgical options include total proctocolectomy with end ileostomy, total abdominal colectomy with IRA, or restorative proctocolectomy with ileal pouch anal anastomosis (IPAA). Total abdominal colectomy with IRA has a low complication rate, provides good functional results, and is a viable option for patients with low rectal adenoma burden (e.g., fewer than 20 adenomas). These patients must be followed postoperatively with 6- to 12-month endoscopic examinations for adenoma clearance. If rectal polyps become too numerous or undergo malignant transformation, completion proctectomy is warranted. Restorative proctocolectomy with IPAA has the advantage of removing all, or nearly all, colorectal mucosa at risk for cancer while preserving transanal defecation. Complication rates are low when this procedure is done in large centers. Studies report the mortality rate to be between 0.2% and 1.5%. Morbidity from the procedure includes incontinence, multiple loose stools, impotence, retrograde ejaculation, dyspareunia. Pouch-specific complications include pouchitis, pelvic sepsis, stricture, and fistula. A meta-analysis reported that approximately 7% of patients have to be converted to permanent ileostomy due to complications after IPAA. The Cleveland Clinic Foundation recently evaluated their registry of patients with FAP who were treated with IRA or IPAA. Prior to the use of IPAA for patients with high rectal polyp burdens, the risk of cancer in the retained rectum was 12.9% at a median follow-up of 212 months. Because of the use of IPAA for patients with large rectal polyp burdens and the selected use of IRA for those with low rectal polyp burdens, no patient had developed rectal cancer in the remaining rectum at a median follow-up of 60 months.

Obstructing or Perforated CRCs

Obstructing or perforated left-sided CRCs are complicated clinical scenarios that require careful surgical planning. The principles of oncologic resection should be followed, but consideration must be given to the patient's comorbidities, hemodynamics, and septic status. These considerations may require a two-stage operation with resection and Hartmann procedure, followed by restoration of gastrointestinal continuity or diverting loop colostomy based on the clinical scenario. Contraindications for primary anastomosis include advanced peritonitis, hemodynamic instability, poor general health, steroid therapy, or immunosuppressed state. Endoscopic stenting of obstructive lesions can be used as a bridge therapy to allow for bowel preparation and subsequent single-step resection. A meta-analysis of 7 randomized prospective trials comparing endoscopic stenting with resection found stenting to be technically successful in 77% of patients. Additionally, patients had higher rates of primary anastomosis, decreased use of permanent ostomy, and fewer wound infections following the resection after the stent was successfully placed. Of note, perforation is a possible complication of endoscopic stenting of an obstructing tumor, and receipt of an antiangiogenic agent such as bevacizumab has been found to confer a significantly higher risk of perforation compared to patients not treated with an antiangiogenic agent (12.5% vs. 7%). Obstructing right-sided cancers can typically be treated with resection and anastomosis in one stage.

Treatment of Locally Advanced Colon Cancer

Approximately 10% of all colon cancers present with direct extension into adjacent structures (T4b). Preoperative imaging and planning must carefully elucidate an operative approach that removes the tumor and all adjacent involve structures en bloc without violation of malignant tissue planes, in order to minimize the chance of local failure and optimize long-term disease control. Importantly, all adhesions between the carcinoma and adjacent structures should be assumed to be malignant and not taken down. Thirty-three to 84% of these adhesions are found to be malignant when examined histologically. The affected organ should have resection limited to the involved area with a margin of normal tissue. A patient who has a margin-negative multivisceral resection has a chance of attaining the same survival as a patient with no adjacent organ involvement on a stage-matched basis.

Historically, there were considerations for postoperative radiation. Previously retrospective series had shown subsets of patients who benefited from postoperative radiation therapy with or without 5-FU–based chemotherapy. Thus far however, there is no level 1 evidence for recommendations of adjuvant radiation following resection of locally advanced colon cancer. With improvements in preoperative imaging modalities, greater attention has been centered on a neoadjuvant approach. In the recently completed FOxTROT randomized controlled trial, 1,053 patients treated in the United Kingdom, Denmark, and Sweden were allocated to either neoadjuvant chemotherapy followed by surgery and adjuvant chemotherapy or upfront surgery and adjuvant chemotherapy. The study noted significant histologic downstaging with lower pT and pN stages and a reduction in incomplete (R1/R2) resections in the neoadjuvant chemotherapy arm. Neoadjuvant chemotherapy was therefore associated with greater disease control without significant increases in perioperative morbidity and facilitates multivisceral, en-bloc resections with R0 margin. Neoadjuvant treatment most commonly consists of chemotherapy regiments such as FOLFOX, but radiation therapy can also be used in the management of highly selected patients with locally advanced colon cancer.

Survival

Five-year OS and DFS of patients with colon cancer varies by pathologic stage. Nodal involvement is the primary determinant of OS. In node-negative disease, the 5-year survival rate is 90% for patients with T1 and T2 lesions and 80% for those with T3 lesions. For node-positive cancers, the 5-year survival ranges from 74% with N1 disease to 51% with N2 disease. These figures also vary depending on the total number of lymph nodes retrieved and evaluated in the surgical specimen, with improved survival associated with a higher number of lymph nodes evaluated. Other factors that are proven prognostic indicators include grade, bowel perforation, and obstruction. Patients who present with unresectable metastatic disease have poor OS with 5-year survival at 11%. In patients who undergo resection of distant metastasis, 5-year survival approaches 40% in some series.

Adjuvant Therapy

Most patients with colon cancer present with disease that appears localized and can be completely resected with surgery. The risk of locoregional recurrence as the primary site of recurrence following a curative resection of a localized colon cancer is approximately 2% to 3%, thought to be secondary to untreated occult microscopic metastasis. Adjuvant therapy is administered to treat and hopefully eradicate such residual micrometastatic disease. Adjuvant systemic therapy is recommended for all patients with stage III disease where their risk of recurrence approaches 50%. The first-line chemotherapy regimen should include a fluoropyrimidine (5-FU/leucovorin or capecitabine) and oxaliplatin. In the recently published IDEA collaboration, six randomized phase 3 trials compared patients receiving 3 months or 6 months of adjuvant FOLFOX (fluorouracil, leucovorin, and oxaliplatin) or CAPOX (capecitabine and oxaliplatin). Given the significant reduction in potential treatment toxicities, cost, and improvement in patient adherence, the results supported the administration of 3 months of adjuvant chemotherapy following resection of stage III colon cancer. Currently, there is no evidence to support biologic agents such as bevacizumab in the adjuvant treatment of stage III colon cancer.

The role of adjuvant therapy in stage II CRC is more controversial. Several adjuvant trials included both stage II and III diseases. Subgroup analysis of stage II patients in the NSABP C-07 and MOSAIC trials showed trends toward benefit without reaching statistical significance, as these trials were underpowered to see a difference in this subgroup. However, three meta-analyses from the NSABP, NCCTG, and International Multi-Center Pooled Analysis of Colon Cancer Trials suggest only marginal improvements in DFS and OS with 5-FU and LV in stage II colon cancer patients. Adjuvant chemotherapy in stage II patients provides a relative improvement in overall 5-year survival that was comparable to that seen in stage III patients (approximately 30% relative improvement). However, the absolute improvement in OS is only 2% to 7%.

Multi-gene testing platforms for recurrence risk stratification have shown more robust utility in breast cancer than colon cancer, where they have not been able to deliver added prognostic or predictive power to guide the choice of chemotherapy agents. Current recommendations reserve adjuvant chemotherapy for high-risk stage II colon cancers, which are defined by T4 lesions, <12 harvested lymph nodes, lymphovascular invasion, bowel obstruction or bowel perforation, and poorly differentiated histology.

Surgical Management of Rectal Cancer

The rectum can be generally divided into thirds: lower, middle, and upper. The upper rectum extends above 12 cm from the anal verge; however, the length of the rectum varies significantly depending on the size of the individual, and therefore these distinctions should be individualized. Tumors of the upper rectum, at the level of the sacral promontory are labeled "rectosigmoid" because they can behave similarly to colon cancers. Their surgical management is analogous to the management of colon cancer previously discussed. The remainder of this discussion will outline the management of rectal cancer within 12 cm of the anal verge.

The primary goal of rectal cancer surgery is to achieve a negative margin resection of the primary tumor with resection of all draining lymph nodes. Additional goals include restoration of intestinal continuity and preservation of anorectal sphincter, sexual, and urinary function when possible. Achieving these targets can be difficult due to the anatomical constraints of the bony pelvis. There is also significant surgeon- and center-related variation in patient outcomes after treatment for rectal cancer. The Stockholm Rectal Cancer Study Group found that specialists and high-volume centers had lower local failure rates and improved survival rates when compared to low-volume practitioners. As such, it is not unusual to see wide ranges of local recurrence rates from 3.7% to 43% in various series for curative surgical resection, with or without multimodal therapy.

Clinical Staging

At the time of diagnosis, all rectal cancer patients should undergo total colonoscopy to assess for synchronous tumors. Surgeons should perform proctoscopy at initial evaluation to confirm location of the tumor from the anal verge as well as the anorectal ring which is the top of the anal sphincters. A CT of the chest, abdomen, and pelvis should be performed and baseline CEA levels acquired. Assessment of clinical T and N stages can be performed using MRI or ERUS. Meta-analysis of studies investigating the accuracy of CT, MRI, or ERUS for preoperative staging in rectal cancer show MRI and ERUS with similar T-stage sensitivity, with a slight increase in specificity with ERUS. MRI and ERUS have equivalent sensitivity for N stage, but only MRI provides excellent assessment of the circumferential margin. For this reason, high-resolution MRI is the preferred modality for clinical rectal cancer staging.

Resection Margins

Low rectal cancers are at an increased risk for positive proximal, distal, and especially CRMs. In 1986, Quirke et al. were the first to characterize the critical importance of the negative radial margin in preventing rectal cancer recurrence. In their series, the rate of local recurrence was 86% in the setting of a positive radial resection margin. The proximal margin is rarely a problem in rectal cancer. In low rectal cancers however, the distal and circumferential margins require good judgment and technique. Histologic examination of the bowel wall distal to grossly resected rectal cancers show that only 2.5% of patients will have submucosal spread of disease greater than 2.5 cm.

It has been well documented that negative radial margins are major determinants of local recurrence and survival. Radial margin clearance can be maximized by sharp dissection between the fascia propria of the mesorectum and the endopelvic fascia. Positive CRM typically is due to an incomplete TME from medial violation of the mesorectal envelope and disruption of the mesorectum. TME involves sharp excision and extirpation of the mesorectum by dissecting outside the investing fascia of the mesorectum. During an abdominal perineal resection (APR), however, the last portion of the rectum just above the anorectal ring that abuts the

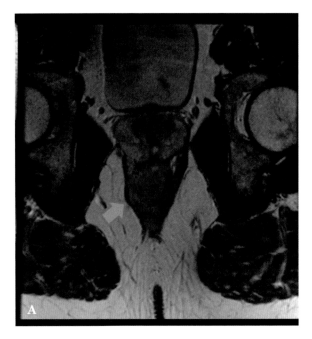

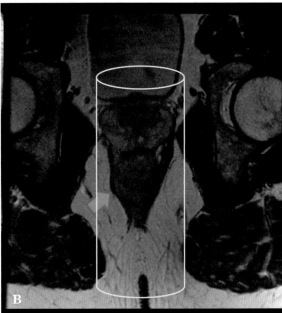

FIGURE 13.4   A: Failure of the total mesorectal excision plane for low rectal cancers. **B:** Cylindrical approach to total mesorectal excision.

levator muscle should not be dissected in a "coning" in fashion, but rather, a cylindrical approach should be undertaken (Fig. 13.4). The cylindrical approach requires a standard TME to the level of the levators and a wide extralevator resection. It has been shown to improve oncologic outcomes by reducing CRM positivity in patients with low anorectal cancers. At MDACC, tumor-specific TME is performed for cases where restoration of GI continuity is anticipated. This would include the entire mesorectum for the lower and lower-middle rectal cancers, while preserving a portion of the mesorectum for upper and upper-middle rectal cancers. The mesorectum is transected 5 cm distal to the distal aspect of the tumor arising in the mid to upper rectum. A distal margin of 2 cm is the aim for low-lying tumors. Shorter distances can be considered in individual cases particularly with a demonstrated excellent response to preoperative therapy in this location. This tumor-specific mesorectal excision does not compromise an adequate oncologic operation and may decrease the risk for anastomotic dehiscence from devascularization of the rectum. Disease-related contraindications for sphincter preservation include involvement of the anal sphincter complex and/or the levator ani muscle. For abdominoperineal resections, TME with a cylindrical approach is performed.

Lymphadenectomy

Adequate lymphadenectomy should be performed for accurate staging and local control. Proximal vascular ligation at the origin of the superior rectal vessels from the IMA should be considered a minimum standard. High ligation of the IMA at its takeoff from the aorta has been advocated for complete lymphadenectomy, although its oncologic value remains controversial. High ligation of the IMA should be performed when clinically suspicious nodes are present and/or when additional reach is needed for the colonic conduit. Nodal spread from the primary tumor occurs along the mesorectum. Therefore, the mesorectal margin should be at least 5 cm distal to the inferior aspect of the tumor or to the end of the mesorectum at the pelvic floor. The technique of TME provides adequate lymphadenectomy for most rectal cancers. TME optimizes the oncologic operation by not only removing draining lymph nodes but also maximizing lateral resection margins around the tumor. There is overwhelmingly comparative observational evidence that demonstrates a significant decrease in the local recurrence rate (in the range of 6.3% to 7.3%) compared with conventional surgery (15% to 30%).

Ligation of the IMA, with or without parallel ligation of the IMV at or near its origin ("high ligation") allows for maximal mobilization of the proximal bowel to facilitate a tension-free low pelvic or coloanal anastomosis (CAA).

Lateral pelvic lymphadenectomy is controversial. In 2017, a randomized controlled trial JCOG 0212 was published in Japan testing the noninferiority of TME versus TME with routine lateral pelvic lymph node dissection (LPLND) in patients without any clinical evidence of lateral pelvic lymph node metastasis. Of note, the patients did not receive neoadjuvant chemoradiation therapy, which is not a mainstay of treatment in locally advanced rectal cancer in Japan as it is in the United States and Europe. The trial found that local recurrence rates in the TME group (13%) were higher compared to the TME with LPLND group (7%). Ultimately the trial determined that the noninferiority of TME alone compared with TME with LPLND was not confirmed. Similarly, a multicenter study analyzed the role of LPLND in 1216 patients with cT3/T4 rectal cancers. The study found that patients with LLNs with a short-axis of at least 7 mm on pretreatment MRI were at significantly higher risk of lateral local recurrence compared to patients with nodes less than 7 mm in size.

Most recently, a retrospective comparative cohort was published comparing patients in the United States who received neoadjuvant chemoradiation therapy with a lateral lymph node dissection compared to patients in the Netherlands and Australia who were treated with neoadjuvant cRT and TME alone. Patients included were those with clinically positive lateral pelvic lymph nodes with a diameter >5 mm in the obturator, internal iliac, external iliac, or common iliac basins. Ultimately, the study did not identify any significant differences in local recurrence, DFS, and OS between the two cohorts, but in subgroup analysis, they did note decreased local recurrence and lateral local recurrence in the adjuvant chemotherapy cohort for patients who received nCRT and an LPLND. Currently, a randomized controlled trial based in China is recruiting patients that randomizes patients with clinically positive lymph nodes for either TME or a TME with LPLND after receipt of nCRT.

At MDACC, management of patients with a lateral pelvic lymphadenectomy can be determined based on the risk of that patient having LPLN disease. Patients at low risk include patients cT1/T2/early T3 with clinically negative LPLN on MRI, and these patients can be managed with TME surgery alone. Patients at moderate risk of LPLN disease are those cT3/T4 with clinically negative LPLN on MRI, and they typically can be managed with neoadjuvant therapy and TME or TME with LPLND. Patients at high risk of LPLN disease are those with any abnormal LPLN on MRI (>5 mm in short-axis in the obturator or iliac chains following nCRT or >7 mm in short-axis before nCRT), and these patients will require neoadjuvant chemoradiation therapy with TME and LPLND.

Surgical Approaches to Rectal Cancer

Surgical approaches to the rectum include transabdominal procedures (LAR, CAA, APR), transanal approaches (local excision, LE), and transsacral approaches (York-Mason, Kraske). The latter two approaches will be discussed in detail in the section Local Approaches to Rectal Cancer. Historically, APR, an operation devised by Ernest Miles in the 1930s, was the treatment for all rectal cancers. With the advent of better preoperative staging, neoadjuvant therapy, and improved surgical techniques and stapler technology, the use of APR has decreased significantly. APR is now reserved for patients with primary sphincter dysfunction and incontinence, patients with direct tumor invasion into the sphincter complex or levator ani, and patients with large or poorly differentiated lesions in the lower third of the rectum that do not have adequate tumor clearance for sphincter preservation.

Sphincter Preservation Procedures

Besides local excision, sphincter preservation procedures include LAR and proctectomy/CAA. Gastrointestinal continuity can be restored with a direct end-to-end anastomosis; sometimes the addition of a colonic reservoir is considered for improved short-term function. Sphincter preservation should only be performed if the oncologic result is not compromised and the functional results are anticipated to be acceptable. It was demonstrated more than 20 years ago that there is no difference in local recurrence rate or survival in patients with midrectal cancers who undergo LAR rather than APR. The technical feasibility of LAR in this setting was increased with the advent of circular stapling devices and the knowledge that distal mucosal margins of resection of 2 cm were adequate in the setting of TME. An alternative to LAR is proctectomy with CAA. It is used in low rectal cancers, with the stapled or hand-sewn anastomosis just above or at the dentate line. Temporary fecal diversion is routinely performed for low rectal or CAA. Using either LAR or proctectomy with CAA (and adjuvant therapy), MDACC and others have reported recurrence rates of 5.3% to 7.9%. Functional results have been good, with 60% to 86% of patients attaining continence by 1 year, 10% to 15% requiring laxative use, and some patients with mild soiling at night. Preoperative chemoradiation does not seem to have a negative impact on these functional results. The lower the anastomosis the greater the potential for bowel dysfunction. Many patient factors are related to the decision to avoid a colostomy; however, there have been no randomized comparative studies of quality of life after CAA versus APR.

Colonic J-Pouch

Although continence can be maintained in patients with CAA, there is a degree of incontinence in some patients, and many require antidiarrheal agents. This is partly due to the lack of a compliant reservoir after proctectomy. This led to the introduction of the colonic J-pouch for low rectal cancers that resulted in better outcomes in terms of stool frequency, urgency, nocturnal bowel movements, and continence compared to straight CAAs. A recent retrospective study examined patients in the National Surgical Quality Improvement Program database who underwent sphincter-preserving resection with CAA versus colonic J-pouch anal anastomosis. 746 patients were included in the colonic J-pouch group and 624 patients were in the coloanal straight anastomosis group. The study found that major complications including deep surgical site infections, septic shock, and return to the operating room were more frequent in the straight anastomosis group, even after adjusting for covariates. These advantages of the colonic J-pouch are principally during the first 12 to 24 months after which time the functional improvements of the straight anastomosis begin to equal those of the J-pouch. One potential problem, especially when the pouch is longer than 5 or 6 cm, is difficulty in pouch evacuation (approximately 20% of patients). As in anterior resection, the functional outcome of patients with CAA (with or without a J-pouch) may take 1 to 3 years to stabilize and is related to the level of the anastomosis (lower anastomoses tend to have poorer function). Unfortunately, many, particularly male patients with low rectal cancers, do not have enough room within the pelvis to accommodate a colonic J-pouch. An alternative approach of a transverse coloplasty pouch has been proposed but it has not been shown to demonstrate significant benefit over a straight anastomosis. Postoperative radiation therapy has not been shown to have a significant adverse effect on pouch function. Thus, at MDACC, the decision for a J-pouch versus a CAA requires an individualized approach with shared decision making between the patient and surgical team regarding the feasibility and advantages of each procedure.

Proximal Diversion

Proximal diversion after sphincter preservation is generally performed in the following circumstances: (a) low anastomosis (i.e., less than 5 to 8 cm above the anal verge), (b) patients who have received preoperative radiation therapy, (c) patients on corticosteroids, (d) when the integrity of the anastomosis is in question, and (e) any case of intraoperative hemodynamic instability.

Intraoperative Radiation Therapy

Intraoperative radiation therapy (IORT) can be used for both recurrent and locally invasive rectal cancer. Its advantages include increased local control in high-risk cancers, accurate treatment of focal areas at risk, and the ability to shield sensitive structures. Even in the setting of adequate preoperative chemoradiation, high-risk tumors will still have a high local recurrence rate in large part due to locoregional extension. IORT allows treatment of areas with close or microscopically positive margins in this situation. Dosing depends on the clinical situation and the total preoperative radiotherapy dose: 12 to 13 Gy is given for close margins (<3 mm), 15 Gy is given for microscopically positive margins, and 17 to 20 Gy is used for areas of gross residual disease. An alternative approach is intraoperative brachytherapy. This allows radiation access in areas where the IORT beam cannot be focused due to anatomical constraints of the pelvis. At MDACC, intraoperative brachytherapy (10 to 20 Gy) is used selectively in patients with locally advanced or recurrent disease where there is a close or microscopically positive margin as demonstrated by frozen section. A recent systematic review found that when comparative studies were evaluated, IORT had a significant effect on improvement of local control, DFS, and OS without a significant increase in total or anastomotic complications.

Minimally Invasive Approaches to CRC

Studies have confirmed that laparoscopic colectomy for colon cancer is technically feasible and safe, yielding an equivalent number of resected lymph nodes and length of resected bowel when compared with open colectomy. Early concerns regarding port-site metastases have been largely addressed due to its rarity. A number of landmark-randomized trials have demonstrated oncologic noninferiority of laparoscopic versus open surgery for colon cancer.

The National Cancer Institute–sponsored multicenter clinical outcomes of surgical therapy (COST) trial enrolled nearly 800 patients and validated the oncologic safety and equivalency of laparoscopy for colon cancer with the exceptions of transverse colon cancer and T4 disease. Laparoscopic-assisted colectomy for cancer was associated with equivalent recurrence-free and OS when compared with open surgery with no increase in wound infections. Statistically significant patient-related benefits included reduced length of hospital stay (1 day shorter in the laparoscopic group, 5 vs. 6 days, $P < .001$) and decreased pain (1 day less each of parenteral narcotics [3 vs. 4 days, $P < .001$] and oral analgesics [1 vs. 2 days, $P = .02$]). There was a small improvement in short-term quality of life, and a small benefit in long-term quality of life could be documented for the patients treated with laparoscopic resection. More recently, a systematic review and meta-analysis of 5 observational studies including 1,268 patients with locally advanced pT4 colon cancer found no significant differences in OS, DFS, or positive surgical margins between the laparoscopic and open resection cohorts. These results, though obtained through nonrandomized and retrospective studies, indicate that even locally advanced colon cancer can be treated via laparoscopic resection without any significant tradeoffs in survival or positive margins.

In rectal cancer however, laparoscopic resection has had mixed results. The Colon Carcinoma Laparoscopic or Open Resection (COLOR) II trial included a subgroup of patients with rectal cancer who were randomized to laparoscopic versus open surgery for rectal cancer. The primary endpoints were locoregional recurrence rates at 3 years, and secondary endpoints included OS and DFS. Laparoscopic surgery in patients with rectal cancer was associated with rates of locoregional recurrence and DFS and OS similar to those for open surgery. ACOSOG Z6051 was a phase 3 randomized controlled trial with a noninferiority design and 1:1 randomization of laparoscopic versus open rectal resection. Primary endpoints included CRM, distal margins, number of lymph nodes recovered, and integrity of the mesorectum. Secondary endpoints included DFS and local recurrence at 2 years. This trial failed to meet the criterion for noninferiority in terms of short-term primary endpoints. In the recent follow-up to the trial, there was no significant difference in the 2-year DFS for laparoscopic versus open resection patients (79.5% vs. 83.2%). Additionally, laparoscopic resection did not increase the risk of local or distant recurrence compared to open resection (80.6% vs. 83.9%).

Minimally invasive techniques result in faster recovery and have the putative benefits of improved quality of life and lower overall health care costs when compared with open surgery. When considering colectomy, reduction in postoperative pain and narcotic use, faster resolution of ileus, and shorter duration of hospitalization are purported benefits of the laparoscopic approach. Added benefits may include the potential for improved short- and long-term complications and a reduction in costs. Further investigation will be required to determine whether the small statistical benefits that have been seen in the randomized clinical trials are clinically significant as well. Furthermore, the importance of these effects may in part depend on the underlying diagnosis. Most patients with colon cancer are candidates for laparoscopic-assisted techniques. Transverse colon tumors require extensive bilateral colonic mobilization and therefore are technically more difficult. Factors associated with an increased need for conversion include tumor-related factors such as proximal left-sided lesions and large bulky tumors, as well as patient obesity, adhesions, and the presence of an associated abscess that was not preoperatively identified. Cancers with perforation, obstruction, or invasion of the retroperitoneum or abdominal wall are not approached laparoscopically.

Since its introduction, the robotic interface has grown popular among colorectal surgeons. Its improved dexterity, range of motion, and better visualization offer significant advantages over laparoscopy and are of particular interest in rectal surgery. Most studies have focused on elucidating the clinical benefits of robotic rectal cancer surgery. However, no clear advantage has been shown to support any one technology over the other. One meta-analysis of the current study suggests that the robotic interface may offer a lower conversion rate, better TME, and earlier recovery of voiding and sexual function over laparoscopic rectal surgery. A more recent meta-analysis found that robot-assisted surgery was associated with longer operative time but also with a shorter length of stay, faster bowel function recovery, and lower postoperative complications. Additionally, the study found no significant differences in estimated blood loss, anastomotic leak rate, lymph node retrieval, distal resection margin positivity, and CRM positivity between the two groups. While these results are positive, more rigorous investigation is warranted in order to adequately evaluate the safety, efficacy, and long-term oncologic and functional benefits of robotic rectal cancer surgery.

Complications of Surgical Therapy for Rectal Cancer

Complications of surgical therapy for rectal cancer include all complications associated with major abdominal surgery (e.g., bleeding, infection, ureteral or adjacent organ injury, and bowel obstruction), with the addition of some complications unique to pelvic surgery. Specifically, anastomotic leak occurs in 5% to 15% of cases overall, with increased rates in association with lower anastomoses, immunocompromised states, and preoperative radiation. A defunctioning stoma will decrease the morbidity of such a leak and may decrease the leak incidence. At MDACC, a diverting loop ileostomy is typically constructed for all patients who have received preoperative radiation. Additional factors which, if present, should make the surgeon strongly consider a diverting ileostomy include: low anastomosis (i.e., within 5 to 8 cm of the anal verge), CAA, or suboptimal tissue quality. Autonomic nerve preservation is always performed during pelvic dissections unless tumor involvement necessitates the sacrifice of these structures. With careful dissection during TME, 75% to 85% of patients have a return to preoperative sexual and urinary function. Other complications include urinary dysfunction, stoma dysfunction, perineal wound complications, hemorrhage from presacral vessels, and anastomotic stricture. The mortality rate from surgical resection varies from less than 2% to 6%.

Local Approaches to Rectal Cancer

Local treatment alone as definitive therapy of rectal cancer was first applied to patients with severe coexisting medical conditions unable to tolerate radical surgery. Currently, local approaches are being more widely considered and have the benefits of potentially sparing major perioperative risks and obtaining favorable functional results. Local excision has been associated with up to 97% local control rate and 92% disease-specific survival for properly selected individuals with early cancers. Local treatment is best applied to rectal cancers within 10 cm of the anal verge, less than 3 cm in diameter involving less than one-third of the circumference of the rectal wall, tumors staged as T1 by ERUS, highly mobile and of low histologic grade. The decision to use local excision (with negative margins) alone or to employ adjuvant therapy after local excision is based on the pathologic characteristics of the primary cancer and the potential for micrometastases in the draining lymph nodes. T1 lesions have been associated with positive lymph nodes in up to 18% of cases, whereas the rate for T2 and T3 lesions is up to 38% and 70%, respectively. T2 tumors treated with local resection alone have local recurrence rates of 25% to 62%. Local excision alone is not considered adequate therapy for T1 lesions with poor prognostic features and all T2 tumors. However, when local excision is performed due to medical comorbidities, neoadjuvant or adjuvant chemoradiation and close surveillance should also be considered. Two phase 2 cooperative group studies evaluated local excision for T1 lesions and local excision with adjuvant chemoradiation using a 5-FU–based regimen for T2 lesions. The CALGB 8984 trial evaluated 177 patients who underwent transanal excision for T1 or T2 lesions. T2 patients were given adjuvant chemoradiation and T1 patients were followed for recurrence and survival. At a median follow-up of 7.1 years, 4 of 59 patients with T1 lesions (2 local, 1 local and distant, and 1 distant) and 10 of 51 patients with T2 lesions (5 local, 2 local and distant, and 3 distant) had recurrences. OS rates were 84% and 66% and DFS 75% and 64%, respectively. Local recurrence rates for patients with T1 and T2 lesions were 8% and 18%, respectively. The Radiation Therapy Oncology Group (RTOG) protocol 89–02 used a similar strategy with a median follow-up of 6.1 years in 52 patients with T1/T2 rectal cancers and demonstrated a 4% local failure rate for T1 lesions and 16% local failure rate for T2 lesions. An additional 3 of 13 (23%) patients with T3 disease treated with local excision and chemoradiation were noted to have local failure. These data should be considered in the background of data from other studies demonstrating a recurrence rate of 18% and 37% in patients undergoing local excision alone for T1 and T2 tumors, respectively. The ACOSOG Z6041 trial is a phase 2 trial of neoadjuvant chemoradiation (capecitabine, oxaliplatin, and radiation) followed by local excision for uT2N0 rectal cancers (uT reflects T category determined using TRUS). The primary endpoint was 3-year DFS, which was 88.2% among 79 patients after a median follow-up of 56 months.

Transanal excision is the conventional approach to removing distal rectal cancers. In order to ensure a full-thickness excision, the deep plane of dissection is the perirectal fat. Tumors should be excised in a non-piecemeal fashion, with a 1-cm circumferential margin.

Transanal minimally invasive surgery (TAMIS) provides accessibility to tumors of the middle and upper rectum, which would otherwise require a laparotomy or transsacral approach, through improved visibility and instrumentation. This approach can be used for selected lesions up to 15 cm from the anal verge. Caution must be taken with higher lesions because full-thickness excision can result in perforation into the abdominal cavity that will result in intraoperative leakage of gas and potential for injury to intraperitoneal organs. The procedure is technically demanding and requires special equipment and is not recommended for tumors within 5 cm of the anal verge.

Other local approaches are mentioned here for historical interest and are rarely performed in clinical practice today. *Posterior proctotomy* involves a posterior incision along the paracoccygeal plane above the anus (Kraske procedure) or to the anus (York-Mason procedure), the coccyx is removed, and the levator is divided. The rectum can then be mobilized for a sleeve resection, or a proctotomy is performed for excision of the tumor. This procedure presently has limited application for rectal tumors.

Patient selection for local procedures is important, and it is recommended that patients have preoperative MRI and/or EUS to accurately identify T category and to select superficial lesions. Patients with deeper lesions could only be considered potential candidates if there is concurrent metastatic disease or significant comorbid conditions. Although local procedures have become more commonly used, few randomized prospective trials have evaluated oncologic and functional outcomes compared with anterior resection or APR. In 1996, Winde et al. prospectively randomized 50 patients with T1 adenocarcinoma of the rectum to either anterior resection or transanal endocsopic microsurgery (TEM). Similar local recurrence and survival rates, as well as decreased morbidity rates for local excision, were found in the two study arms.

Though these additional new platforms for tumor resection are becoming more widely available, patient selection remains critically important. At MDACC, transanal excision is used for highly selected early T1 tumors with favorable features, while radical resection is preferred for other rectal lesions. Optimal specimens from local excision are characterized by nonpiecemeal full-thickness excision, at least a 1-cm mucosal margin circumferentially, and are not fragmented. An inadequate local excision mandates an alternative resection strategy, not merely the addition of adjuvant therapy. If preoperative T category is increased after pathologic evaluation following local excision, the appropriate standard resection is recommended. T1 tumors with any poor prognostic features identified (e.g., tumor greater than 4 cm, poorly differentiated histologic type, lymphatic or vascular invasion, or clinical or radiologic evidence of enlarged lymph nodes) are not appropriate for local excision. For patients with T2 tumors, local excision should only be considered when radical resection is contraindicated and should be performed in conjunction with neoadjuvant or adjuvant therapies ideally in the context of a clinical protocol.

The Role of External Beam Radiation in Management of Rectal Cancer

In addition to high-quality surgery, external beam radiation plays an important role in the modern management of rectal cancer. Historically, there was debate regarding the sequence of radiation therapy, with the initial preference being receipt of radiation in the postoperative setting. However, over the past few decades, there has been a shift in standards of care, with many patients now receiving preoperative radiation or chemoradiation prior to surgical resection. This historical trend from a focus on adjuvant therapy to treatment in the neoadjuvant setting can be traced to several randomized trials conducted over the past three decades.

The Stockholm I and II trials demonstrated a decreased risk of pelvic recurrence in rectal cancer patients who underwent neoadjuvant short course radiation therapy. The Medical Research Council CR07 trial demonstrated that, compared with selective postoperative chemoradiation, preoperative short course radiation reduced 3-year local recurrence rates and improved 3-year DFS among patients with operable rectal cancer. The German Rectal Cancer Study Group (CAO/ARO/AIO-94) trial demonstrated a significant reduction in local recurrence and radiation related toxicity in stage II/III rectal cancer patients undergoing preoperative radiation versus postoperative chemoradiation. Though there was no difference in OS or DFS between groups; the difference in local recurrence persisted at 10-year follow-up. This trial firmly established the role of neoadjuvant chemoradiation in the treatment of locally advanced rectal cancer and was instrumental in the current shift toward neoadjuvant therapy.

The Swedish Rectal Cancer Trial randomized stage I/II/III rectal cancer patients to surgery alone versus preoperative short course radiation (25 Gy in 5 fractions) followed by surgery. At 13-year follow-up, they demonstrated persistent improved local recurrence rate, DFS, and OS in the preoperative radiation arm. The findings further supported the recommendation for preoperative radiation in patients with high-risk (T ≥3, node positive) rectal cancers.

Currently, national consensus guidelines recommend neoadjuvant radiation or chemoradiation for any locally advanced rectal cancers (T ≥3, node positive). In patients with a clear CRM by MRI, they may receive either short-course radiotherapy (SCRT) or long-course chemoradiation with capecitabine or infusional 5-FU. An alternative treatment regimen provided is total neoadjuvant therapy (TNT), which will be subsequently discussed in detail.

For patients with locally invasive rectal cancer (T ≥3, node positive) and an involved/threatened CRM based on MRI or for patients who are medically inoperable or whose tumors are deemed locally unresectable, national consensus guidelines recommend TNT.

Several advantages to the use of preoperative compared with postoperative radiation therapy have been identified, including the following:

1. There is a decreased risk of local failure due to improved compliance with the chemoradiation regimen and improved tumor response in the preoperative setting. There is a decreased risk of toxicity because the small bowel can more readily be excluded from the radiation field in a preoperative setting.
2. There is less bowel dysfunction because the colon used for reconstruction is not in the radiation field.
3. A reduction in tumor size increases rates of sphincter preservation in those patients initially deemed to require APR and improves overall resectability.
4. There is no delay of therapy as in some cases of postoperative therapy due to operative morbidity.

In the United States, preoperative radiation therapy trials have usually included chemotherapy in a more protracted course rather than using SCRT alone. Concurrent chemotherapy with long-course radiation has two benefits. Chemotherapy primarily serves as a sensitizer to radiation, aiding its delivery and effectiveness. A Cochrane systematic review of stage III rectal cancer patients randomized to preoperative concurrent chemoradiation versus radiation only showed a decrease in local recurrence in the patients receiving chemoradiation without a difference in OS. Other studies have shown that concurrent preoperative chemoradiation is more likely to exhibit significant reduction in tumor size and achieve pathologic complete response (pathCR) when compared to preoperative radiation only. Two randomized trials, the Polish trial and the Trans-Tasman Radiation Oncology Group (TROG) trial, reported long-term oncologic outcomes in patients receiving SCRT versus long course chemo-radiation therapy (LCCRT). These trials demonstrated no significant differences in local recurrence and OS between the two treatment arms. However, SCRT was associated with less acute toxicity than LCCRT in both trials.

The complications associated with chemoradiation treatment include radiation enteritis and dermatitis, autonomic neuropathy, hematologic toxicity, stomatitis (mostly with continuous 5-FU infusions), and venous access infections. The frequency and intensity of these complications depend on multiple factors, including radiation therapy total dosing, fractionation, field technique, and whether the radiation therapy is given preoperatively or postoperatively. There are no good predictors of which patients will have these complications and to what degree they will have them.

The Role of Systemic Chemotherapy in Management of Rectal Cancer

Many of the initial guidelines for systemic therapy in rectal cancer were borrowed from those for colon cancer. Currently, national consensus guidelines recommend 6 months of adjuvant chemotherapy for all stage II and III rectal cancers patients. However, strong evidence for use of systemic chemotherapy after neoadjuvant chemoradiation is lacking. In the CAO/ARO/AIO-04 trial, adjuvant chemotherapy was administered to nearly all (89%) patients who received preoperative chemoradiation but only 50% of the patients who received postoperative chemoradiation. Despite these significantly different rates of adjuvant chemotherapy administration, there was no difference in OS or in distant recurrence rates, calling into question the benefit from systemic chemotherapy. The EORTC Radiotherapy Group Trial 22921 investigated the addition of 5-FU–based adjuvant chemotherapy to preoperative radiation or preoperative chemoradiation in stage II/III rectal cancer. The addition of adjuvant 5-FU–based therapy was not associated with any difference in local recurrence, distant metastases, or OS. The CHRONICLE, I-CNR-RT, and PROCTOR-SCRIPT trials also did not demonstrate a clear benefit to systemic therapy among patients undergoing TME after chemoradiation.

However, some patients may benefit from systemic therapy. In the ADORE trial from Korea, 321 patients with pathologic stage II or III rectal cancer after having undergone neoadjuvant long-course chemoradiation and standard resection, were randomized to receive adjuvant 5-FU and leucovorin or adjuvant FOLFOX. FOLFOX therapy was associated with improved DFS among pathologically node-positive patients but not among node-negative patients.

Of particular interest is the question of adjuvant therapy in patients undergoing neoadjuvant chemoradiation followed by surgical resection with a complete pathologic response (ypT0N0). Current national consensus guidelines recommend adjuvant systemic treatment in this setting. A 2019 meta-analysis examining 2,948 patients with rectal cancer who had a complete pathologic response (ypCR) showed a significant improvement in OS for patients who received adjuvant therapy compared to those who were observed. However, a recent Korean study demonstrated that, among patients who received preoperative chemoradiation followed by TME and had ypT0–1 disease on final pathology, the receipt of adjuvant chemotherapy did not significantly impact 5-year OS or RFS.

With regard to the timing of the adjuvant therapy, studies have shown that the interval between resection and initiation of therapy impacts the survival benefit of the treatment. One meta-analysis featuring 6 studies with a total of 12,584 patients showed that for every 4-week increase in time to adjuvant treatment, patients were found to have a decrease in both DFS and OS.

Total Neoadjuvant Therapy

Recently, the concept of TNT has emerged in management of patients with locally advanced rectal cancer. This treatment strategy, which involves delivery of both radiation or chemoradiation and systemic chemotherapy prior to surgery, seeks to maximize the response of the primary tumor, improve treatment tolerance and completion, and improve survival.

The publication of results from two randomized controlled trials has established the standard for TNT protocols. The RAPIDO (Rectal Cancer and Preoperative Induction Therapy Followed by Dedicated Operation) trial, which randomized patients with high-risk tumors to short-course radiation followed by either FOLFOX or CAPEOX followed by TME (TNT) or long-course chemoradiation, TME, and postop FOLFOX or CAPEOX (standard therapy), demonstrated that TNT could be used safely compared to standard therapy and was associated with improved rates of pCR (28.4% TNT vs. 14.3% standard therapy) and decreased rates of developing distant metastases (20.0% TNT vs. 26.8% standard therapy) and disease-related treatment failure (23.7% TNT vs. 30.4% standard therapy). The PRODIGE 23 (Partenariat de Recherche en Oncologie Digestive) trial, meanwhile, randomized patients with T3 or T4 M0 tumors to either preoperative mFOLFIRINOX then long-course chemoradiation then TME then postoperative FOLFOX or CAPEOX (TNT) or long-course chemoradiation then TME then postoperative FOLFOX or CAPEOX (standard therapy). TNT severe adverse event rate was 45%, but >90% of patients were able to comply with therapy. Compared to standard therapy, TNT conferred improved 3-year DFS (75.7% vs. 68.5% standard therapy). As in RAPIDO, TNT resulted in higher rates of pCR (27.8% vs. 12.1% standard therapy) and lower rates of developing distant metastases (17% vs. 25% standard therapy). Importantly, in both trials, OS did not differ between TNT and standard therapy groups.

It is important to note that optimal use of TNT remains a topic of ongoing investigation. While TNT provides potential benefits as outlined above, it is not without morbidity. Thus, a risk-benefit analysis should be performed for each patient taking into account both patient and tumor-related factors. Indeed, guidelines differ among the United States, Europe, and Japan. US guidelines support TNT as a possible treatment strategy for any patient with T3 or higher or node-positive disease. Meanwhile, European guidelines support the use of TNT in patients with high-risk tumors, low tumors, or lateral pelvic lymph node involvement, and Japanese guidelines suggest TNT in patients with tumors below the peritoneal reflection or situations in which resectability and sphincter preservation would be optimized with maximum pretreatment. The MD Anderson approach to utilization of TNT will be discussed subsequently in the context of our treatment approach to rectal cancer.

Treatment of Locally Invasive Rectal Cancer

Approximately 10% of rectal cancer patients will present with involvement of adjacent structures (bladder, vagina, ureters, seminal vesicles, and sacrum). Locally invasive rectal cancers are historically difficult to treat. Recurrence rates can be high with surgery alone, but outcomes have significantly improved with the use of multimodality treatment. Although preoperative and adjuvant therapy is important in these patients, the mainstay treatment in rectal cancer is R0 resection of the tumor with complete TME and en-bloc resection of involved structures. The confines of the pelvis and the proximity of critical nerves and blood vessels are frequent challenges. IORT or brachytherapy has been shown to provide additional potential benefit.

Improved resectability and decreased locoregional recurrence have been demonstrated for locally invasive rectal cancers after preoperative chemoradiation treatment. As reported by the Mayo Clinic, the addition of IORT to standard external beam radiation therapy with 5-FU in patients with locally invasive rectal cancer has been associated with improved local disease control and possibly some improvement in survival. Preoperative chemoradiation has also been shown to improve rates of sphincter preservation in patients who were initially believed to need APR for curative resection by as much as twofold when compared with postoperative chemoradiation regimens. The best chance of cure in patients with locally invasive disease appears to involve preoperative chemoradiation treatment, maximal surgical resection, with IORT used in selected cases.

MD Anderson Experience

Our treatment approach to patients with rectal cancer involves first appropriately staging and risk-stratifying patients with digital rectal examination, high-quality colonoscopy, high-quality rectal MRI, and CT chest, abdomen, and pelvis. Based on T category, distance of the tumor from the anal verge, CRM status, the presence or absence of EMVI, and the presence or absence of locoregional nodal disease, patients can be classified as low, intermediate, or high risk. This risk stratification informs our decision regarding utilization and sequencing of chemotherapy, radiation, and surgery in treating patients with rectal cancer. This framework can be found in a 2022 review in *Cancer* by Bhutiani, Peacock, and Chang.

Organ Preservation ("Watch and Wait") Strategy for Rectal Cancer

Up to 20% of patients who receive nCRT have been found to have a pathologic complete response. For this reason, in a selected group of patients with a complete clinical response, an organ preservation ("watch and wait") approach can be implemented. Compete clinical response has been defined as no palpable tumor on digital rectal examination, no evidence of disease on cross-sectional imaging, and no visible pathology other than a flat scar on endoscopic examination. Subsequent studies have found that the pooled 2-year local recurrence rate in "watch and wait" patients was up to 30% and that salvage surgery was feasible in up to 95% of patients who presented with a recurrence after this management approach. Recently, the OPRA (Organ Preservation in Rectal Adenocarcinoma) trial demonstrated a 43% to 58% rate of organ preservation at 3 years among patients with stage II or III distal rectal cancer treated with either long-course chemoradiation followed by consolidation FOLFOX or CAPEOX or induction FOLFOX or CAPEOX followed by long-course chemoradiation. Interestingly, rates of organ preservation were higher in the group that received consolidation rather than induction chemotherapy.

Surveillance

Patients with a history of colorectal carcinoma require close surveillance. However, data to demonstrate a survival advantage from an intensive surveillance program has been limited. In a Danish prospective study, 597 CRC patients were randomized to either close follow-up (every 6 months for the first 3 years) or routine follow-up (every year) for 3 years, using examination, stool heme test, colonoscopy, laboratory testing, and chest radiograph. The frequency of recurrent cancer was the same in both groups, but it was diagnosed earlier in the close follow-up group. The close follow-up group had more resections for curative intent (local and distant), but cancer-specific survival (CSS) differences have been more difficult to demonstrate. More recently, the CEA Watch Study, a multicenter, crossover randomized trial based in the Netherlands, compared intensive CEA follow-up (every 2 months for 3 years followed by every 3 months for the next 2 years) with a less-intensive follow-up (checked every 3 to 6 months for 3 years and then annually for 2 years). The study found no significant differences in terms of OS and DFS, although the more intensive surveillance did identify significantly more recurrences (55.2% vs. 41.9%). In a more recent systematic review and meta-analysis including studies with different follow-up strategies after curative resection in nonmetastatic CRC, the more intensive follow-up strategies resulted in a higher likelihood of detection of asymptomatic recurrences, survival after recurrences, and a shorter period of time in detecting recurrences. A recent retrospective cohort examined stage I–III CRC patients receiving surveillance at high-intensity and low-intensity facilities. The study found imaging and CEA surveillance intensity were not associated with a significant difference in time to detection of cancer recurrence. Furthermore, there were no differences in rates of resection for those with recurrences. Table 13.4 outlines current endoscopic guidelines for CRC patients. In general, close follow-up including regularly scheduled CEA level determination during the first 2 years followed by less intensive follow-up during years 3 to 5 are advocated.

At MDACC, the surveillance intensity and frequency are tailored to individual patients, and key factors are considered including disease stage, comorbidities, eligibility for salvage treatment, and the priorities and preferences of the patient. In general, history, physical examination, and laboratory tests including CEA are performed every 3 to 4 months for the first 2 to 3 years after surgery, and every 6 months during years 3 or 4 through 5, and yearly thereafter for a total of 5 to 8 years. Colonoscopy is performed after 1 year if the proximal colon had been examined preoperatively or after 6 months if the proximal colon had not been examined preoperatively. If normal, it is then repeated after an interval of 3 years, with a life-long interval of every 3 to 5 years. CT scans of the chest abdomen and pelvis are also obtained every 3 to 6 months for 2 to 3 years and every 6 to 12 months for up to 5 years.

Recurrent and Metastatic Disease

Among the patients who develop recurrences, 85% do so during the first 2.5 years after surgery. The remaining 15% experience recurrence during the subsequent years. Recurrence develops in less than 5% of patients who are disease-free at 5 years. The risk of recurrence is higher with higher-stage disease. Other recurrence risk modifiers include race, grade of tumor, aneuploidy, as well as environmental factors such as smoking and obesity. Recurrences may be local, regional, or distant. Distant recurrence, the most common presentation, occurs either alone or concomitantly with locoregional recurrence. Local recurrence can develop in up to 15% of the patients undergoing initial curative intent resection for rectal cancer and the risk is increased with non-R0 resections. When local recurrence is isolated, complete salvage resection with R0 margins in combination with multimodality therapy can result in a 5-year survival rate of between 37% and 60% after salvage. Recurrence isolated to the anastomosis (intramural) is rare but is typically technically easier to salvage than recurrences that involve the lateral pelvis.

The most common sites of distant metastases from rectal cancer are the lung and liver depending on the distance of the tumor to the anal verge. Retroperitoneal nodal disease and peritoneal disease are two additional patterns of distant failure. Recurrences can present with a constellation of symptoms ranging from the vague and nonspecific to the clinically overt. Serum CEA level provides added insight in postoperative monitoring. Elevated preoperative CEA levels (>5 ng/mL) have been found to associated with an increase in recurrence rates and disease-related mortality. CEA levels are most useful in patients in whom levels were increased preoperatively and returned to normal following surgery. Levels should be determined preoperatively, 6 weeks postoperatively, and then according to the schedule described in the surveillance section. The absolute level and rate of increase in CEA and the patient's clinical status are important factors to consider. Postoperative CEA levels that do not normalize within 4 to 6 weeks suggest incomplete resection or recurrent disease, although false-positive results do occur. CEA levels that normalize postoperatively and then start to increase are suggestive of recurrence. This may represent occult or clinically obvious disease. A rapidly increasing CEA level may more likely suggest liver or lung involvement, whereas a slow, gradual rise is more likely to be associated with locoregional disease. Despite the reliability of an increased CEA level in predicting tumor recurrence, 20% to 30% of patients with locoregionally recurrent tumors have a normal CEA level. Poorly differentiated tumors may not make CEA, which is one explanation for such false-negative results.

In contrast, CEA is increased in 80% to 90% of patients with hepatic recurrences. A prospective randomized trial evaluated the significance of CEA in follow-up in 311 asymptomatic patients. Patients with increased CEA levels were followed until symptoms developed; then a full workup was initiated. The sensitivity, specificity, and positive predictive values of an increased CEA level were 58%, 93%, and 79%, respectively. The median lead-time of the increased CEA to detection by other means was 6 months. Seven percent of patients who had an increased CEA failed to have identifiable recurrent disease on workup. Two meta-analyses have been performed pooling results from five randomized studies and a survival advantage in patients allocated to intensive follow-up with CEA has been shown. The German CRC Study Group evaluated follow-up CEA levels in 1,321 patients after curative resection and determined that CEA monitoring was beneficial in 47% of patients with recurrence and 11% of patients overall; however, only 2.3% underwent a curative R0 resection of recurrent disease. Results from a UK multicenter randomized prospective trial of protracted infusion 5-FU versus bolus 5-FU in the adjuvant setting demonstrated that both CT and CEA were valuable components for postoperative follow-up and resulted in improved survival.

PET scan with 2-(^{18}F)fluorodeoxy-D-glucose (FDG) has been reported to have 89% positive predictive value and excellent negative predictive value in patients who had a rising CEA and normal conventional radiographic imaging.

In the era prior to modern imaging technology, if the metastatic evaluation was negative in the face of increased CEA level, a second-look laparotomy would be indicated. Studies from that time period have reported that approximately 60% to 90% of patients with asymptomatically increased CEA levels were found to have recurrent disease at laparotomy; 12% to 60% of whom had resectable disease.

Treatment of the asymptomatic patient with an increased CEA level can be challenging. An increased level should be confirmed by a repeat CEA evaluation. A thorough clinical investigation should include transaminases, serum bilirubin, coagulation profile, CT scan of the chest, abdomen, pelvis, and colonoscopy. At

MDACC, we routinely monitor CEA values because of the potential to detect site of disease relapse that may be amenable for salvage therapy, especially within the liver. This allows for the potential identification of a subgroup of patients who may benefit from salvage intervention. PET scans are not routinely performed for surveillance; rather they are utilized to evaluate patients with rising CEA values where conventional cross-sectional imaging does not identify the site of recurrence. Early detection of asymptomatic disease results in a higher resectability rate than when resection is attempted for symptomatic disease (60% vs. 27%). The liver is the most common site of recurrence, followed by adjacent organs, the anastomotic site, and the mesentery. Resectability rates correspond to the level of CEA elevation, with CEA levels less than 11 ng/mL being associated with higher resectability rates.

Of recent interest is assessing for other potential tumor markers as an indicator for relapse risk. Circulating tumor DNA (ctDNA) is the fraction of circulating DNA that is shed into the bloodstream by a patient's cancer. In two separate cohort studies evaluating stage I–III CRC patients, recurrence rate in ctDNA positive patients was between 77% and 87.5%, and ctDNA positive patients were found to be 40 times more likely to experience a disease recurrence than their ctDNA negative counterparts. These findings have yet to be validated in a randomized prospective trial, and thus the utilization of assessing for ctDNA in standard practice is pending further evidence.

Treatment of Recurrent Locoregional CRC

The appropriate treatment of resectable recurrent disease depends largely on the location of the disease. Potentially resectable recurrent disease is treated in a multimodal fashion using preoperative chemotherapy (with or without radiation or re-irradiation), surgery, and IORT (if available). In a recent systematic review evaluating survival in patients with locally recurrent colon cancer, the median OS for patients undergoing resection was between 14 and 42 months, with patients who had R0 resections having a survival between 19 and 66 months. The study found that R0 resection was achieved in 50.6% of patient and found the re-recurrence rate following resection to be 25%.

For recurrence involving the sacrum, en-bloc sacral resection can sometimes result in 4-year survival rates of 30%. Contraindications to sacral resection include pelvic sidewall involvement, sciatic notch or ala involvement, bilateral S2 involvement, encasement of common or external iliac vessels, and extra pelvic disease. Given the extent of surgery required and the high rates of morbidity associated with salvage resections, resection for the sole purpose of palliation should be carefully deliberated and alternative procedures that may alleviate symptoms without the high risk for complications should be considered first.

At MDACC, patients presenting with locally recurrent rectal cancer are evaluated by CT chest, abdomen, pelvis, MRI pelvis, and PET/CT. Potentially resectable pelvic recurrences are evaluated for potential re-irradiation. Those who are candidates typically undergo preoperative chemotherapy and re-irradiation, while others are considered for preoperative systemic chemotherapy. Every effort is made to achieve an R0 resection, and IORT is utilized for close or R1 resection margins. Using this approach in 229 patients with locally recurrent and re-recurrent rectal cancer, multimodality salvage therapy resulted in a 5-year OS of 50%. A subsequent study examining patients with both locoregional and distant recurrences found that salvage surgery following locoregional recurrence was not associated with any survival benefit as it was in distal recurrences in either the lungs or liver. In this group, distant recurrence was the most common re-recurrence site for patients who received salvage surgery for locoregional recurrence. Although the usual surgical procedure for resectable recurrent rectal cancer is salvage APR or pelvic exenteration, very selected cases can be treated with sphincter preservation.

Surgical Treatment of Metastatic Disease

Liver

The liver is the most common site of visceral metastases. Liver metastases occur in upward of 25% to 30% of CRC patients and it is the only site affected in up to 20% of patients with recurrent CRC. Recent data from MDACC demonstrates that surgical resection of hepatic metastases now offers the potential for 5-year survival up to 58%. Colorectal liver metastases are discussed in detail in Chapter 14, Hepatobiliary Cancers.

Lung

Pulmonary metastases occur in 10% to 20% of patients with CRC. They are typically found in association with concurrent hepatic metastases. Isolated pulmonary metastases occur most commonly with distal rectal lesions because the venous drainage of the distal rectum bypasses the portal system and allows metastasis to travel directly to the lungs.

The finding of a solitary lesion on a chest radiograph should prompt evaluation with thoracic CT scanning and, for a centrally located lesion, bronchoscopy with biopsy. Peripheral lesions may be amenable to

CT-guided needle biopsy or video-assisted thoracoscopic surgery. A less invasive approach includes stereotactic body radiation therapy (SBRT). Fifty percent of patients with solitary pulmonary nodules will have primary lung tumors rather than colorectal metastases.

Patients with locally controlled primary tumors, no evidence of metastases elsewhere, good pulmonary reserve, and low medical risk are candidates for resection. Patients with solitary metastases experience the best survival, but patients with as many as three lesions (unilateral or bilateral) can experience up to a 40% 5-year survival. In the recently discontinued PulMiCC multicenter randomized clinical trial comparing patients with pulmonary metastasectomy versus continued active monitoring, the estimated survival in the metastasectomy group was 38%, whereas the survival was 29% in the well-matched cohorts. The trial was discontinued due to poor recruitment, and given the small sample size, cannot provide conclusive answers regarding the improvement in OS between the two courses of management. As in liver resection for metastatic disease, the optimum surgery includes achievement of negative margins at resection without the routine use of pneumonectomy.

The 5-year survival rate following resection of pulmonary metastases can approach 40%. There is very limited evidence comparing metastasectomy with a noninvasive approach such as SBRT. A recent study showed no difference in OS between the two modalities, but it did show improved lung progression-free survival (PFS) at 2.5 years in the group of patients with surgical intervention compared to those who received SBRT. Age, gender, location of the primary disease, disease-free interval, and involvement of hilar or mediastinal lymph nodes do not seem to influence survival. The number of metastases in most series is inversely correlated with 5-year survival. Recurrence confined to the lung after resection is an indication in selected patients, for repeat resection.

Bone and Brain

Metastatic disease to the brain is uncommon and usually occurs after established lung involvement. Symptomatic solitary lesions can be treated by palliative craniotomy and resection. In a very small subpopulation of patients, cranial disease may be the only site of involvement, and excision in this setting may increase survival. Bone metastases are uncommon but are best managed with radiation therapy, especially when symptomatic.

Ovary

Because 1% to 8% of women who undergo potentially curative CRC resections subsequently develop ovarian metastases, prophylactic oophorectomy at the time of colectomy has been considered for postmenopausal patients. However, prophylactic oophorectomy has not been shown to improve survival and therefore is not routinely performed, but grossly abnormal ovaries should be removed. When isolated metastatic disease to the one ovary is identified, bilateral oophorectomy is the procedure of choice even if the contralateral ovary appears grossly normal, because there is a high risk for bilateral involvement.

Peritoneum

Among patients with CRC, approximately 2% to 19% will develop peritoneal disease. For selected patients, cytoreduction may provide survival benefit in the context of a multimodal treatment regimen. The management of colorectal peritoneal carcinomatosis is covered in detail in Chapter 14, Hepatobiliary Cancers.

Targeted Therapies for CRC

Dramatic improvements have been seen in overall and DFS for CRC with the introduction of cytotoxic chemotherapy agents such as fluorouracil, oxaliplatin, and irinotecan. However, not all patients and their tumors respond to these drugs, leaving some individuals to suffer the severe side effects of these therapies without significant benefit. Precision medicine aims to shift treatment regimens from a population approach based on TNM staging to a personalized approach based on a patient's unique tumor characteristics. Recent advances in molecular biology and epigenetics have identified several biomarkers of prognostic and predictive significance in CRC that will be briefly described below.

Vascular Endothelial Growth Factor

VEGF signaling via the VEGFR2 receptor is a potent regulator of angiogenesis. Signaling results in endothelial cell proliferation and migration. Consequently, VEGF overexpression has been associated with worse outcomes related to tumor progression and poor OS in patients with CRC. Bevacizumab was the first antiangiogenic targeted drug to be FDA approved for the treatment of metastatic CRC. The drug is a recombinant monoclonal antibody against VEGF-A. When added to traditional cytotoxic chemotherapy bevacizumab results in an increased response rate in metastatic CRC patients and leads to longer PFS and OS. Additionally, bevacizumab in combination with FOLFOX (5-FU, oxaliplatin, leucovorin)/FOLFIRI (5-FU, leucovorin, irinotecan) has been found to enhance response in patients with potentially resectable metastases and has increased the number of patients able to undergo curative-intent hepatic metastasectomy. Of note, the drug is associated with impaired wound healing and should be discontinued at least 4 weeks prior to elective surgery.

Epidermal Growth Factor Receptor

Epidermal growth factor receptor (EGFR) signaling activates the Ras/Raf/MAPK and the phosphatidylinositol 3-kinase (*PI3K*) signaling pathways leading to cellular proliferation, inhibiting apoptosis, and promoting cellular invasion. EGFR activation likely not only contributes to CRC tumorigenesis, but also to CRC metastasis. Two classes of anti-EGFR therapies were developed to target this mechanism; tyrosine kinase inhibitors (TKIs) and monoclonal antibodies targeting EGFR. TKIs, such as gefitinib and erlotinib, block EGFR activity and preferentially suppress PI3K signaling in CRC. They are, however, associated with severe GI toxicity and are typically poorly tolerated. Cetuximab was the first anti-EGFR monoclonal antibody (mAb) to be FDA approved for the treatment of metastatic CRC. The drug binds to EGFR and inhibits both MAPK and PI3K cell signaling. Cunningham et al. reported improved PFS and OS with single agent cetuximab or when used in conjunction with irinotecan in mCRC patients with refractory disease. Panitumumab, another anti-EGFR mAb, showed a similar response and was FDA approved soon after.

KRAS/NRAS

The RAS family of proteins (KRAS, NRAS, and HRAS) act downstream of EGFR-mediated cellular signaling (Fig. 13.5). KRAS mutations occur in 30% to 40% of CRCs, while NRAS mutations are rare at 5% and HRAS is not seen in CRC. In retrospective analysis of several clinical trials of anti-EGFR mAbs, wild type–KRAS was found to be required for anti-EGFR antibody-mediated response. Because these proteins act downstream of EGFR, KRAS/NRAS mutations result in constitutive activation of the Ras-Raf-MAPK pathway and confers tumor resistance to anti-EGFR therapies. Current guidelines require testing for KRAS and NRAS prior to initiating anti-EGFR therapy. KRAS mutations appear to also confer poor prognosis in metastatic CRC.

BRAF

The BRAF oncogene is another modulator of the MAPK pathway downstream from RAS. BRAF mutations result in the development of CRC via the serrated pathway. BRAF mutant tumors are more prevalent in women and older patients (>70 years). These tumors are usually right-sided, MSI-high, mucinous, and poorly differentiated. BRAF mutant CRCs exhibit a unique pattern of metastatic spread, often bypassing the liver and developing lung or peritoneal disease. BRAF-mutated metastatic CRC is associated with poorer OS likely because metastatic disease sites are not amenable to resection. BRAF mutations also contribute to

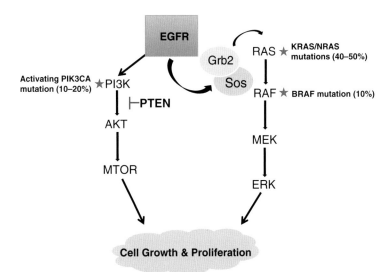

FIGURE 13.5 EGFR signaling pathway.

cetuximab resistance, though perhaps not as potently as KRAS. Studies are ongoing to investigate the role of targeted BRAF therapy in CRC using drugs previously approved for treatment in melanoma. The recent BEACON trial investigated the effects of encorafenib, binimetinib, and cetuximab on patients with BRAF V600E-mutated metastatic CRC. In this phase 3 trial, patients in the experimental arm received triplet-therapy of encorafenib, binimetinib, and cetuximab or doublet-therapy of encorafenib and cetuximab, and the control arm received either cetuximab and irinotecan or cetuximab and FOLFIRI. OS was 9 months in the experimental arm, and 5.4 months in the control group. Ultimately, this study showed the promise that triplet-therapy had over standard regimens in treating metastatic CRC patients with the BRAF V600E mutation.

Human Epidermal Growth Factor 2 (HER2) Gene Status

HER2 gene amplification and protein overexpression occurs in 5% to 12% of colon cancer and as high as 26% of rectal cancers. Its prognostic and predictive relevance in CRC is currently being investigated. One study demonstrated improved CSS in patients with advanced HER2-positive rectal cancers while others have shown HER2-amplified CRC do worse. The recent HERACLES trial investigated the effect of dual anti-HER2 therapy in mCRC. In this small phase 2 study, after a median follow-up of 94 weeks, 8 patients (30%) responded to therapy, 1 patient (4%) had a complete response, and 12 patients (44%) had stable disease suggesting a novel therapeutic target for CRC albeit in only a small percentage of patients.

Mismatch Repair and Tumor Immunity

Until recently, tumor immunity was not considered a major driver of CRC outcomes. However, recent studies have demonstrated that CRC that display high lymphocyte infiltration, in particular with cytotoxic T lymphocytes/T helper 1 lymphocytes (CTL/Th1), are associated with improved PFS and OS. MSI-high tumors are especially immune driven with significant lymphocyte infiltration and overexpressed PD1 and PD-L1 immune checkpoints. Pembrolizumab, a monoclonal antibody against PD-L1 and PD-L2, has demonstrated promising responses in patients with advanced CRC and is being further investigated. The KEYNOTE-177 trial, a phase 3, open label trial including 307 patients with metastatic MSI-H-dMMR CRC, was recently completed, with one treatment arm receiving pembrolizumab and the other receiving traditional chemotherapy (5-FU with or without bevacizumab or cetuximab). The study showed a significantly improved PFS (16.5 months vs. 8.2 months) in the pembrolizumab group. Additionally, there were fewer treatment-related adverse events in the pembrolizumab arm compared with the conventional chemotherapy arm. Additionally, Overman et al. reported results of the combination immune checkpoint blockade (nivolumab plus ipilimumab once every 3 weeks for four doses then nivolumab once every 2 weeks) group of the CheckMate 142 trial. They demonstrated that, among patients with MSI-H dMMR CRC who had progressed or were unable to tolerate at least one line of standard of care therapy, treatment with combination immune checkpoint blockade resulted in 71% 12-month PFS and 85% 12-month OS with manageable toxicity. Subsequent work, also from CheckMate 142, has demonstrated the safety and efficacy of nivolumab and low-dose ipilimumab in first-line treatment for MSI-H dMMR metastatic CRC.

Uncommon Colorectal Tumors

Lymphoma

Lymphoma is uncommon in the colon/rectum, occurring in 0.4% of patients; intestinal lymphoma can present anywhere between the second and eighth decades of life and almost all are non-Hodgkin lymphomas. Twenty-five percent of patients may present with fever, occult blood loss, anemia, a palpable mass, or an acute abdomen. A history of abdominal pain, fever, and weight loss in a patient who is younger than the expected age for a colorectal tumor should raise the suspicion of intestinal lymphoma.

Abdominal CT and endoscopy with biopsy are the most useful diagnostic tests. A thickened bowel segment, adjacent organ extension, or nodal enlargement may be seen. If the lesion is intraluminal, endoscopic biopsy will facilitate the diagnosis. Most of these lesions are intermediate- to high-grade B-cell lymphomas. If a diagnosis is made preoperatively in an otherwise asymptomatic patient, bone marrow biopsy should be performed. A primary lesion is defined as a lesion with no associated organ or lymphatic involvement, negative chest CT, and a negative peripheral blood smear and bone marrow biopsy.

Surgery is performed in the clinical setting of obstruction, bleeding, perforation, or an uncertain diagnosis. In rare cases, surgery may be performed for complete resection of a primary lesion. A thorough exploration is performed, and all suspicious nodes or organs are biopsied to assess the stage of disease. The primary intestinal lesion should be resected with negative margins whenever possible. The bowel mesentery should be resected with the tumor so regional nodes can be assessed pathologically. Intestinal continuity should be restored whenever possible. If a large tumor is found to be unresectable and is obstructing the bowel, a bypass can be performed. Surgical clips should be placed to facilitate identification of the tumor by the radiation oncologist.

Intestinal lymphoma is mainly treated by chemotherapy, with or without radiation, and surgery is performed to avoid complications. For rectal lymphoma, complete resection is followed by external beam radiation to the pelvis. Chemoradiation is used if the resection was incomplete. The OS for stage I and II diseases is approximately 80%. This decreases to 35% with advanced disease.

Gastrointestinal Stromal Tumors

Gastrointestinal stromal tumors (GISTs) account for most mesenchymal tumors arising in the wall of the colon or rectum. Primary colorectal GISTs are rare and comprise less than 1% of colonic tumors. GISTs have recently been characterized and historically classified as leiomyomas, leiomyosarcomas, neurofibromas, and schwannomas and are further discussed in Chapter 6, Soft Tissue and Bone Sarcoma. In a review of 1,458 cases of malignant GISTs from 1992 to 2000 in the SEER database, 7% were located in the colon and 5% in the rectum. These tumors can present as small submucosal lesions or as large intramural masses. Patients can present with pain, bleeding, obstruction, nausea, vomiting, anemia, tenesmus, or hematuria. Ulceration may be present in 30% to 50% of patients. A thorough clinical evaluation should be conducted to exclude metastatic disease. Significant prognostic factors for GISTs include mitotic index of activity, tumor location, and tumor size. Excision with negative surgical margins represents the mainstay of treatment. Colonic tumors are excised with adjacent mesentery. Extended nodal excision is not indicated in the absence of clinically evident disease. Small tumors of the rectum and anal canal can be removed transrectally or endoscopically. Abdominoperineal resection should be considered in patients with high-risk or large low-risk rectal GISTs. Criteria similar to GISTs elsewhere in the GI tract, are used for determining the need for adjuvant therapy with imatinib mesylate (STI-571, Gleevec), a monoclonal antibody to the tyrosine kinase receptor.

Neuroendocrine Tumors

Neuroendocrine tumors classified as low grade (carcinoid) or high grade are uncommonly found in the colon and rectum. Approximately 18% to 30% of intestinal carcinoids occur in the rectum or rectosigmoid, 4% to 15% occur in the colon, and 4% to 50% have been reported to occur in the appendix. They are usually discovered incidentally unless they are large. After histologic grade, size and depth of invasion are the best predictors of clinical behavior. A commonly used grading system for neuroendocrine tumors is based on the degree of formation of glandular structures, nuclear pleomorphism, and number of mitoses. Grade 1 tumors have the most developed glandular structures with the fewest mitoses, grade 3 is the least differentiated with a high incidence of mitoses, and grade 2 is intermediate between grades 1 and 3. Hindgut carcinoids are almost never biochemically active and therefore do not cause carcinoid syndrome. Although large tumors may present with bleeding, obstruction, or constipation, tumors less than 2 cm are frequently asymptomatic. Diagnosis is made by endoscopic biopsy. In general, tumors less than 1 cm rarely metastasize, with some reports noting rates as low as 2%, whereas those greater than 2 cm have increased metastatic potential between 60% and 80%; in the 1- to 2-cm range, 10% to 20% will metastasize. This makes treatment decisions for tumors in the 1- to 2-cm range challenging. Small lesions (<1 cm) are commonly well differentiated and can be adequately treated with endoscopic excision. Lesions less than 2 cm can be treated with full-thickness local excision. High-grade tumors have a poorer overall prognosis, with 5-year survival for high-grade rectal NETs approximating 32% for grade 3 compared to 91% for grade 1. For this reason, the role of radical resection as well as of any neoadjuvant chemo/chemoradiation therapy must be deliberated in a coordinated and multidisciplinary fashion.

Anal Cancer

Epidemiology and Etiology

Approximately 9,000 new cases and 1,400 deaths from anal cancer occur annually in the United States. Although anal carcinoma has been considered an uncommon cancer, the incidence in the United States has increased by 2.7% for women between 2000 and 2015 and 1.1% for men between 200 and 2018. According to data obtained from the HIV/AIDS Cancer Match Study, between 1980 and 2005, HIV had a strong impact on the incidence of anal cancer in man, with incidence rates being increased by 3.4% annually in men with HIV, compared to 1.7% of those men without HIV during that same time period. Other causes of immunocompromise such as transplantation or immunotherapy for autoimmune diseases are additional risk factors. Kidney transplant patients have at least a fourfold increased incidence of the disease. In the general population, elderly women and men in their 60s are at the highest risk for anal cancer, with women having the greater risk.

Population-based evidence has established that anal cancer is a sexually transmitted disease (STD) in much the same way that cervical cancer is an STD. Women with anal cancer are more likely to have had a history of genital warts or other STDs, and men with anal cancer are more likely to have reported homosexual activity or to have had a history of genital warts or gonorrhea. As with cervical cancer, anal cancer has been linked to human papillomavirus (especially HPV-16 and HPV-18) infection. Studies have shown that 40% to 95% of anal cancers harbor HPV DNA, with the strongest association seen with nonkeratinizing squamous cell types originating from the squamous mucosa of the anal canal. This association has proven to be even stronger with advances in HPV detection techniques showing the presence of HPV-16 and HPV-18 in up to 88% of patients with anal carcinoma.

The national cancer registries in Denmark and Sweden identified 417 patients with anal cancer between 1991 and 1994 and compared them with 534 controls with rectal adenocarcinoma and 554 population controls. Using multivariate analysis while adjusting for smoking and education, this study found that in women, the lifetime number of sexual partners especially those with STDs, a history of anal intercourse, a history of anogenital warts, gonorrhea, or cervical neoplasia, and testing for HIV were associated with a significantly increased risk for anal cancer. Risk factors for men included lifetime number of sexual partners, homosexuality, history of anal warts or syphilis, and being unmarried with or without a current sexual partner. The associations were similar when data from Denmark and Sweden were considered separately or together. When polymerase chain reaction for HPV DNA was performed on archived tissue specimens from these patients, 88% of patients overall were positive for HPV, with 83% HPV-16 positive. In comparison, HPV-16 is responsible for about 50% of cervical cancer cases, and additional HPV types such as HPV 18, 31, and 45 are responsible for an additional 30%. Analysis of the data from the SEER program revealed that the relative risks of anal cancer in women who had been diagnosed with invasive cervical cancer was 4.6 when compared to general population. This increased risk for anal cancer in women with cervical dysplasia or cancer, and their sexual partners, is likely through autoinoculation by the virus that caused the cervical dysplasia.

Anal cancers can be located within the anal canal or in the perianal skin (anal margin). Anal canal cancers are three to four times more common in women than in men. Anal margin cancers (tumors of the hair-bearing perianal skin) are more common in males. There are significantly more cases of anal margin cancers in homosexual males.

Pathologic Characteristics

More than 60% of malignant anal lesions are histologically SCCs. With the exception of melanoma, small cell carcinoma, and anal adenocarcinoma, all other histologic subtypes behave similarly and are treated according to their anatomical location. Basaloid carcinoma (basal cell carcinoma with a massive squamous component), mucoepidermoid carcinoma (originating in anal crypt glands), and cloacogenic carcinoma are all variants of squamous carcinoma. As with cervical cancer, SCC of the anus may be preceded by or coexist with premalignant dysplasia or anal intraepithelial neoplasia (AIN).

The prognosis of anal margin cancers is favorable. The rate of local recurrence is higher than the rate of distant metastases, which are rare. When they do occur, metastases are most commonly found in the superficial inguinal lymph nodes (approximately 15% of cases). It is unusual for anal margin cancers to metastasize to mesenteric or internal iliac nodes.

Anal canal cancers are associated with aggressive local growth and if untreated will extend to the rectal mucosa and submucosa, subcutaneous perianal tissue and perianal skin, ischiorectal fat, local skeletal muscle, perineum, genitalia, lower urinary system, and the broad ligament. Historically, mesenteric lymph node metastases have been detected in 30% to 50% of surgical specimens. More than 50% of patients will present with locally advanced disease. The most common sites of distant metastases are the liver, lung, and abdominal cavity. However, most cancer-related morbidities are due to uncontrolled pelvic or perineal disease.

Diagnosis

The initial symptoms of anal cancer include bleeding, pain, local fullness, and other symptoms consistent with a malignant fistula. The more common benign anal diseases, which accompany anal cancer in more than 50% of cases, can present with similar symptoms. A detailed history, including previous anal pathology and sexual habits, should precede a meticulous physical examination. Physical examination should attempt to identify the lesion, its size and anatomical boundaries, and any associated scarring or condylomata. It is also important to determine the resting and voluntary anal sphincter tone. Occasionally, an examination under general anesthesia may be necessary to complete the local evaluation. Cross-sectional imaging of the chest, abdomen, and pelvis is important in assessing extent of local disease and distant spread. Proctosigmoidoscopy is essential to assess the proximal extent of disease and to obtain tissue for biopsy. Palpable inguinal lymph nodes should be evaluated by fine-needle aspiration. PET–CT may be helpful in the workup for lesions in the anal canal to evaluate for distant metastases.

| TABLE 13.10 | American Joint Committee on Cancer Staging of Anal Cancer |

Primary Tumor (T)

TX	Primary tumor cannot be assessed
T0	No evidence of primary tumor
Tis	High-grade squamous intraepithelial lesion
T1	Tumor no larger than 2 cm
T2	Tumor >2 cm but ≤5 cm
T3	Tumor > 5 cm
T4	Tumor of any size invading other organs (urethra, bladder, vagina, etc.)

Regional Lymph Nodes (N)

NX	Regional lymph nodes cannot be assessed
N0	No regional lymph node metastasis
N1	Metastasis to inguinal, mesorectal, internal iliac, or external iliac nodes
N1a	Metastasis in inguinal, mesorectal, or internal iliac lymph nodes
N1b	Metastasis in external iliac lymph nodes
N1c	Metastasis in external iliac lymph nodes with any N1a nodes

Distant Metastases (M)

MX	Distant metastasis cannot be assessed
M0	No distant metastasis
M1	Distant metastases present

Stage	T	N	M
0	Tis	N0	M0
I	T1	N0	M0
IIA	T2	N0	M0
IIIA	T1–T3	N1	M0
IIB	T3	N0	M0
IIIB	T4	N0	M0
IIIC	T3–T4	N1	M0
IV	Any T	Any N	M1

Staging

The current AJCC staging system for anal margin and anal canal cancers is depicted in Table 13.10.

Treatment

Anal Canal

Until the 1980s, APR with permanent colostomy was the recommended treatment for all SCCs of the anal canal. This treatment, however, was associated with low survival rates as a result of distant failure. Radiation therapy in the range of 50 to 60 Gy was also used as definitive treatment of these cancers, with recurrence and survival rates similar to those seen using APR. The pioneering chemoradiation protocol developed by Nigro et al. (1974), which has since been confirmed and modified by others, radically changed the approach to this disease.

Currently, well-differentiated anal margin lesions characterized as T1N0 are treated with wide local excision to grossly negative margins. For anal canal tumors, surgical intervention is reserved for the following indications: (a) APR for salvage treatment in patients with persistent disease (within 6 months of chemoradiation) or recurrent disease (after 6 months); (b) APR or exenerative procedures for severely symptomatic patients (perineal sepsis, intractable urinary or fecal fistulae, and intolerable incontinence); (c) inguinal lymph node dissection for persistent inguinal disease, recurrent inguinal disease (treated first with radiation therapy unless associated with local recurrence), or for bulky or fungating or symptomatic primary disease in the inguinal basin; and (d) palliative fecal diversion in patients with obstructing, fistulizing, nearly obstructing lesions.

TABLE 13.11	Current and Classic Treatment Protocols for Anal Canal Cancer
Current	External beam radiation therapy 5 d/wk for total dose of 45–55 Gy
	5-FU, 250 mg/m²/day, M–F for the entire duration of radiation
	Cisplatin, 4 g/m²/day, M–F for the entire duration of radiation
Classic	5-FU, 750–1,000 mg/m² over 24-hour continuous IV infusion
Days 1–4	Mitomycin C, 10–15 mg/m², IV bolus
Day 1	Radiation therapy 5 d/wk for total dose of 45–55 Gy; boosts of up to 60 Gy may be given to the anus and/or
Days 1–35	inguinal basins 5-FU, 5-fluorouracil; IV, intravenous
Days 29–32	5-FU, 750–1,000 mg/m² over 24-hour continuous IV infusion

5-FU, 5-fluorouracil; IV, intravenous.

Since the initial work of Nigro et al. (1974), studies have been performed to dissect out the vital components and doses of the chemoradiation in order to optimize treatment. There is evidence that (a) higher doses of radiation produce better local control rates using a constant mitomycin-C dose (Rich, 1997); (b) 5-FU and mitomycin-C with radiation therapy produces better local control rates than radiation therapy alone; (c) 5-FU and mitomycin-C with radiation therapy produces better local control rates than 5-FU alone with radiation therapy; and (d) 5-FU and cisplatin with radiation therapy produces local control and survival rates similar to 5-FU, mitomycin-C, and radiation therapy with less toxicity. The randomized intergroup RTOG 98-11 trial investigated the use of mitomycin or cisplatin with 5-FU–based chemoradiation therapy in patients with SCC of the anus. Patients were randomly assigned to receive either concurrent chemoradiation therapy with 5-FU/mitomycin or induction chemotherapy with 5-FU and cisplatin for two cycles followed by concurrent chemoradiation therapy with 5-FU/cisplatin. No significant differences were seen in 5-year OS or DFS. Moreover, the colostomy rate was significantly increased in the cisplatin-containing arm. However, the mitomycin arm of this study was compared the cisplatin arm which included both induction chemotherapy and chemoradiation. Therefore, the trial has been criticized with respect to its generalizability to all cisplatin-based strategies. The phase 3 UK ACT II trial was designed to compare 5-FU/mitomycin to 5-FU/cisplatin with concurrent radiation of 50.4 Gy with or without additional systemic chemotherapy. No significant difference was observed in 5-year colostomy-free survival rates among any of the four arms. Additionally, these investigators showed that the optimal time for assessing clinical response to chemoradiation was 26 weeks after its initiation.

The current regimen for primary treatment of SCC of the anal canal is chemoradiation therapy (Table 13.11). At MDACC we utilize a 5-FU and cisplatin-based chemoradiation protocol because of decreased toxicity and similar response, survival, and colostomy data. Complete responses with this treatment can be expected in up to 90% of patients, with 5-year survival rates approaching 85%.

The presence of a persistent mass on examination 12 to 14 weeks after chemoradiation is an indication for biopsy given that a persistent mass after therapy will demonstrate cancer on biopsy in 18% to 34% of cases. The timing of the assessment for determining whether there is persistent disease is critical. There are reports of positive biopsy results taken at 6 to 8 weeks after therapy (persistent disease) reverting to negative biopsy results when taken later in patients who refused surgery. This implies that there may be a delayed radiation effect for up to several months after treatment. At MDACC, we do not routinely obtain a biopsy specimen of the treated tumor site unless gross abnormalities are present; the first assessment occurs at approximately 8 weeks after completing chemoradiation but up to 24 weeks is given before operating on persistent disease.

Patients with persistent or locally recurrent disease are typically salvaged with APR with or without adjacent organ resection, with a resultant 50% 5-year survival. Additionally, cisplatin-based chemotherapy with re-irradiation therapy has been used successfully to salvage up to one-third of patients with recurrent disease.

Anal Margin

SCC of the perianal skin is defined currently by the AJCC as a lesion originating in an area between the anal margin and 5 cm in any direction onto the perianal skin and is classified with skin tumors. The terms anal margin and perianal skin have often been used synonymously, but the most recent AJCC staging manual classifies these tumors as perianal cancers. Note that the data supporting the treatment of these uncommon, heterogeneous lesions derive from small, single-institution, mostly retrospective studies. Moreover, many of these studies include lesions of the lower anal canal (dentate line to anal verge) that were included previously in older definitions of the anal margin. The rationale for any modality of therapy derives from the proportional increase in chance of metastases with increasing tumor size; in tumors less than 2 cm, lymph node metastases are rarely found. For lesions between 2 and 5 cm, and those greater than 5 cm, the rates are 24% and 25% to 67%, respectively.

Small (<2 cm), superficial T1, well-differentiated anal margin cancers that do not invade the sphincter complex can be treated by a negative-margin wide local excision alone, with a 5-year survival rate greater than 80%. Wide local excision may include parts of the superficial internal and external anal sphincters without compromising anal continence. Positive margins can be re-excised or considered for treatment with radiation therapy with or without 5-FU–based chemotherapy.

Larger T2 to T4 or N-positive lesions are best treated with multimodality therapy using chemoradiation, as in anal canal cancers, given the higher local recurrence rate. Inclusion of bilateral inguinal/low pelvic nodal regions in the radiation field should be considered. Lymph node dissection is reserved for those patients with residual or recurrent disease. It is not known whether the treatment of inguinal disease translates into improved survival. Patients with T3 to T4 and poor sphincter function may require APR. For all patients, the 5-year disease-specific survival is 71% to 88%, and the local control rate after initial therapy is 70% to 100%. Platinum-based chemotherapy is recommended for metastatic disease.

Surveillance

Patients should be followed for detection of local and systemic failures and treatment complications. Local inspection, digital examination, and anoscopy are recommended between 8 and 12 weeks after chemoradiation treatment and every 3 to 6 months for 5 years. A biopsy is performed only if gross disease is suspected after serial digital examinations. Biopsy-proven persistent disease should be re-evaluated in 8 to 12 weeks, and if regression is seen, continued observation and re-evaluation in 3-month intervals with yearly CT scans is appropriate. If there is no regression or there is progression of disease, the patient should be restaged and APR offered if the disease is locoregional. Distant failures of epidermoid cancer are responsive to radiation therapy, and up to 30% of patients respond to second-line chemotherapy. Therefore, at a minimum, chest radiography, transaminases, serum bilirubin, coagulation markers, and pelvic CT are recommended every 6 to 12 months for 2 to 3 years after initial therapy. Patients with anal margin cancers should have careful, close follow-up, given the indolent nature of these tumors and the benefits of further local therapy.

Anal Intraepithelial Neoplasia

AIN is a term used to describe squamous intraepithelial lesions (SILs) of the anus. This is an increasingly prevalent condition associated with HPV infection and condylomata that can occur both externally on the perianal skin and internally within the anal canal. Dysplasia in SILs may be low grade or high grade (HSIL); the latter is an intermediate stage in the malignant transformation to SCC of the anus. Anal HSIL represents cytopathologic and histopathologic findings that had been referred to as AIN II/III, severe dysplasia, carcinoma in situ, or Bowen disease, in the past. The presence of HPV infection is the principal risk factor for anal neoplasia. Cofactors include anal-receptive intercourse and immunocompromise. Paralleling observations in the cervix, infection by oncogenic strains of HPV are causally related to the development of the precursor lesion, HSIL, and later of anal cancer. Under the microscope, cervical SIL and anal SIL are virtually indistinguishable. The anatomical region at risk includes the anal transition zone and the distal rectum extending up to 8 cm proximal to the dentate line where immature squamous metaplastic cells are the most susceptible to oncogenic HPV, although the nonkeratinizing and keratinizing squamous epithelium of the surrounding tissues are also susceptible. There is also morphologic and histologic similarity between cervical and anal cancers.

The populations at greatest risk for AIN are the same as those for anal cancer. Natural history studies have demonstrated that in HIV-negative men who have sex with men (MSM), the 4-year incidence of HSIL was 17%. It is higher in HIV-positive men, with receptive anal intercourse, the presence of condylomata, multiplicity of HPV serotype infections, injection drug abuse, cigarette smoking, depressed host immunity, and the presence of cervical, vulvar, or penile neoplasia.

Treatment

Patients with anal SIL often present with minor complaints related to anal condylomata, hemorrhoids, or pruritus ani. Physical examination may reveal anything from typical condylomatous lesions to normal-appearing anal and rectal mucosa. The perianal skin and the entire surgical anal canal, as defined by the AJCC and by the World Health Organization, as extending through the length of the internal anal sphincter from the anal verge (2 to 4 cm in women, up to 6 cm in men), should be thoroughly examined. The application of dilute acetic acid allows lesions in the distal rectum, anal canal, and keratinized skin to become more visible. The use of high-resolution anoscopy has also been advocated.

Patients with LSIL typically do not need treatment but should be followed by high-resolution anoscopy every 6 months. Patients with low-volume HSIL external to the anal canal and no history of dysplasia may be treated with topical agents in the office, regardless of risk factors, with surveillance anoscopy. Eradication of dysplasia can be achieved with topical cytokine stimulator imiquimod (Aldara) or antimetabolite 5-FU (Efudex). Patients with large-volume disease are treated in the operating room with a combination of excisional biopsy or cautery destruction under monitored anesthetic care with a standard perianal block. This can be achieved with infrared coagulation (IRC) and photodynamic therapy (PDT). "Mapping" of the lesions can be performed and is a strategy that is safe and well tolerated and has been shown to eradicate HSIL in HIV-negative patients. In HIV-positive patients, recurrence is high and treatment may need to be repeated; however, with close follow-up, transformation to invasive cancer can be prevented.

Bowen Disease

Bowen disease is an intraepithelial SCC (carcinoma in situ or intraepithelial high-grade dysplasia) that develops most commonly in middle-aged women and is often discovered during histologic evaluation of an anal specimen obtained for an unrelated diagnosis. The lesion is raised, irregular, scaly, and plaque like, with eczematoid features. Histologically, large atypical haloed cells (Bowenoid cells) are seen that stain periodic-acid–Schiff negative. Although it has previously been believed to have an association with other invasive carcinomas, the evidence for this is weak. The risk of progression to invasive cancer has been reported to be approximately 10%. Bowen disease has traditionally been treated with random biopsies and wide excision with flap reconstruction. However, even if normal tissue is sacrificed to obtain clear margins, the recurrence rate is 23%, and the patient may still be at risk for cancer development. This aggressive approach is associated with complications such as anal stenosis and fecal incontinence. Thus, the extent of excision is typically only to grossly normal tissue.

Bowen disease is histologically and immunohistochemically indistinguishable from anal HSIL and has also been associated with HPV infection. There is increasing agreement that Bowen disease and anal HSIL should be treated in a similar fashion. Local recurrence may occur, but re-excision provides excellent local control. Other therapeutic modalities include topical 5-FU cream, topical imiquimod, PDT, radiation therapy, laser therapy, and combinations of these. Published reports are generally small series with limited follow-up, but there has been anecdotal success with each approach, and all options should be considered for challenging cases.

Paget Disease

Paget disease is an intraepithelial adenocarcinoma that occurs mostly in elderly women. The lesion (a well-demarcated, eczematoid plaque) is usually characteristic; however, morphologic variations can occur, making the diagnosis difficult by inspection alone. The diagnosis is made histologically by the presence of large, vacuolated Paget cells, which stain periodic-acid–Schiff positive (from high mucin content). There is some evidence for the association of perianal Paget disease with other invasive carcinomas, but this relationship is not as strong as that seen with Paget disease of the breast. Invasion can develop in these lesions, and the prognosis is poor in those cases. Perianal Paget disease should be treated with wide local excision.

Anal Melanoma

Primary melanoma of the anus or rectum is a rare tumor, accounting for 0.4% to 1.6% of all melanomas and less than 1.0% of all anal canal tumors. The overall prognosis for patients with anorectal melanoma is very poor. Several reports in the literature have shown 5-year survival rates that are less than 25% and the median survival time is about 15 months. Mucosal melanoma is further discussed in Chapter 3. This discussion focuses on anal melanoma.

Pathologic Characteristics

The primary tumor may arise from the skin of the anal verge or the transitional epithelium of the anal canal. Inguinal nodal metastases are common at presentation. Prognosis is related to tumor thickness, as with cutaneous melanomas.

Diagnosis

Patients most commonly present with rectal bleeding. The incidental finding of a mass on digital examination may also lead to a workup that establishes the diagnosis. Melanoma may be an incidental pathologic finding after hemorrhoidectomy. Physical examination should include evaluation of the rectal mass and palpation of the inguinal nodes. Radiographic staging should be performed as for melanomas elsewhere.

Treatment

Historically, APR has been the treatment of choice, but high failure rates have called into question the benefit of this radical approach. Wide local excision with at least 2 cm of normal surrounding tissue and sentinel lymph node biopsy of the inguinal lymph nodes is now performed whenever possible, reserving APR for large bulky tumors that cannot be locally excised. Therapeutic inguinal node dissection or external radiation therapy is indicated for nodal disease. Using this approach with hypofractionated adjuvant radiation therapy (30 Gy in five fractions) to the primary site and nodal beds, MDACC has reported a 5-year actuarial survival of 31%, local control rate of 74%, and a nodal control rate of 84% in 23 patients after a median follow-up of 32 months. Patients presenting with unresectable disease can be treated with neoadjuvant chemo/immunotherapy. Responders can be offered transanal excision or APR with postoperative radiation therapy with or without additional chemotherapy. Nonresponders can be offered palliative surgery.

Anal Adenocarcinoma

Adenocarcinoma of the anal canal is a rare malignancy representing less than 20% of all anal cancers with limited data regarding treatment and outcomes. In a recent retrospective consecutive cohort study at MDACC, the OS and recurrence outcomes were evaluated in 34 patients identified with anal adenocarcinoma. Six patients underwent palliative treatment, and in the remaining 28 patients, 13 (46%) were treated with local excision followed by radiotherapy or chemoradiotherapy. Fifteen patients (54%) underwent radical surgery and neoadjuvant or adjuvant chemoradiotherapy. Median DFS was 13 months after local excision and 32 months after radical surgery. OS at 5 years was 43% for patients treated with local excision and 63% for patients treated with radical surgery. High risk for distant failure emphasizes the need for effective adjuvant therapy regimens. Recently, a retrospective study was conducted using the National Cancer Database (NCDB) to analyze outcomes of 1,729 patients with anal adenocarcinoma from 2004 to 2015. The study found that patients treated without surgery had worse OS, with a median OS of 45 months compared to 87 months for those who did receive surgery. Additionally, 5-year survival was 42% in the nonsurgical cohort and 55% in the surgical cohort.

CASE SCENARIO

Case Scenario 1

Presentation

A 45-year-old African American male presents with abdominal pain, nausea, and vomiting over the past 3 days. He has not passed flatus in the past 24 hours, and he has no prior history of colonoscopy or surgery. The patient notes a family history of a brother diagnosed with colon cancer 5 years ago at the age of 48 years. On examination, his abdomen is moderately distended, and he is severely tender to palpation. Computed tomography of the abdomen and pelvis reveals an obstructing mass in the rectum. Given his age and presentation, he is taken to the operating room for a laparoscopic diverting loop colostomy. Following the surgery and an uncomplicated postoperative course, the patient arrives to your surgical oncology office for further workup and management.

Confirmation of Diagnosis and Treatment

During workup, the patient is found to have a CEA of 2.1, and rigid proctoscopy shows an obstructing mass 7 cm from the anal verge. Tissue diagnosis is obtained and sent to pathology, confirming moderately differentiated rectal adenocarcinoma. Pelvic MRI is obtained, showing a T4b, N1b tumor 5 cm in cranio-caudal length with invasion of the CRM. The patient is then discussed at multidisciplinary tumor board and referred to medical and radiation oncology for total neoadjuvant therapy prior to definitive resection.

Surgical Approach—Key Steps

Diverting colostomy is typically able to be completed laparoscopically in patients without an extensive prior abdominal surgical history. The patient should be evaluated by an enterostomal therapist and marked prior to diversion. After lateral mobilization of the colon a fascial and skin defect able to accommodate two fingers is formed and the colon is delivered through this defect. After closure of any port sites or laparotomy incision as needed, a colotomy is made and the colostomy is matured ensuring that the full extent of the mucosa is above the level of the skin. Use of an ostomy rod or skin bridge is left to the surgeon's discretion.

Common Curve Balls

- Synchronous colon cancers should be considered and ruled out if possible prior to definitive surgical intervention. This may require colonoscopy through the patient's diverting colostomy.
- Sigmoid colon will not reach to the level of the skin necessitating a transverse colostomy.
- Distance from anal verge should be confirmed by operating surgeon along with potential involvement of surrounding structures including the anal sphincters.

Take Home Points

- Patients with a first-degree relative diagnosed with CRC ≤60 are considered to be at higher risk and undergo screening colonoscopy beginning at age 40 years or 10 years prior to age of youngest affected immediate family member and every 5 years thereafter. See Table 13.4 for full screening guidelines.
- Locally advanced rectal cancer is managed in a multidisciplinary fashion and treated with neoadjuvant therapy prior to resection.

Case Scenario 2

Presentation

A 51-year-old Caucasian female presents to her PCP for routine examination. History and physical examination are unremarkable except for no prior colonoscopy and labs consistent with iron-deficiency anemia. Patient is promptly referred to an endoscopist for further workup. At the time of colonoscopy, the patient is found to have a tubular adenoma 2 cm in size in the ascending colon. The polyp is removed via endoscopic mucosal resection, but in a piecemeal fashion. Pathology is reported to be notable for high-grade dysplasia.

Confirmation of Diagnosis and Treatment

As a part of staging workup, the patient undergoes a CT scan of the chest, abdomen, and pelvis showing a 3-cm intraluminal mass in the ascending colon and a 1-cm mass in the left lobe of the liver, concerning for metastasis. Baseline labs notable for CEA of 15.1 and Hgb of 9.5. CT of the abdomen and pelvis with liver protocol is obtained and demonstrates a single, resectable left-sided liver lesion. After multidisciplinary discussion the patient undergoes four cycles of neoadjuvant FOLFOX followed by synchronous resection of their primary tumor and liver metastasis.

Surgical Approach—Key Steps

For synchronous lesions undergoing resection during a single operation, any hepatectomy is typically performed first under volume-restricted anesthesia protocols. Both surgical teams as well as anesthesia should discuss resection of the primary lesion prior to undertaking its resection. Intraoperative complications including extended operative time, unexpected blood loss, or hemodynamic instability should lead to strong consideration for a staged resection. Colectomy or proctectomy should be performed following a standard resection and lymphadenectomy. In selected centers, a minimally invasive approach can be considered but should not jeopardize a complete oncologic resection.

Common Curve Balls

- Synchronous resection should only be considered in medically fit patients with clearly resectable liver metastases.
- Peritoneal disease found at the time of operation should be considered in light of the patient's overall disease state, biology, and extent of peritoneal disease. Data on synchronous resections are limited.

Take Home Points

- Following piece-meal resection of adenoma, surveillance colonoscopy is indicated within 2 to 6 months to verify complete excision of polyp.
- Multidisciplinary discussion between surgical services, oncologist, and patient is recommended for patients with resectable primary and metastatic disease, given the variety of approaches that are available.
- Surveillance following resection of pathologic stage II+ disease typically includes a combination of routine history and physical examinations, cross-sectional imaging, and serial laboratory measurements over the course of 5 years, with specific intervals noted in the surveillance section of this chapter.

CASE SCENARIO REVIEW

Questions

1. A 46-year-old patient with multiple family members with colon cancer at a young age, is concerned about the risk of colorectal cancer in his young adult children. He asks for recommendations for what test they should obtain for screening and when this should occur. What test would you recommend, and at what age should the patient's children receive it?

   A. FIT or FOBT at the age of 50 years
   B. Thorough H&P including DRE and CEA level at the age of 45 years
   C. Screening colonoscopy at the age of 35 years
   D. Flexible sigmoidoscopy with FIT/FOBT at the age of 45 years

2. A patient with a T4b N1 M0 rectal cancer 7 cm from the anal verge with circumferential margin involvement reports he would like his tumor resected as soon as possible. Given this patient's imaging and laboratory findings, what are the appropriate next steps for this patient?

   A. Surgical resection via low anterior resection (LAR), followed by adjuvant FOLFOX chemotherapy regimen for 12 to 16 weeks
   B. Neoadjuvant chemoradiation with capecitabine and long-course radiation followed by 12 to 16 weeks of systemic chemotherapy and subsequent surgical resection via LAR
   C. Surgical resection via abdominoperineal resection (APR), and adjuvant chemotherapy pending pathology results
   D. No surgery indicated at this time. Provide short-course radiation therapy (25 Gy in 5 days) and reassess for complete clinical response

3. Following a piecemeal polypectomy of a lesion with high-grade dysplasia, what is the recommended follow-up examination/procedure, and when should this take place?

   A. FIT/FOBT in conjunction with Flexible Sigmoidoscopy in 5 years
   B. Diagnostic colonoscopy in 3 to 5 years
   C. FIT/FOBT every year until repeat colonoscopy in 3 years
   D. Colonoscopy in 6 months to verify complete excision of polyp

4. What are the appropriate next steps in the management of a patient with a solitary colorectal liver metastasis in segment II and a right-sided primary tumor?

   A. Right hemicolectomy with intraoperative ultrasound of the liver followed by 2 to 3 months of adjuvant FOLFOX and staged hepatic resection
   B. Neoadjuvant CAPEOX, synchronous right hemicolectomy and partial lobectomy of liver, and adjuvant CAPEOX after surgical resection
   C. Synchronous right hemicolectomy and partial lobectomy of liver followed by adjuvant CAPEOX
   D. All of the above are acceptable treatment regimens

5. The patient tolerates the surgery and adjuvant therapy without any complications. Pathology confirms colonic adenocarcinoma in both the colon and liver specimens with negative margins. Following completion of her treatment regimen, she inquires how frequently she will need to follow up to identify any possible recurrences. What is the ideal surveillance regimen given her clinical history?

   A. Repeat colonoscopy at annual intervals following surgery for a total of 5 years
   B. History and physical every year for 2 years followed by CEA measurements every 6 months for the following 3 years
   C. CEA every 3 to 6 months for 2 years, then every 6 months for a total of 5 years along with concurrent CT CAP every 3 to 6 months for 2 years, then every 6 to 12 months for a total of 5 years
   D. Colonoscopy, CEA, and CT CAP every 6 months for a total of 5 years

Answers

1. **The correct answer is C**. *Rationale:* Per screening guidelines, average-risk patients would normally begin screening at age 45 ideally with a screening colonoscopy or flexible sigmoidoscopy with FIT/FOBT. For individuals with a first-degree relative with a diagnosed CRC, screening begins either at age

40 or 10 years prior to the diagnosis of the first-degree relative. In the case of this particular patient with a diagnosis of CRC at the age of 45, the patient's children should have initial screening at age 35.

2. **The correct answer is B.** *Rationale:* A, B, C: Per national consensus guidelines, a patient with locally invasive rectal cancer (T ≥ 3, node positive) and a threatened/involved CRM should receive total neoadjuvant therapy (chemoradiation followed by systemic chemotherapy or vice versa) and subsequent resection after restaging. Given this patient's presentation, immediate surgical resection via either LAR or APR should be delayed until after the patient receives neoadjuvant treatment.

   D: While the patient may be eligible for watch-and-wait management, the patient should ideally receive total neoadjuvant therapy (TNT) rather than only short-course radiation therapy (SCRT) prior to reassessment for complete clinical response (cCR). Compete clinical response is defined as no palpable tumor on digital rectal examination, no evidence of disease on cross-sectional imaging, and no visible pathology other than a flat scar on endoscopic examination. Following TNT and noted cCR, the decision to undergo this nonoperative management approach should only take place after a multidisciplinary discussion between the treatment team and the patient.

3. **The correct answer is D.** *Rationale:* A, B, C: Colonoscopy after 3 years would be indicated following polypectomy of polyp >1 cm in size, but not in a piece-meal fashion.

   D: Following polypectomy, for patients with tubular adenoma >1 cm in size, repeat colonoscopy within 2 to 6 months is indicated to verify complete excision of polyp. Colonoscopy would be indicated in 3 years if the polyp had been removed en bloc.

   Unfortunately, the patient is lost to follow-up. Several years later, she presents back to clinic with concern for fatigue, intermittent episodes of dizziness, and unintentional weight loss over the past year. The patient is taken to the endoscopic suite for a colonoscopy, during which an abnormal mass is found in the ascending colon. Photographs and biopsies are obtained, and tissue diagnosis confirms colon adenocarcinoma. The patient presents to your surgical oncology office for further management.

4. **The correct answer is D.** *Rationle:* Per national consensus guidelines, for patients with resectable synchronous liver (and/or lung metastases) only, patients can receive any of the above treatment regimens. The procedure can be staged or synchronous, and patients can receive neoadjuvant CAPEOX or FOLFOX. Almost all patients should receive adjuvant CAPEOX or FOLFOX—only patients with dMMR/MSI-H can receive nivolumab +/− ipilimumab or pembrolizumab.

   A, B, C: All of these are acceptable next steps for this patient. CAPEOX or FOLFOX is the preferred chemotherapy regimen, per national consensus guidelines. The variety of treatment options illustrates the importance of multidisciplinary discussions, particularly in patients such as this one with resectable primary and metastatic disease.

5. **The correct answer is C.** *Rationale:* As discussed in the section on surveillance, patients ideally receive cross-sectional imaging and laboratory measurements as a part of postresection surveillance. Per national consensus guidelines, for pathologic stage IV colon cancer patients, they are to obtain CT chest, abdomen, and pelvis every 3 to 6 months for 2 years followed by every 6 to 12 months for the next 3 years. At the same time, CEA measurements are obtained every 3 to 6 months for 2 years followed by every 6 months for the next 3 years.

Recommended Readings

Bruening W, Sullivan N, Paulson EC, et al. Imaging Tests for the Staging of Colorectal Cancer [Internet]. Rockville (MD): Agency for Healthcare Research and Quality (US); 2014 Sep.

Ng KS, Gonsalves SJ, Sagar PM. Ileal-anal pouches: a review of its history, indications, and complications. *World J Gastroenterol.* 2019;25(31):4320–4342.

Aarons CB, Shanmugan S, Bleier JI. Management of malignant colon polyps: current status and controversies. *World J Gastroenterol.* 2014;20(43):16178–16183.

Abdalla EK, Vauthey JN, Ellis LM, et al. Recurrence and outcomes following hepatic resection, radiofrequency ablation, and combined resection/ablation for colorectal liver metastases. *Ann Surg.* 2004;239(6):818–825, discussion 825–827.

Ajani JA, Winter KA, Gunderson LL, et al. Fluorouracil, mitomycin and radiotherapy vs. fluorouracil, cisplatin and radiotherapy for carcinoma of the anal canal. A randomized controlled trial. *JAMA.* 2008;299:1714–1721.

Ajani JA, Winter KA, Gunderson LL, et al. US Intergroup Anal Carcinoma Trial: tumor diameter predicts for colostomy. *J Clin Oncol.* 2009;27:1116–1121.

Al-Tassan N, Chmiel NH, Maynard J, et al. Inherited variants of MYH associated with somatic G:C→T:A mutations in colorectal tumors. *Nat Genet.* 2002;30(2):227–232.

André T, Meyerhardt J, Iveson T, et al. Effect of duration of adjuvant chemotherapy for patients with stage III colon cancer (IDEA collaboration): final results from a prospective, pooled analysis of six randomised, phase 3 trials. *Lancet Oncol.* 2020;21(12):1620–1629.

André T, Shiu KK, Kim TW, et al. Pembrolizumab in microsatellite-instability-high advanced colorectal cancer. *N Engl J Med.* 2020;383(23):2207–2218.

Baer, C, Menon R, Bastawrous S, Bastawrous A. Emergency presentations of colorectal cancer. *Surg Clin N Am.* 97 (2017) 529–545

Bahadoer RR, Dijkstra EA, van Etten B, et al; Short-course radiotherapy followed by chemotherapy before total mesorectal excision (TME) versus preoperative chemoradiotherapy, TME, and optional adjuvant chemotherapy in locally advanced rectal cancer (RAPIDO): a randomised, open-label, phase 3 trial. *Lancet Oncol.* 2021;22(1):29–42.

Ballo MT, Gershenwald JE, Zagars GK, et al. Sphincter-sparing local excision and adjuvant radiation for anal-rectal melanoma. *J Clin Oncol* 2002;20(23):4555–4558.

Bedrosian I, Rodriguez-Bigas MA, Feig B, et al. Predicting the node-negative mesorectum after preoperative chemoradiation for locally advanced rectal carcinoma. *J Gastrointest Surg* 2004;8(1):56–62, discussion 62–63.

Bertagnolli M, Miedema B, Redston M, et al. Sentinel node staging of resectable colon cancer: results of a multicenter study. *Ann Surg.* 2004;240(4):624–628, discussion 628–630.

Bertelsen CA, Neuenschwander AU, Jansen JE, et al; Danish Colorectal Cancer Group. Disease-free survival after complete mesocolic excision compared with conventional colon cancer surgery: a retrospective, population-based study. *Lancet Oncol.* 2015;16(2):161–168.

Body A, Prenen H, Latham S, et al. The role of neoadjuvant chemotherapy in locally advanced colon cancer. *Cancer Manag Res.* 2021;13:2567–2579.

Bonjer HJ, Deijen CL, Abis GA, et al. A randomized trial of laparoscopic versus open surgery for rectal cancer. *N Engl J Med.* 2015;372(14):1324–1332.

Bonnen M, Crane C, Vauthey JN, et al. Long-term results using local excision after preoperative chemoradiation among selected T3 rectal cancer patients. *Int J Radiat Oncol Biol Phys.* 2004;60(4):1098–1105.

Bouchard P, Efron J. Management of recurrent rectal cancer. *Ann Surg Oncol.* 2010;17(5);1343–1356

Bowne WB, Lee B, Wong WD, et al. Operative salvage for locoregional recurrent colon cancer after curative resection: an analysis of 100 cases. *Dis Colon Rectum.* 2005;48(5):897–909.

Brown S, Margolin DA, Altom LK, et al. Morbidity following coloanal anastomosis: a comparison of colonic J-pouch vs straight anastomosis. *Dis Colon Rectum.* 2018;61(2):156–161.

Burn J, Sheth H, Elliott F, et al; Cancer prevention with aspirin in hereditary colorectal cancer (Lynch syndrome), 10-year follow-up and registry-based 20-year data in the CAPP2 study: a double-blind, randomised, placebo-controlled trial. *Lancet.* 2020;395(10240):1855–1863.

Burt RW. Colon cancer screening. *Gastroenterology.* 2000;119(3):837–853.

COLOR II Study Group, Buunen M, Bonjer HJ, et al. Color II. A randomized trial comparing laparoscopic and open surgery for rectal cancer. *Dan Med Bull.* 2009;56:89–91.

Callender GG, Das P, Rodriguez-Bigas MA, et al. Local excision after preoperative chemoradiation results in an equivalent outcome to total mesorectal excision in selected patients with T3 rectal cancer. *Ann Surg Oncol.* 2010;17(2):441–447.

Cancer Genome Atlas N. Comprehensive molecular characterization of human colon and rectal cancer. *Nature.* 2012;487(7407):330–337.

Casadaban L, Rauscher G, Aklilu M, Villenes D, Freels S, Maker AV. Adjuvant chemotherapy is associated with improved survival in patients with stage II colon cancer. *Cancer.* 2016;122(21):3277–3287.

Cawthorn SJ, Parums DV, Gibbs NM, et al. Extent of mesorectal spread and involvement of lateral resection margin as prognostic factors after surgery for rectal cancer. *Lancet.* 1990;335(8697):1055–1059.

Chablaney S, Zator ZA, Kumta NA. Diagnosis and management of rectal neuroendocrine tumors. *Clin Endosc.* 2017;50(6):530–536.

Chang DZ, Kumar V, Ma Y, Li K, Kopetz S. Individualized therapies in CRC: KRAS as a marker for response to EGFR-targeted therapy. *J Hematol Oncol.* 2009;2:18.

Chang GJ, Berry JM, Jay N, Palefsky JM, Welton ML. Surgical treatment of high-grade anal squamous intraepithelial lesions: a prospective study. *Dis Colon Rectum.* 2002;45(4):453–458.

Chang GJ, Gonzalez RJ, Skibber JM, Eng C, Das P, Rodriguez-Bigas MA. A twenty-year experience with adenocarcinoma of the anal canal. *Dis Colon Rectum.* 2009;52(8):1375–1380.

Chang GJ, Rodriguez-Bigas MA, Skibber JM, Moyer VA. Lymph node evaluation and survival after curative resection of colon cancer: systematic review. *J Natl Cancer Inst.* 2007;99(6):433–441.

Chau I, Allen MJ, Cunningham D, et al. The value of routine serum carcino-embryonic antigen measurement and computed tomography in the surveillance of patients after adjuvant chemotherapy for CRC. *J Clin Oncol.* 2004;22(8):1420–1429.

Chesney TR, Nadler A, Acuna SA, Swallow CJ. Outcomes of resection for locoregionally recurrent colon cancer: a systematic review. *Surgery.* 2016;160:54–66

Church J, Simmang C. Practice parameters for the treatment of patients with dominantly inherited CRC (familial adenomatous polyposis and hereditary nonpolyposis CRC). *Dis Colon Rectum.* 2003;46(8):1001–1012.

Compton C, Fenoglio-Preiser CM, Pettigrew N, Fielding LP. American Joint Committee on Cancer Prognostic Factors Consensus Conference: Colorectal Working Group. *Cancer.* 2000;88(7):1739–1757.

Cooper HS. Pathologic issues in the treatment of endoscopically removed malignant colorectal polyps. *J Natl Compr Canc Netw.* 2007;5:991–996.

Cotton PB, Durkalski VL, Pineau BC, et al. Computed tomographic colonography (virtual colonoscopy): a multicenter comparison with standard colonoscopy for detection of colorectal neoplasia. *JAMA.* 2004;291(14):1713–1719.

Crane CH, Skibber JM, Birnbaum EH, et al. The addition of continuous infusion 5-FU to preoperative radiation therapy increases tumor response, leading to increased sphincter preservation in locally advanced rectal cancer. *Int J Radiat Oncol Biol Phys.* 2003;57(1):84–89.

Crane CH, Skibber JM, Feig BW, et al. Response to preoperative chemoradiation increases the use of sphincter-preserving surgery in patients with locally advanced low rectal carcinoma. *Cancer.* 2003;97(2):517–524.

Cunningham D, Humblet Y, Siena S, et al. Cetuximab monotherapy and cetuximab plus irinotecan in irinotecan-refractory metastatic CRC. *N Engl J Med.* 2004;351(4):337–345.

Das P, Crane CH. Staging, prognostic factors, and therapy of localized rectal cancer. *Curr Oncol Rep* 2009;11(3):167–174.

de Gramont A, Figer A, Seymour M, et al. Leucovorin and fluorouracil with or without oxaliplatin as first-line treatment in advanced CRC. *J Clin Oncol.* 2000;18(16):2938–2947.

de Haan MC, van Gelder RE, Graser A, Bipat S, Stoker J. Diagnostic value of CT-colonography as compared to colonoscopy in an asymptomatic screening population: a meta-analysis. *Eur Radiol.* 2011;21(8):1747–1763.

Di Nicolantonia F, Martini M, Molinari F, et al. Wild-type BRAF is required for response to panitumumab or cetuximab in metastatic CRC. *J Clin Oncol.* 2008;26:5705–5712.

Engstrand J, Nilsson H, Strömberg C, Jonas E, Freedman J. Colorectal cancer liver metastases—a population-based study on incidence, management and survival. *BMC Cancer.* 2018;18(1):78.

Enker WE. Sphincter-preserving operations for rectal cancer. *Oncology.* 1996;10(11):1673–1684, 1689, discussion 1690–1692.

Farouk R, Nelson H, Gunderson LL. Aggressive multimodality treatment for locally advanced irresectable rectal cancer. *Br J Surg.* 1997;84(6):741–749.

Filippi AR, Guerrera F, Badellino S, et al. Exploratory analysis on overall survival after either surgery or stereotactic radiotherapy for lung oligometastases from colorectal cancer. *Clin Oncol (R Coll Radiol).* 2016;28(8):505–512

Fisher B, Wolmark N, Rockette H, et al. Postoperative adjuvant chemotherapy or radiation therapy for rectal cancer: results from NSABP protocol R-01. *J Natl Cancer Inst.* 1988;80(1):21–29.

Fleshman J, Branda M, Sargent DJ, et al. Effect of laparoscopic-assisted resection vs open resection of stage II or III rectal cancer on pathologic outcomes the ACOSOG Z6051 randomized clinical trial. *JAMA.* 2015;314(13):1346–1355.

Fleshman J, Branda ME, Sargent DJ, et al. Disease-free survival and local recurrence for laparoscopic resection compared with open resection of stage II to III rectal cancer: follow-up results of the ACOSOG Z6051 randomized controlled trial. *Ann Surg*. 2019;269(4):589–595.

Frisch M, Glimelius B, Van Den Brule AJ, et al. Sexually transmitted infection as a cause of anal cancer. *N Engl J Med*. 1997;337(19):1350–1358.

Garcia-Aguilar J, Mellgren A, Sirivongs P, Buie D, Madoff RD, Rothenberger DA. Local excision of rectal cancer without adjuvant therapy: a word of caution. *Ann Surg*. 2000;231(3):345–351.

Gastrointestinal Tumor Study Group. Prolongation of the disease-free interval in surgically treated rectal carcinoma. *N Engl J Med*. 1985;312(23):1465–1472.

Gerard A, Buyse M, Nordlinger B, et al. Preoperative radiotherapy as adjuvant treatment in rectal cancer. Final results of a randomized study of the European Organization for Research and Treatment of Cancer (EORTC). *Ann Surg*. 1988;208(5):606–614.

Gill S, Sinicrope FA. CRC prevention: is an ounce of prevention worth a pound of cure? *Semin Oncol*. 2005;32(1):24–34.

Guillem JG, Chessin DB, Cohen AM, et al. Long-term oncologic outcome following preoperative combined modality therapy and total mesorectal excision of locally advanced rectal cancer. *Ann Surg*. 2005;241(5):829–836, discussion 836–838.

Guinney J, Dienstmann R, Wang X, et al. The consensus molecular subtypes of CRC. *Nat Med*. 2015;21(11):1350–1356.

Gunderson LL, Nelson H, Martenson JA, et al. Locally advanced primary CRC: intraoperative electron and external beam irradiation ± 5-FU. *Int J Radiat Oncol Biol Phys*. 1997;37(3):601–614.

Habr-Gama A, Perez RO, Nadalin W, et al. Operative versus nonoperative treatment for stage 0 distal rectal cancer following chemoradiation therapy: long-term results. *Ann Surg*. 2004;240(4):711–717, discussion 717–718.

Haggitt RC, Glotzbach RE, Soffer EE, Wruble LD. Prognostic factors in colorectal carcinomas arising in adenomas: implications for lesions removed by endoscopic polypectomy. *Gastroenterology*. 1985;89(2):328–336.

Hahnloser D, Haddock MG, Nelson H. Intraoperative radiotherapy in the multimodality approach to CRC. *Surg Oncol Clin N Am*. 2003;12(4):993–1013, ix.

Hall C, Clarke L, Pal A. A review of the role of carcinoembryonic antigen in clinical practice. *Ann Coloproctol*. 2019; 35(6):294–305

Hardiman K, Felder S, Friedman G. The American Society of Colon and Rectal Surgeons Clinical Practice Guidelines for the Surveillance and Survivorship Care of Patients After Curative Treatment of Colon and Rectal Cancer. *Dis Colon Rectum*. 2021;64:517–533.

Harewood GC. Assessment of publication bias in the reporting of EUS performance in staging rectal cancer. *Am J Gastroenterol*. 2005;100(4):808–816.

Havenga K, Enker WE. Autonomic nerve preserving total mesorectal excision. *Surg Clin North Am*. 2002;82(5):1009–1018.

Heald RJ, Ryall RD. Recurrence and survival after total mesorectal excision for rectal cancer. *Lancet*. 1986;1(8496):1479–1482.

Hida J, Yasutomi M, Maruyama T, Fujimoto K, Uchida T, Okuno K. Lymph node metastases detected in the mesorectum distal to carcinoma of the rectum by the clearing method: justification of total mesorectal excision. *J Am Coll Surg*. 1997;184(6):584–588.

Hohenberger W, Weber K, Matzel K, et al. Standardized surgery for colonic cancer: complete mesocolic excision and central ligation–technical notes and outcome. *Colorectal Dis*. 2009;11(4):354–364; discussion 364–365.

Hoots BE, Palefsky JM, Pimentz JM, Smith JS. Human papillomavirus type distinction in anal cancer and anal intraepithelial lesions. *Int J Cancer*. 2009;124:2375–2383.

Hueting WE, Buskens E, van der Tweel I, Gooszen HG, van Laarhoven CJ. Results and complications after ileal pouch anal anastomosis: a meta-analysis of 43 observational studies comprising 9,317 patients. *Dig Surg*. 2005;22:69–79

Ikoma N, You YN, Bednarski BK, et al. Impact of recurrence and salvage surgery on survival after multidisciplinary treatment of rectal cancer. *J Clin Oncol*. 2017;35(23):2631–2638.

James R, Wan S, Glynne-Jones D, et al. A randomized trial of chemoradiation using mitomycin or cisplatin with or without maintenance cisplatin/5-FU in squamous cell carcinoma of the anus. ACT II. *J Clin Oncol.* 2009;27:LBA4009.

Janney A, Powrie F, Mann EH. Host-microbiota maladaptation in colorectal cancer. *Nature.* 2020;585(7826):509–517.

Johnson CD, Chen MH, Toledano AY, et al. Accuracy of CT colonography for detection of large adenomas and cancers. *N Engl J Med.* 2008;359(12):1207.

Kaltenbach T, Anderson JC, Burke CA, et al. Endoscopic removal of colorectal lesions-recommendations by the US Multi-Society Task Force on Colorectal Cancer. *Gastroenterology.* 2020;158(4):1095–1129.

Kasi A, Abbasi S, Handa S, et al. Total neoadjuvant therapy vs standard therapy in locally advanced rectal cancer: a systematic review and meta-analysis. *JAMA Netw Open.* 2020;3(12):e2030097.

Kesmodel SB, Ellis LM, Lin E, et al. Preoperative bevacizumab does not significantly increase postoperative complication rates in patients undergoing hepatic surgery for CRC liver metastases. *J Clin Oncol.* 2008;26(32):5254–5260.

Kim NK, Kim YW, Han YD, et al. Complete mesocolic excision and central vascular ligation for colon cancer: principle, anatomy, surgical technique, and outcomes. *Surg Oncol.* 2016;25(3):252–262.

Kopetz S, Grothey A, Yaeger R, et al. Encorafenib, binimetinib, and cetuximab in BRAF V600E-mutated colorectal cancer. *N Engl J Med.* 2019;381(17):1632–1643.

Korner H, Soreide K, Stokkeland PJ, Söreide JA. Systematic follow-up after curative surgery for CRC in Norway: a population-based audit of effectiveness, costs, and compliance. *J Gastrointest Surg.* 2005;9(3):320–328.

Koura AN, Giacco GG, Curley SA, Skibber JM, Feig BW, Ellis LM. Carcinoid tumors of the rectum: effect of size, histopathology, and surgical treatment on metastasis-free survival. *Cancer.* 1997;79(7):1294–1298.

Kroon HM, Malakorn S, Dudi-Venkata NN, et al. Local recurrences in western low rectal cancer patients treated with or without lateral lymph node dissection after neoadjuvant (chemo)radiotherapy: an international multi-centre comparative study. *Eur J Surg Oncol.* 2021;47(9):2441–2449.

Kuebler JP, Wieand HS, O'Connell MJ, et al. Oxaliplatin combined with weekly bolus fluorouracil and leucovorin as surgical adjuvant chemotherapy for stage II and III colon cancer: results from NSABP C-07. *J Clin Oncol.* 2007;25:2198–2204.

Kwak JM, Kim SH. Robotic surgery for rectal cancer: an update in 2015. *Cancer Res Treat.* 2016;48(2):427–435.

Le Voyer TE, Sigurdson ER, Hanlon AL, et al. Colon cancer survival is associated with increasing number of lymph nodes analyzed: a secondary survey of intergroup trial INT-0089. *J Clin Oncol.* 2003;21(15):2912–2919.

Libutti SK, Alexander HR, Jr, Choyke P, et al. A prospective study of 2-[18F]fluoro-2-deoxy-D-glucose/positron emission tomography scan, 99mTc-labeled arcitumomab (CEA-scan), and blind second-look laparotomy for detecting colon cancer recurrence in patients with increasing carcinoembryonic antigen levels. *Ann Surg Oncol.* 2001;8(10):779–786.

Lightner, AL, Vogel JD, Carmichael JC. The American Society of Colon and Rectal Surgeons Clinical Practice Guidelines for the Surgical Management of Crohn's Disease. *Dis Colon Rectum.* 2020;63:1028–1052

Lowy AM, Rich TA, Skibber JM, Dubrow RA, Curley SA. Preoperative infusional chemoradiation, selective intraoperative radiation, and resection for locally advanced pelvic recurrence of colorectal adenocarcinoma. *Ann Surg.* 1996;223(2):177–185.

Mamounas E, Wieand S, Wolmark N, et al. Comparative efficacy of adjuvant chemotherapy in patients with Dukes' B versus Dukes' C colon cancer: results from four National Surgical Adjuvant Breast and Bowel Project adjuvant studies (C-01, C-02, C-03, and C-04). *J Clin Oncol.* 1999;17(5):1349–1355.

Menahem B, Alves A, Regimbeau JM, Sabbagh C. Lynch syndrome: current management in 2019. *J Visc Surg.* 2019;156:507–514.

Mendenhall WM, Zlotecki RA, Vauthey JN, Hochwald SN, Riggs CE, Mendenhall WM. Squamous cell carcinoma of the anal margin. *Oncology (Williston Park).* 1996;10(12):1843–1848, discussion 1848, 1853–1854.

MERCURY Study Group. Diagnostic accuracy of preoperative magnetic resonance imaging in predicting curative resection of rectal cancer: prospective observational study. *BMJ.* 2006;333:779–785.

Merg A, Lynch HT, Lynch JF, Howe JR. Hereditary colorectal cancer-part II. *Curr Probl Surg.* 2005;42(5):267–333.

Merg A, Lynch HT, Lynch JF, Howe JR. Hereditary colon cancer-part I. *Curr Probl Surg.* 2005;42(4):195–256.

Meterissian SH, Skibber JM, Giacco GG, El-Naggar AK, Hess KR, Rich TA. Pelvic exenteration for locally advanced rectal carcinoma: factors predicting improved survival. *Surgery.* 1997;121(5):479–487.

Meyerhardt JA, Mayer RJ. Systemic therapy for CRC. *N Engl J Med.* 2005; 352(5):476–487.

Meyerhardt JA, Tepper JE, Niedzwiecki D, et al. Impact of hospital procedure volume on surgical operation and long-term outcomes in high-risk curatively resected rectal cancer: findings from the Intergroup 0114 Study. *J Clin Oncol.* 2004;22(1):166–174.

Middleton PF, Sutherland LM, Maddern GJ. Transanal endoscopic microsurgery: a systematic review. *Dis Colon Rectum.* 2005;48(2):270–284.

Mirnezami R, Chang GJ, Das P. Intraoperative radiotherapy in colorectal cancer: systematic review and meta-analysis of techniques, long-term outcomes, and complications. *Surg Oncol.* 2013; 22(1):22–35.

Moertel CG, Fleming TR, Macdonald JS, et al. Levamisole and fluorouracil for adjuvant therapy of resected colon carcinoma. *N Engl J Med.* 1990;322(6):352–358.

Mohamed F, Kallioinen M, Braun M, Fenwick S, Shackcloth M, Davies RJ; Guideline Committee. Management of colorectal cancer metastases to the liver, lung or peritoneum suitable for curative intent: summary of NICE guidance. *Br J Surg.* 2020;107(8):943–945.

Molska M, Reguła J. Potential mechanisms of probiotics action in the prevention and treatment of colorectal cancer. *Nutrients.* 2019;11(10):2453.

Morton D. FOxTROT: An international randomised controlled trial in 1053 patients evaluating neoadjuvant chemotherapy (NAC) for colon cancer. On behalf of the FOxTROT Collaborative Group. *Annals of Oncology.* 2019;30:v198.

Nascimbeni R, Burgart LJ, Nivatvongs S, Larson DR. Risk of lymph node metastasis in T1 carcinoma of the colon and rectum. *Dis Colon Rectum.* 2002;45(2):200–206.

Nelson H, Petrelli N, Carlin A, et al. Guidelines 2000 for colon and rectal cancer surgery. *J Natl Cancer Inst.* 2001;93(8):583–596.

Neilson LJ, Rutter MD, Saunders BP, Plumb A, Rees CJ. Assessment and management of the malignant colorectal polyp. *Frontline Gastroenterol.* 2015;6(2):117–126.

Nigro ND, Vaitkevicius VK, Considine B, Jr. Combined therapy for cancer of the anal canal: a preliminary report. *Dis Colon Rectum.* 1974;17(3):354–356.

NIH Consensus Conference. Adjuvant therapy for patients with colon and rectal cancer. *JAMA.* 1990;264(11):1444–1450.

Nishihara R, Wu K, Lochhead P, et al. Long-term colorectal cancer incidence and mortality after lower endoscopy. *N Engl J Med.* 2013;369(12):1095–1105.

Nivatvongs S. Surgical management of malignant colorectal polyps. *Surg Clin North Am.* 2002;82(5):959–966.

O'Connell MJ, Martenson JA, Wieand HS, et al. Improving adjuvant therapy for rectal cancer by combining protracted-infusion fluorouracil with radiation therapy after curative surgery. *N Engl J Med.* 1994;331(8):502–507.

Ogura A, Konishi T, Cunningham C, et al; Neoadjuvant (chemo)radiotherapy with total mesorectal excision only is not sufficient to prevent lateral local recurrence in enlarged nodes: results of the multicenter lateral node study of patients with low cT3/4 rectal cancer. *J Clin Oncol.* 2019;37(1):33–43.

Olen O, Erichsen R, Sachs MC, et al. Colorectal cancer in ulcerative colitis: a Scandinavian population-based cohort study. *Lancet.* 2020;395(10218):123.

Papillon J. Intracavitary irradiation of early rectal cancer for cure. A series of 186 cases 1975. *Dis Colon Rectum.* 1994;37(1):88–94.

Patel P, Hanson DL, Sullivan PS, et al. Incidence of types of cancer among HIV-infected persons compared with the general population in the United States, 1992–2003. *Ann Intern Med.* 2008;148:728–736.

Peacock O, Chang GJ. The landmark series: management of lateral lymph nodes in locally advanced rectal cancer. *Ann Surg Oncol.* 2020;27(8):2723–2731.

Pickhardt PJ, Choi JR, Hwang I, et al. Computed tomographic virtual colonoscopy to screen for colorectal neoplasia in asymptomatic adults. *N Engl J Med.* 2003;349(23):2191–2200.

Pignone M, Rich M, Teutsch SM, Berg AO, Lohr KN. Screening for CRC in adults at average risk: a summary of the evidence for the U.S. Preventive Services Task Force. *Ann Intern Med.* 2002;137(2):132–141.

Pisano M, Zorcolo L, Merli C, et al. 2017 WSES guidelines on colon and rectal cancer emergencies: obstruction and perforation. *World J Emerg Surg*. 2018;13:36.

Pita-Fernández S, Alhayek-Aí M, González-Martín C, López-Calviño B, Seoane-Pillado T, Pértega-Díaz S. Intensive follow-up strategies improve outcomes in nonmetastatic colorectal cancer patients after curative surgery: a systematic review and meta-analysis. *Ann Oncol*. 2015;26(4):644–656.

Quintero E, Castells A, Bujanda L, et al; COLONPREV Study Investigators. Colonoscopy versus fecal immunochemical testing in colorectal-cancer screening. *N Engl J Med*. 2012;366(8):697–706.

Quirke P, Durdey P, Dixon MF, Williams NS. Local recurrence of rectal adenocarcinoma due to inadequate surgical resection. Histopathological study of lateral tumour spread and surgical excision. *Lancet*. 1986;1(2):996–999.

Rabkin CS, Yellin F. Cancer incidence in a population with a high prevalence of infection with human immunodeficiency virus type 1. *J Natl Cancer Inst*. 1994;86(22):1711–1716.

Randel KR, Schult AL, Botteri E, et al. Colorectal cancer screening with repeated fecal immunochemical test versus sigmoidoscopy: baseline results from a randomized trial. *Gastroenterology*. 2021;160(4):1085–1096.e5.

Repici A, Pellicano R, Strangio G, Danese S, Fagoonee S, Malesci A. Endoscopic mucosal resection for early colorectal neoplasia: pathologic basis, procedures, and outcome. *Dis Colon Rectum*. 2009;52:1502–1515.

Rodriguez-Bigas MA, Boland CR, Hamilton SR, et al. A National Cancer Institute Workshop on Hereditary Nonpolyposis CRC Syndrome: meeting highlights and Bethesda guidelines. *J Natl Cancer Inst*. 1997;89(23):1758–1762.

Rodriguez-Bigas MA, Chang GJ, Skibber JM. Surgical implications of CRC genetics. *Surg Oncol Clin N Am*. 2006;15(1):51–66.

Rosen M, Chan L, Beart RW Jr, van Houwelingen HC, Habbema JD, van de Velde CJ. Follow-up of CRC: a meta-analysis. *Dis Colon Rectum*. 1998;41(9):1116–1126.

Ross, H. Steele SR, Varma M, et al. Practice parameters for the surgical treatment of ulcerative colitis. *Dis Colon Rectum*. 2014;57:5–22

Roth AD, Tejpar S, Delorenzi M, et al. Prognostic role of KRAS and BRAF in stage II and III resected colon cancer: results of the translational study on the PETACC-3, EORTC 40993, SAKK 60-00 trial. *J Clin Oncol*. 2010;28:466–474.

Rullier E, Rouanet P, Tuech JJ, et al. Organ preservation for rectal cancer (GRECCAR 2): a prospective, randomised, open-label, multicentre, phase 3 trial. *Lancet*. 2017;390(10093):469–479.

Saltz LB, Cox JV, Blanke C, et al. Irinotecan plus fluorouracil and leucovorin for metastatic CRC. Irinotecan Study Group. *N Engl J Med*. 2000;343(13):905–914.

Sanfilippo NJ, Crane CH, Skibber J, et al. T4 rectal cancer treated with preoperative chemoradiation to the posterior pelvis followed by multivisceral resection: patterns of failure and limitations of treatment. *Int J Radiat Oncol Biol Phys*. 2001;51(1):176–183.

Sartore-Bianchi A, Trusolino L, Martino C, et al. Dual-targeted therapy with trastuzumab and lapatinib in treatment-refractory, KRAS codon 12/13 wild-type, HER2-positive metastatic CRC (HERACLES): a proof-of-concept, multicentre, open-label, phase 2 trial. *Lancet Oncol*. 2016;17(6):738–746.

Sauer R, Becker H, Hohenberger W, et al. Preoperative versus postoperative chemoradiotherapy for rectal cancer. *N Engl J Med*. 2004;351(17):1731–1740.

Schaffzin DM, Wong WD. Endorectal ultrasound in the preoperative evaluation of rectal cancer. *Clin CRC*. 2004;4(2):124–132.

Scott N, Jackson P, al-Jaberi T, Dixon MF, Quirke P, Finan PJ. Total mesorectal excision and local recurrence: a study of tumour spread in the mesorectum distal to rectal cancer. *Br J Surg*. 1995;82(8):1031–1033.

Seitz V, Bohnacker S, Seewald S, et al. Is endoscopic polypectomy an adequate therapy for malignant colorectal adenomas? Presentation of 114 patients and review of the literature. *Dis Colon Rectum*. 2004;47:1789–1797.

Shiels MS, Pfeiffer RM, Chaturvedi AK, Kreimer AR, Engels EA. Impact of the HIV epidemic on the incidence rates of anal cancer in the United States. *J Natl Cancer Inst*. 2012;104(20):1591–1598.

Siegel RL, Miller KD, Jemal A, Cancer statistics, 2016. *CA Cancer J Clin*. 2016;66(1):7.

Silberfein EJ, Kattepogu KM, Hu CY, et al. Long-term survival and recurrence outcomes following surgery for distal rectal cancer. *Ann Surg Oncol*. 2010;17(11): 2863–2869.

Skibber J, Rodriguez-Bigas MA, Gordon PH. Surgical considerations in anal cancer. *Surg Oncol Clin N Am*. 2004; 13(2):321–338.

Smith JJ, Strombom P, Chow OS, et al. Assessment of a watch-and-wait strategy for rectal cancer in patients with a complete response after neoadjuvant therapy. *JAMA Oncol.* 2019;5:e185896.

Snyder RA, Hu CY, Cuddy A, et al;; Alliance for Clinical Trials in Oncology Network Cancer Surveillance Optimization Working Group. Association between intensity of posttreatment surveillance testing and detection of recurrence in patients with colorectal cancer. *JAMA.* 2018;319(20):2104–2115.

Soetikno RM, Kaltenbach T, Rouse RV, et al. Prevalence of nonpolypoid (flat and depressed) colorectal neoplasms in asymptomatic and symptomatic adults. *JAMA.* 2008;299(9):1027–1035.

Steele GD Jr, Herndon JE, Bleday R, et al. Sphincter-sparing treatment for distal rectal adenocarcinoma. *Ann Surg Oncol.* 1999;6(5):433–441.

Stidham, R, Higgins PD, Colorectal cancer in inflammatory bowel disease. *Clin Colon Rectal Surg.* 2018;31:168–178.

Stuckey CC, Pockaj BA, Novotny PJ, et al. Long-term follow-up and individual item analysis of quality of life assessments related to laparoscopic-assisted colectomy in the COST trial 93–46-53 (INT 0146). *Ann Surg Oncol.* 2011;18(9):2422–2431.

Swedish Rectal Cancer Trial, Cedermark B, Dahlberg M, Glimelius B, et al. Improved survival with preoperative radiotherapy in resectable rectal cancer. *N Engl J Med.* 1997;336(14):980–987.

Tepper JE, O'Connell M, Niedzwiecki D, et al. Adjuvant therapy in rectal cancer: analysis of stage, sex, and local control—final report of intergroup 0114. *J Clin Oncol.* 2002;20(7):1744–1750.

The Clinical Outcomes of Surgical Therapy Study Group. A comparison of laparoscopically assisted and open colectomy for colon cancer. *N Engl J Med.* 2004;350(20):2050–2059.

The SCOTIA Study Group. Single-stage treatment for malignant left-sided colonic obstruction: a prospective randomized clinical trial comparing subtotal colectomy with segmental resection following intraoperative irrigation. Subtotal colectomy versus on-table irrigation and anastomosis. *Br J Surg.* 1995;82(12):1622–1627.

Theodoropoulos DG. Gastrointestinal tumors of the colon and rectum. *Clin Colon Rectal Surg.* 2011;24(3):161–170.

Treasure T, Farewell V, Macbeth F, et al. Pulmonary metastasectomy versus continued active monitoring in colorectal cancer (PulMiCC): a multicentre randomised clinical trial. *Trials.* 2019;20(1):718.

Tsukamoto S, Fujita S, Ota M, et al. Long-term follow-up of the randomized trial of mesorectal excision with or without lateral lymph node dissection in rectal cancer (JCOG0212). *Br J Surg.* 2020;107(5):586–594.

U.S. Preventative Task Force. Screening for CRC: recommendation and rationale. *Ann Intern Med.* 2002;137(2):129–131.

Umar A, Boland CR, Terdiman JP, et al. Revised Bethesda guidelines for hereditary nonpolyposis CRC (Lynch syndrome) and microsatellite instability. *J Natl Cancer Inst.* 2004;96(4):261–268.

Van Cutsem E, Kohne CH, Hitre E, et al. Cetuximab and chemotherapy as initial treatment for metastatic CRC. *N Engl J Med.* 2009;360:1408–1417.

Vieira AR, Abar L, Chan DSM, et al. Foods and beverages and colorectal cancer risk: a systematic review and meta-analysis of cohort studies, an update of the evidence of the WCRF-AICR Continuous Update Project. *Ann Oncol.* 2017;28(8):1788–1802.

Vogel J, Eskicioglu C, Weiser M. The American Society of Colon and Rectal Surgeons Clinical Practice Guidelines for the Treatment of Colon Cancer. *Dis Colon Rectum.* 2017;60:999–1017.

Vogelsang H, Haas S, Hierholzer C, Berger U, Siewert JR, Präuer H. Factors influencing survival after resection of pulmonary metastases from CRC. *Br J Surg.* 2004;91(8):1066–1071.

Vogelstein B, Fearon ER, Hamilton SR, et al. Genetic alterations during colorectal-tumor development. *N Engl J Med.* 1988;319:525–532.

Walsh JM, Terdiman JP. CRC screening: scientific review. *JAMA.* 2003;289(10):1288–1296.

Walsh JM, Terdiman JP. CRC screening: clinical applications. *JAMA.* 2003;289(10):1297–1302.

Wang X, Cao G, Mao W, Lao W, He C. Robot-assisted versus laparoscopic surgery for rectal cancer: A systematic review and meta-analysis. *J Cancer Res Ther.* 2020;16(5):979–989.

Ward E, Jemal A, Cokkinides V, et al. Cancer disparities by race/ethnicity and socioeconomic status. *CA Cancer J Clin.* 2004;54(2):78–93.

Wegner RE, White RJ, Hasan S, et al. Anal adenocarcinoma: treatment outcomes and trends in a rare disease entity. *Cancer Med.* 2019;8(8):3855–3863.

Weisenberger DJ, Siegmund KD, Campan M, et al. CpG island methylator phenotype underlies sporadic microsatellite instability and is tightly associated with BRAF mutation in CRC. *Nat Genet.* 2006;38(7):787–793.

Wibe A, Eriksen MT, Syse A, et al. Effect of hospital caseload on long-term outcome after standardization of rectal cancer surgery at a national level. *Br J Surg.* 2005;92(2):217–224.

Wilson SM, Beahrs OH. The curative treatment of carcinoma of the sigmoid, rectosigmoid, and rectum. *Ann Surg.* 1976;183(5):556–565.

Winawer SJ, Zauber AG. Colonoscopic polypectomy and the incidence of CRC. *Gut* 2001;48(6):753–754.

Winde G, Nottberg H, Keller R, Schmid KW, Bünte H. Surgical cure for early rectal carcinomas (T1). Transanal endoscopic microsurgery vs. anterior resection. *Dis Colon Rectum.* 1996;39(9):969–976.

Wolf AMD, Fontham ETH, Church TR, et al. Colorectal cancer screening for average-risk adults: 2018 guideline update from the American Cancer Society. *CA Cancer J Clin.* 2018;68(4):250–281.

Wolmark N, Rockette H, Fisher B, et al. The benefit of leucovorin-modulated fluorouracil as postoperative adjuvant therapy for primary colon cancer: results from National Surgical Adjuvant Breast and Bowel Project protocol C-03. *J Clin Oncol.* 1993;11(10):1879–1887.

World Cancer Research Fund and American Institute for Cancer Research Food, Nutrition, Physical Activity, and the Prevention of Cancer: A Global Perspective. Washington, DC: American Institute for Cancer Research; 2007.

Xue K, Li FF, Chen YW, Zhou YH, He J. Body mass index and the risk of cancer in women compared with men: a meta-analysis of prospective cohort studies. *European J Cancer Prev.* 2017;26(1):94–105.

You YN, Hardiman KM, Bafford A. The American Society of Colon and Rectal Surgeons Clinical Practice Guidelines for the Management of Rectal Cancer. *Dis Colon Rectum.* 2020;63:1191–1222

You YN, Skibber JM, Hu CY, et al. Impact of multimodal therapy in locally recurrent rectal cancer. *Br J Surg.* 2016;103:753–762.

Young-Fadok TM, Wolff BG, Nivatvongs S, Metzger PP, Ilstrup DM. Prophylactic oophorectomy in colorectal carcinoma: preliminary results of a randomized, prospective trial. *Dis Colon Rectum.* 1998;41(3):277–283, discussion 283–285.

Zaheer S, Pemberton JH, Farouk R, Dozois RR, Wolff BG, Ilstrup D. Surgical treatment of adenocarcinoma of the rectum. *Ann Surg.* 1998;227(6):800–811.

Hepatobiliary Cancers

Caitlin A. Hester, Anai N. Kothari, Harufumi Maki, Steven Wei, Rebecca A. Snyder, and Jean-Nicolas Vauthey

INTRODUCTION

This chapter outlines treatment approaches to the major hepatobiliary cancers, addresses issues of anatomy, and describes preoperative preparation and the operative approach. For each disease type, the current literature is reviewed to provide an explanation of epidemiology, pathology, clinical presentation, diagnosis, staging, and issues regarding resection and multimodal therapy.

Surgical Anatomy of the Liver: Considering Differences in Morphologic and Functional Anatomy
Morphological Anatomy
"Lobe" literally translates as "parenchyma limited by fissures or grooves." Thus, morphologically the liver is comprised of two main lobes and two accessory lobes. The umbilical fissure and the falciform ligament separate the right and the left lobe. Along the inferior surface of the liver is a transverse hilar fissure, and the portion of the right lobe located anteriorly to this fissure is called the quadrate lobe. Posterior to the hilar transverse fissure is the Spiegel lobe.

Functional Anatomy
The first description of functional anatomy of the liver was introduced by Cantlie in 1898 and was followed by others including Couinaud. The description provided by Couinaud is the most comprehensive and will therefore be adopted for our description. The anatomy is determined by the distribution of the portal pedicles and the location of the hepatic veins.

The functional anatomy of the liver is divided into two livers (or hemi-livers) by the main portal scissura which creates a tangential line from the gallbladder fossa anteriorly to the left side of the vena cava posteriorly, following the position of the middle hepatic vein. This scissura is angled 75 degrees toward the left hemi-liver. It is this functional anatomic location that denotes the proper transection line for a formal right or left hepatectomy.

In 1957, Couinaud first described four sectors and eight anatomical segments. The hepatic veins, or the portal scissurae, provide the surgeon with an anatomic understanding of the four sectors of the liver. The main portal scissura, the line from the middle of the gallbladder fossa anteriorly to the left side of the vena cava posteriorly and following the position of the middle hepatic vein, divides the liver into two hemi-livers: the right and left hemi-livers. Likewise, the right and left portal scissurae divide the hemi-livers into two sectors each. The right scissura, following the plane of the right hepatic vein, delineates the right anterior or paramedian sector from the right posterior or lateral sector, and the left scissura, following the plane of the left hepatic vein, delineates the left lateral or posterior and left anterior or paramedian sectors (Fig. 14.1).

The portal branches provide inflow to the eight segments of the liver, such that any of the eight segments can be resected while preserving the vascular inflow, venous outflow, and biliary drainage of the remaining segments. The right anterior or right paramedian sector is subdivided into segment V inferiorly and segment VIII superiorly, and the right posterior or right lateral sector is subdivided into segment VI inferiorly and segment VII superiorly. The left anterior or left paramedian sector is subdivided into segments III and IV, and the left posterior or left lateral sector is segment II. The left hepatic vein defines these sectors based on its course between segment II and segment III (Fig. 14.1).

The right liver typically comprises two-thirds of the total liver volume (TLV), and the left liver one-third. The caudate lobe (segment I), which is a single anatomical unit, represents approximately 1% to 2% of the TLV. Three segments comprise the caudate lobe: the caudate process, paracaval caudate, and Spiegel's lobe. The caudate lobe has highly variable biliary and portal anatomy, as well as its own venous drainage, with short veins draining directly into the vena cava.

It is essential that surgeons understand the many anatomical variations of the liver that can be identified on preoperative cross-sectional imaging and intraoperative ultrasound (IOUS). Surgical techniques, including the Glissonian approach or dissection along the fibrous sheath that surrounds the portal veins, bile ducts, and hepatic arteries (portal triads), may enable the surgeon to identify important elements of the anatomy intrahepatically, and thereby minimize the risk of injury to the remaining liver during the resection

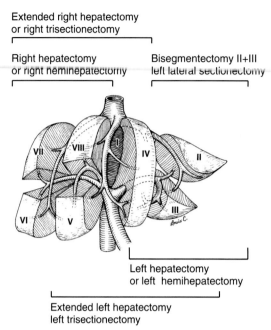

Extended right hepatectomy
or right trisectionectomy

Right hepatectomy
or right hemihepatectomy

Bisegmentectomy II+III
left lateral sectionectomy

Left hepatectomy
or left hemihepatectomy

Extended left hepatectomy
left trisectionectomy

FIGURE 14.1 Segmental liver anatomy as originally described by Claude Couinaud, with the terminology that should be used to describe liver resection according to the Brisbane 2000 International Consensus Conference. (Adapted from Abdalla EK, Denys A, Chevalier P, et al. Total and segmental liver volume variations: implications for liver surgery. *Surgery* 2004;135:405, with permission from Elsevier.)

of anatomical segments. IOUS is essential for safe liver surgery and permits real-time identification of the intrahepatic anatomy.

Terminology for Hepatic Resection

Terminology for hepatic resection has changed over time. Accordingly, the Brisbane 2000 International Conference was held to establish a consensus on terminology used for liver resection. That revised terminology is used throughout this chapter (Fig. 14.1).

The terminology for hepatectomy is as follows: (a) resection of the right liver (or segments V to VIII) is termed a right hepatectomy or right hemihepatectomy; (b) resection of the left liver (or segments II to IV) is termed a left hepatectomy or left hemihepatectomy; (c) resection of the left lateral liver (or segments II and III) is termed a bisegmentectomy II + III or a left lateral sectionectomy; and (d) extended right hepatectomy, or right trisectionectomy, is the resection of segments IV to VIII, whereas extended left hepatectomy, or left trisectionectomy, is resection of segments II to V and VIII.

Predicting Liver Remnant Function

Liver Volume Determination

Careful analysis of outcomes based on liver remnant volume stratified by underlying liver disease has led to recommendations regarding the safe limits of resection. The residual liver remnant following formal resection is termed the future liver remnant (FLR). For patients with a normal underlying liver, complications, extended hospital stay, admission to the intensive care unit, and hepatic insufficiency are rare when the standardized FLR is >20% of the total liver volume (TLV). For patients with tumor-related cholestasis or marked underlying liver disease, a 40% liver remnant is necessary to avoid cholestasis, fluid retention, and liver failure. Among patients who have been treated with preoperative systemic chemotherapy for more than 8 to 12 weeks, FLR >30% reduces the rate of postoperative liver insufficiency and subsequent mortality (Fig. 14.2).

When the liver remnant is normal or has only mild disease, the volume of liver remnant can be measured directly and accurately with three-dimensional computed tomography (CT) volumetry. However, inaccuracy may arise because the liver to be resected is often diseased, particularly in patients with cirrhosis or biliary obstruction. When multiple or large tumors occupy a large volume of the liver that is to be resected,

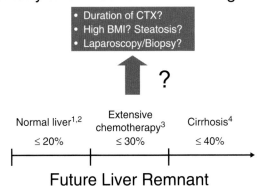

Volumetry and Assessments of Surgical Risk

- Duration of CTX?
- High BMI? Steatosis?
- Laparoscopy/Biopsy?

?

Normal liver[1,2]   Extensive chemotherapy[3]   Cirrhosis[4]

≤ 20%   ≤ 30%   ≤ 40%

Future Liver Remnant

1. Abdalla EK *Arch Surg* 2002
2. Vauthey JN *Ann Surg* 2004
3. Azoulay D *Ann Surg* 2000
4. Kubota K *Hematology* 1997

FIGURE 14.2 Diagram of the future liver remnant required for hepatectomy depending on the parenchymal quality and any pre-existing liver injury. CTX, chemotherapy; BMI, body mass index. (Adapted from Tzeng CW, Vauthey JN. Liver anatomy, physiology, and preoperative evaluation. In: Zyromski NJ, ed. *Handbook of Hepato-Pancreato-Biliary Surgery*, 2015, with permission.)

subtracting tumor volumes from liver volume further decreases accuracy of CT volumetry. The calculated TLV, which has been derived from the association between body surface area (BSA) and liver size, provides a standard estimate of the TLV. The following formula is used:

$$\text{TLV (cm}^3) = -794.41 + 1{,}267.28 \times \text{BSA (square meters)}$$

Thus, the standardized FLR (sFLR) volume calculation uses the *measured* FLR volume from CT volumetry as the numerator and the *calculated* TLV as the denominator:

$$\text{Standardized FLR (sFLR)} = \text{measured FLR volume/TLV}$$

Calculating the standardized TLV corrects the actual liver volume to the individual patient's size and provides an individualized estimate of that patient's postresection liver function. This approach has been validated and used at the MD Anderson Cancer Center. In the event of an inadequate FLR prior to major hepatectomy, preoperative liver preparation may include portal vein embolization (PVE), which will be discussed in detail in the following section.

Portal Vein Embolization

PVE is a preoperative procedure designed to increase the safety of major liver resections. The portal flow is diverted from the liver segments to be resected to the FLR resulting in hypertrophy of the FLR prior to resection. PVE was refined by Makuuchi after Kinoshita observed that embolization of the portal vein (PV) to prevent tumor extension led to hypertrophy of the contralateral liver. Since then, PVE techniques and indications have been standardized to increase the safety of major hepatectomy in patients with both normal and diseased livers.

Patients requiring an extended right hepatectomy often have inadequate sFLR and require preoperative PVE (Fig. 14.3). In a study by Shindoh et al. of 265 patients undergoing extended right hepatectomy, 52.5% ($N = 139$) had inadequate sFLR and underwent preoperative PVE. Of these, 62.6% ($N = 87$) underwent curative resection, increasing the resection rate from 46.2% at baseline to 79.2% following PVE. Outcomes, including complication and mortality rates as well as disease free and overall survival (OS), were equivalent among the PVE and non-PVE groups.

The kinetic growth rate (KGR) is a dynamic measure of the degree of hypertrophy at initial volume assessment divided by the number of weeks elapsed after PVE, and it has been shown to more effectively predict postoperative morbidity and mortality after liver resection compared to the one-dimensional, conventional measure of sFLR. A KGR of <2% per week versus ≥2% correlates with higher rates of hepatic insufficiency (21.6% vs. 0%; $P = .0001$) and liver-related 90-day mortality (8.1% vs. 0%; $P = .04$). Additionally, patients who had a right PVE + segment IV PVE experienced a higher degree of hypertrophy (9.5% vs. 6.2%, $P = .07$) and

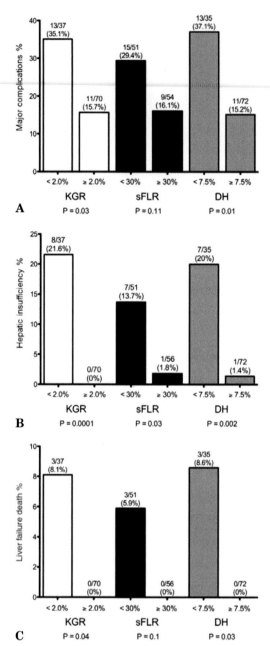

FIGURE 14.3 Rates of (**A**) major complications, (**B**) hepatic insufficiency, and (**C**) 90-day liver-related mortality based on best cut-off values determined with receiver operating characteristics analysis. DH, degree of hypertrophy; KGR, kinetic growth rate, defined as DH at first volume assessment after PVE divided by weeks between PVE and first post-PVE volume assessment; PVE, portal vein embolization; sFLR, standardized future liver remnant. (Adapted from Shindoh J, Truty MJ, Aloia TA, et al. Kinetic growth rate after portal vein embolization predicts posthepatectomy outcomes: toward zero liver-related mortality in patients with colorectal liver metastases and small future liver remnant. *J Am Coll Surg.* 2013;216(2):201–209, with permission.)

Optimize Portal Vein Embolization (PVE) MD Anderson Approach

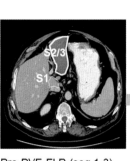
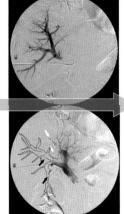
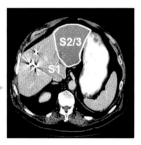

Pre-PVE FLR (seg 1-3)
10% vs. Total Liver Volume

Post-PVE FLR (seg 1-3)
33% vs. Total Liver Volume

Transhepatic Ipsilateral Right PVE Extended to Segment 4 Branches and Spherical Microspheres

FIGURE 14.4 Representative images from contrast-enhanced computed tomography of the liver before and after right portal vein embolization (PVE) extended to segment IV resulting in increase of the standardized future liver remnant (sFLR) from 10% to 33%. Portogram captured during PVE shows contrast in the right portal vein and its branches before PVE (*top image*) and contrast in the main and left portal veins, except segment IV branches, after PVE (*lower image*). Coils in segment IV branches are marked with *white arrows,* and the embolized right portal vein is outlined with *dashed lines. Black arrows* indicate anterior and posterior branches of the right portal vein.

KGR (1.4%/week vs. 2.3%/week, $P = .02$) of segments II and III compared to right PVE alone. Patient factors that are associated with inability to hypertrophy include BMI, previous hepatectomy, and PVE in the setting of two-stage hepatectomy.

At MD Anderson, we recommend that patients undergoing an extended right hepatectomy with a preoperative FLR ≤20% be considered for PVE. These recommendations are based on institutional findings that death and major complications were independently associated with a preoperative FLR of ≤20%, but not with 20% to 30% or >30%. We recommend selective use of PVE for patients with FLR 20.1% to 30.0% if there is prolonged preoperative chemotherapy (more than 8 to 12 weeks) or suspicion of hepatic injury, chronic liver disease or in patients undergoing complex or combined operations.

At the MD Anderson Cancer Center, we use the percutaneous ipsilateral approach to avoid puncturing or injuring the liver remnant. Using spherical microspheres followed by larger coils, the portal branches supplying the entire tumor-bearing liver, including segment IV (if this is to be resected), are occluded (Fig. 14.4). This procedure diverts portal flow to the FLR. Hypertrophy occurs quite rapidly, and the normal liver can be reassessed by volumetry within 3 or 4 weeks. However, hypertrophy may occur more slowly in cirrhotics, diabetics, and patients with other types of chronic liver injury; therefore, an interval of 5 or 6 weeks may be required to achieve the desired degree of hypertrophy.

Attention to the liver remnant, systemic volumetry for major resection, use of PVE, and measurement of KGR based on carefully prescribed indications has enabled very safe extended hepatic resection in patients with normal liver function and major hepatectomy in patients with underlying liver disease.

Increasingly, the combination method of portal + hepatic vein embolization (PHVE) has been used. Nagino et al. first described this technique as an additional venous isolation technique to induce further hypertrophy in the FLR and stimulate development of inferior hepatic veins to the remaining liver. In the majority of reported cases, HVE was performed following failed hypertrophy after PVE, and the question of whether HVE should be performed simultaneously or sequentially remains open. At the MD Anderson Cancer Center, we do consider the use of simultaneous PHVE in patients who are considered to be at high risk of failure with PVE alone.

Among patients with HCC and Child's A cirrhosis secondary to underlying viral hepatitis or alcoholic fibrosis, PVE is indicated to achieve an sFLR of >40%. Because the rate of liver regeneration may be slower in these patients, sequential use of transarterial chemoembolization (TACE) and PVE can prevent tumor progression during liver regeneration prior to resection. Ogata et al. demonstrated that sequential TACE and PVE leads to improved FLR regeneration rates and DFS when compared to PVE alone in patients with HCC and cirrhosis. At MD Anderson, direct PV pressure measurement is performed routinely prior to PVE in order to avoid performing PVE in patients with occult portal hypertension.

Associating Liver Partition with Portal Vein Ligation for Staged Hepatectomy

The technique of associating liver partition surgery with PV ligation for staged hepatectomy (ALPPS) has been promoted as an alternative to PVE for patients undergoing extended right hepatectomy. With this technique, PV ligation and in situ splitting of the liver along the falciform ligament is performed to induce rapid hypertrophy of the left lateral section. After a short interval (median 9 days; range 5 to 28 days) patients undergo completion hepatectomy. The proposed benefits include early abdominal exploration for intra- or extrahepatic disease that might preclude curative resection as well as a shortened interval of hypertrophy prior to resection. However, major morbidity rates (40%) and liver-related mortality (12%) are significantly higher after ALPPS compared to PVE, and the long-term oncologic outcomes are not yet known. As a result, PVE remains the preferred technique to induce hypertrophy of the FLR when indicated prior to liver resection.

Metastases to the Liver

Most liver metastases originate from gastrointestinal primary tumors, and of these, most are from the colon and rectum. In general, 5-year survival is rare among patients who undergo resection for noncolorectal metastases to the liver. The exceptions are selected patients with neuroendocrine tumors, Wilms tumor, and to a lesser extent, renal cell carcinoma; 5-year survival rates of 40% to 70% have been reported after resection in these cases. Hepatic resection may also provide excellent palliation in selected patients with hormone-secreting neuroendocrine tumors.

Recently, there has been increased interest in resection of breast cancer liver metastases. Our group led by Chun et al. demonstrated that the intrinsic subtype was the strongest independent predictor of survival, even more so than number and size of liver metastases. We found that patients with luminal B and HER2– enriched subtypes experienced an OS of 75 and 81 months, significantly longer than patients with basal-like and luminal A subtypes with 17 and 53 months, respectively. More data are needed to determine the role of hepatectomy within this pathology, however surgical resection should be considered in selected cases.

Given that the vast majority of liver metastases considered for resection are secondary to colorectal primary tumors (CRLM), the remainder of this discussion is focused on their management.

Epidemiology and Etiology

Colorectal cancer represents the third most common type of cancer for both men and women in the United States, with an estimated incidence of 135,000 cases per year. Approximately 80% of the patients will have malignancies that are amenable to surgical cure, but approximately 20% of the resected cancers will recur within 5 years. Only 20% of these recurrences will be solely or predominantly in the liver, and fewer still will be amenable to surgical resection. It has been estimated that 15,000 to 20,000 patients per year are potential candidates for resection of their liver metastases.

Clinical Presentation and Diagnosis

In the vast majority of patients, metastases to the liver are found during routine postoperative carcinoembryonic antigen (CEA) screening or radiologic imaging after resection of a colorectal primary tumor. Patients with increasing CEA levels should undergo thorough diagnostic evaluation, including contrast-enhanced CT scan of the chest, abdomen, and pelvis. A slowly increasing CEA level usually indicates local or regional recurrence, whereas a rapidly increasing CEA level suggests hepatic metastases. Overall, 75% to 90% of patients with hepatic colorectal cancer metastases have an increased CEA level.

Preoperative Staging

High-quality imaging is critical to assessment of CRLM resectability. We favor CT scanning at our institution; our published survival rates are equal to the best reported for resection of metastases from colorectal cancer, validating this approach. CT not only permits assessment of extrahepatic structures, but also accurately provides liver volumetry, accurate localization of the tumors within the liver, and accurate detection of extrahepatic disease. Multiphase, thin-cut, spiral, hepatic CT is our modality of choice, and the information thus gained has been superior to that afforded by MRI and other approaches. MRI is used selectively in patients with metastases poorly visualized on CT and in patients with a significant degree of underlying steatosis.

Careful pre-laparotomy staging must also include colonoscopy to rule out local recurrence as well as CT of the chest. Although [^{18}F]fluoro-2-deoxy-D-glucose PET has been proposed as necessary for staging, no study has shown that PET improves outcome or changes therapy when high-quality cross-sectional imaging is used. Additionally, false-negative PET is common after chemotherapy, limiting the utility of this technique alone.

Determining Resectability and Operative Planning

The definition of resectable liver metastases has evolved over time. Whereas previous definitions considered the size, number, and location of lesions, colorectal liver metastases are now considered resectable if all of the disease can be completely resected with a negative margin and an adequate FLR remains.

The planned hepatic resection should encompass all metastases detectable on prechemotherapy imaging. Benoist et al. showed that a complete radiographic response cannot be equated with a complete pathologic response; in fact, 83% of metastases suggestive of a complete radiographic response harbor viable tumor cells or develop early intrahepatic recurrence. Conversely, patients with imaging suggestive of viable tumor after preoperative chemotherapy may demonstrate evidence of a complete pathologic response at the time of resection.

The use of fiducial markers in very small lesions may be considered prior to initiation of chemotherapy in order to preserve localization of the site of disease at the time of resection. Passot et al. reviewed 32 patients who underwent fiducial placement in 41 metastatic lesions. Median size was 12 mm and 83% ($N = 34$) were located >10 mm deep within the liver parenchyma. After chemotherapy, nearly half (46%) disappeared on cross-sectional imaging. All were treated with resection ($N = 31$) or ablation ($N = 10$), and no local recurrences were identified at median follow-up of 14 months. Consideration of fiducial marker placement should be made for all lesions that are <20 mm in size or >10 mm in depth.

In cases of bilateral disease, multistage approaches to surgery should be considered. Preoperative systemic chemotherapy can reduce the size and volume of tumors such that all tumor sites can be resected safely and provide long-term survival. At the first stage, wedge or limited resection clears the planned FLR, preserving the major portion of the parenchyma in preparation for resection of the remaining liver. At the second stage, major hepatectomy or extended hepatectomy removes all remaining disease. Staged resection usually requires interval PVE to increase the volume and function of the FLR after the first-stage resection.

The safety and efficacy of this approach has been recently reported by Passot et al. Of 109 patients in whom two-stage hepatectomy for CRLM was planned, 82% ($N = 89$) underwent second stage resection. The cumulative rate of major complications during the first and second stages was 15% with 3-year survival of 68%. A recent series reported marked improvement in survival among patients who underwent two-stage resection for CRLM, with 5-year overall of 51% compared to 15% among patients with liver-only disease who had a good response to chemotherapy but did not undergo resection. Although this difference may partly represent patient selection, complete resection of disease is associated with an excellent outcome.

Highly selected patients with *resectable* extrahepatic disease—whether limited peritoneal carcinomatosis, minimal hilar lymphadenopathy, or metastatic disease to the lung—can also undergo resection with acceptable survival. Nearly all of these patients have received a significant amount of systemic chemotherapy with either response or stabilization of disease thereby selecting for "favorable" biology.

Controversy remains surrounding the decision making for optimal management of patients with synchronous disease to determine the order of resection of the primary colorectal cancer and liver metastases. The complexity of the operation necessary to remove the primary tumor and the extent of hepatic resection required will affect decision making because the risk of adverse events from hepatic resection increases when the procedure is associated with extrahepatic surgery. Solitary, small, peripherally located lesions in a healthy, hemodynamically stable patient that can be resected by nonanatomical resection or segmentectomy may be resected at the same time as the primary tumor. Lesions that are larger or that will require major hepatic resection are best approached during a separate operation.

A recent study by Snyder et al. compared 30-day surgical morbidity in a national cohort of 31,697 patients with colorectal liver metastases undergoing isolated or simultaneous resection. Simultaneous resection was associated with increased overall complications (OR 1.64 [1.36 to 1.96]) and procedure-specific complications (OR 1.80, 95% CI 1.26 to 2.57). The METASYNC trial published in 2021 was the first randomized trial comparing simultaneous versus staged resection of synchronous colorectal cancer liver metastases. The primary outcome of major perioperative complications was similar between groups (49% vs. 46%, $P = .70$). However, the high rate of perioperative morbidity seen in the study, variability in chemotherapy use, and imbalance in randomization makes interpreting the results difficult. An individualized strategy based on extent of liver disease, location of primary tumor, and biologic assessment remains the favored approach at our institution.

Specifically, patients with synchronous CRLM and an asymptomatic primary tumor are treated with neoadjuvant chemotherapy followed by resection of the liver disease first. We have found that this results in an earlier recovery due to the fact that infectious complications are less common following liver resection compared to resection of the colorectal primary. Additionally, we consider disease progression in the liver to be the greatest risk to the patient, which is eliminated with resection of the liver disease first. In the specific setting of synchronous liver metastases and rectal cancer, patients are treated with preoperative chemotherapy and liver resection, followed by chemoradiation and then resection of the primary rectal cancer.

Survival and Prognostic Factors

Modern reports of patients undergoing hepatic resection for CRLM reveal that the 5-year survival rate is 53% to 58%. The 5-year survival rate has improved from earlier reported rates of 25% to 40%. These improvements are likely related to refinements in technique for surgical resection, expanded indications for resection, advances in systemic chemotherapy, and adoption of multigene testing in this population. For example, chemotherapy regimens included irinotecan and/or oxaliplatin in the majority of patients beginning in 2001 and anti-VEGF and/or anti-EGFR agents in 2006. When comparing patients across these eras (2006–2014 vs. pre-2001), there is a stepwise increase in the rate of multiple resected CRLM, size of largest CRLM, and utilization of parenchymal-sparing approach (Fig. 14.5).

An optimal morphologic response, defined as homogeneous low attenuation with a thin, sharply defined tumor–liver interface on post-chemotherapy, preoperative imaging has been demonstrated to be predictive of both pathologic response and improved OS. This assessment is distinct from RECIST, and is not a measure of downstaging, but rather imaging features representative of pathologic response to chemotherapy. Among 209 patients with CRLM treated with preoperative chemotherapy with either oxaliplatin- or irinotecan-based regimens with or without bevacizumab, major pathologic response rates were 92% among patients with an

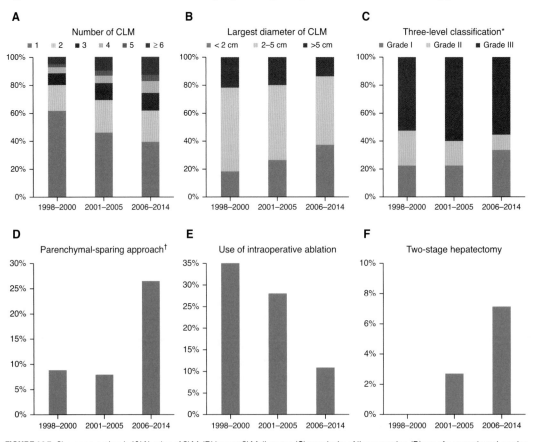

FIGURE 14.5 Changes over time in (**A**) Number of CLM, (**B**) largest CLM diameter, (**C**) complexity of liver resection, (**D**) use of a parenchymal-sparing approach, (**E**) concomitant use of intraoperative ablation, and (F) two-stage hepatectomy. *Grade I, low complexity; grade II, intermediate complexity; grade III, high complexity. †Defined as frequency of multiple resections (≤1 Couinaud segment) for multiple CLM. (Adapted from Kawaguchi Y, Kopetz S, Panettieri E, et al. Improved survival over time after resection of colorectal liver metastases and clinical impact of multigene alteration testing in patients with metastatic colorectal cancer. *J Gastroint Surg*. 2022;26:583–593, with permission.)

Pathologic Response to Chemotherapy and Survival (n = 305)

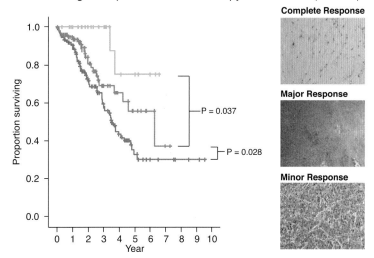

FIGURE 14.6 Representative photomicrographs of metastases demonstrating complete response (0% residual tumor cells), major response (1% to 49% residual tumor cells), and minor response (≥50% residual tumor cells). Overall survival cures by the degree of pathologic response. (Adapted from Blazer DG, Kishi Y, Maru DM, et al. Pathologic response to preoperative chemotherapy: a new outcome end point after resection of hepatic colorectal metastases. *J Clin Oncol.* 2008;25(33):5344–5351, with permission.)

optimal morphologic response compared to 59% among patients with suboptimal response. Additionally, the 3- and 5-year OS rates were higher in the group with an optimal morphologic response ([82% and 74%] and [60% and 45%]; $P < .001$]). The improved prognosis associated with an optimal morphologic response has also been validated in medical patients with advanced colorectal liver metastases not amenable to resection.

One of the most widely quoted studies to outline prognostic factors is from Fong et al. who evaluated a series of 1,001 consecutive patients who underwent hepatic resection for metastatic colorectal cancer at the Memorial Sloan-Kettering Cancer Center (MSKCC). Seven independent factors were associated with poor outcome: disease at the surgical margin, presence of extrahepatic disease, metastatic disease in the lymph nodes of the primary lesion, a short disease-free interval from resection of the primary tumor to detection of metastases, the number of hepatic tumors, hepatic tumor diameter >5 cm, and an elevated CEA level. These factors contribute to outcome with varying degrees and scoring of these factors is helpful in predicting prognosis after resection, *but not in selecting patients for surgery*.

The notion that a 1-cm margin is necessary to ensure long-term survival has been dispelled. Analysis of nearly 500 patients in a multi-institutional database showed that the pattern and probability of disease recurrence and the rates of disease-free and OS were identical in patients with 1-mm and 1-cm resection margins. A recent international multidisciplinary consensus statement on the management of synchronous CRLM advocates for minimal surgical clearance margin of 1 mm.

A study from the MD Anderson Cancer Center by Pawlik et al. clarified the importance of a margin-negative resection by examining the site of recurrence after resection for CRLM based on surgical margin status in a multi-institutional database. Patients with surgical margins positive for tumor cells had an overall recurrence rate of 52%, compared with 39% for patients with negative margins. Only 3.8% of patients had a recurrence at the surgical margin. The recurrence rates were similar in patients with negative margins of 1 and 4 mm (39%), 5 and 9 mm (41%), and ≥1 cm (39%). The majority of patients who had recurrences developed them at an extrahepatic site (66%), whether alone (30%) or with simultaneous intrahepatic recurrence (36%).

In addition to margin status, the pathologic response to preoperative chemotherapy has emerged as an important prognostic factor after resection of colorectal liver metastases. Blazer et al. showed that the 5-year OS for patients with no residual tumor cells in the resected specimen is 75% versus 33% for patients whose resected specimens contain ≥50% residual tumor cells (Fig. 14.6).

The Impact of Mutational Status on Oncologic Outcomes

The role that the mutational profile of a tumor contributes to outcomes is an evolving understanding among oncologists. Mutations in RAS genes were the first to be linked to worse oncologic outcomes and were reported

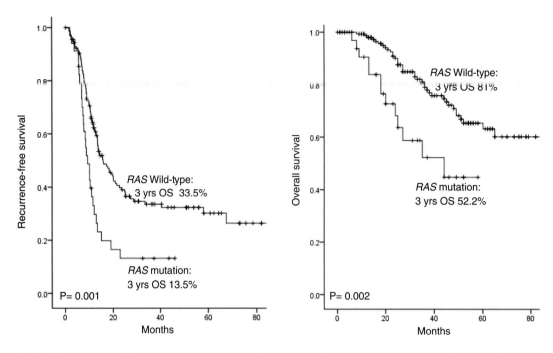

FIGURE 14.7 Overall survival (OS) and recurrence-free survival (RFS) according to RAS mutation status. (Adapted from Vauthey JN, Giuseppe Z, Kopetz S et al. RAS mutation status predicts survival and patterns of recurrence in patients undergoing hepatectomy for colorectal liver metastases. *Ann Surg.* 2013;258:619–626, with permission.)

by Nash et al. and Vauthey et al. Vauthey et al. demonstrated that in 193 patients treated with neoadjuvant chemotherapy with subsequent hepatectomy at MD Anderson, 3-year OS rates of patients with RAS mutation (including KRAS and NRAS) were 52.2% compared to 81% among RAS wild-type patients (Fig. 14.7). With an HR of 2.3 ($P = .002$), RAS mutational status independently was a strong predictor of worse survival. It is hypothesized that this difference in survival is secondary to improved morphologic and major pathologic response to neoadjuvant chemotherapy among RAS wild-type patients. Additionally, Brudvik et al. demonstrated in a study of 633 patients, 229 (36%) of whom had mutant RAS, RAS-mutant tumors were independently associated with higher risk of positive margin (OR 2.4, $P = .005$).

It appears that somatic mutational burden plays an important role in prognosis for patients undergoing resection for CRLM. Multiple somatic mutations in RAS, TP53, and SMAD4 are associated with a worse prognosis than any one gene. Coexisting mutations in all three (RAS, TP53, SMAD4) confer a worse OS than double mutations (HR 3.21 [1.72 to 5.99]), single mutation (HR 6.04 [3.21 to 11.3]), and all wild-type (HR 8.61 [3.80 to 19.5]). These results further emphasize the critical need to characterize tumor biology when considering resection for CRLM (Fig. 14.8).

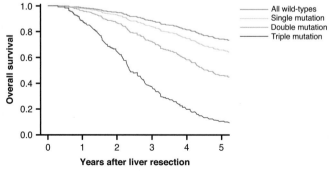

FIGURE 14.8 OS by RAS, TP53, and SMAD4 mutation status after adjustment for BRAF mutation status, largest liver metastasis diameter, and surgical margin status.

Ablative Therapy

Radiofrequency ablation (RFA) is used widely as a treatment for CRLM. Its use was widespread before consistent indications for ablation were established. Initial, well-designed studies proved the safety, excellent side-effect profile, and efficacy of RFA for CRLM. Studies from our institution and later from Europe and the Cleveland Clinic suggested a 78% 1-year survival rate could be attained by RFA, with 3-year survival at 46%. Unfortunately, >12% of patients had disease recurrence at 1 year. Abdalla et al. demonstrated that although RFA provides a modest survival benefit over chemotherapy alone for CRLM at 4 years (22% vs. 7%), the outcome after RFA is vastly inferior to that after resection in terms of both overall and disease-free survival, whether single or multiple tumors are treated, and regardless of tumor size. Furthermore, the overall recurrence rate after RFA (84%) in our study was much greater than that after resection (52%); intrahepatic-only recurrence was four times higher with RFA (44%) than with resection (11%), and the frequency of true local recurrences at the RFA site (9%) was 4.5 times that of margin recurrences after resection (2%). Although we ablated only unresectable tumors, these data strongly suggest RFA is inferior to resection as a treatment for CRLM and subsequent studies have supported these findings.

In our practice, RFA is used as the primary treatment modality in patients deemed unresectable due to the patient comorbidity profile or underlying liver disease, or as an alternative option at the time of recurrence. It is important to note that though we sometimes consider ablation as an adjunct to resection when further resection would pose a risk to the FLR, this does not prove to be equal to complete resection in any of our prior studies, and when possible, we prefer complete resection utilizing a second stage approach as described above.

An important consideration when using ablation is the tumor's proximity to the confluence of the bile ducts, as thermal injury to the ducts may lead to biloma or biliary fistula. We consider distance within 1-cm of a bile duct to be a contraindication for ablation.

Chemotherapy

One of the advantages of preoperative chemotherapy is the potential for rendering unresectable tumors resectable. Giacchetti et al. and subsequently Adam et al. demonstrated that approximately 13% of patients who present with unresectable CRLM, with or without extrahepatic disease, can undergo resection after chemotherapy.

The first standard chemotherapy used for CRLM was single agent 5-FU with leucovorin, which provided modest pathologic response rates of 12% to 40% and median OS of 10 to 17 months. Subsequent combination therapies using oxaliplatin or irinotecan (5-FU or LV, with or without oxaliplatin, FOLFOX [5-FU, LV, folinic acid, and oxaliplatin], and FOLFIRI [5-FU, LV, folinic acid, and irinotecan]) have yielded significant improvement compared to monotherapy with response rates >50% and median OS >20 months in the general population of patients with stage IV disease. The addition of biologic agents (including bevacizumab and cetuximab) has increased response rates by 10% and increased median survival to 25 to 27 months.

The EORTC 40983 randomized controlled trial is the only study aimed to evaluate the efficacy of preoperative chemotherapy (FOLFOX) in the setting of resectable CRLM. Patients in this trial who received chemotherapy were more likely to undergo resection than patients with an upfront surgery approach. Though there was no difference in reported OS at the 3-year analysis, patients who were resected following neoadjuvant FOLFOX had improved progression-free survival compared to those who were resected *de novo* (35.4% vs. 28.1%, $P < .001$). Long-term results of this trial were recently reported and confirmed no difference in OS (61.3 months vs. 54.3 months, $P = .34$), but it is important to understand that the trial was not powered to detect a difference in OS. The difference in PFS remained significant with a median PFS of 20.9 months in the neoadjuvant chemotherapy group and 12.5 months in the surgery *de novo* group ($P = .035$). MD Anderson's multidisciplinary approach to colorectal liver metastasis is provided in Figure 14.9.

It is important to consider the risk of hepatotoxicity with different regimens. Steatosis is manifested by a grossly yellow appearance to the liver and is associated with the use of 5-FU. This type of parenchymal injury does not appear to increase postoperative morbidity. In contrast, steatohepatitis, characterized by inflammatory features such as hepatocyte ballooning and lobular inflammation, has been associated with the use of irinotecan and shown to result in an increase in 90-day mortality following liver resection (15% vs. 2% in patients without steatohepatitis). Consequently, major hepatic resection in the setting of steatohepatitis is a relative contraindication. Sinusoidal injury is associated with oxaliplatin, which results in a grossly blue hue to the liver surface. Histologically these changes can be recognized by the presence of hepatic sinusoidal congestion and dilatation. Sinusoidal injury may increase the risk of hepatic resection, but the conflicting nature of the published data suggests that this entity is of lesser clinical concern than steatohepatitis.

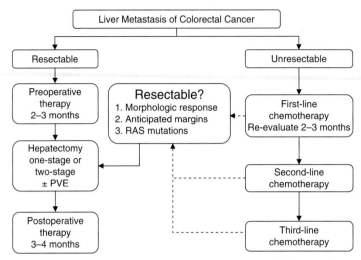

FIGURE 14.9 Multidisciplinary approach to colorectal liver metastases at MD Anderson Cancer Center. PVE, portal vein embolization. (Adapted by permission from Springer: Shindoh J, Zimmitti G, Vauthey JN, et al. Management of liver metastases from colorectal cancer. In: Chu Q, ed. *Surgical Oncology: A Practical and Comprehensive Approach.* 2015, with permission.)

Hepatic Arterial Infusion

Regional chemotherapy via hepatic arterial infusion (HAI) was originally investigated for the treatment of hepatic metastases based on the idea that infusion of chemotherapy directly into the hepatic artery would increase drug availability at the site of disease while minimizing systemic toxicity. The best reported response rates using HAI chemotherapy are 50% to 62% in studies that date from the late 1980s. However, two separate European trials that used 5-FU delivered via HAI in patients with unresectable liver disease failed to demonstrate an improvement in survival and reported high complication rates.

More recently, the use of HAI has been proposed as a method to downstage CRLM from clinically unresectable to resectable disease. Although there is no level 1 evidence to defend HAI in this setting, some data suggest that HAI may allow for conversion to surgery and improved survival in a selected group of patients. In a phase II trial from MSKCC by D'Angelica et al., 49 patients with unresectable liver metastases were treated with combined systemic chemotherapy and HAI. Nearly half ($N = 23$) achieved conversion to resection at a median of 6 months. In multivariable analysis, conversion to resectability was the only factor associated with prolonged PFS and OS (HR 0.26 [95% CI 0.15 to 0.48] and HR 0.17 [95% CI 0.05 to 0.52]). Other studies have also demonstrated improved macroscopic complete resection and median OS of patients treated with HAI, however the HAI regimen varied significantly across studies, as did the use of concomitant systemic chemotherapy.

The advantage of systemic chemotherapy is that it effectively addresses all metastatic sites, including not only the liver, but also extrahepatic occult disease. However, HAI may have a role in the conversion of unresectable liver metastases to surgery in selected patients. Further studies are necessary to better understand the benefit of HAI with or without standard systemic chemotherapy.

Hepatocellular Carcinoma

Epidemiology

Worldwide, hepatocellular carcinoma (HCC) is the fifth most common malignant neoplasm in men and the ninth in women, accounting for approximately 780,000 cancer cases annually. In the United States, HCC is comparatively rare, with an annual incidence of approximately 6 cases per 100,000 persons in 2010.

HCC arises in the background of steatohepatitis or cirrhosis and the three most common etiologies are viral-related cirrhosis (hepatitis B virus [HBV] and hepatitis C virus [HCV]), alcohol-related cirrhosis, and nonalcoholic steatohepatitis (NASH) associated with metabolic syndrome. Other less prevalent etiologies are metabolic disorders such as hemochromatosis, Wilson disease, hereditary tyrosinemia, type I glycogen storage disease, familial polyposis coli, alpha-1 antitrypsin deficiency, and Budd–Chiari syndrome. There is considerable variation in the prevalence of HCC and the underlying etiology of HCC depending on a patient's country of origin.

HCC occurs with greater frequency in regions of the world where viral hepatitis is endemic. In many Eastern countries where both HBV and HCV are prevalent, the vast majority of HCC patients are seropositive for either HBV or HCV. However, in the United States and Western Europe, only 40% of patients are positive for HBV or HCV, and there is a higher incidence of NASH-related and alcohol-related HCC. Alcohol-related HCC is often confounded by coinciding rates of viral hepatitis, so it is difficult to ascertain the contribution of alcohol consumption on cirrhosis and HCC. NASH is an emerging cause of HCC and has a prevalence that is estimated between 3% and 5% in the U.S. population with a 2.6% annual incidence of HCC among patients with NASH-related cirrhosis. Given the rising rates of obesity within the United States, it is likely that NASH will become an even more prominent risk factor for HCC in the general population.

Pathology
The histologic variations of HCC are of little importance in determining treatment and prognosis, except for fibrolamellar HCC which is found in younger patients without cirrhosis, carries a better prognosis than standard HCC, and can be cured by resection. HCC is a locally aggressive tumor with frequent local extension to the diaphragm and adjacent organs and into the portal and hepatic veins. Metastatic spread occurs most often to the lungs, bone, adrenal glands, and brain.

Clinical Presentation
In countries with systematic screening programs, HCC may be detected at an earlier stage. In Eastern countries, including Taiwan, Hong Kong, Japan, and Korea, HCC is often diagnosed by surveillance abdominal US, helical CT scan, magnetic resonance imaging (MRI), or routine screening of blood for features such as elevated serum alpha-fetoprotein (AFP) before clinical symptoms are apparent. Patients with HBV infection or no serologic evidence of hepatitis infection tend to present with larger tumors in the setting of less advanced cirrhosis.

In the United States, where there is no systematic screening for HCC, patients usually present at a later stage, often with upper abdominal pain or discomfort, a palpable right upper quadrant mass, weight loss, ascites, or other sequelae of portal hypertension. Jaundice is relatively uncommon but is a poor prognostic sign if present. The triad of abdominal pain, weight loss, and an abdominal mass is the most common clinical presentation in the United States. Rarely, patients present with tumor rupture.

Diagnosis
AFP is increased in 50% to 90% of all patients with HCC, with levels greater than 400 ng/mL usually found in patients with large or rapidly growing tumors. Despite these general correlations, AFP is neither sensitive nor specific for HCC. A patient with a small HCC tumor may have minimal or no elevation of AFP. Moreover, transient increases in AFP may be seen with inflammatory hepatic disease or cirrhosis. Several studies have reported a correlation between AFP elevation, advanced tumor stage, and poor patient prognosis, or an association between highly elevated AFP and metastatic disease; AFP >200 ng/mL in association with characteristic imaging findings is nearly 100% sensitive for HCC.

Several imaging modalities can be used to diagnose HCC, including helical CT scanning, ultrasound (US), and MRI. Both CT and MRI permit dynamic contrast-enhanced imaging. Each imaging modality has advantages and disadvantages. US is an inexpensive screening tool, but its sensitivity and specificity are low, with an overall false-negative rate of more than 50%.

At the MD Anderson Cancer Center, helical thin-slice CT scanning is the preferred imaging technique. The liver is imaged in four phases of contrast enhancement: precontrast, early vascular or arterial phases, a portal phase, and a delayed phase. LI-RADS (Liver Imaging Reporting And Data System) is used to characterize the probability that a patient has radiographic evidence of HCC in a patient at high risk for HCC and who is untreated without pathologic proof of HCC. Radiographic features that are diagnostic of HCC are arterial hyperenhancement, washout in the delayed phase, capsular enhancement, and growth ≥50% size increase in ≤6 months. Figure 14.10 is provided as a scoring system and algorithm for radiographic diagnosis of HCC.

When the diagnosis of HCC is uncertain (e.g., when imaging findings are equivocal and AFP is normal), the histologic diagnosis of HCC can be obtained by US-guided percutaneous needle biopsy or fine-needle aspiration (FNA) biopsy of the mass. Tumor seeding along the biopsy needle track rarely occurs when using modern techniques (<1% of cases). The risks of significant bleeding are low. The risks associated with major resection or transplantation for benign disease may be outweighed by the benefit of FNA biopsy in cases where the diagnosis is uncertain.

Staging of HCC: Considering Tumor Stage and Liver Synthetic Function
The eighth edition American Joint Committee on Cancer (AJCC) staging system for HCC updated the T stage. The T classification is based on several pathologic features that impact prognosis after resection: the presence

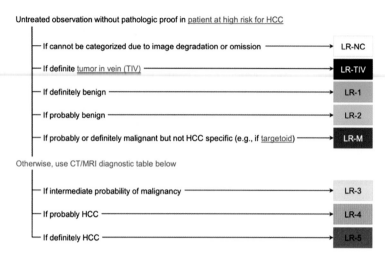

Untreated observation without pathologic proof in <u>patient at high risk for HCC</u>

- If cannot be categorized due to image degradation or omission ⟶ LR-NC
- If definite <u>tumor in vein (TIV)</u> ⟶ LR-TIV
- If definitely benign ⟶ LR-1
- If probably benign ⟶ LR-2
- If probably or definitely malignant but not HCC specific (e.g., if <u>targetoid</u>) ⟶ LR-M

Otherwise, use CT/MRI diagnostic table below

- If intermediate probability of malignancy ⟶ LR-3
- If probably HCC ⟶ LR-4
- If definitely HCC ⟶ LR-5

CT/MRI Diagnostic Table

Arterial phase hyperenhancement (APHE)		No APHE		Nonrim APHE		
Observation size (mm)		< 20	≥ 20	< 10	10-19	≥ 20
Count additional major features:	None	LR-3	LR-3	LR-3	LR-3	LR-4
• Enhancing "capsule" • Nonperipheral "washout"	One	LR-3	LR-4	LR-4	LR-4 / LR-5	LR-5
• Threshold growth	≥ Two	LR-4	LR-4	LR-4	LR-5	LR-5

LR-4 / LR-5 Observations in this cell are categorized based on one additional major feature:
- LR-4 – if enhancing "capsule"
- LR-5 – if nonperipheral "washout" **OR** threshold growth

FIGURE 14.10 The 2018 Liver Imaging Reporting and Data System's comprehensive system for standardizing the terminology, technique, interpretation, reporting, and data collection of liver imaging. This figure provides LI-RADS classifications for patients at high risk for HCC and who are untreated without pathologic proof of HCC. (From Kanmaniraja D, Dellacerra G, Holder J, Erlichman D, Chernyak V. Liver Imaging Reporting and Data System (LI-RADS) v2018: Review of the CT/MRI Diagnostic Categories. *Can Assoc Radiol J.* 2021;72(1):142–149. Reprinted by Permission of SAGE Publications.)

or absence of vascular invasion (either radiographically or microscopically), the number of tumor nodules (single vs. multiple), and the size of the dominant nodule. A study by Shindoh et al. of 1,109 patients with solitary HCC <2 cm found no difference in long-term survival based on the presence of microvascular invasion. Therefore, the new staging system includes tumors less than 2 cm irrespective of microvascular invasion (T1a) and tumors >2 cm without invasion (T1b) within the same T1 category. Similarly, patients with tumors >2 cm with vascular invasion and <5 cm without vascular invasion are both considered T2. HCC with vascular invasion of a major branch of the portal or hepatic vein are designated T4. N1 disease designates any regional lymph node metastasis.

HCC is unique in that fibrosis or cirrhosis scores are just as important in prognosis as tumor stage. The presence of severe fibrosis of the underlying liver has a negative impact on OS, regardless of the T classification. For stage I disease, the 5-year survival rate is 64% with no to moderate fibrosis (F0) and 49% with severe fibrosis or cirrhosis present (F1). The 5-year survival rate for F0 disease is 46% for stage II and 17% for stage III, compared to 30% and 9% for F1 disease. The AJCC staging manual recommends notation of fibrosis but has not yet formally incorporated the F classification into the staging system.

The most widely used classification system for the assessment of liver function is the Child–Pugh score. The parameters measured in this classification system are the total bilirubin and albumin levels, presence or absence of ascites, presence or absence of encephalopathy, and prothrombin time/international normalized ratio (INR). Together, these parameters give a rough estimate of the gross synthetic capacity of the liver. Numerous studies have validated this system as an overall predictor of survival after surgery in cirrhotic patients. Patients with Child–Pugh class A liver function generally tolerate hepatic resection. Patients with class B liver function may tolerate minor resection, but typically do not tolerate major resection. Patients with class C liver function are at significant risk from anesthesia and laparotomy and are only considered candidates for potential orthotopic liver transplantation (OLT).

The model for end-stage liver disease (MELD) score provides a more objective measure of the extent of liver disease, relying only on quantifiable laboratory values without consideration of subjective physical examination findings such as ascites or encephalopathy. The MELD score combines serum creatinine, total bilirubin, and INR to calculate an overall score which is most helpful in determining allocation of organs for liver transplant.

For anatomically resectable HCC without extrahepatic metastases, our approach to patient selection for major hepatectomy is first based on clinical parameters (performance status, Child–Pugh classification) and degree of portal hypertension. We require a platelet count ≥100,000 and exclude patients with gastric or esophageal varices. Next, systematic determination of the sFLR volume and consideration of PVE, as described previously, is necessary. This approach enables resection in patients with liver cirrhosis with a low incidence of hepatic insufficiency and death. In patients with normal liver function, this approach enables extended hepatectomy with <1% mortality and very low morbidity.

A number of staging systems have been developed outside of the classic AJCC staging system and incorporate both tumor characteristics and underlying liver function, including the Okuda staging, the Cancer of the Liver Italian Program (CLIP), and the Barcelona Clinic Liver Cancer (BCLC) systems. The BCLC is widely used and incorporates tumor stage, Child-Pugh cirrhosis classification, and performance status to guide treatment options.

Surgical Resection

The standard treatment for HCC is surgical resection or OLT. However, not all patients with HCC are candidates for surgical resection; of those presenting with HCC, only 10% to 30% will be eligible for surgery, and of those patients who undergo exploratory surgery, only 50% to 70% will achieve resection with curative intent. Patients with cirrhosis may be candidates for limited surgical resection, OLT, or locoregional ablative treatment, depending on the severity of the cirrhosis.

The only absolute criterion that initially renders a tumor unresectable is the presence of extrahepatic disease (and even this exclusion has caveats in highly selected cases). Other relative contraindications to resection are evidence of severe hepatic dysfunction, inadequate sFLR, and tumor involvement of the main PV or vena cava. Patients with normal liver parenchyma are usually eligible for extensive resection. Patients with compensated cirrhosis may be candidates for minor or major hepatectomy in selected cases. As previously described, when indicated, PVE can be a useful preoperative maneuver in patients with HCC. Palavecino et al. compared the outcomes of patients who did and did not undergo PVE prior to major hepatic resection for HCC. Patients who underwent preoperative PVE for predicted inadequate sFLR had equivalent overall- and disease-free survival and were less likely to experience major complications than patients who did not undergo PVE. No deaths occurred in the PVE group compared to 18% in the non-PVE group, re-emphasizing the importance of FLR volume analysis.

Diagnostic laparoscopy may have a role in the staging of some patients with HCC. We feel its utilization is best fit for patients with cirrhosis and visualization of the liver may better characterize the quality of the parenchyma or if there are indeterminate nodules with the FLR.

Once the tumor has been deemed resectable, the next decision is the extent of liver resection necessary, which depends on tumor size, the number of nodules, proximity to vascular structures, and the severity of any underlying liver disease. Formerly, a 1-cm surgical margin was believed to be necessary to ensure long-term survival after resection. However, Poon et al. analyzed outcomes based on resection margin in 288 patients who underwent hepatectomy for HCC and found that recurrence rates were similar between groups with narrow (<1 cm) and wide (≥1 cm) margins; only patients with histologically positive margins or satellite nodules separate from the main tumor had relatively higher recurrence rates. The authors noted that patients with margins positive for HCC had a higher incidence of intratumoral microvascular invasion than other patients. In addition, recurrences did not always occur at the margin, but also in the remaining liver distant from the margin, indicating that tumor biology is a more likely determinant of recurrence risk than is a positive margin.

Anatomic resections are preferred over segmental resections, when feasible, based on the extent of underlying liver disease and because of the tendency of HCC to spread along portal tracts. In addition, portal-oriented resections have been shown to be associated with lower morbidity, mortality, and blood loss, as well as higher survival rates, than segmental resections. Regimbeau et al. demonstrated that the overall 5-year survival rate in patients who underwent anatomic resections (54%) exceeded that of those who had segmental resections (35%).

A major pattern of recurrence after hepatic resection is intrahepatic failure with development of new disease. In the setting of underlying viral hepatitis or alcohol-related cirrhosis, the tendency of the remaining liver to generate new HCCs partially explains the 30% to 70% recurrence rate after hepatic resection. The most potent predictors of poor survival and high-risk recurrence of HCC are vascular invasion in the tumor and severe fibrosis in the underlying liver. Other correlates with poor outcome are absence of a tumor capsule and high-grade or poor tumor differentiation.

Although some classification systems, such as the BCLC system, and some groups in the United States, propose that patients with large tumors should not be considered for surgery, tumor size alone does not predict biology. In fact, multiple studies have shown that patients with T1 tumors >10 cm in diameter have similar survival after resection as those with tumors <3 cm. We analyzed 300 patients undergoing resection for tumors >10 cm and found that, for the entire group, including some patients with vascular invasion, the 5-year survival was 27% and the 10-year survival was 18%. Perioperative mortality was 5%. There were long-term (≥10 years) survivors among patients who had more than one tumor in which the largest exceeded 10 cm in diameter. The best survival was achieved in patients who had tumors without vascular invasion and who did not have severe fibrosis.

In the event of recurrence after resection, selected patients can be considered for repeat resection or ablation, depending on the pattern of recurrence. A recent randomized controlled trial by Xia et al. demonstrated no statistically significant difference in survival outcomes after repeat hepatectomy versus RFA for patients with early-stage recurrent HCC (5-year survival rate was 43.6% for repeat hepatectomy and 38.5% for RFA, $P = .17$). However, RFA was associated with worse local disease control and long-term survival for patients with recurrent HCC if tumor diameter was greater than 3 cm (HR 1.72, 95% CI 1.05 to 2.84) or AFP greater than 200 ng/mL (HR 1.85, 95% CI 1.15 to 2.96). Solitary extrahepatic metastases at sites such as the lung, diaphragm, and abdominal wall can also be resected in highly selected patients. In all of these cases, median survival may be as high as 50 months, compared with survival on the order of 10 months for those treated without surgery.

Orthotopic Liver Transplantation

Even after margin-negative resection of HCC, recurrence remains a problem. For these reasons, some have proposed that the only definitive treatment for HCC is OLT to remove both the HCC tumors and the damaged liver parenchyma.

Once liver transplantation was established as a safe treatment for cirrhosis, it began to be considered as a treatment option for unresectable tumors of the liver; however, early recurrence was common. Improved outcomes following transplantation for liver failure in patients found *incidentally* to have small HCC suggested that better selection criteria might improve outcomes for liver transplantation performed for HCC. These criteria were formalized after analysis of a study by Mazzaferro et al. who evaluated patients with Child's B or C cirrhosis and either a single tumor ≤5 cm or three tumors ≤3 cm in maximum diameter who underwent liver transplantation. Survival at 5 years after transplantation exceeded 60%, with disease-free survival exceeding 50%. These criteria, based on the Milan Meeting, were then adopted as the criteria for appropriate selection of patients for OLT for HCC even though the study was small (48 patients) and no tumors had vascular invasion.

On the basis of 70 cirrhotic patients who underwent OLT for HCC during a 12-year period at the University of California–San Francisco (UCSF), some groups now advocate OLT for solitary tumors <6.5 cm, or three nodules with the largest lesion ≤4.5 cm and total tumor diameter ≤8 cm, commonly referred to as the extended "UCSF criteria."

Locoregional Therapies

For selected patients with HCC confined to the liver whose disease is not amenable to surgical resection or OLT, locoregional ablative therapies can be considered. Although these therapies may also be used in patients with resectable HCC, their efficacy has not been established as equivalent to resection.

The advantages of ablation techniques include destruction of tumors and preservation of a maximal volume of liver, with the potential to combine ablation of small lesions with resection of larger lesions. The major disadvantages of any ablation technique are the limited ability to evaluate treatment margins and the need to obtain negative treatment margins in three dimensions. All ablation techniques have higher local recurrence rates than resection for virtually all tumors. Percutaneous ablation is particularly attractive for treatment of patients with severe underlying liver disease, for treatment of patients with a contraindication to laparotomy, or as a bridge to more definitive therapy, such as OLT.

Percutaneous Ethanol Injection

Percutaneous ethanol injection (PEI) is a treatment administered under US that induces cellular dehydration, necrosis, and vascular thrombosis, causing tumor cell death. Several studies have documented post-PEI survival rates similar to those obtained with hepatic resection for extremely small tumors in well-selected patients, but HCC recurrence in the liver is frequent, with an incidence of 50% at 2 years; the majority of recurrences are new lesions in distant segments of the liver. Randomized trials suggest PEI is appropriate for tumors ≤2 cm in diameter because it has lower rates of morbidity but equivalent efficacy when compared with other ablation techniques, such as RFA.

Radiofrequency Ablation

RFA uses heat to destroy tumors. Using US or CT guidance, a needle electrode with an uninsulated tip is inserted into the tumor and delivers a high-frequency alternating current, generating rapid vibration of ions, which leads to frictional heat and, ultimately, coagulative tissue necrosis. RFA can be performed percutaneously, laparoscopically, or through an open incision and is most effective in tumors <3 cm in diameter. Early tumor recurrence after RFA treatment is associated with large tumor size, poor histologic differentiation, advanced stage of presentation, elevated serum AFP, and the presence of hepatitis. RFA cannot be safely performed in tumors adjacent to a segmental bile duct due to the risk of bile leak. For tumors adjacent to a major vessel, the vessel acts as a heat sink, diminishing the efficacy of RFA.

Several studies have suggested that RFA may be effective for unresectable tumors. Two reports have directly compared percutaneous RFA and surgery for treatment of HCC. Hong et al. reported a series of 148 patients who presented with solitary small (<4 cm diameter) HCCs and either no or Child–Pugh class A cirrhosis. The patients selected for RFA either refused surgery or were predicted to have insufficient postoperative hepatic reserve to justify the high operative risks and were significantly older than those in the comparative resection group. The overall recurrence rates for RFA and surgery were 41.8% and 54.8%, respectively, but the rate of local recurrence was higher in the RFA group (7.3% vs. 0.0%). Rates of remote recurrence (defined as distant metastasis or intrahepatic metastasis separate from the original tumor site) and of simultaneous local and remote recurrence were similar between the two treatment groups. The 1- and 3-year OS rates were 97.9% and 83.9%, respectively, in the surgery group and 100% and 72.7%, respectively, in the RFA group.

Vivarelli et al. reported 158 patients who underwent either RFA or surgical resection. The majority of patients in the surgery group had Child–Pugh class A liver function, whereas most patients treated with RFA had class B function. 1- and 3-year rates of OS were 78% and 33%, respectively, for surgical patients and 60% and 20%, respectively, for RFA patients. Patients with Child–Pugh class A liver function and with solitary lesions, as well as lesions <3 cm in maximum diameter, had significantly higher rates of survival with surgery (overall 3-year survival = 79%) than with RFA (overall 3-year survival = 50%).

The high rate of HCC recurrence following RFA is supported by studies that evaluate the explanted liver following OLT. Mazzaferro et al. observed that among a group of patients with HCC and cirrhosis who underwent RFA followed by OLT, 45% had evidence of residual HCC in the explanted liver. Likewise, Pompili et al. studied a similar cohort and found that 53% of the ablated HCC nodules showed incomplete necrosis. A recent meta-analysis of 13 randomized, controlled trials found higher 3- and 5-year OS rates among patients treated with surgery compared to RFA. Consequently, RFA is unattractive as the sole modality for treatment of HCC in patients without evidence of underlying cirrhosis. However, RFA may be the preferred treatment for small HCCs in patients whose tumor cannot be resected safely due to tumor location or due to underlying cirrhosis. For patients who have a tumor recurrence after treatment and who are not candidates for resection, RFA is a satisfactory "salvage technique" and may enable extended remission. Therefore, ablation techniques such as RFA clearly have an important role in the treatment of this HCC patient subset.

Systemic Therapy

In general, systemic chemotherapy has little activity against HCC. Single-agent chemotherapy with 5-fluorouracil (5-FU), doxorubicin, cisplatin, vinblastine, etoposide, and mitoxantrone provides response rates of 15% to 20%, and the responses are usually transient. Combination chemotherapy does not seem to improve these results. The most active agent appears to be doxorubicin, with an overall response rate pooled from several trials of 19%.

Investigational regimens for unresectable HCC combine conventional chemotherapy (specifically 5-FU) with immunomodulatory agents, such as alpha-interferon. Preclinical and clinical studies have demonstrated that the two drugs have synergistic activity against colorectal cancer. Despite its considerable toxic effects, including myelosuppression, the combination of doxorubicin, 5-FU, and alpha-interferon (PIAF) downstaged initially unresectable tumors to a size amenable for resection, and increased the overall median survival rate in an important study by Lau et al. conducted in Hong Kong. The same investigators have reported sufficient tumor regression for subsequent resection, enabling long-term survival after PIAF.

The SHARP trial demonstrated that in patients with advanced HCC and preserved liver function (Child's A status), the oral multikinase inhibitor sorafenib was associated with a 3-month increase in median OS compared to placebo. However, a recent phase III randomized controlled trial evaluated the efficacy and safety of sorafenib in the adjuvant setting after resection or ablation of HCC and found no difference in recurrence-free survival between sorafenib versus placebo (median 33.3 vs. 33.7 months).

A small phase I trial demonstrated that sorafenib is feasible and tolerable in the posttransplant setting for patients with high-risk HCC. It does not appear that sorafenib provides a benefit in the neoadjuvant setting prior to transplant. A phase III trial found no difference in time to progression among patients treated with preoperative sorafenib and TACE compared to placebo and TACE prior to OLT.

In 2020, Finn et al. presented a phase Ib trial demonstrating improved OS and progression-free survival with combination therapy atezolizumab-bevacizumab as compared to sorafenib (1-year OS 67% vs. 55%, $P = .01$) among patients with unresectable HCC. This has created enthusiasm for using atezolizumab-bevacizumab in the neoadjuvant and adjuvant settings and we are awaiting results of ongoing clinical trials.

Transcatheter Arterial Embolization and Transarterial Chemoembolization

TACE is a combination of intra-arterially infused chemotherapy and hepatic artery occlusion, whereas transcatheter arterial embolization (TAE) omits doxorubicin, the most common chemotherapeutic agent. Chemotherapeutic agents may be either infused into the liver before embolization or impregnated in the gelatin sponges used for the embolization. Lipiodol also has been used in conjunction with TACE because this agent will remain selectively in HCCs for an extended period, allowing the delivery of locally concentrated therapy.

Two randomized control trials have shown that TACE provides a survival advantage for patients with unresectable HCC; thus, TACE is the standard of care for patients who are not candidates for resection, transplantation, or ablation. Furthermore, TACE can be used in combination with ablation or resection or as a bridge to transplantation.

Despite the favorable results of TACE therapy, this treatment modality has limitations. Morbidity rates have been reported to be as high as 23%, especially among patients with HCCs >10 cm in diameter. Moreover, postembolization syndrome, including fever, nausea, and pain, is common. Other adverse reactions, such as fatal hepatic necrosis and liver failure, have rarely been reported. TACE is generally contraindicated in patients with ascites.

Lo et al. presented a randomized controlled trial of TACE and Lipiodol for unresectable HCC in patients with compensated liver failure and in patients with advanced disease (including segmental portal invasion). The chemotherapeutic agent was an emulsion of cisplatin in Lipiodol and gelatin-sponge particles, which was injected through the hepatic artery. The chemoembolization group (40 patients) received a median of 4.5 courses per patient and showed significant tumor response. For the chemoembolization group, the 1-, 2-, and 3-year survival rates were 57%, 31%, and 26%, respectively, while for the control group the rates were 32%, 11%, and 3%, respectively ($P = .005$).

Another investigator from the BCLC group performed a randomized trial comparing either TAE or TACE with symptomatic treatment in a much more selected group of patients, who had favorable characteristics compared with those studied by Lo et al. The 112 nonsurgical candidates with HCC and cirrhosis had Child–Pugh class A or B liver functional reserve. The TACE group received doxorubicin combined with Lipiodol and Gelfoam. The trial was stopped when data review demonstrated that chemoembolization yielded survival rates significantly higher than those of conservative treatment. One- and 2-year survival rates were, respectively, 75% and 50% for the embolization group, 82% and 63% for the chemoembolization group, and 63% and 27% for the control group. Since publication of these trials, TACE has secured a role in the treatment of selected patients with HCC.

A recent phase II trial demonstrated safety of TACE using doxorubicin drug-eluting beads (DEBs) for unresectable HCC although the technique has not been proven to be superior to standard TACE.

Radiation Therapy

Historically, external beam radiation therapy has had limited utility in the treatment of HCC. The dose that can be safely delivered to the liver is approximately 30 Gy; higher doses cause radiation hepatitis and liver failure. Among patients with unresectable HCC (or other tumors such as cholangiocarcinoma or metastatic adenocarcinoma), tumor-related liver failure—secondary to either biliary obstruction or vascular compromise—is a common cause of mortality. Radiation therapy is therefore most beneficial for patients with unresectable tumors in the hilum or adjacent to the main PV or inferior vena cava (IVC) who cannot undergo local ablative therapies. At the MD Anderson Cancer Center, modified stereotactic radiation techniques including hypofractionation; administration of high, ablative doses to the center of the tumor while sparing nearby organs at risk; and controlling for respiratory motion are utilized to effectively treat unresectable, large liver tumors.

More recently, radioembolization with yttrium-90–labeled microspheres (Y90) has emerged as a local therapy. The advantage of this modality compared to external beam radiation relates to the delivery of a higher radiation dose that is confined within a more precise liver volume. The target lesion is identified and isolated using catheter-based techniques identical to TACE. The radiolabeled particles are delivered into tumoral arterial feeding vessels. The 25-μm spheres lodge at the distal arteriolar level and the emitted radiation penetrates approximately 10 mm, delivering a dose of about 150 Gy.

Summary

To summarize, patient selection, in the context of accounting for the extent of underlying liver disease, is critical when considering resection for HCC. Patients with normal liver function or Child's A cirrhosis are good candidates for major or minor resection. Minor resection may be considered among patients with Child's B cirrhosis; however, more extensive resection is not typically tolerated. Patients with HCC in the setting of Child's C cirrhosis may be considered for OLT if the Milan criteria are met. Prior to resection for HCC, determination of the sFLR is critical, and PVE is often necessary. Among patients who are not candidates for resection, locoregional therapy such as RFA, TACE, or Y90 radioembolization, may be an effective bridge to transplantation, and in some cases, can result in improvements in time to progression or OS. At select centers, stereotactic ablative radiation can be used to treat unresectable tumors at risk for local progression and liver failure. In general, systemic chemotherapy provides little benefit for patients with HCC. Based on the current data, there is a role for sorafenib but only in the metastatic setting. Emerging evidence has demonstrated a role for atezolizumab and bevacizumab in combination for advanced HCC with regorafenib and cabozantinib as options in refractory disease.

Cholangiocarcinoma

Intrahepatic Cholangiocarcinoma

Epidemiology and Etiology

Intrahepatic cholangiocarcinomas (ICCAs) arise from the intrahepatic bile ducts and can be grouped according to their growth patterns, which can be mass-forming (MF), periductal-infiltrating (PI), or can grow within the duct lumens (intraductal growth). The MF type presents as a round mass within the liver parenchyma and can recur in the remnant liver after hepatic resection. The PI type of intrahepatic CCA grows longitudinally along the bile duct, often causing an obstruction or stricture. A worse outcome is associated with tumor infiltration of the bile duct serosa, lymph node metastases, and vascular and perineural invasion. ICCAs have a higher propensity to metastasize to regional lymph nodes than perihilar cholangiocarcinomas (PCCAs).

The incidence in the United States appears to be rising, at least in part secondary to the increasing prevalence of nonalcoholic steatohepatitis. However, OS rates remain low, with less than 5% overall 5-year survival, and little is known about outcomes related to specific treatment types.

In a recent series by Yamashita et al. of 362 patients treated at the MD Anderson Cancer Center from 1997 to 2015, 160 patients were initially considered to be candidates for surgery, including up-front resection ($N = 79$) or neoadjuvant chemotherapy followed by resection ($N = 43$). An additional 38 patients were found to have unresectable disease either due to intraoperative findings or progression on preoperative chemotherapy. Of the remaining 202 with unresectable disease, most were treated with systemic chemotherapy ($N = 116$), radiation ($N = 81$), or supportive care ($N = 5$).

The most common cause of death was liver failure secondary to local tumor progression. Patients treated with definitive chemotherapy died from liver failure more often ($N = 71/99$, 72%) compared to patients treated with resection ($N = 14/47$, 30%) or radiation ($N = 18/44$, 41%). On multivariable analysis, the only independent predictor of death without liver failure was local therapy (either resection or radiation) (OR 4.11 [95% CI 2.1 to 8.2]). Therefore, we advocate liver-directed therapies for all stages of disease in order to maximize intrahepatic disease control.

Survival rates in this study improved over time among patients treated with local therapies. Although it is difficult to compare outcomes by treatment times due to selection bias, resection appears to provide the best potential for long-term disease-free status in patients with ICC.

Perihilar Cholangiocarcinoma

Epidemiology and Etiology

The etiology of PCCA is unknown. Several diseases are associated with an increased risk, including sclerosing cholangitis, ulcerative colitis, choledochal cysts, and Caroli disease (a congenital disease characterized by multiple intrahepatic biliary cysts). The common cancer-causing factor in these conditions is unclear, although chronic inflammation of the bile duct probably plays a role.

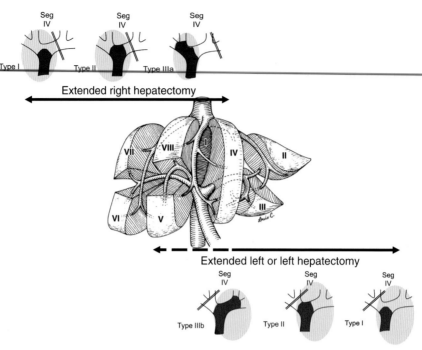

FIGURE 14.11 Classification of extrahepatic bile duct tumors according to the Bismuth–Corlette system, which describes the common patterns of hilar CCA within the biliary tree. The figure displays the surgical strategy for each tumor type and provides the language used to describe such tumors. Types I, II, and IIIa are treated by extended right hepatectomy, whereas types I, II, and IIIb are treated by left or extended left hepatectomy.

Pathologic Characteristics

Adenocarcinoma is the most common histologic type of biliary cancer; morphologically, PCCA can be classified as papillary (<5% of cases), nodular (20%), or sclerosing (70%). Most papillary tumors are well differentiated and present with multiple lesions within the duct. Virtually all long-term survivors have papillary-type PCCA. Conversely, most sclerosing-type PCCAs are poorly differentiated, and this type is associated with a poor prognosis. A tumor arising at the confluence of the right and left hepatic ducts is termed a Klatskin tumor, following the description of 13 such lesions by Klatskin in 1965.

PCCA is typically classified according to the Bismuth–Corlette classification. This classification defines the longitudinal extension of the tumor and helps define the surgical strategy (Fig. 14.11). Type I tumors are below the confluence of the left and right hepatic ducts without involvement of the "roof" of the biliary confluence. Type II tumors are similar to type I tumors but *extend* to the roof. Type III lesions extend through the intrahepatic bile ducts to involve second-order ducts to the right (type IIIa) or left (type IIIb) only, sparing contralateral ducts. Type IV tumors extend to second-order ducts on both the right and the left. Treatment is defined by anatomic location since curative resection entails removal of all liver drained by diseased ducts.

PCCAs are slow growing and most often spread by local intrabiliary ductal extension, peritoneal metastasis, or intrahepatic metastasis. Metastasis to regional lymph nodes occurs less frequently (30% to 50% of cases), and perineural extension occurs as well. Distant metastases are present in approximately 25% to 30% of patients at the time of diagnosis, but hematogenous spread is rare. Lesions of the proximal and middle thirds of the extrahepatic bile duct can compress, constrict, or invade the underlying PV or hepatic artery. In addition, proximal tumors can invade the liver parenchyma. PCCAs will involve the parenchyma of the caudate lobe in as many as 36% of patients; their appearance at this site usually occurs by means of biliary extension through the short caudate ducts that drain to the confluence, although they may emanate from a tumor located near the biliary confluence.

Clinical Presentation

The most common presenting symptoms in patients with PCCA are obstructive jaundice (which occurs in 90% of patients) and pruritus. Rarely, a very proximal tumor may block a segmental or lobar bile duct without causing jaundice. Other symptoms that may occur are weight loss (29% of cases), vague abdominal pain (20%), fatigue, and nausea. A patient may also present with cholangitis and sepsis resulting from bacterial contamination of the obstructed bile duct. In the case of middle or distal duct obstruction, a distended gallbladder may be palpable on abdominal examination; conversely, hilar PCCA is typically associated with a nondistended gallbladder. In addition to having elevated serum total bilirubin, patients with PCCA will present with elevated alkaline phosphatase, and possibly elevated tumor markers (carbohydrate antigen 19-9 [CA19-9] and CEA).

Diagnosis

The first radiologic test that should be performed when extrahepatic bile duct obstruction is suspected is an US, which can provide information about the level and nature of an obstructing lesion. US also provides information about the morphology of the lesions, possible dilation of extra- and intrahepatic bile ducts, PV and hepatic artery patency, and the presence of gallstones and gallbladder dilation.

Further imaging is necessary to delineate the cross-sectional and longitudinal (intrabiliary) extent of the tumor. At MD Anderson, multiphase helical thin-cut CT scanning is used in combination with endoscopic retrograde cholangiopancreatography (ERCP). Helical CT scanning has an overall accuracy of 76% to 100%, and MRI has an overall accuracy of 89% for staging PCCA. We prefer CT because it allows assessment of vascular encasement, cross-sectional assessment of the tumor's biliary extent, and assessment for distant metastatic disease in a single study.

In the absence of distant disease, the precise location of the tumor and its proximal and distal extent must be defined before any intervention is planned. This information can be obtained using ERCP, magnetic resonance cholangiopancreatography (MRCP), or percutaneous transhepatic cholangiography (PTC). Both ERCP and MRCP overestimate the extent of bile duct involvement in about 40% of cases, and both imaging modalities may fail to define the extent of intrabiliary tumor proximally. If the point of obstruction is believed to be proximal to the perihilar region, PTC is the preferred method for defining the biliary tract. PTC also allows brush biopsies of the tumor, external drainage of obstructed biliary ducts, and palliative stent placement when indicated.

Despite improved pre-laparotomy imaging, 25% to 40% of patients are found to have unresectable disease at the time of surgery. DL is recommended in most patients with large or extensive hilar tumors because the frequency of peritoneal metastases. For resectable PCCA, obtaining tissue to confirm the diagnosis of bile duct cancer is not essential and often proves difficult. In most instances, the decision to operate is based on the preoperative radiologic findings, not histologic confirmation. The sensitivity of brush biopsies is poor (well below 50%), although newer techniques such as endoscopic US-guided FNA of the bile duct may improve diagnostic accuracy. Treatment is guided by anatomical findings (e.g., biliary obstruction, vascular encasement, liver atrophy).

Resectability Criteria

The definitive therapy for all extrahepatic bile duct carcinomas is complete resection. Overall resectability rates range from 10% to 85%. Lesions of the lower third of the bile duct have the best rates of resectability by pancreatoduodenectomy (discussed in Chapter 15, Pancreatic Ductal Adenocarcinoma); middle-third obstructions of the bile duct are almost always due to gallbladder cancer, which is considered separately. PCCAs are technically more challenging to resect, giving them the lowest rate of resectability among bile duct tumors. Standard criteria used to determine resectability relate to the biliary extent and vascular encasement by the tumor. Involvement of secondary bile ducts necessitates hepatic resection on the side involved. Vascular involvement of the PV or hepatic artery necessitates hepatic resection of the anatomical side involved as well. However, if secondary bile ducts are involved on one side and vascular encasement occurs on the opposite side, complete resection is not possible. Lymph node involvement outside the hepatic pedicle (N2) and distant metastases preclude resection. Intrahepatic CCAs are treated by hepatic resection with tumor-free margins.

Surgical treatment of PCCA is subject to several controversies, which are described briefly: biliary drainage, extent of hepatic and caudate resections, and PV resection (PVR). Other factors in selecting patients for resection, such as patient performance status, are common between this disease and any others, and assessment of the FLR volume is a mandatory part of PCCA treatment because most patients require major or extended hepatectomy with resection of the extrahepatic bile duct.

Studies from our own institution, as well as that of the largest series of patients in the world (from Nagino et al.), show that FLR volume must be considered and PVE used to increase the FLR volume prior to extended hepatectomy for PCCA. Because the confluence of the bile ducts sits at the base of segment IV, this segment must often be resected, regardless of whether the tumor is central, left-sided, or right-sided. Hepatic resection is usually to the right, to include extended right hepatectomy, because 97% of the described variations in biliary anatomy include preservation of a long left hepatic duct. Thus, hilar disease extending even slightly to the left or significantly to the right can be cleared by means of extended right hepatectomy, taking advantage of the longer left hepatic duct. However, the problem with this approach is the higher risk of liver failure secondary to inadequate FLR even after PVE.

Disease to the left requires a left hepatectomy, which necessarily includes resection of segment IV or extended left hepatectomy. In general, obtaining a negative margin is more difficult for Bismuth type IIIb tumors involving the left hepatic duct due to the need for biliary reconstruction using the shorter right hepatic duct. Further, the right hepatic artery may be involved in this scenario and may require arterial reconstruction. Nagino et al. have reported performing an increasing number of extended left hepatectomies, comprising 30% of the total number of hepatectomies for PCCA from 2006 to 2010. Additionally, his group has demonstrated an improvement in overall mortality (from 11.1% from 1977 to 1990 to 1.4% from 2006 to 2010).

On the basis of these principles, we next discuss several controversial issues and provide our recommendations for those situations, which attend closely to the principles of preoperative preparation of the patient and liver for surgery.

Biliary Drainage

The need for preoperative biliary drainage has been debated at length in the literature, but most consider resolution of jaundice as a critical element in preparing the patient and liver for major hepatectomy. The procedure itself is safe and does not appear to increase operative complications. In a Japanese series by Ebata et al. of 160 patients with PCCA, percutaneous intrahepatic biliary drainage was performed in 50 of the 52 patients who underwent combined liver and PVR without complications.

At the MD Anderson Cancer Center, we routinely place preoperative biliary drainage catheters to drain the FLR. The liver to be resected is not typically drained unless it is necessary to resolve jaundice. Hyperbilirubinemia impairs liver regeneration and reduces resistance to systemic infection. Hepatic resection in a jaundiced patient is associated with increased rates of mortality (36% vs. 16% for those with bilirubin <2 mg/dL) and complications (50% vs. 15%).

Preoperative placement of biliary drainage catheters also facilitates the identification and dissection of the bile duct during surgery. In a study of 133 patients with PCCA who underwent major hepatectomy, Ribero et al. found a higher rate of preoperative cholangitis among patients treated with endoscopic retrograde biliary drainage as compared to percutaneous transhepatic drainage (64% vs. 13%, $P = .002$). Therefore, we typically prefer percutaneous drainage in the preoperative setting.

Finally, the degree of cholestasis in the FLR impacts not only the need for preoperative biliary drainage, but also may impact the threshold to pursue PVE. On multivariable analysis, preoperative cholangitis (OR 7.5, $P = .016$) and FLR volume <30% (OR 7.2, $P = .019$) predicted postoperative liver failure-related death. Therefore, we advocate PVE in order to ensure FLR >30% among patients with cholestasis.

Extent of Hepatic Resection

Resection of PCCA should be performed only when negative surgical margins (R0) can be achieved. Anatomically, resection of hilar cholangiocarcinoma should be considered to include the caudate lobe for two reasons. First, preoperative imaging inadequately defines the precise caudate drainage, which is quite variable among the general population. Second, the boundary between the posterior caudate and the anterior right or left hemi-liver is often difficult to appreciate intraoperatively. Attempts at preserving the caudate parenchyma may unintentionally result in incomplete tumor resection. Pathologic examination of resected specimens demonstrates direct invasion of tumor into the liver parenchyma or bile ducts of the caudate lobe in as many as 35% of patients. In addition, the caudate lobe is often the site of tumor recurrence following bile duct resection.

Jarnagin et al. reported a series of 80 patients who underwent resection for PCCA; the operative mortality and 5-year survival rates were 10% and 27%, respectively. However, the 5-year survival after resection including hepatectomy (28% with caudate resection) was 37% versus 0% after resection of the bile duct without hepatectomy. Ebata et al. later reported a series of 160 patients, all of whom underwent hepatic resection with caudate resection and reported a similar operative mortality (10%) and 5-year survival (37%), despite the need for portal resection in 52/160 patients.

At MD Anderson Cancer Center, type I and II PCCAs are treated with extended right hepatectomy or (extended) left hepatectomy along with resection of the caudate process and paracaval caudate. Type IIIa PCCAs are treated with an extended right hepatectomy, along with resection of the caudate process and paracaval caudate. Spiegel's lobe is resected if the duct is involved. Type IIIb PCCAs are treated with a left or extended left hepatectomy, along with resection of the entire caudate liver.

Type IV lesions previously considered as unresectable are now selectively considered for resection. Several studies have reported OLT as a treatment option for CCA as a part of a multimodality protocol-based approach. The results have been consistently disappointing, with high tumor recurrence rates and low OS (5-year survival rate of 23%). The sequence of open laparotomy for staging, intensive chemoradiation, and then OLT has been investigated primarily at the Mayo Clinic. Approximately 80% of patients satisfying the strict entrance criteria eventually undergo transplantation. The 5-year survival for all patients after the start of chemoradiation therapy is 55%, and 71% for those patients who undergo transplantation. Patients entering this protocol need not have biopsy-proven cholangiocarcinoma; instead, the inclusion criteria accommodate for other radiographic and biochemical surrogates. Consequently, the possibility exists that a portion of the patients may not have definitively had cholangiocarcinoma prior to initiation of neoadjuvant therapy and subsequent transplantation.

Lesions of the lower third of the bile duct do not require hepatic resection, but rather pancreatoduodenectomy (Whipple procedure). The proximal bile duct should be resected to the point that the surgical margin is negative for tumor. Occasionally, this may require removal of most of the extrahepatic biliary tract with a high hepaticojejunostomy. The operative approach for pancreatoduodenectomy at the MD Anderson Cancer Center is outlined in Chapter 15, Pancreatic Ductal Adenocarcinoma.

Lesions of the middle third of the bile duct (termed type 0 tumors by Akeeb and Pitt) are exceedingly rare. Because of these tumors' proximity to the hepatic artery and the PV, these structures are typically involved. When a type 0 tumor is deemed resectable, it is best treated by either hilar resection or pancreatoduodenectomy. Clinically, most mid-duct obstructions are due to gallbladder cancer.

Limited regional lymphadenectomy is generally indicated for PCCAs during extrahepatic bile duct resection to allow for proper staging in order to determine appropriate postoperative therapy and prognosis.

Portal Vein Resection

There are two general approaches to PV invasion when considering resection of hilar CCA. Although some would consider portal invasion a contraindication to resection, long-term survival can be achieved by complete resection, including PVR.

Neuhaus et al. in Germany proposed a systematic approach to PVR; the "no touch technique." It involves PVR in all cases of hilar CCA. Although a better 5-year survival rate was attained with PVR (65%) than without (0%), most patients with PVR underwent right-sided margin-negative resection (which, as described previously, enables a tumor-negative margin because of the longer left hepatic duct). Furthermore, the operative mortality rate was significant (17%). A second approach was proposed by Nimura et al. and updated by their group in a report from Ebata et al. This group recommended evaluating portal adherence to the region of the tumor at surgery. They validated their selective PVR approach (used in 52/160 patients) by demonstrating that 69% of those who underwent PVR had microscopic evidence of tumor invasion in the resected PV. Those in this series, patients who did not undergo PVR had a better 5-year survival rate (37%) than those who did (10%), which most likely reflects a difference in biology in these cases and supports a selective approach.

At the MD Anderson Cancer Center, the PV is resected and reconstructed when the vein is inseparable from the tumor and when vein resection will enable a negative margin resection. Routine PVR is not performed at our institution.

Surgical Outcomes

Despite aggressive surgical management, most patients with bile duct carcinoma will succumb to their tumors. Survival after resection of distal bile duct tumors has generally been better than that after resection of PCCAs. Reported 5-year survival rates range from 9% to 18% for proximal CCAs and 20% to 30% for distal CCAs. Median survival is 18 to 30 months for patients without hilar involvement but only 12 to 24 months in patients with hilar involvement. Factors predictive of long-term survival after hepatic resection for CCA are T1 tumor stage, N0 lymph node status, non–mass-forming histology, and R0 resection. Vascular invasion, N2 lymph node metastases, and lobar atrophy are all associated with worse outcomes. Lymph node metastases are found in 3% to 53% of patients; there are no data to support extended lymphadenectomy.

The optimal palliation for patients with unresectable tumors is unclear. If the tumor has been deemed unresectable before exploration, the bile duct can be drained either percutaneously or endoscopically. The use of metallic in-dwelling stents, which are more durable than traditional stents, has made this option more appealing. Unresectable lesions at the bile duct confluence, especially Bismuth type III and IV lesions, can be particularly difficult to palliate and usually require percutaneous stenting.

Chemotherapy

No chemotherapeutic agents have been definitely shown to be effective against CCA. Single-agent trials using 5-FU have demonstrated response rates less than 15%. Other agents, such as doxorubicin, mitomycin C, and cisplatin, used alone or in combination with 5-FU, have been no more successful.

The SWOG S0809 phase II Intergroup trial evaluated the efficacy of postoperative capecitabine and gemcitabine followed by concurrent radiation and capecitabine in patients with extrahepatic cholangiocarcinoma and gallbladder cancer. A total of 79 patients were treated, and the combination of chemotherapy followed by chemoradiation was generally well tolerated, with grade 3 and 4 toxicities observed in 52% and 11% of patients, respectively.

An ongoing randomized multinational phase III trial (ACTICCA-1) is investigating adjuvant chemotherapy with gemcitabine and cisplatin compared to observation after resection of cholangiocarcinoma and gallbladder cancer. The study was initiated in 2014 and will require accrual of 271 patients to assess the primary outcome of DFS.

Radiation Therapy

Several studies have investigated the role of adjuvant radiation therapy after bile duct resection. Two separate studies from The Johns Hopkins University found no benefit from adjuvant radiation therapy. Kamada et al., however, showed radiation to be beneficial in patients with surgical margins histologically positive for disease. At MD Anderson, if pathologic analysis reveals positive margins or nodes, or peritoneal invasion, patients receive a continuous infusion of 5-FU concomitantly with 54 Gy of radiation to the tumor bed. A review by Borghero et al. of 65 patients who underwent resection for extrahepatic CCA at the MD Anderson Cancer Center from 1984 to 2005 compared patients considered high risk for locoregional recurrence (R1 and/or pN1) who received adjuvant chemoradiation with either 5-FU or capecitabine ($N = 42$) with those at standard risk (R0pN0) treated with surgery alone. Five-year locoregional recurrence and OS were similar between groups, demonstrating that adjuvant chemoradiation may offset the locoregional recurrence risk in high-risk patients.

Radiation therapy has also been found to be effective in the palliation of unresectable bile duct cancers. Doses of 40 to 60 Gy have resulted in a median survival of 12 months, as well as reduced symptoms, probably because of improved stent patency. Palliative photodynamic bile duct therapy is also emerging as a potential palliative treatment option.

Gallbladder Cancer

Epidemiology and Etiology

Although carcinoma of the gallbladder is rare, it is the sixth most common cancer of the gastrointestinal tract. The tumor has been reported in all age groups but occurs most often in patients in their 50s and 60s. There is a striking difference in incidence of the tumor between genders: females are affected three to four times as often as males. Examination of the SEER database reveals an incidence of 1.2 cases per 100,000 people per year in the United States.

The exact etiology of carcinoma of the gallbladder is not known; however, it has been associated with several conditions. Cholelithiasis is present in 75% and 92% of gallbladder carcinoma cases. Patients with larger stones (>3 cm in diameter) have a 10 times greater risk of cancer than patients with small stones (<1 cm). In addition, gallbladder carcinoma can be found in 1% to 2% of all cholecystectomy specimens, a rate several times higher than that reported in autopsy studies. Chronic cholecystitis, including cases in which the gallbladder is calcified ("porcelain" gallbladder), is not associated with an increased risk of cancer, as was once believed.

Other factors linked to gallbladder carcinoma include cholecystoenteric fistulas, anomalous pancreaticobiliary junction, chemical carcinogens, inflammatory bowel disease, familial predisposition, chronic salmonella carrier status, and Mirizzi syndrome.

Pathologic Characteristics

Adenocarcinoma of the gallbladder is a slow-growing tumor that arises from the fundus in 60% of cases. On gross examination, the gallbladder appears firm with a thickened wall. The papillary adenocarcinoma subtype characteristically grows intraluminally and spreads intraductally. It is a less aggressive tumor that, consequently, carries a better prognosis when compared with other histologic subtypes. Adenosquamous cancer is very rare and is treated like adenocarcinoma.

Gallbladder carcinoma spreads by metastasis to the lymph nodes and direct invasion of the adjacent liver. It can spread to the peritoneal cavity after bile spillage, and cells may be implanted in biopsy tracts or at laparoscopic port sites. Lymph node metastases are found in 56% of T2 gallbladder carcinomas and peritoneal disease has been found in 79% of patients with T4 gallbladder carcinoma. The cystic duct node, at the confluence of the cystic and hepatic ducts, is the usual initial site of regional lymphatic spread. Invasion of the liver, either by direct extension or via draining veins that empty into segments IV and V, is seen in >50% of patients. The most common site of distant extra-abdominal metastasis is the lung.

Clinical Presentation

In most series, abdominal pain is the most common presenting symptom. Nausea, vomiting, weight loss, and jaundice are other frequent symptoms. On physical examination, patients may have right upper quadrant pain with hepatomegaly or a palpable, distended gallbladder. Laboratory results are unremarkable unless the patient has developed obstructive jaundice. The tumor markers CEA and CA19-9 may be elevated in patients with gallbladder carcinoma but are neither sensitive nor specific for the disease.

Diagnosis

No laboratory or radiologic tests have shown consistent sensitivity in the diagnosis of gallbladder carcinoma. Furthermore, the paucity of clinical signs and symptoms makes preoperative diagnosis of this cancer difficult. The disease is usually diagnosed either incidentally after cholecystectomy or at an advanced stage, when presenting with a mass, jaundice, ascites, or peritoneal disease. A correct preoperative diagnosis of gallbladder carcinoma is made in fewer than 10% of cases in most series. In the Roswell Park experience, none of the 71 cases reported were diagnosed correctly preoperatively. The most common preoperative diagnoses are acute or chronic cholecystitis and malignancies of the bile duct or pancreas. Jaundice with a mid-left bile duct stricture (type 0) is almost always related to gallbladder cancer.

In the case of gallbladder carcinoma, US may demonstrate an abnormally thickened gallbladder wall or the presence of a mass. Additional imaging by contrast-enhanced CT or MRI will help determine resectability and provide information about the local extent of disease, including PV or hepatic artery invasion, lymphadenopathy, and distant metastases.

Staging

Numerous staging systems have been described for gallbladder carcinoma. The original staging system, as described by Nevin, is based on the depth of invasion and the spread of tumor. The AJCC staging system for gallbladder carcinoma was recently revised. This included the addition of stage T2h and T2p to characterize the location of the tumor based on data from a recent international review by Shindoh et al. of 252 patients with T2 gallbladder cancer found that tumors on the hepatic side (T2h) had higher rates of vascular invasion, neural invasion, and nodal metastases than tumors on the peritoneal side (T2p) of the gallbladder ($P < .001$). T2h tumors were independently associated with worse survival on multivariate analysis (HR 2.7, [95% CI 1.7 to 4.2]) and higher rates of locoregional recurrence after resection.

Laparoscopy has a clear role in prelaparotomy staging of gallbladder carcinoma as peritoneal disease is common with this cancer. Gallbladder carcinoma also spreads locally, metastasizing to the locoregional (N1) and distant peripancreatic/aortocaval lymph nodes (N2), often encasing the PV and hepatic artery precluding surgical resection. Two studies demonstrated that DL could prevent nontherapeutic laparotomy in 33% to 55% of patients with metastatic disease. Laparoscopy was more accurate than CT in detecting peritoneal disease in patients with locally advanced tumors, suggesting that patients with T3 and T4 lesions may benefit from DL prior to surgery.

Surgical Therapy

Standard features that make a gallbladder tumor unresectable include (a) the presence of distant hematogenous or lymphatic metastases; (b) the presence of peritoneal implants; and (c) invasion of tumor into major vascular structures such as the celiac or superior mesenteric arteries, vena cava, or aorta.

Gallbladder carcinoma in situ (Tis) and carcinoma limited to the mucosa (T1) can be treated adequately with a cholecystectomy alone, provided that the cystic duct margin is negative for disease. This approach can give 5-year survival rates as high as 100%. When carcinoma is suspected before surgery, open cholecystectomy with hepatoduodenal lymphadenectomy is advocated because the T stage cannot be accurately determined at the time of surgery and because bile spillage is a significant risk factor for peritoneal or wound recurrence.

The most common site of spread from gallbladder cancer is to the periportal lymph nodes (LN) and then to aortocaval LN. Celiac LN can also be involved. Long-term survival has not been demonstrated for patients who undergo resection in the setting of positive extraregional (para-aortic, celiac, or SMA) lymph nodes (N2). The most recent AHPBA/SSAT/SSO/ASCO Consensus Conference published a consensus statement recommending aortocaval LN sampling at the initiation of intended resection for gallbladder cancer. If these LN are positive on frozen section, there is no benefit to proceeding with radical resection.

Surgical treatment for T2 tumors is somewhat controversial. Because the incidence of lymph node spread in the case of T2 tumors is 56%, optimal surgical treatment for these patients would consist of at least an extended cholecystectomy that includes resection of the gallbladder en bloc along with the portal lymph nodes.

Therefore, at MD Anderson, we recommend extended cholecystectomy that includes a resection of the gallbladder en bloc along with the portal lymph nodes, and wedge or anatomical resection of the gallbladder bed (segments IVb and V) for all T2 tumors.

Locally advanced tumors (T3 and T4) often present with lymph node metastases (75% of cases) and peritoneal metastases (79%) and are often associated with long-term (>5 year) survival rates in the range of 0% to 5%. However, recent studies have reported 5-year survival rates of 21% to 44% for series of patients with T3 and T4 tumors without metastatic disease who underwent radical resection. The extent of hepatic resection is determined by the extent of tumor invasion into the gallbladder fossa and involvement of the right portal triad. To achieve a tumor-free margin, a right hepatectomy, extended right hepatectomy, or pancreatoduodenectomy may be necessary. Pancreatoduodenectomy is generally not warranted unless the tumor extends into the head of the pancreas. Tumors involving the hepatic artery or PV can be resected en bloc, but such an extensive procedure is not considered standard due to the associated high morbidity and mortality rates.

Multimodality Therapy

Historically, the use of single and multiple chemotherapeutic agents, either as primary or adjuvant therapy, has been disappointing. The response rate of locally advanced gallbladder cancer to 5-FU regimens is approximately 12%. 5-FU combined with doxorubicin has produced response rates of 30% to 40%. A Japanese study of adjuvant 5-FU and mitomycin C found improvement in 5-year OS among patients with gallbladder cancer who received chemotherapy (26% vs. 14%; $P = .037$), however this regimen has not been routinely implemented in the United States.

More recently, systemic chemotherapy in the adjuvant setting for resected biliary tract cancers (including invasive gallbladder cancer) has shown promise. The BILCAP trial, a randomized phase III study comparing adjuvant capecitabine with observation after resection of biliary tract cancer demonstrated improved survival in the per-protocol population. It should be noted that the trial was negative based on the primary endpoint, OS by intention to treat. Still, the 14.7-month improvement seen in the trial is clinically meaningful and has changed practice. For those with unresectable or metastatic disease, the reference regimen is gemcitabine and cisplatin based on the 410-patient UK ABC-02 study which showed a survival improvement of 3 months (11.7 vs. 8.1, $P < .001$) compared to gemcitabine monotherapy. Immunotherapy and molecular profiling (i.e., fibroblast growth factor receptor, FGFR or isocitrate dehydrogenase-1, IDH1) offer the potential for novel targets and improved treatment options.

Radiation therapy has shown some promise in the postoperative adjuvant setting, although most series have been small. External beam radiation therapy at a dose of 45 Gy can reduce the tumor size in 20% to 70% of cases and relieves jaundice in up to 80% of patients. At the MD Anderson Cancer Center, patients with gallbladder cancer are treated postoperatively with a combination of continuous-infusion chemotherapy with gemcitabine and cisplatin in an approach similar to that used in patients with CCA.

Conclusion

Many advances have been made in the surgical treatment of diseases of the liver. Advances in imaging, patient selection, and patient preparation for major hepatectomy have translated into longer and better survival of patients who undergo surgery. In particular, careful attention to liver volume measurement prior to major resection in patients with liver disease and extended resection in patients with a normal liver, using such techniques as PVE or HPVE, have enabled much lower morbidity and very low mortality for liver surgery. For HCC, the spectrum of treatments reflects the spectrum of the disease and/or underlying liver disease complex. Treatments range widely, including hepatic resection, OLT, tumor ablation, transarterial embolization, Y90 embolization, and external beam radiation or proton therapy. For this disease, systemic therapy has a relatively small role in a highly selected group of patients.

For patients with CRLM, criteria for resection have expanded to include larger, multiple, and bilateral tumors. Despite these expanded indications, survival continues to improve.

Furthermore, rapidly evolving effective chemotherapy is expanding the population of patients eligible for definitive surgical treatment. Understanding a specific tumor's phenotypic profile, driven by its individual genetic sequence, is imperative to understand prognosis and will likely lead to individual tailoring of both systemic and surgical treatment in the future.

The benefits of perioperative therapies have, unfortunately, not extended to patients with biliary tract cancer. Although a small group of patients with hilar CCA and gallbladder carcinoma benefit from major hepatic resection, most patients present with unresectable disease and face limited treatment options, despite therapeutic advances in other areas.

In summary, the multidisciplinary approach to patients with liver tumors requires the involvement of specialists in hepatobiliary surgery; surgical, medical, and radiation oncology; gastroenterology; and radiology to enable optimal treatment today and advancement of multimodality treatment in the future.

CASE SCENARIO

Case Scenario 1: Colorectal Liver Metastasis

Presentation

A 64-year-old woman presented with anemia. Workup included a colonoscopy that demonstrated a near-obstructing ascending colon mass. A pre-referral right colectomy was performed, and pathology was pT4N0 (0/28). Staging CT abdomen and pelvis revealed synchronous liver and lung metastases. She had bulky metastases in her right liver (16.3 cm in size and abutting the right portal vein) and in segment IV (8.5 cm in size and abutting S3 and S4 portal triads) (Fig. 14.12). She had a solitary lung metastasis. Genetic analysis showed alterations of KRAS and APC.

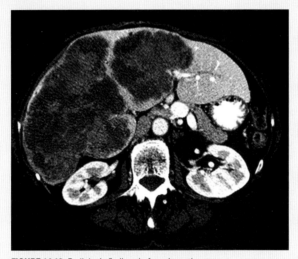

FIGURE 14.12 Radiologic findings before chemotherapy.

The patient underwent five cycles of FOLFOX + bevacizumab with restaging (Fig. 14.13).

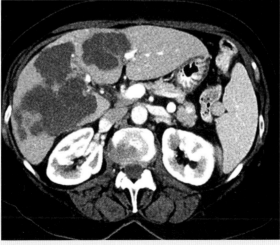

FIGURE 14.13 Morphologic response after FOLFOX + bevacizumab.

She was considered to have an optimal morphologic response to chemotherapy (Fig. 14.13). Her preoperative FLR was 31.8%, and the decision was made to proceed with right portal vein and S4 portal vein embolization. Following PVE, the KGR was 4.2% per week, and FLR increased to 44.4%. She underwent an extended right hepatectomy.

Figure 14.14 represents her postoperative imaging that demonstrates her liver remnant following extended right hepatectomy including the left portal vein branch to segments II and III. She subsequently underwent resection of her lung metastasis. She has no evidence of disease recurrence on surveillance imaging 4 years after hepatectomy.

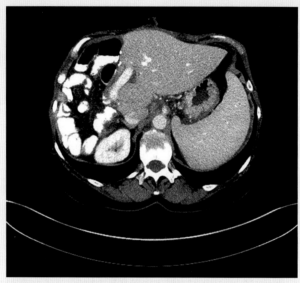

FIGURE 14.14 After extended right hepatectomy.

CASE SCENARIO 1 REVIEW

Case Scenario 1 Questions

1. What is considered an optimal morphologic response?
   A. Decrease in size of all tumors
   B. Heterogeneous attenuation within the tumor
   C. Homogeneous low attenuation of tumors with a thin, sharply defined tumor–liver interface
   D. None of the above

2. What is the minimal target kinetic growth rate (KGR)?

   A. At least 1% per week
   B. At least 2% per week
   C. At least 3% per week
   D. At least 4% per week

3. What segments are resected in an extended right hepatectomy?

   A. Segments V–VIII
   B. Segments VI and VII
   C. Segments V–VIII + at least part of segments IVa and IVb

Case Scenario 1 Answers

1. **The correct answer is C.** *Rationale:* An optimal morphologic response occurs when a postchemotherapy scan demonstrates the lesions are homogeneous and have a thin, sharply defined

tumor–liver interface. This is distinct from RECIST which is a measure of downstaging. Morphologic response to therapy is considered a more accurate predictor of pathologic response and survival.

2. **The correct answer is B.** *Rationale:* The kinetic growth rate is a dynamic functional measurement of the degree of hypertrophy divided by the number of weeks following PVE. It is associated with a more effective prediction of postoperative morbidity and mortality. A KGR of <2% per week versus a KGR of ≥2% per week is associated with higher rates of hepatic insufficiency (21.6% vs. 0%, $P < .01$) and liver-related 90-day mortality (8.1% vs. 0%, $P = .04$). Thus, a KGR of at least 2% per week is the target following portal vein embolization.

3. **The correct answer is C.** *Rationale:* A formal right hepatectomy is defined as resecting all parenchyma to the *right* of the middle hepatic vein. Since this patient has disease in segments IVa and IVb, she would require an extended right hepatectomy which includes an extension of parenchymal resection to the left of the middle hepatic vein and would include segments IVa and IVb, in addition to the right liver.

CASE SCENARIO

Case Scenario 2: Colorectal Liver Metastasis

Presentation

A 67-year-old man had a prior history of T4N1 (1/14) right colon adenocarcinoma that was resected 2 years ago. Mutational status revealed mutant APC, and wild-type RAS, TP53, and SMAD4. He completed 12 cycles of adjuvant FOLFOX. Surveillance scans revealed a solitary liver metastasis 2 years later. On imaging, the lesion measured 8.0 cm in size and was abutting the middle hepatic vein and the right hepatic vein and the hepatic hilum (Fig. 14.15).

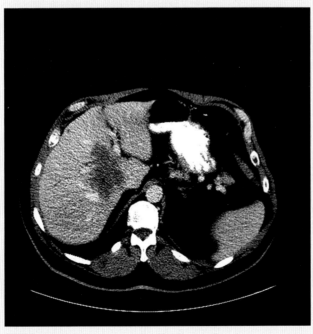

FIGURE 14.15 Radiologic findings before FOLFIRI + bevacizumab.

The patient was deemed a candidate for extended right hepatectomy, and his FLR was 16.7%. He underwent four cycles of FOLFIRI + bevacizumab followed by right portal vein embolization (Fig. 14.16).

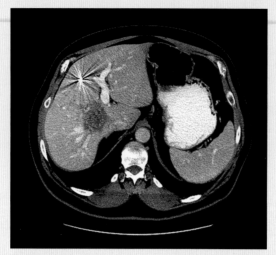

FIGURE 14.16 Radiologic findings after FOLFIRI + bevacizumab and portal vein embolization.

He underwent an extended right hepatectomy with extrahepatic bile duct resection with hepaticojejunostomy (Fig. 14.17). One year later he developed a left lower lobe lung recurrence and underwent a thoracoscopic wedge resection. He is alive without evidence of disease 5 years following resection.

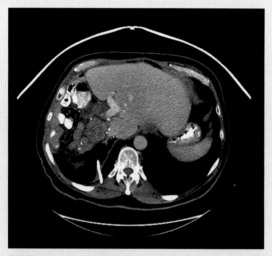

FIGURE 14.17 After extended right hepatectomy with extrahepatic bile duct resection.

CASE SCENARIO 2 REVIEW

Case Scenario 2 Questions

1. Which mutations are associated with poorer prognosis?

    A. RAS, TP53, APC

    B. TP53, APC, SMAD4

    C. TP53, RAS, SMAD4

    D. RAS, SMAD4, APC

Case Scenario 2 Answers

1. **The correct answer is C.** *Rationale:* Single mutations of RAS, TP53, and SMAD 4 are poor prognosticators. APC mutations are associated with improved survival.

CASE SCENARIO

Case Scenario 3: Hepatocellular Carcinoma

Presentation

A 53-year-old man with a history hepatitis B and C was found to have a 10-cm right liver mass (Fig. 14.18). On four phase CT scan, the tumor was enhancing on arterial phase with washout on delayed phases. He had preserved liver function and his Child–Pugh class was A. His portal pressure was measured 14 mmHg.

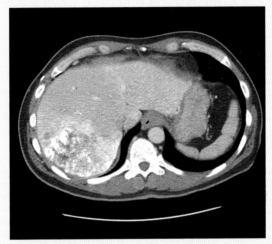

FIGURE 14.18 After transarterial chemoembolization.

He underwent sequential TACE and PVE (Fig. 14.19).

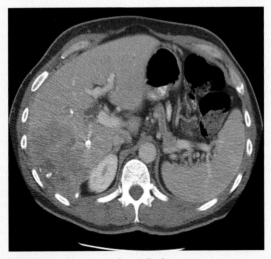

FIGURE 14.19 After portal vein embolization.

Right hepatectomy was performed with evidence of right liver atrophy and left liver hypertrophy 6 weeks following PVE (Fig. 14.20).

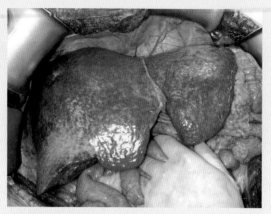

FIGURE 14.20 Intraoperative findings after ligation the right hepatic artery shows atrophy of the right liver (ischemic blue liver) and hypertrophy of the left liver prior to hepatic transection.

He was without evidence of recurrence on surveillance imaging 4 years following resection. After 4 years he developed an intrahepatic recurrence and underwent liver transplantation. He has been recurrence-free for 9 years.

CASE SCENARIO 3 REVIEW

Case Scenario 3 Questions

1. Is a biopsy necessary in this primary liver tumor?

   A. Yes
   B. No

2. What is the minimum FLR for a patient with cirrhosis and HCC?

   A. 20%
   B. 30%
   C. 40%
   D. 50%

Case Scenario 3 Answers

1. **The correct answer is B.** *Rationale:* Hepatocellular carcinoma is a radiographic diagnosis based on the LI-RADS criteria and calculates the risk for HCC in a patient at high risk for HCC. Radiographic features that are diagnostic of HCC are arterial enhancement, washout in the delayed phase, capsular enhancement, and growth ≥50% size in ≤6 months. Given this patient's history of hepatitis B and C with the radiographic findings described in the scenario, biopsy is unnecessary to confirm a diagnosis of HCC.

2. **The correct answer is C.** *Rationale:* In patients with HCC and Child's A cirrhosis secondary to viral hepatitis, alcohol, or NASH, a minimum FLR of at least 40% is recommended. Because the rate of liver regeneration may be slower among patients with chronic liver disease, sequential use of TACE and PVE can prevent tumor progression during liver regeneration prior to resection. Sequential TACE and PVE also leads to improved FLR regeneration rates and disease-free survival when compared to PVE alone in patients with HCC and cirrhosis.

Recommended Readings

Abdalla EK, Denys A, Chevalier P, Nemr RA, Vauthey J-N. Total and segmental liver volume variations: implications for liver surgery. *Surgery*. 2004;135(4):404–410.

Abdalla EK, Vauthey JN, Couinaud C. The caudate lobe of the liver: implications of embryology and anatomy for surgery. *Surg Oncol Clin N Am*. 2002;11(4):835–848.

Abdalla EK, Vauthey J-N, Ellis LM, et al. Recurrence and outcomes following hepatic resection, radiofrequency ablation, and combined resection/ablation for colorectal liver metastases. *Ann Surg*. 2004;239(6):818–825.

Adam R, de Gramont A, Figueras J, et al. Managing synchronous liver metastases from colorectal cancer: a multidisciplinary international consensus. *Cancer Treat Rev*. 2015;41:729–741.

Adam R, Wicherts DA, de Haas RJ, et al. Complete pathologic response after preoperative chemotherapy for colorectal liver metastases: myth or reality? *J Clin Oncol*. 2008;26(10):1635–1641.

Ahmad SA, Bilimoria MM, Wang XM, et al. Hepatitis B or C virus serology as a prognostic factor in patients with hepatocellular carcinoma. *J Gastrointest Surg*. 2001;5(5):468–476.

Aloia TA, Jarufe N, Javle M, et al. Gallbladder cancer: expert consensus statement. *HPB (Oxford)*. 2015;17:681–690.

American College of Radiology. LI-RADS Core v2018. Released June 2018. Accessed August 29, 2021. https://www.acr.org/Clinical-Resources/Reporting-and-Data-Systems/LI-RADS/CT-MRI-LI-RADS-v2018

Amin MB, Edge SE, Green FL, et al. *AJCC Cancer Staging Manual*. 8th ed. Springer; 2016.

Ascha MS, Hanouneh IA, Lopez R, Tamimi TA-R, Feldstein AF, Zein NN. The incidence and risk factors of hepatocellular carcinoma in patients with nonalcoholic steatohepatitis. *Hepatology*. 2010;51:1972–1978.

Bartlett DL, Fong Y, Fortner JG, Brennan MF, Blumgart LH. Long-term results after resection for gallbladder cancer. Implications for staging and management. *Ann Surg*. 1996;224(5):639–646.

Belghiti J, Cortes A, Abdalla EK, et al. Resection prior to liver transplantation for hepatocellular carcinoma. *Ann Surg*. 2003;238(6):885–892.

Ben-Josef E, Guthrie KA, El-Khoueiry AB, et al. SWOG S0809: A Phase II Intergroup Trial of adjuvant capecitabine and gemcitabine followed by radiotherapy and concurrent capecitabine in extrahepatic cholangiocarcinoma and gallbladder carcinoma. *J Clin Oncol*. 2015;33:2617–2622.

Benoist S, Brouquet A, Penna C, et al. Complete response of colorectal liver metastases after chemotherapy: does it mean cure? *J Clin Oncol*. 2006;24(24):3939–3945.

Bismuth H. Surgical anatomy and anatomical surgery of the liver. *World J Surg*. 1982;6:3–9.

Bismuth H, Corlette MB. Intrahepatic cholangioenteric anastomosis in carcinoma of the hilus of the liver. *Surg Gynecol Obstet*. 1975;140(2):170–178.

Bismuth H, Nakache R, Diamond T. Management strategies in resection for hilar cholangiocarcinoma. *Ann Surg*. 1992;215(1):31–38.

Blazer DG, Kishi Y, Maru DM, et al. Pathologic response to preoperative chemotherapy: a new outcome end point after resection of hepatic colorectal metastases. *J Clin Oncol*. 2008;25(33):5344–5351.

Blumgart LH, Kelley CJ. Hepaticojejunostomy in benign and malignant high bile duct stricture: approaches to the left hepatic ducts. *Br J Surg*. 1984;71(4):257–261.

Borghero Y, Crane CH, Szklaruk J, et al. Extrahepatic bile duct adenocarcinoma: patients at high-risk for local recurrence treated with surgery and adjuvant chemoradiation have an equivalent overall survival to patients with standard-risk treated with surgery alone. *Ann Surg Oncol*. 2008;15:3147–3156.

Brouquet A, Abdalla EK, Kopetz S, et al. High survival rate after two-stage resection of advanced colorectal liver metastases: response-based selection and complete resection define outcome. *J Clin Oncol*. 2011;29:1083–1090.

Brouquet A, Mortenson MM, Vauthey JN, et al. Surgical strategies for synchronous colorectal liver metastases in 156 consecutive patients: classic, combined or reverse strategy? *J Am Coll Surg*. 2010;210:934–941.

Brudvik KW, Mise Y, Chung MH, et al. RAS mutation predicts positive resection margins and narrower resection margins in patients undergoing resection of colorectal liver metastases. *Ann Surg Oncol*. 2016;23(8):2635–2643.

Burke EC, Jarnagin WR, Hochwald SN, Pisters PW, Fong Y, Blumgart LH. Hilar cholangiocarcinoma: patterns of spread, the importance of hepatic resection for curative operation, and a presurgical clinical staging system. *Ann Surg*. 1998;228(3):385–394.

Chan DL, Alzahrani NA, Morris DL, Chua TC. Systematic review and metaanalysis of hepatic arterial infusion chemotherapy as bridging therapy for CRLM. *Surg Oncol*. 2015;24:162–171.

Choti MA, Sitzmann JV, Tiburi MF, et al. Trends in long-term survival following liver resection for hepatic colorectal metastases. *Ann Surg*. 2002;235(6):759–766.

Chun YS, Mizuno T, Cloyd J, et al. Hepatic resection for breast cancer liver metastases: Impact of intrinsic subtypes. *Eur J Surg Oncol*. 2020;46(9):1588–1595.

Chun YS, Vauthey JN, Boonsirikamchai P, et al. Association of computed tomography morphologic criteria with pathologic response and survival in patients treated with bevacizumab for colorectal liver metastases. *JAMA*. 2009;302(21):2338–2344.

Chun YS, Vauthey JN, Ribero D, et al. Systemic chemotherapy and two-stage hepatectomy for extensive bilateral colorectal liver metastases: perioperative safety and survival. *J Gastrointest Surg*. 2007;11(11):1498–1505.

Cillo U, Vitale A, Bassanello M, et al. Liver transplantation for the treatment of moderately or well-differentiated hepatocellular carcinoma. *Ann Surg*. 2004;239(2):150–159.

Corvera CU, Weber SM, Jarnagin WR. Role of laparoscopy in the evaluation of biliary tract cancer. *Surg Oncol Clin N Am*. 2002;11(4):877–891.

Crane CH, Koay EJ. Solutions that enable ablative radiotherapy for large liver tumors: fractionated dose painting, simultaneous integrated protection, motion management, and computed tomography image guidance. *Cancer*. 2016;122:1974–1986.

D'Angelica MI, Correa-Gallego C, Paty PB, et al. Phase II trial of hepatic artery infusional and systemic chemotherapy for patients with unresectable hepatic metastases from colorectal cancer: conversion to resection and long-term outcomes. *Ann Surg*. 2015;261:353–360.

Ebata T, Nagino M, Kamiya J, Uesaka K, Nagasaka T, Nimura Y. Hepatectomy with portal vein resection for hilar cholangiocarcinoma: audit of 52 consecutive cases. *Ann Surg*. 2003;238(5):720–727.

Esnaola N, Vauthey JN, Lauwers G. Liver fibrosis increases the risk of intrahepatic recurrence after hepatectomy for hepatocellular carcinoma (Br J Surg 2002;89:57–62). *Br J Surg*. 2002;89(7):939–940.

Esposito F, Lim C, Lahat E, et al. Combined hepatic and portal vein embolization as preparation for major hepatectomy: a systematic review. *HPB*. 2019;21(9):1099–1106.

Figueras J, Jaurrieta E, Valls C, et al. Resection or transplantation for hepatocellular carcinoma in cirrhotic patients: outcomes based on indicated treatment strategy. *J Am Coll Surg*. 2000;190(5):580–587.

Figueras J, Valls C, Rafecas A, Fabregat J, Ramos E, Jaurrieta E. Resection rate and effect of postoperative chemotherapy on survival after surgery for colorectal liver metastases. *Br J Surg*. 2001;88(7):980–985.

Finn R, Qin S, Ikeda M, et al. Atezolizumab plus bevacizumab in unresectable hepatocellular carcinoma. *N Engl J Med*. 2020;382:1894–1905.

Fong Y, Fortner J, Sun RL, Brennan MF, Blumgart LH. Clinical score for predicting recurrence after hepatic resection for metastatic colorectal cancer: analysis of 1001 consecutive cases. *Ann Surg*. 1999;230(3):309–318.

Groupe d'Etude et de Traitement du Carcinome Hepatocellulaire. A comparison of lipiodol chemoembolization and conservative treatment for unresectable hepatocellular carcinoma. *N Engl J Med*. 1995;332:1256–1261.

Han S, Zhang X, Zou L, et al. Does drug-eluting bead transcatheter arterial chemoembolization improve the management of patients with hepatocellular carcinoma? A meta-analysis. *PLoS One*. 2014;9:e102686.

Hester CA, Rich NE, Singal AG, Yopp AC. Comparative analysis of nonalcoholic steatohepatitis- versus viral hepatitis- and alcohol-related liver disease-related hepatocellular carcinoma. *J Natl Compr Canc Netw*. 2019;17(4):322–329.

Hoffmann K, Ganten T, Gotthardtp D, et al. Impact of neo-adjuvant sorafenib treatment on liver transplantation in HCC patients—a prospective, randomized, double-blind, phase III trial. *BMC Cancer*. 2015;15:392.

Hong TS, Wo JY, Yeap BY, et al. Multi-institutional phase II study of high-dose hypofractionated proton beam therapy in patients with localized, unresectable hepatocellular carcinoma and intrahepatic cholangiocarcinoma. *J Clin Oncol*. 2016;34:460–468.

Iwatsuki S, Starzl TE, Sheahan DG, et al. Hepatic resection versus transplantation for hepatocellular carcinoma. *Ann Surg*. 1991;214(3):221–228.

Jarnagin WR, Bodniewicz J, Dougherty E, Conlon K, Blumgart LH, Fong Y. A prospective analysis of staging laparoscopy in patients with primary and secondary hepatobiliary malignancies. *J Gastrointest Surg*. 2000;4(1):34–43.

Jarnagin WR, Fong Y, Dematteo RP, et al. Staging, resectability, and outcome in 225 patients with hilar cholangiocarcinoma. *Ann Surg*. 2001;234(4):507–517.

Jia N, Liou I, Halldorson J, et al. Phase I adjuvant trial of sorafenib in patients with hepatocellular carcinoma after orthotopic liver transplantation. *Anticancer Res*. 2013;33:2797–2800.

Kawaguchi Y, Kopetz S, Kwong L, et al. Genomic sequencing and insight into clinical heterogeneity and prognostic pathway genes in patients with metastatic colorectal cancer. *J Am Coll Surg*. 2021;233(2):272–284.

Kawaguchi Y, Kopetz S, Newhook TE, et al. Mutation status of RAS, TP53, and SMAD4 is superior to mutation status of RAS alone for predicting prognosis after resection of colorectal liver metastases. *Clin Cancer Res*. 2019;25(19):5843–5851.

Kawaguchi Y, Kopetz S, Panettieri E, et al. Improved survival over time after resection of colorectal liver metastases and clinical impact of multigene alteration testing in patients with metastatic colorectal cancer. *J Gastroint Surg*. 2022;26:583–593.

Kawai S, Okamura J, Ogawa M, et al. Prospective and randomized clinical trial for the treatment of hepatocellular carcinoma—a comparison of lipiodol-transcatheter arterial embolization with and without adriamycin (first cooperative study). The Cooperative Study Group for Liver Cancer Treatment of Japan. *Cancer Chemother Pharmacol*. 1992;31(Suppl):S1–S6.

Kemeny N, Huang Y, Cohen AM, et al. Hepatic arterial infusion of chemotherapy after resection of hepatic metastases from colorectal cancer. *N Engl J Med*. 1999;341(27):2039–2048.

Kishi Y, Abdalla EK, Chun YS, et al. Three hundred and one consecutive extended right hepatectomies. *Ann Surg*. 2009;250(4):540–548.

Kishi Y, Zorzi D, Contreras C, et al. Extended preoperative chemotherapy does not improve pathologic response and increases postoperative liver insufficiency after hepatic resection for colorectal liver metastases. *Ann Surg Oncol*. 2010;17:2870–2876.

Klatskin G. Adenocarcinoma of the hepatic duct at its bifurcation within the porta hepatis. An unusual tumor with distinctive clinical and pathological features. *Am J Med*. 1965;38:241–256.

Lau WY, Leung TW, Lai BS, et al. Preoperative systemic chemoimmunotherapy and sequential resection for unresectable hepatocellular carcinoma. *Ann Surg*. 2001;233(2):236–241.

Llovet JM, Bruix J. Systematic review of randomized trials for unresectable hepatocellular carcinoma: chemoembolization improves survival. *Hepatology*. 2003;37(2):429–442.

Llovet JM, Real MI, Montana X, et al. Arterial embolisation or chemoembolisation versus symptomatic treatment in patients with unresectable hepatocellular carcinoma: a randomised controlled trial. *Lancet*. 2002;359(9319):1734–1739.

Llovet JM, Ricci S, Mazzaferro V, et al. Sorafenib in advanced hepatocellular carcinoma. *N Engl J Med*. 2008;359(4):378–390.

Lo C-M, Ngan H, Tso W-K, et al. Randomized controlled trial of transarterial lipiodol chemoembolization for unresectable hepatocellular carcinoma. *Hepatology*. 2002;35(5):1164–1171.

Madoff DC, Hicks ME, Abdalla EK, Morris JS, Vauthey J-N. Portal vein embolization with polyvinyl alcohol particles and coils in preparation for major liver resection for hepatobiliary malignancy: safety and effectiveness—study in 26 patients. *Radiology*. 2003;227(1):251–260.

Madoff DC, Hicks ME, Vauthey JN, et al. Transhepatic portal vein embolization: anatomy, indications, and technical considerations. *Radiographics*. 2002;22(5):1063–1076.

Mazzaferro V, Regalia E, Doci R, et al. Liver transplantation for the treatment of small hepatocellular carcinomas in patients with cirrhosis. *N Engl J Med*. 1996;334(11):693–699.

Mise Y, Passot G, Wang X, et al. A nomogram to predict hypertrophy of liver segments 2 and 3 after right portal vein embolization. *J Gastrointest Surg*. 2016;20(7):1317–1323.

Mise Y, Zimmitti G, Shindoh J, et al. RAS mutations predict radiologic and pathologic response in patients treated with chemotherapy before resection of colorectal liver metastases. *Ann Surg Oncol*. 2015;22:834–842.

Moulton C-A, Gu C-S, Law CH, et al. Effect of PET before liver resection on surgical management for colorectal adenocarcinoma metastases: a randomized clinical trial. *JAMA*. 2014;311:1863–1869.

Nagino M, Ebata T, Yokoyama Y, et al. Evolution of surgical treatment for perihilar cholangiocarcinoma: a single-center 34-year review of 574 consecutive resections. *Ann Surg*. 2013;258(1):129–140.

Nagino M, Kamiya J, Kanai M, et al. Right trisegmentectomy portal vein embolization for biliary tract carcinoma: technique and clinical utility. *Surgery*. 2000;127(2):155–160.

Nagino M, Kamiya J, Uesaka K, et al. Complications of hepatectomy for hilar cholangiocarcinoma. *World J Surg.* 2001;25(10):1277–1283.

Nagino M, Yamada T, Kamiya J, Uesaka K, Arai T, Nimura Y. Left hepatic trisegmentectomy with right hepatic vein resection after right hepatic vein embolization. *Surgery.* 2003;133:580–582.

Nash GM, Gimbel M, Shia J, et al. KRAS mutation correlates with accelerated metastatic progression in patients with colorectal liver metastases. *Ann Surg Oncol.* 2010;17:572–578.

Nathan H, Aloia TA, Vauthey J-N, et al. A proposed staging system for intrahepatic cholangiocarcinoma. *Ann Surg Oncol.* 2009;16(1):14–22.

Neuhaus P, Jonas S, Settmacher U, et al. Surgical management of proximal bile duct cancer: extended right lobe resection increases resectability and radicality. *Langenbecks Arch Surg.* 2003;388(3):194–200.

Nevin JE, Moran TJ, Kay S, King R. Carcinoma of the gallbladder: staging, treatment, and prognosis. *Cancer.* 1976;37(1):141–148.

Nordlinger B, Sorbye H, Glimelius B, et al. Perioperative chemotherapy with FOLFOX4 and surgery versus surgery alone for resectable liver metastases from colorectal cancer (EORTC Intergroup trial 40983): a randomised controlled trial. *Lancet.* 2008;371(9617):1007–1016.

Nordlinger B, Sorbye H, Glimelius B, et al. Perioperative FOLFOX4 chemotherapy and surgery versus surgery alone for resectable liver metastases from colorectal cancer (EORTC 40983): long-term results of a randomised, controlled, phase 3 trial. *Lancet Oncol.* 2013;14:1208–1215.

Ogata S, Belghiti J, Farges O, Varma D, Sibert A, Vilgrain V. Sequential arterial and portal vein embolizations before right hepatectomy in patients with cirrhosis and hepatocellular carcinoma. *Br J Surg.* 2006;93(9):1091–1098.

Oshowo A, Gillams A, Harrison E, Lees WR, Taylor I. Comparison of resection and radiofrequency ablation for treatment of solitary colorectal liver metastases. *Br J Surg.* 2003;90(10):1240–1243.

Parikh AA, Gentner B, Wu T-T, Curley SA, Ellis LM, Vauthey J-N. Perioperative complications in patients undergoing major liver resection with or without neoadjuvant chemotherapy. *J Gastrointest Surg.* 2003;7(8):1082–1088.

Passot G, Odisio BC, Zorzi D, et al. Eradication of missing liver metastases after fiducial placement. *J Gastrointest Surg.* 2016;20:1173–1178.

Pawlik TM, Esnaola NF, Vauthey JN. Surgical treatment of hepatocellular carcinoma: similar long-term results despite geographic variations. *Liver Transpl.* 2004;10(2 suppl 1):S74–S80.

Pawlik TM, Poon RT, Abdalla EK, et al. Hepatectomy for hepatocellular carcinoma with major portal or hepatic vein invasion: results of a multicenter study. *Surgery.* 2005;137(4):403–410.

Pawlik TM, Scoggins CR, Zorzi D, et al. Effect of surgical margin status on survival and site of recurrence after hepatic resection for colorectal metastases. *Ann Surg.* 2005;241(5):715–722.

Poon RT, Fan ST, Lo CM, et al. Improving survival results after resection of hepatocellular carcinoma: a prospective study of 377 patients over 10 years. *Ann Surg.* 2001;234(1):63–70.

Poon RT, Fan ST, Ng IO, Wong J. Significance of resection margin in hepatectomy for hepatocellular carcinoma: a critical reappraisal. *Ann Surg.* 2000;231(4):544–551.

Poon RT, Fan ST, Wong J. Selection criteria for hepatic resection in patients with large hepatocellular carcinoma larger than 10 cm in diameter. *J Am Coll Surg.* 2002;194(5):592–602.

Poon RT, Ng IO, Fan ST, et al. Clinicopathologic features of long-term survivors and disease-free survivors after resection of hepatocellular carcinoma: a study of a prospective cohort. *J Clin Oncol.* 2001;19(12):3037–3044.

Reddy SK, Pawlik TM, Zorzi D, et al. Simultaneous resections of colorectal cancer and synchronous liver metastases: a multi-institutional analysis. *Ann Surg Oncol.* 2007:14(12):3481–3491.

Regimbeau JM, Abdalla EK, Vauthey JN, et al. Risk factors for early death due to recurrence after liver resection for hepatocellular carcinoma: results of a multicenter study. *J Surg Oncol.* 2004;85(1):36–41.

Regimbeau JM, Kianmanesh R, Farges O, Dondero F, Sauvanet A, Belghiti J. Extent of liver resection influences the outcome in patients with cirrhosis and small hepatocellular carcinoma. *Surgery.* 2002;131(3):311–317.

Reyes DK, Vossen JA, Kamel IR, et al. Single-center phase II trial of transarterial chemoembolization with drug-eluting beads for patients with unresectable hepatocellular carcinoma: initial experience in the United States. *Cancer J.* 2009;15:526–532.

Ribero D, Wang H, Donadon M, et al. Bevacizumab improves pathologic response and protects against hepatic injury in patients treated with oxaliplatin-based chemotherapy for colorectal liver metastases. *Cancer.* 2007;110(12):2761–2767.

Ribero D, Zimmitti G, Aloia TA, et al. Preoperative cholangitis and future liver remnant volume determine the risk of liver failure in patients undergoing resection for hilar cholangiocarcinoma. *J Am Coll Surg.* 2016;223(1):87–97.

Sala M, Varela M, Bruix J. Selection of candidates with HCC for transplantation in the MELD era. *Liver Transpl.* 2004;10(10 suppl 2):S4–S9.

Salem R, Gordon AC, Mouli S, et al. Y90 radioembolization significantly prolongs time to progression compared with chemoembolization in patients with hepatocellular carcinoma. *Gastroenterology.* 2016;151(6):1155–1163.

Schnitzbauer AA, Lang SA, Goessmann H, et al. Right portal vein ligation combined with in situ splitting induces rapid left lateral liver lobe hypertrophy enabling 2–staged extended right hepatic resection in small-for-size settings. *Ann Surg.* 2012;255:405–414.

Shindoh J, de Aretxabala X, Aloia TA, et al. Tumor location is a strong predictor of tumor progression and survival in T2 gallbladder cancer: an international multicenter study. *Ann Surg.* 2015;261:733–739.

Shindoh J, Loyer EM, Kopetz S, et al. Optimal morphologic response to preoperative chemotherapy: an alternate outcome end point before resection of hepatic colorectal metastases. *J Clin Oncol.* 2012;30:4566–4572.

Shindoh J, Truty MJ, Aloia TA, et al. Kinetic growth rate after portal vein embolization predicts posthepatectomy outcomes: toward zero liver-related mortality in patients with colorectal liver metastases and small future liver remnant. *J Am Coll Surg.* 2013;216:201–209.

Shindoh J, Tzeng C-WD, Aloia TA, et al. Optimal future liver remnant in patients treated with extensive preoperative chemotherapy for colorectal liver metastases. *Ann Surg Oncol.* 2013;20:2493–2500.

Shindoh J, Tzeng C-WD, Aloia TA, et al. Portal vein embolization improves rate of resection of extensive colorectal liver metastases without worsening survival. *Br J Surg.* 2013;100:1777–1783.

Shindoh J, Vauthey JN, Zimmitti G, et al. Analysis of the efficacy of portal vein embolization for patients with extensive liver malignancy and very low future liver remnant volume, including a comparison with the associating liver partition with portal vein ligation for staged hepatectomy approach. *J Am Coll Surg.* 2013;217:126–133; discussion 133–134.

Shirabe K, Shimada M, Gion T, et al. Postoperative liver failure after major hepatic resection for hepatocellular carcinoma in the modern era with special reference to remnant liver volume. *J Am Coll Surg.* 1999;188(3):304–309.

Shirai Y, Yoshida K, Tsukada K, Muto T. Inapparent carcinoma of the gallbladder. An appraisal of a radical second operation after simple cholecystectomy. *Ann Surg.* 1992;215(4):326–331.

Siegel AB, El-Khoueiry AB, Finn RS, et al. Phase I trial of sorafenib following liver transplantation in patients with high-risk hepatocellular carcinoma. *Liver Cancer.* 2015;4:115–125.

Snyder RA, Hao S, Irish W, Zervos EE, Tuttle-Newhall JE, Parikh AA. Thirty-day morbidity after simultaneous resection of colorectal cancer and colorectal liver metastasis: American College of Surgeons NSQIP analysis. *J Am Coll Surg.* 2020;230(4):617–627.e9.

Stein A, Arnold D, Bridgewater J, et al. Adjuvant chemotherapy with gemcitabine and cisplatin compared to observation after curative intent resection of cholangiocarcinoma and muscle invasive gallbladder carcinoma (ACTICCA-1 trial)—a randomized, multidisciplinary, multinational phase III trial. *BMC Cancer.* 2015;15:564.

Takada T, Amano H, Yasuda H, et al. Is postoperative adjuvant chemotherapy useful for gallbladder carcinoma? A phase III multicenter prospective randomized controlled trial in patients with resected pancreaticobiliary carcinoma. *Cancer.* 2002;95:1685–1695.

Valle JW, Kelley RK, Nervi B, Oh DY, Zhu AX. Biliary tract cancer. *The Lancet.* 2021;397(10272):428–444.

Vauthey JN, Abdalla EK, Doherty DA, et al. Body surface area and body weight predict total liver volume in Western adults. *Liver Transpl.* 2002;8(3):233–240.

Vauthey JN, Chaoui A, Do KA, et al. Standardized measurement of the future liver remnant prior to extended liver resection: methodology and clinical associations. *Surgery.* 2000;127(5):512–519.

Vauthey JN, Lauwers GY, Esnaola NF, et al. Simplified staging for hepatocellular carcinoma. *J Clin Oncol.* 2002;20(6):1527–1536.

Vauthey JN, Pawlik TM, Lauwers GY, et al. Critical evaluation of the different staging systems for hepatocellular carcinoma. *Br J Surg.* 2004;91(8):1072.

Vauthey JN, Pawlik TM, Ribero D, et al. Chemotherapy regimen predicts steatohepatitis and an increase in 90-day mortality after surgery for hepatic colorectal metastases. *J Clin Oncol.* 2006;24:2065–2072.

Vauthey JN, Sobin LH. On the uniform use of the AJCC/UICC staging system for hepatocellular carcinoma. *Surgery.* 2000;128(5):870.

Vauthey JN, Zimmitti G, Kopetz SE, et al. RAS mutation status predicts survival and patterns of recurrence in patients undergoing hepatectomy for colorectal liver metastases. *Ann Surg.* 2013;258:619–626; discussion 626–627.

Xia Y, Li J, Liu G, et al. Long-term effects of repeat hepatectomy vs percutaneous radiofrequency ablation among patients with recurrent hepatocellular carcionma: a randomized clinical trial. *JAMA Oncol.* 2020;6(2):255–263.

Yamamoto J, Sugihara K, Kosuge T, et al. Pathologic support for limited hepatectomy in the treatment of liver metastases from colorectal cancer. *Ann Surg.* 1995;221(1):74–78.

Yamashita S, Koay EJ, Passot G, et al. Local therapy reduces the risk of liver failure and improves survival in patients with intrahepatic cholangiocarcinoma: a comprehensive analysis of 362 consecutive patients. *Cancer.* 2017;123:1354–1362, http://dx.doi.org/10.1002/cncr.30488

Yao FY, Ferrell L, Bass NM, et al. Liver transplantation for hepatocellular carcinoma: expansion of the tumor size limits does not adversely impact survival. *Hepatology.* 2001;33(6):1394–1403.

Younossi ZM. Review article: current management of non-alcoholic fatty liver disease and non-alcoholic steatohepatitis. *Aliment Pharmacol Ther.* 2008;28:2–12.

15 Pancreatic Ductal Adenocarcinoma

Cameron E. Gaskill, Michael P. Kim, and Matthew H.G. Katz

Epidemiology

Pancreatic ductal adenocarcinoma (PDAC) is the most common invasive carcinoma of the pancreas. The disease is the third most common cause of cancer-related deaths in the United States with 48,220 estimated cases in 2021 and a yearly incidence of 13.2 cases per 100,000 people. The overall risk of developing pancreatic cancer rises after age 50 years, and the median age of diagnosis is 70 years. Despite recent advances in the treatment of PDAC, the 5-year overall survival rate remains a dismal 10.8%, in part because most patients present with advanced disease that precludes curative therapy. Identifying patient populations at increased risk for PDAC, enabling earlier diagnosis and application of evolving targeted therapies, is therefore imperative.

Multiple risk factors have been identified that increase the risk for development of PDAC, including genetically inherited cancer syndromes and diverse environmental factors. Inherited cancer syndromes associated with pancreatic cancer include Peutz–Jeghers syndrome (up to 132-fold risk), hereditary breast–ovarian cancer syndrome (associated with *BRCA1* or *BRCA2* mutations, up to four-fold risk), familial atypical multiple mole melanoma syndrome (FAMM, up to 22-fold risk), and hereditary nonpolyposis colon cancer syndrome (HNPCC, 30-fold risk). Up to 10% of all pancreatic cancers are familial, and a person's risk of developing pancreatic cancer appears to increase with its penetrance among related family members. Identification of patient populations with genetic predispositions to PDAC may therefore improve patient outcomes through aggressive disease surveillance and early detection.

Significant risk factors for sporadic pancreatic cancer include cigarette smoking, obesity, and chronic pancreatitis. One case-control study of more than 1,600 patients revealed that smoking and diabetes acted synergistically with family history to increase the risk of PDAC. Another major study revealed that diabetes mellitus and elevated insulin concentrations were associated with a twofold higher risk of PDAC. Despite the identification of several risk factors for this disease, PDAC screening in the general population is logistically and financially impractical because of its relatively low prevalence and the lack of well-defined patient subgroups at high risk for the disease.

Whole exome sequencing of tumor genomes across a spectrum of patients have defined the PDAC mutational landscape. Activating missense mutations in *KRAS,* the most commonly altered oncogene in human cancers, are present in ~95% of patients with PDAC and represent a prevalent and critical therapeutic target in pancreatic cancer biology. Subsequent mutations in key tumor suppressor genes including *TP53*, *CDKN2A*, and *SMAD4* lead to unopposed mitogenic signaling, impaired oncogene-induced senescence, and the promotion of tumor cell proliferation and metastasis. Interactions of tumor cells with diverse cellular and noncellular constituents of the tumor microenvironment (TME) are extensive and result in immunosuppression, epithelial-to-mesenchymal transition, and chemoresistance. Much attention has therefore been focused on understanding underlying biology of the PDAC TME to improve the delivery of chemotherapy while reversing immunosuppression and promoting T cell activation. To date, efforts to target various drivers of the malevolent TME (failed hyaluronidase inhibitor trial, checkpoint+chemo trials, etc.) have not resulted in widespread improvements in patients' survival, However, the recent success of oncogenic KRAS inhibition (G12C) in the treatment of lung cancer, combined with other KRAS inhibitors reported to be in the drug development pipeline that target prevalent isoforms of oncogenic KRAS in PDAC, continue to inspire hope that transformational KRAS-based therapies will set a new standard of care and improve survival metrics in PDAC.

Clinical Presentation

The clinical presentation of pancreatic cancer is variable and nonspecific. The most common symptom at presentation is jaundice related to extrahepatic biliary obstruction, which occurs in up to 50% of all patients with PDAC and is more common in patients with cancers of the pancreatic head. Nonspecific complaints include constitutional symptoms, weight loss, and abdominal pain that often radiates to the back. Many patients diagnosed with pancreatic cancer have been recently diagnosed with diabetes, which may be related to β-cell dysfunction and/or peripheral insulin resistance induced by tumor-derived factors, such as adrenomedullin or islet amyloid polypeptide.

Symptoms associated with PDAC are often indicative of the stage of disease and overall prognosis. Pain, for example, is generally indicative of advanced cancer. Kelsen et al. found that patients who presented with pain had a shorter median overall survival than did patients who did not, regardless of the resectability status of their tumors. Patients may also present with physical findings that may be helpful in assessing disease stage and prognosis. Patients who present with cachexia are less likely to undergo resection and have shorter survival than patients who are not cachectic at presentation. Other subtle signs of metastatic disease include enlargement of left supraclavicular lymph nodes (Virchow node) or periumbilical lymph nodes (Sister Mary Joseph node). Rectal examination may reveal a Blumer shelf, which may indicate intraperitoneal tumor deposits. Ascites, a more common finding, may indicate carcinomatosis. Rarely, patients with advanced disease present with cutaneous nodules.

Diagnosis and Staging

The fundamental goals of the initial evaluation of a patient with a pancreatic mass suspicious for PDAC are: (a) to secure the histopathologic diagnosis, (b) to stage the disease, and (c) to estimate the patient's physiologic profile. It is only once these fundamental goals have been met that rational treatment recommendations can be delivered.

Cross-Sectional Imaging

Computed tomography (CT) remains the most important imaging modality in the diagnostic workup of patients with suspected pancreatic cancer. CT may identify a pancreatic mass, delineate important anatomic relationships between the mass and mesenteric vasculature, and identify sites of metastatic disease.

At the MD Anderson Cancer Center (MDACC), a pancreas protocol CT scan uses water as a negative oral contrast agent and starts with precontrast imaging from the dome of the liver extending caudally to include the entire liver reconstructed to 2.5-mm slice thickness. Next, 125 mL of iodinated contrast is administered intravenously at a rate of 3 to 5 mL/s. The arterial phase uses bolus tracking and images are obtained 10 seconds after a Hounsfield unit value of 100 is reached in the aorta at the level of the celiac axis, from the dome of the liver to the iliac crests. Images for the portal venous phase are obtained at a 20-second delay from the arterial phase. Delayed images are obtained 15 seconds after the portal venous phase. The images are reconstructed to 2.5-mm slice thickness for imaging review and at 0.625- or 1.25-mm slice thickness to create coronal and sagittal reformatted images.

The primary pancreatic tumor is best seen on the arterial phase of the CT scan and typically appears as a hypodense mass against the relatively contrast-enhancing normal pancreatic parenchyma that surrounds it. Significant attention should be paid to the precise vascular anatomy and the anatomic relationships between the mesenteric vasculature and the primary pancreatic tumor. As many as 40% to 45% of patients have variants of "normal" hepatic arterial anatomy, and it is of vital importance to appreciate such variants on preoperative imaging as they directly impact operative planning. Notable examples include a replaced or accessory right hepatic artery that is present in up to 15% of patients, and most commonly arises from the SMA and courses posterior to the pancreas and posterolateral to the bile duct. An additional 2.5% of patients have a replaced common hepatic artery that arises from the SMA and follows a similar path as a replaced or accessory right hepatic artery.

The superior mesenteric vein (SMV) and portal vein (PV), as well as their major venous tributaries, are best evaluated on the portal venous phase. The initial staging CT scan has great sensitivity and specificity for determining venous involvement by tumor, and the surgeon should carefully estimate the circumferential extent of the tumor–vein interface, as well as note the vein contour and the presence or absence of deformity. Tran Cao et al. evaluated the preoperative CT scan of 254 patients who underwent pancreatoduodenectomy for PDAC and measured the tumor–vein interface as none, ≤180 degrees, >180 degrees, or associated with venous occlusion. The need for vein resection was associated with the extent of circumferential interface; for example, 34 of 38 patients (89%) with a tumor–vein interface >180 degrees or venous occlusion required a vein resection at pancreatectomy. The surgeon should also identify the location and anatomic relationships of the gastroepiploic vein, colic veins, inferior mesenteric vein (IMV), and jejunal/ileal branches of the SMV as these have variable courses and the drainage pattern directly impacts surgical options for reconstruction of the superior mesenteric–portal vein (SMV–PV) confluence, which can be expected in as many as 40% to 60% of cases performed at high-volume centers.

Hepatic metastases are usually best visualized on the portal venous phase of CT. Liver metastases may be better characterized using magnetic resonance imaging (MRI), which is most useful as an adjunct to CT imaging. MRI should not replace a pancreas-protocol CT scan in the workup/staging of patient with suspected PDAC, although it may be a better option in patients with chronic kidney disease.

	MDACC	AHPBA/SSO/SSAT	National Consensus Guidelines	Intergroup
CA	Abutment	No abutment or encasement	Contact ≤180 degrees	Interface <180 degrees
CHA	Abutment of short-segment encasement	Short-segment abutment or encasement amenable to reconstruction	Contact without extension to celiac axis or hepatic artery bifurcation amenable to resection and reconstruction	Short-segment interface of any degree amenable to reconstruction
SMA	Abutment <180 degrees	Abutment <180 degrees	Contact ≤180 degrees	Interface <180 degrees
SMV-PV	Short-segment occlusion amenable to resection and reconstruction	Abutment >180 degrees or occlusion amenable to resection and reconstruction	Contact of >180 degrees, contact of ≤180 degrees with irregularity of vein, or thrombosis amenable to resection and reconstruction	Interface ≥180 degrees and/or occlusion amenable to reconstruction

TABLE 15.1 Definitions of Borderline Resectable PDAC[a]

[a]Absence of extrapancreatic disease.

CA, celiac axis; CHA, common hepatic artery; HA, hepatic artery; PDAC, pancreatic ductal adenocarcinoma; SMA, superior mesenteric artery; SMV-PV, superior mesenteric vein-portal vein.

Definitions of Surgical Resectability

Over the years, the multidisciplinary team at MDACC has defined imaging criteria that characterize tumors as clinically resectable, borderline resectable (BR), and locally advanced (LA) based on the anatomic relationship between the primary tumor and adjacent mesenteric vasculature. Several other groups and societies have offered similar definitions; a summary of various radiographic definitions of BR PDAC can be found in Table 15.1. Tumors anatomically less infiltrative than these are considered resectable, and those more infiltrative are considered LA and generally unresectable.

Endoscopic Ultrasound

Endoscopic ultrasonography (EUS) may aid in diagnosis and is particularly valuable in the evaluation of smaller pancreatic lesions: EUS has an overall sensitivity of 99% and a sensitivity of 96% for tumors <2 cm in diameter. EUS can also be used to help assess the primary tumor's relationship to the mesenteric vasculature and regional lymph node involvement.

EUS-guided fine-needle aspiration biopsy is the preferred method to secure a tissue diagnosis of the primary tumor and any suspicious regional lymph nodes. Although confirmation of the diagnosis may not always be necessary in patients with suspected PDAC who are anticipated to undergo immediate surgery, we typically recommend it to exclude other diagnoses (e.g., focal pancreatitis, lymphoma, idiopathic pancreatitis) that may masquerade as PDAC but which would be best treated nonsurgically. Further, a tissue diagnosis is required prior to the administration of chemotherapy or chemoradiation.

Serum CA 19-9

The serum tumor marker assayed most frequently in the workup of patients with suspected pancreatic cancer is carbohydrate antigen (CA) 19-9, a ganglioside Lewis blood group–associated antigen. Patients who are Lewis antigen negative (about 10% of the population) do not express CA 19-9. CA 19-9 levels have been correlated to tumor size and have limited sensitivity to detect small lesions. Although CA 19-9 is not beneficial as a screening tool, it does have value as a diagnostic tool and can also be used to monitor response to therapy. Biliary obstruction from any cause may result in an elevation in the CA 19-9 level; therefore, serum bilirubin should always be measured alongside serum CA 19-9.

The diagnostic specificity of CA 19-9 may increase in the presence of other diagnostic findings. For example, a retrospective analysis of 150 patients who underwent surgery for suspected pancreatic cancer revealed that the combination of a serum CA 19-9 level >37 U/mL, weight loss of >20 lb, and a serum bilirubin level >3 mg/dL was associated with 100% sensitivity and a 100% positive predictive value for pancreatic cancer. The CA 19-9 level should therefore always be interpreted in light of the other clinical and radiographic findings.

CA 19-9 may help to clinically stage PDAC and its level in the blood should influence treatment recommendations. Ferrone et al. analyzed CA 19-9 levels in a series of pancreatic cancer patients with serum bilirubin levels <2 mg/dL, who underwent surgery de novo, and found that preoperative CA 19-9 levels correlated with the T stage, N stage, and survival. Using the National Cancer Database, Bergquist et al. found that an elevated CA 19-9 was associated with decreased stage-specific survival, which was most dramatic in patients with early stage (I/II) cancer. Maithel et al. found that an elevation of CA 19-9 was associated with identification of radiographically occult unresectable disease. A high-serum CA 19-9 is therefore suggestive of advanced disease irrespective of imaging findings. At MDACC, a high level of CA 19-9 would prompt the administration of preoperative systemic chemotherapy to a patient with localized PDAC, even in the absence of radiographic evidence of metastatic disease.

Once treatment has been initiated, the change in CA 19-9 in response to therapy can be used as an indicator of treatment efficacy. In a study done by Perri et al, normalized CA 19-9 levels after neoadjuvant therapy was associated with increased odds of achieving a major pathologic response.

Staging Laparoscopy

Several studies have validated the use of staging laparoscopy to identify subcentimeter hepatic and peritoneal metastases not detected by CT. Although some studies have found that laparoscopy altered the management of up to 44% of patients with radiographically resectable PDAC, the yield of laparoscopy for cancer staging has decreased as imaging techniques have improved. A 2001 study showed that laparoscopic findings enabled laparotomy to be avoided in only 4% to 13% of patients who had disease that was radiographically determined to be resectable. More recently, a large study of more than 1,000 patients revealed that laparoscopy was of even less benefit, especially among patients in whom high-quality CT had been recently performed.

At MDACC, we generally reserve laparoscopy for patients with large primary tumors, patients with cancers in the pancreatic body or tail, patients with markedly elevated CA 19-9 levels, patients with a history of severe weight loss and hypoalbuminemia, and patients with radiographic findings equivocal for the presence of metastatic disease or carcinomatosis. We may perform staging laparoscopy as a separate procedure. However, given its simplicity and low associated morbidity, staging laparoscopy often precedes planned laparotomy under the same anesthetic. We also use staging laparoscopy selectively in patients with radiographic evidence of LA disease (i.e., to exclude metastases prior to the administration of radiotherapy to the primary tumor and regional lymph nodes).

Biliary Drainage

Historically, it was thought that jaundiced patients were at higher risk of perioperative complications, so biliary drainage was often performed prior to pancreatectomy to improve postoperative outcomes. Several studies have since shown that infectious complications occur more frequently in patients who undergo biliary drainage procedures prior to surgery. In 2010, a multicenter randomized trial from the Netherlands found that the rate of serious perioperative complications was higher in patients who underwent biliary decompression with plastic biliary stents compared to those who did not undergo biliary decompression (74% vs. 39%, P < .001). A few years later, a Cochrane review confirmed that preoperative biliary drainage is associated with higher rates of serious adverse events. Thus, routine biliary drainage for patients with resectable pancreatic cancer is not routinely recommended for patients undergoing surgery de novo.

In contrast, an obstructed biliary system mandates urgent biliary drainage prior to the preoperative administration of chemotherapy or chemoradiation. In this scenario, we use short metal biliary stents to decompress the biliary tree. We have found that when compared to plastic stents, short metal stents have longer patency, require fewer ERCP sessions, and have fewer episodes of cholangitis without increasing perioperative complications. Recently, the group from the Netherlands that performed the multicenter randomized trial cited above compared a cohort of patients who underwent biliary drainage with a metal stent to the patients from the trial, who underwent biliary drainage with a plastic stent, and found that metal stents had a lower rate of PBD-related complications (24% vs. 46%, P = .01).

Surgical Treatment

Surgical Considerations

The majority of primary PDAC tumors arise in the proximal gland and are treated surgically with pancreatoduodenectomy. In contrast, distal lesions are treated with distal pancreatectomy, which typically includes splenectomy given the required perisplenic vessel lymphadenectomy. Total pancreatectomy is generally avoided because of the high morbidity associated with the procedure and its adverse effects on pancreatic endocrine function. The surgical approach should be selected with the primary goal of achieving microscopically negative surgical margins (R0 resection).

Pancreatoduodenectomy

Patients who have a good functional status and who have a radiographic potentially resectable primary tumor are eligible for resection. If staging laparoscopy does not reveal extrapancreatic disease, the surgeon makes either a midline or bilateral subcostal incision and carefully inspects the liver and the peritoneum for

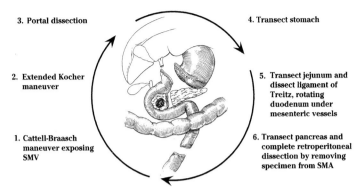

FIGURE 15.1 Six surgical steps of standard pancreaticoduodenectomy (clockwise resection). SMA, superior mesenteric artery; SMV, superior mesenteric vein. (From Tyler DS, Evans DB. Reoperative pancreaticoduodenectomy. *Ann Surg.* 1994;219(2):211–221, reprinted with permission.)

evidence of radiographically occult metastatic disease. At MDACC, we do not routinely perform intraoperative frozen-section analysis of regional lymph nodes. Instead, frozen-section analysis is done on an individual basis. For example, intraoperative frozen-section analysis of regional or extraregional lymph nodes (e.g., aortocaval nodes) may be performed in high-risk patients (patients with advanced age, significant medical comorbidities, high CA 19-9 serum levels, etc.). In such patients, the finding of metastatic disease in regional lymph nodes may suggest that pancreatoduodenectomy is unjustified, even in the absence of visceral metastases.

To help organize a complex operation, minimize operative time, and provide a clear operative plan, we divide pancreatoduodenectomy into six well-defined steps (Fig. 15.1).

1. The lesser sac is entered through the avascular plane between the omentum and transverse mesocolon/colon, the right colon is mobilized, and the visceral peritoneum to the ligament of Treitz is divided, which facilitates retraction of the right colon and small bowel. The duodenum is exposed. The infrapancreatic SMV is identified by following the course of the gastrocolic trunk or the middle colic vein to the root of the mesentery.
2. A Kocher maneuver is performed to mobilize the duodenum and head of the pancreas to the level of the left renal vein.
3. Portal dissection is performed to expose the hepatic artery both proximal and distal to the origin of the gastroduodenal artery. The gastroduodenal artery is then ligated and divided. The gallbladder is dissected from the liver, and the common hepatic duct is transected just cephalad to its junction with the cystic duct. The PV is exposed by dividing the common hepatic duct and performing cephalad retraction of the common hepatic artery; during this step, any variant hepatic artery anatomy must be identified to avoid injury.
4. If the pylorus is to be preserved, the duodenum is transected 1 to 2 cm distal to the pylorus to preserve a cuff for anastomosis. Otherwise, a standard antrectomy is performed.
5. The jejunum is transected approximately 10 cm distal to the ligament of Treitz. The jejunal and duodenal mesenteries are sequentially ligated and divided to the level of the aorta. The duodenum and jejunum are then rotated beneath the mesenteric vessels.
6. The pancreas is transected using electrocautery at the level of the PV. The specimen is separated from the SMV by ligating and dividing the small venous tributaries to the uncinate process and the pancreatic head. The SMA is completely exposed, and the lateral aspect of the vessel is skeletonized in the periadventitial plane to its origin at the aorta. This step is crucial for achieving a negative SMA margin, which is one of the main drivers of good oncologic outcome. The specimen is then removed from the abdomen.

Reconstruction is initiated in a similar, but reverse, stepwise fashion (Fig. 15.2). The four steps of reconstruction are: (a) end-to-side pancreaticojejunostomy; (b) end-to-side hepaticojejunostomy; (c) end-to-side duodenojejunostomy or gastrojejunostomy; and (d) placement of a gastrostomy tube, a jejunostomy tube, and drains according to surgeon's preference. At MDACC, we do not typically place a gastrostomy tube, and we reserve jejunostomy tubes for the rare patient at high risk of nutritional deficiency following surgery.

Laparoscopic and robotic-assisted pancreatectomies are gaining in popularity across the country. These minimally invasive techniques are best reserved for well selected patients with amenable anatomy and minimal preoperative concern for threatened surgical margins. For distal pancreatectomy, several postoperative

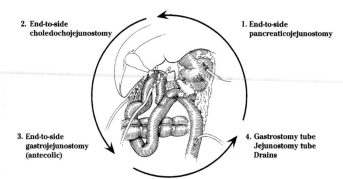

FIGURE 15.2 Four surgical steps of counterclockwise reconstruction following standard pancreaticoduodenectomy. (From Tyler DS, Evans DB. Reoperative pancreaticoduodenectomy. *Ann Surg.* 1994;219(2):211–221, reprinted with permission.)

metrics, including mortality, pancreatic fistula, and other major complications, are near equal to that of open operations. Early data on robotic pancreatoduodenectomy has demonstrated the safety of the technique with suggestion of similar perioperative outcomes. However, the lack of randomized trials limits any definitive comparison and these procedures should be performed only at high volume centers with such expertise. At MDACC, we have developed techniques meant to replicate the open procedure as above, including extracorporeal retraction of the portosplenic confluence for uncinate dissection, 180-degree periadvential skeletonization of the SMA, and intracorporeal duct-to-mucosal pancreaticojejunostomy and hepaticojejunostomy anastomoses.

Lymphadenectomy

PDAC commonly metastasizes through extrapancreatic lymphatics to regional lymph nodes, and lymph node involvement is a dominant prognostic factor. The primary goal of a lymphadenectomy at the time of pancreatectomy is to ensure adequate staging; although higher lymph node counts have been correlated with better outcomes, it has been difficult to prove that extensive lymphadenectomy significantly impacts survival given PDAC's high rate of early systemic dissemination.

Lymphadenectomy at the time of pancreatectomy is guided by vascular and visceral anatomy. The regional nodal basins that are included in a standard pancreatoduodenectomy are located along the bile duct, common hepatic artery, PV, pancreatoduodenal arterial arcades, SMV, and along the lateral wall of the SMA. Studies have evaluated the role of extended lymphadenectomy and have failed to demonstrate a survival benefit compared to a less extensive, "standard" lymphadenectomy. This high-level data notwithstanding, the standard lymphadenectomy performed with pancreatoduodenectomy at MDACC includes lymph nodes (numerical stations): anterior and posterior to the common hepatic artery (8a/p), along the proper hepatic artery (12a1/2), common bile duct and hepatic duct (12b1/2), PV (12p1/2), gallbladder (12c), posterior superior and posterior inferior pancreatic head (13a/b), superior mesenteric artery (14a/b), and anterior superior and anterior inferior pancreatic head (17a/b), while a distal pancreatectomy and splenectomy includes lymph node stations in the splenic hilum (10), along the splenic artery (11p/d), and superior margin of the pancreas (18).

Mesenteric Vascular Resection

Vascular involvement by cancer, particularly involvement of the SMV–PV, does not represent a contraindication to pancreatectomy. We have found that resecting and reconstructing the SMV–PV confluence and the major first order venous branches at pancreatoduodenectomy is both safe and associated with an overall survival rate similar to that of patients who do not require venous resection to achieve negative surgical margins. At MDACC, most patients with tumors that appear on cross-sectional imaging to involve the SMV or PV receive preoperative chemotherapy and/or chemoradiation. Venous resection should be performed only to achieve a negative resection margin and not as part of an en bloc regional pancreatectomy.

Cross-sectional imaging can predict the need for vascular resection. On the other hand, evidence for histologic vein invasion is not needed to justify a venous resection; pancreatitis and/or tumor- or treatment-related fibrosis may mandate venous resection, even though true invasion of the vessel may not exist. In the series by Tran Cao et al., 98 of 254 patients with resectable or BR PDAC underwent venous resection, among whom only 69% had histopathologic evidence for vein invasion.

The strategy used for venous reconstruction should be dictated by the patient's venous anatomy and the location and extent of venous involvement. The surgical objective is to preserve portal venous flow from the stomach, spleen, and intestines while minimizing the risk of sinistral portal hypertension.

Unlike venous resection and reconstruction, we believe that superior mesenteric artery resection is typically unjustified during pancreatoduodenectomy. In contrast, arterial resection may be justified when the tumor appears to extend along the gastroduodenal artery to involve the proper or common hepatic artery, or when a replaced right hepatic artery or replaced common hepatic artery arising from the SMA appears to be involved by tumor. Resection of the celiac axis and common hepatic artery en bloc with distal tumors (DP-CAR) may also be appropriate. In such cases, however, careful patient selection is paramount and we usually offer patients an extended course of preoperative therapy before considering pancreatectomy.

Adjuvant (Postoperative) Therapy for Resected PDAC

The first study of adjuvant chemoradiation in patients with resected pancreatic cancer was performed by the Gastrointestinal Study Group and reported in 1985. The patients who received postoperative 5-FU–based chemoradiation had significantly longer median overall survival (21.0 months) than patients who underwent surgery alone (10.9 months), thus establishing 5-FU as the standard for postoperative chemoradiation. However, subsequent trials conducted by the European Organization for Research and Treatment of Cancer (EORTC) and the European Study Group for Pancreatic Cancer (ESPAC) did not confirm that there was a survival advantage associated with adjuvant chemoradiation. Indeed, the ESPAC-1 trial suggested that chemoradiation was actually harmful. The Radiation Therapy Oncology Group study 0848 randomized patients to adjuvant gemcitabine or gemcitabine plus radiotherapy and final results are pending. This study should help clarify the role of adjuvant chemoradiation therapy in patients with resected pancreatic cancer.

In 2008, the Charite Onkologie and the Radiation Therapy Oncology Group evaluated the role of adjuvant gemcitabine for resected pancreatic cancer. The CONKO-001 trial determined that adjuvant gemcitabine was associated with an increased disease-free and overall survival (22.8 vs. 20.2 months, P = .005) relative to surgery alone. The ESPAC-3 trial compared adjuvant gemcitabine to infusional 5-FU and found similar median survival (23.6 vs. 23.0 months) but noted that gemcitabine had fewer treatment-related serious adverse events (7.5% vs. 14%, P < .001). ESPAC-4 randomized patients with resected pancreatic cancer to receive either adjuvant gemcitabine and capecitabine or gemcitabine monotherapy. The median survival was longer for patients treated with gemcitabine and capecitabine than gemcitabine alone (28.0 vs. 25.5 months, P = .03), and there was no significant difference in adverse events between the two groups.

These were followed by the 2018 PRODIGE-24 study, a phase III trial that randomized patients who had previously undergone pancreatectomy to receive 6 months of either mFOLFIRINOX or single-agent gemcitabine. Although associated with significant toxicity, mFOLFIRINOX was associated with an improved median survival of 54.4 months compared to 35.0 months with gemcitabine. Most recently, the multicenter phase III APACT trial compared adjuvant gemcitabine plus nab-paclitaxel to gemcitabine alone. While the study did not meet its primary endpoint of independently assessed disease-free survival, the overall survival data suggested improved outcomes with the combined agents. The 2021 updated findings demonstrated an overall survival benefit of gemcitabine plus nab-paclitaxel over gemcitabine alone (41.8 vs. 37.7 months, P = .023). Treatment emergent adverse events (grade ≥3) occurred in 86% of patients in the gemcitabine plus nab-paclitaxel group. While the gemcitabine group outperformed historical data (e.g., PRODIGE-24 above), the modest survival improvement of the gemcitabine plus nab-paclitaxel led investigators to propose this regimen as a potential alternative regimen for those patients unable to tolerate mFOLFIRINOX.

To date, there is high-level evidence indicating that adjuvant chemotherapy improves survival over surgery alone. The American Society of Clinical Oncology (ASCO) recommends that all patients with resected pancreatic cancer who did not receive preoperative therapy be offered 6 months of postoperative therapy, initiated within 8 weeks of surgical resection.

Preoperative (Neoadjuvant) Therapy

Resectable Tumors

The argument for administering preoperative therapy to patients with resectable pancreatic cancer begins with the fact that 80% to 90% of patients who undergo potentially curative resection develop recurrence. Additionally, up to 50% of patients who undergo surgery for resectable pancreatic cancer ultimately do not receive postoperative adjuvant therapy for reasons related to the surgery (i.e., complications or nutritional impairment) and/or the disease itself (i.e., disease progression). Administering preoperative therapy enables patients to receive requisite "adjuvant" therapy immediately and ensures that all patients who undergo resection receive systemic therapy. Preoperative therapy also facilitates the selection of patients for surgery who are most likely to benefit from it; patients with clinically occult but progressive systemic disease can often be identified during the preoperative therapy period and spared the potential morbidity associated with pancreatic resection.

Prospective data demonstrate the safety of preoperative systemic chemotherapy and suggest a favorable therapeutic impact. The phase II trial SWOG S1505, for example, compared perioperative chemotherapy regimens (12 weeks preoperative and 12 weeks postoperative) of mFOLFIRINOX and gemcitabine plus nab-paclitaxel. The study demonstrated that both preoperative regimens were well tolerated; 85% of patients in both arms completed neoadjuvant therapy and more than 70% went on to surgical resection. Of patients who underwent resection, 42% of the gemcitabine plus nab-paclitaxel group had a complete or major pathologic response, compared to 25% of the mFOLFIRINOX group. Overall, the study found equivalent survival among patients in the mFOLFIRINOX and gemcitabine plus nab-paclitaxel groups, with median overall survival of 22.4 and 23.6 months, respectively.

The phase III PREOPANC-1 trial compared neoadjuvant gemcitabine-based chemoradiation with 36 Gy followed by surgery and adjuvant gemcitabine to upfront surgery and adjuvant gemcitabine alone. While the study included BR patients, long-term results from subgroup analysis of resectable cases reported a nonstatistically significant improved overall survival (HR 0.79; 95% CI 0.54 to 1.16; $P = .23$).

Currently, there are several ongoing phase I/II studies evaluating the role of immunologic agents and kinase inhibitors in combination with chemoradiation, as well as some studies that are investigating the role of new radiotherapy modalities (intensity-modulated radiation therapy [IMRT] and stereotactic body radiation therapy) in patients with resectable pancreatic cancer.

Phase III randomized trails comparing the addition of neoadjuvant chemotherapy to adjuvant therapy alone are needed to further clarify the role of neoadjuvant chemotherapy for patients with resectable PDAC. One such study currently in progress is Alliance A021806, a phase III randomized control trial comparing perioperative versus adjuvant only mFOLFIRINOX. This study began in July 2020; however, final results are not anticipated until late 2030.

Borderline Resectable Tumors

MDACC has defined and developed multidisciplinary treatment strategies for patients with BR pancreatic cancer (Table 15.1). In 2008, Katz et al. proposed a definition for BR pancreatic cancer based upon strict anatomic imaging criteria, but also included other clinical factors. Patients were classified as BR-A, BR-B, or BR-C, where A refers to tumor "anatomy," B stands for cancer "biology," and C refers to the patient's "condition" or performance status. BR-A tumors meet specific anatomic imaging criteria (Table 15.1). BR-B tumors have associated clinical findings suspicious for extrapancreatic disease such as indeterminate liver lesions, serum CA 19-9 ≥1,000 U/mL in the setting of a normal bilirubin, or biopsy-proven metastasis to regional lymph nodes. BR-C patients are advanced in age (≥80 years old) or have severe comorbidities requiring extensive evaluation or optimization, or depressed performance status (ECOG ≥2). In a series of 160 patients with BR cancers using this scheme who were treated with preoperative chemotherapy and/or chemoradiation, 41% of patients underwent resection. The resection rates for patients with BR-A, BR-B, and BR-C disease were 38%, 50%, and 38%, respectively. The median overall survival for the entire cohort was 18 months with a 5-year survival of 18%. For the 66 patients who completed all therapies, the median survival was 40 months with a 5-year survival of 36%. This classification system has been adopted by the International Study Group of Pancreas Surgery (ISGPS) in their 2014 consensus statement and has led to further trials investigating the importance of a multidisciplinary approach.

Although older consensus statements advocate the administration of both systemic chemotherapy and chemoradiation to patients with BR PDAC, most of the data used to support this approach are based on relatively low-level data. Among BR patients included in the PREOPANC-1 study, patients who received preoperative chemoradiation demonstrated improved overall survival compared to the those who underwent immediate surgery (HR 0.67; 95% CI 0.45 to 0.99; $P = .045$). The Alliance Trial A021101, conducted by Katz et al. was a prospective, multicenter trial of this approach. Twenty-two patients initiated therapy, which consisted of modified FOLFIRINOX (four cycles) and chemoradiation (50.4-Gy external beam radiation and capecitabine) prior to pancreatectomy. Fifteen of 22 (68%) patients underwent resection; 12 (80%) required vascular resection, 14 (93%) had microscopically negative margins, and 5 (33%) had less than 5% residual cancer cells. Patients had an overall survival rate of 55% at 18 months. Following the success of this trial, a second phase II trial (Alliance A021501) was undertaken which randomized patients with BR pancreatic cancer to modified FOLFIRINOX (eight cycles), surgery and adjuvant FOLFOX (four cycles), or modified FOLFIRINOX (seven cycles), short course radiation therapy, surgery and adjuvant FOLFOX (four cycles). The median overall survival duration of patients who received modified FOLFIRINOX alone was almost 30 months. The modified FOLFIRINOX plus SBRT arm closed at interim analysis for futility. Further trials are needed to more clearly define the optimal treatment strategy for patients with BR PDAC.

Surgical Outcomes

In 2006, Winter et al. reported the Johns Hopkins experience of 1,423 pancreatoduodenectomies for pancreatic cancer from 1970 to 2006. The perioperative mortality rates in the 1970s, 1980s, 1990s, and 2000s were 30%, 5%, 2%, and 1%, respectively. Forty-two percent of patients had a margin-positive resection. The median survival durations in the 1970s, 1980s, 1990s, and 2000s were 8, 14, 17, and 19 months, respectively. The 5-year survival rates for the 1970s, 1980s, 1990s, and 2000s also improved over time—5%, 11%, 18%, and 20%, respectively. Of note, the median and 5-year survival rates for the 1990s and 2000s were not significantly different, suggesting that the maximum impact of surgery on survival had been realized.

In 2009, Katz et al. published the cumulative MDACC experience of the surgical treatment of patients with localized pancreatic cancer. Three hundred and twenty-nine patients treated between 1990 and 2002 were evaluated. Two hundred and fifty-three (77%) patients received preoperative chemotherapy and/or chemoradiation. Most patients (92%) underwent pancreatoduodenectomy. A total of 108 (33%) patients underwent vascular resection and reconstruction. Regional lymph node metastases were identified in 157 (48%) of patients and margins were microscopically positive in 52 (16%) patients. The median and 5-year overall survival was 23.9 months and 27%, respectively. Recently, a more inclusive 25-year MDACC experience of preoperative therapy and pancreatoduodenectomy was published, which included 622 patients. Over that time, a larger proportion of patients who underwent resection had BR and LA tumors. The use of induction systemic chemotherapy and postoperative adjuvant chemotherapy increased over time. R0 resection and vascular resection rates increased over time, and were 94% and 66%, respectively, in the most recent time period. Over the 25-year time period, the median overall survival increased from 24 to 43 months, and the 5-year overall survival increased from 23% to 35%. These results are a testament to the evolution of multidisciplinary care in the setting of advances in chemotherapeutic regimens, selection of surgical patients, and the optimization of surgical therapy. Further improvements in patient outcomes will come from improved systemic therapy and treatment sequencing.

Postoperative Oncologic Surveillance

There is little evidence to guide the frequency or intensity of surveillance strategies after potentially curative resection for PDAC. Tzeng et al. performed a cost-effectiveness analysis comparing no follow-up to 3- or 6-month intervals with or without CA 19-9 testing and routine CT scans. A clinical evaluation every 6 months with CA 19-9 testing and no imaging seemed to be the most cost-effective strategy and provided a similar survival benefit when compared to more frequent and intense surveillance strategies. ASCO recommends that patients who have completed treatment of potentially curable pancreatic cancer be offered follow-up visits at 3- to 6-month intervals, admitting that there is little evidence to support this recommendation. Nonetheless, we typically see patients every 6 months for the first 2 years following potentially curative resection with a CT scan of the abdomen, chest x-ray, and CA 19-9 level. Visits are spread out to yearly after 5 years.

Locally Advanced Tumors

LA pancreatic cancer is defined as anatomically unresectable. Building on the experience in the treatment of metastatic disease, chemotherapy and radiation therapy have been applied to LA in an attempt to achieve disease response and conversion to surgical resectability.

Chemotherapy

The ACCORD-11/PRODIGE-4 trial, a phase III randomized trial, compared FOLFIRINOX to gemcitabine in patients with metastatic pancreatic cancer, and found that FOLFIRINOX had a higher response rate with increased progression-free and overall survival. Based upon the efficacy of FOLFIRINOX in patients with metastatic disease, it seemed rational to also use it for patients with LA pancreatic cancer. Marthey et al. reported a prospective cohort study conducted at multiple institutions in France that administered FOLFIRINOX to patients with LA pancreatic cancer. Seventy-seven patients were enrolled. Grade III–IV toxicities occurred in 26% of patients, but only five patients had to stop therapy due to toxicities. According to RECIST criteria, disease progression, stable disease, and partial response were seen in 16%, 56%, and 16% of patients, respectively. Fifty-five patients (75%) underwent consolidation therapy. Twenty-five of 28 patients (89%) who underwent surgical resection achieved an R0 resection. The median progression-free and overall survivals for the entire cohort were 13 and 22 months, respectively, leading to the conclusion that surgery may also be applied selectively following chemotherapy in patients with LA disease.

The use of gemcitabine plus nab-paclitaxel has also been evaluated in LA disease. Building on the phase III MPACT trial in metastatic pancreatic cancer that suggested potential benefit, the LAPACT trial was a multicenter phase II study evaluating gemcitabine plus nab-paclitaxel. Patients with LA pancreatic cancer underwent an induction period six cycles of therapy, followed by either continued chemotherapy, chemoradiation, or surgery. Of the 107 enrolled patients, 58% completed the induction cycles and 44% went on to additional therapy; 11% continued gemcitabine plus nab-paclitaxel, 17% received chemoradiation, and 16% underwent surgery. During induction therapy, 83 patients achieved disease control and 36 patients had a partial response. Median overall survival was 18.8 months and global quality of life was maintained in most patients.

Following this, the phase II German multicenter NEOLAP randomized trial sought to investigate the optimal preoperative treatment for LA pancreatic cancer, comparing four cycles of nab-paclitaxel plus gemcitabine with two cycles of nab-paclitaxel plus gemcitabine followed by four cycles of FOLFIRINOX as multidrug induction therapy. Grade 3 or higher treatment-emergent adverse events during induction chemotherapy occurred in 55% in the nab-paclitaxel plus gemcitabine group and in 53% the sequential FOLFIRINOX group. Following induction, 23 of 64 and 29 of 66 patients enrolled in respective arms successfully underwent surgical resection (OR 0.72, $P = .38$). Median overall survival was 18.5 months in the nab-paclitaxel plus gemcitabine group and 20.7 months in the sequential FOLFIRINOX group ($P = .53$). This study concluded that the two regimens were similar in efficacy and safety.

Chemoradiation

LAP07 was an international phase III trial that randomized patients with LA PDAC to chemotherapy or chemoradiotherapy, if there was no evidence of disease progression after 4 months of gemcitabine with or without erlotinib. After 4 months of chemotherapy (gemcitabine ± erlotinib), 269 of 442 patients had no evidence of disease progression and were randomized to chemoradiotherapy or two more months of the same chemotherapy. Three-dimensional conformal radiation therapy was used with a total planned dose of 54 Gy in 30 fractions over 6 weeks with concurrent capecitabine. There was no difference in progression-free survival (9.9 vs. 8.4 months) or overall survival (15.2 vs. 16.5 months), between patients treated with chemoradiation or chemotherapy, respectively. Locoregional progression occurred less frequently in the chemoradiation group (32%) than in the chemotherapy group (46%), whereas distant progression occurred more often in patients treated with chemoradiation than chemotherapy (60% vs. 44%).

The phase II SCALOP trial tested gemcitabine-based and capecitabine-based chemoradiation therapy (CRT) for LA PDAC. Patients completed four cycles of gemcitabine and capecitabine induction therapy, before being randomized to either gemcitabine- or capecitabine-based chemoradiation with 50.4 Gy over 28 fractions. Thirty-six patients completed radiation in the gemcitabine group with twenty-four (67%) having stable disease and seven (19%) with demonstrating partial response. Thirty-five patients completed therapy in the capecitabine group with twenty-two (63%) having stable disease, six (17%) with demonstrating partial response, and two (6%) with complete response. Long-term results showed a median overall survival of 14.6 months in the gemcitabine arm and 17.6 months in the capecitabine arm (P = .19). The study thus did not detect a significant survival benefit of capecitabine-based consolidation chemoradiotherapy after a course of induction chemotherapy for LA pancreatic cancer. Building on these results and further exploring the utility of chemoradiation in LA PDAC, the SCALOP-2 trial is investigating the addition of nelfinavir to capecitabine-based chemoradiation following gemcitabine plus nab-paclitaxel induction therapy. These results are expected to be available early in 2022.

High-dose radiation therapy may also have a role in the treatment of patients with advanced disease. Krishnan et al. reported a series of 200 consecutive MDACC patients with LA PDAC who received induction chemotherapy (gemcitabine or FOLFIRINOX) for a median of 3.5 months followed by chemoradiation. Forty-seven patients with unresectable tumors >1 cm from the closest GI mucosa were treated with dose-escalated IMRT that delivered a biologically effective dose (BED) >70 Gy. The patients who received a BED >70 Gy had improved local–regional recurrence-free and overall survival when compared to those who received a BED ≤70 Gy.

Ablative Therapies

Over the years, several ablative therapies have been investigated for the treatment of LA pancreatic cancer. Radiofrequency and microwave ablation use thermal damage to destroy the cancer cells, but can also damage vital structures in the surrounding area like the bile duct or mesenteric vessels and have reported morbidity rates of 28% to 40% and mortality rates of 7.5%.

Irreversible electroporation (IRE) has gained increasing interest in recent years. IRE uses two electrodes to deliver electrical pulses that disrupt the cell wall lipid bilayer leading to apoptosis but does not affect the structure of the extracellular matrix. In 2015, Paiella et al. reported a prospective safety and feasibility study in patients with LA PDAC. That same year, Martin et al. reported a series of 200 patients with LA pancreatic cancer that were treated with IRE alone ($N = 150$) or in combination with surgical resection ($N = 50$). Fifty-four of the 150 patients who underwent IRE alone suffered a complication—32% of the complications were at least grade III in severity. The median overall survival following IRE alone was 18 months. The PANFIRE study was a phase I/II study designed to evaluate the safety and efficacy of percutaneous CT-guided IRE for LA pancreatic cancer, which found a 40% rate of grade III/IV complications. It is clear that ablative therapy for LA PDAC is associated with a significant risk of severe complications, and as of yet has not been proven to be more efficacious than systemic chemotherapy or consolidative strategies, such as high-dose chemoradiation.

CASE SCENARIO

Case Scenario 1

Presentation

A 63-year-old man is referred to you from his primary care physician with a history of amber urine, diarrhea, and an unintentional weight loss of 15 pounds over the past month. He otherwise feels well, with no fatigue and a normal performance status. His past medical history is notable for hypertension and type 2 diabetes. He has no history of surgery and no family history of malignancies. On examination you note mild jaundice and a scaphoid nontender abdomen. Outside CT images reveal extrahepatic biliary distension with narrowing of the distal common bile duct. The main pancreatic duct measures 1 cm; however, no discrete pancreatic mass is visualized, and no other abnormalities are noted in the abdomen or pelvis. Basic metabolic panel and complete blood count laboratory studies are normal.

Differential Diagnosis

Pancreatic adenocarcinoma
Distal cholangiocarcinoma
Immunoglobulin G4-related disease
Pancreatic mass
Duodenal adenocarcinoma
Ampullary mass

Confirmation of Diagnosis

Dedicated imaging, endoscopy, and tumor markers are essential for the evaluation of suspected pancreatic malignancies. CT imaging should be repeated with a dedicated pancreas protocol. Liver function tests should be obtained, as well as CA 19-9; however, CA 19-9 may be falsely elevated in the setting of hyperbilirubinemia or normal in the 10% of patients who are Lewis antigen negative. Endoscopic evaluation with upper endoscopy and endoscopic ultrasound can aid in the differentiation of painless jaundice etiology, as well as provide tissue diagnosis through fine-needle aspiration (FNA) of identified masses. Endoscopic retrograde cholangiopancreatography with common bile duct cytologic brushings can be used to establish an alternative diagnosis of distal cholangiocarcinoma. Finally, serum IgG4 could suggest a nonmalignancy autoimmune etiology for distal bile duct stricture.

In this case, the patient was found to have an elevated total bilirubin of 11, with otherwise normal liver function tests. CT pancreas imaging demonstrated a 2-cm mass in the head of the pancreas, with abutment of the common hepatic artery, no involvement of the superior mesenteric artery, and <180-degree abutment of the superior mesenteric vein (SMV) with contour irregularity. He underwent endoscopic biliary drainage with metal stent placement. Endoscopic FNA confirmed pancreatic adenocarcinoma. After normalization of his bilirubin, CA 19-9 was elevated at 356. CT staging of the chest, abdomen, and pelvis revealed no other evidence of disease.

The patient's case was discussed at multidisciplinary tumor board and germline testing was completed, revealing no hereditary mutations.

Treatment

While the patient has no SMA involvement, the abutment of the common hepatic artery and SMV contour irregularity each defines this as borderline respectable per national consensus guidelines. Per MD Anderson nomenclature, he is BR-A (based on the potential common hepatic artery involvement), but otherwise a good surgical candidate with no major comorbidities (not BR-C) and a moderate but not extreme elevation in his tumor markers (not BR-C). As such, he goes on to receive neoadjuvant chemotherapy. There is limited evidence to recommend any specific neoadjuvant regimen; however, modified FOLFIRINOX is often preferred over gemcitabine/nab-paclitaxel for patients with a good performance status. He undergoes four cycles of chemotherapy with stable imaging on restaging and improvement of his CA 19-9 to 100. He goes on to complete an additional four cycles with a decrease in the size of his primary tumor and normalization of his CA 19-9 to 10.

The patient then undergoes surgical resection with a diagnostic laparoscopy and pancreaticoduodenectomy requiring SMV resection. The surgical margins including SMA, pancreatic neck, and bile duct are negative by immediate pathology examination. The SMV is reconstructed using patch veinoplasty. A JP drain is positioned near the pancreaticojejunostomy and he is transferred postoperatively to the surgical floor. He is started on an ERAS protocol, nasogastric tube removed, diet initiated, and ambulated by post-operative day 1. He met with the nutritionist and started on pancreatic enzyme replacement. On postoperative day 3, the JP drain is removed after the measured drain amylase is 80 and output is minimal. He is discharged to home on post-operative day 5 on daily aspirin and to complete 28 days of low-molecular weight heparin.

On his 2-week postoperative clinic visit, he is doing well aside from complaints of diarrhea; however, complaining of diarrhea. Pathology report indicates an R0 resection with a pathologic response (10% to 49% remaining viable tumor cells). He undergoes repeat CT scan imaging to serve as a postoperative baseline scan and started adjuvant chemotherapy with modified FOLFIRINOX by 12 weeks after surgery. He is planning to return to clinic with repeat CT imaging and tumor markers every 4 to 6 months for the first 2 years, and every 6 to 12 months following this.

Common Curve Balls

- Preoperative increase in CA 19-9 on neoadjuvant therapy
- Obstructed biliary stent
- Gastric outlet obstruction
- Peritoneal or liver nodules found at diagnostic laparoscopy
- Positive intraoperative margins
- Unexpected major arterial involvement
- Positive celiac or common hepatic lymph nodes
- Postoperative nausea and emesis
- Pancreatic fistula
- Acute postoperative hemorrhage (GDA, staple lines, etc.)
- Early disease recurrence on imaging

Take Home Points

- Evaluation of painless jaundice should include dedicated pancreas cross-sectional imaging, with adjunct endoscopy as needed for tissue diagnosis or evaluation of alternative etiologies.
- Understanding defined resectability, including anatomic, biochemical, and comorbidity factors will ultimately dictate treatment.
- Multidisciplinary evaluation of the patient is essential for consideration of neoadjuvant and adjuvant therapies.
- Surgical evaluation should include restaging in the preoperative period and be mindful of anatomic considerations with surgical resection.

Case Scenario 2

Presentation

A 79-year-old woman is referred to you after an incidental finding of a pancreatic body cystic mass on cross-sectional imaging for lung cancer screening. She has an ongoing 25 pack-year history of tobacco use and lives a sedentary lifestyle with a performance status of 2. She has no surgical history and no family history of malignancies. Laboratory studies including a complete blood count, comprehensive metabolic panel, and CA 19-9 are all normal.

Differential Diagnosis

Pancreatic adenocarcinoma
Intraductal papillary mucinous neoplasm
Mucinous cystic neoplasm

Confirmation of Diagnosis

Dedicated CT imaging shows a 3-cm mass with cystic components, and a 12 mm dilated distal main pancreatic duct consistent with pancreatic adenocarcinoma with cystic degeneration. The cystic mass is distant from major vasculature, and without any lymphadenopathy or other abnormalities in the abdomen or pelvis. Upper endoscopy with fine-needle aspiration confirms adenocarcinoma.

Treatment and Surgical Considerations

While the patient meets resection criteria from an anatomic and biochemical criteria, her ongoing tobacco use, deconditioning, and performance status call into question her ability to tolerate surgery. Her case is discussed at multidisciplinary tumor board and she is started on neoadjuvant gemcitabine and nab-paclitaxel while initiating smoking cessation and an exercise regimen.

Following 2 months of neoadjuvant therapy, her restaging examinations show a slight decrease in the size of her primary tumor without any evidence of metastatic disease. She has been walking 20 to 40 minutes daily, now with an improved performance status of 0.

She proceeds to the operating room for surgical resection. The mass is identified in the anterior–inferior aspect of the pancreatic body, to the left of the superior mesenteric vein (SMV), without apparent vascular involvement. The remainder of the arterial and venous anatomy is identified, the branches of the celiac axis are distant, and vessel loops are placed around the SMV trunk, portal vein, splenic vein, and gastric coronary vein. A tunnel is created between the pancreas and the SMV. The pancreas is then transected between the mass and the head of the pancreas. A margin is sent for immediate pathologic examination and found to be free of malignancy or dysplasia. The operation proceeds to complete a distal pancreatectomy with splenectomy and adjacent lymphadenectomy.

Common Curve Balls

- Presence of multiple cysts meeting resection criteria
- Pancreatic mass with indeterminate histology
- Pancreatic mass location or positive margins dictating operation
- Other patient factors impacting surgical candidacy

Take Home Points

- Tumor location dictates operative care
- Patient candidacy for resection depends on anatomic and biochemical aspects of the tumor, but also patient comorbidities and performance status
- Choice of chemotherapy should consider patient performance status

CASE SCENARIO REVIEW

Questions

1. Which of the following patients does <u>not</u> meet resectable or borderline resectable criteria according to accepted criteria?
   - **A.** Pancreatic head mass with short segment encasement of the superior mesenteric vein and associated occlusion
   - **B.** Pancreatic neck mass with 90-degree abutment of the common hepatic artery
   - **C.** Pancreatic head mass with more than 180-degree contact with the superior mesenteric artery
   - **D.** Pancreatic head mass with 360-degree encasement of the gastroduodenal artery

2. Which of the following therapies has been associated most with increased survival in pancreatic cancer patients?

   A. Neoadjuvant chemoradiation
   B. Neoadjuvant chemotherapy
   C. Adjuvant chemoradiation
   D. Adjuvant chemotherapy

3. Which of the following genetically inherited cancer syndromes is <u>least</u> associated with development of pancreatic adenocarcinoma?

   A. BRCA1
   B. MEN2a
   C. FAP
   D. HNPCC

4. Which of the following patients would benefit least from diagnostic laparoscopy?

   A. 2-cm pancreatic tail tumor without evidence of extra pancreatic disease on imaging and CA 19-9 of 3500
   B. 2-cm resectable pancreatic neck tumor with CA 19-9 of 120
   C. 4-cm pancreatic neck tumor with possible invasion into the stomach
   D. 4-cm borderline resectable pancreatic head tumor with several indeterminate hepatic nodules that have remained stable over neoadjuvant therapy

5. Pathologic margin assessment of pancreaticoduodenectomy specimen for pancreatic head adenocarcinoma does not include which of the following?

   A. Superior mesenteric artery margin
   B. Pancreatic neck margin
   C. Bile duct transection margin
   D. Celiac artery margin

Answers

1. **The correct answer is C.** *Rationale*: While definitions of resectability vary slightly by organization, none accept more than 180 degrees of contact with the superior mesenteric artery.

2. **The correct answer is D.** *Rationale*: While the utility of neoadjuvant chemotherapy has proposed advantages of increased chemotherapy course completions compared to post-operative delivery, adjuvant chemotherapy is currently the only adjunct to surgery recognized to improve pancreatic cancer patient survival. The role of radiation therapy remains unclear in the treatment of pancreatic cancer.

3. **The correct answer is B.** *Rationale*: MEN2a is typically associated with medullary thyroid cancer, parathyroid adenomas, and pheochromocytomas. BRCA1, FAP, and HNPCC are associated with a 3.5-fold, 4-fold, and 9-fold increased risk of pancreatic adenocarcinoma, respectively.

4. **The correct answer is B.** *Rationale*: Diagnostic laparoscopy provides additional information in suspected but unconfirmed metastatic disease as it will preclude pancreatic resection. Large primary tumors, concern for invasion into additional organs, grossly elevated CA 19-9, and otherwise indeterminate nodules all increase suspicion for occult or underlying advanced disease that may alter the patient's treatment course.

5. **The correct answer is D.** *Rationale*: Pathologic reporting of margin status in a uniformed and defined manner is critical. National consensus guidelines recommend that the following anatomic locations undergo circumferential pathologic evaluation as part of the standard pathologic assessment of a Whipple specimen: SMA margin, portal vein margin, pancreas transection margin, and bile duct margin. Additional margins examined include the proximal (gastric or duodenal) and distal enteric margins. The celiac artery margin is not routinely assessed.

Recommended Readings

Abrams RA, Lowy AM, O'Reilly EM, Wolff RA, Picozzi VJ, Pisters PW. Combined modality treatment of resectable and borderline resectable pancreas cancer: expert consensus statement. *Ann Surg Oncol.* 2009;16(7):1751–1756.

Bachmann J, Heiligensetzer M, Krakowski-Roosen H, Büchler MW, Friess H, Martignoni ME. Cachexia worsens prognosis in patients with resectable pancreatic cancer. *J Gastrointest Surg.* 2008;12(7):1193–1201.

Balachandran A, Darden DL, Tamm EP, Faria SC, Evans DB, Charnsangavej C. Arterial variants in pancreatic adenocarcinoma. *Abdom Imaging.* 2008;33(2):214–221.

Bergquist JR, Puig CA, Shubert CR, et al. Carbohydrate antigen 19-9 elevation in anatomically resectable, early stage pancreatic cancer is independently associated with decreased overall survival and an indication for neoadjuvant therapy: a national cancer database study. *J Am Coll Surg.* 2016;223(1):52–65.

Bockhor M, Uzunoglu F, Adham M, et al. Borderline resectable pancreatic cancer: a consensus statement by the International Study Group of Pancreatic Surgery (ISGPS). *Surgery.* 2014;155(6):977–988.

Breslin TM, Hess KR, Harbison DB, et al. Neoadjuvant chemoradiotherapy for adenocarcinoma of the pancreas: treatment variables and survival duration. *Ann Surg Oncol.* 2001;8(2):123–132.

Callery MP, Chang KJ, Fishman EK, Talamonti MS, William Traverso L, Linehan DC. Pretreatment assessment of resectable and borderline resectable pancreatic cancer: expert consensus statement. *Ann Surg Oncol.* 2009;16(7):1727–1733.

Cancer Genome Atlas Research Network. Integrated genomic characterization of pancreatic ductal adenocarcinoma. *Cancer Cell.* 2017;32(2):185–203.e13.

Canto MI, Harinck F, Hruban RH, et al. International cancer of the pancreas screening (CAPS) consortium summit on the management of patient with increased risk for familial pancreatic cancer. *Gut.* 2013;62: 339–347.

Cloyd JM, Crane CH, Koay EJ, et al. Impact of hypofractionated and standard fractionated chemoradiation before pancreatoduodenectomy for pancreatic ductal adenocarcinoma. *Cancer.* 2016;122(17):2671–2679.

Cloyd JM, Crane CH, Koay EJ, et al. Preoperative therapy and pancreatoduodenectomy for pancreatic ductal adenocarcinoma: a 25-year single-institution experience. *J Gastrointest Surg.* 2017;21(1):164–174.

Conroy T, Desseigne F, Ychou M, et al. FOLFIRINOX versus gemcitabine for metastatic pancreatic cancer. *N Engl J Med.* 2011;364(19):1817–1825.

Corsini MM, Miller RC, Haddock MG, et al. Adjuvant radiotherapy and chemotherapy for pancreatic carcinoma: the Mayo Clinic experience (1975-2005). *J Clin Oncol.* 2008;26(21):3511–3516.

Denbo JW, Bruno ML, Cloyd JM, et al. Preoperative chemoradiation for pancreatic adenocarcinoma does not increase 90-day postoperative morbidity and mortality. *J Gastrointest Surg.* 2016;20(12):1975–1985.

Evans DB; Multidisciplinary Pancreatic Cancer Study Group. Resectable pancreatic cancer: the role for neoadjuvant/preoperative therapy. *HPB (Oxford)* 2006;8(5):365–368.

Evans DB, Rich TA, Byrd DR, et al. Preoperative chemoradiation and pancreaticoduodenectomy for adenocarcinoma of the pancreas. *Arch Surg.* 1992;127(11):1335–1339.

Evans DB, Varadhachary GR, Crane CH, et al. Preoperative gemcitabine-based chemoradiation for patients with resectable adenocarcinoma of the pancreatic head. *J Clin Oncol.* 2008;26(21):3496–3502.

Fang Y, Gurusamy KS, Wang Q, et al. Pre-operative biliary drainage for obstructive jaundice. *Cochrane Database Syst Rev.* 2012;9(9):CD005444.

Ferrone CR, Finkelstein DM, Thayer SP, Muzikansky A, Fernandez-delCastillo C, Warshaw AL. Perioperative CA 19-9 levels can predict stage and survival in patients with resectable pancreatic adenocarcinoma. *J Clin Oncol.* 2006;24(18):2897–2902.

Ferrone CR, Marchegiani G, Hong TS, et al. Radiological and surgical implications of neoadjuvant treatment with FOLFIRINOX for locally advanced and borderline resectable pancreatic cancer. *Ann Surg.* 2015;261(1):12–17.

Gaskill CE, Maxwell J, Ikoma N, et al. History of preoperative therapy for pancreatic cancer and the MD Anderson experience. *J Surg Onc.* 2021;123(6):1414–1422.

Goonetilleke KS, Siriwardena AK. Systematic review of carbohydrate antigen (CA 19-9) as a biochemical marker in the diagnosis of pancreatic cancer. *Eur J Surg Oncol.* 2007;33(3):266–270.

Hammel P, Huguet F, van Laethem JL, et al. Effect of chemoradiotherapy vs chemotherapy on survival in patients with locally advanced pancreatic cancer controlled after 4 months of gemcitabine with or without erlotinib: the LAP07 randomized clinical trial. *JAMA.* 2016;315(17):1844–1853.

Hassan MM, Dundy ML, Wolff RA, et al. Risk factors for pancreatic cancer: case-control study. *Am J Gastroenterol.* 2007;102(12):2696–2707.

Hoffman JP, Lipsitz S, Pisansky T, Weese JL, Solin L, Benson AB 3rd. Phase II trial of preoperative radiation therapy and chemotherapy for patients with localized, resectable adenocarcinoma of the pancreas: an Eastern Cooperative Oncology Group Study. *J Clin Oncol.* 1998;16(1):317–323.

Katz MH, Pisters PW, Evans DB, et al. Borderline resectable pancreatic cancer: the importance of this emerging stage of disease. *J Am Coll Surg.* 2008;206(5):833–846; discussion 846–848.

Katz MH, Shi Q, Ahmad SA, et al. Preoperative modified FOLFIRINOX treatment followed by capecitabine-based chemoradiation for borderline resectable pancreatic cancer: alliance for clinical trials in oncology trial A021101. *JAMA Surg.* 2016;151(8):e161137.

Katz MH, Varadhachary GR, Fleming JB, et al. Serum CA 19-9 as a marker of resectability and survival in patients with potentially resectable pancreatic cancer treated with neoadjuvant chemoradiation. *Ann Surg Oncol.* 2010;17(7):1794–1801.

Katz MH, Wang H, Fleming JB, et al. Long-term survival after multidisciplinary management of resected pancreatic adenocarcinoma. *Ann Surg Oncol.* 2009;16(4):836–847.

Kelsen DP, Portenoy R, Thaler H, Tao Y, Brennan M Pain as a predictor of outcome in patients with operable pancreatic carcinoma. *Surgery.* 1997;122(1):53–59.

Khorana AA, Mangu PB, Berlin J, et al. Potentially curable pancreatic cancer: American Society of Clinical Oncology clinical practice guideline update. *J Clin Onc.* 2019;37(23):2082–2088.

Klinkenbijl JH, Jeekel J, Sahmoud T, et al. Adjuvant radiotherapy and 5-fluorouracil after curative resection of cancer of the pancreas and periampullary region: phase III trial of the EORTC gastrointestinal tract cancer cooperative group. *Ann Surg.* 1999;230(6):776–782; discussion 782–784.

Krishnan S, Chadha AS, Suh Y, et al. Focal radiation therapy dose escalation improves overall survival in locally advanced pancreatic cancer patients receiving induction chemotherapy and consolidative chemoradiation. *Int J Radiat Oncol Biol Phys.* 2016;94(4):755–765.

Kunzmann V, Siveke JT, Agul H, et al. Nab-paclitaxel plus gemcitabine versus nab-paclitaxel plus gemcitabine followed by FOLFIRINOX induction chemotherapy in locally advanced pancreatic cancer (NEOLAP-AIO-PAK-0113): a multicentre, randomised, phase 2 trial. *The Lancet.* 2021;6(2):128–138.

Ikoma N, Kim MP, Tran Cao HS, et al. Early experience of a robotic foregut surgery program at a cancer center: video of shared steps in robotic pancreatoduodenectomy and gastrectomy. *Ann Surg Onc.* 2022;29(1):285.

Maithel SK, Maloney S, Winston C, et al. Preoperative CA 19-9 and the yield of staging laparoscopy in patients with radiographically resectable pancreatic adenocarcinoma. *Ann Surg Onc.* 2008;15(12):3512–3520.

Marten A, Debus J, Harig S, et al. CapRI: final results of the open-label, multicenter, randomized phase III trial of adjuvant chemoradiation plus interferon-a2b (CRI) versus 5-FU alone for patients with resected pancreatic adenocarcinoma (PAC). *J Clin Oncol.* 2010;28(suppl 18):LBA4012.

Marthey L, Sa-Cunha A, Blanc JF, et al. FOLFIRINOX for locally advanced pancreatic adenocarcinoma: results of an AGEO multicenter prospective observational cohort. *Ann Surg Oncol.* 2015;22(1):295–301.

Martin RC, Kwon D, Chalikonda S, et al. Treatment of 200 locally advanced (stage III) pancreatic adenocarcinoma patients with irreversible electroporation: safety and efficacy. *Ann Surg.* 2015;262(3):486–494.

Mukherjee S, Hurt CN, Bridgewater J, et al. Gemcitabine-based or capecitabine-based chemoradiotherapy for locally advanced pancreatic cancer (SCALOP): a multicentre, randomised, phase 2 trial. *Lancet Oncol.* 2013;14(4):317–326.

Mullen JT, Lee JH, Gomez HF, et al. Pancreaticoduodenectomy after placement of endobiliary metal stents. *J Gastrointest Surg.* 2005;9(8):1094–1104; discussion 1104–1105.

Neoptolemos JP, Stocken DD, Friess H, et al. A randomized trial of chemoradiotherapy and chemotherapy after resection of pancreatic cancer. *N Engl J Med.* 2004;350(12):1200–1210.

Neuhaus P, Riess H, Post S, et al. CONKO-001: final results of the randomized, prospective, multicenter phase III trial of adjuvant chemotherapy with gemcitabine versus observation in patients with resected pancreatic cancer (PC). *J Clin Oncol.* 2008;26(suppl 15):LBA4504.

Nukui Y, Picozzi VJ, Traverso LW. Interferon-based adjuvant chemoradiation therapy improves survival after pancreaticoduodenectomy for pancreatic adenocarcinoma. *Am J Surg.* 2000;179(5):367–371.

Oettle H, Post S, Neuhaus P, et al. Adjuvant chemotherapy with gemcitabine vs observation in patients undergoing curative-intent resection of pancreatic cancer: a randomized controlled trial. *JAMA.* 2007;297(3):267–277.

Perri G, Prakash L, Wang H, et al. Radiographic and serologic predictors of pathologic major response to peroperative therapy for pancreatic cancer. *Ann Surg.* 2021;273(4):806–813.

Pingpank JF, Hoffman JP, Ross EA, et al. Effect of preoperative chemoradiotherapy on surgical margin status of resected adenocarcinoma of the head of the pancreas. *J Gastrointest Surg.* 2001;5(2):121–130.

Pisters PW, Hudec WA, Hess KR, et al. Effect of preoperative biliary decompression on pancreaticoduodenectomy-associated morbidity in 300 consecutive patients. *Ann Surg.* 2001;234(1):47–55.

Pisters PW, Hudec WA, Lee JE, et al. Preoperative chemoradiation for patients with pancreatic cancer: toxicity of endobiliary stents. *J Clin Oncol.* 2000;18(4):860–867.

Philip PA, Lacy J, Portales F, et al. Nab-paclitaxel plus gemcitabine in patients with locally advanced pancreatic cancer (LAPACT): a multicentre, open-label phase 2 study. *The Lancet.* 2020;5(3):285–284.

Rahib L, Smith BD, Aizenberg R, Rosenzweig AB, Fleshman JM, Matrisian LM. Projecting cancer incidence and deaths to 2030: the unexpected burden of thyroid, liver, and pancreas cancer in the United States. *Cancer Res.* 2014;74(11):2913–2921.

Raut CP, Tseng JF, Sun CC, et al. Impact of resection status on pattern of failure and survival after pancreaticoduodenectomy for pancreatic adenocarcinoma. *Ann Surg.* 2007;246(1):52–60.

Regine WF, Winter KA, Abrams RA, et al. Fluorouracil vs gemcitabine chemotherapy before and after fluorouracil-based chemoradiation following resection of pancreatic adenocarcinoma: a randomized controlled trial. *JAMA.* 2008;299(9):1019–1026.

Reni M, Riess H, O'Reilly EM, et al. Phase III APACT trial of adjuvant nab-paclitaxel plus gemcitabine versus gemcitabine alone for patients with resected pancreatic cancer: outcomes by geographic region. 2020 ASCO Annual Meeting. Abstract 4515. Presented May 25, 2020.

Singal AK, Ross WA, Guturu P, et al. Self-expanding metal stents for biliary drainage in patients with resectable pancreatic cancer: single-center experience with 79 cases. *Dig Dis Sci.* 2011;56(12):3678–3684.

Skoulidis F, Li BT, Dy GK. Sotorasib for lung cancers with KRAS p.G12C mutation. *N Engl J Med.* 2021;384(25):2371–2381.

Smeenk HG, van Eijck CH, Hop WC, et al. Long-term survival and metastatic pattern of pancreatic and periampullary cancer after adjuvant chemoradiation or observation: long-term results of EORTC trial 40891. *Ann Surg.* 2007;246(5):734–740.

Sohal D, Duong MT, Ahmad SA, et al. SWOG S1505: results of perioperative chemotherapy (peri-op CTx) with mfolfirinox versus gemcitabine/nab-paclitaxel (Gem/nabP) for resectable pancreatic ductal adenocarcinoma (PDA). *J Clin Oncol.* 2020;15(38):4504.

Stessin AM, Meyer JE, Sherr DL. Neoadjuvant radiation is associated with improved survival in patients with resectable pancreatic cancer: an analysis of data from the surveillance, epidemiology, and end results (SEER) registry. *Int J Radiat Oncol Biol Phys.* 2008;72(4):1128–1133.

Tamm EP, Balachandran A, Bhosale PR, et al. Imaging of pancreatic adenocarcinoma: update on staging/resectability. *Radiol Clin of North Am.* 2012;50(3):407–428.

Tempero M, Reni M, Riess H, et al. APACT: phase III, multicenter, international, open-label, randomized trial of adjuvant nab-paclitaxel plus gemcitabine (nab-P/G) vs gemcitabine (G) for surgically resected pancreatic adenocarcinoma. *J Clin Oncol.* 2019;15(37):4000.

Tran Cao HS, Balachandran A, Wang H, et al. Radiographic tumor-vein interface as a predictor of intraoperative, pathologic, and oncologic outcomes in resectable and borderline resectable pancreatic cancer. *J Gastrointest Surg.* 2014;18(2):269–278.

Tseng JF, Raut CP, Lee JE, et al. Pancreaticoduodenectomy with vascular resection: margin status and survival duration. *J Gastrointest Surg.* 2004;8(8):935–949; discussion 949–950.

Tzeng CWD, Abbott DE, Cantor SB, et al. Frequency and intensity of postoperative surveillance after curative treatment of pancreatic cancer: a cost-effectiveness analysis. *Ann Surg Onc.* 2013;20:2197–2203.

van der Gaag NA, Rauws EA, van Eijck CH, et al. Preoperative biliary drainage for cancer of the head of the pancreas. *N Engl J Med.* 2010;262(2):129–137.

Varadhachary GR, Tamm EP, Abbruzzese JL, et al. Borderline resectable pancreatic cancer: definitions, management, and role of preoperative therapy. *Ann Surg Oncol.* 2006;13(8):1035–1046.

Varadhachary GR, Wolff RA, Crane CH, et al. Preoperative gemcitabine and cisplatin followed by gemcitabine-based chemoradiation for resectable adenocarcinoma of the pancreatic head. *J Clin Oncol.* 2008;26(21):3487–3495.

Versteijne E, Suker M, Groothuis K, et al. Preoperative chemoradiotherapy versus immediate surgery for resectable and borderline resectable pancreatic cancer: results of the dutch randomized phase III PREOPANC trial. *J Clin Oncol.* 2020;16(38):1763–1773.

White R, Winston C, Gonen M, et al. Current utility of staging laparoscopy for pancreatic and peripancreatic neoplasms. *J Am Coll Surg.* 2008;206(3):445–450.

White RR, Xie HB, Gottfried MR, et al. Significance of histological response to preoperative chemoradiotherapy for pancreatic cancer. *Ann Surg Oncol.* 2005;12(3):214–221.

Winter JM, Cameron JL, Campbell KA, et al. 1423 pancreaticoduodenectomies for pancreatic cancer: a single-institution experience. *J Gastrointest Surg.* 2006;10(9):1199–1210; discussion 1210–1211.

Yekebas EF, Bogoevski D, Cataldegirmen G, et al. En bloc vascular resection for locally advanced pancreatic malignancies infiltrating major blood vessels: perioperative outcome and long-term survival in 136 patients. *Ann Surg.* 2008;247(2):300–309.

16 Pancreatic Neuroendocrine Tumors and Multiple Endocrine Neoplasia

Natalia Paez Arango and Jessica E. Maxwell

Sporadic Pancreatic Neuroendocrine Tumors

Pancreatic neuroendocrine tumors (PNETs) are a heterogeneous group of neoplasms that arise from pancreatic islet cells and account for 1% to 3% of pancreatic malignancies. PNETs may be classified as functional or nonfunctional, depending on their ability to secrete hormones and elicit characteristic symptoms (Table 16.1). PNETs exhibit a wide range of biologic behavior, from indolent to aggressive. While PNETs have their own TNM staging system according to the American Joint Committee on Cancer (AJCC), independent from that of pancreatic adenocarcinoma, PNETs are more commonly classified according to a proliferation-based grading system (Table 16.2) which influences diagnostic modalities, treatment decisions, and prognosis. PNETs comprise approximately 7% of all neuroendocrine tumors, and the incidence appears to be increasing, presumably in part due to the increased use of high-quality cross-sectional imaging. Fortunately, there have been significant advances in diagnostic imaging, tumor localization, and therapeutic options in recent years.

Nonfunctional Pancreatic Neuroendocrine Tumors

Sixty to 90% of PNETs are nonfunctional (NF-PNETs), and they occur most commonly in the pancreatic head. Increasingly, NF-PNETs are identified incidentally on cross-sectional imaging performed for other indications. NF-PNETs are often diagnosed late in the course of the disease, with up to 64% of patients presenting with distant metastasis, mainly because symptoms do not become evident until the primary tumor grows large enough to compress adjacent structures or large-volume metastatic disease develops. Patients with NF-PNETs who present with symptoms may endorse abdominal pain, weight loss, obstructive jaundice, bleeding, and/or intestinal obstructive symptoms, particularly gastric outlet obstruction. The vast majority of metastases occur in the liver; other less common sites include bone, peritoneum, adrenal glands, and spleen. The median overall survival (OS) duration among all patients with NF-PNETs is approximately 3.2 years: 7.1 years in patients with resectable disease, 5.2 years in patients with locally advanced and unresectable disease, and 2.1 years in patients with unresectable metastatic disease.

TABLE 16.1 Functional Pancreatic Neuroendocrine Tumors

Pancreatic Tumor	% of PNETs	Malignant (%)	Pancreatic Cell Type	Clinical Manifestation	Diagnostic Tests
Insulinoma	40–60	<10	Beta	Hypoglycemia with symptomatic relief after glucose administration	• Monitored 72-hr fast • Insulin, proinsulin, C-peptide
Gastrinoma	20–50	60–90	Delta	Abdominal pain, food intolerance, peptic ulcers uncontrolled with conventional medical therapy	• Fasting gastrin (off PPI) • Basal to maximal acid output ratio • Basal acid output >15 mEq/hr • Nocturnal (12 hrs) gastric acid secretion test • Secretin stimulation test
VIPoma	Rare	40–70	A–D	Watery diarrhea, hypokalemia, achlorhydria, dehydration	Fasting VIP
Glucagonoma	Rare	50–80	Alpha	Diabetes, necrolytic migratory erythema, weight loss, depression, psychosis, venous thrombosis	Fasting glucagon
Somatostatinoma	Rare	>70	Delta	Mild diabetes, cholelithiasis, steatorrhea, weight loss, anemia, diarrhea	Fasting somatostatin

TABLE 16.2	WHO 2019 Grading System For Neuroendocrine Masses			
Terminology	Grade	Differentiation	Ki-67 Index (%)	Mitotic Rate (Mitosis/2 mm²)
NET, G1	Low	Well	<3	<2
NET, G2	Intermediate	Well	3–20	2–20
NET, G3	High	Well	>20	>20
NEC, small-cell type	High	Poorly	>20	>20
NEC, large-cell type	High	Poorly	>20	>20

NEC, neuroendocrine carcinoma; NET, neuroendocrine tumor.

Diagnosis

NF-PNETs are usually detected with computed tomography (CT) or magnetic resonance imaging (MRI), where they characteristically appear as well-circumscribed hyperenhancing lesions on contrast-enhanced scans. Hypoenhancement, cystic changes, and calcifications can also be seen. Imaging features may overlap with other entities including pancreatic adenocarcinoma and benign processes. At our institution, the preferred imaging modality is a pancreatic protocol CT with an arterial and portal venous phase to help identify the relevant anatomy, as well as possible lymphadenopathy and metastatic disease. MRI can also assist in characterizing liver lesions; generally liver metastases are best seen on T1 hepatic arterial phase and T2 fat-suppressed images. Endoscopic ultrasound (EUS) is the method of choice to confirm the diagnosis via fine-needle aspiration, evaluate the relationship with critical structures, and define the extent and distribution of the often multiple PNETs associated with patients who have inherited endocrine tumor syndromes.

Somatostatin receptor (SSTR) scintigraphy may be used selectively to help identify occult metastases, particularly in regional lymph nodes or the liver. SSTR-based positron emission tomography (PET) imaging using ^{68}Ga-DOTATATE is an FDA-approved imaging modality that has demonstrated improved image quality, sensitivity, shorter scan time, and lower radiation dose and is preferred over the traditional ^{111}In-octreotide SPECT (Octreoscan). One must keep in mind the potential for false positive uptake, as up to 50% patients can have physiologic uptake in the pancreas, particularly the uncinate and some in the tail of the pancreas (Fig. 16.1). Adrenal adenomas are also avid and thus these findings should be characterized further using CT or MRI.

NF-PNETs may secrete a variety of factors whose effects are often not clinically apparent. For example, as many as 75% of patients with NF-PNETs have elevated fasting pancreatic polypeptide levels, whereas chromogranin A (CgA) levels are elevated in 60% to 100% of patients. While there are studies that have shown that higher CgA levels correlate with more advanced disease, it is important to remember that the levels may be elevated in patients even in the absence of a PNET, due to advanced age, heavy alcohol use, inflammatory conditions, renal failure, or chronic proton pump inhibitor (PPI) use. Pancreastatin is another marker that may be more sensitive and specific than CgA, with higher levels correlating with shorter survival in patients with NF-PNETs. As such, neuroendocrine markers are used for surveillance and in monitoring response to

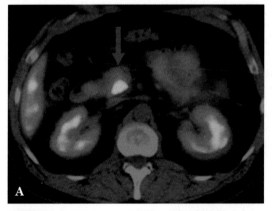
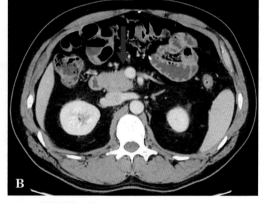

FIGURE 16.1 Physiologic uptake in PNET on 68Ga-DOTATATE. **A:** Strong physiologic DOTATATE avidity in the uncinate process of the pancreas can be easily misinterpreted as a tumor. **B:** The correlating pancreas protocol CT scan clearly demonstrates lack of tumor in that area.

treatment; they are not diagnostic for NF-PNET. In contrast, a prebiopsy-elevated CA19-9 and/or carcinoembryonic antigen (CEA) level in a patient with a hypodense pancreatic tumor and normal bilirubin level suggests that the tumor represents an adenocarcinoma rather than a PNET.

Treatment

Surgical resection with regional lymph node dissection (at least 11 to 15 nodes) is recommended for patients with localized, well-differentiated sporadic NF-PNETs, particularly if the tumor is >2 cm in diameter, growing rapidly (>0.5 cm/year) or causing symptoms, and if the patient is relatively young with a good performance status. There is growing consensus that small (i.e., 1 cm) PNETs identified incidentally that are not associated with nodal metastasis or other symptoms can safely be monitored without immediate surgery in many patients, particularly in older adults and in those with significant comorbidities. Modestly sized PNETs (1 to 2 cm) without radiographic or clinical evidence of involved regional lymph nodes may be selectively considered for primary resection without lymph node dissection. The anatomic considerations for determining the resectability and appropriate surgical approach in patients with sporadic NF-PNETs are generally the same as those for pancreatic adenocarcinomas. However, since PNETs are much less likely to demonstrate local invasiveness, limited resections (e.g., central pancreatectomy, spleen-preserving distal pancreatectomy, enucleation) and minimally invasive resection (e.g., robotic and laparoscopic surgery) can be selectively applied to patients with PNETs when appropriate. In contrast, since patients with locally advanced NF-PNETs (e.g., surrounding the celiac axis or superior mesenteric artery) often have relatively favorable survival duration with an intact primary tumor, incomplete resection or primary tumor debulking is not recommended. The potential morbidity associated with palliative pancreatic resection is high and there is no demonstrable survival or palliative benefit to incomplete resection of a primary NF-PNET. Resection of a primary PNET with concomitant or staged resection of oligometastatic disease (e.g., liver metastases) can be indicated in well-selected patients. There is no standard adjuvant systemic therapy for patients who undergo potentially curative surgical resection. Long-term follow-up after surgery is essential, as up to 50% of patients who undergo complete resection develop liver metastases, for which surgery or systemic therapy can be indicated.

Functioning Pancreatic Neuroendocrine Tumors

Insulinoma

In 1935, Whipple and Frantz first described the clinical manifestations of insulinoma as a triad of hypoglycemic symptoms while fasting, blood glucose levels <50 mg/dL, and symptomatic relief after glucose administration (Whipple triad). Insulinomas are the most common type of functioning PNET. Approximately 10% exhibit malignant behavior, 10% are associated with MEN1, and 10% are multifocal. Importantly, most patients with malignant insulinomas have distant metastases at the time of initial presentation. Insulinomas oversecrete insulin, and the resultant hypoglycemic episodes are exacerbated during periods of fasting or exercise. During an insulin surge, patients may develop a sympathetic overdrive characterized by sweating, weakness, tremors, hyperphagia, and palpitations. Neuroglycopenic symptoms including confusion, visual changes, altered consciousness, and convulsions may also occur.

Diagnosis The most reliable test for diagnosing insulinomas is a monitored 72-hour fast, during which the patient's plasma glucose, C-peptide, proinsulin, and insulin levels are measured every 4 to 6 hours. The test is continued until the plasma glucose level is <45 mg/dL and the patient develops hypoglycemic symptoms. It is helpful to remember that 33% of patients become symptomatic within 12 hours, 80% within 24 hours, 90% within 48 hours, and 100% within 72 hours. The diagnosis of insulinoma is established by a serum insulin concentration ≥6 μU/mL (50% of patients with an insulinoma will have an insulin level >24 μU/mL), an insulin-to-glucose ratio >0.3, a C-peptide level ≥0.2 nmol/L, a proinsulin level ≥5 pmol/L, and an absence of plasma sulfonylurea. An insulin level >7 μU/mL after a prolonged fast in the presence of a blood sugar <40 mg/dL is highly suggestive of an insulinoma, and virtually all patients with an insulinoma have an insulin-to-glucose ratio of >0.3. Patients who self-administer exogenous forms of insulin usually have low C-peptide and proinsulin levels because commercial insulin does not contain insulin precursor or cleavage fragments. Patients who surreptitiously consume oral hypoglycemic agents may be identified by the presence of plasma sulfonylurea.

Depending on the size of the tumors, insulinomas may be visualized by CT, MRI, or EUS. 68Ga-DOTATATE PET/CT is a useful adjunct for localizing insulinomas; and with the combination of a high-quality pancreas protocol CT scan, the need for more invasive procedures for localization purposes has fallen out of favor and is not currently recommended.

Treatment The primary treatment for sporadic insulinoma is surgical resection. Before surgery, glucose levels should be controlled with frequent small meals, intravenous dextrose infusion, or diazoxide, a drug that inhibits insulin release and promotes glycogenolysis. During surgery, intraoperative ultrasound is encouraged in order to localize small tumors deep in the pancreatic parenchyma, locate the main pancreatic duct (important if enucleation is planned), and exclude the presence of parenchymal liver metastases. Enucleation is appropriate for many smaller insulinomas, whereas larger lesions (> 2 cm) require formal pancreatectomy. If no tumor can be localized at the time of operative intervention, the surgeon may consider pancreatic biopsy to rule out beta cell hyperplasia or adult nesidioblastosis; however, blind distal pancreatectomy is not recommended. Instead, the surgeon should abandon attempts at resection and repeat biochemical testing, imaging, and possibly regionalization studies. Enlarged regional lymph nodes, especially if suspicious on preoperative imaging or DOTA-avid, should be resected even if a primary tumor cannot be located as these may be a source of ectopic insulin secretion and can provide the patient with symptom control. Additionally, these lymph nodes occasionally harbor ectopic pancreas tissue and may represent the primary tumor. Most patients with insulinoma are cured after resection; local recurrence, even after enucleation, is rare; and the median disease-free survival after resection of malignant insulinoma is approximately 5 years.

Gastrinoma

In 1955, Zollinger and Ellison described the first series of atypical peptic ulcerations, gastric hypersecretion with hyperacidity, and a noninsulin-producing islet tumor of the pancreas. Gastrinomas secrete gastrin, a hormone that induces hyperchlorhydria and parietal cell hyperplasia. Patients with sporadic gastrinoma often present at about 45 years of age with abdominal pain (75% to 100%), diarrhea (35% to 73%), heartburn (44% to 64%), duodenal and prepyloric ulcers (71% to 91%), and complications of peptic ulcer disease (PUD). Gastrinomas account for <1% of all cases of PUD. Approximately 75% of gastrinomas are sporadic; the remaining 25% are associated with MEN1. Most gastrinomas are located in the duodenum (70% to 90%) or the pancreas (2% to 30%) in what is typically known as the "gastrinoma triangle," which is delineated by the junction of the second and third portion of the duodenum, the junction of the body and neck of the pancreas, and the junction of the cystic and common bile ducts. However, primary gastrinomas have been identified at other sites including the stomach, jejunum, peripancreatic tissue, lymph nodes, ovaries, heart, and liver. The majority of gastrinomas are malignant, and the most important predictor of survival is the presence of liver metastases.

Diagnosis Patients with a suspected gastrinoma should be evaluated with a fasting gastrin level and gastric pH at 1 to 2 weeks after discontinuation of PPIs. Withdrawing PPIs in patients with suspected gastrinoma should be done carefully because bowel perforation can occur. A fasting gastrin level >1,000 pg/mL with a gastric pH of <2.5 is highly suggestive of a gastrinoma. Other causes of hypergastrinemia include PPI use, vagotomy, fundectomy, gastric outlet obstruction, resection of the large bowel, chronic renal failure, and autoimmune or *Helicobacter pylori* gastritis with atrophy and associated achlorhydria.

The majority of patients with gastrinomas have a basal–maximal acid output ratio ≥0.6, or a 12-hour nocturnal gastric acid secretion >100 mEq. To establish the diagnosis in the setting of an occult disease, a basal acid output of 15 mEq/hr and a positive secretin stimulation test have traditionally been used, although such testing is now rarely employed. Importantly, secondary neuroendocrine tumors, referred to as "type I gastric carcinoids" and pathologically indistinguishable from gastrinomas, occur in patients with achlorhydria due to atrophic gastritis, apparently due to the relentless stimulation of the very high gastrin levels in such patients. The gastrinomas in such patients are indolent, typically presenting as multiple small (<1 cm) tumors in the gastric fundus, and should almost always be treated conservatively, for example, with endoscopic monitoring and excision.

Serum CgA is usually elevated in patients with gastrinomas and several studies have shown that higher levels correlate with worse prognosis; however, it is less sensitive than serum gastrin levels, is not specific to gastrinomas, and can be falsely elevated due to PPI use.

Once a biochemical diagnosis of gastrinoma has been established, tumor localization studies are performed: esophagogastroduodenoscopy with EUS should be performed and cross-sectional imaging with either thin-slice pancreatic protocol CT or MRI. 68Ga-DOTATATE scan is useful for identifying primary tumors and metastases. Liver metastases from gastrinoma are most commonly limited to patients with primary tumors ≥2 cm in diameter.

Treatment Before surgery, acid hypersecretion must be controlled, typically with twice-daily administration of full-dose PPI. Surgical resection for sporadic gastrinomas can provide a biochemical cure in up to 60% of cases and has been shown to improve survival. For this reason, resection along with regional lymph node dissection is recommended. At least 30% to 50% of gastrinoma patients have regional lymph node metastases at the time of operative intervention. Previous studies have shown that excision of more than 10 lymph nodes may result in higher rates of biochemical cure. On the other hand, patients with MEN1 with gastrinomas that are <2 cm have excellent long-term prognosis and gastric hypersecretion can be controlled medically; thus, routine surgical exploration or resection at this size is not recommended.

Despite the number of imaging modalities available, (e.g., CT, MRI, EGD, EUS, 68Ga-DOTA) there are rare situations where the primary tumor is not found. For nonlocalizable gastrinomas in patients for whom symptoms are not controlled medically, surgical exploration should include the following: exploration of the lesser sac to evaluate the pancreatic body and tail; intraoperative ultrasound of the liver and pancreas; Kocher maneuver to inspect the pancreatic head; lateral duodenotomy with digital palpation to identify small duodenal wall tumors; periduodenal, peripancreatic head, portal, and hepatic arterial lymph node dissection (primary lymph node gastrinomas have been reported in up to 10% of sporadic cases); and exploration of extrapancreatic locations including the ovary, stomach wall, small bowel, omentum, and intestinal mesentery. Intraoperative endoscopy with transillumination may help localize duodenal wall tumors; if done, it should be performed prior to exploratory duodenotomy.

Vasoactive Intestinal Polypeptidoma

Vasoactive intestinal polypeptide (VIP)-secreting tumors (VIPomas) are associated with Verner–Morrison syndrome or watery diarrhea, hypokalemia, and achlorhydria (WDHA) syndrome. These are very rare PNETs characterized by large-volume secretory diarrhea that can be life threatening, with 70% of patients having over 3 L of stool volume per day. This is often accompanied by electrolyte imbalance (hypokalemia and hypercalcemia), dehydration, hypochlorhydria or achlorhydria, hyperglycemia, and flushing. More than 80% of VIPomas are found in the pancreas with 75% located in the pancreatic tail. Extrapancreatic primary tumors that secrete VIP have been identified in the chest and retroperitoneum and have included such tumors as ganglioneuroblastomas, ganglioneuromas, and neuroblastomas.

At presentation, 60% to 80% of VIPomas are metastatic. The 5-year OS rate for patients with VIPomas (all stages) is 69%. The 5-year survival rate is 60% for patients with metastatic disease and 94% for patients without metastasis.

Diagnosis A fasting plasma VIP level >500 pg/mL along with high-volume diarrhea is suggestive of a VIPoma. These tumors are usually identified on CT, MRI, EUS, or SSTR-PET scans as part of an evaluation for diarrhea.

Treatment VIPomas are usually treated with surgical resection and regional lymph node dissection. Before operative intervention, patients should be hydrated, their electrolytes should be normalized, and they should receive somatostatin analogues (SSAs), which inhibit the secretion of VIP, to control the diarrhea prior to resection. In patients whose diarrhea is refractory to SSAs, the use of steroids may be considered. In select patients with metastatic disease, cytoreduction may help improve symptoms.

Glucagonoma

Glucagonomas arise from the alpha cells of the pancreas and are characterized by excess glucagon secretion that results in glucose intolerance (occurring in >90% of patients), weight loss, neuropsychiatric disturbances (e.g., depression or psychosis), and venous thrombosis. Approximately 70% to 80%% of glucagonoma patients develop necrolytic migratory erythema (NME), a rash that occurs on the lower abdomen, perineum, perioral area, and/or feet. The diagnosis of NME can be made with a biopsy showing superficial necrolysis and perivascular infiltration with lymphocytes. The majority of glucagonomas arise in the body or tail of the pancreas, are malignant, and frequently present with metastases. The characteristic patient with a glucagonoma is elderly, ill, and has a large pancreatic tail mass.

Diagnosis An inappropriately elevated fasting glucagon level >500 to 1,000 pg/mL is diagnostic of a glucagonoma. However, elevated glucagon levels may occur in patients with cirrhosis, pancreatitis, diabetes mellitus, prolonged fasting, renal failure, burns, sepsis, familial glucagonemia, and acromegaly. While NME is not specific for glucagonoma and has been reported in association with other disorders, glucagonoma should be suspected in patients with NME even in the absence of symptoms. Glucagonomas are commonly >5 cm in diameter, making them easily identifiable on cross-sectional imaging.

Treatment Management of localized glucagonomas includes surgical resection and regional lymph node dissection. Metastatic disease should be resected when possible to alleviate symptoms. Necrolytic migratory erythema (NME) secondary to unresectable glucagonoma can be effectively treated with somatostatin.

Somatostatinoma

Somatostatinomas, which arise from the delta cells of the pancreas, are extremely rare and have an estimated incidence of 1 in 40 million. To date, only about 200 cases of somatostatinomas have been reported. Ninety percent of somatostatinomas are malignant. Although the majority (90%) of somatostatinomas are sporadic, some have been linked to familial disorders such as neurofibromatosis type 1 (NF1), MEN1, and Von Hippel–Lindau (VHL) disease.

Somatostatinomas are most frequently located in the pancreas or duodenum; however, there have been reports of somatostatinomas occurring in other locations such as the jejunum. Patients with duodenal somatostatinomas commonly present with symptoms of obstruction, whereas patients with pancreatic somatostatinomas frequently present with diabetes mellitus, cholelithiasis, steatorrhea, weight loss, anemia, and/or diarrhea. Five-year OS rates for patients with somatostatinoma are 100% for patients with localized disease and 60% for patients with distant metastatic disease.

Diagnosis Because of their rarity and nonspecific symptoms, patients with somatostatinomas are often diagnosed late in the course of the disease. A somatostatin level >100 pg/mL and a tumor identified on CT, MRI, SSTR-PET, or EUS suggest a diagnosis of somatostatinoma. Pancreatic somatostatinomas are typically solitary, large, and located in the head of the pancreas. Duodenal somatostatinomas are generally smaller than pancreatic somatostatinomas and can be directly visualized with esophagogastroduodenoscopy.

Treatment Somatostatinoma patients frequently present with metastatic disease; nevertheless, these patients should undergo surgical resection when possible. Given the high incidence of cholelithiasis in somatostatinoma patients, cholecystectomy should be performed at the time of surgery. As with other functional PNETs, tumor debulking of metastatic disease may be selectively considered for palliation.

Management of Liver Metastases

All patients with liver metastases from PNETs should be considered for surgical resection once an understanding of overall disease biology has been ascertained. Although associated with high recurrence rates, surgical resection of neuroendocrine metastases is associated with improved survival outcomes, with studies reporting 5-year OS from 60% to 80% in carefully selected patients. Predictors of poor outcomes included extrahepatic disease, incomplete resection, and poor histologic grade. Previous studies reported that cytoreduction of liver metastasis for either palliation or improved survival is only helpful when over 90% of tumor burden can be resected safely; however, there have been several recent studies that have shown that >70% cytoreduction can improve progression free survival, overall survival, and symptom control. Palliative treatment for hepatic metastasis should be individualized, taking into account the patient's comorbidities, symptoms, tumor grade, and rate of disease progression.

When patients are not candidates for surgical resection of liver metastases, alternative therapies should be considered. Microwave or radiofrequency ablation, transarterial chemoembolization (TACE), and yttrium-90 radioembolization are helpful strategies that may improve local control and palliate symptoms, although there is insufficient evidence to recommend one strategy over another. The RETNET trial (ClinicalTrials.gov; identifier: NCT02724540) is currently underway and seeks to determine the optimal strategy by comparing bland embolization, TACE, and embolization by drug-eluding beads (DEBs) in metastatic gastroenteropancreatic NET patients. Of note, the DEB-TACE arm closed early due to toxicity concerns. Finally, although reasonable outcomes have been described in well-selected patients with metastatic neuroendocrine tumors who underwent liver transplantation, worse results have been observed in patients with tumors of pancreatic origin; with reported recurrence rates of up to 60%, therefore, transplantation is typically not recommended and should only be considered in highly selected patients.

Systemic Therapy

Systemic therapy may be considered for patients with symptomatic, advanced, or metastatic disease. The decision to start treatment should be considered on an individual basis, keeping in mind that patients with stable and asymptomatic disease may be observed. The goal of systemic therapy in these settings is to prolong survival and improve quality of life by controlling symptoms. The mainstay of treatment is somatostatin analogs. Evaluation with somatostatin receptor imaging can assess receptor status and guide treatment options. The PROMID and CLARINET double-blind randomized controlled trials demonstrated significant improvements in PFS in patients with enteropancreatic neuroendocrine neoplasms who received lanreotide.

Increasingly, PNETs are being treated with targeted therapies. As an example, the RADIANT-3 trial demonstrated improved PFS in patients with nonfunctional PNETs who received the mTOR inhibitor everolimus. Similar results have been shown with the VEGF inhibitor sunitinib. Traditional cytotoxic chemotherapy is typically reserved for patients with high-grade tumors, since most well-differentiated tumors are indolent and response rates are low. Streptozocin was one of the first systemic agents to demonstrate activity in the setting of metastatic PNETs and its use in combinations with doxorubicin and 5-fluorouralcil (5-FU) has shown modest response rates. Similarly, in the past 10 years, the use of temozolomide regimens, particularly in combination with capecitabine, have been shown to improve survival in patients. Temozolomide use in an adjuvant setting is currently under investigation (ClinicalTrials.gov; identifier: NCT05040360).

More recent research has focused on the use peptide receptor radionuclide therapies (PRRTs). The NETTER-1 trial, a phase III randomized control trial of ^{177}Lu-DOTATATE in metastatic midgut NETs, demonstrated significant improvement in overall survival. Multiple other single arm studies suggest PRRT with ^{177}Lu-DOTATATE to be an effective treatment modality for unresectable metastatic PNETs. Currently, the NETTER-2 trial is recruiting to evaluate the use of PRRT as a first-line treatment for patients with both gastrointestinal and pancreatic NETs (ClinicalTrials.gov; identifier: NCT03972488). Its use as a means to reduce liver tumor burden, with the goal of reducing the size and number of lesions to facilitate resection, is under investigation.

Surveillance

Surveillance should be tailored to patients based on the treatment given, symptoms, and tumor burden. According to NANETS guidelines, asymptomatic patients, or those with stable and minimal disease well controlled on SSAs, should be seen every 3 to 6 months with CT scan of abdomen and pelvis. The timing interval may be lengthened based on stability of the patient's disease. Routine chest CT scan is not indicated. SSTR PET at initial staging can be used as baseline; however, it is not indicated for surveillance of PNETs unless there is a particular clinical concern. For patients who undergo resection of NF-PNETS, the timing of imaging has been debated with some recommending baseline imaging 3 to 6 months after surgery followed by every 6 to 12 months annually. At MD Anderson, patients undergoing pancreatectomy are often evaluated with CT scan 1 month after surgery for the purposes of obtaining a baseline examination and then followed every 3 months for the first 3 years if high risk or metastatic disease was found versus every 6 months if disease was confined to the pancreas and regional lymph nodes. Patients are followed up annually thereafter.

Multiple Endocrine Neoplasia and Other Hereditary Syndromes Associated with Pancreatic Neuroendocrine Tumors

Even though the majority of PNETs are sporadic, several hereditary syndromes are associated with an increased incidence of PNETs. Although surgical resection is generally indicated, as is the case for sporadic PNETs, a unique aspect of PNETs in the setting of an inherited tumor syndrome is their multiplicity. Therefore, surgical treatment of patients with inherited PNETs may be influenced by the need to preserve pancreatic parenchyma and avoid the long-term sequela of pancreatectomy (i.e., diabetes), particularly when the identified tumors are relatively small and distributed throughout the pancreas.

Multiple Endocrine Neoplasia Type 1

Multiple endocrine neoplasia type 1 (MEN1), also known as Wermer syndrome, is an autosomal dominant disorder caused by germline mutations in the *MEN1* gene. Located on chromosome 11q13, *MEN1* is a tumor suppressor gene that encodes menin, a protein involved in DNA replication, repair, transcription, and chromatin modification. Individuals with MEN1 commonly develop tumors in the anterior pituitary gland, parathyroid glands, and pancreas. More than 20 other endocrine tumors (e.g., foregut neuroendocrine tumors and adrenocortical and medullary lesions) and nonendocrine tumors (e.g., facial angiofibromas and collagenomas) have been described in MEN1. Thyroid nodules, meningiomas, ependymomas, leiomyomas, and lipomas are also associated with MEN1.

Parathyroid Tumors in MEN1

The most common first clinical manifestation associated with MEN1, primary hyperparathyroidism (PHPT), is also the most common endocrinopathy overall. The age of onset for PHPT ranges from 20 to 25 years, which is approximately 30 years earlier than that for sporadic PHPT. Nearly all MEN1 patients develop multiglandular PHPT by the age of 50 years. Therefore, all patients younger than 40 years who are diagnosed with multiglandular PHPT should be considered for genetic counseling and testing. Patients with PHPT may be completely asymptomatic or they may develop nephrolithiasis, osteoporosis, myopathy, fatigue, PUD, and neurocognitive deficits such as depression and difficulty sleeping.

Two major operative strategies for MEN1 patients with PHPT include subtotal parathyroidectomy and total parathyroidectomy. Because MEN1 patients are at increased risk of thymic carcinoid and because supernumerary parathyroid glands are often located in the thymus, cervical thymectomy is recommended as a component of both strategies. At MD Anderson, we favor subtotal parathyroidectomy (3.5-gland resection) with cervical thymectomy and parathyroid cryopreservation at the initial operation. In the event of recurrent hyperparathyroidism, which occurs in 30% to 40% of patients who undergo subtotal parathyroidectomy, we recommend performing completion (total) parathyroidectomy with autografting and cryopreservation of the remaining parathyroid tissue. We avoid total parathyroidectomy as the initial approach because as many as one-third of patients treated in this way develop permanent postoperative hypoparathyroidism.

Pituitary Tumors in MEN1

More commonly identified in women, anterior pituitary adenomas are diagnosed in 10% to 60% of MEN1 patients at an average age of 35 years (the same age as seen in sporadic tumors). Pituitary adenomas are the first clinical manifestation of MEN1 in approximately 10% of patients. The most common pituitary adenomas are prolactinomas (60%), nonfunctioning pituitary tumors (15%), somatotropinomas (10% to 15%), and corticotropin-secreting tumors (5%). Up to 85% of MEN1-associated pituitary tumors are macroadenomas that often present with symptoms of local compression such as headache, visual field deficits, hypopituitarism, temporal lobe epilepsy, mild hyperprolactinemia from stalk compression, and cranial nerve III or VI dysfunction. Pituitary adenomas are best detected by MRI with and without gadolinium at 3-mm intervals.

Women with prolactinomas may present with amenorrhea or galactorrhea, whereas men with prolactinomas may present with sexual dysfunction or gynecomastia. A serum prolactin level >200 ng/mL and an associated adenoma on MRI are diagnostic for prolactinoma. Patients with an adenoma on MRI and who have an elevated prolactin level <100 ng/mL most likely have a nonfunctional tumor leading to mildly elevated prolactin from stalk compression. The treatment of prolactinomas begins with long-acting dopamine agonists such as cabergoline or bromocriptine, although patients with MEN1-associated prolactinomas generally have a poor response to treatment. Surgical resection is indicated for symptomatic or growing tumors.

Somatotropinomas produce excess insulin-like growth factor 1 (IGF-1) and/or growth hormone, leading to gigantism in prepubescent children and acromegaly in adults. The diagnosis is rendered with an elevated IGF-1 level and a tumor on MRI; serum growth hormone levels may or may not be elevated. Inability to suppress growth hormone levels to <5 ng/dL after administering 1.75 g/kg (max 100 g) of oral glucose is diagnostic of a somatotropinoma. Corticotropin-secreting pituitary tumors lead to the development of Cushing disease. The clinical manifestations of corticotropin-secreting tumors include central weight gain, mood changes, thinning of the skin, easy bruising, diabetes, hypertension, and osteoporosis. Excess cortisol production can be detected by measuring the urinary free cortisol level. The diagnosis may also be confirmed by obtaining a plasma adrenocorticotrophic hormone level, a midnight salivary cortisol level, or by performing the dexamethasone suppression test. Inferior petrosal sinus sampling is the most invasive but also the most definitive test. The treatment of choice for both somatotropinomas and Cushing disease is surgical resection.

Pancreatic Neuroendocrine Tumors in MEN1

PNETs develop in 50% to 75% of patients with MEN1, and metastatic PNETs are the most frequent cause of death among MEN1 patients. PNETs associated with MEN1 are usually diagnosed at an earlier age than in sporadic cases. They may be solitary or multifocal, functional or nonfunctional, or both simultaneously (functional PNET 20% to 80% and NF-PNET 80% to 100%) and solid or cystic. Microscopically, the pancreas in MEN1 patients demonstrates multiple microadenomas, islet cell hypertrophy, hyperplasia, and dysplasia. Tumor localization strategies in patients with MEN1-associated PNETs are the same as in patients with sporadic PNETs. In general, early diagnosis and surgical excision of MEN1-associated PNETs is associated with improved OS.

Timing of surgical intervention in MEN1 patients with NF-PNETs must be individualized. Due to the frequent multiplicity of tumors, the relatively rare presence of liver metastases in patients with small primary PNETs, and the desire to maintain endocrine and exocrine function, surgery is often delayed in MEN1 patients until the largest tumor is ≥2 cm in size. When surgery is performed, an attempt is usually made to resect all identified pancreatic tumors; for example, enucleation of a superficial pancreatic head tumor is sometimes combined with formal distal pancreatectomy. Splenic preservation is a reasonable goal in most patients with moderately sized distal pancreatic tumors, and minimally invasive distal pancreatectomy is appropriate in selected patients.

Although several types of functional PNETs can occur within the same patient, one hormonal syndrome usually dominates. Gastrinoma, which has been identified in as many as 60% of MEN1 patients, is the most common functional pancreaticoduodenal endocrine tumor in MEN1 patients. More than 80% of MEN1-associated gastrinomas are located in the duodenum. Duodenal gastrinomas are usually very small tumors that are often not readily apparent on standard imaging modalities or upper endoscopy. Therefore, in MEN1 patients with an elevated gastrin level and a radiographically evident PNET, it should not be assumed that the visible PNET is the source of the elevated gastrin. Furthermore, patients with MEN1-associated hypergastrinemia and concomitant PHPT should usually undergo parathyroidectomy first because achieving normocalcemia may decrease serum gastrin levels.

The surgical management of gastrinoma in MEN1 patients is controversial. Unlike gastrinomas in patients with sporadic Zollinger–Ellison syndrome (ZES), MEN1-associated gastrinomas are significantly more likely to recur, and long-term cure is less likely after surgical resection. Therefore, current recommendations include surgical exploration for gastrinoma only in patients with biochemically confirmed ZES and a radiographically apparent primary tumor that is ≥2.0 cm or with apparent lymph node spread. Management of ZES in patients without an identifiable tumor consists of medical control of acid hypersecretion, although a regional operation (duodenotomy and regional lymph node dissection) can be selectively considered as part of the comprehensive surgical treatment of an MEN1 patient with hypergastrinemia in whom open distal pancreatectomy is planned for treatment of PNETs.

MEN1-associated insulinomas, which are diagnosed in 10% to 20% of patients with MEN1, are often multifocal, present earlier than sporadic insulinomas, and may be located throughout the pancreas. Although 85% to 95% of MEN1-associated insulinomas are benign, they have a higher recurrence rate after surgical resection than do sporadic insulinomas. As many as 5% of MEN1 patients with PNETs have other functioning tumors such as glucagonomas, VIPomas, or somatostatinomas. The diagnosis and treatment of these rare tumors are similar to that of their sporadic counterparts.

Screening of MEN1 Patients

Given the high penetrance of the previously mentioned disorders, patients with positive genetic testing or those at high risk of MEN1 should undergo regular screening. Screening for pituitary tumors begins with annual serum prolactin and IGF-1 levels as early 5 years of age. Brain MRI every 2 to 3 years may also be considered. Screening for PHPT may begin as early as 8 years of age and involves annual serum calcium and parathyroid hormone (PTH) levels. An elevated serum calcium level with an inappropriately elevated PTH level confirms the diagnosis of PHPT. Screening for functional PNETs includes annual serum fasting glucose, insulin, gastrin, chromogranin-A, glucagon, and proinsulin, whereas surveillance for NF-PNETs requires CT or MRI of the abdomen every 1 to 3 years. Patients with new, growing, or intermediate-size tumors (2 to 3 cm) in whom surgery is not immediately planned may require more frequent imaging (e.g., every 6 months).

Diagnosis of MEN1 and the Role of Genetic Testing

Obtaining a thorough and accurate family history is key to identifying MEN1 patients. Patients are clinically diagnosed with MEN1 if they develop two or more of the classic MEN1-associated tumors—pituitary, parathyroid, or endocrine tumors of the pancreas or duodenum—or have one of the classic tumors and at least one close relative with a clinical diagnosis of MEN1. Genetic counseling and the option of genetic testing should be offered to all patients with a clinical diagnosis of MEN1, to patients with one classic feature and a nonclassic tumor, and to patients with one of the classic tumors plus a family history of a classic tumor.

As many as 90% of MEN1 patients have an identifiable *MEN1* mutation although multiple mutations have been identified within the *MEN1* gene, and specific mutations may be unique to each family. Early genetic testing for MEN1 has many potential advantages: facilitating early identification and treatment of disease, preventing complications associated with long-term hormonal excess, allowing for consideration of preimplantation or prenatal genetic testing to assist in family planning, and allowing mutation-negative relatives to be spared unnecessary clinical screening.

Multiple Endocrine Neoplasia Type 2

MEN2 is an autosomal dominant disorder characterized by the development of medullary thyroid carcinoma (MTC), pheochromocytomas, and PHPT. MEN2 is divided into three different subtypes: MEN2A, familial MTC, and MEN2B. About 95% of MEN2 patients have germline activating missense mutations of the *RET* protooncogene. The *RET* gene encodes a tyrosine kinase receptor that is expressed in neuroendocrine and neural cells and consists of 21 exons located on chromosome 10q11.2. The specific RET mutation in MEN2 patients can be used to predict the MEN2 subtype as well as the aggressiveness of MTC. MTC is usually the first manifestation of MEN2, and the age of presentation ranges from the first to fourth decade of life.

MEN2A

MEN2A, the most common subtype of MEN2, is associated with the MTC in 90% of patients, PHPT in 20% to 30%, and pheochromocytoma in up to 50% of patients. *RET* mutations are identified in more than 95% of MEN2A patients. Patients who test negative for a *RET* mutation may be diagnosed with MEN2A if at least two of the classic features of the disease (i.e., MTC, pheochromocytoma, and PHPT) are present. Recently, familial MTC has been classified as a clinical variant of MEN2A, in which MTC is the only manifestation. Even though these patients are at low risk of developing pheochromocytoma and PHPT, families once thought to have familial MTC have later developed clinical manifestations of MEN2A and therefore must be monitored for the development of these tumors.

MEN2B

Less common than MEN2A, MEN2B is a condition characterized by MTC (nearly 100%), a marfanoid habitus, medullated corneal nerve fibers, ganglioneuromatosis, and pheochromocytoma (50%). Patients with MEN2B typically develop MTC approximately 10 years earlier than patients with MEN2A. MEN2B patients commonly have an elongated face with enlarged, nodular lips; thickened and everted eyelids; and neuromas of the tongue and oral mucosa. Patients may also develop skeletal abnormalities such as genu valgum, pes cavus, club foot, and kyphoscoliosis. Neuromas are frequently identified in the gastrointestinal tract but may also occur in organs with a submucosa, such as the bronchi and bladder. In addition, abdominal distention, megacolon, constipation, and diarrhea may develop in MEN2B patients as a result of the ganglioneuromatosis of the GI tract.

Medullary Thyroid Carcinoma in MEN2

MTC develops from the parafollicular cells (C cells) of the thyroid gland that produce calcitonin, a hormone that decreases plasma calcium levels by inhibiting osteoclastic bone absorption and stimulating urinary excretion of calcium and phosphate. In MEN2 patients, MTC is preceded by the development of C-cell hyperplasia, leading to an increase in serum calcitonin levels. Because the majority of C cells are located in the superior one-third of the thyroid gland, MTC is most commonly concentrated in this location. MTC in patients with MEN2 is usually bilateral and multicentric. A serum calcitonin level >1,000 pg/mL and an elevated CEA level suggest MTC. A positive pentagastrin stimulation test and the identification of a thyroid mass with positive cytologic evidence of MTC on ultrasonography-guided fine-needle aspiration biopsy are diagnostic.

MTC is a relatively aggressive disease. Patients may present with neck pain, a palpable neck mass, or diarrhea due to elevated serum calcitonin levels. Patients who have dysphagia or hoarseness likely have advanced disease. Metastasis first develops in cervical or mediastinal lymph nodes, followed by the lungs, liver, and bones. Surgical resection is the treatment of choice for MTC. The timing and extent of surgery should be individualized according to the patient's specific *RET* mutation to achieve the best overall outcome (Table 16.3). The disease is generally resistant to chemotherapy, and radioactive iodine is ineffective. Targeted therapies, with tyrosine kinase inhibitors (TKIs) such as vandetanib and cabozantinib are associated with improved PFS in patients with advanced MTC but are associated with significant toxicity and therefore usually reserved for patients with large tumor burden and documented disease progression. The role of CDKN2C mutations has also been studied, with reports demonstrating that loss of CDKN2C may be associated with worse prognosis. CDK inhibitors are currently under investigations as potential targeted agents for MTC treatment.

The initial evaluation of patients diagnosed with MTC includes performing cervical neck ultrasonography and measuring serum CEA, calcium, and calcitonin levels. Before operative intervention, serum PTH and plasma metanephrines should be measured to rule out pheochromocytoma and PHPT. If a pheochromocytoma is present, it should be resected before thyroidectomy to prevent a hypertensive crisis. Total

TABLE 16.3			
Aggressiveness of MTC Based on *RET* Mutation			

American Thyroid Association Level	RET Mutation	Aggressiveness of MTC	Timing of Prophylactic Thyroidectomy
A	768, 790, 791, 804, 891	Lowest risk of aggressiveness (lower serum calcitonin, lower tumor stage, and higher rate of cure than level B tumors)	May be delayed beyond 5 yrs of age if serum *calcitonin* and neck ultrasound are normal[a]
B	609, 611, 618, 620, 630	Lower risk of aggressiveness	Consider prophylactic thyroidectomy before age 5 yrs (may be delayed beyond 5 years of age if serum calcitonin and neck ultrasound are normal[a])
C	634	High risk of aggressiveness	Before 5 yrs of age
D	883, 918	Highest risk of aggressiveness and youngest age at onset	Within the first yr of life

[a]Must be screened with annual serum calcitonin levels and cervical ultrasonography; if abnormal, thyroidectomy is indicated at that time.
RET, rearranged during transfection.

thyroidectomy with prophylactic central neck dissection is recommended for patients with no evidence of local invasion or lymph node metastasis. In patients who have calcitonin levels >400 pg/mL or evidence of lymph node metastasis, a triple phase CT of the neck, chest, and liver is necessary to rule out distant metastasis. Patients who demonstrate lateral cervical lymph node metastasis should undergo a lateral neck dissection of levels IIA, III, IV, and V on the affected side. In patients with established distant metastatic disease, limited surgical resection to preserve speech and swallowing may be considered.

Thyroid hormone suppression therapy is not effective for patients with MTC, so patients should only receive thyroid hormone replacement therapy after total thyroidectomy. Baseline serum calcitonin and CEA levels should be measured 2 to 3 months after operative intervention and every 6 to 12 months thereafter. Cervical ultrasonography should be performed 6 months after surgical resection. The detection of calcitonin after total thyroidectomy indicates that residual or persistent disease is present. Patients in whom serum calcitonin and CEA levels are undetectable may be monitored with biochemical assessments alone.

Primary Hyperparathyroidism in MEN2A

PHPT occurs in 10% to 35% of patients with MEN2A. Although the diagnosis and the clinical presentation of PHPT in MEN2A are similar to those seen in sporadic or MEN1-associated cases, surgical intervention for MEN2A-associated PHPT differs in several important ways. MEN2A patients who have PHPT at the time of initial thyroidectomy should undergo resection of visibly enlarged parathyroid glands with possible forearm autograft, subtotal parathyroidectomy (leaving one or a piece of one gland in situ), or total parathyroidectomy with forearm autograft. In patients who develop PHPT after initial thyroidectomy, surgical intervention should be guided by the identification of abnormal parathyroid glands on preoperative imaging, and the use of forearm autografting should be considered. During thyroidectomy for patients with MEN2A, especially those with a strong family history of PHPT, normal devascularized parathyroid glands should be implanted into the forearm.

Pheochromocytoma in MEN2

Pheochromocytomas—catecholamine-secreting tumors of the adrenal medulla—develop in up to 50% of MEN2A patients during their lifespan and typically 10 to 20 years earlier than in patients with sporadic pheochromocytomas. Patients with pheochromocytomas typically present with headache, sweating, palpitations, hypertension, and anxiety. Pheochromocytomas may be unilateral or bilateral, and synchronous or metachronous. Elevated plasma-free metanephrines and normetanephrines or urinary metanephrines are necessary for the diagnosis. Once biochemical diagnosis is established, CT or MRI of the abdomen should be performed to identify an adrenal tumor. Metaiodobenzylguanidine (MIBG) scanning may be used for localization in difficult cases.

The treatment of choice for pheochromocytoma is surgical resection. At least 1 to 2 weeks before surgery, patients should be well hydrated and treated with an alpha antagonist. The recommended initial dose of phenoxybenzamine is 10 mg twice a day with a goal to achieve a blood pressure of 130/80 mm Hg while sitting and 100 mm Hg systolic while standing. Other alpha-1-adrenergic blocking agents such as prazosin, terazosin, or doxazosin may be used instead of phenoxybenzamine. When needed, beta blockers may be used to obtain a target heart rate of 60 to 70 beats per minute while sitting and 70 to 80 beats per minute while standing. Beta-1 blockers (atenolol 12.5 to 25 mg three times per day, or metoprolol 25 to 50 mg two to three times per day) are preferred and must always be used with alpha-adrenergic blockade. Beta blockers should never be used alone or before the initiation of alpha blockade, due to the risk of exacerbating hypertension in these patients.

The most common operative approach in patients with a unilateral pheochromocytoma is minimally invasive adrenalectomy. At MD Anderson, we prefer retroperitoneoscopic adrenalectomy over a transperitoneal laparoscopic approach for patients with modestly sized, clinically benign pheochromocytomas. This approach avoids the need for intra-abdominal solid-organ mobilization and for repositioning in patients with bilateral tumors. If possible, cortical sparing adrenalectomy should be performed in MEN2 patients with bilateral pheochromocytomas because the procedure can prevent postoperative corticosteroid dependence in up to 65% of patients. Otherwise, patients who undergo bilateral adrenalectomy will require lifelong corticosteroid supplementation. With careful preoperative planning and meticulous surgical technique, including minimizing unnecessary dissection to preserve remnant blood supply, cortical-sparing adrenalectomy can be performed successfully with use of minimally invasive techniques, including via a retroperitoneoscopic approach.

Diagnosis of MEN2 and the Role of Genetic Testing

Genetic counseling and testing are recommended for patients who are diagnosed with MTC, primary C-cell hyperplasia, cutaneous lichen amyloidosis, or early-age-of-onset pheochromocytoma. *RET* genetic testing should also be suggested to patients who have a positive family history of MEN2 or MTC. Patients at risk of developing MEN2A should undergo genetic testing before 5 years of age, and patients at risk of MEN2B should be tested shortly after birth. If possible, all first-degree relatives should be offered genetic testing before the age of recommended prophylactic thyroidectomy when a specific *RET* mutation is identified within a family.

Von Hippel–Lindau Disease

VHL is an autosomal dominant disease characterized by mutations of the *VHL* gene and is associated with pancreatic pathology in 20% to 75% of patients. VHL patients most commonly develop pancreatic cysts, but 15% to 20% will develop PNETs and it may be difficult to differentiate between these two processes. For this reason, SSTR-PET can be helpful in establishing a diagnosis when a pancreatic mass is found. Other characteristics of this disease include hemangioblastomas of the nervous system, retinal angiomas, clear cell renal carcinomas, pheochromocytomas, and endolymphatic sac tumors. PNETs associated with VHL are usually nonfunctional and solitary. In cases of multifocal disease, they can be located anywhere in the pancreas (52% present in the head) and are typically diagnosed at an earlier age than in sporadic PNETs. PNETs associated with VHL may be more indolent than PNETs associated with MEN1, with distant disease only seen in about 10% of patients. Factors associated with higher risk of distant metastasis include lesions >3 cm or larger, rate of tumor growth with doubling time <500 days, as well as germline mutations in exon 3. Patients with these characteristics should be considered for resection. Patients with lesions that are <2 cm can be safely observed.

Tuberous Sclerosis

Tuberous sclerosis is a rare, autosomal dominant disorder associated with mutations in the *TSC1* gene on the 9q34 chromosome or the *TSC2* gene on the 16p13.3 chromosome. Tuberin, a *TSC2* gene product associated with cell growth and proliferation, has been associated with the development of malignant PNETs in tuberous sclerosis patients.

von Recklinghausen Disease

Associated with a mutation of the *NF1* tumor suppressor gene, von Recklinghausen disease, also known as NF1, is manifested by the development of neurofibromas, café-au-lait macules, optic gliomas, Lisch nodules, bony lesions, short stature, learning disabilities, and macroencephaly. Malignant pheochromocytomas are the most common endocrine malignancy associated with NF1; however, a few case reports of pancreatic insulinomas and duodenal somatostatinomas have been published.

CASE SCENARIO

Case Scenario 1

Presentation

A 65-year-old female presents with diarrhea and facial flushing for the past year. She states that she has been having liquid bowel movements shortly after eating and it has been progressively getting worse. She is otherwise healthy and does not have any major comorbidities.

Additional Workup

She underwent colonoscopy which demonstrated diverticulosis but no polyps or signs of malignancy. An EDG with EUS was performed and a 4-cm hyper enhancing lesion was found in the body of the pancreas. Biopsies revealed an intermediate grade, well-differentiated neuroendocrine carcinoma. She underwent CT scan of the abdomen and pelvis which demonstrated a hyperenhancing lesion at the body of the pancreas, as well as a 3-cm lesion in segment 6 of the liver, consistent with metastatic disease. She was started on octreotide for control of her symptoms and then scheduled for a distal pancreatectomy with partial hepatectomy of segment 6 of the liver.

Surgical Approach—Key Steps

The primary treatment of PNETs is surgical resection with lymph node dissection for patients with tumors >1 cm, are growing, or are symptomatic. All patients with liver metastasis from PNETs should be considered for surgical resection when a complete resection is feasible. Predictors of poor outcome include extrahepatic disease, incomplete resection, and poor histologic grade. When a complete resection of hepatic lesions is not feasible, alternative options including radiofrequency or microwave ablation, transarterial chemoembolization, and yttrium-90 radioembolization should be considered.

CASE SCENARIO REVIEW

Questions

1. A 65-year-old female with history of severe chronic obstructive pulmonary disease on supplemental oxygen and chronic kidney disease presents with a 5-cm liver lesion. Percutaneous biopsy is performed and demonstrates a well-differentiated neuroendocrine tumor. Which of the following is the most appropriate next step in management?

   A. Extended right hepatectomy
   B. Streptozocin
   C. Fluorouracil
   D. Yttrium-90 radioembolization

2. A 63-year-old male with widely metastatic neuroendocrine tumor to the liver has had liver-directed therapy and stable disease for the past 5 years on octreotide. He presents to the emergency department with a small bowel obstruction that seems to be associated with a new, isolated 2-cm lesion at the mesenteric border of the mid jejunum. What is the best course of action?

   A. Treatment with somatostatin analog
   B. Palliative gastrostomy tube
   C. Minimally invasive resection of isolated lesion
   D. Debulking of small bowel lesion in conjunction with hepatectomy

Answers

1. **The correct answer is D.** *Rationale:* For patients with unresectable liver metastasis, whether due to anatomical location of the lesions or comorbidities that preclude major surgical resection, yttrium-90 microspheres are a great treatment option, particularly for patients with symptomatic disease.

2. **The correct answer is C.** *Rationale:* For patients with metastatic PNET that have demonstrated a favorable tumor biology, complete resection of isolated lesions in select patients may be considered for palliative purposes. However, incomplete resection or primary tumor "debulking" is not recommended due to morbidity associated with cytoreduction in nonresectable disease.

CASE SCENARIO

Case Scenario 2

Presentation

A 48-year-old female presents with repeated bouts of dizziness, palpitations, and with reported episodes of hypoglycemia. Her symptoms improve after eating and she reports significant weight gain in the past year. She presents to her primary doctor and her fasting glucose level comes back as 35 mg/dL.

Additional Workup

A monitored fast is performed, and the patient develops symptoms of hypoglycemia within the first 10 hours of the test. Further testing revealed an elevated fasting insulin level of 55 mg, as well as elevated C-peptide and proinsulin levels. A CT scan is performed and a 3-cm hyperenhancing lesion is found in the tail of the pancreas. Surgical resection is recommended.

Surgical Approach

For patients with insulinomas, complete surgical resection is the treatment of choice. Given that 90% of insulinomas are benign, enucleation should be considered for smaller lesions if anatomically feasible. Larger lesions or lesions that are within 2 mm of the main pancreatic duct should undergo formal anatomical resection according to the location of the lesion. If the tumor cannot be localized on imaging studies preoperatively, a blind pancreatectomy should not be performed and further localizing studies should be done. In the rare situation where a tumor cannot be localized with preoperative or intraoperative techniques, random pancreatic biopsies should be taken to evaluate for nesidioblastosis or beta cell hyperplasia. Most patients with insulinomas are cured after surgical resection.

CASE SCENARIO REVIEW

Questions

1. A 52-year old male presents with repeated bouts of hypoglycemia. After further workup, a 1-cm mass is found in the tail of the pancreas. The most appropriate next course of treatment is:

   A. treatment with molecular inhibitor of mTOR (everolimus)
   B. distal pancreatectomy and splenectomy
   C. enucleation of lesion
   D. observation

2. A 48-year-old female presents to her primary care clinic with hyperglycemia and skin lesions. CT scan is obtained which demonstrates a 3-cm mass in the tail of the pancreas. The most appropriate definitive treatment is:

   A. distal pancreatectomy with lymphadenectomy
   B. enucleation of the lesion
   C. total pancreatectomy
   D. 5-fluorouracil and radiation therapy

3. A 56-year-old female is incidentally found to have a 1-cm lesion in the tail of pancreas on a CT scan obtained after a motor vehicle accident. She is asymptomatic with regard to pain, skin changes, bowel habit changes, or endocrinopathies. An EGD with EUS confirms presence of the lesion and biopsy demonstrates a low grade, well-differentiated neuroendocrine tumor with Ki-67 proliferation index of 3%. Next course of action should be:

   A. observation
   B. distal pancreatectomy with lymphadenectomy
   C. somatostatin analogues
   D. sunitinib

Answers

1. **The correct answer is C.** *Rationale:* Complete resection is the treatment of choice for all insulinomas; however, given that 90% of insulinomas are benign, consideration for enucleation is reasonable in lesions that are less than 1 cm. For lesions that are large or within 2 mm of the main pancreatic duct, anatomical resection should be performed. mTOR inhibitors are considered a treatment option for unresectable, metastatic PNETs according to the RADIANT-3 trial.

2. **The correct answer is A.** *Rationale:* Resection of PNET with regional lymphadenectomy should be the goal of treatment in patients with resectable lesions that are ≥3 cm or symptomatic.

3. **The correct answer is A.** *Rationale:* Observation of select pancreatic neuroendocrine tumors can be considered for lesions under <2 cm, those that are nonfunctioning, and those with lower risk features such as low grade, well-differentiated tumors and those with a low Ki-67 index.

Recommended Readings

Agarwal SK, Lee BA, Sukhodolets KE, et al. Molecular pathology of the MEN1 gene. *Ann NY Acad Sci.* 2004;1014:189–198.

Bartsch DK, Waldmann J, Fendrich V, et al. Impact of lymphadenectomy on survival after surgery for sporadic gastrinoma. *Br J Surg.* 2012;99(9):1234–1240.

Caplin ME, Pavel M, C´wikła JB, et al. Lanreotide in metastatic enteropancreatic neuroendocrine tumors. *N Engl J Med.* 2014;371(3):224–233.

Cloyd JM, Poultsides GA. Non-functional neuroendocrine tumors of the pancreas: advances in diagnosis and management. *World J Gastroenterol.* 2015;21(32):9512–9525.

Cloyd, J M, Ejaz A, Konda B, Makary MS, Pawlik TM Neuroendocrine liver metastases: a contemporary review of treatment strategies. *Hepatobiliary Surg Nutr.* 2020; 9(4): 440–451.

Dasari A, Shen C, Halperin D, et al. Trends in the incidence, prevalence, and survival outcomes in patients with neuroendocrine tumors in the United States. *JAMA Oncol.* 2017;3(10):1335–1342.

Dickson PV, Rich TA, Xing Y, et al. Achieving eugastrinemia in MEN1 patients: both duodenal inspection and formal lymph node dissection are important. *Surgery*. 2011;150(6):1143–1152.

Eng C, Clayton D, Schuffenecker I, et al. The relationship between specific RET proto-oncogene mutations and disease phenotype in multiple endocrine neoplasia type 2. International RET Mutation Consortium analysis. *JAMA*. 1996;276(19):1575–1579.

Falconi M, Eriksson B, Kaltsas G, et al. ENETS consensus guidelines update for the management of patients with functional pancreatic neuroendocrine tumors and non-functional pancreatic neuroendocrine tumors. *Neuroendocrinology*. 2016;103(2):153–171.

Fendrich V, Ramaswamy A, Slater EP, Bartsch DK. Duodenal somatostatinoma associated with Von Reckling-hausen's disease. *J Hepatobiliary Pancreat Surg*. 2004;11(6):417–421.

Ferolla P, Falchetti A, Filosso P, et al. Thymic neuroendocrine carcinoma (carcinoid) in multiple endocrine neoplasia type 1 syndrome: the Italian series. *J Clin Endocrinol Metab*. 2005;90(5):2603–2609.

Gedaly R, Daily MF, Davenport D, et al. Liver transplantation for the treatment of liver metastases from neuro-endocrine tumors: an analysis of the UNOS database. *Archives of Surgery*. 2011;146(8):953–958.

Gauger PG, Scheiman JM, Wamsteker EJ, Richards ML, Doherty GM, Thompson NW. Role of endoscopic ultra-sonography in screening and treatment of pancreatic endocrine tumours in asymptomatic patients with multiple endocrine neoplasia type 1. *Br J Surg*. 2003;90(6):748–754.

Guettier JM, Kam A, Chang R, et al. Localization of insulinomas to regions of the pancreas by intraarterial calcium stimulation: the NIH experience. *J Clin Endocrinol Metab*. 2009;94(4):1074–1080.

Jensen RT, Berna MJ, Bingham DB, Norton JA. Inherited pancreatic endocrine tumor syndromes: advances in molecular pathogenesis, diagnosis, management, and controversies. *Cancer*. 2008;113(suppl 7):1807–1843.

Jensen RT, Norton JA. Treatment of pancreatic neuroendocrine tumors in multiple endocrine neoplasia type 1: some clarity but continued controversy. *Pancreas*. 2017;46(5):589–594.

Kindmark H, Sundin A, Granberg D, et al. Endocrine pancreatic tumors with glucagon hypersecretion: a retro-spective study of 23 cases during 20 years. *Med Oncol*. 2007;24(3):330–337.

Klimstra DS, Klöppel G, La Rosa S, et al. Classification of neuroendocrine neoplasms of the digestive system. In: *WHO Classification of Tumours Editorial Board. Digestive System Tumours*. 5th ed. International Agency for Research on Cancer. 2019:16–19.

Lairmore TC, Piersall LD, DeBenedetti MK, et al. Clinical genetic testing and early surgical intervention in patients with multiple endocrine neoplasia type 1 (MEN 1). *Ann Surg*. 2004;239(5):637–645.

Mayo SC, de Jong MC, Pulitano C, et al. Surgical management of hepatic neuroendocrine tumor metastasis: results from an international multi-institutional analysis. *Ann Surg Oncol*. 2010;17(12):3129–3136.

Maxwell J E, Sherman SK, O'Dorisio TM, Bellizzi AM, Howe JR. Liver-directed surgery of neuroendocrine metastases: what is the optimal strategy? *Surgery*. 2016;159(1):320–333.

Maxwell JE, Gule-Monroe MK, Subbiah V, et al. Novel use of a clinical laboratory improvements amendments (CLIA)-certified cyclin-dependent kinase N2C (CDKN2C) loss assay in sporadic medullary thyroid carci-noma. *Surgery*. 2020;167(1):80–86.

Moertel CG, Lefkopoulo M, Lipsitz S, Hahn RG, Klaassen D. Streptozocin-doxorubicin, streptozocin-fluoroura-cil or chlorozotocin in the treatment of advanced islet-cell carcinoma. *N Engl J Med*. 1992;326(8):519–523.

Moris D, Tsilimigras DI, Ntanasis-Stathopoulos I, et al. Liver transplantation in patients with liver metastases from neuroendocrine tumors: a systematic review. *Surgery*. 2017;162(3):525–536.

Nagtegaal ID, Odze RD, Klimstra D, et al. The 2019 WHO classification of tumours of the digestive system. *Histopathology*. 2020;76(2):182–188.

Norton JA, Alexander HR, Fraker DL, Venzon DJ, Gibril F, Jensen RT. Possible primary lymph node gastrinoma: occurrence, natural history, and predictive factors: a prospective study. *Ann Surg*. 2003;237(5):650–657; dis-cussion 657–659.

Norton JA, Foster DS, Blumgart LH, et al. Incidence and prognosis of primary gastrinomas in the hepatobiliary tract. *JAMA Surgery*. 2018;153(3):e175083–175083.

Norton JA, Fraker DL, Alexander HR, Jensen RT. Value of surgery in patients with negative imaging and spo-radic Zollinger-Ellison syndrome. *Ann Surg*. 2012;256(3):509–517.

Norton JA, Krampitz G, Zemek A, Longacre T, Jensen RT. Better survival but changing causes of death in patients with multiple endocrine neoplasia type 1. *Ann Surg*. 2015;261(6):e147–e148.

Perrier ND, Kennamer DL, Bao R, et al. Posterior retroperitoneoscopic adrenalectomy: preferred technique for removal of benign tumors and isolated metastases. *Ann Surg.* 2008;248(4):666–674.

Raymond E, Dahan L, Raoul JL, et al. Sunitinib malate for the treatment of pancreatic neuroendocrine tumors. *N Engl J Med.* 2011;364(6):501–513.

Rinke A, Muller HH, Schade-Brittinger C, et al. Placebo-controlled, double-blind, prospective, randomized study on the effect of octreotide LAR in the control of tumor growth in patients with metastatic neuroendocrine midgut tumors: a report from the PROMID Study Group. *J Clin Oncol.* 2009;27(28):4656–4663.

Saxena A, Chua TC, Bester L, Kokandi A, Morris DL. Factors predicting response and survival after yttrium-90 radioembolization of unresectable neuroendocrine tumor liver metastases: a critical appraisal of 48 cases. *Ann Surg.* 2010;251(5):910–916.

Saxena A, Chua TC, Perera M, Chu F, Morris DL. Surgical resection of hepatic metastases from neuroendocrine neoplasms: a systematic review. *Surg Oncol.* 2012;21(3):e131–e141.

Strosberg JR, Fine RL, Choi J, et al. First-line chemotherapy with capecitabine and temozolomide in patients with metastatic pancreatic endocrine carcinomas. *Cancer.* 2011;117:268–275.

Strosberg J, El-Haddad G, Wolin E, et al. Phase 3 trial of 177Lu-DOTATATE for midgut neuroendocrine tumors. *N Engl J Med.* 2017;376(2):125–135.

Squires MH, Worth PJ, Konda B, et al. Neoadjuvant capecitabine/temozolomide for locally advanced or metastatic pancreatic neuroendocrine tumors. *Pancreas.* 2020;49(3):355–360.

Tran CG, Sherman SK, Chandrasekharan C, Howe JR. Surgical management of neuroendocrine tumor liver metastases. *Surg Oncol Clin N Am.* 2021;30(1):39–55.

Yao JC, Shah MH, Ito T, et al. Everolimus for advanced pancreatic neuroendocrine tumors. *N Engl J Med.* 2011;364(6):514–523.

Yip L, Cote GJ, Shapiro SE, et al. Multiple endocrine neoplasia type 2: evaluation of the genotype-phenotype relationship. *Arch Surg.* 2003;138(4):409–416.

17

Adrenal Tumors

Andrew D. Newton and Jeffrey E. Lee

INTRODUCTION

Proper surgical evaluation and treatment of adrenal tumors can be complex and includes the application of appropriate diagnostic imaging, selective endocrine hormone evaluation, and, when indicated, either minimally invasive or open surgery. Advances in diagnostic imaging have facilitated early detection and accurate surgical treatment planning, whereas advances in minimally invasive and open surgical techniques have improved the surgeon's ability to minimize surgical morbidity while optimizing outcomes.

Evaluation of a patient presenting with an adrenal mass requires an understanding of relevant adrenal endocrine physiology. Appropriate biochemical evaluation and radiographic assessment of an identified adrenal mass are crucial prior to any surgical intervention. In the case of biochemical evaluation, this helps determine the functional status of the tumor and directs the management, algorithm including the potential role for surgery. Common functioning adrenal tumors include cortisol-producing adrenal adenomas, pheochromocytomas, aldosteronomas, and adrenal cortical carcinomas. Nonfunctioning adrenal tumors include nonfunctioning adrenal adenomas or "incidentalomas," metastases to the adrenal gland, and uncommon primary tumors including angiomyelolipomas. Recent developments in genetics (reviewed later in this chapter), especially for patients with pheochromocytomas, are being increasingly incorporated into the management of patients with adrenal tumors and their families.

Anatomy

The adrenal glands are paired, pyramid-shaped structures located in the retroperitoneum atop the superior–medial aspect of each kidney. The normal adult adrenal gland weighs approximately 4 to 5 g, spanning approximately 4 to 5 cm vertically, 3 cm transversely, and 1 cm in the anteroposterior plane. The adrenal glands are soft and highly vascular structures with two discrete embryologic, anatomic, and functional layers: the cortex (outer) and the medulla (inner). The cortex is normally a thin (1 to 2 mm), bright yellow layer which produces steroid hormones. From superficial to deep, it is subdivided into the zona glomerulosa which produces the mineralocorticoid aldosterone, the zona fasciculata which produces the glucocorticoid cortisol, and the zona reticularis which produces the sex steroids, primarily androgens. The medulla is a dark red-gray layer which produces norepinephrine and epinephrine.

The arterial blood supply to the adrenal glands is derived from branches of the inferior phrenic artery, the renal artery, and contributions directly from the aorta. Nutrient arteries coalesce and form a capsular arterial plexus that sends capillaries throughout the cortex, which subsequently combine to form a venous portal system that drains into the adrenal medulla. In the medulla, the vessels come together to join the central adrenal vein. The adrenal medulla is also supplied by arteriae medullae that penetrate directly into the medullary substance. Although there are some small veins draining the surface of the adrenal cortex, the central vein drains most of the blood from the medulla stemming from the cortex via the capsular plexus. The right adrenal vein is short and wide as it exits the gland and immediately enters the posterolateral aspect of the inferior vena cava at an acute angle. The left adrenal vein exits anteriorly and usually drains into the left renal vein, although it occasionally may enter the inferior vena cava directly. It is therefore typically easier to obtain vascular control of the left adrenal vein. Vascular control and cannulation of the right adrenal vein can be particularly challenging with increasing size of the adrenal tumor (Fig. 17.1).

Aldosteronoma

Primary aldosteronism was first described by J. W. Conn in 1955 in the setting of a 4-cm aldosterone secreting adenoma in association with hypertension and hypokalemia (Conn syndrome). Since then, it has been recognized that primary aldosteronism may have multiple etiologies; the condition has been declared a "major public health issue" by the Endocrine Society, with recommendations for physicians to "substantially ramp up the screening of hypertensive patients." The two major causes are a unilateral aldosterone-producing adenoma (60%) and bilateral adrenal hyperplasia or idiopathic aldosteronism (40%). Other rare causes of primary aldosteronism include unilateral primary adrenal hyperplasia, aldosterone-producing adrenal cortical carcinoma,

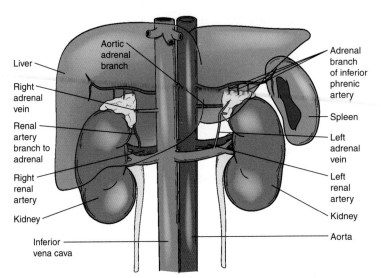

FIGURE 17.1 Adrenal vascular anatomy. (From the Anatomical Chart Company and Nolan T, Kawamura D. *Abdomen and Superficial Structures.* 5th ed. Wolters Kluwer; 2023. Figure 15.2.)

familial aldosteronism (glucocorticoid-suppressible and idiopathic aldosteronism), and aldosterone-secreting ovarian tumors. Primary aldosteronism was historically thought to be responsible for approximately 0.5% to 2.0% of all cases of hypertension, but with the recent utilization of more extensive and sensitive diagnostic testing, it is now estimated to be the causative factor in up to 15% of cases of hypertension. Moreover, primary aldosteronism represents 5% to 10% of surgically correctable cases of hypertension. Patients with primary aldosteronism have been shown to have cardiac, cerebrovascular, and renal dysfunction, which may be improved or reversed with appropriate treatment, thus supporting aggressive workup and treatment of patients suspected of having this disease.

Clinical Manifestations

Symptoms of primary aldosteronism are usually mild and nonspecific. The most common symptoms are headache, muscle weakness, fatigue, polydipsia, polyuria, and nocturia. Hypertension is almost always present but is often mild, with diastolic blood pressures less than 120 mm Hg in more than 70% of cases. Patients are characteristically on multiple antihypertensive medications.

Current Endocrine Society Clinical Practice Guidelines, released in May 2016, recommend biochemical evaluation for primary aldosteronism in patients with blood pressure above 150/100 mm Hg resistant to three antihypertensive medications, patients with controlled blood pressure (defined as <140/90 mm Hg) on four or more antihypertensives, and those with hypertension and one of the following: hypokalemia (spontaneous or diuretic-induced), adrenal incidentaloma, sleep apnea, or a family history of early-onset hypertension or cerebrovascular accident at a young age (<40 years old). In addition, it is recommended that all first-degree relatives of patients with known primary aldosteronism are recommended to be screened.

Diagnosis

Initial findings that support a diagnosis of primary aldosteronism include hypertension and spontaneous hypokalemia. However, hypokalemia has been noted to occur in less than 50% of patients with primary aldosteronism. Half of patients with an aldosterone-secreting adenoma and only 17% of patients with idiopathic aldosteronism have been shown to have a serum potassium concentration less than 3.5 mmol/L. Additional electrolyte abnormalities may include hypernatremia and a hypochloremic metabolic alkalosis. Prior to endocrine evaluation, diuretics should be discontinued for at least 2 weeks. Plasma aldosterone/renin ration (ARR) is the initial screening test of choice and is most accurate when performed in the morning after patients have been out of bed for at least 2 hours and have been seated for 5 to 15 minutes. A plasma aldosterone/renin ratio greater than 30 (ng/dL: ng/mL/h) along with a plasma aldosterone level greater than 20 ng/dL is sensitive and specific in the screening for, and diagnostic of, primary aldosteronism.

If aldosterone and renin determination is equivocal, confirmation of the diagnosis can be obtained using the saline suppression test or the 3-day sodium loading test; these additional diagnostic steps are unnecessary in the straightforward situation (i.e., patient with spontaneous hypokalemia, undetectable plasma renin levels, and plasma aldosterone level greater than 20 ng/dL). In the saline suppression test, 2 L of normal saline is infused intravenously over 4 hours and plasma aldosterone is measured. Confirmation of aldosteronism is obtained when the plasma aldosterone level is greater than 10 ng/dL (in the absence of primary aldosteronism, aldosterone secretion should be suppressed with saline infusion). In the 3-day sodium loading test (100 mmol NaCl per day), a 24-hour urine collection is obtained on the third day of the test to measure aldosterone, sodium, and potassium, and serum sodium and potassium are drawn simultaneously. Confirmation of aldosteronism is obtained when the urinary aldosterone is greater than 14 μg per 24 hours. In the latter test, it is important to demonstrate adequate salt loading; therefore, urinary sodium should be greater than 200 mEq per 24 hours. Choice of confirmatory testing depends on patient compliance, cost, laboratory availability, and local expertise.

Imaging

Once the diagnosis of aldosteronism is established biochemically, it is critical to differentiate unilateral adrenal adenoma (60% of cases) from bilateral hyperplasia of the zona glomerulosa (idiopathic aldosteronism, 40% of cases). In patients with an aldosterone-producing adenoma, unilateral adrenalectomy corrects the hypokalemia and decreases the blood pressure in 70% of surgically treated patients. However, surgery is of little value in patients with idiopathic aldosteronism, curing hypertension in only 19% of patients. Patients with a unilateral adenoma are usually younger and have more severe hypertension, lower renin levels, higher atrial natriuretic peptide levels, higher plasma aldosterone levels, and therefore more profound hypokalemia than patients with idiopathic aldosteronism. However, these findings alone cannot accurately differentiate patients with unilateral adenoma from those with idiopathic aldosteronism.

Endocrine Society Clinical Guidelines recommend adrenal computed tomography (CT) scan as the initial imaging modality to localize the source of aldosterone secretion. Magnetic resonance imaging (MRI) has not been shown to have an advantage over CT in determining the subtype of aldosteronism, while also being more costly and having less spatial resolution than CT. An aldosterone secreting adrenal adenoma may appear on CT as a small hypodense nodule with washout of contrast in the delayed phase at 15 minutes; however, what appears to be a microadenoma may in fact be adrenal hyperplasia or a nonfunctioning adrenal cortical nodule. Idiopathic adrenal hyperplasia (IAH) can also appear normal on CT. Rare aldosterone-producing adrenal cortical carcinomas are typically large (>4 cm) and have findings on imaging suspicious for malignancy. Young patients (<35 years old) with straightforward and unequivocal findings (markedly elevated aldosterone, spontaneous hypokalemia, and a unilateral lesion on CT consistent with an adenoma) can proceed straight to adrenalectomy without confirmatory testing.

In patients with no nodules, small nodules, bilateral nodules, or where the biochemical picture is not clear-cut, adrenal venous sampling (AVS) can be helpful in selecting the appropriate patients for surgical intervention and confirming the side of the functioning tumor. AVS is an invasive test that requires special expertise to perform. Furthermore, difficulty in cannulating the short, right adrenal vein can lead to results that are difficult or impossible to interpret. In experienced hands, complications of AVS, such as adrenal vein thrombosis, hemorrhage, adrenal infarction, and back pain, occur in approximately 2.5% of cases, and typically resolve with conservative management.

In a classic retrospective study performed at the Mayo Clinic, Young et al. selected 203 patients with primary aldosteronism and prior CT imaging for selective venous sampling. An infusion of 50 μg of cosyntropin per hour was initiated 30 minutes before catheterization of the adrenal veins by the percutaneous femoral approach. Continuous infusion of cosyntropin is utilized in order to minimize stress-induced fluctuation in aldosterone levels, maximize the gradient in cortisol between the adrenal vein and the inferior vena cava, and maximize the secretion of aldosterone from an adenoma. Venous samples were obtained from both adrenal veins (the left-sided sample was obtained from the inferior phrenic vein near the entrance of the adrenal vein) and the inferior vena cava below the level of the renal veins. Concentrations of cortisol and aldosterone were measured in order to confirm correct catheter placement. Sampling was considered successful if the plasma level of cortisol in the adrenal vein was greater than five times that of the inferior vena cava. Aldosterone concentrations of each adrenal vein were divided by the respective cortisol concentrations to correct for an asymmetric dilutional effect between the adrenal veins. Bilateral adrenal cannulation was successful in 194 of the 203 patients. Of these 194 patients, CT correctly identified unilateral or bilateral disease in 53%. On the basis of CT findings alone, 21.7% of patients may have been incorrectly bypassed as candidates for surgery, while 24.7% may have had an unnecessary adrenalectomy. In a systematic review examining 38 studies including 950 patients, all of whom had CT or MRI in addition to AVS, CT, or MRI was inaccurate in 37.8% of patients. This study concluded that treatment decisions based on CT or MRI would have led to an inappropriate adrenalectomy in 14.6% of patients, exclusion from adrenalectomy in 19.1% of patients, and

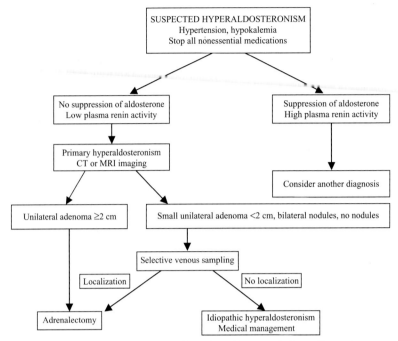

FIGURE 17.2 An algorithm for the evaluation of the patient with suspected primary aldosteronism.

adrenalectomy on the incorrect side in 3.9% of patients. In light of these results and others, AVS can contribute to treatment decisions in as many as 50% of patients. A cortisol-corrected aldosterone ratio from "high-side" to "low-side" of greater than 4:1 indicates unilateral aldosterone secretion, while a ratio of less than 3:1 (or elevated ratios on both sides and a similar response to ACTH stimulation) suggests bilateral aldosterone hypersecretion. Factors that have been shown to be associated with successful lateralization by AVS include a low plasma renin level, high plasma aldosterone: renin ratio, and a lesion on CT of at least 3 cm in size. The use of ACTH stimulation and confirmation of catheter positioning by an adrenal: peripheral cortisol level of >5 are associated with the highest rates of lateralization. Using these criteria, a sensitivity of 95% and a specificity of 100% has been reported.

AVS is technically unsuccessful in approximately 20% of cases, although this number improves with increasing radiologist experience. This is largely due to difficulty in cannulating the right adrenal vein, the rate of which can be as low as 30% in low-volume centers. Despite this, Pasternak et al. demonstrated that cannulation of the left adrenal vein only can still often predict laterality; patients with a left adrenal vein to inferior vena cava (LAV/IVC) aldosterone ratio of greater than 5.5 are likely to have left-sided hypersecretion, while those with a ratio less than 0.5 are likely to have right-sided hypersecretion (due to suppression of the contralateral gland).

Our current approach to the evaluation of patients suspected of having primary aldosteronism is shown in Figure 17.2.

Treatment

The treatment of primary aldosteronism depends on the etiology. Bilateral adrenal hyperplasia is usually best managed medically using the aldosterone antagonist spironolactone. Side effects of spironolactone, including gynecomastia, erectile dysfunction, menstrual disturbances, and muscle cramps can limit patient compliance. Most patients can achieve adequate control of their blood pressure with this medication alone or in conjunction with other antihypertensives.

When an aldosterone-producing adenoma or unilateral adrenal hyperplasia is diagnosed, the appropriate treatment remains surgical resection. Unilateral adrenal hyperplasia cannot be differentiated from an adenoma preoperatively; nevertheless, the treatment is the same. Preoperatively, patients should be placed on spironolactone and given potassium supplementation to help normalize fluid and electrolyte balance over a 3- to 4-week period.

Normalization of hypokalemia, aldosterone levels, and plasma aldosterone: renin ratio occurs in nearly 100% of patients with a unilateral aldosteronoma postoperatively. Up to 70% of patients will have resolution of hypertension after adrenalectomy, while 30% will require continued management with antihypertensive medications. Even those who require continued antihypertensive therapy will usually require fewer medications for adequate blood pressure control compared to preoperatively. Factors predictive of improvement or cure of hypertension after adrenalectomy include female gender, younger age, lower preoperative renin levels, shorter duration of hypertension (indicating that long-standing cardiovascular effects occur independent of aldosterone levels), and fewer antihypertensive medications preoperatively. Patients with primary aldosteronism have been shown to be at increased risk of cardiovascular and renal complications, including arrhythmias, myocardial infarction, stroke, chronic kidney disease, and death. Adrenalectomy decreases left ventricular diameter, volume, and workload, improves carotid artery stiffness, and reverses albuminuria. Adrenalectomy has also been shown to be more cost-effective than lifelong medical therapy in patients with primary aldosteronism amenable to surgical resection.

Since nearly all patients with aldosteronomas have relatively small tumors which are universally benign, they are usually excellent candidates for a minimally invasive approach. Surgical resection can be performed either through a transabdominal laparoscopic or a retroperitoneoscopic approach. While the standard surgical approach for patients with an aldosteronoma is unilateral adrenalectomy, adrenal-sparing surgery (partial adrenalectomy) has been applied in selected patients with good results. Approximately 2% or less of adrenal cortical carcinomas cause isolated aldosteronism. In the very rare situation of a patient presenting with aldosteronism and a large adrenal mass, an open anterior approach should be used to facilitate complete resection (see the section on adrenal cortical carcinoma).

Cortisol-Producing Adrenal Adenoma

Cushing syndrome was first described by Harvey W. Cushing in 1932 and refers to a state of hypercortisolism that can result from several different pathologic processes (Table 17.1). Cortisol regulation involves feedback loops through the pituitary gland and hypothalamus. The most common cause of Cushing syndrome is exogenous steroid administration. After exclusion of patients taking exogenous steroids, approximately 70% of the remaining cases of hypercortisolism are secondary to hypersecretion of adrenocorticotropic hormone (ACTH) from the pituitary gland, a condition known as Cushing disease. Cushing disease is usually caused by a small pituitary adenoma (<1 cm). Ectopic secretion of ACTH, referred to as ectopic ACTH syndrome, is the cause of approximately 15% of cases of Cushing syndrome. Ectopic ACTH syndrome is caused by malignant tumors in 80% of cases. Carcinoma of the lung accounts for nearly three-quarters of cases, with the remaining cases being caused by carcinoma of the pancreas, carcinoid tumors, medullary thyroid cancer, pheochromocytoma, and other neuroendocrine tumors. Ectopic secretion of corticotropin-releasing factor is exceedingly rare but has been reported in a few cases.

Hypersecretion of cortisol from the adrenal glands (ACTH-independent) accounts for approximately 10% to 20% of cases of Cushing syndrome. The underlying cause is an adrenal adenoma 50% to 60% of the time and adrenal cortical carcinoma 20% to 25% of the time. Bilateral adrenal hyperplasia accounts for the remaining 20% to 30% of cases.

Clinical Manifestations

Weight gain is the most common feature of hypercortisolism and occurs predominantly in the truncal area. This centripetal obesity, combined with muscle wasting in the extremities, fat deposition in the head and neck region ("moon facies"), and dorsal kyphosis ("buffalo hump") gives the patient a characteristic body habitus. Abdominal striae, hypertension, hyperglycemia, depression, bruising, osteoporosis and menstrual

TABLE 17.1 Common Causes of Cushing Syndrome

Exogenous steroids
Cushing disease (due to pituitary adenoma)
Adrenal tumors
Adrenal cortical adenoma
Adrenal cortical carcinoma
Primary adrenal cortical hyperplasia
Ectopic adrenocorticotropin syndrome
Ectopic corticotropin-releasing factor syndrome

irregularities can also occur. Children with Cushing syndrome have weight gain in association with decreased linear growth. Several studies have demonstrated that 2% to 3% of patients with poorly controlled diabetes mellitus have confirmed Cushing syndrome, while 5.8% of patients seen in endocrinology clinics for diabetes, hypertension, or polycystic ovarian syndrome are eventually shown to have Cushing syndrome. Similarly, approximately 10% of patients with osteoporosis and a vertebral fracture were found to have Cushing syndrome. In some patients with Cushing syndrome due to an adrenal cortical tumor, these signs may be subtle or even absent altogether ("mild autonomous cortisol excess," discussed later in this section). Adrenal cortical carcinomas can produce cortisol but often also produce androgens, resulting in virilization and hirsutism.

Diagnosis

Patients with Cushing syndrome have been shown to have an increased risk of cardiovascular and infectious complications, thus stressing the importance of early diagnosis and treatment.

The evaluation for Cushing syndrome should be aimed at establishing the diagnosis first and then determining the etiology. To establish the diagnosis, a state of hypercortisolism must be documented. Endocrine Society Clinical Practice Guidelines currently recommend first taking a thorough medication history, followed by testing of any patient with unusual features for age or multiple and progressive features (described above), in children with decreasing height and increasing weight, and in patients with an incidentally discovered adrenal mass.

The adult adrenal glands secrete on average 10 to 30 mg of cortisol each day. The secretion follows a diurnal variation: cortisol levels tend to be high early in the morning and low in the evening. The most sensitive initial screening test for hypercortisolism in patients with an adrenal mass is an overnight 1-mg dexamethasone suppression test (described below). Documentation of lack of cortisol suppression following 1 mg of dexamethasone should be followed by measurement of 24-hour urinary-free (unmetabolized) cortisol; the normal level is generally below 80 µg/day. In addition, to determine the etiology of an elevated cortisol level, plasma ACTH levels should be checked. Secretion of ACTH also follows a diurnal variation, preceding that of cortisol by 1 to 2 hours. Suppressed levels of ACTH are seen in patients with functioning adrenal adenomas, adrenal cortical carcinomas, or autonomously functioning adrenal hyperplasia. In such cases, autonomous secretion of cortisol by the pathologic process within the adrenal gland inhibits pituitary ACTH release ("ACTH-independent Cushing syndrome"). Patients with Cushing disease (i.e., a pituitary adenoma-secreting ACTH) usually have plasma ACTH levels that are elevated or within the upper limits of normal ("ACTH-dependent Cushing syndrome"). When there is an ectopic source of ACTH secretion, for example, with a metastatic tumor process, the plasma ACTH level is usually markedly increased.

The most sensitive standard method for detecting hypercortisolism is the overnight 1-mg dexamethasone suppression test. One milligram of dexamethasone is taken orally at 10:00 or 11:00 PM. The vast majority of normal individuals will suppress their cortisol level to <5 µg/dL at 8:00 AM the following morning. Failure to suppress the 8:00 AM cortisol level to less <5 µg/dL is consistent with hypercortisolism. This test has a false-negative rate of only 3% but unfortunately a false-positive rate of up to 30%. While a normal overnight dexamethasone suppression test excludes clinically significant hypercortisolism, an abnormal test result does not necessarily establish the presence of hypercortisolism but does require further investigation. Many experts currently propose further testing even in patients with serum cortisol values between 1.8 and 5 µg/dL to increase the detection of subclinical hypercortisolism (see below). Naturally, when lower cutoffs are used, specificity decreases, yielding more false positives. Since false-positive results are common, patients with elevated cortisol levels following overnight testing should undergo further evaluation by obtaining 8 AM cortisol and ACTH levels along with 24-hour urine collection for urinary-free cortisol. The 24-hour urinary-free cortisol is somewhat less sensitive than overnight dexamethasone suppression but more specific. In patients who have obvious signs or symptoms of hypercortisolism, a timed urinary collection should be obtained for cortisol determination. It is recommended that patients submit at least two urine collections and the first morning void should be discarded. Again, the normal level of urinary-free cortisol is <80 µg/day. This test is not as accurate in patients with renal failure and those in the second and third trimesters of pregnancy. Importantly, dehydroepiandrosterone sulfate levels will typically be low in patients with ACTH suppression from autonomous cortisol secretion by an adrenal mass.

In equivocal cases, a formal 2-day low-dose dexamethasone test may be performed to detect the presence of cortisol overproduction by an adrenal tumor. A dose of 0.5 mg of dexamethasone is administered every 6 hours for 2 days with pre- and postdexamethasone 24-hour urinary-free cortisol levels. Alternatively, individuals with failure of suppression after the 1-mg overnight dexamethasone test may be subjected to a higher

Surgical Stress	Examples	Hydrocortisone Equivalent (mg)	Duration (days)
Minor	Inguinal herniorrhaphy	25	1
Moderate	Open cholecystectomy Lower-extremity revascularization Segmental colon resection Total joint replacement Abdominal hysterectomy	50–75	1–2
Major	Pancreaticoduodenectomy Esophagogastrectomy Total proctocolectomy Cardiac surgery with cardiopulmonary bypass	100–150	2–3

TABLE 17.2 Recommendations for Perioperative Glucocorticoid Coverage

dose (3 or 8 mg overnight suppression). Patients with true autonomous secretion of cortisol should continue to exhibit nonsuppression with these higher doses of dexamethasone.

In patients who are found to have ACTH-independent Cushing syndrome, CT or MRI of the adrenal gland should be performed to localize the source of hypercortisolism. In patients with ACTH-dependent Cushing syndrome (ACTH levels not suppressed with dexamethasone), chest CT and MRI can be performed, followed by bilateral petrosal sinus sampling. CT or MRI of the sella turcica can also be used prior to surgical resection of a pituitary tumor.

Treatment

The appropriate management of Cushing syndrome depends on the underlying etiology. Patients with Cushing disease should undergo transsphenoidal hypophysectomy of the pituitary adenoma when it is believed to be resectable. Pituitary irradiation may also be used when resection is not curative, or otherwise judged not to be indicated. Patients with ectopic ACTH syndrome should have the underlying malignant condition identified and treated. Bilateral adrenalectomy is only occasionally indicated for patients with Cushing syndrome and should be reserved for those who fail to respond to standard management, including medical therapy and transsphenoidal hypophysectomy, in those with an unresectable primary or metastatic cancer causing ectopic ACTH production, and in those who experience end-organ injury from the consequences of overt hypercortisolism. Data from our institution demonstrate that in patients with ACTH-dependent hypercortisolism (either from a pituitary lesion or ectopic secretion) resistant to other treatment options, bilateral adrenalectomy can improve metabolic disturbances and minimize adverse effects related to medical therapies. However, careful patient selection is essential, as these patients typically have poor performance status prior to surgery and limited overall survival. Patients with autonomously functioning bilateral adrenal hyperplasia usually require bilateral total adrenalectomy. If bilateral adrenalectomy is performed, patients require not only perioperative steroid coverage (Tables 17.2 and 17.3) but also lifelong replacement of both glucocorticoids and mineralocorticoids. Bilateral adrenalectomy can be performed laparoscopically, retroperitoneoscopically, via an open posterior retroperitoneal approach, or via open laparotomy. Our current preferred approach for the majority

TABLE 17.3 Comparison of Common Steroid Preparations

Steroid	Half-Life (hours)	Glucocorticoid Activity (Relative to Cortisol)	Mineralocorticoid Activity (Relative to Cortisol)
Cortisol	8–12	1	1
Cortisone	8–12	0.8	0.8
Prednisone	12–36	4	0.25
Prednisolone	12–36	4	0.25
Methylprednisolone	12–36	5	0
Triamcinolone	12–36	5	0
Betamethasone	36–72	25	0
Dexamethasone	36–72	30–40	0

of these patients is via a minimally invasive retroperitoneoscopic approach when body habitus and adrenal size will permit.

Patients with a cortisol-producing neoplasm of the adrenal gland, whether the tumor represents an adenoma or a carcinoma, should undergo resection of the involved adrenal gland. Although almost all adenomas can be resected, adrenal cortical carcinomas that secrete cortisol are resectable in only 25% to 35% of patients. Combination chemotherapy, as well as adrenolytic treatment with mitotane, has demonstrated activity in patients with unresectable or metastatic adrenal cortical carcinoma, but neither treatment is considered curative. Symptoms related to hypercortisolism in patients with metastatic or unresectable functioning tumors can sometimes be minimized with a variety of agents that are toxic to adrenal tissue or interfere with steroid hormone synthesis, including mitotane as well as aminoglutethimide, metyrapone, or ketoconazole.

Mild Autonomous Cortisol Excess

Mild autonomous cortisol excess, variously called "mild autonomous cortisol syndrome," "subclinical Cushing syndrome," or "subclinical autonomous glucocorticoid hypersecretion," is a state of hypercortisolism without the associated overt clinical findings or phenotype of Cushing syndrome. Mild autonomous cortisol excess may occur in up to 20% of patients with apparently incidental adrenal tumors. Although these patients do not have overt signs and symptoms of Cushing syndrome, further questioning often elucidates a history of hypertension, weight gain, and hyperlipidemia. There are currently no "gold standard" criteria to diagnose mild autonomous cortisol excess, but the best screening test to identify the possible presence of the condition remains an overnight 1-mg dexamethasone suppression test. A morning serum cortisol level of <1.8 µg/dL indicates appropriate suppression and excludes hypercortisolism, while a level above that indicates the possible presence of mild autonomous cortisol excess in patients without typical signs and symptoms. Late-night salivary cortisol testing is an alternative for patients suspected of having mild autonomous cortisol excess, and as a confirmatory test is currently more popular than the 48-hour dexamethasone test. Changes in serum cortisol are mirrored in salivary cortisol levels within minutes. This test is easy to perform, noninvasive, and has been shown to be particularly useful in children with suspected Cushing syndrome. In this test, patients are asked to give a saliva sample on two separate evenings between 11:00 PM and midnight. Saliva is collected via either passive drooling into a tube or having the patient chew on a cotton pledget for 1 to 2 minutes. Patients without autonomous cortisol excess should exhibit a normal circadian variation in cortisol secretion, with a salivary cortisol level of less than 145 ng/dL at midnight, while patients with autonomous, abnormal cortisol secretion should have higher salivary levels.

General recommendations are for adrenalectomy in young patients with a unilateral adrenal nodule with imaging characteristics consistent with an adrenal adenoma and documented or suspected mild autonomous cortisol excess, particularly in the presence of suggestive metabolic disturbances (hypertension, hyperlipidemia, obesity, diabetes, osteoporosis). Several studies have demonstrated trends toward improvement and/or resolution of these comorbidities after surgical resection, in addition to an improvement in reported quality of life. Importantly, patients with mild autonomous cortisol excess may require peri- and postoperative glucocorticoid replacement (Tables 17.2 and 17.3), as the ACTH suppression secondary to the hypercortisolism can result in atrophy of the contralateral adrenal gland, often resulting in symptoms of adrenal insufficiency upon removal of the affected gland. Steroids, if required postoperatively, can typically be tapered within 6 to 12 months postoperatively.

Pheochromocytoma

Pheochromocytomas represent a potentially curable form of endocrine hypertension that, if untreated, places patients at high risk for morbidity and mortality, particularly during surgery and pregnancy. Pheochromocytomas are neuroectodermal tumors that arise from the chromaffin cells of the adrenal medulla. Ten percent of neuroectodermal chromaffin-cell tumors are in an extra-adrenal site (carotid bulb, mediastinum, abdomen, pelvis, urinary bladder, renal hilum, and organ of Zuckerkandl [located between the inferior mesenteric artery and aortic bifurcation]) and are called paragangliomas. The estimated incidence of pheochromocytoma and paraganglioma is between 0.005% and 0.1% of the general population and between 0.1% and 0.6% of the adult hypertensive population. Approximately 10% of adrenal pheochromocytomas are bilateral, with some patients presenting with multiple tumors. Pheochromocytomas represent 5% of incidentally discovered adrenal masses.

Histologic evidence of malignancy can be demonstrated in 2% to 13% of pheochromocytomas and 2.4% to 50% of paragangliomas. Invasion of adjacent organs and/or the presence of metastatic disease are the defining features of malignancy, which can be difficult or impossible to distinguish histologically. Metastatic disease

Syndrome	Gene	Features	Frequency of Pheo/PGL	Malignant Potential
NF1	*NF1*	Von Recklinghausen disease: peripheral nervous system tumors, gastrointestinal stromal tumors, malignant gliomas, breast cancer, leukemia	1–14%	1–9%
VHL	*VHL*	Von Hippel–Lindau disease: retinal and cerebellar hemangioblastoma, renal cell carcinoma, pheo/PGL (multiple, bilateral), pancreatic neuroendocrine tumors	20%	1–9%
MENIIA/B	*RET*	MENIIA: medullary thyroid carcinoma, pheochromocytoma (bilateral), hyperparathyroidism MENIIB: medullary thyroid carcinoma, pheochromocytoma (bilateral), mucosal neuromas	50%	<1%
PGL1	*SDHD*	Multiple pheo and PGL (particularly head and neck), nonmedullary thyroid carcinoma, gastrointestinal stromal tumors	>50%	1–9%
PGL2	*SDHAF2*	Pheo and PGL	1–9%	Not reported
PGL3	*SDHC*	Pheo and PGL (particularly head and neck), nonmedullary thyroid carcinoma, gastrointestinal stromal tumors	1–9%	Not reported
PGL4	*SDHB*	Solitary pheo and PGL, renal cell carcinoma, nonmedullary thyroid carcinoma, gastrointestinal stromal tumors	25–50%	25–50%
PGL5	*SDHA*	Pituitary adenoma, GIST, renal cell carcinoma	25–50%	1–12%
No name	*MAX*	Renal cell carcinoma	>50%	1–9%
No name	*TMEM127*	Not reported	>50%	10–24%

TABLE 17.4 Major Genetic Alterations Associated with Pheochromocytoma/Paraganglioma

Pheo, pheochromocytoma; PGL, paraganglioma.

most commonly occurs in the bones, liver, lungs, kidneys, and lymph nodes. Local recurrence after surgical resection occurs in 6.5% to 16.5% of patients. Metastatic disease, if it occurs, is most commonly present at diagnosis, but has been documented to occur as late as 40 years after the original diagnosis. The 8th Edition of the American Joint Committee on Cancer Staging Manual is the first to include staging for pheochromocytomas and paragangliomas (Adrenal—Neuroendocrine Tumors).

Genetics
Historically, familial pheochromocytomas have been estimated to account for approximately 10% of cases ("the 10% rule"); however, recent data suggest that 40% or more of unselected cases of apparently sporadic pheochromocytomas are in fact hereditary. Genetic alterations associated with pheochromocytoma are listed in Table 17.4.

Multiple endocrine neoplasia (MEN) type IIA and IIB are associated with pheochromocytomas. MEN IIA is characterized by medullary thyroid carcinoma (MTC), pheochromocytoma, and hyperparathyroidism; up to one-half of patients with MEN IIA will develop a clinically significant pheochromocytoma. It is recognized that many patients with MEN IIA will develop small, subclinical pheochromocytomas or bilateral adrenal medullary hyperplasia. Mutations in codon 634 (C634) of exon 11 of the RET proto-oncogene are particularly associated with this feature. The penetrance of pheochromocytoma (either unilateral or bilateral) in patients with C634 mutations in MEN IIA is nearly 100%, indicating that MEN IIA patients with an RET C634 mutation should be screened for pheochromocytoma early and often. Fortunately, the risk of malignant pheochromocytoma in these patients is very low. The risk for inherited pheochromocytoma in patients with MEN I is very low but has been observed (<1% of patients with MEN I).

Neuroectodermal dysplasias consisting of neurofibromatosis, tuberous sclerosis, Sturge–Weber syndrome, and von Hippel–Lindau disease are also associated with pheochromocytomas. The risk for pheochromocytoma in neurofibromatosis type 1 is low. Pheochromocytoma can also occur in hereditary paraganglioma syndromes (mutations in succinate dehydrogenase *SDHD*, *SDHB*, *SDHC*, and *SDH5* genes), with those tumors with mutations in subunit B (SDHB) having a particularly high risk of malignancy. Hereditary paraganglioma syndromes can predispose to both PGL and pheochromocytomas. Patients with familial pheochromocytoma/PGL syndromes require follow-up and periodic screening, especially before any planned surgical procedure.

The tumor suppressor genes nm23-H1, TIMP-4, BRMS-1, TXNIP, CRSP-3, and E-Cad, have been demonstrated to be downregulated in malignant pheochromocytomas. Ki-67, a nuclear antigen used as a marker of proliferation in a variety of tumors, has been examined in pheochromocytoma. A Ki-67 index of greater than 3% can help distinguish between benign and malignant pheochromocytomas and may predict malignant potential.

As mentioned above, recent and evolving data suggest that up to 40% or more of cases of pheochromocytomas or paragangliomas are hereditary. A hereditary syndrome should be suspected when patients are found to have a pheochromocytoma at a young age, bilateral or recurrent disease, or extra-adrenal disease. Several authors recommend genetic screening, or at least referral to a trained genetic counselor, for all patients with pheochromocytoma. Patients who have a family history of pheochromocytoma or paraganglioma or an associated clinical syndrome based on evaluation by a genetic counselor are found to have a mutation in up to 90% of cases. Priority for genetic testing should be based on any familial or syndromic features, particularly RET, VHL, NF-1, and SDH genes. In the case of malignant disease, SDHB testing should be performed. For bilateral tumors, VHL and RET genes should be tested first, and in patients with extra-adrenal disease, testing for SDHD and SDHB genes should be performed. Once a mutation is found, no further testing is recommended, as the chance of two genetic mutations occurring is uncommon. Once a mutation is identified, family members should be tested. High-risk patients in whom a genetic mutation is suspected but not identified should still be followed regularly with annual physical examination, biochemical testing, and imaging; repeat genetic testing can be considered as technologies improve and new mutations are identified.

Clinical Manifestations

Hypertension, sustained or paroxysmal, is the most common clinical presentation of pheochromocytoma. Paroxysmal elevations in blood pressure can vary markedly in frequency and duration and can be initiated by a variety of events, including heavy physical exertion and eating foods high in tyramine (e.g., chocolate, cheese, red wine). Other common symptoms include excessive sweating, palpitations, arrhythmias, tremulousness, anxiety, headache, chest pain, nausea, and vomiting. Half of patients with pheochromocytomas may have impaired glucose tolerance and may have symptoms of diabetes mellitus, including polydipsia or polyuria. These signs and symptoms are secondary to the excess catecholamine secretion by the tumors and resolve with tumor resection. Patients with functioning tumors are infrequently asymptomatic (<10% of patients); an exception is patients with hereditary pheochromocytomas. Nonfunctioning adrenal pheochromocytomas are rare; extra-adrenal paragangliomas, however, may be nonfunctioning. Patients with incidentally discovered pheochromocytoma tend to have higher rates of nonspecific symptoms (abdominal and back pain), lower rates of "classic" pheochromocytoma symptoms, are older than symptomatic patients, and are less likely to have an associated genetic syndrome.

Diagnosis

The diagnosis of pheochromocytoma is made by documenting excess secretion of catecholamines. Increased levels of catecholamines or their metabolites are seen in more than 90% of patients with pheochromocytoma. The adrenal glands and the organ of Zuckerkandl produce the enzyme phenylethanolamine-*N*-methyltransferase, which converts norepinephrine to epinephrine. Pheochromocytomas that arise elsewhere do not contain this enzyme and thus do not produce much, if any, epinephrine. As a result, extra-adrenal pheochromocytomas (paragangliomas) secrete predominantly dopamine and norepinephrine.

Plasma-free metanephrine determination is a very sensitive screen for the presence of catecholamine elevation and is more convenient than timed urine collection. Plasma normetanephrines have also been shown to correlate with a diagnosis of pheochromocytoma. Twenty-four-hour urine collection for free catecholamine levels (dopamine, epinephrine, and norepinephrine) and their metabolites (normetanephrine, metanephrine, vanillylmandelic acid) was the original test of choice; it can still be useful in confirming suspected catecholamine elevation identified by plasma screen. A scoring system has been proposed by Carr et al., which includes elevated levels of normetanephrine (>1.7 times greater than normal) and metanephrine (>1.34 times greater than normal), age less than 50 years, and tumor size larger than 3.3 cm on imaging; a score of 4 or higher has a specificity and positive predictive value of 100% in diagnosing pheochromocytoma. Patients with incidentally discovered pheochromocytoma have lower values in all markers, both plasma and urine. Patients with malignant pheochromocytoma tend to have significantly increased levels of dopamine in their 24-hour urine collection. Clinicians should be aware of common agents and medications that can cause false-positive results, including caffeine, nicotine, tricyclic antidepressants, monoamine oxidase inhibitors, phenoxybenzamine, calcium channel blockers, levodopa, alpha-methyldopa, ephedrine, and acetaminophen.

Once the diagnosis of pheochromocytoma is made, localization studies can be carried out. A review of preoperative imaging in a large series of histologically confirmed pheochromocytomas found that MRI was the most sensitive modality (98%), followed by CT imaging (89%) and ^{131}I-metaiodobenzylguanidine (MIBG) scanning (81%). High-quality CT can detect up to 95% of adrenal masses larger than 6 to 8 mm and is usually the initial imaging study of choice; it is rare for a clinically significant primary pheochromocytoma to not be imaged by CT. On CT, a pheochromocytoma will typically be distinguished from a cortical adenoma in part by having a greater overall tissue density (precontrast Hounsfield units of >10). MRI may be useful in selected cases because the T2-weighted images can identify chromaffin tissue; the T2-weighted adrenal mass-to-liver ratio of pheochromocytomas or paragangliomas is usually more than 3. In contrast, MRI findings consistent with an adrenal adenoma are a high T1 and low T2 signals relative to the liver and spleen. This ratio is also higher than that typical of adrenal cortical carcinomas and metastases to the adrenal gland.

Functional imaging studies including MIBG scan, ^{18}F-Fluorodeoxyglucose (^{18}F-FDG) positron emission tomography (FDG PET), and ^{68}Ga-DOTATATE positron emission tomography (DOTATATE PET) are primarily helpful in localizing extra-adrenal, metastatic, or bilateral pheochromocytomas. These functional imaging studies are useful for patients with biochemical evidence of pheochromocytoma whose tumors cannot be localized by CT or MRI and in the follow-up evaluation of patients with suspected or documented recurrent or metastatic disease. Timmers et al. found that FDG PET was equally effective in detecting nonmetastatic pheochromocytomas and paragangliomas when compared to MIBG but was more sensitive in detecting metastatic disease. The authors also found that FDG PET was superior in localizing bone metastases when compared to both CT and MRI. Tumors with SDHB mutations, which are particularly prone to malignancy and metastases, are frequently identified on FDG PET. ^{68}Ga-DOTATATE PET targets somatostatin receptors, which are expressed in high levels on pheochromocytomas and paragangliomas, and has a higher lesion-to-background contrast than FDG PET. ^{68}Ga-DOTATATE PET and FDG PET have become the imaging modalities of choice for staging of patients with recurrent or metastatic pheochromocytoma or paraganglioma.

There are two histopathology-defined scores that attempt to separate benign and malignant tumors, the Pheochromocytoma of the Adrenal Gland Scaled Score (PASS) and the Grading System for Adrenal Pheochromocytoma and Paraganglioma (GAPP). PASS includes 12 histopathologic characteristics, including large nests of diffuse growth, necrosis, cellularity, spindling, mitotic figures, vascular and capsular invasion, and nuclear pleomorphism and hyperchromasia. Components of the PASS were more common in larger tumors and patients with higher levels of metanephrines and normetanephrines. A PASS greater than 4 (and especially greater than 6), has been associated with malignancy and suggests a patient should be followed closely for recurrence. The criteria included in GAPP are histologic pattern, cellularity, comedo-type necrosis, capsular/vascular invasion, Ki67 index, and catecholamine type. Higher GAPP scores correlate with increased risk of metastasis.

Treatment

After diagnosis and localization of the pheochromocytoma, careful preoperative preparation is required to prevent a cardiovascular crisis during surgery caused by excess catecholamine secretion. The focus of preoperative preparation is adequate alpha-adrenergic blockade and restoration of fluid and electrolyte balance. The practice of alpha blockade originated in 1956, when Priestly and colleagues resected 51 pheochromocytomas using intraoperative alpha blockade without mortality. Alpha blockade is typically achieved with either the nonselective alpha-adrenergic blocking agent phenoxybenzamine or the selective alpha-adrenergic blocking agent doxazosin. Calcium channel blockade may be added in cases of resistant hypertension. Beta blockade following alpha blockade may help prevent tachycardia and other arrhythmias. Beta blockade should not be instituted unless alpha blockade has been established; otherwise, the beta blocker will inhibit epinephrine-induced vasodilation, leading to more significant hypertension and left heart strain. In addition to requiring pharmacologic preparation, patients with pheochromocytoma require correction of volume depletion as well as any concurrent electrolyte imbalances. We encourage patients to salt-load the week prior to operation. While not routinely recommended, some experienced clinical teams have had success with selectively avoiding preoperative alpha blockade in good-risk patients, with excellent outcomes and the suggestion of fewer associated side effects, less postoperative hypotension, and quicker postoperative recovery.

The perioperative management of patients with pheochromocytoma can be challenging but is generally safely accomplished in experienced centers. Rarely is alpha-adrenergic blockade complete prior to surgical resection. The anesthesiologist should be prepared to treat a hypertensive crisis with sodium nitroprusside, nitroglycerine, or nicardipine, while tachyarrhythmias should be treated with either a beta blocker or anti-arrhythmics. Hypotension should first be treated with volume expansion, followed by vasopressor agents such as norepinephrine, phenylephrine, and vasopressin. Magnesium results in vasodilatation and inhibits catecholamine release from the adrenal medulla while blocking catecholamine receptors. Lower preoperative dose of phenoxybenzamine or preoperative use of selective alpha blockade, larger tumors, open procedures, and intraoperative use of vasopressin are associated with increased intraoperative hemodynamic instability. Commonly used preoperative and perioperative medications are listed in Table 17.5.

TABLE 7.5 Common Medications Used in the Management of Pheochromocytoma

Medication	Standard Dosage	Contraindication	Main Drug Interaction	Main Side Effects	Comments
Phenoxybenzamine (nonselective α-blocker)	10 mg BID-TID	Conditions compromised by hypotension	Reports of hypertensive episodes when used in combinations with β-blockers	Orthostatic hypotension, nasal stuffiness, tachycardia, hypoglycemia, miosis, sexual dysfunction, somnolence	May be increased to 20–40 mg/day to total dose of 1–2 mg/kg/day BID-TID; start 10–14 days before surgery
Doxazocin (selective α1-blocker)	5 mg daily	Hypersensitivity to product or quinazolines	β-blockers, verapamil	Hypotension, tachycardia, dizziness	Less expensive, more readily available than phenoxybenazmine
Metyrosine (tyrosine hydroxylase inhibitor)	250 mg TID-QID, with doses titrated by 250–500 mg to maximum of 1.5–4 g/d	Hypersensitivity to metyrosine products	Minimal	Crystalluria, extrapyramidal effects, diarrhea, anxiety, drowsiness, sedation, depression, nightmares. Long-term use can result in heart failure.	Best used for epinephrine-only secreting tumors, or in patients with contraindications to β-blockade. Best to limit use to the perioperative period due to cardiac toxicity. Given as a half dose the morning of surgery.
Propranolol (nonselective β-blocker)	10–40 mg BID-TID	Lack of α-blockade, second- or third-degree atrioventricular block, congestive heart failure, myocarditis, hypersensitivity, asthma	Can interact with other cardiac medications, antidiabetic medications, cimetidine, fentanyl, rifampin, theophylline	Bradycardia, bronchospasm, depression, diarrhea	Should only be used to treat tachyarrhythmias once α-blockade complete
Nicardipine (calcium channel blocker)	20 mg TID or 30 mg BID	Aortic stenosis, angina, congestive heart failure	β-blockers	Heart block/bradycardia, hypotension, dizziness, edema, drowsiness	Used in patients with inadequate blood pressure control with α-blockade or in those who cannot tolerate α-blockade, also decreases coronary vasospasm
Nitroprusside (direct vasodilator)	2–4 µg/kg/min	Hypersensitivity, anemia, optic atrophy, head trauma, tobacco amblyopia	Sildenafil (a phosphodiesterase inhibitor, which potentiates hypotensive effects)	Hypotension, headache, methemoglobinemia, cyanide toxicity	Dilute in D5W only. With prolonged infusion (>24 hours), patients can develop cyanide toxicity. Dose reduced in patients with liver or renal impairment
Esmolol (β-blocker)	Titrate to effect (12–200 µg/kg/min)	Hypersensitivity, bradycardia, atrioventricular block, and cardiogenic shock	Fentanyl, cardiac medications	Hypotension, bradycardia	Short duration of action (half-life 10 minutes)
Norepinephrine (α-agonist)	4–16 µg/min as an infusion	Hypovolemia	Tricyclic antidepressants, cardiac medications	Hypertension, decreased visceral perfusion, anxiety, nausea, vomiting, urinary retention, cardiac arrhythmias	Avoid subcutaneous extravasation
Epinephrine (β-agonist)	0.1–0.2 mg/kg	Hypersensitivity, dilated cardiomyopathy, coronary artery disease, narrow-angle glaucoma, hypovolemic shock, intra-arterial injection, labor	Cardiac medications, halothane, tricyclic antidepressants	Hypertension, nausea, vomiting, headache, cardiac arrhythmias, tachycardia	Limited utility

If preoperative imaging suggests a modestly sized, benign-appearing unilateral pheochromocytoma with a radiographically normal contralateral gland, we currently prefer a unilateral laparoscopic or posterior retroperitoneoscopic approach. A minimally invasive approach is also appropriate for patients with MEN II or von Hippel–Lindau disease with a small, unilateral pheochromocytoma less than approximately 6 cm in size. For patients with MEN II or von Hippel–Lindau disease with bilateral disease, a bilateral minimally invasive approach may also be appropriate. Cortical-sparing adrenalectomy, either open or laparoscopic, has been performed successfully in patients with MEN II or von Hippel–Lindau disease with bilateral pheochromocytomas, avoiding chronic steroid hormone replacement and the risk of addisonian crisis in most patients. In general, at least one-third of one adrenal gland must be preserved with its blood supply in order to reliably prevent adrenal insufficiency. For tumors greater than 6 cm in size open adrenalectomy is generally preferred, although experienced surgeons may apply an individualized approach. Obesity and concern for malignancy based on imaging are relative contraindications to a minimally invasive procedure. Paragangliomas may also be approached in a minimally invasive fashion from either a retroperitoneoscopic approach or an anterior approach, depending on the details of the tumor and patient anatomy and surgeon experience and preference. Whatever the approach, the surgeon should manipulate the tumor as little as possible and ligate the tumor's venous outflow via the adrenal vein as early in the procedure as practical (while recognizing that early division of the vein without concomitant division of arterial inflow may increase venous congestion of the tumor and back-bleeding).

Postoperatively, patients should be monitored carefully at least overnight so that they can be observed for arrhythmias, as well as hypotension secondary to compensatory vasodilation. Hypoglycemia may result from decreased glucose production from a drop in circulating catecholamines. Hypertension may persist postoperatively in 25% of patients, especially in those with sustained hypertension preoperatively.

While follow-up after resection of pheochromocytoma or paraganglioma has not been completely standardized, Press et al. recommend measurement of plasma-free metanephrines at 1, 6, and 12 months postoperatively, then annually thereafter, in addition to yearly cross-sectional imaging. Biochemical testing should include a plasma-free metanephrine level or timed urine collection for catecholamine determination to exclude recurrence. If recurrence is suspected based on biochemical evaluation, localizing studies should be performed as discussed above, and resection of recurrent tumor is indicated when feasible.

The most common sites of metastases from malignant pheochromocytoma are bone, liver, and lungs, and less commonly, regional lymph nodes. Patients with known or suspected malignant pheochromocytoma should be staged with standard imaging studies as well as MIBG scanning. Therapy should be individualized based upon the extent of disease. Resection of malignant pheochromocytoma, including resection of metastases, may be considered in good-risk individuals if the metastases are limited in extent. Surgical debulking can be used to achieve biochemical control, improve response to systemic therapies with diminished tumor burden, and palliate symptoms. However, when extra-abdominal disease is present, a sustained biochemical response is unlikely after resection, stressing the importance of patient selection and determination of treatment goals preoperatively. Palliative therapy may include treatment with alpha-methyltyrosine, which inhibits catecholamine synthesis, as well as alpha- and beta-blockades. Somatostatin analogs have also been used for symptomatic relief. The most commonly used systemic chemotherapy regimen for pheochromocytoma is the combination of cyclophosphamide, vincristine, and dacarbazine. The overall response rate with this regimen is approximately 37%. Radiation therapy has been effective only for symptomatic relief of bony metastases. Targeted radionuclide therapy with modern high specific activity, carrier-free ^{131}I-MIBG is currently recommended as first-line treatment for patients with metastatic pheochromocytoma/paraganglioma and MIBG-avid slowly growing tumors. Fifty percent of patients with metastatic pheochromocytoma/paraganglioma have tumors that concentrate MIBG and can potentially benefit from this therapy. The newer formulation has a much higher reported overall response rate (92%) than the older, less specific agent (30% to 40%), while also avoiding cardiovascular toxicity, although high-dose regimens may result in bone marrow suppression. Other alternative options for the treatment of metastatic disease include arterial embolization, chemoembolization, cryoablation, and radiofrequency ablation. The 5-year survival rate for patients with malignant pheochromocytoma is approximately 43%, with no significant difference in survival between adrenal and extra-adrenal pheochromocytomas. Patients with benign pheochromocytoma have a 97% 5-year survival rate.

Since the molecular pathogenesis of malignant pheochromocytoma/paraganglioma importantly includes hypoxia-inducible factors and angiogenesis, there has been significant interest in the potential utility of tyrosine kinase inhibitors including sunitinib, carbozantanib, and lenvatinib. The results of a recent phase 2 trial of sunitinib in patients with progressive pheochromocytoma/paraganglioma found a low overall response rate (13%), with all objective responses occurring in patients with germline *RET* or *SDH* mutations, suggesting that molecularly defined subgroups of patients with pheochromocytoma/paraganglioma are more likely to benefit from TKI therapy. Evaluation of axitinib and cabozantanib are ongoing (NCT03839498, NCT02302833).

Since molecularly defined cluster-1 pheochromocytomas/paragangliomas, including SDH- and VHL-associated tumors demonstrate an immunosuppressive molecular phenotype, investigators have been interested in the potential role of immune checkpoint inhibitors in these patients. A trial of pembrolizumab that includes patients with metastatic pheochromocytoma and paraganglioma is under way (NCT02721732).

Pheochromocytomas and paragangliomas express high levels of somatostatin receptor, however organized investigation of the potential efficacy of somatostatin analogs has not previously been carried out. A trial of lanreotide in patients with advanced or metastatic pheochromocytoma/paraganglioma has been initiated.

Pheochromocytoma in pregnancy deserves special mention. Pheochromocytoma occurs in 1 among 50,000 pregnancies. Historically, maternal and fetal mortality was approximately 50%; however, with improvements in detection and treatment, mortality rates have decreased to 5% and 15%, respectively. Plasma and urine metanephrines should be used for screening. MRI is the preferred imaging modality during pregnancy rather than CT or MIBG. Surgical resection of a pheochromocytoma is recommended during the first or second trimester, while those that are diagnosed during the third trimester can be resected after delivery. Cesarean delivery is recommended due to the decreased risk of maternal mortality compared to a vaginal delivery in the setting of an in situ pheochromocytoma. Prior to delivery, preoperative alpha and beta blockade should be used. Of note, phenoxybenzamine poses a risk of hypotension and respiratory depression in the newborn during the first 48 hours of life. Genetic testing is indicated in these patients, as 30% of pregnant women with a pheochromocytoma have a hereditary syndrome.

Adrenal Cortical Carcinoma

Adrenal cortical carcinoma is a rare endocrine malignancy with an incidence of 0.5 to 2 cases per 1 million people each year in the United States. There is a bimodal age distribution, with incidence peaking in young children less than 5 years old and then again between 40 and 50 years of age. Prognosis tends to be poor because the diagnosis is usually delayed, with one-third of patients presenting with metastatic disease, and there is a dearth of effective systemic chemotherapy options. Surgical resection remains the mainstay of curative therapy. Even after surgical resection, rates of locoregional recurrence and metastasis are as high as 85%. Five-year survival rates range from 16% to 50%.

Advances in molecular biology have identified several genetic alterations associated with adrenal cortical carcinoma. Driver genes identified include *TP53, CTNNB1, ZNRF3, PRKAR1, CCNE1, TERF2, CDKN2A, RB1, MEN1, DAXX, TERT, MED12, RPL22,* and *NF1*. The two most common mutations found in adrenal cortical carcinoma are the overexpression of IGF-2, occurring in nearly 90% of cases, and overactivation of the Wnt/β-catenin pathway. The presence of β-catenin nuclear staining is associated with worse overall survival in patients with adrenal cortical carcinoma. Mutations in the tumor suppressor gene TP53 are seen in 60% to 80% of pediatric adrenal cortical carcinomas but in only 4% of adult cases. Sporadic mutations of TP53 are associated with a poor prognosis. Ki-67 has been demonstrated to be a prognostic marker and may be useful in treatment planning.

Clinical Manifestations

Patients with adrenal cortical carcinoma commonly present with vague abdominal symptoms secondary to an enlarging retroperitoneal mass and/or with clinical manifestations of overproduction of one or more adrenal cortical hormones. At least one-third are hormonally functional, most commonly secreting cortisol and producing Cushing syndrome. Another 10% to 20% of adrenal cortical carcinomas produce androgens, estrogens, or aldosterone, often in combination with cortisol, which can cause virilization in females, feminization in males, or hypertension, respectively.

Diagnosis

The preoperative evaluation of these patients involves biochemical screening for hormone overproduction as detailed above. With a cortisol-secreting tumor, the results of these tests serve to guide perioperative glucocorticoid replacement therapy. Screening to exclude pheochromocytoma should also be performed. Standard preoperative staging in patients with suspected adrenal cancer includes high-resolution abdominal CT or MRI. MRI may be especially helpful in delineating tumor extension into the inferior vena cava. Positron emission tomography when combined with CT imaging may be helpful in detecting metastasis or recurrence in patients with adrenal cortical cancer. Chest CT is used to rule out pulmonary metastasis. The median size of these tumors is 11 cm. Preoperative biopsy is not typically recommended (see discussion in

TABLE 17.6	American Joint Committee on Cancer 8th Edition Staging System for Adrenal Cortical Carcinoma

Stage	TNM Status
I	T1 (≤5 cm, no extra-adrenal invasion), N0, M0
II	T2 (>5 cm, no extra-adrenal invasion), N0, M0
III	T1 or T2, N1 (regional lymph node metastasis), M0
	T3 (tumor of any size with local invasion, but not invading adjacent organs), any N, M0
	T4 (tumor of any size that invades adjacent organs or large blood vessels), any N, M0
IV	Any T, any N, M1 (distant metastasis)

Adrenal Incidentaloma section) when the initial treatment plan would be surgery. However, fine-needle aspiration biopsy can be safely performed when necessary to establish a tissue diagnosis and guide treatment when surgery is not planned, or systemic therapy is preferred prior to consideration for surgery (neoadjuvant approach). Pheochromocytoma should always be clinically excluded prior to biopsy. Staging of patients with adrenal cortical carcinoma is now internationally concordant, as the 8th edition update of the AJCC Staging System for adrenal cortical carcinoma brought the AJCC staging system into alignment with the European Network for the Study of Adrenal Tumors (ENSAT) staging system (Table 17.6).

Treatment

Complete surgical resection is the only potentially curative therapy for localized adrenal cortical cancer. Approximately 50% of the tumors are localized to the adrenal gland at the time of initial presentation.

Several studies have examined the issue of minimally invasive versus open resection for adrenal cortical carcinoma. Donatini et al. propose that laparoscopic resection for stage I and II tumors (≤10 cm with no extra-adrenal invasion) can be performed without compromising oncologic outcomes. However, several other centers, including our own, have reported that laparoscopic resection is associated with higher rates of local and peritoneal recurrence, positive margins, shorter time to recurrence, and worse overall survival compared to open resection. These results are likely due to high rates of tumor fracture and peritoneal contamination of the typically soft adrenal cancers during the laparoscopic procedure, despite the procedure apparently appearing technically feasible to the operating surgeon based on preoperative imaging assessment. For this reason, we continue to prefer open adrenalectomy for patients with known or suspected adrenal cortical carcinoma. An open transabdominal approach facilitates adequate exposure to ensure complete resection, minimizes the risk of tumor spillage, and allows for vascular control of the inferior vena cava, aorta, and renal vessels when necessary. Radical en bloc resection of adrenal cortical carcinoma that includes adjacent organs, if involved by tumor, provides the only chance for long-term survival, and should be performed when possible. Routine nephrectomy or resection of other adjacent organs, however, without radiographic or macroscopic evidence of invasion, is generally not warranted. Tumor thrombectomy of the renal vein or inferior vena cava may be required. Lymph node invasion is common in patients with adrenal cortical carcinoma and is associated with worse overall survival. Patients who undergo lymphadenectomy have been reported to have improved survival and recurrence rates, and therefore, lymphadenectomy of radiographically or clinically suspicious lymph nodes should be performed at the time of adrenalectomy, and formal lymph node dissection (potentially including celiac, renal hilum, and ipsilateral aortic lymph nodes) should be at least selectively considered.

Risk factors for local recurrence include the center at which surgery is performed (tertiary referral center vs. other), age, stage at presentation, and incomplete resection. Patients who undergo a complete resection of their tumor have a 5-year survival rate of approximately 40% and a median survival of 43 months; those who undergo incomplete resection have a median survival less than 12 months. Therefore, the strongest predictor of outcome in this disease is the ability to perform a complete resection. The importance of complete resection has been highlighted in a study of 113 patients treated for adrenal cortical cancer at Memorial Sloan–Kettering Cancer Center. Patients with complete primary resections had improved 5-year survival rates compared to patients with incomplete resections (55% vs. 5%). Moreover, the benefit of complete resection was demonstrated in selected patients who underwent repeat surgery. Patients with a complete second resection demonstrated improved 5-year survival rates compared to patients with an incomplete second resection (57% vs. 0%).

Common sites of metastasis of adrenal cortical carcinoma include lungs, lymph nodes, liver, peritoneum, and bone. Complete resection of recurrent disease, including pulmonary metastases, is associated with prolonged survival in selected patients and can help control symptoms related to excess hormone production. Surveillance after surgical resection for adrenal cortical carcinoma is typically by CT or MRI of the abdomen and CT of the chest, in addition to biochemical testing, every 3 to 4 months. After 2 years of follow-up, the frequency of surveillance may be decreased, but should continue for at least 10 years.

Mitotane has been one of the most commonly used systemic agents in patients with advanced adrenal cortical carcinoma. This drug is an isomer of dichlorodiphenyltrichloroethane (DDT) and not only inhibits steroid production but also leads to atrophy of adrenal cortical cells. Mitotane is associated with a number of side effects, most notably gastrointestinal and neuromuscular symptoms. In addition, the drug has a relatively narrow therapeutic range (ideal plasma level >14 to 20 mg/L), and it requires close monitoring of serum levels to minimize toxicity as well as provision of exogenous steroid hormone replacement to avoid symptoms associated with adrenal insufficiency due to suppression of cortisol production by the normal contralateral gland. The role of mitotane in the adjuvant setting after radical resection of adrenal cortical carcinoma remains controversial. A 2007 nonrandomized retrospective study by Terzolo et al. examined the role of adjuvant mitotane postoperatively with respect to overall and recurrence-free survival. The authors examined 177 patients with adrenal cortical carcinoma who had undergone resection in 55 centers in Italy and Germany over a period of 20 years. The study included a group of 47 Italian patients treated at a single center with adjuvant mitotane and compared these patients to a group of 55 Italian patients as well as another group of 75 German patients who had not received adjuvant mitotane. While there was no significant difference in overall survival, recurrence-free survival was prolonged in the mitotane group (median 42 months) compared to the Italian (10 months) and German (25 months) controls. The recurrence rates were 49% in the mitotane group, 91% in the Italian control group, and 73% in the German control group. Limitations of the study included lack of details regarding the mitotane regimen and potential inconsistencies in surgery and follow-up evaluation among the various institutions over the span of two decades, resulting in an ascertainment or lead-time bias in the detection of recurrences. Importantly, the high recurrence rate of the Italian control group suggests that some patients may not have had a complete resection.

Our group has examined 218 patients with adrenal cortical carcinoma who underwent primary resection either at our MD Anderson Cancer Center institution (28 patients) or an outside institution (190 patients). After a median follow-up of 7.3 years, patients who had undergone surgery at MD Anderson had superior overall survival compared with outside patients (median not reached vs. 44 months) as well as superior disease-free survival (median of 25 months vs. 12 months). The overall survival rates were 68% versus 32%, and the recurrence rates were 50% versus 86% for the MD Anderson and outside patients, respectively. Twenty-two of the 218 patients (10%) in this series received adjuvant mitotane. A subset analysis demonstrated a prolonged disease-free survival in the mitotane group (median of 30 months vs. 12 months) without a benefit in overall survival. Importantly, the outcomes of the index and outside patient groups in our study compare favorably to the outcomes of the mitotane and control groups in the Terzolo et al. study. Based on these results, differences in outcomes between the patient groups in the European mitotane study may be related at least in part to quality and completeness of surgery rather than adjuvant mitotane therapy. We and others therefore have advocated individualizing adjuvant mitotane therapy in the postoperative management of patients with resected adrenal cortical carcinoma; we generally favor adjuvant mitotane in the postoperative management of relatively young healthy patients with a good performance status.

The US Adrenocortical Carcinoma Group examined the outcomes of 207 patients who received adjuvant mitotane after surgical resection. After adjusting for tumor factors, the receipt of mitotane was not associated with improved recurrence-free or overall survival. The Efficacy of Adjuvant Mitotane Treatment (ADIUVO) trial is currently underway and will provide additional insight into the utility of adjuvant mitotane in patients with resected ACC. Until then, Kim et al. have created a nomogram to accurately predict recurrence and survival after resection of adrenal cortical carcinoma; variables included are tumor size, nodal status, T stage, cortisol secretion, capsular invasion, and resection margins. This nomogram can help select high-risk patients who may be candidates for adjuvant therapy following resection of adrenal cortical carcinoma.

While no chemotherapeutic agent or combination of agents has been shown to be consistently effective against unresectable or metastatic adrenal cortical cancer, the FIRM-ACT trial has established combination chemotherapy with mitotane as the standard of care for patients with unresectable adrenal cortical carcinoma. This study randomized 304 patients to receive etoposide, doxorubicin, cisplatin, and mitotane (EDP-M) or streptozocin and mitotane (Sz-M). Response rates were higher with EDP-M compared to Sz-M (23.2% vs. 9.2%, $P < .001$), and median time to progression with EDP-M was longer (5.0 months vs. 2.1 months; hazard ratio 0.55; 95% confidence interval, 0.43 to 0.69; $P < .001$). The median survival of the EDP-M group was 14.8 months versus 12 months for patients in the Sz-M group, which was not statistically significant (hazard ratio 0.79; 95% confidence interval, 0.61 to 1.02; P = .07), emphasizing the need for improved systemic therapies for patients with adrenal cortical carcinoma. Gemcitabine-based chemotherapy (gemcitabine plus capecitabine) represents an alternative, second-line treatment regimen for adrenal cortical carcinoma. It is well tolerated, modestly active, and can be administered with or without mitotane.

The potential role of radiation therapy as adjuvant treatment following primary resection for adrenal cortical carcinoma remains controversial; it is more commonly used selectively (delivered via external beam or as brachytherapy) following resection for locoregional recurrence. Radiation therapy has an established role for treatment of isolated metastasis from adrenal cortical carcinoma, including as palliative therapy for bone metastasis.

Our group has examined the use of preoperative chemotherapy in patients with borderline resectable adrenal cortical carcinoma. Fifteen patients evaluated between 1995 and 2012 were deemed borderline resectable for one of three reasons: perceived requirement of multivisceral or vascular resection with high associated risk for a margin-positive resection; radiographic suspicion of metastatic disease or potentially resectable confirmed oligometastatic disease; or patient condition or comorbidities not amenable to an extensive surgical procedure. Based on standard RECIST criteria, 38% of evaluable patients had a partial response to neoadjuvant therapy, and six of seven patients with a vena caval tumor thrombus experienced at least a 30% reduction in the extent of the tumor thrombus. Eighty-seven percent of patients (13 of 15) were able to undergo surgical resection, with a 92.3% negative margin rate (R0). Median disease-free survival was 27.6 months for patients who underwent neoadjuvant chemotherapy compared to 12.6 months for patients with adrenal cortical carcinoma who underwent upfront surgery (P = .48), while actuarial 5-year overall survival was 65% and 57%, respectively. Based on this early experience, neoadjuvant chemotherapy may be an attractive option for selected patients with borderline resectable adrenal cortical carcinoma who are considered good candidates for initial chemotherapy followed by surgery.

Especially with the emergence of integrated molecular information revealing driver mechanisms in adrenal cortical carcinoma, there has been increased investigation of targeted therapies. Unfortunately, results to date have been generally discouraging. The IGF1R inhibitors cixutumumab, figitumumab, and linsitinib have been investigated with modest or no benefit documented. The antiangiogenic VEGF inhibitor bevacizumab did not show benefit. The multikinase inhibitors sorafenib, sunitinib, dovitinib, and axitinib, have all been evaluated, with very few or no objective responses. In the phase II study of sunitinib, an inverse correlation was identified between mitotane levels and the active metabolite of sunitinib. Mitotane induces the CYP34A hepatic metabolism which leads to rapid clearance of most targeted agents. A trial with the multikinase inhibitor cabozantinib is ongoing (NCT03370718). The EGFR inhibitors gefitinib and erlotinib have been investigated, without demonstrated benefit. The mTOR inhibitor temsirolimus (in combination with the immunomodulatory agent lenalidomide or cixutumumab) has been evaluated without clear benefit.

Multiple clinical trials are currently evaluating the role of immune checkpoint inhibitors in adrenal cortical carcinoma. The rationale for pursuing such treatment includes the observation of adrenalitis in patients receiving immune checkpoint inhibitors, the presence of programmed death-ligand 1 (PD-L1) and tumor-infiltrating lymphocytes (TIL) in adrenal cortical cancers.

In a phase 1b trial of avelumab (anti–PD-L1) in patients with previously treated adrenal cortical carcinoma, 3 of 50 patients had an objective response (6%) and an additional 21 patients (42%) had stable disease. Importantly, almost half of study participants were on concomitant mitotane therapy that could have influenced the findings of this trial. In a phase 2 trial of nivolumab (anti-PD1) in 10 patients with metastatic adrenal cortical carcinoma, 2 patients had stable disease for 11 and 48 weeks. In a phase 2 trial of pembrolizumab (anti-PD1) in patients with previously treated, advanced rare cancers including a prespecified cohort of adrenal cortical carcinoma, among 14 previously evaluable patients with adrenal cortical carcinoma, there were 2 partial responses (14%) and an additional 7 with stable disease (50%). A second phase 2 study with pembrolizumab reported 9 of 39 evaluable patients (23%) experienced a partial or complete response. Toxicities have generally been in line with that seen with these treatments in other cancers (84, 85). Ipilimumab (anti–CTLA-4) in combination with nivolumab is being evaluated in two phase 2 trials that include patients with adrenal cortical carcinoma (NCT03333616 and NCT02834013).

Since IL-13Rα2 is overexpressed on adrenal cortical carcinoma, a trial of IL-13-PE, a recombinant cytokine consisting of human interleukin-13 (IL-13) and a truncated form of pseudomonas endotoxin A (PE) was administered in a phase 1 trial of patients with adrenal cortical carcinoma and IL-13Rα2 expression; 1 of 5 patients treated had stable disease.

Since 30% of adrenal cortical carcinomas demonstrate significant iodometomidate uptake, treatment with [131]Iiodometomidate may offer a targeted radionuclide therapeutic option. In 11 patients with advanced adrenal cortical carcinoma who had high [123]Iiodometomidate uptake on diagnostic scans, administration of [131]Iiodometomidate resulted in partial response in one patient and stable disease in five. Toxicities included adrenal insufficiency and bone marrow suppression.

Adrenal Incidentaloma

With the widespread use of abdominal CT imaging, asymptomatic and unanticipated adrenal lesions are discovered with increasing frequency. These lesions, termed incidentalomas, are seen in up to 5% of routinely performed abdominal imaging studies and in up to 9% of autopsy series. Incidentalomas are more commonly found in white, obese, diabetic, hypertensive, and elderly patients, and are rare in children and adolescents. Although most of these lesions represent benign adenomas, some are hormonally active, and only a small minority represents an invasive malignancy. The risk of an incidentaloma being associated with hypercortisolism is approximately 5%, a pheochromocytoma 3% to 5%, aldosteronism 1%, adrenal cortical carcinoma 2% to 5%, and metastasis to the adrenal gland 2.5%. In contrast, in patients with a known extra-adrenal malignancy with biologic behavior that includes adrenal metastasis (e.g., lung cancer, melanoma, renal cell carcinoma), up to 50% to 75% of adrenal tumors are metastases. Fifteen percent of adrenal incidentalomas will be bilateral.

The European Society of Endocrinology Clinical Practice Guideline states that patients identified with an incidental adrenal mass >1 cm in size should be screened to rule out a hormonally active adenoma or pheochromocytoma. Evaluation of patients with an incidentally identified adrenal mass includes measurement of serum electrolyte levels, an overnight 1-mg dexamethasone suppression test (described previously), and measurement of plasma metanephrine levels. Patients with hypertension and an adrenal incidentaloma should also have plasma aldosterone and renin levels drawn in order to calculate the plasma aldosterone: renin ratio. DHEAS may be helpful in evaluating for mild autonomous cortisol excess, but levels of other sex hormones and steroid precursors are not routinely checked unless the patient is found to have symptoms of hormone excess (hirsutism, virilization) or if imaging findings are suspicious for adrenal cortical carcinoma. In general, any hormonally active lesion, regardless of size, should be resected. Furthermore, surgery is indicated if the adrenal mass demonstrates radiographic characteristics suggestive of malignancy or if the tumor enlarges during follow-up. Fine-needle aspiration biopsy is rarely indicated in the evaluation of an adrenal incidentaloma. If percutaneous biopsy is felt to be indicated (e.g., to assist with treatment planning in a patient with known or suspected metastatic cancer), a diagnosis of pheochromocytoma should be excluded prior to performing the biopsy to avoid inducing paroxysmal hypertension.

If the incidentaloma is nonfunctioning, the risk of malignancy is related to its size and radiographic characteristics. CT is ideal for the characterization of adrenal incidentalomas. A benign adrenal adenoma typically has high lipid content, resulting in low attenuation on CT ($\leq$10 HU). Adenomas also demonstrate rapid washout of contrast medium on adrenal protocol CT compared to pheochromocytomas, carcinomas, or adrenal metastases. Adrenal adenomas on MRI lose signal on out-of-phase images in relation to the spleen. However, it is important to recognize that up to 30% of benign adenomas do not contain high levels of lipid, making MRI and CT less useful in the diagnosis.

Size remains the single best clinical indicator of primary malignancy in patients who present with an incidental adrenal mass. Adrenal cortical carcinoma accounts for 2% of tumors less than 4 cm in size compared to 25% or more of tumors more than 6 cm in size. In addition, 90% of adrenal cortical carcinomas are larger than 6 cm. In general, lesions larger than 6 cm should be resected because of the relatively high risk of malignancy. Data from our own institution and elsewhere have identified rare patients with adrenal cortical carcinomas arising in tumors smaller than 5 cm. The overwhelming majority of these small tumors had CT or MRI characteristics suspicious for carcinoma such as heterogeneity and irregular borders. Recent recommendations for resection of nonfunctioning adrenal masses have ranged from 5 cm down to 3 cm. A cost-effectiveness analysis by Wang et al. supports the American Association of Clinical Endocrinologists (AACE) and American Association of Endocrine Surgeons (AAES) recommendation that tumors $\geq$4 cm be resected. The recent success and advantages of laparoscopic adrenalectomy have led some investigators to suggest operative removal of even relatively small incidentalomas. However, the decision to operate on a nonfunctioning adrenal incidentaloma must also take into account the patient's comorbidities, life expectancy, and personal wishes.

At MD Anderson, we recommend adrenalectomy for all biochemically confirmed functioning adrenal tumors and those with suspicious radiographic findings regardless of size. Nonfunctioning tumors between 3 and 6 cm in diameter are most appropriately managed on an individual basis, taking into consideration patient age and comorbidities. For example, a 3-cm tumor in an otherwise healthy 40-year-old patient is

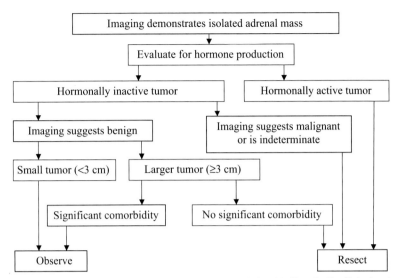

FIGURE 17.3 An algorithm for the evaluation of patients with isolated, incidentally identified adrenal tumors.

probably most appropriately managed by adrenalectomy, whereas the same tumor in a 75-year-old patient with multiple comorbidities might be observed. Figure 17.3 provides an overview of our approach to patients with adrenal incidentalomas.

Small, hormonally inactive adrenal incidentalomas can be observed. In this scenario, the NIH Consensus statement and AACE/AAES guidelines recommend repeat imaging at 6, 12, and 24 months. Biochemical testing is recommended annually for 4 to 5 years. If the mass enlarges by more than 20% in largest diameter or becomes hormonally active, consideration for resection is recommended. In patients whose tumors remain stable in size and biologically nonfunctioning, no further follow-up is recommended after 5 years. Table 17.7 outlines a variety of recommended regimens for the radiographic surveillance of an adrenal incidentaloma.

Adrenal Metastases

Cancer metastasis to the adrenal glands is relatively common, occurring in up to 27% of patients with extra-adrenal malignancies at autopsy. Based on these studies, 42% of lung cancers, 16% of gastric cancers,

TABLE 17.7 Examples of Recommended Follow-Up Regimens for a Patient with a Nonfunctioning, Benign-Appearing Adrenal Incidentaloma

Author, Publication	Who to Image	How to Image	When to Image
European Society of Endocrinology Clinical Practice Guidelines/European Network for the Study of Adrenal Tumors, 2016	Benign-appearing, <4 cm Indeterminate-appearing	No routine imaging Noncontrast CT or MRI	No routine imaging 6–12 months after diagnosis
Italian Association of Clinical Endocrinologists (AME) Position Statement, 2011	Benign-appearing	CT	3–6 months after diagnosis, once
Boland, AJR, 2011	Benign-appearing	CT	6 months after diagnosis, then no further imaging if stable
White Paper of the ACR, 2010	<4 cm	Noncontrast CT Or MRI	12 months after diagnosis
AACE/AAES Guidelines, 2009	Benign-appearing, <4 cm	Noncontrast CT Or MRI	3–6 months after diagnosis, then annually for 1–2 years
Young, NEJM 2007	<4 cm	CT	6, 12, and 24 months after diagnosis, then consider no further imaging if stable
NIH Consensus, 2002	Benign-appearing, <4 cm	CT	6–12 months after diagnosis, then consider no further imaging if stable

58% of breast cancers, 50% of malignant melanomas, and a high percentage of renal and prostate cancers have metastasized to the adrenal glands by the time of death. The adrenal gland is the sole site of metastatic disease in 75% to 85% of patients, and the majority present with metachronous disease (>6 months after diagnosis of the primary malignancy). Most patients are asymptomatic from the standpoint of their adrenal metastasis, and adrenal insufficiency is encountered only occasionally (e.g., bilateral adrenal metastases from lung cancer). In general, more than 90% of normal adrenal cortical tissue in both adrenal glands must be replaced before clinically detectable adrenal cortical hypofunction is appreciated. When adrenal insufficiency does occur, it is usually in the setting of gross bilateral enlargement of the adrenal glands as detected by CT. Bilateral adrenal metastases occur in 4% of patients.

Evaluation of the patient with an adrenal mass and a history of malignancy includes an evaluation for hormone production, since as many as 50% of these patients will have occult, functioning adrenal tumors unrelated to their prior malignancy, for example, pheochromocytoma (Fig. 17.4). Functional assessment for

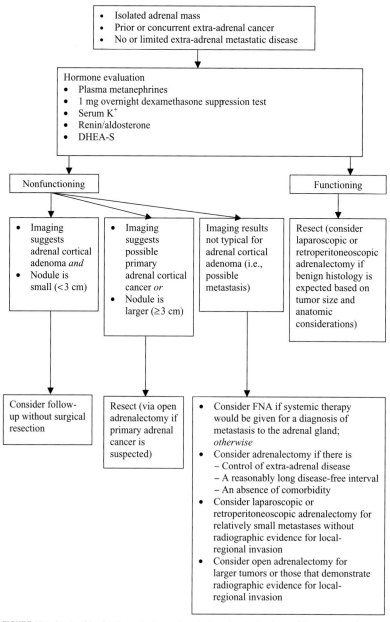

FIGURE 17.4 An algorithm for the evaluation and surgical treatment of patients with extra-adrenal cancer presenting with an adrenal mass.

hormone overproduction is performed as for patients without malignancy who are found to have an incidentaloma and should include an overnight 1-mg dexamethasone suppression test, plasma metanephrines, and plasma renin and aldosterone levels in hypertensive patients. As mentioned earlier, CT is the preferred imaging modality for an incidentaloma, as benign adenomas have low attenuation on non-contrast CT and rapid washout on contrast CT images. PET/CT is more frequently used in patients with a known malignancy and can be used to help differentiate between benign and malignant adrenal lesions. Adrenal adenomas are usually not FDG-avid, while malignant lesions are FDG-avid, although PET/CT has a false-positive rate of 20% in detecting malignancy.

Once a functional adrenal mass is ruled out, fine-needle aspiration biopsy may be helpful in selected patients with suspected adrenal metastasis when the results would influence the treatment plan; for example, to confirm the diagnosis of metastasis in those who are not surgical candidates. Percutaneous biopsy can be done under CT or ultrasound guidance and has been shown to be 89% sensitive in the diagnosis of malignancy. A nondiagnostic sample is obtained in 5% of cases. Complication rates of adrenal biopsy range from 3% to 13%, with the most common complications being adrenal hematoma, abdominal pain, pancreatitis, hematuria, pneumothorax, abscess, and tumor seeding of the biopsy tract. Percutaneous biopsy should not be performed in patients suspected of having primary adrenal cortical carcinoma when the initial treatment plan would be surgery, and pheochromocytoma should always be excluded by biochemical testing prior to biopsy. In selected patients, surgical treatment of a suspected adrenal metastasis may be planned solely based on the patient's history and on noninvasive studies without preoperative needle biopsy. A history of a malignancy that commonly metastasizes to the adrenal glands, with favorable tumor biology, negative biochemical screening for hormone production, and a mass that either fulfills size criteria for surgical excision or is radiographically suspicious for metastasis, may be considered for resection without preoperative tissue diagnosis.

Surgery for isolated metastases to the adrenal gland can be considered in highly selected patients. Appropriate selection criteria include good-risk individuals in whom there is a prolonged disease-free interval and evidence of favorable underlying tumor biology. Favorable tumor biology is implied in those who have had a significant progression-free interval, those who have responded to systemic therapy, and those who have a history of isolated metachronous metastases. Primary tumor site also appears to affect survival, in that longer median survival times are observed following resection of metastases from primary renal, melanoma, colon, and lung cancers, and poorer survival in patients with esophageal, liver, unknown primary tumors, and high-grade sarcomas. Metachronous disease, disease-free interval of >12 months, complete resection of the adrenal metastasis (R0 vs. R1/R2), and smaller tumor size are associated with prolonged survival after adrenal metastasectomy. Several studies have shown that open and laparoscopic adrenalectomy for metastasis are feasible and have equivalent rates of positive margins, local recurrence, and overall survival, as long as sound judgment is used in determining the safest approach for each patient based on tumor characteristics and surgeon experience.

Surgical Approach

When choosing an operative approach for a patient with an adrenal tumor, several factors must be considered: the size and site of the tumor, the malignant potential of the disease, the laterality or bilaterality of the disease, the presence of multiple or extra-adrenal tumors, the presence of additional intra-abdominal disease or extra-abdominal extension, history of prior abdominal surgery, the patient's body habitus, and the surgeon's experience. Generally, large tumors and tumors suspected to represent a primary malignancy are best approached with an open operation.

Open Adrenalectomy

An open adrenalectomy is indicated for known or suspected primary adrenal cancer, large tumors, recurrent disease, and for tumors that involve adjacent viscera. Open adrenalectomy can be performed by four approaches: anterior, posterior, lateral (flank), and thoracoabdominal.

The anterior approach is the preferred method for resection of most adrenal cortical carcinomas. The patient is placed in a supine or semi-lateral position. Access is accomplished via a midline incision, a bilateral subcostal incision, or a Makuuchi (hockey stick-shaped) incision. For an open left adrenalectomy, the splenic flexure and descending colon are mobilized inferiorly, and the retroperitoneum is entered by incising along the inferior border of the pancreas. Medial visceral rotation of the spleen and tail of the pancreas is usually helpful and necessary when dealing with large tumors. The adrenal gland can be visualized by exposing the renal hilum and then following the left renal vein to the junction of the adrenal vein. The left adrenal gland lies lateral to the aorta, just above the left renal vein. The adrenal vein can be ligated early in the procedure to limit the release of catecholamines when dealing with a pheochromocytoma; it should be recognized, however, that early venous ligation may increase venous congestion and bleeding from the tumor. Small arterial perforators from the aorta, inferior phrenic, and renal arteries are identified and ligated with sutures or with energy alone. Open adrenalectomy of the right adrenal gland is approached similarly; on the right side, mobilization of the right triangular ligament of the liver allows anteromedial rotation of the liver and access to the right adrenal gland. A Kocher maneuver facilitates exposure of the right kidney and vena cava and is helpful when the adrenal tumor is large. The right adrenal vein generally drains directly into the vena cava and is very short. Care is taken to control it appropriately with suture ligation or a vascular stapler. Drains are used selectively but are usually unnecessary, especially in the absence of multiorgan resection.

The open posterior approach, formerly commonly used in the resection of small, benign adrenal tumors (e.g., aldosteronomas), is now rarely employed. The procedure begins with the patient in a prone position with the table flexed about 35 degrees. An oblique incision is made over the 12th rib with retraction of sacrospinalis muscle medially, resection of the 12th rib, and reflection of the pleura superiorly. On the left, the superior extent of the dissection is the diaphragm. The perirenal fat and soft tissues are reflected downward with the diaphragm exposed superomedially. Medially, a vertically coursing inferior phrenic vein can be encountered indicating the adrenal gland is nearby, laterally. On the right, care is taken to preserve the subcostal nerve and exposure is facilitated by transecting the free edge of the diaphragm medially to the spine. The adrenal gland is located against the bare area of the liver with exposure of the liver delineating the superior extent of the dissection.

In the lateral (flank) approach, the patient is placed in a lateral decubitus position with an extraperitoneal approach to the involved side. The lateral approach can be helpful in obese patients with gravity assisting the retraction. The lateral approach, like the posterior approach, can obviate the need to perform extensive adhesiolysis in a patient with previous abdominal surgery. However, vascular control of large vessels may be difficult.

The thoracoabdominal approach provides the broadest exposure and is occasionally useful for tumors that may require en bloc resection of adjacent organs or extensive lymph node dissection. The patient is placed in the decubitus position and the incision is carried over the 10th rib on the right or over the 11th rib on the left, followed by resection of the rib. For tumors with significant extension into the IVC, the hepatic veins, or the right atrium, a median sternotomy may be necessary.

Laparoscopic Adrenalectomy

Since the first description of laparoscopic adrenalectomy in 1992, this approach has been expanded and is considered now the standard approach for modestly sized benign adrenal tumors as well as selected metastases to the adrenal gland. Patients who undergo laparoscopic adrenalectomy have a more rapid recovery, less discomfort, faster return to preoperative activity level, and better cosmetic results compared to patients who undergo open adrenalectomy.

Patients who are good candidates for laparoscopic adrenalectomy include those with aldosterone-producing adenomas; other small (<4 cm) functioning or nonfunctioning but presumably benign cortical neoplasms; those with unilateral, benign-appearing sporadic pheochromocytomas; MEN II or von Hippel–Lindau syndrome patients with a unilateral pheochromocytoma; and selected patients with adrenal metastasis. Bilateral laparoscopic adrenalectomy can be performed in selected patients with bilateral adrenal hyperplasia. Laparoscopic cortical-sparing partial adrenalectomy has been successfully performed in patients with bilateral pheochromocytomas in the familial setting. We continue to urge caution in the use of laparoscopic adrenalectomy for patients with malignant or potentially malignant primary adrenal tumors. This includes the occasional patient with cortical neoplasms (functioning or nonfunctioning) 4 cm in size or greater with radiographic features suggesting malignancy.

For a standard, 4-port transperitoneal laparoscopic left adrenalectomy, the patient is placed in the right lateral decubitus position, with the table appropriately padded and flexed. The abdomen and chest are prepped from the nipple to below the iliac crest, and from the right of the umbilicus to the vertebral column. An infracostal 12-mm port, 10 to 15 cm anterior to the anterior axillary line, is placed using the open technique, abdominal insufflation achieved, and the 30-degree laparoscope is inserted. Three additional trocars are then placed under direct vision. One is placed at the anterior axillary line (12 mm), one is placed at the posterior axillary line (5 mm), and one is placed 5 cm posterior to the posterior axillary port, just medial to the left kidney (5 mm). Dissection begins by mobilizing the splenic flexure of the colon, and gravity is used to carry it inferiorly and medially. Mobilization of the spleen is performed by incising the peritoneum lateral to the spleen. This incision is developed around to the level of the short gastric vessels. This allows the spleen to rotate medially. It is often helpful to move the laparoscope to the posterior port as dissection proceeds to maximize visualization of the adrenal bed. The adrenal gland is dissected from the retroperitoneal fat; the Harmonic Scalpel (Ethicon Endo-Surgery, Inc.) works well for this dissection. In contrast to the open approach, technical considerations in laparoscopic adrenalectomy often result in delaying ligation of the adrenal vein to the penultimate step in the procedure, following complete mobilization of the tumor and the adrenal gland, and just prior to specimen removal. Vein division on the left side can be safely accomplished with either the vascular stapler or with two titanium clips placed on the proximal side of the vein. The specimen is removed in a sterile plastic retrieval bag through the umbilical port site. Laparoscopic right adrenalectomy is performed with similar positioning in the left lateral decubitus position. Abdominal access is obtained through placement of four ports, placed similar to those on the left side. The most medial port is used to assist in retraction of the liver. The surgeon begins the operation through the two lateral ports; the right lateral hepatic attachments and the right triangular ligament of the liver are divided to allow for medial retraction of the liver. The adrenal gland is then dissected inferiorly along the renal vein and medially along the vena cava. The right adrenal vein is usually short and wide and drains directly into the vena cava. Again, either the vascular stapler or titanium clips may be used to secure the vein on the right side.

Posterior Retroperitoneoscopic Adrenalectomy

The posterior retroperitoneoscopic adrenalectomy (PRA) has become the preferred technique at our institution for resection of small, benign adrenal masses and isolated metastases to the adrenal gland. The technique of PRA was first reported by Mercan et al. in 1995 and further modified by Walz et al. in Essen, Germany. This method offers the advantage of a minimally invasive approach to the adrenal glands, obviating the need for adhesiolysis while minimizing hemodynamic or respiratory instability from CO_2 insufflation. In addition, this approach allows the surgeon to address bilateral disease without the need for patient repositioning. Contraindications include suspicion of adrenal cortical carcinoma, adjacent organ invasion, lesions greater than approximately 6 cm, morbid obesity, and limited distance between the ribs and iliac crest. Barczyński et al. performed a randomized clinical trial comparing PRA and lateral transperitoneal laparoscopic adrenalectomy for adrenal lesions less than 7 cm in size. In this investigation, PRA was associated with decreased operative time and blood loss, decreased postoperative pain and nausea, improved time to ambulation, shorter length of stay and lower hospital costs. In contrast, a meta-analysis by Nigri et al. did not show any differences in these same outcomes between PRA and laparoscopic adrenalectomy. Thus, surgeon experience and preference can continue to dictate the technical approach to minimally invasive adrenalectomy in most situations.

With the patient placed in a prone jackknife position on a Cloward table saddle (Fig. 17.5), the 12th rib is palpated and a 1.5-cm transverse incision is made just beneath the tip of the rib. This will be the eventual site of the middle (12 mm) trocar. The soft tissues are divided sharply and the retroperitoneal space

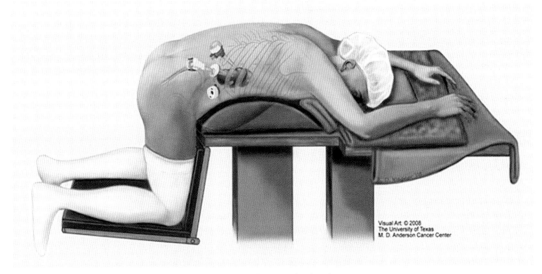

Visual Art © 2008
The University of Texas
M. D. Anderson Cancer Center

FIGURE 17.5 Patient positioning for a right-sided posterior retroperitoneoscopic adrenalectomy.

is entered. Using the index finger, a small space is created, and the index finger is then used to guide the placement of the medial (12 mm) and lateral (5 mm) trocars into this space. The medial trocar is placed approximately 5 cm medial to the middle trocar site, just lateral to the paraspinal musculature. This trocar is angled at 45 degrees and aimed slightly laterally toward the adrenal gland. The lateral trocar is placed approximately 5 cm lateral to the middle trocar site, beneath the 11th rib, and aimed medially. A blunt 12-mm trocar with an inflatable balloon and an adjustable sleeve is then placed into the retroperitoneal space through the middle incision. Pneumoretroperitoneum is then created with CO_2 insufflation to a pressure of up to 24 mm Hg.

A 30-degree 10-mm videoscope is first inserted through the middle trocar, allowing for a combination of blunt and sharp dissection to establish the retroperitoneal space beneath the diaphragm. The videoscope can then be switched to the medial trocar, and the middle and lateral trocars used as the working ports. Gerota fascia is entered and the superior pole of the kidney is identified. The psoas muscle, the posterior surface of the liver or spleen which is visible through the peritoneum, and the superior pole of the kidney serve as landmarks. On the right side, the inferior vena cava is a key landmark.

The adrenal gland is allowed to retract superiorly with gentle downward retraction on the kidney. Division of the tissue along the superior border of the kidney is performed using the Harmonic Scalpel, the EnSeal device (Ethicon Endo-Surgery, Inc.), or laparoscopic scissors. It is important to dissect the adrenal gland from the kidney before dividing the superior and medial attachments of the gland. This maneuver minimizes direct manipulation of the fragile adrenal gland and allows the gland to be suspended from its superior attachments until late in the procedure, greatly facilitating dissection.

On the left side, the adrenal vein drains inferiorly into the renal vein. On the right side, the adrenal vein is identified coursing medially to drain into the inferior vena cava. The inferior vena cava must be carefully identified. Due to high insufflation pressures, it loses its normal tubular appearance and its lateral border appears as a flat white line. The adrenal vein is dissected and divided between clips, while simultaneously retracting the gland on the distal side of the adrenal vein. Bleeding tends to be very modest due in part to the high insufflation pressures.

The adrenal gland is then completely mobilized medially and superiorly. A retrieval bag is used to remove the specimen through the middle trocar site. The retroperitoneal space is then inspected for hemostasis. Insufflation is gradually decreased to pressures of 8 to 12 mm Hg, facilitating visualization of any venous bleeding that may have been tamponaded by the high insufflation pressures. Ports are then removed, and the skin is closed with absorbable suture.

We have updated and published our experience with PRAs performed at MD Anderson between 2005 and 2010. One hundred and eighteen PRAs were performed for indications which included functioning tumors (pheochromocytomas, Cushing syndrome, failure of medical management of Cushing disease, etc.), nonfunctioning cortical adenomas, and isolated adrenal metastasis. Mean tumor size was 2.7 cm. Complications occurred in 11.2% of patients, with a significant decrease in the complication rate during the second half of the study. There was no perioperative mortality. Longer operative times were encountered in male patients, obese patients, and in patients with a right-sided lesion. Conversion to an open procedure was necessary in 6.6% of cases. Of note, 48% of the patients had a body mass index greater than 30. We have thus found PRA to be a safe and, in our hands, the preferred approach for resection of benign tumors and small adrenal metastases, generally avoiding difficulties encountered in patients with obese habitus or extensive adhesions secondary to prior abdominal surgery.

CASE SCENARIO

Case Scenario 1

Presentation

A 20-year-old female presented with left leg pain and abdominal discomfort. X-ray showed a lytic bone lesion. MRI of the femur demonstrated multiple lytic bone lesions. Biopsy was obtained and identified a metastatic paraganglioma. A CT of the abdomen and pelvis (Fig. 17.6A) demonstrated a 17-cm borderline resectable retroperitoneal mass with long segment abutment of the superior mesenteric artery and involvement of multiple adjacent organs. A ^{68}Ga-DOTATATE PET/CT confirmed a PET avid left retroperitoneal mass and multiple bone metastases.

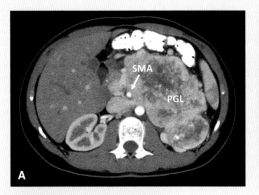
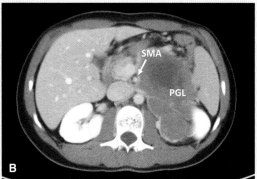
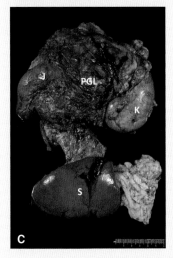

FIGURE 17.6 **(A)** CT of the abdomen and pelvis demonstrating a 17-cm borderline resectable retroperitoneal mass (PGL, paraganglioma) with long segment abutment of the superior mesenteric artery (SMA) and involvement of multiple adjacent organs. **(B)** Partial radiographic response after neoadjuvant therapy. **(C)** Resected left retroperitoneal tumor (PGL) en bloc with the involved adjacent organs including the left adrenal gland and kidney (K), spleen (S), tail of pancreas (P), and proximal jejunum (J); the SMA was preserved.

Confirmation of Diagnosis and Treatment

In this case, the patient presented with established metastatic paraganglioma confirmed via percutaneous biopsy. The next step is to determine whether the tumor is functional. This can be confirmed with plasma normetanephrines and 24-hour urine catecholamines (dopamine and norepinephrine) and metabolites (normetanephrine and vanillylmandelic acid). Paragangliomas secrete predominantly dopamine and norepinephrine because phenylethanolamine-N-methyl-transferase, which converts norepinephrine to epinephrine, is only produced in the adrenal glands and the organ of Zuckerkandl. When a patient presents with a retroperitoneal mass suspicious for pheochromocytoma or paraganglioma, a percutaneous biopsy should not be performed at least until hormone evaluation is performed and appropriate adrenergic blockade established due to the risk of hypertensive crisis.

Patients with a family history of pheochromocytoma or paraganglioma or an associated clinical syndrome based on evaluation by a genetic counselor are found to have a pathogenic mutation in 90% of cases. Genetic testing should be based on the presence of familial or syndromic features, particularly those associated with RET, VHL, NF-1, or SDH mutation. In cases of malignant disease, SDHB testing should be prioritized. For those with bilateral tumors, VHL and RET genes should be tested first, and in patients with extra-adrenal disease, testing for SDHD and SDHB genes should be prioritized. Once a mutation is identified, no further testing is recommended, as the chance of two genetic mutations occurring in a single patient is rare. Once a mutation is identified, family members should be tested. Hereditary paraganglioma syndromes result from mutations in succinate dehydrogenase (*SDHD, SDHB, SDHC,* and *SDH5*) genes. This patient had a mutation in subunit B (*SDHB*), which carries a particularly high risk of malignancy (34% to 83%). Hereditary paraganglioma syndromes predispose to both extra-adrenal and adrenal tumors. Patients with a familial pheochromocytoma syndrome require follow-up and periodic screening, especially before any planned surgical procedure.

Neoadjuvant chemotherapy was recommended for this patient because she had metastatic disease at presentation and her primary tumor was borderline resectable. She received a total of 7 cycles of cisplatin/vinblastine/doxorubicin with stable disease, then treatment was initiated with the tyrosine kinase inhibitor cabozantinib, with partial biochemical and radiographic response (Fig. 17.6B).

Resection of malignant pheochromocytoma or paraganglioma, including resection of metastases, may be considered in good-risk individuals if the metastases are limited in extent. Surgical debulking can be used to achieve biochemical control, improve response to systemic therapies with diminished tumor burden, and palliate symptoms. However, when extra-abdominal disease is present, a sustained biochemical response is unlikely after resection, stressing the importance of patient selection and determination of treatment goals preoperatively. In this patient, surgical resection was performed given the patient's young age and to decrease the tumor burden in an attempt to improve response to systemic therapies.

Surgical Approach—Key Steps

For patients with functioning paragangliomas or pheochromocytoma, appropriate alpha blockade with phenoxybenzamine or doxazosin is important prior to surgical resection. A calcium channel blocker can help manage those with refractory hypertension, and a beta blocker may help prevent tachyarrhythmias. Beta blockade should not be instituted unless alpha blockade has been established; otherwise, the beta blocker will inhibit epinephrine-induced vasodilation, leading to more significant hypertension and left heart strain. Given that this patient's tumor was demonstrated to be nonfunctioning, she did not require alpha blockade prior to surgery.

Small paragangliomas may be approached in a minimally invasive fashion from either a retroperitoneoscopic approach or an anterior approach, depending on the details of the tumor and patient anatomy and surgeon experience and preference, while larger tumors such as the one described here require an open approach. Whatever the approach, the surgeon should manipulate the tumor as little as possible and ligate the tumor's venous outflow as early in the procedure as practical (while recognizing that early division of the vein without concomitant division of arterial inflow may increase venous congestion of the tumor and back-bleeding). In this patient, resection of the primary left retroperitoneal tumor (Fig. 17.6C) was performed en bloc with the involved adjacent organs including the left adrenal gland and kidney, spleen, tail of pancreas, and proximal jejunum; the SMA was preserved.

Postoperative Management

Postoperatively, patients with functioning tumors should be monitored carefully for 24 to 48 hours for arrhythmias, as well as hypotension secondary to compensatory vasodilation. Hypoglycemia may result from decreased glucose production from a drop in circulating catecholamines. Hypertension may persist postoperatively, especially in those with sustained hypertension preoperatively.

While follow-up after resection of pheochromocytoma or paraganglioma has not been completely standardized, we typically measure plasma-free metanephrines at 1, 6, and 12 months postoperatively, then annually thereafter, and do yearly cross-sectional imaging. Biochemical testing should include a plasma-free metanephrine level or timed urine collection for catecholamine determination to exclude recurrence. If recurrence is suspected based on biochemical evaluation, localizing studies ^{68}Ga-DOTATATE PET or FDG PET should be obtained, and resection of recurrent tumor is indicated when feasible. This patient has been followed with alternating CT and ^{68}Ga-DOTATATE PET/CT with overall relatively stable metastatic disease and control of the prior intra-abdominal and retroperitoneal tumor process.

Common Curve Balls

- Falsely elevated catecholamines from common medications including caffeine, nicotine, tricyclic antidepressants, monoamine oxidase inhibitors, phenoxybenzamine, calcium channel blockers, levodopa, alpha-methyldopa, ephedrine, and acetaminophen
- Intraoperative hypertension or hypotension or postoperative hypotension are common in functioning tumors
- Other neoplasms that may also require surgery can occur in patients with inherited pheochromocytoma

Take Home Points

- Adequate alpha blockade prior to surgery and intraoperative monitoring with preparation for hypertension or hypotension is critical for patients with functioning pheochromocytomas and paragangliomas.

- Genetic testing is important in patients with pheochromocytoma or paraganglioma as at least 40% are associated with a genetic syndrome, and results of genetic testing can affect preoperative and operative planning as well as long-term surveillance strategies.
- Functioning tumors should be manipulated as little as possible, and the venous drainage should be ligated as early as possible, to minimize hemodynamic instability.

Case Scenario 2

Presentation

A 30-year-old woman presented with bilateral leg swelling, amenorrhea, and thinning of the hair. Biochemical evaluation demonstrated elevated testosterone, DHEA, and cortisol levels. A CT was performed demonstrating a large left adrenal tumor with involvement of the inferior vena cava and a suspected metastasis in segment VIII of the liver (Fig. 17.7A,B).

Differential Diagnosis

- Adrenal cortical adenoma
- Adrenal cortical carcinoma
- Metastasis from unknown primary cancer
- Metastatic pheochromocytoma

Confirmation of Diagnosis and Treatment

This patient's large adrenal tumor with suspected hepatic metastasis is suspicious for adrenal cortical carcinoma. Patients with adrenal cortical carcinoma commonly present with vague abdominal symptoms secondary to an enlarging retroperitoneal mass and/or with clinical manifestation of overproduction of one or more adrenal cortical hormones. At least one-third of tumors are hormonally functional, most commonly secreting cortisol and leading to Cushing syndrome. Another 10% to 20% of adrenal cortical carcinomas produce androgens, estrogens, or aldosterone, often in combination with cortisol, which can cause virilization in females, feminization in males, or hypertension, respectively. The preoperative

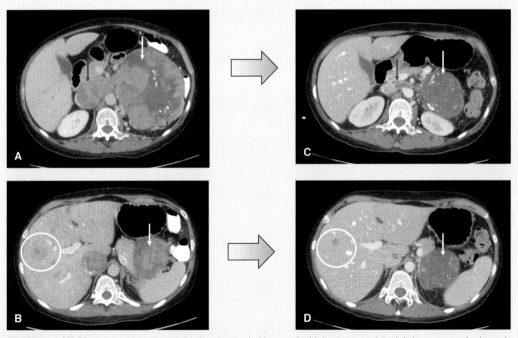

FIGURE 17.7 (A) CT demonstrating a large left adrenal tumor (*white arrow*) with involvement of the inferior vena cava (*red arrow*). **(B)** Suspected metastasis in segment VIII of the liver. **(C)** Decreased size of the primary tumor (*white arrow*) and IVC component (*red arrow*), and **(D)** decreased size of the segment VIII liver metastasis following neoadjuvant treatment.

evaluation of these patients involves biochemical screening for hormone overproduction. With a cortisol-secreting tumor, the results of these tests serve to guide perioperative glucocorticoid replacement therapy. Screening to exclude pheochromocytoma should also be performed. This patient had an elevated testosterone and DHEA, and her examination was consistent with mild Cushing syndrome with facial fullness and thinning of the skin.

Standard preoperative staging in patients with suspected adrenal cancer includes high-resolution abdominal CT or MRI. MRI may be especially helpful in delineating tumor extension into the inferior vena cava. Positron emission tomography when combined with CT imaging may be helpful in detecting metastasis or recurrence in patients with adrenal cortical cancer. Chest CT is used to rule out pulmonary metastasis. When adrenal cortical carcinoma is suspected and upfront surgery is planned, preoperative biopsy is not typically recommended. However, when the diagnosis is in question or neoadjuvant therapy is planned, then a fine needle aspiration can be performed after ruling out pheochromocytoma.

This patient underwent FNA, which was consistent with adrenal cortical carcinoma. Complete surgical resection is the only potentially curative treatment for adrenal cortical carcinoma; however, given that the primary tumor was borderline resectable and that she had suspected metastatic disease, the patient initially received 9 cycles of neoadjuvant therapy consisting of etoposide, doxorubicin, and cisplatin together with mitotane. With this treatment, the primary tumor decreased in size from 11×8.4 cm to 7.8×6.6 cm, the liver metastasis also responded (Fig. 17.7C), and the burden of tumor thrombus improved with delineation of the renal vein (Fig. 17.7D), thus allowing for subsequent en bloc resection of the left kidney together with vena cava tumor thrombectomy and segment VIII liver resection.

Surgical Approach—Key Steps

Some centers would consider laparoscopic or robotic resection of small adrenal cortical carcinomas. However, minimally invasive resection of adrenal cortical carcinoma has been associated with higher rates of local and peritoneal recurrence, positive margins, shorter time to recurrence, and worse overall survival compared to open resection in several series. These results are likely due to high rates of tumor fracture and peritoneal contamination of the typically soft adrenal cancers during the laparoscopic procedure, despite the procedure apparently appearing technically feasible to the operating surgeon based on preoperative imaging assessment. For this reason, we continue to prefer open adrenalectomy for patients with known or suspected adrenal cortical carcinoma.

This patient underwent en bloc resection of the left kidney together with vena cava tumor thrombectomy and segment VIII liver resection. Radical en bloc resection of adrenal cortical carcinoma that includes adjacent organs, if involved by tumor, provides the only chance for long-term survival, and should be performed when possible. Routine nephrectomy or resection of other adjacent organs, however, without radiographic or macroscopic evidence of invasion, is generally not warranted. Tumor thrombectomy of the renal vein or inferior vena cava, as in this case, may be required. Lymph node invasion is common in patients with adrenal cortical carcinoma and is associated with worse overall survival. Patients who undergo lymphadenectomy have been reported to have improved survival and recurrence rates, and therefore, lymphadenectomy of radiographically or clinically suspicious lymph nodes should be performed at the time of adrenalectomy, and formal lymph node dissection (potentially including celiac, renal hilum, and ipsilateral aortic lymph nodes) should be at least selectively considered.

Postoperative Management

While adjuvant therapy decisions for adrenal cortical carcinoma patients should continue to be individualized, we generally favor adjuvant mitotane in the postoperative management of relatively young patients with a good performance status. Tumor size, nodal status, T stage, cortisol secretion, capsular invasion, and resection margins are also associated with recurrence risk and can be used to select high-risk patients who may be candidates for adjuvant therapy following resection of adrenal cortical carcinoma. Radiation is typically used only selectively following resection for locoregional recurrence and can be used as palliative therapy for bone metastasis.

Surveillance after surgical resection for adrenal cortical carcinoma is typically by CT or MRI of the abdomen and CT of the chest, in addition to biochemical testing, every 3 to 4 months. After 2 years of follow-up, the frequency of surveillance may be decreased, but it should continue for at least 10 years.

Common Curve Balls

- Failure to rule out pheochromocytoma prior to biopsy
- Invasion of adjacent organs requiring careful surgical planning
- Postoperative adrenal insufficiency if corticosteroids are not given in the perioperative period for patients with cortisol secreting tumors

Take Home Points

- Complete surgical resection is the only potentially curative treatment for adrenal cortical carcinoma, and long-term disease-free survival is occasionally observed following complete resection of metastatic disease. Palliative resection may be indicated to alleviate symptoms in patients with advanced disease, particularly in those with functioning tumors.
- Neoadjuvant therapy can be an excellent option particularly for patients with borderline resectable adrenal cortical carcinoma that will require multivisceral resection and for those presenting with potentially resectable oligometastases.
- We continue to favor an open surgical approach for patients with known or suspected adrenal cortical carcinoma to minimize the risk of intraoperative tumor fracture and associated early postoperative recurrence.

CASE SCENARIO REVIEW

Questions

1. A patient with a previously resected malignant pheochromocytoma has elevated serum metanephrines on surveillance laboratory studies. What is the most sensitive imaging study to detect recurrence?

   A. MRI of the abdomen and pelvis
   B. CT of the abdomen and pelvis
   C. (68)Ga-DOTATE PET/CT
   D. MIBG scan

2. A 30-year-old woman presents with a 14-cm right adrenal tumor with direct invasion into the liver and extensive tumor thrombus in the inferior vena cava. Hormone evaluation documents markedly elevated cortisol levels. Imaging documents multiple small pulmonary emboli. What is the most appropriate next step?

   A. Preoperative radiation followed by surgical resection
   B. Anticoagulation and vena cava filter, followed by en bloc adrenalectomy and partial hepatectomy with resection of inferior vena cava tumor thrombus.
   C. Referral to palliative care
   D. Percutaneous FNA of the tumor, anticoagulation, and systemic chemotherapy; reconsideration for surgery if emboli resolve, hypercortisolism is controlled, and the tumor responds to systemic therapy

3. A 60-year-old man with a newly diagnosed sigmoid colon cancer discovered on screening colonoscopy has lymphadenopathy along the inferior mesenteric artery and an intermediate density and inhomogeneous 2 cm right adrenal mass on staging CT scan. His CEA is 6.0. There is no other evidence of disease. What is the most appropriate next step?

   A. Minimally invasive sigmoid colectomy and right adrenalectomy
   B. Percutaneous fine needle aspiration biopsy of the right adrenal mass
   C. Initiate chemotherapy with FOLFOX
   D. Biochemical evaluation including plasma metanephrines

4. All of the following are important principles of a retroperitoneoscopic adrenalectomy except:

   A. The inferior and lateral attachments of the adrenal gland are divided before the superior and medial attachments
   B. The inferior vena cava appears as a thin white line
   C. The retroperitoneal space is initially entered with a finger just lateral to the paraspinal muscles
   D. Gradual desufflation at the end of the case to visualize any bleeding that was tamponaded by high insufflation pressures

5. A 50-year-old woman presents with a heterogeneous, irregular 7-cm mass in the left adrenal gland that enhances with intravenous contrast and retains contrast on delayed images. There appears to be no involvement of adjacent organs. What is the recommended next step?

   A. Surgical resection via an open approach
   B. Fine needle aspiration biopsy
   C. Surgical resection via a laparoscopic transabdominal approach
   D. Neoadjuvant mitotane

Answers

1. **The correct answer is C.** *Rationale*: If recurrence of resected pheochromocytoma is suspected based on biochemical evaluation, a ^{68}Ga-DOTATATE PET or FDG PET is the most sensitive imaging test to evaluate for recurrence.

2. **The correct answer is D.** *Rationale:* For patients with borderline resectable adrenal cortical carcinoma, and especially in patients with associated potentially correctable comorbidities, we typically recommend neoadjuvant chemotherapy, which can help make subsequent surgery safer and more straightforward, including as in this case by shrinking the primary tumor and reducing the extent of vena cava tumor thrombus. Radiation is not typically used in the neoadjuvant setting but can be used for locoregional recurrence or as palliation for bone metastasis. Adrenal cortical carcinomas are typically large and often require multivisceral resection, but long-term survival is possible with complete surgical resection.

3. **The correct answer is D.** *Rationale:* In any patient with a newly diagnosed adrenal tumor, including a patient with another malignancy, pheochromocytoma should be ruled out first. While this patient may have an adrenal metastasis from his colorectal cancer, it is possible that the adrenal tumor represents a pheochromocytoma, which should be ruled out prior to either resection or biopsy.

4. **The correct answer is C.** *Rationale:* For a retroperitoneoscopic adrenalectomy, the patient is placed in the prone jackknife position on a Cloward table. The middle port site is positioned below the 12th rib. After digital entry into the retroperitoneal space at this site, the index finger is used to create a small space and guide the placement of first the medial (12 mm) and then the lateral (5 mm) trocars. Thus entry into the retroperitoneal space is most safely and conveniently obtained beneath the 12th rib, rather than just lateral to the paraspinal muscles. The medial trocar is placed approximately 5 cm medial to the middle trocar site, just lateral to the paraspinal muscles, and aimed slightly cephalad. The lateral trocar is placed approximately 5 cm lateral to the middle trocar site, beneath the 11th rib, and aimed medially and superiorly. A blunt 12-mm trocar with an inflatable balloon and an adjustable sleeve is then placed into the retroperitoneal space at the middle port site. Pneumoretroperitoneum is then created with CO_2 insufflation to a pressure of up to 24 mm Hg.

   A 30-degree 10-mm videoscope is first inserted through the middle port and then switched to the medial port, and the middle and lateral ports used as the working ports. Gerota fascia is entered and the superior pole of the kidney is identified. The psoas muscle, the posterior surface of the liver or spleen which is visible through the peritoneum, and the superior pole of the kidney serve as landmarks. On the right side, the inferior vena cava is a key landmark. The adrenal gland is allowed to retract superiorly with gentle downward retraction on the kidney. It is important to dissect the adrenal gland from the kidney before dividing the superior and medial attachments of the gland to minimize direct manipulation of the fragile adrenal gland and allow the gland to be suspended from its superior attachments until late in the procedure.

   On the left side, the adrenal vein drains inferiorly into the renal vein. On the right side, the adrenal vein is identified coursing medially to drain into the inferior vena cava. The inferior vena cava must be carefully identified. Due to high insufflation pressures, the vena cava loses its normal tubular appearance and its lateral border appears as a flat white line. The adrenal vein is dissected and divided between clips, while simultaneously retracting the gland on the distal side of the adrenal vein. The adrenal gland is then completely mobilized medially and superiorly. A retrieval bag is used to remove the specimen through the middle port site. Insufflation is gradually decreased to pressures of 8 to 12 mm Hg, facilitating visualization of any venous bleeding that may have been tamponaded by the high insufflation pressures. Ports are then removed, and the skin is closed with absorbable suture.

5. **The correct answer is A.** *Rationale*: The only potentially curative treatment for adrenal cortical carcinoma is complete surgical resection. Neoadjuvant combination chemotherapy can be considered for borderline resectable tumors with involvement of adjacent organs, but it is not typically given for patients with resectable tumors. Furthermore, the radiographic response rate to single agent mitotane for a primary adrenal cancer would be anticipated to be low. We continue to favor an open approach for suspected adrenal cortical carcinomas given the anticipated higher risk of fracture with minimally invasive approaches. A biopsy is not indicated in this case as it would not be expected to change management.

Recommended Readings

Primary Aldosteronism

Citton M, Viel G, Rossi GP, Mantero F, Nitti D, Iacobone M. Outcome of surgical treatment of primary aldosteronism. *Langenbecks Arch Surg*. 2015;400(3):325–331.

Funder JW, Carey RM, Mantero F, et al. The management of primary aldosteronism: case detection, diagnosis, and treatment: An Endocrine Society Clinical Practice Guideline. *J Clin Endocrinol Metab*. 2016;101(5):1889–1916.

Harvey A, Pasieka JL, Kline G, So B. Modification of the protocol for selective adrenal venous sampling results in both a significant increase in the accuracy and necessity of the procedure in the management of patients with primary hyperaldosteronism. *Surgery*. 2012;152(4):643–649; discussion 649–651.

Mathur A, Kemp CD, Dutta U, et al. Consequences of adrenal venous sampling in primary hyperaldosteronism and predictors of unilateral adrenal disease. *J Am Coll Surg*. 2010;211(3):384–390.

Oh EM, Lee KE, Yoon K, Kim SY, Kim HC, Youn YK. Value of adrenal venous sampling for lesion localization in primary aldosteronism. *World J Surg*. 2012;36(10):2522–2527.

Pasternak JD, Epelboym I, Seiser N, et al. Diagnostic utility of data from adrenal venous sampling for primary aldosteronism despite failed cannulation of the right adrenal vein. *Surgery*. 2016;159(1):267–273.

Pirvu A, Naem N, Baguet JP, Thony F, Chabre O, Chaffanjon P. Is adrenal venous sampling mandatory before surgical decision in case of primary hyperaldosteronism? *World J Surg*. 2014;38(7):1749–1754.

Sawka AM, Young WF, Thompson GB, et al. Primary aldosteronism: factors associated with normalization of blood pressure after surgery. *Ann Intern Med*. 2001;135(4):258–261.

Webb R, Mathur A, Chang R, et al. What is the best criterion for the interpretation of adrenal vein sample results in patients with primary hyperaldosteronism? *Ann Surg Oncol*. 2012;19(6):1881–1886.

Weigel RJ, Wells SA, Gunnells JC, Leight GS. Surgical treatment of primary hyperaldosteronism. *Ann Surg*. 1994;219(4):347–352.

Weinberger MH, Fineberg NS. The diagnosis of primary aldosteronism and separation of two major subtypes. *Arch Intern Med*. 1993;153(18):2125–2129.

Young WF, Stanson AW, Thompson GB, Grant CS, Farley DR, van Heerden JA. Role for adrenal venous sampling in primary aldosteronism. *Surgery*. 2004;136(6):1227–1235.

Cushing Syndrome

de La Villeon B, Bonnet S, Gouya H, et al. Long-term outcome after adrenalectomy for incidentally diagnosed subclinical cortisol-secreting adenomas. *Surgery*. 2016;160(2):397–404.

Iacobone M, Citton M, Viel G, et al. Adrenalectomy may improve cardiovascular and metabolic impairment and ameliorate quality of life in patients with adrenal incidentalomas and subclinical Cushing's syndrome. *Surgery*. 2012;152(6):991–997.

Morris LF, Harris RS, Milton DR, et al. Impact and timing of bilateral adrenalectomy for refractory adrenocorticotropic hormone-dependent Cushing's syndrome. *Surgery*. 2013;154(6):1174–1183; discussion 1183–1184.

Nieman LK, Biller BM, Findling JW, et al. The diagnosis of Cushing's syndrome: an Endocrine Society Clinical Practice Guideline. *J Clin Endocrinol Metab*. 2008;93(5):1526–1540.

Orth DN Cushing's syndrome. *N Engl J Med.* 1995;332(12):791–803.

Terzolo M, Pia A, Reimondo G. Subclinical Cushing's syndrome: definition and management. *Clin Endocrinol (Oxf).* 2012;76(1):12–18.

Pheochromocytoma

Agarwal A, Mehrotra PK, Jain M, et al. Size of the tumor and pheochromocytoma of the adrenal gland scaled score (PASS): can they predict malignancy? *World J Surg.* 2010;34(12):3022–3028.

Amar L, Bertherat J, Baudin E, et al. Genetic testing in pheochromocytoma or functional paraganglioma. *J Clin Oncol.* 2005;23(34):8812–8818.

Chang CA, Pattison DA, Tothill RW, et al. (68)Ga-DOTATATE and (18)F-FDG PET/CT in paraganglioma and pheochromocytoma: utility, patterns and heterogeneity. *Cancer Imaging.* 2016;16(1):22.

Chouaib S, Noman MZ, Kosmatopoulos K, Curran MA. Hypoxic stress: obstacles and opportunities for innovative immunotherapy of cancer. *Oncogene.* 2017;36(4):439–445.

Ellis RJ, Patel D, Prodanov T, et al. Response after surgical resection of metastatic pheochromocytoma and paraganglioma: can postoperative biochemical remission be predicted? *J Am Coll Surg.* 2013;217(3):489–496.

Fishbein L, Merrill S, Fraker DL, Cohen DL, Nathanson KL. Inherited mutations in pheochromocytoma and paraganglioma: why all patients should be offered genetic testing. *Ann Surg Oncol.* 2013;20(5):1444–1450.

Goffredo P, Adam MA, Thomas SM, Scheri RP, Sosa JA, Roman SA. Patterns of use and short-term outcomes of minimally invasive surgery for malignant pheochromocytoma: a population-level study. *World J Surg.* 2015;39(8):1966–1973.

Han S, Suh CH, Woo S, Kim YJ, Lee JJ. Performance of (68)Ga-DOTA-conjugated somatostatin receptor-targeting peptide PET in detection of pheochromocytoma and paraganglioma: a systematic review and metaanalysis. *J Nucl Med.* 2019;60(3):369–376.

Harari A, Inabnet WB. 3rd. Malignant pheochromocytoma: a review. *Am J Surg* 2011;201(5):700–708.

Iacobone M, Schiavi F, Bottussi M, et al. Is genetic screening indicated in apparently sporadic pheochromocytomas and paragangliomas? *Surgery.* 2011;150(6):1194–1201.

Jimenez C, Erwin W, Chasen B. Targeted radionuclide therapy for patients with metastatic pheochromocytoma and paraganglioma: from low-specific-activity to high-specific-activity Iodine-131 Metaiodobenzylguanidine. *Cancers (Basel).* 2019;11(7).

Kiernan CM, Solorzano CC. "Pheochromocytoma and paraganglioma: diagnosis, genetics, and treatment." *Surg Oncol Clin N Am.* 2016;25(1):119–138.

Kimura N, Takayanagi R, Takizawa N, et al. Pathological grading for predicting metastasis in phaeochromocytoma and paraganglioma. *Endocr Relat Cancer.* 2014;21:405–414

Koh JM, Ahn SH, Kim H, et al. Validation of pathological grading systems for predicting metastatic potential in pheochromocytoma and paraganglioma. *PLoS One.* 2017;12(11):e0187398.

Lee JE, Curley SA, Gagel RF, Evans DB, Hickey RC. Cortical-sparing adrenalectomy for patients with bilateral pheochromocytoma. *Surgery.* 1996;120(6):1064–1070; discussion 1070–1071.

Mittendorf EA, Evans DB, Lee JE, Perrier ND. Pheochromocytoma: advances in genetics, diagnosis, localization, and treatment. *Hematol Oncol Clin North Am.* 2007;21(3):509–525; ix.

Niemeijer ND, Alblas G, van Hulsteijn LT, Dekkers OM, Corssmit EP. Chemotherapy with cyclophosphamide, vincristine and dacarbazine for malignant paraganglioma and pheochromocytoma: systematic review and meta-analysis. *Clin Endocrinol (Oxf).* 2014;81(5):642–651.

O'Kane GM, Ezzat S, Joshua AM, et al. A phase 2 trial of sunitinib in patients with progressive paraganglioma or pheochromocytoma: the SNIPP trial. *Br J Cancer.* 2019;120(12):1113–1119.

Patel D, Phay JE, Yen TWF, et al. Update on pheochromocytoma and paraganglioma from the SSO Endocrine/ Head and Neck Disease-Site Work Group. Part 1 of 2: advances in pathogenesis and diagnosis of pheochromocytoma and paraganglioma. *Ann Surg Oncol.* 2020;27(5):1329–1337.

Pederson LC, Lee JE. Pheochromocytoma. *Curr Treat Options Oncol.* 2003;4(4):329–337.

Press D, Akyuz M, Dural C, et al. Predictors of recurrence in pheochromocytoma. *Surgery.* 2014;156(6):1523–1527; discussion 1527–1528.

Pryma DA, Chin BB, Noto RB, et al. Efficacy and safety of high-specific-activity (131)I-MIBG therapy in patients with advanced pheochromocytoma or paraganglioma. *J Nucl Med.* 2019;60(5):623–630.

Rana HQ, Rainville IR, Vaidya A. Genetic testing in the clinical care of patients with pheochromocytoma and paraganglioma. *Curr Opin Endocrinol Diabetes Obes.* 2014;21(3):166–176.

Timmers HJ, Chen CC, Carrasquillo JA, et al. Staging and functional characterization of pheochromocytoma and paraganglioma by 18F-fluorodeoxyglucose (18F-FDG) positron emission tomography. *J Natl Cancer Inst.* 2012;104(9):700–708.

Yip L, Lee JE, Shapiro SE, et al. Surgical management of hereditary pheochromocytoma. *J Am Coll Surg.* 2004;198(4):525–534; discussion 534–535.

Adrenocortical Masses and Carcinoma

Agcaoglu O, Sahin DA, Siperstein A, Berber E. Selection algorithm for posterior versus lateral approach in laparoscopic adrenalectomy. *Surgery.* 2012;151(5):731–735.

Asare EA, Wang TS, Winchester DP, Mallin K, Kebebew E, Sturgeon C. A novel staging system for adrenocortical carcinoma better predicts survival in patients with stage I/II disease. *Surgery.* 2014;156(6):1378–1386.

Asari R, Koperek O, Niederle B. Endoscopic adrenalectomy in large adrenal tumors. *Surgery.* 2012;152(1):41–49.

Barczyński M, Konturek A, Nowak W. Randomized clinical trial of posterior retroperitoneoscopic adrenalectomy versus lateral transperitoneal laparoscopic adrenalectomy with a 5-year follow-up. *Ann Surg.* 2014;260(5):740–747; discussion 747–748.

Bednarski BK, Habra MA, Phan A, et al. "Borderline resectable adrenal cortical carcinoma: a potential role for preoperative chemotherapy." *World J Surg.* 2014;38(6):1318–1327.

Birsen O, Akyuz M, Dural C, et al. A new risk stratification algorithm for the management of patients with adrenal incidentalomas. *Surgery.* 2014;156(4):959–965.

Carneiro BA, Konda B, Costa RB, et al. Nivolumab in metastatic adrenocortical carcinoma: results of a phase 2 trial. *J Clin Endocrinol Metab.* 2019;104(12):6193–6200.

Cooper AB, Habra MA, Grubbs EG, et al. Does laparoscopic adrenalectomy jeopardize oncologic outcomes for patients with adrenocortical carcinoma? *Surg Endosc.* 2013;27(11):4026–4032.

Delivanis DA, Erickson D, Atwell TD, et al. Procedural and clinical outcomes of percutaneous adrenal biopsy in a high risk population for adrenal malignancy. *Clin Endocrinol (Oxf).* 2016;85:710–716.

Dickson PV, Jimenez C, Chisholm GB, et al. Posterior retroperitoneoscopic adrenalectomy: a contemporary American experience. *J Am Coll Surg.* 2011;212(4):659–665; discussion 665–667.

Donatini G, Caiazzo R, Do Cao C, et al. Long-term survival after adrenalectomy for stage I/II adrenocortical carcinoma (ACC): a retrospective comparative cohort study of laparoscopic versus open approach. *Ann Surg Oncol.* 2014;21(1):284–291.

Dy BM, Strajina V, Cayo AK, et al. Surgical resection of synchronously metastatic adrenocortical cancer. *Ann Surg Oncol.* 2015;22(1):146–151.

Dy BM, Wise KB, Richards ML, et al. Operative intervention for recurrent adrenocortical cancer. *Surgery.* 2013;154(6):1292–1299.

Eichhorn-Wharry LI, Talpos GB, Rubinfeld I. Laparoscopic versus open adrenalectomy: another look at outcome using the Clavien classification system. *Surgery.* 2012;152(6):1090–1095.

Fassnacht M, Arlt W, Bancos I, et al. Management of adrenal incidentalomas: European Society of Endocrinology Clinical Practice Guideline in collaboration with the European Network for the Study of Adrenal Tumors. *Eur J Endocrinol.* 2016;175(2):G1–G34.

Fassnacht M, Kroiss M, Allolio B. Update in adrenocortical carcinoma. *J Clin Endocrinol Metab.* 2013;98(12):4551–4564.

Fassnacht M, Terzolo M, Allolio B, et al. Combination chemotherapy in advanced adrenocortical carcinoma. *N Eng J Med.* 2012;366(23):2189–2197.

Gaujoux S, Al-Ahmadie H, Allen PJ, et al. Resection of adrenocortical carcinoma liver metastasis: is it justified? *Ann Surg Oncol.* 2012;19(8):2643–2651.

Gaujoux S, Brennan ME. Recommendation for standardized surgical management of primary adrenocortical carcinoma. *Surgery.* 2012;152(1):123–132.

Grubbs EG, Callender GG, Xing Y, et al. Recurrence of adrenal cortical carcinoma following resection: surgery alone can achieve results equal to surgery plus mitotane. *Ann Surg Oncol.* 2010;17(1):263–270.

Habra MA, Stephen B, Campbell M, et al. Phase II clinical trial of pembrolizumab efficacy and safety in advanced adrenocortical carcinoma. *J Immunother Cancer.* 2019;7(1):253.

Hahner S, Kreissl MC, Fassnacht M, et al. [131I]iodometomidate for targeted radionuclide therapy of advanced adrenocortical carcinoma. *J Clin Endocrinol Metab.* 2012;97(3):914–922.

Hauch A, Al-Qurayshi Z, Kandil E. Factors associated with higher risk of complications after adrenal surgery. *Ann Surg Oncol.* 2015;22(1):103–110.

Henning JEK, Deutschbein T, Altieri B, Steinhauer S, Kircher S, Sbiera S, et al. Gemcitabine-based chemotherapy in adrenocortical carcinoma: a multicenter study of efficacy and predictive factors. *J Clin Endocrinol Metab.* 2017;102(11):4323–4332.

Howell GM, Carty SE, Armstrong MJ, et al. Outcome and prognostic factors after adrenalectomy for patients with distant adrenal metastasis. *Ann Surg Oncol.* 2013;20(11):3491–3496.

Kazaure HS, Roman SA, Sosa JA. Adrenalectomy in older Americans has increased morbidity and mortality: an analysis of 6,416 patients. *Ann Surg Oncol.* 2011;18(10):2714–2721.

Kim Y, Margonis GA, Prescott JD, et al. Curative surgical resection of adrenocortical carcinoma: determining long-term outcome based on conditional disease-free probability. *Ann Surg.* 2017;265(1):197–204.

Kim Y, Margonis GA, Prescott JD, et al. Nomograms to predict recurrence-free and overall survival after curative resection of adrenocortical carcinoma. *JAMA Surg.* 2016;151(4):365–373.

Kroiss M, Quinkler M, Johanssen S, et al. Sunitinib in refractory adrenocortical carcinoma: a phase II, single-arm, open-label trial. *J Clin Endocrinol Metab.* 2012;97(10):3495–3503.

Kuritzkes B, Parikh M, Melamed J, Hindman N, Pachter HL. False-positive rate of positron emission tomography/computed tomography for presumed solitary metastatic adrenal disease in patients with known malignancy. *Ann Surg Oncol.* 2015;22(2):437–440.

Lang BHH, Cowling BJ, Li JYY, Wong KP, Wan KY. High false positivity in positron emission tomography is a potential diagnostic pitfall in patients with suspected adrenal metastasis. *World J Surg.* 2015;39(8):1902–1908.

Lee JE. Adjuvant mitotane in adrenocortical carcinoma. *N Engl J Med.* 2007;357(12):1258; author reply 1259.

Lee JE, Berger DH, el-Naggar AK, et al. Surgical management, DNA content, and patient survival in adrenal cortical carcinoma. *Surgery.* 1995;118(6):1090–1098.

Lee JE, Evans DB, Hickey RC, et al. Unknown primary cancer presenting as an adrenal mass: frequency and implications for diagnostic evaluation of adrenal incidentalomas. *Surgery.* 1998;124(6):1115–1122.

Le Tourneau C, Hoimes C, Zarwan C, et al. Avelumab in patients with previously treated metastatic adrenocortical carcinoma: phase 1b results from the JAVELIN solid tumor trial. *J Immunother Cancer.* 2018;6(1):111.

Liu-Chittenden Y, Jain M, Kumar P, et al. Phase I trial of systemic intravenous infusion of interleukin-13-Pseudomonas exotoxin in patients with metastatic adrenocortical carcinoma. *Cancer Med.* 2015;4(7):1060–1068.

Livhits M, Li N, Yeh MW, Harari A. Surgery is associated with improved survival for adrenocortical cancer, even in metastatic disease. *Surgery.* 2014;156(6):1531–1541.

Miller BS, Gauger PG, Hammer GD, Doherty GM. Resection of adrenocortical carcinoma is less complete and local recurrence occurs sooner and more often after laparoscopic adrenalectomy than after open adrenalectomy. *Surgery.* 2012;152(6):1150–1156.

Mir MC, Klink JC, Guillotreau J, et al. Comparative outcomes of laparoscopic and open adrenalectomy for adrenocortical carcinoma: single, high-volume center experience. *Ann Surg Oncol.* 2013;20(5):1456–1461.

Moreno P, Basarrate AD, Musholt TJ, et al. Adrenalectomy for solid tumor metastases: results of a multicenter European study. *Surgery.* 2013;154(6):1215–1222.

Naing A, Meric-Bernstam F, Stephen B, et al. Phase 2 study of pembrolizumab in patients with advanced rare cancers. *J Immunother Cancer.* 2020;8(1).

Nigri G, Rosman AS, Petrucciani N, et al. Meta-analysis of trials comparing laparoscopic transperitoneal and retroperitoneal adrenalectomy. *Surgery.* 2013;153(1):111–119.

Nilubol N, Patel D, Kebebew E. Does lymphadenectomy improve survival in patients with adrenocortical carcinoma? A population-based study. *World J Surg.* 2016;40(3):697–705.

Postlewait LM, Ethun CG, Tran TB, et al. Outcomes of adjuvant mitotane after resection of adrenocortical carcinoma: A 13-Institution Study by the US Adrenocortical Carcinoma Group. *J Am Coll Surg.* 2016;222(4): 480–490.

Raj N, Zheng Y, Kelly V, et al. PD-1 blockade in advanced adrenocortical carcinoma. *J Clin Oncol* 2019:JCO1901586.

Reibetanz J, Jurowich C, Erdogan I, et al. Impact of lymphadenectomy on the oncologic outcome of patients with adrenocortical carcinoma. *Ann Surg.* 2012;255(2):363–369.

Sancho JJ, Triponez F, Montet X, Sitges-Serra A. Surgical management of adrenal metastases. *Langenbecks Arch Surg.* 2012;397(2):179–194.

Strong VE, D'Angelica M, Tang L, et al. Laparoscopic adrenalectomy for isolated adrenal metastasis. *Ann Surg Oncol.* 2007;14(12):3392–3400.

Suman P, Calcatera N, Wang CH, Moo-Young TA, Winchester DJ, Prinz RA. Preoperative adrenal biopsy does not affect overall survival in adrenocortical carcinoma. *Am J Surg.* 2017;214(4):748–751.

Terzolo M, Angeli A, Fassnacht M, et al. Adjuvant mitotane treatment for adrenocortical carcinoma. *N Engl J Med.* 2007;356(23):2372–2380.

Terzolo M, Stigliano A, Chiodini I, et al. Italian Association of Clinical Endocrinologists. AME position statement on adrenal incidentaloma. *Eur J Endocrinol.* 2011;164(6):851–870.

Vazquez BJ, Richards ML, Lohse CM, et al. Adrenalectomy improves outcomes of selected patients with metastatic carcinoma. *World J Surg.* 2012;36(6):1400–1405.

Walz MK, Alesina PF, Wenger FA, et al. Posterior retroperitoneoscopic adrenalectomy—results of 560 procedures in 520 patients. *Surgery.* 2006;140(6):943–948; discussion 948–950.

Wang TS, Cheung K, Roman SA, Sosa JA. A cost-effectiveness analysis of adrenalectomy for nonfunctional adrenal incidentalomas: is there a size threshold for resection? *Surgery.* 2012;152(6):1125–1132.

Young WF, Jr. Clinical practice. The incidentally discovered adrenal mass. *N Engl J Med.* 2007;356(6):601–610.

18

Carcinoma of the Thyroid Gland and Neoplasms of the Parathyroid Glands

Aditya S. Shirali and Elizabeth G. Grubbs

Thyroid Gland

Introduction

Thyroid cancer is the most common endocrine malignancy and represented the most rapidly increasing cancer diagnosis worldwide in 2016. After 30 years of rising incidence rates in differentiated thyroid cancer (DTC), particularly papillary thyroid cancer (PTC), these rates peaked in 2015 at 14.9 per 100,000, and between 2015 and 2017, a decline was observed for the first time in three decades. Although the observed increase in thyroid cancer incidence is thought to be due, in large part, to "overdiagnosis" of small microcarcinomas (<1 cm) from the increased use of imaging and diagnostic tests, data from the past decade suggest an increasing incidence of both low-risk thyroid cancer that cannot be explained by overdiagnosis alone as well as advanced-stage PTC with concomitant increase in incidence-based mortality. Patients with DTC usually have an excellent long-term prognosis, with 5-year survival rates approaching 100% for localized disease.

The diagnosis, management, and surveillance of malignant thyroid disease are evolving as consensus guidelines continue to be published regarding extent of surgical resection, role of lymphadenectomy, and adjuvant medical therapies for thyroid cancer. Significant advances in the fields of molecular and genetic testing and targeted therapies have offered new avenues for the management of advanced disease.

Pathology

Thyroid cancers are categorized by the cell of origin. Those derived from follicular cells are well-differentiated thyroid cancer, broadly categorized as PTC, follicular cancer (FTC) and Hürthle cell cancer (HCC), poorly differentiated thyroid cancer (PDTC) and anaplastic thyroid cancer (ATC). DTC makes up greater than 95% of thyroid cancer diagnosed each year with the most common subtype being PTC. Medullary thyroid cancer (MTC) is derived from the parafollicular or C cell. Rare primary tumors of the thyroid gland can include lymphoma, squamous cell carcinoma and sarcoma. In addition, the thyroid may serve as a metastatic site for other malignancies (most commonly renal cell, lung, or breast). Table 18.1 lists the various categories of thyroid carcinomas.

PTC affects people with a peak incidence in the third and fourth decades and a female predominance (3:1). It is the predominate histology seen in patients exposed to ionizing radiation. Microscopically, PTC is characterized by papillary architecture, calcifications, psammoma bodies, and large overlapping nuclei that are optically clear, known as Orphan Annie nuclei. The classical variant makes up 75% to 80% of PTC variants. Histopathologic variants include follicular-variant PTC (FVPTC), which include infiltrative (or nonencapsulated) and encapsulated (EFVPTC), along with the hobnail, tall cell, columnar morular, diffuse sclerosing and solid variants that are associated with more aggressive clinical behavior (Table 18.1). In 2016, EFVPTC that is characterized by lack of capsular or vascular invasion was reclassified as a nonmalignant entity and called "noninvasive follicular thyroid neoplasm with papillary-like nuclear features" (NIFTP). PTC is characterized by multifocality in up to 80% of patients and is associated with an increased risk of lymph node metastasis (30% to 80% cervical lymph node metastasis). Despite the high incidence of lymph node metastases, the 10-year survival rate is still 85%.

Follicular thyroid cancer is the second most common thyroid cancer which represents approximately 10% to 15% of all thyroid malignancies. These tumors are most common in the fifth decade of life, similar to PTC, such as PTC, have a female predominance with a 3:1 ratio. FTCs are usually unifocal, well-encapsulated lesions containing highly cellular follicles, and are easily confused with benign follicular adenomas on FNA. Pathologic diagnosis of this malignancy can only be made by permanent sectioning and is categorized by capsular and vascular invasion. The 2017 World Health Organization (WHO) Classification groups FTC into minimally invasive (capsular invasion only), grossly encapsulated, angioinvasive and widely invasive FTC. While metastasis to the cervical lymph nodes is uncommon and found in 5% to 10% of cases at initial presentation, distant disease may be seen in 10% to 33% of patients, most often with hematologic spread to the lungs or bone. Ten-year disease-free survival rates of 97% to 98% have been reported for minimally invasive FTC and <50% for widely invasive FTC.

Pathologic Classification of Thyroid Malignancies	
Subtype	**Variants/Classifications**
Well-Differentiated	
Papillary (80%)	Conventional
	FVPTC: infiltrative and invasive EFVPTC
	Tall Cell
	Hobnail
	Diffuse sclerosing
	Cribiform morular
	Columnar cell
Follicular (10%)	Minimally invasive
	Grossly encapsulated angioinvasive
	Widely invasive
Hürthle cell (5%)	Minimally invasive
	Grossly encapsulated angioinvasive
	Widely invasive
Medullary	
Poorly Differentiated	
Anaplastic	
Other	Lymphoma
	Metastatic

FVPTC, follicular-variant papillary thyroid carcinoma; EFVPTC, encapsulated follicular-variant papillary thyroid carcinoma.

Hürthle cell carcinoma, previously described as a variant of FTC, is now considered distinct from FTC due to its unique mutational profile. HCCs are characterized by the presence of oncocytic cells, abundant eosinophilic granular cytoplasm and hyperchromatic nuclei. Classification of invasion for HCC is similar to the 2017 WHO Classification for FTC. HCC may have a higher risk for local recurrence and be less iodine-avid than FTC. Ten-year survival for HCC is lower than FTC at 76% versus 85%.

MTC represents less than 5% of all thyroid malignancies and is distinguished from DTCs by its origin from calcitonin-producing parafollicular C cells of the thyroid neuroendocrine-type cells. Although the majority of MTC cases are sporadic, approximately 25% are hereditary due to germline alterations in the *RET* proto-oncogene, which gives rise to multiple endocrine neoplasia (MEN) type 2 syndrome (Table 18.2). MEN2 is covered in Chapter 16 (Pancreatic Endocrine Tumors and Multiple Endocrine Neoplasia). When associated with familial syndromes, MTC presents in the third to fourth decades of life and is frequently multifocal. Sporadic MTC, on the other hand, tends to present slightly later and is most commonly unifocal in nature. These tumors tend to be localized to the upper poles of the thyroid gland where the C cells reside. The presence of C-cell hyperplasia is thought to be a harbinger for the development of hereditary MTC. Tumor cells often possess round or oval regular nuclei with nonprominent nucleoli and scant mitotic figures. The important immunohistochemical markers used to identify MTC are calcitonin and carcinoembryonic antigen (CEA). Patients with MTC confined to the thyroid and/or cervical lymph nodes and with low levels of postoperative

Hereditary Syndromes Associated with Increased Risk of Thyroid Cancer		
Syndrome	**Susceptibility Genes**	**Thyroid Cancer**
Cowden syndrome	*PTEN*	PTC, FV-PTC, FTC
Carney complex type 1	*PRKAR1a*	PTC, FTC
DICER1 syndrome	*DICER1*	FV-PTC, FTC
Familial adenomatous polyposis	*APC*	PTC FV-PTC, CMV-PTC
Werner syndrome	*WRN*	PTC, FTC, ATC
Multiple endocrine neoplasia 2A and 2B	*RET*	MTC

PTC, papillary thyroid carcinoma; FV-PTC, follicular variant papillary thyroid carcinoma; FTC, follicular thyroid carcinoma; CMV-PTC, cribiform morular variant papillary thyroid carcinoma; ATC, anaplastic thyroid carcinoma; MTC, medullary thyroid carcinoma.

tumor markers have excellent prognoses, with >90% 10-year disease-specific survival (DSS). In patients with advanced MTC, progression most commonly involves the liver, lungs, and bone. Overall, the 10-year DSS rate in patients with stage IV MTC is less than 30%.

PDTCs are heterogeneous, advanced thyroid cancers with a higher risk of relapse and higher mortality. PDTCs occupy a morphologically intermediate position between DTC and ATC. The Turin classification of PDTC is that of a solid, insular, or trabecular growth pattern lacking papillary nuclear features with mitoses and/or necrosis. Patients with PDTCs experience frequent locally invasive disease in the trachea and/or esophagus as well as distant progression to the lungs, liver, bone and brain.

ATC represents only 1% of all thyroid cancers but accounts for 40% of thyroid cancer death due to its alarmingly aggressive features. The peak incidence is in the seventh decade of life, and survival is very poor with 25% survival at 1 year. Microscopically, ATCs are described as high-grade cancers and are often composed of giant cells or cells with squamous-like features with high levels of mitosis and necrosis. These histologic features may lead to a nondiagnostic FNA and require a core biopsy to secure a diagnosis. At presentation, 90% will have regional metastases and 50% will have distant spread, most commonly to the lungs. ATC is the most aggressive of any human malignancy. Death due to asphyxiation caused by a rapidly progressing primary tumor may be prevented with emergent and aggressive multimodal therapies with or without primary tumor resection. While previously surgery rarely played a role in definitive management of ATC, the emergence of targeted systemic therapies have increased the role of surgery for potentially curative purposes.

Primary thyroid lymphoma (PTL), most commonly non-Hodgkin lymphomas of B-cell origin, comprises <5% of thyroid malignancies and <2% of extranodal lymphomas. PTL is seen more frequently in women and particularly in those with a history of Hashimoto thyroiditis. This disease may present with a rapidly growing mass, dysphagia, or dysphonia and may be confused with ATC. The role of surgical intervention is limited for diagnostically challenging cases. Definitive therapy involves chemotherapy and radiation.

Genetics and Molecular Markers

Over the past two decades, next-generation, high-throughput deep sequencing genomic interrogations of thyroid cancer have generated comprehensive molecular signatures of the major thyroid cancer subtypes. The varying molecular signatures identified in each major thyroid cancer subtype likely accounts for the range of biologic behavior observed among thyroid cancers. Investigators with The Cancer Genome Atlas (TCGA) examined nearly 500 PTCs and demonstrated that nonoverlapping alterations within the MAPK (MAPK kinase [MEK]/ERK) signaling pathway dominate, with point mutations in *BRAF* (60%) and *RAS* (10%), as well as *RET* fusions (5%) contributing to approximately 80% of the known alterations in PTCs. A constitutive activation of the BRAF kinase, usually from a V600E amino acid substitution, results in potent downstream phosphorylation of MEK/ERK that results in thyroid tumorigenesis and activation of thyroid-specific genes that impact responses to therapy in patients with advanced disease. In a minority of PTCs without MAPK pathway alterations, mutations in *EIF1AX* and fusions within *PPARγ, NTRK1/3,* and *THADA* may be found in well-differentiated PTCs.

Oncogenic drivers in FTC are primarily *RAS* point mutations and *PAX8-PPARγ* rearrangements. *Ras* mutations (*H-, K-, N-Ras*) were identified in 66% of advanced FTCs, with mutations in *NRAS* being the most frequent subtype. *PAX8-PPARγ* fusions may be found in 30% to 40% of FTCs. FTCs also demonstrate enrichment in *TERT* alterations, similar to those observed in advanced PTCs and PDTCs, as well as *PTEN* mutations and *RB1* mutations. Mutations in *Ras* may result in allelic loss or in chromosomal rearrangements leading to increased rates of FTC formation. Chromosomal instability occurs in up to 65% of FTC, including extra copies, unbalanced rearrangements, complex karyotypes and chromosomal losses.

Two large comprehensive data sets have clearly demonstrated that HCC is a distinct clinicopathologic subtype of thyroid cancer. HCCs harbor a high frequency of mitochondrial DNA mutations along with duplications of chromosomes 5 and 7 and widespread loss of heterozygosity. Interestingly, HCCs do not harbor *BRAF* alterations, whereas 10% harbor *NRAS* alterations. Similar to other advanced thyroid cancers, 22% of advanced or widely invasive HCCs contain *TERT* promoter mutations. Alterations within the PI3K/AKT/mTOR pathways play a dominant role in driving HCC-related tumorigenesis and may also serve as therapeutic targets for the treatment of advanced disease.

The *RET* proto-oncogene is a tyrosine kinase receptor that is mainly expressed in tumors of neural crest origin, explaining the high incidence of *RET* mutations in MTC which originate from the C cells. *RET* mutations are present in >95% of hereditary MTC. Germline *RET* 634 and 918 point mutations give rise to MEN2A and MEN2B syndromes, respectively, with 100% penetrance of MTC. Screening for germline *RET* mutations has been invaluable in the early identification of patients who have a genetic basis for their disease. Even in patients with suspected sporadic MTC, 6% to 10% of these patients will have a *RET* proto-oncogene germline mutation, revealing a new kindred of patients with previously diagnosed MTC. Mutational analysis of sporadic MTC has found alterations in *RET* and *Ras* in 40% and 15% of patients, respectively.

Next-generation sequencing studies of PDTCs and ATCs have given evidence suggesting that DTC may progress to PDTC and ATC. Similar to PTC, alterations in oncogenic *BRAF* (35% to 40%), *RAS* (18% to 27%), and *RET* fusions dominate the genomic landscape in PDTCs and ATCs. In addition, mutations within *TERT* and *TP53* are highly enriched in ATCs, present in 65% to 75% of cases, and are frequently absent in well-differentiated low-risk tumors. This observation suggests that *TERT* and *TP53* mutations play a role later in thyroid tumor pathogenesis, specifically in the dedifferentiating transition to the anaplastic phenotype. Mutations in other tumor suppressors, such as *MEN1, RB1,* and *ATM,* have been identified at higher frequencies in ATCs, highlighting the involvement of multiple other pathways in the process of dedifferentiation.

Diagnosis
Clinical Presentation
Thyroid nodules are most frequently diagnosed incidentally by cervical imaging performed for unrelated reasons or identified during routine physical examination. The prevalence of thyroid nodules identified by palpation is estimated to be approximately 5% with up to 10 times more identified by imaging studies. High-resolution ultrasound can detect thyroid nodules in up to 68% of randomly selected individuals. With the increasing use of positron emission tomography (PET) during cancer staging and surveillance, FDG-avid thyroid nodules are increasingly being identified with an estimated malignancy rate of 30% to 40%.

Patients may seek treatment for symptoms of a palpable neck mass or compressive symptoms, such as hoarseness, dysphagia, or dyspnea. Significant compressive symptoms, odynophagia or hemoptysis may result from local invasion and suggest aggressive pathology. Particular attention to a prior history of ionizing radiation exposure, family history of thyroid or other endocrine malignancies (including familial syndromes associated with thyroid cancer, Table 18.2), or prior neck surgeries should be noted in the initial clinical encounter. Examination for any palpable cervical adenopathy, particularly along the mid to lower jugular chains, serves as an adjunct to high-resolution ultrasound imaging. The degree of neck extension should be evaluated prior to any surgical planning, as should vocal cord function. If a patient has any history of prior neck surgery or hoarseness, flexible laryngoscopy or videostroboscopy should be performed to evaluate vocal fold mobility.

Radiographic Studies and Fine Needle Aspiration
Radiographic evaluation of the thyroid gland and the central and lateral cervical compartments is an essential part of the workup for a thyroid nodule. Radiographic studies included in the initial workup of thyroid cancer usually include ultrasonography and computed tomography (CT) with intravenous contrast. Ultrasonography is the preferred modality during initial workup for thyroid cancer. The objectives of diagnostic ultrasound are to assess the nodule or tumor size, location, and suspicious features, and to identify and characterize abnormal lymph nodes in the central and lateral neck which may be involved in thyroid cancer. Neck CT with intravenous contrast may be performed if ultrasound demonstrates features concerning for local invasion or to further characterize bulky adenopathy, including if there is a concern for mediastinal involvement that is not well visualized by ultrasound.

Fine needle aspiration (FNA) and biopsy of nodules with suspicious sonographic features should be performed to exclude the presence of malignancy. The 2015 American Thyroid Association (ATA) Guidelines recommend FNA biopsy based on the size and sonographic appearance of nodules (Fig. 18.1). Similarly, the American College of Radiology published the Thyroid Imaging, Reporting and Data System (TI-RADS) which uses nodule composition, echogenicity, shape, margin and echogenic foci to assign a predictive score from TR1 to TR5 to guide decision-making regarding FNA. Taken together, these guidelines are used to direct FNA of suspicious-appearing thyroid nodules in order to determine if there is evidence of malignancy.

FNA provides direct diagnostic information on a lesion and is an invaluable tool, however it needs to be performed by experienced clinicians. The accuracy of FNA to diagnose a thyroid malignancy can be as high as 90% with a false-negative rate of less than 5% when performed by an experienced clinician and evaluated by an experienced cytopathologist. FNA has the greatest accuracy for lesions that are 1 to 4 cm, as smaller and larger lesions have a greater chance of sampling error. In addition to the use of FNA for cytologic assessment of thyroid nodules, FNA should be used for suspicious central and lateral neck adenopathy to help guide extent of surgery. Any suspicious central or lateral neck adenopathy should be biopsied to determine whether patients require therapeutic central or lateral neck dissection. For nondiagnostic FNAs, samples should be sent for thyroglobulin washout or calcitonin to assess for the presence of metastatic DTC or MTC, respectively.

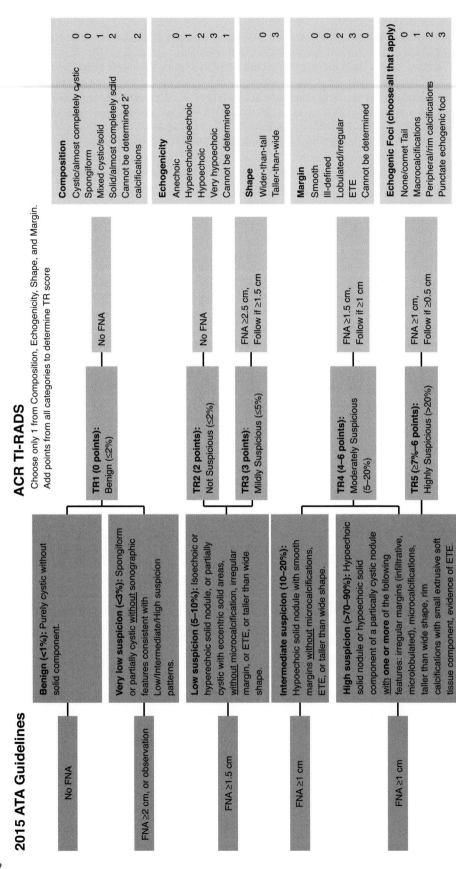

FIGURE 18.1 Comparison of the American Thyroid Association 2015 Guidelines and American College of Radiology 2017 TI-RADS Classification System for recommending Fine Needle Aspiration of Thyroid Nodules. (Reprinted with permission from Patel KN, Yip L, Lubitz CC, et al. The American Association of Endocrine Surgeons guidelines for the definitive surgical management of thyroid disease in adults. *Ann Surg.* 2020;271:e1-e93.)

TABLE 18.3	The Bethesda System for Reporting Thyroid Cytology		

Category		Clinical Management	Proposed Risk of NIFTP or Malignancy
I	Nondiagnostic	Repeat FNA with US guidance	5–10%
II	Benign	Clinical follow-up	0–3%
III	Follicular lesion/atypia of undetermined significance	Observation, with or without molecular testing, and/or lobectomy	6–18%
IV	Follicular neoplasm/suspicious for follicular neoplasm	Lobectomy, with molecular testing and or observation employed in select situations	10–40%
V	Suspicious for malignancy	Lobectomy or total thyroidectomy[a]	45–60%
VI	Malignant	Lobectomy or total thyroidectomy[a]	94–96%

FNA, fine needle aspiration; US, ultrasound.
[a]Based on tumor size, histopathologic characteristics, and potential need for adjuvant radioactive iodine therapy.
Adapted with permission from Patel KN, Yip L, Lubitz CC, et al. The American Association of endocrine surgeons guidelines for the definitive surgical management of thyroid disease in adults. *Ann Surg.* 2020;271:e21–e93.

Cytologic Assessment

FNA cytology results should be reported using the Bethesda System for Reporting Thyroid Cytopathology, a consensus recommendation created from the National Cancer Institute State of the Science Conference in 2007 that was most recently updated in 2017. As described in Table 18.3, the system describes six diagnostic categories and an estimation of cancer risk for each lesion. These classifications include: nondiagnostic (I), benign (II), follicular lesion of undetermined significance/atypia of undetermined significance (including Hürthle cell lesion, III), follicular neoplasm/suspicious for follicular neoplasm (including Hürthle cell neoplasm, IV), suspicious for malignancy (V), and malignant (VI). The recent reclassification of some neoplasms as NIFTP, which requires surgical excision for diagnosis, has altered the risk of malignancy for all cytology categories and resulted in malignancy risk being reported either with or without NIFTP. Importantly, true rates of malignancy are institution-specific and dependent on the experience of the physician performing the FNA as well as the cytopathologist interpreting the specimen.

The risk of malignancy for a specimen categorized as "benign" on FNA is <1% while those labeled "malignant" have close to 100% risk of malignancy. Nodules that are categorized as Bethesda III, IV, and V are considered cytologically indeterminate and require a combination of clinical decision making, knowledge of malignancy and patient preference to guide management. Bethesda III lesions have a 6% to 18% risk of malignancy and may undergo repeat FNA with or without molecular testing (discussed later), which leads to a more definitive reclassification in 60% to 65% of nodules, or diagnostic lobectomy in the event of suspicious sonographic findings. Bethesda IV lesions have a 10% to 40% risk of malignancy and usual management involves either molecular testing or surgical intervention. Bethesda V lesions have a 45% to 60% risk of malignancy and routinely undergo thyroid lobectomy or total thyroidectomy.

Although PTC, MTC, PDTC, and ATC can often by diagnosed by FNA or core biopsy, the distinction between FTC/HCC and a follicular/Hürthle cell adenoma requires the ability to determine the presence of vascular or capsular invasion. This cannot be achieved with FNA alone and usually requires diagnostic thyroid lobectomy in order to ascertain whether malignancy is present. Intraoperative frozen section evaluation of follicular neoplasms at the time of lobectomy is usually not definitive and we do not recommend this practice due to the high rate of false-negative results.

Molecular Testing

Molecular testing helps refine the cancer risk of cytologically indeterminate thyroid nodules to guide surgical decision making. Multiple molecular panels, which use gene expression classification with or without additional evaluation for specific mutations or fusions associated with thyroid cancer, are commercially available. The two most commonly used tests in the United States currently are Afirma and Thyroseq. The Afirma Gene Sequencing Classifier (GSC, Veracyte, South San Francisco, CA) assesses mRNA expression and uses machine learning to provide a binary result—either benign or suspicious. In addition to its original assay (The Afirma Gene Expression Classifier), which assesses the expression of 167 genes, the GSC has added cassettes to aid in the detection of follicular and Hürthle cell neoplasms, RET fusion transcripts, BRAF[V600E] mRNA, MTC, and parathyroid tissue, which has resulted in improved sensitivity (91%) and specificity (68%) with an overall cancer prevalence of 20%. Thyroseq v3 (CBLPath, Rye Brook, NY) uses next-generation sequencing to test specific oncogenic mutations and five classes of molecular alterations: point mutations, insertions/deletions, copy number variations, gene fusions, and gene expression variations. Unlike Afirma GSC, which provides a binary result, Thyroseq v3 reports specific mutation profiles with numeric risks of malignancy. Multi-institution validation has shown improved sensitivity (94%) and specificity (82%) when compared to prior versions. When the need for thyroidectomy is unclear after consideration of clinical, imaging and cytologic features, molecular testing may be considered as a diagnostic adjunct for cytologically indeterminate nodules.

Treatment

Surgical resection, in the form of thyroid lobectomy or total thyroidectomy with or without lymph node dissection, should be considered once a thyroid malignancy is definitively diagnosed or for cytologically indeterminate thyroid nodules. The initial extent of surgery for thyroid cancer or cytologically indeterminate nodules is determined by multiple factors including primary etiology, presence of contralateral nodular disease, comorbidities, family history, surgical risk and patient preferences. Appropriate surgical treatment will allow careful postoperative screening and adjuvant therapies, if necessary, and minimizes the chance of disease recurrence.

Papillary thyroid carcinomas ≤1 cm may be considered for active surveillance in a selected group of patients. Active surveillance, which involves serial physical examination, ultrasound, and laboratory assessment may be considered in patients with PTCs <1 cm located away from vital structures without evidence of extrathyroidal extension (ETE) or lymph node involvement in patients who wished to avoid surgery. Although studies in North America have showed tumor growth in 3.8% of patients over 25 months with no regional or distant metastases in patients undergoing active surveillance, the oncologic safety of such an approach warrants further evaluation.

Thyroidectomy

Patients should be considered for some extent of thyroidectomy if their FNA demonstrates DTC, MTC, isolated secondary metastasis to the thyroid, or cytologically indeterminate nodules with suspicious sonographic features or molecular testing. Total thyroidectomy is favored in patients in whom postoperative radioactive iodine (RAI) is planned (i.e., those with ATA intermediate or high risk of recurrence). These include patients with malignant FNA with lesions greater than 4 cm, gross ETE on ultrasound or intraoperatively and clinical or radiographic evidence of cervical lymph node metastasis or distant metastasis. Total thyroidectomy may also be considered in patients with low-risk DTC in the setting of bilateral disease, history of ionizing radiation, or familial predisposition. In addition, total thyroidectomy is favored with MTC and struma ovarii.

The 2015 ATA guidelines were revised to state that in WDTC 1 to 4 cm in size without ETE or lymph node metastases, either a lobectomy or total thyroidectomy is acceptable treatment. Several studies have demonstrated that lobectomy for WDTC 1 to 4 cm yields disease-specific mortality and recurrence outcomes similar to total thyroidectomy. Nevertheless, studies since the adoption of the guidelines have shown the rate of completion thyroidectomy after initial lobectomy for WDTC to be approximately 10% to 20%. The low incidence of recurrent laryngeal nerve (RLN) injury or permanent hypoparathyroidism (2%) in surgeries performed by experienced surgeons makes total thyroidectomy a reasonable choice for 1 to 4 cm WDTC when performed by an experienced surgical group. From a postoperative standpoint, thyroid lobectomy makes RAI of the remaining gland prohibitive. A total thyroidectomy avoids this pitfall and minimizes reoperative surgery, but must be weighed against the absolute requirement for lifelong thyroid hormone replacement and the knowledge that while complications occur less frequently when operations are performed by experienced surgeons, the extent of surgery can increase the risk of complications, irrespective of surgeon volume. Each patient presents with their unique set of risk factors and preferences that must be factored into the treatment discussion.

Thyroid lobectomy and isthmusectomy are favored in patients with unilobar PTC, FTC, or HCC <1 cm. As discussed previously, the diagnosis of FTC or HCC cannot be made utilizing FNA. As such, diagnostic lobectomy is required to obtain the diagnosis. If the diagnosis of FTC or HCC is made postoperatively, a completion thyroidectomy may be performed in high-risk patients that may go on to require RAI. These patients include those with FTC or HCC with >4 foci of vascular invasion or widely invasive disease as defined histologically based on WHO classification.

Nodal Dissection

Lymph node metastasis is often present at the initial diagnosis of thyroid cancer and can occur subclinically. As such, all patients should have sonographic evaluation of the central (levels VI and VII) and lateral (levels I to V) compartments at the time of initial thyroid cancer diagnosis. Initial nodal dissection, whether central and/or lateral, should involve a compartment-oriented clearance of the fibrofatty and lymphoid tissue within the defined anatomic boundaries of the compartment.

The most common site of lymph node metastasis in PTC and MTC is the central compartment. Central lymph node metastasis involving the bilateral (left and right) compartments occurs in 20% to 25% of PTC and is more common with PTC >1 cm, PTC in the isthmus and with concomitant ipsilateral lateral neck compartment involvement. The majority of patients with MTC have central lymph node metastasis that is frequently occult. Conversely, FTC and HCC metastases to central neck lymph nodes are encountered less frequently. Ipsilateral therapeutic central compartment neck dissection (CCND) should be performed for macroscopic lymphadenopathy; if macroscopic disease is seen in the contralateral central compartment, bilateral therapeutic CCND should be performed. The role of contralateral CCND, in the absence of macroscopic contralateral central neck lymphadenopathy, is controversial. However, intraoperative inspection of the central compartment has a poor predictive value for the presence of metastatic disease, and consideration should be given to proceeding with a contralateral CCND in the presence of ipsilateral macroscopic disease. More extensive surgical resection should always be balanced with the goal of preservation of parathyroid tissue and the RLN. Prophylactic CCND is surgeon dependent for PTC. We perform a prophylactic ipsilateral CCND often for primary tumors >4 cm or when ETE is diagnosed either preoperatively or at the time of surgery. Prophylactic bilateral CCND is performed in all patients with a preoperative diagnosis of MTC.

At initial compartment-oriented lateral neck dissection (COLND) for PTC, levels IIa, III, IV and Vb are typically included and their clearance is associated with a lower risk of recurrence. Prophylactic COLND has not shown improvement in survival or recurrence rates in PTC and is therefore only performed for therapeutic purposes for clinically evident disease. Although some advocate for prophylactic selective COLND of the ipsilateral neck for MTC based on preoperative calcitonin level, we perform selective COLND lateral neck dissection in the event of clinically or radiographic evidence of disease.

Surgical Technique
Removal of the thyroid gland and compartment-oriented cervical lymph node dissection requires precision and vigilance in identifying and preserving critical structures in the region. After the induction of general endotracheal anesthesia, the patient's arms are tucked and placed in the semi-Fowler position with the neck hyperextended using a shoulder roll and appropriate support behind the head. The field is then prepped and draped in the usual sterile fashion to include the chin, neck and chest.

A transverse incision is made approximately 1 to 2 fingerbreadths above the suprasternal notch. Dissection is then carried through the subcutaneous tissue and platysma muscle and flaps are created in the subplatysmal plane both superiorly to the level of the thyroid notch and inferiorly to the suprasternal notch. The strap muscles are then separated vertically along the median raphe. Strap muscles adherent to the gland or tumor should be resected en bloc with the specimen.

Once proper exposure has been obtained, the sternothyroid muscle is freed from the underlying thyroid (unless precluded by tumor involvement) and the lobe of interest is retracted medially in order to identify and ligate the middle thyroid vein. This allows further medial mobilization of the lobe in order to enter the tracheoesophageal groove and identify and preserve the RLN as it runs caudally to cephalad. In approximately 1% of patients, a nonrecurrent RLN is present on the right side and can be identified as it originates from the vagus nerve proximally.

Blunt dissection is performed medial to the common carotid artery to delineate the paratracheal groove and is carried from the thoracic inlet to the superior pole vessels to allow exposure of the RLN. Some surgeons prefer to identify the RLN after release of the superior pole, which may allow enhanced identification of the nerve in the paratracheal groove. At the superior pole, the external branch of the superior laryngeal nerve can be injured as it enters the cricothyroid muscle, resulting in difficulty with high-pitched tones. This nerve has a variable course in relation to the superior pole vessels. Therefore, the superior pole vessels must be meticulously dissected close to the thyroid gland and divided individually, being careful to avoid the external branch of the superior laryngeal nerve. Attention is then directed to the paratracheal groove where the RLN and inferior thyroidal artery are encountered. The RLN often runs posterior to this artery but may run between its branches or anterior to the artery. Careful dissection of both the RLN and the inferior thyroid artery is necessary in order to preserve the nerve as well as maintain the blood supply to the parathyroid glands. The parathyroid glands are carefully dissected free from the thyroid paying special attention to preserve the lateral vascular pedicle. Should the vascular supply be compromised, the parathyroid gland should be carefully minced and autotransplanted into the ipsilateral sternocleidomastoid muscle or brachiocephalic muscle in the nondominant forearm after its identity has been confirmed on immediate pathologic evaluation. Resection of the contralateral thyroid lobe, when indicated, proceeds in the same manner as described above.

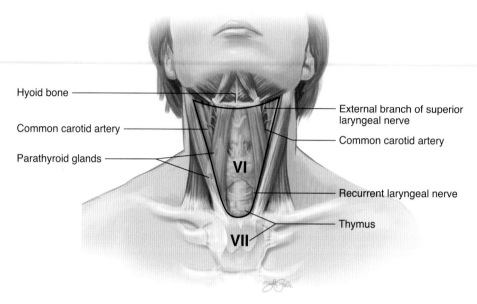

Hyoid bone

External branch of superior laryngeal nerve

Common carotid artery

Common carotid artery

Parathyroid glands

VI

Recurrent laryngeal nerve

Thymus

VII

FIGURE 18.2 Anatomic boundaries of the central neck compartment. (Reprinted with permission from American College of Surgeons, Katz MH. *Operative Standards for Cancer Surgery, Vol 2—Thyroid, Gastric, Rectum, Esophagus, Melanoma.* American College of Surgeons/Wolters Kluwer Health; 2019. Figure 2.3.)

A CCND, usually level VI, is performed to remove lymphatic tissue bordered superiorly by the hyoid bone, inferiorly by the level of the innominate artery, laterally by the carotid arteries, posteriorly by the deep layer of the cervical fascia and anteriorly by the superficial layer of the cervical fascia with special attention to remove all lymphatic and areolar tissue posterior to the RLN (Fig. 18.2). The goal is to clear all prelaryngeal, pretracheal and paratracheal lymphatic tissue on the side of the tumor. Contralateral CCND should also be performed for macroscopic contralateral lymphatic disease. Isolated removal of only grossly involved lymph nodes violates the nodal compartment entered and may be associated with higher recurrence rates. Level VII lymph nodes reside in the superior mediastinum caudal to the innominate artery on the right. The level VII nodal basin is not typically involved in a CCND; however, macroscopic lymph node involvement in level VII should be removed if encountered and may be removed via a transcervical approach or, in some rare cases, partial or complete median sternotomy.

When the removal of lateral lymph nodes is indicated for clinically or radiographically evident metastatic disease, a COLND is performed, generally removing all lymphatic tissue from levels IIa, III, IV and Vb while sparing the sternocleidomastoid muscle, spinal accessory nerve, vagus nerve, phrenic nerve and internal jugular vein when possible (Fig. 18.3). The borders of the lateral COLND are defined posteriorly by the anterior border of the trapezius muscle (posterior aspect of level V), inferiorly by the clavicle (inferior aspect of levels IV and V), medially by the lateral limit of the sternohyoid muscle (medial aspect of levels III and IV) and superiorly by the lower border of the body of the mandible and skull base (superior aspect of level II). Inclusion of levels I, IIb and Va in a lateral COLND is dependent on the presence of metastatic disease in those compartments and the burden of disease in adjacent compartments. The surgeon must be prepared to resect any involved adjacent structures, such as tracheal rings, laryngeal cartilage, vascular structures, or laryngeal or spinal accessory nerves, in the event of ETE or extranodal extension.

Staging

Prognostication of thyroid cancer is most commonly performed using the American Joint Committee on Cancer (AJCC) tumor-node-metastasis (TNM) staging system, which was most recently updated in 2016. Research has demonstrated the superiority of the AJCC TNM staging system in predicting cancer-related mortality. Unfortunately, the TNM system was designed to correlate with survival thus is not as accurate in predicting recurrence.

The 8th edition of the AJCC staging system modified definitions of primary tumor and regional lymph node metastases. For DTCs the following updates to staging were made: (1) increasing the age threshold at diagnosis from 45 to 55 years before stratifying into Stage III/IV disease, (2) removing minimal ETE from

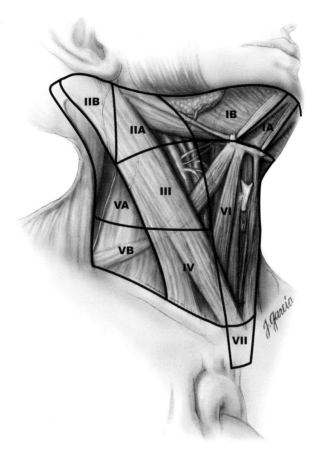

FIGURE 18.3 Anatomic compartments of the lateral neck. (Reprinted with permission from Patel KN, Yip L, Lubitz CC, et al. The American Association of endocrine surgeons guidelines for the definitive surgical management of thyroid disease in adults. *Ann Surg* 2020;271:e21-e93.)

the T3 definition, thus reserving the T3b status to tumors with gross ETE visualized intraoperatively, (3) the definition of central neck was expanded to include both level VI and level VII lymph nodes, and (4) decreasing the assigned stage (from III/IV to II) for tumors <4 cm (T1 and T2) with lymph node metastases. Recent studies using the Surveillance, Epidemiology, and End Results program (SEER) and National Cancer Database (NCDB) databases have shown that the AJCC 8th edition staging system downstaged 23% to 24% of PTC patients and improved staging discrimination for survival.

There is no change to TNM staging for MTC in the 8th edition. A large analysis using the SEER and NCDB databases, however, showed that the current staging system upstages a large proportion of patients with MTC to stage IV and may not accurately stratify groups based on survival. The ATC staging system follows the same definitions for TNM categories as PTC and MTC. However, all patients with ATC are considered to have stage IV disease.

A large retrospective single-institution analysis corroborated 10-year DSS using the AJCC 8th edition for WDTC. They found a 10-year DSS of 99.8%, 88.3%, 72.4%, and 71.9% for stages I to IV, respectively. A large analysis using the AJCC 8th edition for MTC found an overall survival of 95% for stage I, 91% for stage II, 89% for stage III, and 68% for stage IV disease. ATC has one of the worst survival rates of all malignancies with a 1-year survival of 17% and a 5-year survival of approximately 6%.

Adjuvant Therapy

The main goals of adjuvant treatment for thyroid cancer are reducing the future recurrence of disease and prolonging survival. In 2015, the ATA revised an initial risk stratification system for DTC utilizing histology type, pathology characteristics, and mutational status (Fig. 18.4) to assist in decision making for the initiation

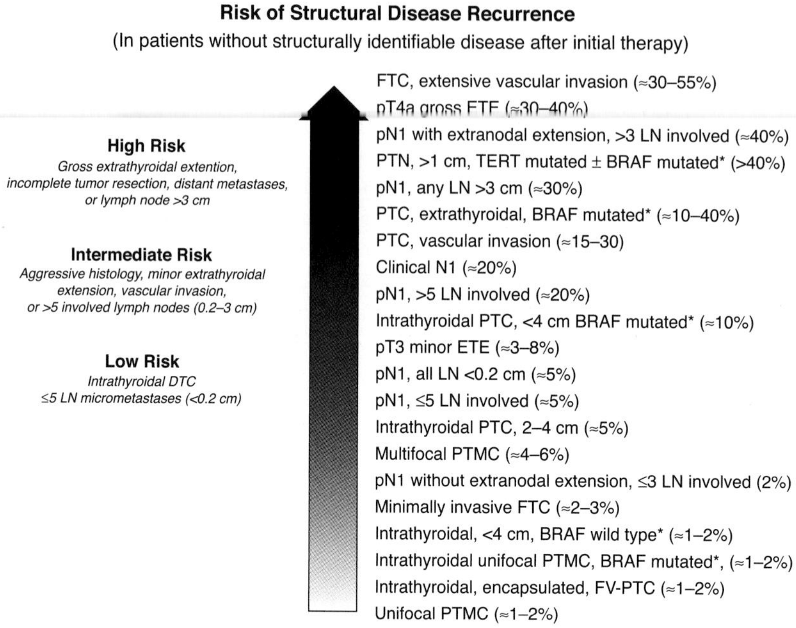

Risk of Structural Disease Recurrence

(In patients without structurally identifiable disease after initial therapy)

High Risk
Gross extrathyroidal extention,
incomplete tumor resection, distant metastases,
or lymph node >3 cm

Intermediate Risk
Aggressive histology, minor extrathyroidal
extension, vascular invasion,
or >5 involved lymph nodes (0.2–3 cm)

Low Risk
Intrathyroidal DTC
≤5 LN micrometastases (<0.2 cm)

FTC, extensive vascular invasion (≈30–55%)
pT4a gross ETE (≈30–40%)
pN1 with extranodal extension, >3 LN involved (≈40%)
PTN, >1 cm, TERT mutated ± BRAF mutated* (>40%)
pN1, any LN >3 cm (≈30%)
PTC, extrathyroidal, BRAF mutated* (≈10–40%)
PTC, vascular invasion (≈15–30)
Clinical N1 (≈20%)
pN1, >5 LN involved (≈20%)
Intrathyroidal PTC, <4 cm BRAF mutated* (≈10%)
pT3 minor ETE (≈3–8%)
pN1, all LN <0.2 cm (≈5%)
pN1, ≤5 LN involved (≈5%)
Intrathyroidal PTC, 2–4 cm (≈5%)
Multifocal PTMC (≈4–6%)
pN1 without extranodal extension, ≤3 LN involved (2%)
Minimally invasive FTC (≈2–3%)
Intrathyroidal, <4 cm, BRAF wild type* (≈1–2%)
Intrathyroidal unifocal PTMC, BRAF mutated*, (≈1–2%)
Intrathyroidal, encapsulated, FV-PTC (≈1–2%)
Unifocal PTMC (≈1–2%)

FIGURE 18.4 Risk stratification system for differentiated thyroid cancer. *Testing not routinely recommended for initial stratification. (Reprinted with permission from Haugen BR, Alexander EK, Bible KC, et al. 2015 American Thyroid Association Management guidelines for adult patients with thyroid nodules and differentiated thyroid cancer: The American Thyroid Association Guidelines Task Force on thyroid nodules and differentiated thyroid cancer. *Thyroid.* 2016;26(1):1–133. The publisher for this copyrighted material is Mary Ann Liebert, Inc. publishers.)

of adjuvant therapy. The mainstay of adjuvant treatment for WDTC is radioactive ^{131}I (RAI) treatment and TSH suppression. There is a limited role for external-beam radiation therapy (EBRT) and systemic therapy in the adjuvant setting.

The use of ^{131}I treatment (radioiodine) after total thyroidectomy improves clinical outcomes including recurrence and survival in selected patients with DTC. RAI is administered at least 4 weeks after surgery and is performed either through thyroid hormone withdrawal or using recombinant human TSH (rhTSH). An initial diagnostic whole-body scan is then performed using ^{123}I or ^{131}I to aid in disease staging and assist with the decision to proceed with, as well as dosing, of ^{131}I therapy. RAI is given for remnant ablation to facilitate surveillance (30 mCi), as adjuvant therapy to treat microscopic disease (up to 150 mCi) and to treat distant metastasis if not surgically resectable (either as an empiric fixed dose or by dosimetry). Indications for adjuvant RAI include patients that are ATA intermediate-risk (including consideration of microscopic ETE, cervical lymph node metastasis, vascular invasion or aggressive tumor histology) or high-risk (gross ETE, incomplete tumor resection, distant metastasis or inappropriate postoperative serum thyroglobulin level).

After surgery and subsequent RAI ablation therapy (if indicated) patients receive thyroid hormonal replacement therapy (levothyroxine) to suppress TSH below physiologic levels. This is performed in patients with DTC with TSH goals dependent on ATA risk stratification. The goal TSH range for patients with high-, moderate- and low-risk disease are <0.1 mU/L, 0.1 to 0.5 mU/L and 0.5 to 2 mU/L, respectively. TSH suppression and RAI are of no use in the management of MTCs and ATCs because these tumors do not show consistent uptake of RAI and generally do not contain TSH receptors, making them insensitive to TSH suppression. The physiologic effects of hyperthyroidism must be balanced with the oncologic benefit of TSH suppression. The extent and duration of TSH suppression is influenced by disease stage, status of recurrence, as well as other comorbidities, with constant reevaluation based on the patients' disease status.

The role of EBRT is limited if complete surgical resection for DTC was performed and should only be used in the neck after all surgical options are exhausted. Currently EBRT is most commonly used to palliate metastatic or locally advanced disease, such as bone metastases or thyroid bed recurrences not amenable to further surgical resection, or in an attempt to avoid a more extensive surgery such as laryngectomy. EBRT does have a role in the palliative management of ATC to improve local control and in some cases survival. Furthermore, there is no role for systemic therapy in the adjuvant setting in the absence of distant metastatic disease.

Surveillance

Most DTC recurrences occur within the first 5 years after initial treatment, but recurrence can also occur several decades later. Patients with PTC often recur locoregionally in the neck, whereas patients with FTC or HCC most commonly recur at distant sites. MTC can recur locoregionally or distantly. The most common site of distant metastases for thyroid cancers are the lungs, bone, soft tissues, brain, liver and adrenal glands with a propensity for lung metastases in young patients and bone metastases in older patients.

Follow-up visits for WDTC patients typically include clinical examination and blood tests measuring serum thyroglobulin (Tg), TSH and free T4 levels as well as cervical ultrasonography every 6 months for 1 to 3 years postoperatively and annually after that. Thyroglobulin values normally drop after thyroidectomy and ablation and serve as a sensitive indicator for recurrent or persistent disease. However, it is important to keep in mind that Tg production and measurement is affected by TSH levels and anti-thyroglobulin antibodies, respectively. Thyroglobulin levels must always be interpreted in the setting of both these values.

Because MTC is derived from parafollicular C cells rather than follicular epithelium, biochemical surveillance differs from DTC. CEA and calcitonin levels are measured in addition to routine cervical ultrasonography. Patients with detectable serum markers should undergo US of the neck and, depending on the level of calcitonin, CT or MRI of the chest, abdomen (with liver protocol) and axial skeleton is performed to detect any evidence of recurrence. If elevated serum markers are identified without structural evidence of disease recurrence, conservative follow-up with repeat biochemical testing every 6 months should be performed.

Locoregional Recurrence and Distant Metastasis

The risk of recurrence and distant metastasis depends largely on tumor biology, extent of initial surgery and other prognostic variables. Approximately 30% of patients with DTC will develop recurrent disease with 66% of patients recurring within the first decade after definitive treatment. Most recurrences (80%) are isolated to the neck and most commonly involve the cervical lymph nodes in 74% of cases. The remaining 20% of patients who recur develop distant metastatic disease, most commonly to the lungs (60%). Half of the patients with distant metastatic disease will die of their disease.

The treatment of recurrent disease depends partly on the iodine avidity of the disease as well as the surgical resectability. In patients with recurrent WDTC in which stimulated Tg levels are 1 to 10 ng/mL, TSH suppression is often the treatment of choice. If stimulated Tg levels are >10 ng/mL and all imaging is negative in detecting recurrence, RAI should be considered. If recurrence is detected locoregionally either by clinical examination or radiographically, surgical resection is the preferred management option. Surgical intervention, however, should be individualized due to the increased risk of RLN injury and hypoparathyroidism. Reoperation may be considered for adenopathy >10 mm, adenopathy in anatomically threatening locations such as immediately adjacent to the trachea or the path of the RLN, excessive rate of nodal growth or rising Tg levels in the setting of radiographic evidence of disease.

Treatment of distant metastatic disease depends on the site of metastases. Central nervous system (CNS) disease may be considered for neurosurgical resection in select patients or RAI ablation and/or stereotactic radiation therapy. Bone and distant metastases other than CNS should be treated surgically in the presence of isolated enlarging lesions or EBRT for patients unable to tolerate surgery. RAI remains an option for iodine-avid disease.

Unfortunately up to 50% of patients with unresectable or metastatic disease develop the inability to uptake iodine and are labeled RAI-refractory. For these patients and patients with MTC with distant metastatic disease, a period of observation may be appropriate as many patients with MTC and DTC have an indolent clinical outcome despite having metastases. If progression is noted, however, redifferentiation therapy and/or targeted systemic therapies of known altered signaling pathways, such as *BRAF, RET/PTC* fusions, or *NTRK1–3*, for example, can be used. Redifferentiation therapy refers to treatment designed to increase or restore RAI uptake in tumors, enabling treatment with RAI. Inhibitors of MEK and BRAF have shown promise in redifferentiation of DTC. Oral multitargeted tyrosine kinase inhibitors, such as sorafenib and lenvatinib are FDA approved for RAI-refractory DTC and PDTC. Patients with $BRAF^{V600E}$ mutated thyroid cancer can be given vemurafenib or dabrafenib. In fact, combination dabrafenib and trametinib has been used in a neoadjuvant fashion to downstage patients with initially unresectable ATC to allow for complete surgical resection with impressive outcomes. Other potential avenues of system therapy include mTOR inhibitors, NTRK inhibitors, and selective RET inhibitors (Table 18.4).

TABLE
18.4

Systemic Therapy Options for Thyroid Cancer

Drug	Mechanism of Action: Target(s)	FDA-Approved Indication	Potential Thyroid Cancer Subtypes
Axitinib	TKI: VEGFR1–3	RCC	DTC, MTC, ATC
Cabozantinib	TKI: VEGFR2, MET, FLT3, RET, c-kit	MTC, RCC, HCC	MTC, DTC (second or third line)
Dabrafenib	STKI: BRAF^{V600E}	BRAF-mutated melanoma	DTC
Dabrafenib + trametinib	STKI: BRAF^{V600E} (dabrafenib), MEK1/2 (trametinib)	BRAF-mutated ATC, melanoma, NSCLC	ATC
Everolimus	STKI: mTOR	RCC, SEGA, TS	DTC, MTC, ATC
Lenvatinib	TKI: VEGFR1–3, FGFR1–4, PDGFR, RET, c-kit	DTC, RCC (in combination with everolimus)	DTC, MTC, ATC
Larotrectinib	Trk1: NTRK fusion	Adult and pediatric patients with solid tumors and NTRK fusions	*NTRK*-fusion thyroid carcinoma
Pazopanib	TKI: VEGFR1–3, PDGFR, FGFR1/2, c-kit	RCC	DTC, MTC, ATC
Pralsetinib	TKI: RET V804	RET-mutated MTC and NSCLC	RET-mutated MTC, *RET* fusion thyroid carcinoma
Selpercatinib	TKI: RET V804	RET-mutated MTC and NSCLC	RET-mutated MTC, *RET* fusion thyroid carcinoma
Sorafenib	TKI: VEGFR1–3, PDGFR, RET, c-kit, BRAF	DTC, HCC, RCC	DTC, MTC, ATC
Sunitinib	TKI: VEGFR1–3, PDGFR, RET, c-kit, CSF-1R, Flt-3	GIST, RCC, pNET	DTC, MTC
Vandetanib	TKI: VEGFR2/3, EGFR, RET	MTC	MTC, DTC
Vemurafenib	STKI: BRAF^{V600E}	BRAF-mutated melanoma	PTC

TKI, tyrosine kinase inhibitor; VEGFR, vascular endothelial growth factor receptor; RCC, renal cell carcinoma; DTC, differentiated thyroid cancer; MTC, medullary thyroid cancer; ATC, anaplastic thyroid cancer; HCC, hepatocellular carcinoma; STKI, serine-threonine kinase inhibitor; NSCLC, non–small cell lung cancer; mTOR, mammalian target of rapamycin; SEGA, subependymal giant cell astrocytoma; TS, tuberous sclerosis; FGFR, fibroblast growth factor receptor; PDGFR, platelet-derived growth factor receptor; Trk1, tropomyosin receptor kinase inhibitor; GIST, gastrointestinal stromal tumor; pNET, pancreatic neuroendocrine tumor; EGFR, epidermal growth factor receptor; PTC, papillary thyroid carcinoma.
Adapted with permission from Cabanillas ME, Ryder M, Jimenez C. Targeted therapy for advanced thyroid cancer: kinase inhibitors and beyond. *Endocr Rev.* 2019;40(6):1573–1604.

Neoplasms of the Parathyroid Glands

Primary Hyperparathyroidism

Primary hyperparathyroidism (PHPT) is most commonly defined as hypercalcemia resulting from the inappropriate, autonomous overproduction of parathyroid hormone (PTH) by one or more parathyroid glands. PHPT has an estimated prevalence of 0.23% among women and 0.085% among men with at least 100,000 new cases diagnosed annually in the United States. A solitary parathyroid adenoma is most commonly responsible for PHPT, present in approximately 85% of patients. PHPT is less commonly caused by multigland hyperplasia (15%). PHPT can occur as a sporadic entity, accounting for at least 85% of cases, or in association with different familial disorders (up to 15% of cases) such as MEN types 1, 2A or 4 (discussed in chapter 16), familial PHPT or hyperparathyroidism-jaw tumor syndrome (HPT-JT).

Presentation

The increased recognition of PHPT as a cause of hypercalcemia by primary care physicians has led to changes in referral patterns of patients with PHPT with an increasing number of patients presenting without classic objective symptoms. Nearly 85% of patients are diagnosed on routine laboratory values obtained for other reasons. These patients are sometimes labeled with 'asymptomatic HPT,' a medical misnomer as many symptoms of hypercalcemia go unrecognized or are attributed to medical conditions other than PHPT. Nonspecific, constitutional symptoms of fatigue, sleep disturbance, memory loss, depression, constipation, nausea, loss of appetite, muscle weakness, bone pain and arthralgias have all shown improvement when hypercalcemia secondary to PHPT is corrected demonstrating that these symptoms may be the initial, subtle presentation of disease. Some patients, however, present with more objective symptoms of hypercalcemia, such as osteoporosis, nephrolithiasis, gastroduodenal ulcers or pancreatitis, triggering a workup for PHPT.

TABLE 18.5	Differential Diagnosis of Hypercalcemia

Primary Hyperparathyroidism • Solitary adenoma • Multigland hyperplasia • Parathyroid carcinoma **Secondary/Tertiary Hyperparathyroidism** **Familial Hypocalciuric Hypercalcemia** **Endocrine Disorders** • Addison disease • Thyrotoxicosis • Hypothyroidism • Pheochromocytoma • Vasoactive intestinal peptide tumor (VIPoma) **Medication** • Thiazide diuretics • Lithium • Calcium supplements	**Malignancy** • Multiple myeloma • Tumors producing PTH-related peptide (ovarian, lung) • Acute or chronic leukemia • Lymphoma **Granulomatous Disorders** • Sarcoidosis • Tuberculosis **Paget Disease** **Increased Dietary Intake** • Milk-alkali syndrome • Vitamin A toxicity • Vitamin D toxicity **Immobilization**

Osteoporosis and nephrolithiasis are among the more common end-organ effects of prolonged hypercalcemia that prompt a formal evaluation for PHPT, particularly in younger patients. Chronic PHPT may cause severe bone demineralization leading to osteoporosis and fragility fractures. Nephrolithiasis may occur secondary to the effect of PTH increasing renal tubular reabsorption of filtered calcium. Finally, severe hypercalcemia (>12 mg/dL) has cardiac implications such as shortened QT interval, hypertension (possibly from concomitant renal insufficiency or calcium-mediated vasoconstriction) and deposition of calcium leading to accelerated atherosclerosis. Given these end-organ manifestations of hypercalcemia, patients presenting with elevated or high-normal levels of serum calcium should undergo an expeditious workup regardless of the presence of objective or subjective symptoms.

A diagnosis of PHPT is made biochemically and is defined by an elevated or high-normal serum calcium level with an inappropriately nonsuppressed PTH level. The initial assessment is made using serum calcium, intact parathyroid hormone (iPTH), phosphorus, creatinine, albumin, 25-OH vitamin D and 24-hour urinary calcium excretion. In the setting of an appropriately suppressed iPTH, other causes of hypercalcemia should be entertained and investigated (Table 18.5), as the diagnosis of PHPT is unlikely in the setting of a suppressed iPTH. If one encounters an elevated iPTH level, secondary hyperparathyroidism must be ruled out before a diagnosis of PHPT can be made. Causes of secondary hyperparathyroidism include vitamin D deficiency, chronic renal insufficiency, hungry bone syndrome and dietary calcium deficiency. A deficiency in vitamin D (usually measured as 25-hydroxyvitamin D), for example, will cause an increase in iPTH that may mimic PHPT. Once the vitamin D level has been corrected with supplementation, repeat serum calcium and iPTH should be measured to ensure the accuracy of the diagnosis of PHPT. Measurement of 24-hour urine calcium should be performed to rule out benign familial hypocalciuric hypercalcemia (FHH), which presents with hypercalcemia and hyperparathyroidism that is not surgically correctable. A 24-hour urine calcium >100 mg/day effectively rules out concern for FHH. Eucalcemic PHPT is a variant of PHPT usually found in patients who are being evaluated for low bone mineral density at which time they are found with elevated serum PTH in the absence of hypercalcemia. The diagnosis of this entity should be considered after all causes of secondary hyperparathyroidism have been excluded. Another recognized variant of primary HPT is that with normal PTH levels. In this group of patients, elevated serum calcium levels are detected, but PTH levels are found within the normal range (i.e., an inappropriately normal PTH).

In addition to establishing the diagnosis of PHPT, the surgeon must also pay close attention to the presence or risk of inherited PHPT. Inherited PHPT is typically characterized by younger age at presentation, the presence of multigland parathyroid disease, lower rates of biochemical cure and higher risks of disease recurrence and parathyroid cancer. Specific genetic mutations influence the clinical manifestations of the disease, indications for surgical intervention, and the risk of disease recurrence. A family history of PHPT (including a history of hypercalcemia and/or nephrolithiasis), in two or more first-degree relatives, age <45 years at diagnosis, recurrent PHPT and the presence of multigland disease should prompt referral to a genetic counselor for genetic testing. The most commonly encountered inherited PHPT syndromes, susceptibility gene, and clinical features are summarized in Table 18.6.

TABLE
18.6   Inherited Primary Hyperparathyroidism

Syndrome	Susceptibility Genes	Clinical Features
FHH	CaSR, GNA11, AP2S1	Mild-to-moderate hypercalcemia with relative hypocalciuria.
FIHP	GCM2	Significant hypercalcemia, nephrolithiasis, and severe osteoporosis
HPT-JT	CDC73	Higher risk (>15%) of parathyroid cancer of one or more parathyroid glands. High risk of multigland disease. In addition to PHPT, may have uterine cancer, renal cysts, ossifying fibromas of the mandible and/or maxilla, and adult Wilms tumor.
MEN1	MEN1	Higher risk of multigland disease, recurrence, and ectopic and supernumerary parathyroid tissue. In addition to PHPT, may have pituitary tumors, duodenopancreatic neuroendocrine tumors, adrenal tumors, thymic carcinoid tumors, bronchopulmonary neuroendocrine tumors, and benign skin lesions.
MEN2A	RET	Higher risk of multigland disease. • Codon 634 mutation associated with ~20% risk of PHPT • Codons 609, 611, 618, 620, 804, and 891 mutations associated with ~5% risk of PHPT
MEN4	CDKN1B (CDKN1A, CDKN2B, CDKN2C)	Higher risk of multigland disease. Similar PHPT presentation as MEN1.
NSHPT	CaSR	Parathyroid hyperplasia. Severe hypercalcemia with relative hypocalciuria in neonates.

FHH, familial hypocalciuric hypercalcemia; FIHP, familial isolated primary hyperparathyroidism; HPT-JT, hyperparathyroidism-jaw tumor syndrome; MEN, multiple endocrine neoplasia; NSHPT, neonatal severe hyperparathyroidism.
Adapted with permission from Alobuia W, Annes J, Kebebew E. Genetic testing in endocrine surgery: Opportunities for precision surgery. *Surgery.* 2020;168(2): 328–334.

Once the diagnosis of PHPT is established and the risk of familial PHPT (and thus multigland disease) is assessed, the indications for parathyroidectomy should then be established.

Surgical Indications

Surgery remains the primary definitive treatment for PHPT, resulting in >95% cure. Parathyroidectomy is indicated in all patients with objective symptoms of hypercalcemia in order to relieve symptoms and prevent complications of chronic hypercalcemia. This category includes patients with overt nephrolithiasis, recent fractures, osteoporosis or deteriorating bone mineral density, bone pain, pancreatitis, mental status changes, or muscle weakness. Patients without overt subjective symptoms of hypercalcemia, who represent the majority of patients referred for surgery, are offered parathyroidectomy based on guidelines written by the American Association of Endocrine Surgeons (AAES) and Fourth International Workshop Guidelines. These include serum calcium >1 mg/dL above the upper limit of normal, age less than 50 years, objective evidence of renal involvement (clinically documented by nephrocalcinosis, hypercalciuria (24-hour urine calcium >400 mg/dL), or impaired renal function (glomerular filtration rate <60 ml/min) and osteoporosis or vertebral compress fracture documented by imaging studies.

Surgical Planning and Preoperative Radiographic Localization

After the diagnosis of PHPT is made and appropriate indications have been met, the most important next step is determination of single or multigland disease. This can be ascertained from one's suspicion for an inherited PHPT as well as preoperative radiographic localization. Patients with any suspicion for an inherited PHPT should be referred for genetic counseling and testing, and if a genetic mutation associated with inherited PHPT is found, the patient has a high likelihood of multigland disease. Patients without concern for inherited PHPT should receive preoperative radiographic localization to evaluate for single gland disease.

Cervical ultrasonography (US), technetium (^{99}Tc) sestamibi-single photon emission computed tomography/computed tomography (sestamibi-SPECT/CT) and four-dimensional multidetector computed tomography (4D-CT) are the preferred initial imaging modalities at our institution. Ultrasonography plays a key role in patients with both suspected single gland and multigland disease because of its cost-effectiveness and added benefit of identifying any concomitant thyroid pathology. Imaging from the submandibular region cephalad to the clavicles caudally is completed with Doppler imaging to assess the vascularity for any suspicious lesions and inform the surgeon of the location of the vascular pedicle. An FNA biopsy of a suspicious lesion is generally not indicated with the exception of a suspicious intrathyroidal lesion, for which both cytologic assessment and PTH biochemical assay may be considered.

The sestamibi-SPECT/CT scan relies on the fact that sestamibi is a lipophilic cation that concentrates in mitochondria. Since parathyroid adenomas and hyperplastic parathyroid glands are metabolically more active when compared to their normal counterparts, the mitochondrial concentration is higher and sestamibi therefore concentrates there, allowing them to be imaged on radionuclide scan. When combined with SPECT imaging, sestamibi scan can more accurately detect smaller parathyroid glands and those that are more posteriorly located. The use of sestamibi radionuclide scan alone has a sensitivity of 65% to 90% in detecting parathyroid adenomas or hyperplastic glands.

4D-CT is a powerful modality for identifying ectopic parathyroid glands, especially those in undescended positions. The study should include multiple views from jaw to aortic arch and with arterial and delayed enhancement phases. 4D-CT allows visualization of differences in perfusion characteristics between hyperfunctioning parathyroid glands (i.e., rapid uptake and quick washout) and normal parathyroid glands and other structures in the neck. This single study provides both anatomic information and a correlation for function (perfusion). 4D-CT has a sensitivity over 90% in identifying single-gland disease initially.

A nomenclature system has been designed that takes into account the pathologic position of the parathyroid glands (Fig. 18.5). Superior and inferior glands are defined by the location of the gland's pedicle and its relationship to the RLN. Superior glands anatomically have a vascular pedicle superior and lateral to the RLN (type A through D glands). Inferior glands have a vascular pedicle inferior and medial to the RLN (type D through F glands). Type G glands represent intrathyroidal parathyroid lesions. This information not only

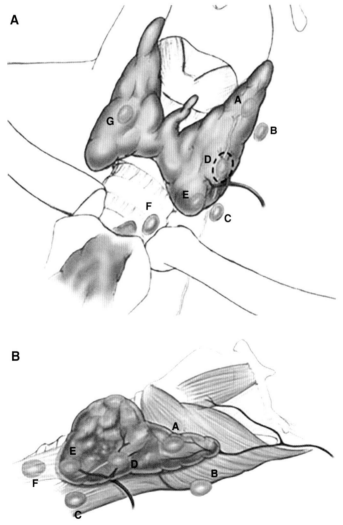

FIGURE 18.5 Schematic representation of the nomenclature system for localization of parathyroid adenomas. Anterior view (**A**); right lateral view (**B**) of the superior thyroid pole is oriented to the left. The *dotted circle* depicts the region where the recurrent laryngeal nerve is most at risk. (Reprinted with permission from Moreno MM, Callendar GG, Woodburn K, et al. Common Locations of Parathyroid Adenomas. *Ann Surg Oncol.* 2011; 18:1047–1051.)

helps radiologists communicate potential parathyroid lesions of interest to surgeons, but also helps surgeons direct their dissection in relation to the RLN.

Patients who are candidates for parathyroidectomy should be referred to an expert clinician trained in parathyroid disease to decide which imaging should be performed based on their regional imaging capabilities.

Surgical Technique

The two main options for parathyroidectomy include standard cervical exploration (SCE) and minimally invasive parathyroidectomy (MIP). An SCE involves four-gland evaluation as the primary procedure and is now often reserved for patients in whom multigland involvement is suspected prior to surgery (i.e., inherited PHPT) or in cases in which preoperative localization was not possible. In the era of preoperative localization, MIP has become the most common surgical treatment for suspected single gland disease given that the majority of PHPT is due to a solitary adenoma that is frequently visualized with high quality preoperative radiographic studies.

The four-gland approach affords the ability to evaluate all four glands and resect as necessary based on the visualized pathology. The patient is brought to the operating room and general endotracheal anesthesia is induced. The patient's neck is extended and the patient is placed in the semi-Fowler position with arms tucked at the side for maximum exposure and surgeon access to the field. A transverse incision is made approximately 2 fingerbreadths above the suprasternal notch and dissection is then carried through the subcutaneous tissue and platysma muscle. The strap muscles are then divided along the median raphe and are elevated off of the posteriorly positioned thyroid gland to retract the gland medially and anteriorly. This facilitates exposure of the carotid sheath, tracheoesophageal groove, and retroesophageal space which are then palpated, prior to any dissection, in order to discover any suspicious parathyroid glands. Attention is generally directed to an area identified as a potential target on preoperative imaging (i.e., largest gland in patients with suspicion for multigland disease) or, in the event no target is identified, the right inferior position as this is statistically where more parathyroid disease is identified. With the thyroid gland rotated medially, the inferior thyroid artery is identified and preserved so as not to devascularize the parathyroid glands. The RLN is then identified and protected as it approaches the inferior thyroid artery. The inferior parathyroid gland, as shown in Figure 18.5, will be found anterior and medial to the RLN, often inferior to the thyroid gland in the thyrothymic tract, but also possibly residing within the capsule of the lower thyroid pole (types E and F). After the inferior gland is identified, the superior parathyroid gland is identified by tracing the RLN superiorly as it enters the cricothyroid membrane. The superior gland will be found posterior and lateral to the RLN and may be found posterior to the thyroid (type A), or either cephalad or caudal in the tracheoesophageal groove (types B and C, respectively). Once both glands are discovered on one side, the contralateral side is explored in the same fashion. Once all four glands have been discovered, the abnormal gland is gently teased from its position, paying special attention to preserving the RLN, and the gland elevated on its vascular pedicle. The pedicle is then ligated and the parathyroid gland is removed. In cases of 4-gland hyperplasia necessitating a 3.5-gland parathyroidectomy, attention should first be turned to partial resection of the most normal (smallest), clearly viable gland in order to preserve 50 to 80 mg of tissue. As resection of the other glands proceeds, the viability of the preserved gland should always be checked prior to resecting the next gland as this allows greater freedom in case the gland becomes nonviable. Less frequently, all four glands can be resected and the smallest one placed on ice in order to mince and reimplant approximately 50 to 80 mg of tissue in the sternocleidomastoid muscle or, in patients at high risk for recurrence (i.e., inherited PHPT), the nondominant brachioradialis muscle. The sternocleido-mastoid muscle is often chosen because it is already exposed during the procedure. However, some surgeons prefer to reimplant into the brachioradialis muscle because if recurrent hyperparathyroidism occurs it would avoid a repeat operation in the neck. In particular, cases of PHPT thought to be due to inherited PHPT should have any reimplantation performed in the nondominant brachioradialis muscle, as recurrent hyperplasia is highly likely. This process, known as autotransplantation, is successful in over 80% of cases.

Minimally invasive parathyroidectomy is now the most common parathyroidectomy performed for PHPT and represents 80 to 85% of cases. The technique targets a specific gland identified on high quality preoperatively radiographic studies and offers potential benefits of improved cosmesis, shorter operation, decreased length of stay, and fever complications, with cure rates comparable to SCE. At our institution, MIP is performed in patients without history suggestive of inherited PHPT and with at least two concordant preoperative radiographic studies identifying a suspicious parathyroid gland. This technique most frequently relies on the use of intraoperative PTH (ioPTH) measurement and intraoperative confirmation of hypercellular parathyroid tissue in the resected specimen. At the time of surgery, the patient is positioned as previously described and a baseline PTH is drawn at the time of incision. The procedure can be performed under gender or locoregional anesthesia. A 2-cm incision is then made on the side of the localized adenoma just medial to the sternocleidomastoid muscle in line with a traditional Kocher incision. An approach medial to the sternocleidomastoid muscle and lateral to the strap muscles is well-suited for patients with targeted superior parathyroid glands (types A, B, or C) and in the reoperative setting. The adenoma is then resected as previously described and a repeat PTH level is drawn 5 and 10 minutes after removal of the gland. A 50% decline in PTH level from baseline is predictive of cure in 96% of cases. Failure of PTH to drop by 50%, a rebound of the PTH level, or a level that plateaus above the normal range indicates residual disease and prompts a four-gland exploration.

A thorough knowledge of parathyroid embryology is required in order to locate pathologic parathyroid glands. One of the most common causes of persistent disease is a missed gland and it is of utmost importance to thoroughly explore the area using a systematic approach with knowledge of embryology and the nomenclature system to help locate the gland. If a superior gland cannot be located, areas posterior and lateral to the RLN should be inspected. The posterior thyroid should first be thoroughly reinspected to identify a gland hidden under investing fascia. The tracheoesophageal groove and retroesophageal spaces may be inspected next followed by the carotid sheath. If an inferior gland cannot be located, areas medial and anterior to the RLN should be inspected, such as the posterior lateral border of the thyroid gland. The thyrothymic tract should be thoroughly explored for an inferior gland and a cervical thymectomy may be required as upward of 17% of inferior glands can be found in the thymus. Lastly, in the rare event of an intrathyroidal parathyroid gland, intraoperative ultrasound may be used with PTH aspirate to identify a parathyroid gland that is situated deeper in the thyroid parenchyma that may necessitate a hemithyroidectomy. It is important to remember that most missed abnormal parathyroid glands are found in the usual anatomic locations.

Parathyroid Carcinoma

Parathyroid carcinoma (PC) is a rare cause of hypercalcemia, accounting for less than 1% of PHPT. Unlike PHPT, which is 3 to 4 times more likely to occur in women, PC has an equal incidence between men and women with presentation usually occurring in the fifth decade. No disproportionate clustering by race, income level, or geographic region has been demonstrated in the literature.

The etiology of PC is unknown. No true risk factors have been identified, largely due to the rarity of the disease. Rare cases of PC have been reported in patients with end-stage renal disease. Although PC is most commonly a sporadic disease, 15% of patients with HPT-JT developed PC and cases, although rare, have been found in FIHP, MEN1 and MEN2A. Germline mutations of the *CDC73* gene are responsible for HPT-JT and somatic *CDC73* mutations have been found in 15% to 70% of sporadic PC cases. Mutations in *CDC73* result in loss of the tumor suppressor role of parafibromin, a protein that interacts with polymerase II/PAFi complex and is involved in transitional and posttranscriptional control pathways. Other somatic gene mutations have been implicated in PC, including *Rb, p53, BRCA2,* and *PRAD1,* although their pathogenetic role is still uncertain.

Presentation

The vast majority (90% to 95%) of PCs are functional and result in severe hypercalcemia. Most patients with PC show markedly elevated levels of serum calcium (>14 mg/dL) and PTH (3 to 10 times the upper limit of normal), and thus frequently present with profound symptoms of hyperparathyroidism such as polydipsia, polyuria, myalgias, nephrolithiasis, fatigue, renal insufficiency, pancreatitis, peptic ulcer disease, bone pain, osteoporosis and pathologic fractures. Renal and skeletal involvement in particular are prominent manifestations of PC, reported in 60% and 50% of patients, respectively. A significant number of patients (40%) with PC will present with a palpable neck mass, which when found in association with PHPT should prompt suspicion for PC. Patients with nonfunctional PC usually present late with symptoms related to compression of adjacent structures, such as hoarseness, dysphagia or dyspnea and can be misdiagnosed with thyroid or thymic carcinoma.

In addition to certain clinical and laboratory findings that may raise clinical suspicion of malignant disease, imaging modalities that provide anatomic information to suggest local invasion should be utilized when one's index of suspicion for PC is high. Although ultrasound cannot definitively detect malignancy, sonographic features concerning for malignancy include a lobulated, hypoechoic and large parathyroid gland with ill-defined borders, local infiltration, calcification, suspicious vascularity and the presence of a thick capsule. In addition, ultrasound imaging may show invasion of the tumor into surrounding structures. 4D-CT may provide a more accurate anatomical description of the lesion including the extent of local invasion into surrounding structures and also map out other involved regions. Functional sestamibi imaging, however, provides little benefit in differentiating benign from malignant parathyroid lesions.

Diagnosis, Staging, and Treatment

PC is particularly challenging to diagnosis preoperatively due to overlapping presentations with benign parathyroid adenomas. If there is clinical, laboratory or radiographic suspicion for PC, preoperative FNA should not be performed for risk of local tumor dissemination. Once the diagnosis of PHPT has been established and PC suspected, the patient is brought to the operating room and an en bloc resection of the parathyroid gland with adjacent involved tissues and avoidance of capsular disruption should be performed. En bloc resection may involve ipsilateral thyroid lobectomy, ipsilateral central compartment lymph nodes and removal of ipsilateral tracheoesophageal soft tissue. In situations where PC was not suspected preoperatively, PC should be suspected intraoperatively if the surgeon encounters a lobulated, gray-white and firm tumor with adherence and invasion of the surrounding neck structures and en bloc resection of the tumor and adherent tissue should be performed.

Histologically, PC may show fibrosis, nuclear atypia, necrosis and atypical mitotic figures. Per WHO criteria, the diagnosis of PC requires lymphovascular invasion, invasion into adjacent structures, or metastatic disease. The cornerstone of accurately diagnosing PC is engaging an experienced pathologist in histopathologic evaluation of the specimen. Immunohistochemistry may improve the diagnostic accuracy of PC. Diagnostic nomograms involving RB, PGP9.5, Ki67, galectin-3 and parafibromin, have been utilized in diagnosing PC with high diagnostic accuracy.

The 8th edition of AJCC guidelines has established a staging system for PC. Multiple studies have demonstrated that the extent of surgery, with en bloc resection of the tumor being the gold standard, has been shown to correlate with improved overall (OS) and disease-free survival (DFS) in multivariate analysis. Estimated 5-year OS rates are 78% to 85% and DFS rates are 60% to 70%. Negative prognostic factors for DFS were higher serum calcium level at presentation, vascular invasion, and older age. Negative prognostic factors for OS were higher calcium level at recurrence, number of recurrences, parathyroidectomy alone at initial presentation, nonfunctioning PC and the presence of lymph node or distant metastases.

Disease Recurrence and Metastasis

Surveillance for disease recurrence is performed using calcium and PTH measurements, in the event of functional disease, at regular intervals and periodic ultrasound and chest CT following surgery. Local recurrence occurs in greater than 50% of patients at varying time periods from the initial surgery but typically occurs 2 to 4 years after surgery. Distant metastases, most commonly to the lungs, bone, or liver, occur in 25% of patients. Local recurrences and localized distant metastatic disease should be considered for reoperation to help curb symptomatic hypercalcemia in addition to disease progression. Reoperation and metastasectomy remain at the cornerstone of treating disease progression due to lack of other effective treatments.

Data remain limited about the effect of adjuvant therapies on disease recurrence and progression. Our experience with a small cohort of patients demonstrated benefit of adjuvant radiation after en bloc resection at initial surgery in preventing disease recurrence versus in those receiving salvage surgery. Chemotherapy has shown no survival benefit in patients with PC and is rarely used in the armamentarium of the endocrine oncologist in this disease. Molecular profiling of advanced PC cases has paved the way for novel treatment opportunities through targeted therapy. Recent studies of genomic alterations in PC have identified TKIs and mTOR pathway inhibitors as potential treatment options for patients with specific mutational profiles. Furthermore, tumors with elevated mutational burdens may benefit from immune checkpoint inhibitor therapy, although further studies are required to assess true therapeutic benefit.

In addition to the use of targeted therapies for patients with widespread metastatic disease or unresectable disease, patients will require medical management of malignant hypercalcemia. In the acute setting, aggressive hydration with saline infusion is the first step in management. Subsequently, the addition of loop diuretics, which increases urinary calcium excretion, and calcitonin, which inhibits both osteoclast-mediated bone resorption and increases urinary calcium excretion, may be used to help further decrease serum calcium levels. Use of antiresorptive drugs, such as bisphosphonates (pamidronate and zoledronate) or a RANK ligand inhibitor (denosumab), has been shown to further decrease serum calcium levels. However, calcimimetic agents have proved to be the most effective agents for the long-term treatment of hypercalcemia secondary to PC. Cinacalcet has been shown to be efficacious in lowering serum calcium levels in patients with inoperable PC.

CASE SCENARIO

Case Scenario 1: Medullary Carcinoma

Presentation

A 45-year-old male was referred to your clinic from his primary care physician who identified a palpable and mobile thyroid nodule during routine physical examination. He reports not noticing it prior to his visit. He denies compressive symptoms. He is clinically euthyroid with normal TSH and free T4 levels. He denies a history of ionizing radiation to the neck. He denies a family history of thyroid cancer or other endocrinopathies. His cervical ultrasound shows a 2.5-cm hypoechoic nodule in the left upper pole with irregular borders and microcalcifications. Fine needle aspiration (FNA) of the nodule demonstrates cytology consistent with medullary thyroid cancer. He is very anxious about the diagnosis and would like expedient care.

Confirmation of Diagnosis and Treatment

Fine needle aspiration (FNA) can provide cytologic confirmation of medullary thyroid cancer. Staining of cytologic specimens for calcitonin or sequencing through molecular testing platforms may also be used to help identify medullary thyroid cancer in cytologically indeterminate nodules. Any patient with a cytologic diagnosis of medullary thyroid cancer should undergo laboratory testing for biomarkers, specifically calcitonin and carcinoembryonic antigen (CEA), and radiographic studies to evaluate for macroscopic central and lateral neck disease. Ultrasonography is usually the first preoperative imaging study to be performed. If there is obvious macroscopic evidence of central or lateral neck disease, a CT of the neck with IV contrast is obtained to delineate the extent of disease and level of invasion in to surrounding structures. If suspicious central or lateral neck adenopathy is seen on imaging studies, patients should undergo image-guided FNA of the adenopathy, especially in the lateral neck, to determine whether a more extensive resection is necessary. In the absence of macroscopic evidence of lateral neck disease, patients should undergo a total thyroidectomy and bilateral central neck dissection. Patients with macroscopic evidence of lateral neck disease will also require a compartment-oriented lateral neck dissection.

Surgical Approach—Key Steps

1. A transverse incision is made approximately one to two fingerbreadths above the suprasternal notch, subplatysmal flaps are created superiorly and inferiorly, and the strap muscles are separated vertically along the median raphe.
2. The sternothyroid muscle is freed from the underlying thyroid (unless precluded by tumor involvement), the thyroid lobe (usually with the primary cancer) is retracted medially, and the RLN is identified in the tracheoesophageal groove.
3. The superior pole vessels must be meticulously dissected close to the thyroid gland and divided individually, being careful to avoid the external branch of the superior laryngeal nerve.
4. The RLN and inferior thyroid artery are carefully dissected off the thyroid lobe to preserve the nerve as well as maintain the blood supply to the parathyroid glands. The thyroid lobe and isthmus is then freed from the trachea.
5. Resection of the contralateral thyroid lobe proceeds in the same manner as described in steps 2–4.
6. A CCND is performed to remove all prelaryngeal, pretracheal, and paratracheal lymphatic tissue between the two carotid sheaths from the hyoid bone superiorly to the brachiocephalic vessels inferiorly.

Common Curve Balls

- The presence of MEN2A or B and the presence of a pheochromocytoma should be ruled out prior to neck surgery. Up to 25% of patients with MTC may have MEN2, which is associated with pheochromocytomas, a catecholamine-producing adrenal tumor that must be diagnosed prior to elective surgery to prevent morbidity associated with hypertensive crises.
- Persistent elevation in serum calcitonin or CEA after total thyroidectomy and bilateral central neck dissection may be due to persistent disease, either in the central neck or lateral neck, particularly adjacent to the superior pole of the thyroid. Patients should have comprehensive evaluation of the bilateral lateral neck lymph node compartments to evaluate for macroscopic evidence of disease before initial surgery.

- Persistent elevation in serum calcitonin or CEA after initial surgery may also be due to distant metastases. Patients with initial serum calcitonin >500 pg/mL or serum calcitonin >150 pg/mL after initial comprehensive surgery should undergo radiographic evaluation for distant metastases.

Take Home Points

- After cytologic confirmation of MTC, patients should have serum calcitonin and CEA obtained in addition to comprehensive radiographic examination of the thyroid and central neck and bilateral lateral neck lymph node basins.
- Patients with MTC should undergo germline *RET* testing and/or biochemical testing for pheochromocytoma prior to elective neck surgery.
- The initial surgical treatment is total thyroidectomy and bilateral central neck dissection with lateral neck dissection in the presence of macroscopic evidence of disease.

CASE SCENARIO 1 REVIEW

Case Scenario 1 Questions

1. What is the next best step in management of this patient?

   A. Proceed to total thyroidectomy
   B. Proceed to total thyroidectomy and bilateral central neck dissection
   C. Further laboratory and radiographic workup
   D. Offer the patient genetic counseling
   E. C and D

2. The patient has normal plasma metanephrines. He underwent total thyroidectomy and bilateral central neck dissection. Pathology was consistent with a 2.6-cm medullary thyroid carcinoma. There was no extrathyroidal extension or angioinvasion and all margins were negative. Three out of 18 central neck lymph nodes were positive for MTC. He then underwent genetic testing which was negative for a germline *RET* mutation. His postoperative calcitonin and CEA are within normal limits. How should you proceed with adjuvant therapy?

   A. Radioactive iodine ablation with 30 mCi and TSH suppression
   B. TSH suppression alone
   C. No adjuvant therapy
   D. Selective *RET* inhibitor (selpercatinib or pralsetinib) therapy
   E. Postoperative external beam radiation

3. The patient moves out of town and returns to you 5 years later with significant dyspnea, abdominal pain and bone pain. Biochemical workup is significant for a profound rise in his calcitonin and CEA levels that prompts a metastatic workup. CT chest, abdomen, and pelvis and bone scan reveals multiple bilateral lung and liver metastases, bilateral iliac crest metastases and cervical, thoracic and lumbar vertebral body metastases. You discuss the patient in multidisciplinary tumor board to devise a plan. What is the next step in management?

   A. Radioactive iodine ablation and EBRT to bone metastases
   B. Percutaneous biopsy with molecular testing of specimen to guide targeted therapy
   C. Selective *RET* inhibitor therapy
   D. Referral to palliative care and hospice
   E. None of the above

Case Scenario 1 Answers

1. **The correct answer is E.** *Rationale:* Any patient with a cytologic diagnosis of medullary thyroid cancer should undergo laboratory testing for biomarkers, specifically calcitonin and CEA, and radiographic studies to evaluate for macroscopic central and lateral neck disease. This patient has radiographic evidence of disease localized to the thyroid with a serum calcitonin <500 pg/mL, decreasing the likelihood of distant metastases, and thus further radiographic studies are not needed.

In addition to calcitonin and CEA, however, one should strongly consider obtaining plasma or urine metanephrines to rule out pheochromocytoma. Up to 25% of patients with MTC may have MEN2, which is associated with pheochromocytomas, a catecholamine-producing adrenal tumor that must be diagnosed prior to elective surgery to prevent morbidity associated with hypertensive crises. This patient should also be offered genetic counseling. A genetic counselor will discuss the role of genetic testing for mutations associated with MTC as well as the implications of a positive result on the patient and the patient's family from a medical and psychosocial standpoint.

Surgery for MTC in this case scenario would involve a total thyroidectomy and bilateral central neck dissection. Choice A is incorrect because patients with MTC should be offered a bilateral central neck dissection due to the risk of occult central neck lymph node metastases. In the presence of confirmed lateral neck metastasis, a compartment-oriented lateral neck dissection would be offered as well. Choice B is incorrect because the surgeon cannot safely proceed to surgery without either ruling out pheochromocytoma or ruling out a hereditary cause for MEN2 that would place the patient at increased risk for having a pheochromocytoma. If an appreciable decrease in calcitonin and CEA are not seen postoperatively, evaluation for distant metastasis should be considered.

2. **The correct answer is C.** *Rationale:* This patient underwent a therapeutic resection with normalization of his calcitonin and CEA, suggestive of resection of all gross disease, thus decreasing the chance of persistent locoregional disease and distant metastasis. In the absence of obvious unresectable and large volume distant metastases, the use of a selective *RET* inhibitor is not indicated. This patient has MTC with evidence of cervical neck metastases. There is no role for radioactive iodine or TSH suppression in patients with MTC. If this patient's pathology were PTC he would be a candidate for TSH suppression. Based on the 2015 ATA guidelines, patients with PTC, are at low/intermediate risk of structural disease recurrence (Fig. 18.4). Based on the size of this patient's lymph node metastases, he would be a potential candidate for radioactive iodine. There is no role for postoperative external beam radiation in this patient, given the absence of gross residual disease not amenable to resection or distant, isolated but unresectable metastases.

3. **The correct answer is B.** *Rationale:* The patient now has widely metastatic disease. Given his symptoms and the extent of disease, he may benefit from systemic therapy. Systemic therapy for MTC includes nontargeted therapies such as cabozantenib or vandetinib, or *RET*-specific therapies, such as pralsetinib or selpercatinib. It is important to determine whether *RET* inhibitor therapies may benefit this patient prior to initiation of systemic therapy. He would therefore, require percutaneous biopsy and molecular testing of the specimen to determine the presence of *RET* or *Ras* mutations. *RET* mutations can be found in 40% of sporadic MTC, while *Ras* mutations, which have few options for targeted therapies, can be found in 15% of sporadic MTC.

Choice (A) is incorrect because there is no role for RAI ablation in patients with MTC. Given his significant bone pain, he would benefit from a consultation with radiation oncology to discuss EBRT to his bone metastases. Choice (D) is incorrect. It is premature to refer the patient to hospice without a discussion of systemic therapy.

CASE SCENARIO

Case Scenario 2: Hypercalcemia

Presentation

A 70-year-old female presents with a history of fatigue, insomnia, constipation, myalgias, nephrolithiasis and osteoporosis. Her serum calcium is 12.0 mg/dL (normal 8.4 to 10.2 mg/dL), iPTH is 290 pg/mL (normal 15 to 65 pg/mL), 25-OH vitamin D 50 ng/mL (normal 30 to 100 ng/mL), eGFR > 60, and 24-hour urine calcium is 550 mg/day. She denies a family history of parathyroid disease, other endocrinopathies or cancers. She is otherwise healthy and does not take any medications. She denies a history of ionizing radiation to the neck. Her preoperative ultrasound, sestamibi-SPECT/CT, and 4D-CT identified a right superior parathyroid gland as a potential target.

Differential Diagnosis

The differential diagnosis is that of hypercalcemia, which is listed in Table 18.5. All patients with hypercalcemia should be evaluated for primary hyperparathyroidism, secondary/tertiary hyperparathyroidism, medication-induced hypercalcemia, hypercalcemia of malignancy, and endocrinopathy-related hypercalcemia.

Confirmation of Diagnosis and Treatment

Primary hyperparathyroidism is a biochemical diagnosis usually defined as hypercalcemia with elevated or inappropriately normal PTH. The presence of a normal 25-OH vitamin D level and eGFR decrease the likelihood of secondary hyperparathyroidism. Absence of a history of endocrinopathies, cancers or other medications rules out other causes of hypercalcemia. Once a biochemical diagnosis of primary hyperparathyroidism is made, surgery involves parathyroidectomy, which may involve minimally invasive parathyroidectomy or standard cervical exploration depending on the surgeon's level of suspicion for multigland disease, concomitant thyroid pathology, and preoperative radiographic findings.

Surgical Approach—Key Steps

The two main options for parathyroidectomy include standard cervical exploration (SCE) and minimally invasive parathyroidectomy (MIP). A standard cervical exploration involves four-gland evaluation as the primary procedure and is now often reserved for patients in whom multigland involvement is suspected prior to surgery (i.e., inherited PHPT) or in cases in which preoperative localization was not possible. In the era of preoperative localization, MIP has become the most common surgical treatment for suspected single gland disease given that the majority of PHPT is due to a solitary adenoma that is frequently visualized with high-quality preoperative radiographic studies.

1. Standard Cervical Exploration.
   a. A transverse incision is made approximately 2 fingerbreadths above the suprasternal notch and the strap muscles are divided along the median raphe.
   b. Attention is generally directed to an area identified as a potential target on preoperative imaging (i.e., largest gland in patients with suspicion for multiglandular disease) or, in the event no target is identified, the right inferior position as this is statistically the most likely place that parathyroid disease is identified. The thyroid lobe is rotated medially, the inferior thyroid artery is identified and preserved so as not to devascularize the parathyroid glands, and the RLN is identified and protected as it approaches the inferior thyroid artery.
   c. Both the superior and inferior parathyroid glands are visualized and evaluated for pathology on the ipsilateral side. Once both glands are discovered on one side, the contralateral side is explored in the same fashion.
   d. Once all four glands have been discovered, the abnormal gland is gently teased from its position, paying special attention to preserving the RLN, and the gland elevated on its vascular pedicle. The pedicle is then ligated and the parathyroid gland is removed.
   e. In cases of 4-gland hyperplasia necessitating a 3.5-gland parathyroidectomy, attention should first be turned to partial resection of the most normal (smallest), clearly viable gland in order to preserve 50 to 80 mg of tissue, before proceeding to resection of the remaining glands.
2. Minimally invasive parathyroidectomy
   a. A PTH level is drawn and a 2-cm incision is made on the side of the localized adenoma just medial to the sternocleidomastoid muscle in line with a traditional Kocher incision. An approach medial to the sternocleidomastoid muscle and lateral to the strap muscles is well suited for patients with targeted superior parathyroid glands (types A, B, or C) and in the reoperative setting.
   b. After mobilization of the thyroid lobe as described during standard cervical exploration, the adenoma is then resected as previously described and a repeat PTH level is drawn 5 and 10 minutes after removal of the gland. A 50% decline in PTH level from baseline is predictive of cure in 96% of cases.
   c. Failure of PTH to drop by 50%, a rebound of the PTH level, or a level that plateaus above the normal range indicates residual disease and prompts a four-gland exploration.

Common Curve Balls

- MIP hinges upon appropriate use of intraoperative PTH with documentation of an adequate decline in the PTH level. Surgeons must have a thorough understanding of its use before consideration of a MIP. Patient-related factors, anatomic factors, or assay factors may influence the intraoperative PTH results and lead to an inadequate decline. In this situation, patients should undergo SCE to identify further evidence of parathyroid disease.
- MIP is considered in the absence of suspicion for multigland disease or concomitant thyroid pathology. During evaluation for hyperparathyroidism, patients are often found with thyroid pathology that

should be addressed at the same time as parathyroidectomy if possible. These patients would undergo unilateral exploration, in the setting of parathyroidectomy and thyroid lobectomy, or SCE, in the setting of parathyroidectomy and total thyroidectomy.

- Although uncommon, surgeons must have a high suspicion for parathyroid carcinoma in the setting of profound hypercalcemia and PTH 3 to 10 times the upper limit of normal. Intraoperatively, parathyroid carcinoma appears gray-white with invasion into surrounding structures. Parathyroidectomy should be performed with en bloc ipsilateral thyroid lobectomy, central neck dissection, and paratracheal dissection.

Take Home Points

- Primary hyperparathyroidism is a biochemical diagnosis. A thorough evaluation of other causes of hypercalcemia should be performed prior to consideration for surgery for primary hyperparathyroidism.
- The type of surgery (SCE or MIP) is dependent on suspicion for multiglandular disease, concomitant thyroid pathology, and preoperative radiographic localization studies.
- Surgeons must have a high index of suspicion for parathyroid carcinoma, which will present with profound hypercalcemia and PTH 3 to 10 times the upper limit of normal.

CASE SCENARIO 2 REVIEW

Case Scenario 2 Questions

1. Which of the following surgical options may be used for this patient?
   A. Standard cervical exploration with four-gland exploration
   B. Minimally invasive parathyroidectomy targeting a right superior gland with intraoperative PTH measurement
   C. Minimally invasive parathyroidectomy targeting a right superior gland and cervical thymectomy
   D. The patient does not meet criteria for surgery
   E. A and B

2. A minimally invasive parathyroidectomy with intraoperative PTH is performed. Her pathology comes back as low grade parathyroid carcinoma with angioinvasion, 5 mitoses/10 HPF and extension into the surrounding soft tissues. At 2 months postoperatively, her labs show serum calcium 9.0 mg/dL (normal 8.4 to 10.2 mg/dL) and iPTH 80 (normal 15 to 65 pg/mL). Which of the following statements regarding future management strategies is true?

   A. The patient has no risk factors for recurrence and has a 2-year recurrence free survival >90%
   B. Adjuvant chemotherapy has a well-established role in management of parathyroid cancer and should be offered to this patient
   C. Reoperative surgery plays an important role in the treatment of locoregional recurrence
   D. The patient has definitive evidence of recurrence at this point and would benefit from reoperation
   E. There is no role for systemic therapy in patients with metastatic parathyroid carcinoma

Case Scenario 2 Answers

1. **The correct answer is B.** *Rationale:* When encountering a patient with suspected primary hyperparathyroidism, one must first determine whether the patient has biochemical evidence of disease. This patient has an elevated serum calcium with an elevated iPTH. Furthermore, she has normal 25-OH vitamin D and normal GFR, decreasing the likelihood of secondary hyperparathyroidism contributing to the iPTH elevation. Taken together, this patient has biochemical evidence of disease. Next, one must determine whether she has indications for surgical intervention. According to the AAES Guidelines, indications for surgical intervention with biochemical evidence of PHPT include serum calcium >1 mg/dL above the upper limit of normal, age <50 years, objective evidence of renal involvement (i.e., nephrolithiasis), osteoporosis or 24-hour urine calcium >400 mg/dL. This patient has elevated serum calcium >1 mg/dL above the upper limit of normal, nephrolithiasis, and 24-hour urine calcium >400 mg/dL, and thus meets criteria for surgical intervention. As such, Choice D is incorrect.

The patient's preoperative imaging studies all localize her parathyroid disease to the right superior parathyroid gland. Given that she has 3 concordant imaging studies and has no family history suggestive of inherited HPT, it is reasonable to offer the patient a minimally invasive parathyroidectomy with intraoperative PTH. Studies have shown that this approach has comparable cure rates to standard cervical exploration with four-gland exploration with the added benefit of decreased operative times, decreased length of stay and improved cosmesis. Standard cervical exploration, however, may also be offered for this patient and has remained the gold standard approach. Furthermore, if there was not an appropriate drop in intraoperative PTH (>50% drop at 10 minutes following excision), the patient would then receive a standard cervical exploration. The patient would not, however, receive a prophylactic cervical thymectomy given the information in this question stem (Choice C). A prophylactic cervical thymectomy would be indicated in patients with MEN1 to remove potential parathyroid rest tissue. A prophylactic cervical thymectomy may also be performed in the event of a standard cervical exploration when a right inferior parathyroid gland cannot be appropriately identified.

2. **The correct answer is C.** *Rationale:* Parathyroid carcinoma is rare and accounts for <1% of PHPT. The parathyroid surgeon must have a high index of suspicion of parathyroid carcinoma in a patient with a high preoperative calcium and PTH and should look for evidence of invasion at the time of operation. If any evidence of invasive disease is identified, the surgeon should perform a parathyroidectomy with en bloc ipsilateral thyroid lobectomy and ipsilateral paratracheal dissection to significantly decrease the chance of recurrence. Silva-Figueroa et al. identified age >65 years, vascular invasion and serum calcium >15 mg/dL at presentation as negatively correlated with recurrence free survival. With two-thirds risk factors for poorer recurrence free survival, this patient has a 27% 2-year recurrence free survival (Choice A is incorrect).

Treatment for parathyroid carcinoma is mainly targeted toward treating hypercalcemia related to recurrence. In patients with functional tumors, which make up the majority of parathyroid carcinoma, the principal morbidity associated with recurrence is related to symptoms of hypercalcemia. Although cinacalcet and bone-modulating therapies have been shown to improve symptoms associated with malignant hypercalcemia, patients benefit most from reoperation and resection of recurrent disease, if possible. Chemotherapy does not play a significant role in management of parathyroid carcinoma (Choice B is incorrect). However, the use of molecular profiling has allowed endocrine oncologists to use targeted therapies to treat grossly metastatic parathyroid carcinoma that is not amenable to surgical resection (Choice E is incorrect).

Patients with significantly high preoperative calcium and PTH are at high risk for postoperative bone hunger. These patients often develop hypocalcemia resulting in elevation of PTH to normalize the patient's serum calcium, thus leading to a postoperative normal serum calcium with an elevated PTH, as is the case in this patient. However, in a patient with parathyroid carcinoma with angioinvasion and extension into surrounding soft tissue who did not undergo en bloc resection with an ipsilateral thyroid lobectomy and paratracheal lymph node dissection, one must always consider persistent or recurrent disease. At 2 months postoperatively, however, the patient may either be suffering from bone hunger or persistent disease (Choice D is incorrect). It would be reasonable to treat the bone hunger with oral calcium supplementation and reevaluate in several weeks to determine whether her PTH normalizes and serum calcium remain within normal limits. If not, one should be suspicious of persistent disease and offer the patient reoperation.

Recommended Readings

Alobuia W, Annes J, Kebebew E. Genetic testing in endocrine surgery: opportunities for precision surgery. *Surgery*. 2020;168(2):328–334.

Asare EA, Sturgeon C, Winchester DJ, et al. Parathyroid carcinoma: an update on treatment outcomes and prognostic factors from the National Cancer Data Base (NCDB). *Ann Surg Oncol*. 2015;22(12):3990–3995.

Bilezikian JP, Brandi ML, Eastell R, et al. Guidelines for the management of asymptomatic primary hyperparathyroidism: Summary Statement from the Fourth International Workshop. *J Clin Endocrinol Metab*. 2014;99(10):3561–3569.

Cabanillas ME, Ryder M, Jimenez C. Targeted therapy for advanced thyroid cancer: kinase inhibitors and beyond. *Endocr Rev*. 2019;40(6):1573–1604.

Cetani F, Pardi E, Marcocci C. Parathyroid carcinoma. *Front Horm Res*. 2019;51:63–76.

Gartland RM, Lubitz CC. Impact of extent of surgery on tumor recurrence and survival for papillary thyroid cancer patients. *Ann Surg Oncol.* 2018;25(9):2520–2525.

Haugen BR, Alexander EK, Bible KC, et al. 2015 American Thyroid Association Management Guidelines for Adult Patients with Thyroid Nodules and Differentiated Thyroid Cancer: The American Thyroid Association Guidelines Task Force on Thyroid Nodules and Differentiated Thyroid Cancer. *Thyroid.* 2016;26(1):1–133.

Landry CD, Wang TS, Asare EA, et al. Parathyroid. In: Amin MB, ed. *AJCC Cancer Staging Manual Eighth Edition.* Springer International Publishing, 2017.

Lim H, Devesa SS, Sosa JA, Check D, Kitahara CM. Trends in thyroid cancer incidence and mortality in the United States, 1974–2013. *JAMA.* 2017;317(13):1338–1348.

Lubitz CC, Sosa JA. The changing landscape of papillary thyroid cancer: epidemiology, management, and the implications for patients. *Cancer.* 2016;122(24):3754–3759.

Molinaro E, Romei C, Biagini A, et al. Anaplastic thyroid carcinoma: from clinicopathology to genetics and advanced therapies. *Nat Rev Endocrinol.* 2017;13(11):644–660.

Moreno MA, Callender GG, Woodburn K, et al. Common locations of parathyroid adenomas. *Ann Surg Oncol.* 2011;18(4):1047–1051.

Nikiforov YE. Thyroid carcinoma: molecular pathways and therapeutic targets. *Mod Pathol.* 2008;21 Suppl 2(Suppl 2):S37–S43.

Operative Standards For Cancer Surgery, *Vol 2—Thyroid, Gastric, Rectum, Esophagus, Melanoma.* American College of Surgeons; Wolters Kluwer Health, 2019.

Patel KN, Angell TE, Babiarz J, et al. Performance of a genomic sequencing classifier for the preoperative diagnosis of cytologically indeterminate thyroid nodules. *JAMA Surg.* 2018;153(9):817–824.

Patel KN, Yip L, Lubitz CC, et al. The American Association of endocrine surgeons guidelines for the definitive surgical management of thyroid disease in adults. *Ann Surg* 2020;271(3):e21-e93

Rosen JE, Lloyd RV, Brierley JD, et al. Thyroid – medullary. In: Amin MB, ed. *AJCC Cancer Staging Manual Eighth Edition.* Springer International Publishing; 2017.

Smallridge RC, Ain KB, Asa SL, et al. American Thyroid Association guidelines for management of patients with anaplastic thyroid cancer. *Thyroid.* 2012;22(11):1104–1139.

Steward DL, Carty SE, Sippel RS, et al. Performance of a multigene genomic classifier in thyroid nodules with indeterminate cytology: a prospective blinded multicenter study. *JAMA Oncol.* 2019;5(2):204–212.

Tuttle RM, Morris LF, Haugen BR, et al. Thyroid—differentiated and anaplastic. In: Amin MB, ed. *AJCC Cancer Staging Manual Eighth Edition.* Springer International Publishing; 2017.

Volante M, Collini P, Nikiforov YE, et al. Poorly differentiated thyroid carcinoma: the Turin proposal for the use of uniform diagnostic criteria and an algorithmic diagnostic approach. *Am J Surg Pathol.* 2007;31(8):1256–1264.

Wells SA, Jr., Asa SL, Dralle H, et al. Revised American Thyroid Association guidelines for the management of medullary thyroid carcinoma. *Thyroid.* 2015;25(6):567–610.

Wilhelm SM, Wang TS, Ruan DT, et al. The American Association of endocrine surgeons guidelines for definitive management of primary hyperparathyroidism. *JAMA Surg.* 2016;151(10):959–968.

Yeh MW, Bauer AJ, Bernet VA, et al. American Thyroid Association statement on preoperative imaging for thyroid cancer surgery. *Thyroid.* 2015;25(1):3–14.

Zafereo M, Yu J, Angelos P, et al. American Head and Neck Society Endocrine Surgery Section update on parathyroid imaging for surgical candidates with primary hyperparathyroidism. *Head Neck.* 2019;41(7):2398–2409.

Hematologic Malignancies and Splenic Tumors

Douglas Swords, David Santos, and Hun Ju Lee

Patients with hematologic malignancies represent a challenging cancer population for the surgical oncologist. Whether to perform an excisional biopsy for a suspicion of lymphoma or a therapeutic splenectomy in a patient with a hematologic malignancy, surgeons in cancer centers are frequently involved in the care of these individuals. Therefore, it is important for surgical oncologists to be familiar with these malignancies and the indications for appropriate interventions. The treatment plan almost always involves the participation of our hematology colleagues and a multidisciplinary approach.

Hematologic disorders are categorized based on the cell type of origin. Leukemia, lymphoma and myeloma account for approximately 10% of new cancer diagnoses in the United States. The National Cancer Institute's Surveillance, Epidemiology, and End Results Program estimated that 186,400 people were diagnosed with these diseases in 2021, and approximately 57,750 people were estimated to have died of these diseases in that year. Leukemia is the most common malignancy in children and young adults younger than 20 years, whereas non-Hodgkin lymphoma (NHL) is the third most common cancer in the same population. For patients less than 35 years, acute leukemia is the leading cause of cancer deaths.

This chapter will review hematologic malignancies and splenic tumors as they relate to the role of a clinical surgical oncologist and describe the therapeutic interventions necessary from a surgeon's perspective.

The Leukemias

Polycythemia Vera and Essential Thrombocythemia

Polycythemia vera (PV) is characterized by an autonomous expansion of red blood cell mass and volume with a variable effect on white blood cells and platelets. The etiologic mechanism is believed to involve a red blood cell clone highly sensitive to erythropoietin. Approximately three-fourths of patients with PV develop palpable splenomegaly and half develop hepatomegaly. Essential thrombocythemia (ET) is associated with an increase in megakaryocytes and platelet count with a variable effect on erythrocytes and white blood cells. Increased risk of thrombosis and hemorrhage occur in both PV and ET.

The primary treatment for both diseases is phlebotomy, low-dose chemotherapy, or the combination of these approaches. The goal of treatment for PV is to maintain a hematocrit less than 45% in men and 42% in women. The goal of treatment for ET is target platelet count of 100 to 400K/μL. Splenectomy has little to no role in the treatment of most patients with PV or ET. Although splenectomy has a minimal role in the treatment of these illnesses, a condition similar to myelogenous metaplasia develops in a few patients who then require splenectomy. The operative risks are greater and the survival is poorer in this group than in patients with myelogenous metaplasia. Patients with PV or ET should be treated with aggressive nonoperative therapy and offered splenectomy only when pain or when anemia and thrombocytopenia are refractory to other treatments. Splenectomy does not increase the survival rate, but it may improve the quality of life.

Myelogenous Metaplasia

Myelogenous metaplasia is a chronic myeloproliferative disease where immature myeloid precursor cells settle in the reticuloendothelial organs, primarily the spleen, liver, and lymph nodes. It is characterized by fibrosis of the bone marrow and extramedullary hematopoiesis, resulting in massive splenomegaly in approximately 75% of patients. Some patients are asymptomatic; however, most present with fatigue, anorexia, or weight loss in addition to symptomatic splenomegaly. Either thrombocytopenia or thrombocytosis can occur. Active splenic destruction may be humoral or cell mediated. Bone marrow biopsy is necessary for diagnosis. Large platelets, nucleated red cells, anisocytosis, and immature myelogenous elements are often seen on peripheral blood smears.

Initial nonoperative management includes transfusions, steroids, androgens, cytotoxic chemotherapy, and splenic irradiation. Hypersplenism refractory to these primary treatments may warrant splenectomy; however, operative mortality is approximately 9%. Nearly a quarter of patients may experience postsplenectomy thrombocytosis and progressive hepatomegaly. At MD Anderson Cancer Center, the indications for splenectomy in patients with myelogenous metaplasia with myelofibrosis are (a) severe anemia due to hypersplenism not responding to medical management; (b) chronically symptomatic splenomegaly; or (c) worsening congestive heart failure due to shunting through the spleen. Prior to splenectomy, adequate bone marrow activity must be documented by bone marrow biopsy and nuclear medicine bone marrow scan. If the major site of hematopoiesis is the spleen, a splenectomy may cause severe pancytopenia in these patients. Coagulation studies should also be performed preoperatively.

Postoperatively, these patients are at increased risk for portal vein thrombosis and thrombocytosis. The Mayo Clinic has published a 30-year review of their splenectomy experience with myeloid metaplasia that suggested that postoperative thrombotic complications may be reduced with the use of platelet-lowering therapy medical therapy with hydroxyurea, aspirin or anagrelide, and platelet apheresis for platelet counts greater than one million/μL. Postoperative portal vein thrombosis may present as a postoperative ileus, hepatic insufficiency, vague abdominal pain, or new-onset ascites. The treatment is 6 months of anticoagulation therapy while collateral circulation develops. To minimize the risk of portal vein thrombosis, the authors recommend ligating the splenic vein at its confluence with the superior mesenteric vein to maintain laminar blood flow.

Once again, splenectomy may improve the quality of life for these patients but does not provide a survival benefit. Following splenectomy, the response rates for anemia are 75% to 95%. For those patients who are poor candidates for surgery, low-dose radiation to the spleen may be used.

Chronic Myelogenous Leukemia

Also known as chronic granulocytic leukemia, chronic myelogenous leukemia (CML) involves the clonal proliferation of myelogenous stem cells. Ninety percent of CML patients have the Philadelphia chromosome, which is the characteristic translocation of chromosomes 9 and 22 and produces an oncoprotein from the fusion of the Abelson (ABL) oncogene with the breakpoint cluster region (BCR) to create unique tyrosine kinase BCR-ABL oncoprotein. Treatment response may be measured using PCR levels of the Philadelphia chromosome.

CML has a chronic benign phase, an accelerated phase, and an acute blastic transformation (i.e., blast crisis). Most patients present with symptoms of the chronic phase, which include fatigue, weakness, night sweats, low-grade fever, and abdominal pain. On physical examination, splenomegaly may be an isolated finding. Anemia or thrombocytopenia may result from hypersplenism. The median duration of the chronic phase is about 45 months and patients should be followed every 3 to 6 months. Approximately 80% of patients with CML will progress from the chronic phase to the acute leukemic phase.

The acute blastic phase may present as progressive fatigue, high fevers, symptomatic splenomegaly, anemia, thrombocytopenia, basophilia, and bone or joint pain. Frequent infections and bleeding episodes may manifest with increased splenic destruction of blood components. Traditional treatments of CML include tyrosine kinase inhibitors (e.g., imatinib), conventional chemotherapy with hydroxyurea or busulfan, and bone marrow transplant. Tyrosine kinase inhibitors are often the initial treatment choice for most newly diagnosed patients with CML.

The indications for splenectomy in CML are to relieve the symptoms of splenomegaly or reduce the need for transfusions. In the rare occasion where medical management fails, our experience with splenectomy for patients in accelerated or blastic phase CML at MD Anderson demonstrates that splenectomy can be performed safely during this phase and thrombocytopenia can be reliably reversed.

Chronic Lymphocytic Leukemia

Chronic lymphocytic leukemia (CLL) is characterized as a low-grade neoplastic disorder involving the accumulation of mature appearing but functionally incompetent B cells. It is the most common leukemia in the Western Hemisphere, and the median age of onset is in the seventh decade of life. Splenomegaly is common in the advanced stages of the disease. Common symptoms of hypersplenism include abdominal pressure, pain, gastric compression, anemia, or thrombocytopenia. Second malignancies develop in 20% of these patients, most commonly lung cancer, melanoma, or sarcoma. Overall survival is highly variable, representing a wide range of indolent to aggressive disease courses. The most common cause of death in patients with CLL is infection from progressive immune system compromise.

The Rai classification system is employed in CLL (Table 19.1). Multiple randomized controlled trials have failed to demonstrate a long-term survival benefit with immediate versus delayed therapy for early stage asymptomatic CLL. Accordingly, treatment is reserved for patients who develop disease-related symptoms or progressive disease (i.e., "active disease"). Treatment options include purine analogues (e.g., fludarabine), alkylating agents (e.g., chlorambucil), monoclonal antibodies (e.g., rituximab), or ibrutinib or venetoclax as single agents or in combination. Splenectomy may be recommended for patients refractory to chemotherapy or with symptomatic splenomegaly. Splenectomy has been shown to improve thrombocytopenia in 70% to 80% and anemia in 60% to 70% of patients with CLL. Our experience at MD Anderson demonstrates that splenectomy provides

TABLE 19.1	Rai Staging of Chronic Lymphocytic Leukemia

Stage	Criteria
0	Lymphocytosis (WBCs >15,000/mL with >40% lymphocytes in the bone marrow)
I	Lymphocytosis with lymphadenopathy
II	Lymphocytosis with enlarged liver or spleen (lymphadenopathy not necessarily present)
III	Lymphocytosis with anemia. Anemia may be due to hemolysis or due to decreased production (lymphadenopathy or hepatosplenomegaly need not be present)
IV	Lymphocytosis with thrombocytopenia (platelet count <100,000/μL), anemia, and lymphadenopathy

WBC, white blood cell.

an excellent hematologic response in patients with either isolated anemia or thrombocytopenia, but a poor response in patients with both. This suggests that hematopoietic reserve is necessary for a significant clinical response to splenectomy. In selected subgroups of patients with advanced-stage CLL, splenectomy demonstrates a significant survival advantage compared with conventional chemotherapy. This selected subgroup of CLL patients includes those with either hemoglobin levels ≤10 g/dL or platelet count ≤50 × 10⁹ L.

Hairy Cell Leukemia

Hairy cell leukemia (HCL) is a monoclonal lymphoproliferative disorder of mature B cells characterized by the pathognomonic cytoplasmic projections that invade the bone marrow and spleen. It is considered a low-grade leukemic disorder that comprises only 2% to 5% of all leukemias with a 3:1 male predominance typically older than the age of 50 years.

Approximately 10% of HCL patients will have mild symptoms and not require treatment. Splenomegaly is almost universally present; other symptoms may include weakness and fatigue. Indications for treatment include neutropenia, splenomegaly, hypersplenism, or bone marrow failure. The most common cause of death is infection in the setting of neutropenia.

Prior to the development of effective chemotherapeutic agents, splenectomy was the traditional treatment of choice for HCL patients and was associated with an increased survival. However, since the discovery of more effective agents, splenectomy is no longer routinely performed in this setting. Pentostatin and cladribine result in complete response rates of 80% to 90% which are also more durable responses compared to splenectomy. Newer therapies such as antibody drug conjugates (e.g. moxetumomab pasudotox targeting CD22), have garnered FDA approval based on a recent trial in chemotherapy refractory HCL patient's achieving 41% complete remission rate with this new antibody drug conjugate. Splenectomy may be considered in rare cases of the pure splenic form of disease or for palliation in HCL patients refractory to medical management.

Acute Lymphocytic Leukemia and Acute Myelogenous Leukemia

In general, there is no role for splenectomy in the treatment of acute lymphocytic leukemia or acute myelogenous leukemia during induction chemotherapy or relapse. Rare exceptions for splenectomy in these patients include cases of splenic rupture or persistent fungal granulomas of the spleen in patients in complete remission.

Splenic Rupture in Leukemia

Splenic rupture is a rare event in patients with leukemia and is almost exclusively the result of a traumatic injury. This is not due to the leukemia but rather the result of splenomegaly. The incidence of splenic rupture in leukemic patients is 0.2% and comprises 3.5% of all cases of spontaneous splenic rupture.

Patients most frequently present with abdominal tenderness, rigidity, and tachycardia. A chest radiograph may demonstrate an elevated hemidiaphragm or pleural effusion. An abdominal computed topography (CT) with intravenous contrast is the diagnostic imaging study of choice. Radiographic findings consist of perisplenic and free peritoneal fluid with possible active extravasation of contrast adjacent to a splenic capsular or hilar injury. For patients who are hemodynamically unstable in the setting of splenic rupture, emergent splenectomy is necessary. For those patients who are hemodynamically stable with evidence of active extravasation of intravenous contrast, emergent arterial embolization by interventional radiology frequently stops further hemorrhage and avoids operative intervention. In evaluating any patient with known splenomegaly and abdominal pain, a clinician must maintain a high index of suspicion for a splenic rupture. Leukemic patients who survive splenectomy after rupture maintain a similar life expectancy as other patients with the same type of leukemia.

The Lymphomas

Hodgkin Lymphoma

Over the past 25 years, the overall survival of patients with Hodgkin lymphoma (HL) has improved significantly. As our understanding of this tumor biology has advanced so has the use of multiple chemotherapy agents and radiation therapy to treat HL. HL is characterized by the presence of a few multinucleated Reed–Sternberg cells or cells of similar morphology and immunotype (Reed-Sternberg like cells) in an abundance of inflammatory cells. In contrast, the predominant cells in non-Hodgkin lymphoma (NHL) are predominantly malignant lymphocytes. The initial symptoms of HL typically include nontender lymphadenopathy, most commonly in the cervical lymph node basins. The axillary, inguinal, mediastinal, and retroperitoneal lymph nodes are less frequently involved at presentation. The presence of B symptoms should also be documented. These include unexplained fever with temperature >38 °C, night sweats, or weight loss of >10% body weight over 6 months.

The initial evaluation includes a comprehensive physical examination focusing on all lymph node basins and palpation for hepatomegaly and splenomegaly. Laboratory workup should include a complete blood count with differential and liver function tests. CT of the chest, abdomen, and pelvis, and bone marrow biopsy are performed to determine the extent of the disease. To confirm the suspected diagnosis of HL, core needle biopsy may be used. In cases where the diagnosis remains unclear, an excisional biopsy of suspected lymph node involvement may be necessary. For a surgical oncologist, selecting an enlarged lymph node in a relatively accessible location for excisional biopsy is the preferred strategy and lends itself to the lowest possible morbidity.

The prognosis of HL depends on the histologic subtype, stage of disease, and response to therapy. The World Health Organization classification of HL identifies two main entities nodular lymphocyte predominant and classical HL. The latter is divided to four subtypes—nodular sclerosis, mixed cellularity, lymphocyte depleted, and lymphocyte-rich cHL.

The Ann Arbor staging system (Table 19.2) was developed in 1971 and staged HL based on the extent of disease. Clinical staging includes data from the history, physical examination, and nonoperative diagnostic studies. Pathologic staging historically involves tissue analysis from staging laparotomy where the stages are designated with "E" or "S" to reflect extranodal involvement or splenic involvement, respectively. The presence of systemic symptoms, B, further subclassifies patients with HL.

Historically, all patients with HL underwent staging laparotomy to define the extent of disease and identify patients with early-stage disease, who could benefit from radiation versus those with extensive disease requiring systemic chemotherapy. A combination of improved noninvasive imaging modalities and more aggressive use of early systemic treatment and radiation therapy has effectively eliminated the role for staging laparotomy for this disease process. At the MD Anderson Cancer Center, nonoperative staging and prognostic factors are used to guide therapy in these patients. This approach is supported by the lack of evidence of a significant survival advantage between clinical and surgical staging. Performing an invasive staging laparotomy or laparoscopy, therefore, provides no benefit to HL patients and may delay the initiation of systemic chemotherapy.

The role for splenectomy, however, does occasionally exist in the HL population for two indications. The first is symptomatic splenomegaly refractory to chemoradiotherapy. Second are rare hematologic disturbances such as thrombocytopenia and leukopenia that may result in chemotherapy delays.

TABLE 19.2 Ann Arbor Staging System for Hodgkin Disease

Stage	Criteria
I	Involvement of a single lymph node region (I) or a single extralymphatic organ or site (IE)
II	Involvement of two or more lymph node regions on the same side of the diaphragm (II) or of an extralymphatic organ and its adjoining lymph node site (IIE)
III	Involvement of lymph node sites on both sides of the diaphragm (III) or localized involvement of an extralymphatic site (IIIE), spleen (IIIS), or both (IIISE)
IV	Diffuse or disseminated involvement of one or more extralymphatic organs with or without associated lymph node involvement
A	Asymptomatic
B	Fever, night sweats, or weight loss of more than 10%

Non-Hodgkin Lymphoma

NHL is the most common type of lymphoma and is characterized by the monoclonal proliferation of lymphocytes. Approximately 80% of NHL is derived from B-cell origin and the remainder 20% are from T cells. B-cell NHL is diagnosed and classified into subsets based on the identification of histopathologic markers using monoclonal antibodies and cellular morphology. These criteria for diagnosis depend on diffuse versus follicular (nodular) pattern of lymph node involvement, small versus large cell type, cell surface marker expression, and molecular/cytogenetic findings. Using these differences and others, patients with NHL may be placed into three categories: mature B-cell, mature T and NK cells, and immunodeficiency-associated lymphomas.

Patients with NHL present with superficial nontender lymphadenopathy, most commonly in the cervical lymph nodes. The Ann Arbor staging system initially developed for HD was adopted for the staging of NHL. It is generally less helpful for NHL because greater than half of NHL patients present with stage III or higher disease and 20% have B symptoms. Hematogenous spread versus lymphatic spread is more common in NHL compared to HL.

Surgical oncologists may be asked to evaluate patients with NHL for a variety of reasons. These include performing a diagnostic biopsy, providing vascular access for chemotherapy or rarely, splenectomy. Staging laparotomy is not indicated for NHL. Splenectomy, on the other hand, is indicated for NHL patients with symptomatic splenomegaly or pancytopenia requiring frequent transfusion requirements as a result of hypersplenism. NHL patients with a persistent isolated splenic focus of disease may also benefit from splenectomy. The prognosis of these selected individuals is similar to other stage I patients. Chimeric antigen receptor (CAR) T-cell therapy represents a significant advance that has allowed dramatically improved outcomes in selected patients with various types of NHL. One limiting factor that can prevent some patients from being able to undergo such therapy is bulky disease that puts them at risk of cytokine release syndrome (CRS) and immune effector cell-associated neurotoxicity syndrome (ICANS). In selected cases of patients with spleen-predominant disease who are otherwise good candidates, debulking splenectomy may improve their chances of tolerating CAR T-cell therapy.

Diagnostic Biopsy for Lymphoma

The pathologic diagnosis of a suspected lymphoma relies on the appropriate planning and communication between the medical oncologist, surgical oncologist, and pathologist. Surgeons are most often involved with excisional lymph node biopsies when core needle biopsies are nondiagnostic or when having nodal architecture will change management. Roughly 21% of lymph node biopsies will yield lymphoma. A large systematic review revealed that combined fine needle aspiration biopsy and core needle biopsy were able to identify subtypes of lymphoma 66% to 74% of the time; however, it was concluded that excisional lymph node biopsy was needed in 25% to 35% of cases to accurately classify lymphomas for treatment. The feasibility of excisional lymph node biopsy, however, depends on several factors in order to increase the chances of successful diagnosis.

Imaging plays a role in guiding excisional lymph node biopsy, and PET-CT has an evolving role in the management of lymphoma. It has been used to not only stage patients, but also provide information of post treatment effect and prognosis after chemotherapy and stem cell transplant. Most patients will present for surgical evaluation after having a PET-CT suspicious for active or residual disease. This combined anatomic and metabolic study is instrumental in the planning of excisional lymph node biopsies. Lymph nodes can be divided into peripheral and central locations, and strategies for biopsy vary by location. The targeted lymph node for excisional biopsy should be the largest node found on physical examination. Lymph nodes larger than 2 cm have the best diagnostic yield whereas nodes less than 1 cm are unlikely to provide a specific diagnosis. If multiple enlarged lymph nodes are present, the preferential biopsy sites are cervical lymph nodes, then axillary lymph nodes, and subsequently inguinal lymph nodes. For cases of matted lymph nodes or extranodal disease, a generous biopsy sample is helpful for diagnosis. The fundamental principle in making the pathologic diagnosis is the preservation of tumor architecture; therefore, sharp dissection is preferred over electrocautery.

Peripheral lymph nodes are located in the cervical, supraclavicular, axillary, and inguinal regions. Historical studies have stated that lymph nodes in the cervical and supraclavicular regions have the highest diagnostic yield, and that the axillary and inguinal regions have the lowest. However, this result has not been reproduced in the era of PET-CT and with improvements in image-guided biopsy. In general, peripheral lymph nodes are accessible with minimal dissection and most surgeons are familiar with the anatomy in these regions given their experience with techniques for sentinel lymph node biopsy from breast and melanoma surgery. At present, no radiotracers, dyes, or fluorescence techniques exist to guide dissection in hematologic malignancy, and palpability of the node is the primary cue to guide dissection. Intraoperative ultrasound is a useful adjunct to locate the node in horizontal and vertical planes into order to guide incision and limit unnecessary dissection. Limited dissection is important in this patient population as they are often neutropenic and prone to impaired healing and infection. Once dissected, the lymph node should immediately be sent fresh and sterile for appropriate studies (touch prep and flow cytometry); thus, having a pathologist readily available is important. It should be clearly communicated to the pathologist that the biopsy is for a suspected lymphoma to further aid in the appropriate processing of the tissue. Needle biopsies may be helpful to rule out a carcinoma or sarcoma or to provide evidence for a suspected relapse of lymphoma; however, they tend not to be as helpful for the initial diagnosis of lymphoma since the histologic architecture is not preserved.

Central lymph nodes are located in the mediastinum, retroperitoneum, and mesentery. These locations are less amenable to surgical biopsy, and core needle biopsies through IR or endoscopy should be utilized before proceeding with surgery. The mediastinum is accessible through mediastinoscopy and should be performed by those familiar with this technique. The retroperitoneum can be accessed through the abdomen or a retroperitoneoscopic approach in the same manner as retroperitoneal adrenalectomy. This technique is novel and still being refined at MD Anderson.

The mesentery can be accessed through laparoscopic techniques, and several case series have been published describing this technique. The mesentery can be accessed with a five port technique (one port in each quadrant, one umbilical camera site). The omentum is first reflected cephalad and tucked under the liver to reveal the colonic mesentery. The small bowel is then run from the ligament of Treitz to the terminal ileum. Evident lymphadenopathy is carefully excised with sharp dissection and electrocautery, and the area of dissection marked with clips. No large studies exist regarding laparoscopic lymph node biopsy; however, multiple smaller case series describe few complications and no mortalities. The primary morbidity is conversion to an open procedure as there is a lack of tactile feedback in minimally invasive techniques. The rate of conversion to open laparotomy ranges from 6% to 33%, and limited information exists regarding the diagnostic sensitivity of laparoscopic biopsy, with one study citing a false negative rate of 6%.

Complications from excisional lymph node biopsy for hematologic malignancy are not well characterized. As many of the procedures for peripheral lymph node biopsy are similar to techniques for sentinel lymph node biopsies for breast and melanoma, risks for lymphedema, lymphocele, vascular and nerve injury, and wound infection likely apply. Central lymph node biopsy complications are not well characterized. Additionally, most lymph nodes are located near major vascular structures and care needs to be taken not to cause major bleeding.

Miscellaneous Splenic Tumors

Splenic Cysts

Splenic cysts are typically classified as either primary (true) or secondary (false or pseudocysts) based on the presence of an epithelial lining. Primary cysts may be further classified as parasitic and nonparasitic. Nonparasitic cysts comprise 75% of splenic cysts in the United States and include both congenital and neoplastic cysts. Congenital cysts are characterized as epidermoid or dermoid cysts. These are usually diagnosed in children and young adults. Approximately 90% of nonparasitic true cysts are epidermoid cysts. Neoplastic cysts include lymphangiomas and cavernous hemangiomas. Parasitic cysts are very rare in the United States and most commonly the result of an echinococcal infection. Secondary cysts are more common than primary cysts and are generally believed to be the result of splenic injury and hematoma formation. Pseudocysts may also develop after acute pancreatitis, infections, or splenic infarcts. Patients with splenic cysts often present with vague symptoms of left upper quadrant pain and early satiety. Splenic cysts are often detected on physical examination as a palpable mass or on CT imaging. For nonparasitic splenic cysts <5 cm, conservative management with ultrasound follow-up is recommended. Indications for surgical management for patients with splenic cysts include size >5 cm, symptoms, hemorrhage, infection, or cyst perforation. The surgical options include complete or partial splenectomy, unroofing or marsupialization of the cyst, and fenestration. These can be performed through an open incision, hand-assisted, or completely laparoscopic techniques. Percutaneous drainage of splenic cysts is generally avoided due to the high incidence of recurrence and difficulty with subsequent operations due to the resulting inflammatory response.

Inflammatory Pseudotumor

Inflammatory pseudotumor, also known as plasma cell granuloma, has features of inflammation and mesenchymal repair. These pseudotumors may be found throughout the body, including the respiratory and gastrointestinal tracts, orbit, and lymph nodes. Similar to pseudocysts, they are believed to result from prior trauma or infection. These lesions are often mistaken for lymphoma, therefore requiring tissue diagnosis with immunohistochemical stains and flow cytometry to differentiate them from lymphoproliferative diseases.

Nonlymphoid Tumors

Nonlymphoid tumors of the spleen may be either benign or malignant. The most common malignant nonlymphoid tumors of the spleen are angiosarcomas, with a worldwide incidence of 0.14 to 0.25/million persons. These tumors tend to have an aggressive biology allowing them to grow quickly and metastasize early in their clinical course. The liver, lung, lymph nodes, and gastrointestinal track are typical sites of metastasis. Angiosarcomas are associated with exposure to thorium dioxide, vinyl chloride, and arsenic. Splenectomy is indicated in these patients but rarely curative. The overall prognosis is poor, with a median survival of only 5 months. Other rare malignant nonlymphoid splenic tumors include Kaposi sarcoma, malignant fibrous histiocytoma, fibrosarcoma, leiomyosarcoma, plasmacytomas, hemangiosarcomas, and lymphangiosarcomas.

Splenic Metastases

Splenic metastases are rare events given the large amount of total blood flow to the spleen. This may be related to the immunologic function of the spleen and its ability to clear microscopic metastatic disease. When they occur, they are usually associated with disseminated disease. The incidence of splenic metastases in autopsy studies ranges from 1.6% to 30%. The most frequently detected metastases originate from melanoma, breast, and lung cancer. Other primary sites include ovarian, endometrial, gastric, colonic, and prostate cancers. Splenectomy may be considered for solitary metastases with stable or treated primary disease such as melanoma or as part of a debulking procedure for ovarian, primary peritoneal, or appendiceal cancers. Novel strategies for patients with predominant bulky splenic disease causing prohibitive cytopenias may consider splenectomy prior to consolidation with CAR T-cell therapy; however, this strategy will require patient selection for their performance status. Other possible indications for splenectomy for metastatic disease include the treatment of complications of perforation of adjacent viscera, hemorrhage, or splenic vein thrombosis.

Splenectomy

Splenectomy for Hypersplenism

Anemia, neutropenia, and thrombocytopenia may occur for a number of reasons in patients with hematologic malignancies. Because only patients with excessive destruction of a blood component will benefit from a splenectomy, a careful workup should be done to identify the etiology of the process. Patients with hypersplenism may present with a normal-sized spleen, and others may have massive splenomegaly without hypersplenism.

Infusion of the patient's or normal donor platelets tagged with [111]indium is helpful in determining whether the spleen is the site of destruction. Patients with an acquired hemolytic anemia generally have a positive Coombs test, and the detection of the warm antibody is a good indication that splenectomy will be beneficial. Although chromium-labeled red blood cell scans may be useful in demonstrating decreases in red blood cell survival, they are not as helpful in identifying the site of sequestration. In cases of suspected splenic sequestration, a bone marrow biopsy is important to determine whether adequate precursor cells are available or whether the patient depends on the hematopoietic activity of the spleen.

Splenectomy in patients with CML has been associated with severe bleeding problems. These may be related to impaired clot formation caused by proteases and serases produced by granulocytes. Patients with CML and severe leukocytosis should receive chemotherapy in an attempt to decrease the WBC count to approximately 20,000 cells/mL. Experience at MD Anderson suggests that splenectomy is best avoided in patients with CML in whom WBC counts cannot be controlled with chemotherapy. Splenectomy should also be avoided in patients with CML who have had splenic irradiation due to significant technical surgical difficulty from the radiation-induced scarring and fibrosis.

Bleeding and infection are the greatest perioperative risks after splenectomy for hypersplenism. Qualitative platelet function should be evaluated rather than relying on a platelet count; however, the presence of thrombocytopenia can make this result inaccurate. The template bleeding time is currently the most widely available laboratory value for identifying adequacy of platelet function. The patient's current and recent medications should be carefully reviewed to identify any drugs that may impair coagulation.

Although splenectomy may be performed through either a midline or a subcostal approach, the midline incision is preferred when coagulation defects, thrombocytopenia, or splenomegaly is present. After the splenic pedicle is clamped, thrombocytopenic patients are transfused with fresh platelets. Careful hemostasis at the conclusion of the procedure is mandatory. Postoperatively, patients should be monitored closely during the first 48 hours for signs of bleeding. A blood cell count with differential and platelet counts should be obtained every 6 hours for the first 24 hours after the operation. Decreasing platelet and blood counts, despite adequate replacement, suggest an ongoing bleeding process.

Open Splenectomy for the Massively Enlarged Spleen

Indications for splenectomy in patients with massively enlarged spleens include debilitating symptoms of splenomegaly, excessive destruction of blood components, and concerns of possible splenic rupture. These patients often complain of chronic severe upper abdominal and back pain, impaired respiration, and early satiety. Hypersplenism may be present. Depending on the size of the spleen and the body habitus, the patient may be judged to be at increased risk of splenic trauma.

Preoperatively, it is important to check quantitative and qualitative platelet function values and coagulation studies because hemorrhage is the major complication of splenectomy in this group. Portal venous contrast studies should be performed in patients with possible portal hypertension.

Adequate blood products must be available preoperatively. The blood of these patients may be difficult to crossmatch because of numerous past transfusions, and fresh single-donor platelets may be required. Patients should undergo routine bowel preparation, and prophylactic antibiotics should be given.

A midline, rather than subcostal, incision is preferred because the rectus muscles are not severed, which limits bleeding. With increasing size, the spleen becomes more of a midline structure and lends itself to this approach. Before mobilization of the spleen, its vessels should be isolated. The gastrocolic omentum is divided, the lesser sac is entered, and the splenic artery is identified along the posterior-superior surface of the pancreas. Preoperative imaging is often helpful in localizing an area where the splenic artery courses most cephalad and superficially where control of it can be gained. The artery is ligated with a tie but left intact. The splenic vein is not disturbed yet. The spleen may decrease 20% to 30% in size at this point and allow platelet transfusion without consumption. The splenic flexure of the colon is mobilized, the splenic ligaments are divided, and the spleen is delivered from the splenic fossa. Many patients with myeloproliferative and lymphoid neoplasms may have undergone numerous chemotherapies that have enlarged or shrunken the spleen, and normally avascular splenic ligaments often contain small vessels or become scarred. Dense adhesions between the spleen and the diaphragm may complicate mobilization; and when dissection is particularly difficult, it is better to resect part of the diaphragm with the spleen than to risk hypertrophy of splenic remnants. Such adhesions are formed in areas of splenic infarction and are the most frequent sites of postoperative bleeding in this group of patients. Small holes in the diaphragm can be repaired primarily, and air can be evacuated from the thoracic cavity using a red rubber catheter.

After the spleen is mobilized, the artery and vein are suture ligated and divided. On rare occasions, scarring from treated lymphadenopathy in the splenic hilum may prevent safe division of the splenic artery and vein necessitating a partial distal pancreatectomy. Liver biopsy may be indicated if involvement by lymphoma is suspected. If an injury to the pancreatic tail is recognized, it should be repaired and drained appropriately. Achieving hemostasis in the splenic bed is crucial and may require suture ligation, cautery, platelet transfusions, and thrombostatic agents. Drains are not routinely used, except in cases of suspected pancreatic injury. Postoperatively, patients should be closely monitored for signs of bleeding or infection.

Minimally Invasive Splenectomy

The minimally invasive approach has several advantages over open splenectomy, most obviously, less morbidity from smaller incisions. Other advantages include shorter length of stay, less pain and need for narcotics, and fewer complications. Overall, a laparoscopic approach has also been associated with lower mortality as compared with open surgery. For benign hematologic disease and splenic tumors, laparoscopic splenectomy has become the standard approach. For malignant conditions without contraindications, its role has been generally accepted, provided that fundamental oncologic surgical principles are observed. The outcomes of robotic surgery in splenectomy are evolving with more surgeons becoming familiar with this platform; however, surgical technique is similar to the laparoscopic approach and the benefit to patients is likely similar.

Absolute contraindications to a minimally invasive approach include emergent conditions such as splenic rupture. Relative contraindications to minimally invasive splenectomy include uncorrected coagulopathy, severe portal hypertension, and pregnancy; however, there have been successful reports in all of these conditions.

A lateral approach, anterior approach, or hand-assisted technique can be used. With the lateral approach, the patient is positioned in right lateral decubitus. It is important to prepare a wide field as conversion to open surgery may be necessary. Pneumoperitoneum is established using either an open cutdown technique or with the use of an optical trochar after insufflation with a Veress needle. Of note, use of the Veress needle is contraindicated in patients with massive splenomegaly and children (due to limited working domain). A total of four trochars are placed; the first in the midclavicular line, 2 to 6 cm below the costal margin. The remaining three ports are placed 3 to 4 cm below the inferior tip of the spleen; one placed in the subxiphoid region (under the left costal margin), another at the anterior axillary line below the left costal edge. The final trochar is usually placed laterally off the tip of the 11th rib once the splenic flexure has been mobilized. Trochar sizes can range from 5 to 12 mm, as per surgeon's preference. Surgery proceeds with a diagnostic laparoscopy to identify accessory spleens, which are present in 12% to 32% of patients. The splenic attachments are then divided in the following order: the splenocolic ligament, splenorenal ligament (inferior pole vessels), gastrosplenic ligament (short gastric vessels), and the splenophrenic ligament. The order can vary, however, according to surgeon's preference. An energy device (e.g., ultrasonic coagulation shears or bipolar sealing device) can facilitate hemostasis when dividing these attachments. Once the spleen has been mobilized, it is elevated to expose the hilum. Care must be taken to avoid the tail of the pancreas when ligating the splenic vasculature with an endoscopic stapler. The spleen can then be placed into a retrieval sac and partially exteriorized via the 12-mm port site where morcellation can ensue. In some instances, extraction of an intact spleen is necessary for pathologic diagnosis. At MD Anderson, retrieval of a whole specimen is preferred by our hematopathologists; however, local preferences should be determined preoperatively. Drains are not necessary unless injury to the pancreatic tail is a concern.

The anterior approach is seldom used except in instances where the spleen is very large or if use of a hand-assist device is anticipated. With the patient in lithotomy position, the surgeon stands between the patient's legs. If no lithotomy is used, the surgeon stands to the patient's right. Access to abdominal cavity is obtained at the umbilicus, usually with an open cutdown approach. Trochars are again placed in a fashion similar to the semicircle in the left upper quadrant described above. The liver and stomach are retracted medially. The splenocolic attachments are released and the lower pole of the spleen is elevated to expose the splenic hilum. The splenic artery is then ligated using clips. The gastrosplenic ligament is released and the remaining splenic attachments are dissected. The stapler is deployed across the hilum staying close to the spleen to avoid damage to the pancreatic tail. Multiple staple loads are often needed to divide the hilar vessels if the spleen is very large. The spleen can then be removed via a retrieval sac.

The hand-assisted laparoscopic surgery (HALS) approach is often used as a bridge between open and laparoscopic splenectomy. This hybrid approach may also be helpful in manipulating a larger spleen. In particular, it can be especially helpful when spleens are >20 cm in size. A hand-port can be used with either in a lateral or anterior approach. Standing on the patient's right, the surgeon's left hand is placed into the abdomen via an incision that is generally 7 to 8 cm long and located 2 to 4 cm caudal to the inferior pole of the spleen. A hand-assist device is then inserted and allows for medial retraction of the spleen. The remainder of the procedure proceeds as described above. Many experts agree that surgical outcomes from HALS and laparoscopic splenectomy are equivalent in regards to complications, hospital length of stay, and patient satisfaction.

Complications of laparoscopic splenectomy are similar to those with open surgery and include bleeding, pancreatic tail injury, portal vein thrombosis, and overwhelming postsplenectomy infection. Postoperative bleeding occurs in approximately 3% of laparoscopic cases. Portal vein thrombosis can occur in 0.7% to 14% of patients and is more common in patients with splenomegaly, myeloproliferative disorders, and hemolysis.

Prophylaxis for Asplenic Sepsis

Patients with hematologic malignancies who undergo splenectomy are at greater risk for asplenic sepsis than those who have the procedure for other indications (i.e., trauma). Some patients with hematologic malignancy, especially those with CML and CLL, are at increased risk for sepsis even before splenectomy. The risk of overwhelming postsplenectomy infection (OPSI) is greatest for children. The expected death rate from OPSI in children is one in every 300 to 350 patient-years; and in adults, one in every 800 to 1,000 patient-years. For all patients, the risk is greatest for the first few years following splenectomy, but deaths attributed to OPSI have occurred 30 or more years after splenectomy. *Streptococcus pneumoniae* is the most common infecting organism.

Following splenectomy, there is loss of the opsonins, tuftsin, and properdin, a decrease in immunoglobulin M production, impaired phagocytosis, and altered cellular immunity. Poorly opsonized bacteria are best cleared by the spleen, and following the spleen's removal, patients are particularly susceptible to encapsulated bacteria.

Vaccination can decrease the risk of postsplenectomy pneumococcal infection. The 23-valent form of the pneumococcal vaccine should be used. The vaccine is most effective when given several weeks preoperatively. Nevertheless, despite the diminished immunity obtained if the vaccine is given after splenectomy, adequate protection is still achieved in most patients if administered after 2 weeks postoperatively. Booster immunizations with the pneumococcal vaccine have no proven benefit, although reimmunization at 3 to 5 years may be required if a decrease in specific antibody levels is documented. Certain subsets of patients are at increased risk of infection with *Haemophilus influenzae* and *Neisseria meningitidis* and, therefore, patients should receive these vaccinations as well. Patients are also instructed to keep a supply of antibiotics such as amoxicillin and Augmentin (amoxicillin; clavulanate potassium) with them, which should be taken at the first sign of a febrile episode. This should also be followed by immediate contact with a physician.

CASE SCENARIO

Case Scenario 1

Presentation

A 68-year-old female presents to clinic after having been diagnosed with myelofibrosis approximately 6 months previously. She had persistent mild thrombocytopenia with a platelet count of 80 to 100. She was started on low-dose ruxolitinib (5 mg twice daily) by her hematologist, who noted an approximately 25-cm spleen. She was referred for consideration of splenectomy with the goal of being able to increase the dose of her ruxolitinib and ultimately to undergo allogeneic stem cell transplant. CT of the abdomen demonstrated that the spleen was 25 in cranial-caudal length, 11 cm in anterior-posterior depth, and did not cross the midline. There were no radiographic findings of portal hypertension. Appropriate vaccines were administered more than 2 weeks preoperatively.

Surgical Approach—Key Steps

The abdomen was explored via a midline laparotomy. The lesser sac was opened by dividing the gastrosplenic ligament. The superior pole of the spleen was mobilized. The splenic artery was visualized coursing superior to and superficial to the junction of the body and tail of the pancreas. The splenic artery was ligated but not divided here. The splenocolic ligament was then mobilized from the inferior pole of the spleen using an energy device, and the posterior spleen was similarly dissected from the splenorenal ligament. The spleen was noted to have substantially reduced in volume by this point. The hilar vessels were well visualized at this point, and they were divided with a vascular stapler. There was good hemostasis. No accessory spleens were noted. Given that the pancreatic tail was protected throughout the operation, no drain was left.

Postoperative Care

The patient was admitted to the hospital and had an uncomplicated course. She demonstrated no evidence of bleeding and was able to be advanced to a regular diet within 2 days. Over 6 months of follow-up, her platelet count remained >300. She was able to be increased to full-dose ruxolitinib because her thrombocytopenia resolved, and she is currently being considered for allogeneic stem cell transplant.

Case Scenario 2

Presentation

A 65-year-old man with history of mantle cell lymphoma that had originally been diagnosed 7 years previously was referred to the surgical oncology clinic with right axillary lymphadenopathy, splenomegaly with splenic lesions, and a small right lung nodule. He had originally been treated with R-Hyper-CVAD for eight cycles with complete remission. He then developed recurrence 4 years later and was treated with ibrutinib and rituximab. He underwent excisional left axillary lymph node biopsy, which showed recurrent pleiomorphic mantle cell lymphoma with a high Ki-67 index. On imaging, his spleen was 18 × 16 × 12 cm in size and it was noted to have increased rapidly in size over a short interval. It was estimated upon review of imaging that over 90% of his visible disease was contained within the spleen. His platelet count was 90. His hematologist assessed his relapsed, aggressive mantle cell lymphoma as incurable with standard therapeutic options, and rapid clinical decline was felt to be likely. The option of a CAR T-cell (Tecartus) clinical trial was discussed. In order for this to be possible, it was necessary for him to undergo splenectomy in order to achieve debulking, which would minimize the risk of CRS and ICANS after initiating the CAR T-cell trial. He was consented for laparoscopic splenectomy and the possibilities of conversion to a hand-assisted or open procedure were also discussed. He was typed and crossed for four units of blood.

Surgical Approach—Key Steps

The patient was positioned on a bump with the left side up. Laparoscopic access to the abdomen was gained with a Hasson port supraumbilically. Upon evaluation, the spleen was 28 × 25 cm—which was larger than his last imaging only 2 weeks prior. There were also many adhesions of the spleen to the abdominal wall. A hand port was placed in the superior midline. The inferior pole of the spleen was freed up by laparoscopically mobilizing the splenic flexure and dividing the splenorenal ligament. The short gastric vessels were then divided heading toward the gastric cardia with the energy device. The lesser sac was inspected and no accessory spleens were noted. The cephalad aspect of the spleen was intimately associated with the short gastric vessels in this area, which were quite friable. Some bleeding was encountered here and the decision was made to convert to an open procedure. After placing a retractor, the splenic artery was ligated at the superior border of the pancreas, which stopped the bleeding from the superior pole of the spleen. The spleen was then carefully mobilized laterally, which allowed exposure of the vessels at the hilum. The splenic artery and vein were ligated and divided near the hilum, taking care to protect the tail of the pancreas. There was a 1-cm hole in the diaphragm where the spleen had been adherent. This was repaired primarily and the air was evacuated with a red rubber catheter. No drain was left. An NG tube was left given the extensive dissection.

Postoperative Care

The patient had an unremarkable postoperative course. His NG was removed on postoperative day 2 and he tolerated a regular diet by postoperative day 4. His Hb trended down to 7.2 by the time of discharge and he was transfused 1 unit of blood. He was discharged on postoperative day 6 and his platelet count at that time was >400. He recovered well but restaging scans approximately 1 month after surgery showed progression of his adenopathy elsewhere. He then enrolled on a CAR T-cell clinical trial and the CAR T-cells were infused approximately 2 months after surgery. He had CRS during this and required management in the intensive care unit, tocilizumab, and a steroid taper. He recovered well and has remained in remission from his mantel cell lymphoma for 5 years after splenectomy.

CASE SCENARIO REVIEW

Questions

1. What is the most reproducible location where early control of the splenic artery can be obtained during an open splenectomy?

    A. The splenic hilum
    B. At the takeoff from the celiac trunk
    C. At the inferior border of the pancreas
    D. At the superior border of the pancreas

2. Which of the following statements on the role of splenectomy in myelofibrosis is correct?

    A. Splenectomy improves thrombocytopenia in over 90% of patients and is associated with improved overall survival.
    B. Splenectomy improves thrombocytopenia in approximately 75% of patients but is associated with decreased overall survival.
    C. Splenectomy improves thrombocytopenia in under 50% of patients and is associated with decreased overall survival.
    D. Splenectomy improves thrombocytopenia in under 50% of patients and is associated with improved overall survival.

3. Which of the statements regarding accessory spleens is true?

    A. Accessory spleens are present in under 5% of patients.
    B. Accessory spleens are rarely a cause of recurrent thrombocytopenia after splenectomy for hematologic malignancy.
    C. Accessory spleens are usually >3 cm in size.
    D. Accessory spleens are commonly found to be associated with the pancreatic tail or splenic vessels, in the greater omentum, in the small bowel mesentery, or in the renal fossa.

4. Which of the following is correct regarding the role of splenectomy in a patient being considered for CAR T-cell therapy for mantle cell lymphoma?

    A. Splenectomy is useful in these patients if there is disseminated disease such that the splenic disease accounts for under half of the overall disease burden.

    B. The purpose of splenectomy in such patients is to reduce the risk of cytokine release syndrome during CAR T-cell therapy.

    C. Careful screening for fitness for CAR T-cell therapy from a medical and performance status standpoint can be undertaken after the splenectomy is completed.

    D. It is worthwhile to persist for long periods of time with a minimally invasive approach in the face of massive with adhesions.

5. A 56-year-old woman with newly diagnosed chronic myomelanocytic leukemia presents with left sided abdominal pain. CT angiogram demonstrates an 18-cm spleen with a 3-cm subcapsular hematoma and an arterial blush from a branch of the splenic artery. The patient has focal left upper quadrant peritonitis on examination. Blood pressure is 135/75 and HR is 85. What is the next best step?

    A. NPO status, serial abdominal examinations, and Q12 hematocrit measurements

    B. Splenic angioembolization

    C. Laparoscopic splenectomy

    D. Open splenectomy

Answers

1. **The correct answer is D.** *Rationale:* CT imaging will often identify where the splenic artery courses above the superior border of the pancreas. The artery can be ligated with a tie here early during the case to decrease blood flow to the spleen, which increases the safety of the rest of the dissection. This is safer than attempting to approach the splenic hilum early (A). There is no need for dissection to proceed near the celiac trunk (B). The splenic artery is most commonly found near the superior border of the pancreas, not the inferior border (C).

2. **The correct answer is B.** *Rationale:* Among a cohort of patients at MD Anderson Cancer Center who underwent splenectomy for myelofibrosis, the thrombocytopenia response rate was 75%. However, patients who required splenectomy had over twofold higher overall mortality and they also had reduced transformation-free survival. Given the development of JAK2 inhibitors as an alternative safe and effective therapy for myelofibrosis, splenectomy should be reserved for patients with refractory cytopenias and large spleens that do not respond to medical management.

3. **The correct answer is D.** *Rationale:* Accessory spleens are present in approximately 10% of patients (A). Accessory spleens are a common cause of recurrent thrombocytopenia after splenectomy for hematologic malignancy (B). Accessory spleens may be of any size but are most commonly approximately 1 cm in size (C).

4. **The correct answer is B.** *Rationale:* Splenectomy is only useful in patients in whom the majority of disease is in the spleen such that they will achieve substantial debulking with splenectomy. C is incorrect. This approach should only be undertaken in carefully selected patients who are thought to be good candidates medically, have adequate family support for CAR T-cell therapy, and have adequate performance status. Such decisions should involve multidisciplinary communication between the surgical and hematology teams. D is incorrect. It is important to balance the benefits of an intended minimally invasive approach with the goal for the patient to have an efficient operation with minimal blood loss. We commonly will set a time limit for conversion to an open procedure if sufficient progress is not being made laparoscopically. Conversion to a hand-assisted approach is often a useful intermediate step, as many cases can be completed in this manner without needing to convert to an open procedure.

5. **The correct answer is B.** *Rationale:* This normotensive patient with an active arterial blush and a subcapsular hematoma would be best served by expedient angioembolization (B). Observation is inappropriate given the presence of an arterial blush and blood counts would need to be checked more often than every 12 hours (A). A minimally invasive approach is contraindicated in cases of splenic rupture (C). Open splenectomy would be appropriate if the patient had hemodynamic instability (D).

Recommended Readings

Berman RS, Yahanda AM, Mansfield PF, et al. Laparoscopic splenectomy in patients with hematologic malignancies. *Am J Surg.* 1999;178:530–536.

Bouvet M, Babiera GV, Termuhlen PM, Hester JP, Kantarjian HM, Pollock RE. Splenectomy in the accelerated or blastic phase of chronic myelogenous leukemia: a single institution, 25-year experience. *Surgery.* 1997;122:20.

Coad JE, Matutes E, Catovsky D. Splenectomy in lymphoproliferative disorders: a report on 70 cases and review of the literature. *Leuk Lymphoma.* 1993;10:245.

Cusack JC, Seymour JF, Lerner S, Keating MJ, Pollock RE. The role of splenectomy in chronic lymphocytic leukemia. *J Am Coll Surg.* 1997;185:237.

Dawes LG, Malangoni MA. Cystic masses of the spleen. *Am Surg.* 1986;52:333.

Fielding AK. Prophylaxis against late infection following splenectomy and bone marrow transplant. *Blood Rev.* 1994;8:179.

Flexner JM, Stein RS, Greer JP. Outline of treatment of lymphoma based on hematologic and clinical stage with expected end results. *Surg Oncol Clin North Am.* 1993;2:283.

Frederiksen JK, Sharma M, Casulo C, Burack WR. Systematic review of the effectiveness of fine-needle aspiration and/or core needle biopsy for subclassifying lymphoma. *Arch Pathol Lab Med.* 2015;139(2):245–251.

Georgia M, Rady K, Prince HM. Inflammatory pseudotumor of the spleen. *Hematol Rep.* 2015;7(2):5905. doi: 10.4081/hr.2015.5905. eCollection 2015 Jun 3.

Harris NL. The pathology of lymphomas: a practical approach to diagnosis and classification. *Surg Oncol Clin North Am.* 1993;2:167.

Harris W, Marcaccio M. Incidence of portal vein thrombosis after laparoscopic splenectomy. *Can J Surg.* 2005;48(5):352–354.

Hubbard SM, Longo DL. Treatment-related morbidity in patients with lymphoma. *Curr Opin Oncol.* 1991;3:852.

Johnson HA, Deterling RA. Massive splenomegaly. *Surg Gynecol Obstet.* 1989;168:131.

Kalhs P, Schwarzinger I, Anderson G, et al. A retrospective analysis of the long-term effect of splenectomy on late infections, graft-versus-host disease, relapse, and survival after allogenic marrow transplantation for chronic myelogenous leukemia. *Blood.* 1995;86:2028.

Kantarjian H, Sawyers C, Hochhaus A, et al. Hematologic and cytogenetic responses to imatinib mesylate in chronic myelogenous leukemia. *N Engl J Med.* 2002;346(9):645.

Klein B, Stein M, Kuten A, et al. Splenomegaly and solitary spleen metastasis in solid tumors. *Cancer.* 1987;60:100.

Kluin-Nelemans HC, Noordijk EM. Staging of patients with Hodgkin's disease: what should be done? *Leukemia.* 1991;4:132.

Kohutek F, Badik L, Bystricky B. Primary angiosarcoma of the spleen: rare diagnosis with atypical clinical course. *Case Rep Oncol Med.* 2016;2016:4905726.

Kojouri K, Vesely SK, Terrell DR, George JN. Splenectomy for adult patients with idiopathic thrombocytopenic purpura: a systematic review to assess long-term platelet count responses, prediction of response, and surgical complications. *Blood.* 2004;104:9.

Kraus MD, Fleming MD, Vonderhide RH. The spleen as a diagnostic specimen: a review of 10 years' experience at two tertiary care institutions. *Cancer.* 2001;91:11.

Kurzrock R, Talpaz M, Gutterman JU. Hairy cell leukaemia: review of treatment. *Br J Haematol.* 1991; 79(suppl 1):17.

Macapinlac HA. FDG PET and PET/CT imaging in lymphoma and melanoma. *Cancer J.* 2004;10(4):262–270.

Mahon D, Rhodes M. Laparoscopic splenectomy: size matters. *Ann R Coll Surg Eng.* 2003;85:248.

McBride CM, Hester JP. Chronic myelogenous leukemia: management of splenectomy in a high-risk population. *Cancer.* 1977;39:653.

Noordijk EM, Carde P, Mandard AM, et al. Preliminary results of the EORTC-GPMC controlled clinical trial H7 in early stage Hodgkin's disease. *Ann Oncol.* 1994;5(suppl 2):107.

Owera A, Hamade AM, Bani Hani OI, Ammori BJ. Laparoscopic versus open splenectomy for massive splenomegaly: a comparative study. *J Laparoendosc Adv Surg Tech A.* 2006;16(3):241–246.

Pittaluga S, Bijnens L, Teodorovic A, et al. Clinical analysis of 670 cases in two trials of the European Organization for the Research and Treatment of Cancer Lymphoma Cooperative Group subtyped according to the Revised European-American Classification of lymphoid neoplasms: a comparison with the working formulation. *Blood*. 1996;10:4358.

Pugalenthi A, Bradley C, Gonen M, et al. Splenectomy to treat splenic lesions: an analysis of 148 cases at a cancer center. *J Surg Oncol*. 2013;108(8):521–525. doi: 10.1002/jso.23433.

Rubin LG, Schaffner W. Clinical practice. Care of the asplenic patient. *N Engl J Med*. 2014;371:349.

Santos FP, Tam CS, Kantarjian H, et al. Splenectomy in patients with myeloproliferative neoplasms: efficacy, complications and impact on survival and transformation. *Leuk Lymphoma*. 2014;55(1):121–127.

Winslow ER, Brunt LM. Perioperative outcomes of laparoscopic versus open splenectomy: a meta-analysis with an emphasis on complications. *Surgery*. 2003;134(4):647.

Yee J, Christou NV. Perioperative care of the immunocompromised patient. *World J Surg*. 1993;17(2):207–214.

Genitourinary Cancer

Jack R. Andrews, Christopher G. Wood, and Jose A. Karam

INTRODUCTION

Global cancer statistics reveals that genitourinary cancers represented approximately 13.1% of new cancers diagnosed worldwide in 2020. These cancers occur in approximately 300,000 patients within the United States each year. Recognizing these facts, practicing physicians require an essential understanding of the diagnosis and treatment of these diseases. In this chapter, we review the current management of prostate, bladder, renal, and testicular neoplasms.

Prostate Cancer

Epidemiology and Etiology

In men, prostate cancer is the most common malignancy and the second leading cause of solid tumor mortality. In the United States, it is estimated that one of seven men will be diagnosed with prostate cancer during their lifetime. In 2021, approximately 248,530 new cases were expected, and 34,130 estimated deaths were attributed to prostate cancer. Nearly 2.4% (1 in 41) of men will die from their disease. Prostate cancer screening was introduced in the United States in 1986. Since this introduction, the pattern of disease incidence has changed. From 1988 to 1992, the annual percent increase of prostate cancer incidence was estimated at 17.5% per year. From 1992 to 1995, the incidence decreased to 10.3% per year. This decrease has leveled off and from 1995 to 1997, the average annual decrease in incidence was 2.1%, and the average annual incidence was 149.7 cases per 100,000. These cancer trends are not equivalent between whites and African Americans. Prostate cancer incidence in white males is 123 per 100,000 compared to 208.7 per 100,000 in African Americans, while the resulting mortality is 19.9 per 100,000 versus 47.2 per 100,000, respectively (2008 to 2012). Furthermore, although the average annual mortality rates have decreased 3.6% per year (2003 to 2012) overall, African Americans have experienced a similar decrease in the average mortality rate compared to white males (3.6% vs. 3.4%), respectively per year, between 2003 and 2012. African Americans used to have 2.4-fold higher mortality rate than white males. It is unclear whether the increased mortality rate of prostate cancer in African Americans is due to unique racial biologic and genetic factors, rather than dietary influences, the existence of confounding medical comorbid conditions, lifestyle differences, and/or access to health care issues. Occupational exposure to cadmium has been associated with increased risk of prostate cancer, but this relationship is not yet proven to be causal.

Over 60% of new cases are diagnosed in men aged 60 years and older, and the mean age at diagnosis is 67 years. Prostate cancer rarely occurs before the age of 50 years, and the incidence increases through the ninth decade of life; however, some of this increase may be attributable to an increase in prostate cancer screening in the later decades. It is estimated that 30% to 50% of men older than 50 years have histologic evidence of prostate cancer at autopsy, while at the age of 75 years or older, it is estimated that this figure increases to 50% to 70%.

Many factors have been proposed to be associated with the development of prostate cancer. The presence of an intact hypothalamic–pituitary–gonadal axis and advanced age are the most universally accepted risk factors. Migration studies support a role for environmental influences on prostate cancer. Higher rates of prostate cancer have been found among populations with higher amounts of fat in the diet. Beneficial dietary associations include isoflavonoids and lycopenes. Until recently, selenium and vitamin E were considered to exert a protective effect against prostate cancer. However, the Selenium and Vitamin E Cancer Prevention Trial (SELECT trial, 2009) showed no difference in prostate cancer incidence in subjects who received selenium and vitamin E. Two large prospective trials have shown that inhibiting 5-alpha reductase (which converts testosterone into dihydrotestosterone [DHT]) can prevent prostate cancer in a subset of patients. The Prostate Cancer Prevention Trial (PCPT trial, 2003 and updated in 2013) reported a 30% decrease in the incidence of prostate cancer in patients on finasteride when followed for 18 years; however, high-grade cancer rates were increased, which was later reported as an artifact resulting from shrinkage of the prostate and selective inhibition of low-grade cancers. Ultimately, there was no difference between the overall survival and prostate cancer–specific survival between the two groups.

Evidence has shown that a man with 1, 2, or 3 first-degree relatives affected with prostate cancer has a 2, 5, or 11 times greater risk, respectively, of the development of prostate cancer than the general population. A Mendelian pattern of autosomal dominant transmission of prostate cancer accounts for 43% of disease occurring before the age of 55 years and 9% of all prostate cancers occurring by the age of 85 years. Recent data have implicated the 8q24 chromosomal locus as a risk factor for prostate cancer.

Anatomy

The normal prostate gland weighs 15 to 20 g and is divided into three major glandular zones. The *peripheral zone* constitutes 70% of the prostate gland and is the area palpated during digital rectal examination (DRE). The area around the ejaculatory ducts is called the *central zone* and accounts for 25% of the gland. The *transitional zone* comprises 5% of the prostate gland around the urethra. In a pathologic review of 104 prostate glands from patients who underwent radical prostatectomy, 68% of the cancers were located in the peripheral zone, 24% in the transitional zone, and only 8% in the central zone. Almost all stage T1 (nonpalpable) cancers in that study were found in the transitional zone, the area most susceptible to benign prostatic hyperplasia, which can be associated with urinary symptoms secondary to bladder neck obstruction. The neurovascular bundle of the prostate runs bilaterally along the posterior–lateral boarder of the prostate at 5 and 7 o'clock.

Screening

Although good screening methods for prostate cancer are available, controversy surrounds the concept of screening for this disease. It is estimated that less than 10% of men with prostate cancer die because of the disease. This leads to a lack of consensus on the optimal management of early-stage disease and to questions regarding the cost-effectiveness of a national screening effort for all men older than 50 years. Two large randomized studies recently questioned the utility of screening for prostate cancer. The Prostate, Lung, Colorectal, and Ovarian Cancer Screening Trial (PLCO, 2009 and updated in 2013) compared one group of men that underwent prostate-specific antigen (PSA) screening with another group that did not undergo screening and found no difference in mortality rates from prostate cancer. However, almost 44% of the patients in both arms of this trial underwent PSA testing prior to enrollment in the trial. On the other hand, the European Randomized Study of Screening for Prostate Cancer (ERSPC, 2009 and updated in 2014) reported that screening with PSA resulted in a 21% reduction in the rate of death from prostate cancer, but was associated with a high risk of overdiagnosis. As such, in 2012 the US Preventive Services Task Force recommended against PSA screening on the grounds that there is no net benefit and that the potential harms outweigh the benefits. In 2018, US Preventive Services Task Force adjusted their stance to recommend a shared decision-making process for PSA screening of men aged 55 to 69 years. Congruently, the American Urological Association (AUA) recommends against routine screening in men between ages 40 and 54 years at average risk of prostate cancer. AUA recommends shared decision-making for men aged 55 to 69 years with a life expectancy of at least 10 years who are considering PSA screening and proceeding based on patients' values and preferences. Routine PSA screening is not recommended in men over age 70 years or any man with less than 10 to 15 years life expectancy. The American Cancer Society recommends discussing screening with patients and offering a DRE and measurement of PSA starting at the age of 50 years for men with a life expectancy of at least 10 years. Screening should begin at age 45 for African-American men or men with one first-degree relative with prostate cancer, and at age 40 for men with even higher risk, such as history of prostate cancer in many first-degree relatives, diagnosed at an early age.

Diagnosis

Patients with low-volume, clinically localized prostate cancer are typically asymptomatic; abnormalities are detected by DRE, increased serum PSA level, or both. Advanced prostate cancer can be asymptomatic; present as local symptoms of urinary hesitancy, frequency, and urgency; or present as systemic symptoms of weight loss, fatigue, and bone pain. Rarely, neurologic sequelae of impending spinal cord compression secondary to bone metastasis or uremia secondary to bilateral ureteral or bladder neck obstruction can be found in the presentation of advanced cases.

PSA is a serine protease produced by the epithelium of the prostate. PSA is not specific for prostate cancer and can be increased in benign conditions of the prostate such as prostatitis, prostatic infarction, and benign prostatic hyperplasia. Traditionally, a PSA threshold of 4 ng/mL was used as a trigger to perform a biopsy. This PSA threshold has been lowered recently to 2.5 ng/mL, although the risk of cancer is also dependent on age, prostate volume, and PSA velocity. In fact, prostate cancer can be found in 6.6% of men with PSA <0.5 ng/mL, 10.1% of men with PSA 0.6 to 1.0 ng/mL, 17% of men with PSA 1.1 to 2.0 ng/mL, 23.9% of men with PSA 2.1 to 3.0 ng/mL, and 26.9% of men with PSA 3.1 to 4.0 ng/mL. It can also be increased as a consequence of recent ejaculation, and patients should be counseled to abstain from sexual activity for periods of up to 1 week prior to PSA screening. Transurethral resection of the prostate (TURP) and prostatic needle biopsy significantly increase the serum PSA level above baseline for up to 8 weeks. DRE (without prostate massage), cystoscopy, and transrectal ultrasound (TRUS) do not alter serum PSA to a clinically significant degree. The positive predictive value of a PSA level greater than 4 ng/mL for the detection of prostate cancer is 34.4%, while the positive predictive value for an abnormal DRE is 21.4%. Detection rates demonstrate that DRE and PSA together (5.8%) are superior to either DRE (3.2%) or PSA (4.6%) alone. Free PSA is a form of PSA not conjugated to protease inhibitors in the serum. Decreased percentage-free PSA (<25%) is associated with prostate cancer, and measurement of free PSA is performed to improve the specificity of PSA testing in the range of 4 to 10 ng/mL and thus eliminate unnecessary biopsies. The primary utility of free PSA is in the patients with a PSA in the 4 to 10 ng/mL range with a history of previously negative prostatic biopsies. In this clinical scenario, the free to total PSA ratio, or alternatively, complexed PSA, can be used to determine the need for repeat biopsies with continued elevation of the serum PSA. A low free to total PSA ratio (<20%) is an indication to repeat a TRUS biopsy of the prostate to rule out the presence of carcinoma.

TRUS is performed using real-time imaging with a 7-MHz transducer, which allows both transverse and sagittal imaging of the prostate gland. Prostate cancer can appear as a hypoechoic region within the prostate, although most experts agree that this is a nonspecific finding. TRUS can also be used to measure the dimensions of the prostate gland to calculate the glandular volume. There is a current trend toward pre-biopsy magnetic resonance imaging (MRI) and classification of lesions with the MRI-based PIRADS classification. PIRADS scores range from 1 to 5, with PIRADS 1 meaning clinically significant prostate cancer is very unlikely, PIRADS 2 meaning clinically significant prostate cancer is unlikely, PIRADS 3 being equivocal, PIRADS 4 meaning clinically significant prostate cancer is likely, and PIRADS 5 meaning clinically significant prostate cancer is very likely. The PIRADS score is helpful in deciding whether a patient requires a biopsy. If a patient does need a biopsy, MRI and ultrasound can allow for a fusion-guided TRUS biopsy of targetable lesions. Clinical trials have shown an increased detection of clinically significant prostate cancer with fusion biopsy compared to standard TRUS systematic biopsy.

Pelvic lymphatic metastases can be detected by computed tomography (CT) or MRI. The risk of pelvic nodal metastasis depends on tumor grade, clinical stage, and PSA level. Nomograms incorporating these three factors have been developed to predict the risk of nodal metastasis. However, the only definitive method for staging pelvic lymph nodes is a pelvic lymphadenectomy.

Radionuclide bone scan remains the most sensitive test to detect skeletal metastases. However, in 1993, Oesterling found the yield of a bone scan was 2% if a patient has a PSA level less than 20 ng/mL and no evidence of skeletal metastasis, while no patients had a positive bone scan with a PSA less than 8 ng/mL. Therefore, based on this data, radionuclide bone scans are not necessary for staging prostate cancer in patients who have a low serum PSA level (<10 ng/mL) and no skeletal symptoms, particularly in cases of low-grade cancers. When bone metastases are present, 80% are osteoblastic, 15% are mixed osteoblastic–osteolytic, and 5% are osteolytic. A chest radiograph is performed to detect the presence of pulmonary metastases, which are extremely rare.

In localized prostate cancer, PET imaging currently has no defined role in staging. In the setting of de-novo metastatic prostate cancer and posttreatment recurrent or metastatic prostate cancer, multiple PET imaging modalities are utilized including C-11 Choline PET, Axumin PET, and PSMA PET. C-11 Choline PET is an FDA-approved PET scan for prostate cancer. However, the biggest limitation of Choline PET is the requirement of an on-site cyclotron which is extremely expensive and cost prohibitive to most hospitals and institutions. The adoption of Axumin PET is variable as it is cheaper and more easily implemented with existing PET systems but is not as specific as C-11 Choline PET or PSMAPET. PSMA PET is likely the future of PET imaging in prostate cancer; it has been shown to be highly sensitive and specific for prostate cancer and does not require a significant institutional cost investment like a cyclotron would. Furthermore, PSMA has theragnostic potential and multiple trials are currently investigating the role Lutetium-177 PSMA PET in the treatment of metastatic prostate cancer.

The diagnosis of prostate cancer is made by the histologic finding of prostate cancer in a prostatic biopsy, in tissue obtained from prostatectomy for benign disease, or in the biopsy of a suspicious metastatic focus. In the past, sextant biopsies of the prostate were considered adequate in the patient with an elevated PSA, with site-specific biopsies directed at palpable or ultrasonographic abnormalities (hypoechoic regions). More recent data based on whole mount step sectioning of radical prostatectomy specimens suggest that sextant biopsies are inadequate, in favor of 12 core strategies that focus on the peripheral zone, but also include the anterior horns of the prostate and the transition zone bilaterally. Adenocarcinoma is the predominant cell type of prostate cancer and is the only type discussed in this chapter.

Grading and Staging

The Gleason grading system is the most widely used grading system. It recognizes five histologic patterns of prostate cancer, graded on a scale of 1 to 5, from most to least differentiated. The Gleason score is arrived at through the addition of the predominant and secondary grade patterns to yield a range of tumor Gleason scores from 2 to 10, with most prostate cancers falling in the Gleason 5 to 10 range. Prostate cancer is well known to be multifocal in nature, so not uncommonly, multiple biopsies from a prostate may be positive, each with a reported Gleason score. The biology of the cancer is frequently dictated by the most aggressive variant found in the prostate.

Recently there has been an attempt to transition from the Gleason grading system to Grade Groups (GGs) in order to simplify prostate cancer grading to increase patient understanding:

- GG 1 includes all Gleason 6 prostate cancer.
- GG 2 includes only Gleason 7 (3+4) prostate cancer.
- GG 3 includes only Gleason 7 (4+3) prostate cancer.
- GG 4 includes all Gleason 8 prostate cancer.
- GG 5 includes all Gleason 9 and 10 prostate cancers.

Currently, both Gleason score and GGs are utilized interchangeably in the guidelines and usage of either system is currently acceptable. The biologic behavior of the tumor can be further categorized by stage, which accounts for tumor volume and location. Prostate cancer typically spreads to the pelvic lymph nodes, bone, and lungs.

Once a diagnosis of prostate cancer is made, risk assessment becomes paramount in guiding treatment decisions and for counseling patients accurately about expected oncologic and functional outcomes. The AUA and national consensus guidelines both have similar risk stratification systems that are primarily based on PSA level, Gleason score, and clinical stage. Prostate cancer risk stratification is shown in Table 20.1.

Management of Early Disease

Active Surveillance

Active surveillance (AS) is defined as a treatment strategy in which men with low-risk prostate cancer are serially monitored for disease progression and then treated definitively (if needed), thereby avoiding or delaying the risk of treatment-related morbidity. Importantly, AS differs from observation/watchful waiting (WW) as the latter indicates a decision to avoid/forgo definitive therapy and palliate only if there is metastatic progression. Entry criteria for AS protocols vary from institution to institution. Typically, men with very low-risk and low-risk prostate cancer per AUA and national consensus guidelines or clinically insignificant disease are candidates for AS. An initial repeat biopsy and/or multiparametric prostate MRI may aid in reclassifying men with higher-risk disease.

TABLE 20.1   Prostate Cancer Risk Stratification

Category Level	AUA Risk Category	National Consensus Risk Category
Very low	N/A	PSA ≤10 ng/mL, Grade Group 1, clinical stage T1c, <3 positive biopsy cores, ≤50% in each core, and PSA density <0.15 ng/mL/g
Low	PSA ≤10 ng/mL, Grade Group 1, clinical stage T1c or T2a	PSA <10 ng/mL, Grade Group 1, clinical stage T1 or T2a
Favorable intermediate	Grade Group 1 (with PSA 10–20) or Grade Group 2	Has all of the following: 1 intermediate-risk factor, Grade group 1 or 2, <50% biopsy cores positive and no high risk or very high-risk group features
Unfavorable intermediate	Grade Group 2 (with either PSA 10–20 or clinical stage T2b-c) or Grade Group 3	Has 1 or more of the following without high risk or very high-risk group features: 2–3 intermediate-risk factors, Grade Group 3, >50% biopsy cores positive
High	PSA >20 ng/mL, Grade Group 4 or 5, or clinical stage ≥T2c	PSA >20 ng/mL, Grade Group 4 or 5, or clinical stage T3a
Very high	N/A	Primary Gleason pattern 5 or >4 cores with Grade Group 4 or 5, or clinical stage T3b–T4

Based on AUA and national consensus risk categories.

In 2005, Bill-Axelson et al. prospectively compared surveillance with radical prostatectomy in patients with PSA <50 and clinical stage T2 or less and found that patients who underwent radical prostatectomy were less likely to develop metastases (15% vs. 25%) and less likely to die of prostate cancer (10% vs. 15%). This reduction in prostate cancer deaths was most significant in patients younger than 65 years of age. The Prostate Cancer Intervention Versus Observation Trial (PIVOT) found that radical prostatectomy did not improve overall or disease-specific mortality. Radical prostatectomy was associated with reduced all-cause mortality among men with a PSA value greater than 10 ng/mL ($P = .04$ for interaction) and possibly among those with intermediate-risk or high-risk tumors ($P = .07$ for interaction). The median 10-year follow-up and less than average health of men in the PIVOT study suggest only men with competing risks may safely be offered AS. Klotz et al. (2015) reported long-term follow-up of 993 men with favorable or intermediate-risk prostate cancer managed with AS. Of these patients, 2.8% developed metastatic disease, and 1.5% ultimately died from their disease. These results are similar with the expected outcomes of invasive treatment and support the use of AS in appropriately selected patients. The PROTECT trial was a randomized control trial of 1,643 men with localized prostate cancer randomized 1:1:1 to AS, radical prostatectomy, or radiotherapy. At a median follow-up of 10 years, surgery and radiotherapy were associated with lower disease progression rates and metastasis rates compared to AS. However, prostate cancer–specific mortality was low and not significantly different between the three groups. Currently, AS is a guideline-based option for patients with very low-risk, low-risk and favorable intermediate-risk prostate cancer.

Cryotherapy

Prostate cryotherapy has been used since 1996. The current third-generation cryotherapy uses high-quality TRUS guidance, an argon-based freezing system, multisensor temperature probes, and a urethral warming device. These features give urologists excellent control of ice ball formation during cryotherapy. Cryotherapy is typically reserved for early-stage, low-volume and low-grade disease. Large contemporary series have shown a 5-year disease-free survival rate of 77% for primary cryotherapy. The incidence of reported complications in the literature after primary cryotherapy for erectile dysfunction, urinary incontinence, and fistula formation range between 49% and 93%, 1% and 8%, 0% and 0.5%, respectively. Focal cryotherapy has been investigated as an alternative treatment but is not widely accepted at present. The main use of cryotherapy though is in patients who have local prostate recurrence after radiation therapy (the so-called salvage cryotherapy for radiorecurrent prostate cancer). In this patient population, the 5-year disease-free survival rate decreases to 58.9%.

Surgery

The surgical excision of prostate cancer by complete removal of the prostate gland, seminal vesicles, and ampullae of the vasa deferentia was first performed in the early 1900s. This procedure, known as a *radical prostatectomy*, can be performed using a perineal or retropubic approach. In the last decade, minimally invasive surgical techniques such as laparoscopic radical prostatectomy and robot-assisted laparoscopic prostatectomy have become mainstream, with similar oncologic and functional outcomes (continence and erectile function), but less blood loss, narcotic and transfusion requirements, and shorter hospital stays compared to open techniques. In 2010, it was estimated that 67% to 85% of all prostatectomies performed in the United States were done using robot-assisted techniques. The PROTECT trial, with a median follow-up of 10 years, reported similar oncologic outcomes between surgery and radiotherapy. Abdel-Rahman et al. (2019) reported on 3,953 patients with localized prostate cancer from the PLCO trial in which 2,044 men underwent radical prostatectomy, and 1,909 men underwent radiation therapy. In a multivariable analysis adjusted for factors affecting overall survival, prostatectomy was associated with a better overall survival (HR 0.548, $P < .001$). Factors that predict for postoperative potency include preoperative erectile function, patient age, and number of cavernosal nerve fibers spared. Factors that influence continence results include nerve sparing, patient age, and obesity. Bilateral pelvic lymph node dissection (PLND) is considered an essential part of radical prostatectomy, especially for high-risk disease. It provides accurate staging, prognostication, and may have a therapeutic benefit. A standard PLND includes removal of lymphatic tissue around the external iliac vein down to the internal iliac artery as well as tissue within the obturator fossa. Proximally, dissection continues up to the bifurcation of the common iliac artery, and distally to Cooper's ligament.

Radiation Therapy

Brachytherapy and external-beam radiation therapy (EBRT) are used for the definitive treatment of localized prostatic adenocarcinoma. Permanent brachytherapy typically uses Palladium-103 (doses of 125 Gy) or

Iodine-125 (doses of 145 Gy) and is mainly reserved for patients with small prostates and low-risk prostate cancer (PSA <10, Gleason 6 or less, and clinical stage T2a or less). For patients with intermediate- or high-risk prostate cancer, brachytherapy should not be given as single-modality therapy and needs to be combined with EBRT. Intensity-modulated radiation therapy (IMRT) is currently used to decrease adverse local side effects of radiation therapy and increase total dosage to the prostate and is the external-beam radiotherapeutic modality of choice due to improved prostate targeting and side-effect profile compared to previous generation radiotherapy. For low-risk patients, IMRT is used alone at doses of up to 75 Gy, while for patients with intermediate- or high-risk disease, doses up to 80 Gy are given, and are combined with androgen deprivation therapy. At the MD Anderson Cancer Center, we recommend radical prostatectomy for the treatment of prostate cancer in the patient with minimal comorbidities, less than 70 years of age. Primary radiation therapy is reserved for patients with significant comorbid medical illnesses or patients older than 70 years of age. Proton beam therapy (PBT) has emerged with potential superiority in sparing organs at risk such as bladder, rectum, and femoral head when compared with photons. PBT is a specific type of EBRT in which a heavy particle (protons) is used instead of photons. While PBT uses image-guided radiation therapy (IGRT), it uses less lateral fields (1 to 2) rather than (5 to 7) fields required for IMRT. The dosimetric advantage of PBT is that it allows a high dose to be delivered to the prostate similar to IMRT, with less pelvic tissue receiving low-to-moderate dose. However, the available, albeit limited evidence, suggests that the use of PBT in treating prostate cancer offers no confirmed advantage over conventional IMRT.

Management of Locally Advanced Prostate Cancer/Lymph Node Metastasis

Locally advanced prostate cancer involves areas outside the prostatic capsule, such as fat, seminal vesicles, levator muscles, or other adjacent structures. Locally advanced prostate cancer is associated with a 53% incidence of lymph node metastases and decreased overall survival rate compared with early-stage disease. Locally advanced disease with or without lymph node metastasis can be treated with primary radiation therapy and androgen ablation with a 6-year biochemical failure rate of 13%, but longer follow-up is still needed. These patients with locally advanced disease at high risk for relapse are frequently enrolled in clinical protocols that use neoadjuvant systemic therapy in combination with surgical extirpation of the prostate followed by adjuvant radiotherapy to improve patient outcome. Our experience at the MD Anderson Cancer Center with locally advanced disease treated with primary radiation therapy demonstrated 5-, 10-, and 15-year uncorrected actuarial survival rates of 72%, 47%, and 17%, respectively. The local control rate was 75% at 15 years of follow-up.

Treatment modalities other than radiation therapy used for locally advanced disease include radical prostatectomy, TURP, and hormonal therapy. However, currently there is paradigm interest in prostatectomy as part of a multidisciplinary approach to provide local control in selected patients with high-risk locally advanced/node positive disease. Tumor grade, stage, bulk of tumor, and seminal vesicle involvement in locally advanced disease are associated with a decreased interval between radical prostatectomy and disease progression. The actuarial 5-year survival rate for patients with locally advanced disease who have undergone TURP is 64%, making TURP an option for patients with short life expectancies who have significant local symptoms associated with their prostate cancer such as urinary obstruction or intractable hematuria. This strategy may be ideal in the elderly and in those with serious coexisting medical problems.

Metastatic Prostate Cancer

Patients with metastatic prostate cancer have a median survival duration of 30 months, with an estimated 5-year survival rate of 20%. The first-line treatment of metastatic prostate cancer is androgen ablation therapy. The hypothalamus produces luteinizing hormone-releasing hormone (LHRH) and corticotropin-releasing factor, which stimulate the anterior pituitary gland to release adrenocorticotropic hormone (ACTH) and luteinizing hormone (LH). LH stimulates testosterone production by the testes, and ACTH stimulates the adrenal glands to produce androstenedione and dehydroepiandrosterone, precursors of testosterone and DHT. Although the testes are the major source of testosterone, the adrenal glands can supply up to 20% of the DHT found in the prostate gland.

Androgen ablation therapy consists of either bilateral orchiectomy or LHRH agonists, which chronically stimulate the pituitary gland, resulting in a decrease in LH release. Direct LHRH antagonists are now also available, but they have not gained widespread acceptance over the agonists that have a more extensive clinical background. Decrease in LH leads to castrate levels of testosterone production by the testes, defined typically as less than 50 ng/mL. Several oral antiandrogens exist that work by blocking uptake or binding of androgen in target tissues. Combination of antiandrogens with either surgical or medical androgen ablation is termed combined androgen blockade.

Bilateral orchiectomy and LHRH agonists appear to have equal efficacy when used as monotherapy for metastatic prostate cancer. The Medical Research Council of the United Kingdom performed a randomized prospective trial with 934 patients and found that immediate androgen ablation delays disease progression and decreases pathologic fractures. We recommend immediate androgen ablation for selected patients. Combined androgen blockade with an LHRH agonist plus an antiandrogen is controversial. Many studies have shown no benefit to combined therapy with an antiandrogen versus LHRH agonist monotherapy. Intermittent androgen therapy has been demonstrated to improve quality of life, but its long-term effects on survival are unknown. Androgen ablation, although useful as first-line therapy in patients with metastatic prostate cancer, has been shown to increase the risk of osteoporosis, metabolic syndrome and cardiovascular disease. The median survival of patients with hormone refractory disease known as castration-resistant prostate cancer (CRPC) is on the order of 12 to 18 months. The median time to castration-resistant state for patients with metastatic prostate cancer treated with hormonal therapy is approximately 2 years. Chemotherapeutic regimens are the mainstay of therapy for metastatic castration-resistant prostate cancer (mCRPC) with taxane-based regimens showing significant activity that includes decreases in PSA, improved quality of life, objective disease regression, and prolonged survival. Docetaxel as a potent inhibitor of microtubule assembly and disassembly showed improved survival in the every 3-week regimen of docetaxel plus prednisone (18.9 months vs. 16.5 months in the mitoxantrone group, HR 0.75; $P = .009$). Cabazitaxel is another tubulin-binding taxane which showed improved overall survival (15.1 months vs. 12.7 months for mitoxantrone group) in patients who had received prior docetaxel. However, targeted therapy has emerged as an important option in mCRPC.

Abiraterone acetate is a steroidal antiandrogen that inhibits CYP17A1 to reduce testosterone production. Prior to docetaxel chemotherapy, 1,088 participants who were randomized to receive 1,000 mg/day of abiraterone plus prednisone 5 mg twice daily had statistically significant improvement in radiographic progression-free survival (16.5 months vs. 8.3 months for placebo and prednisone 5 mg twice daily; HR 0.53; $P < .001$). The final survival analysis of these chemotherapy-naïve 1,088 men revealed a significantly longer overall survival in the abiraterone group than in the placebo group (34.7 months vs. 30.3 months; HR 0.81; $P = .0033$). Similarly, a post-docetaxel randomized phase 3 study showed abiraterone significantly prolonged overall survival in patients with mCRPC who have progressed after docetaxel treatment compared to placebo plus prednisone (15.8 months vs. 11.2 months, respectively; HR 0.74; $P < .0001$). Enzalutamide is another targeted treatment option for men in the pre- and post-docetaxel mCRPC setting and for those who are not candidates for chemotherapy.

Enzalutamide is a competitive inhibitor of androgen binding and also inhibits nuclear translocation of the androgen receptor, DNA binding and coactivator recruitment. The AFFIRM trial randomized 1,199 men with CRPC after chemotherapy to receive enzalutamide 160 mg per day (800 patients) or placebo (399 patients). The study showed that enzalutamide significantly prolonged survival of men with mCRPC (18.4 months vs. 13.6 months in the placebo group; HR 0.63; $P < .001$). The AFFIRM trial also confirmed enzalutamide significantly improved time to first skeletal-related event, pain control, and patient-reported health-related quality of life in post-docetaxel patients with mCRPC. In the phase 3 PREVAIL study which involved 1,717 asymptomatic or mildly symptomatic patients and those who had not received prior chemotherapy, ketoconazole, or abiraterone were randomized to receive either enzalutamide at a dose of 160 mg or placebo once daily. Enzalutamide significantly decreased the risk of radiographic progression at 12 months (65% vs. 14% for patients receiving placebo, 81% risk reduction; HR 0.19; $P < .001$). Chemohormonal trials involving the use of docetaxel and ADT in hormone-sensitive metastatic prostate cancer revealed significantly longer overall survival in combination arms in both the CHAARTED trial (57.6 months vs. 44.0 months for ADT alone; HR 0.61; $P < .001$) and the STAMPEDE trial (5.4 years vs. 3.6 years for ADT alone, $P = .006$).

Apalutamide is a competitive inhibitor of the androgen receptor pathway. Apalutamide prevents androgen receptor translocation, DNA binding and androgen receptor transcription by binding to the androgen receptor ligand-binding domain. The SPARTAN phase 3 clinical trial of 1,207 nonmetastatic castrate-resistant prostate cancer (nmCRPC) patients randomized patients 2:1 to apalutamide versus placebo. Metastasis free survival was significantly improved in the apalutamide arm, 40.5 months compared to 16.2 months (HR 0.28; $P < .001$). Following apalutamide's approval in the nmCRPC space, the TITAN trial assessed its role in metastatic castrate-sensitive prostate cancer (mCSPC). A total of 525 mCSPC men were randomized to receive apalutamide + ADT and 527 mCSPC men were randomized to placebo + ADT. Radiographic progression-free survival at 24 months was 68.2% in the apalutamide versus 47.5% in the placebo group (HR 0.48; $P < .001$). Apalutamide is now approved for both nmCRPC and mCSPC.

The autologous cancer vaccine Sipuleucel-T was approved by the FDA for minimally or asymptomatic patients with CRPC. It is an intravenous immunotherapeutic agent shown to decrease overall mortality by 33%

compared to placebo. In addition to antineoplastic therapy, patients with metastatic prostate cancer typically receive bone-protecting agents (such as the bisphosphonate zoledronic acid), especially when hormone ablation is instituted. Clinical trials continue to be the main and best treatment option for patients; however, some treatment options (primarily taxane-based chemotherapy regimens) now exist that demonstrate objective benefit where none existed previously.

Radium-223 dichloride, an alpha emitter, selectively targets bone metastases with alpha particles. A randomized phase 3 trial was conducted involving 921 patients with histologically confirmed, progressive CRPC with two or more bone metastases detected on skeletal scintigraphy and no known visceral metastases. These patients were not eligible to receive or declined docetaxel, were randomized to receive six injections of radium-223 (at a dose of 50 kBq/kg of body weight intravenously) or matching placebo. Results confirmed the radium-223 survival benefit (median, 14.9 months vs. 11.3 months; HR 0.70; 95% CI, 0.58 to 0.83; $P < .001$).

Bladder Cancer
Epidemiology and Etiology
Bladder cancer is the second most common genitourinary malignancy in the United States. It is the fourth most common cancer in men and the tenth most common cancer in women. In 2021, approximately 83,730 new cases were expected, and 17,020 estimated deaths were attributed to bladder cancer. The lifetime probability of developing bladder cancer is 1 in 27 in males and 1 in 89 in females and is lower for African Americans compared to whites.

The etiology of bladder cancer, of which urothelial (or transitional cell) carcinoma is the most common, is well established. Cigarette smoking has been linked to 30% to 40% of all cases of bladder cancer. The chemicals 1-naphthylamine, 2-naphthylamine, benzidine, and 4-aminobiphenyl have been shown to promote urothelial carcinogenesis. Workers in the textile, leather, aluminum refining, rubber, and chemical industries who are exposed to high levels of these chemicals have an increased incidence of bladder cancer. Other chemicals that have been linked to urothelial cancer are MBUCCA (plastics industry), phenacetin, and the antineoplastic agent cyclophosphamide. In addition, recurrent bladder infections, as well as infections with the parasite *Schistosoma haematobium*, have been associated with squamous cell carcinoma of the bladder.

Pathology
The urinary bladder is a hollow viscus that functions in both the storage and the evacuation of urine. Histologically, the bladder is composed of mucosa, lamina propria, muscularis propria, and serosa (limited to the dome). Localized bladder cancer is classified as *nonmuscle invasive bladder cancer (NMIBC)*, which is limited to the mucosa and lamina propria, or *muscle invasive bladder cancer (MIBC)*, which extends into the muscularis propria and beyond. Approximately 70% of newly diagnosed bladder cancers are NMIBC, whereas the remaining 30% are invasive. Once a bladder cancer extends through the basal layer of the mucosa, it may invade blood vessels and lymphatics, thereby providing a route of metastasis. *Carcinoma in situ (CIS)*, an aggressive form of NMIBC, is composed of flat, high-grade urothelial carcinoma limited to the mucosal layer.

The World Health Organization (WHO) classifies epithelial tumors of the bladder into four histologic types: urothelial carcinoma (91%), squamous cell carcinoma (7%), adenocarcinoma (2%), and other variants of urothelial carcinoma (<1%). However, up to 20% of urothelial carcinomas contain areas of squamous differentiation, and up to 7% contain areas of adenomatous differentiation. The remainder of this section discusses only urothelial carcinomas.

Clinical Presentation
Eighty percent of all patients who present with bladder carcinoma have gross or microscopic hematuria, typically painless and intermittent. Approximately 20% of patients complain of irritative voiding symptoms, including urinary frequency, urgency, dysuria, and stranguria particularly with CIS. Other symptoms include pelvic pain, flank pain (from ureteral obstruction), and lower extremity edema. Patients with systemic disease may present with anemia, weight loss, and bone pain.

Diagnosis
A patient who presents with hematuria or other symptoms of bladder cancer should undergo a thorough urologic evaluation consisting of a history, physical examination, urinalysis, cystoscopic examination of the urinary bladder, voided urine for cytologic examination, and intravenous contrast-enhanced CT scan of the abdomen and pelvis. The most useful of these steps is the direct visual examination of the bladder using a flexible cystoscope in the office. Papillary and sessile tumors are easily visualized through the cystoscope; CIS, however, can appear as normal mucosa or as erythematous patches throughout the bladder. Endoscopic

evaluation has traditionally used white-light cystoscopy but more recently blue-light cystoscopy with intravesical instillation of hexaminolevulinate has emerged as an adjunct with an increased detection rate of bladder cancer particularly for CIS. Fewer than 60% of bladder tumors can be seen on a CT scan, but this examination is obtained primarily to identify other abnormalities that may be present in the upper urinary tract (renal pelvis or ureteral tumors, associated hydronephrosis, etc.) in addition to evaluating the primary bladder tumor, presence of local extension into soft tissues, and presence of regional lymphadenopathy. Urine cytology is reported as positive in ~30% of patients with low-grade tumors, and 65% to 100% of patients with high-grade tumors or CIS (see the next section for definition of grades).

Grading and Staging

The WHO grading system, updated in 2004, is based on the cytologic features of the tumor. Low-grade tumors are well differentiated and high-grade tumors are poorly differentiated.

Once a bladder tumor is diagnosed, the urologist must accurately stage the tumor. The initial transurethral resection of the bladder tumor (TURBT), typically done in association with random biopsies of the bladder and prostatic urethra, will determine the histologic depth of invasion of the tumor and the presence or absence of dysplasia or CIS. A bimanual examination should be performed at the time of resection to determine whether a mass is present and, if so, whether it is fixed or mobile. Further workup for detecting metastasis consists of a CT scan, liver function tests, a chest radiograph, and a bone scan (if the alkaline phosphatase level is elevated or the patient's symptoms suggest systemic disease).

Management

Nonmuscle Invasive Bladder Cancer

Approximately 70% of bladder cancers present as NMIBC (e.g., Ta, T1, or Tis). An estimated 70% of these cancers are Ta and 20% are T1. Ten percent of all bladder cancers present with Tis or CIS. After the initial treatment of NMIBC, the disease can be cured, can recur with the same stage and grade, or can recur with progression of stage or grade. Risk factors associated with both disease recurrence and progression include a high tumor grade, lamina propria invasion, tumor diameter larger than 3 cm, vascular or lymphatic invasion, multiplicity, and expression of either epidermal growth factor or transforming growth factor-alpha. Mutations in *TP53* may also be associated with a significant risk of disease progression.

Initial treatment of NMIBC focuses on eradication of the existing disease using transurethral resection of bladder tumor (TURBT) and chemical prophylaxis against disease recurrence or progression. TURBT has been the standard treatment for existing stage Ta and T1 tumors and visible stage Tis tumors. Laser fulguration is another therapeutic option that results in fewer bleeding complications. The advantage of transurethral resection over laser fulguration is that it provides tissue for histologic examination. Patients with apparently NMIBC at the time of TURBT should receive a single dose of intravesical mitomycin C or gemcitabine within 6 hours of resection if no bladder perforation is evident. This single dose has been shown to decrease the risk of bladder cancer recurrence by about 40%. Patients who have T1 disease should undergo a repeat TURBT 2 to 6 weeks after the initial TURBT, as these patients have a 30% risk of being upstaged into T2 disease or higher.

Patients with NMIBC with high risk of recurrence and progression including those with CIS, high-grade Ta or T1 lesions, multifocal and recurrent tumors, and the rare patient with residual disease may be candidates for adjuvant intravesical therapy. Intravesical agents can be used as therapeutic, adjuvant or prophylactic treatment for bladder cancer. Thiotepa, mitomycin C, and valrubicin are the chemotherapeutic agents used most frequently. Bacillus Calmette—Guérin (BCG), a live attenuated tuberculosis organism, has become the most widely used intravesical agent in NMIBC, typically alone, and less frequently in combination with alpha-interferon. BCG enhances the patient's own immune response against the tumor, providing resistance to disease recurrence thereby potentially delaying progression. BCG is typically started 4 to 6 weeks after TURBT, as starting BCG too soon after TURBT (before urothelial healing occurs) may result in BCG sepsis. Although specific dose scheduling varies, most treatment regimens include intravesical treatment weekly for 6 weeks, followed by a series of maintenance treatments administered over 12 to 36 months. BCG has been shown to eliminate CIS in 80% of patients at a 5-year follow-up, reduce tumor recurrence rate for patients with T1 disease to 30% at 4 years, and eliminate residual tumor in up to 59% of patients. Maintenance therapy regimens with BCG appear to offer the best outcomes for patients. In 2000, Lamm et al. randomized 384 patients with NMIBC to receive induction and maintenance BCG or induction BCG therapy alone. Median recurrence-free survival time was longer for those who received induction and maintenance therapy; however, at 5-year follow-up there was no difference in survival. In 2002, Sylvester et al. performed a meta-analysis of 24 clinical trials and found that only patients who received maintenance BCG after TURBT had a decreased risk of progression into muscle invasive disease.

There is good evidence that a T1 high-grade cancer has a high rate of progression and therefore confers a high risk of death. Therefore, we recommend early radical cystectomy (before developing muscle invasion) for selected patients with high-grade T1 bladder cancer. Furthermore, we also recommend cystectomy for patients who recur within 1 year despite two induction courses of BCG therapy or BCG maintenance because these patients have been shown to be at high risk for disease progression if their bladder remains in situ.

Invasive Bladder Cancer

Tumors that have penetrated the muscularis propria are considered invasive. Several options are available for treatment of patients with invasive tumors. A small subset of patients may be eligible for bladder-sparing therapy. In 2001, Herr demonstrated a 76% overall survival rate, with 57% of the patients preserving their bladders in 45 patients treated with aggressive transurethral re-resection of invasive bladder tumors (median follow-up: 61 months). Patients with an MIBC that is primary and solitary, does not have associated CIS, usually at the dome of the bladder and allows for a 2-cm surgical margin may be candidates for partial cystectomy. At the MD Anderson Cancer Center, data have shown that approximately 5% of patients are actually suitable for bladder-sparing surgery; 5-year survival rates have been comparable to those achieved with radical cystectomy, when negative margins of resection can be achieved.

Primary EBRT has been used to treat MIBC. Treatment protocols advocate doses of 65 to 70 Gy. Five-year survival rates range from 21% to 52% for T2 bladder cancer and from 18% to 30% for T3 tumors. Local recurrence occurs in 50% to 70% of these patients. T4 lesions fare worse, with 5-year survival rates consistently less than 10%. Our experience at the MD Anderson Cancer Center found a 26% 5-year survival rate with primary external-beam radiation. Thus, EBRT may be useful in patients who do not want to have surgery or for whom radical surgery is medically contraindicated; however, the results with radiation therapy, stage for stage, are significantly worse than those seen with radical surgery. EBRT alone is also inferior to EBRT with concurrent chemotherapy following TURBT for MIBC.

In an attempt to improve survival and bladder preservation rates, multimodality strategies have combined TURBT, chemotherapy, and radiation. In 1997, Kachnic et al. from Massachusetts General Hospital reported on 106 patients with T2 to T4 bladder cancers who were treated with TURBT, two cycles of methotrexate, cisplatin, vinblastine (MCV), and 40-Gy radiation therapy plus concurrent cisplatin. Overall 5-year survival was 52%, and overall 5-year survival rate with the bladder intact was 43%. These results are comparable to contemporary radical cystectomy series; however, this regimen involves significant morbidity and patient investment in complex treatment schedules. Moreover, patients are subjected to a considerable risk of eventual cystectomy and superficial bladder cancer recurrence.

Radical cystectomy with pelvic lymphadenectomy is performed with the intent of removing all localized and regional lymphatic disease. There is evidence that an extended pelvic lymphadenectomy (starting cranially from the inferior mesenteric artery takeoff) improves detection of nodal metastasis and could have a therapeutic benefit, especially in patients with minimal nodal disease. In 2001, Stein et al. reported on 1,054 patients who were treated with open radical cystectomy and pelvic lymphadenectomy at a single institution. Perioperative mortality was 2.5% and 28% experienced early complications postoperatively. Ten-year recurrence-free survival in node-negative patients was 86% for pT0, 89% for pTcis, 74% for pTa, 78% for pT1, 87% for pT2, 76% for pT3a, 61% for pT3b, and 45% for pT4. Twenty-four percent of all patients had positive lymph nodes, with a corresponding 10-year recurrence-free survival of 34%. Median time to recurrence in this patient cohort was 12 months (22% of patients had distant recurrence, and 7% had a local pelvic recurrence). In the last decade, several centers have started using laparoscopic and robot-assisted laparoscopic radical cystectomy with extracorporeal or intracorporeal urinary diversion. The recent RAZOR trial compared open and robot-assisted laparoscopic radical cystectomy and the robotic approach was found to be safe and noninferior from an oncologic perspective.

Once a patient undergoes cystectomy, the ureters must be diverted into an alternate drainage system. The most common urinary diversions used today are either an ileal conduit (incontinent diversion), or an orthotopic urinary diversion with an ileal segment (continent diversion). Patients who are unable to undergo an orthotopic diversion include patients with elevated serum creatinine, evidence of lymph node metastasis, prostatic urethral invasive urothelial carcinoma or CIS, inflammatory bowel disease or severe urethral stricture disease in male patients. Furthermore, these patients must be willing and able to undergo a vigorous voiding re-education program. Radiation therapy may render continence difficult; therefore, some patients may not benefit from this type of diversion. Catheterizable cutaneous reservoirs such as an Indiana pouch are also used as methods of continent urinary diversion in selected patients. In the end, if a patient is unable to meet these criteria, then a noncontinent diversion with a cutaneous ileal conduit is recommended.

Grossman et al. led a phase 3 randomized trial through SWOG comparing radical cystectomy alone with neoadjuvant chemotherapy followed by radical cystectomy and reported a 5% overall survival benefit with the latter approach. At the MD Anderson Cancer Center, adjuvant chemotherapy with cisplatin, methotrexate, vinblastine, and doxorubicin (M-VAC) or gemcitabine and cisplatin (GC) is used for selected patients with unfavorable disease characteristics, which include resected nodal metastases, extensive extravesical involvement, or involvement of pelvic viscera. Substituting carboplatin for cisplatin is not recommended and has been shown to reduce response rates and survival. Previously, treatment with adjuvant chemotherapy in selected patients at the MD Anderson Cancer Center resulted in a 70% 5-year survival rate, which is comparable to patients without unfavorable features. Currently, several targeted therapies are being investigated in the neoadjuvant, adjuvant, and metastatic setting. Recently, adjuvant nivolumab was approved by the FDA in high-risk bladder cancer based on the results of the CheckMate 274 phase 3 trial. The trial randomized 709 patients with high-risk bladder cancer after radical cystectomy to receive nivolumab or placebo 1:1. Nivolumab significantly increased median disease-free survival of 20.8 months compared with 10.8 months in the placebo cohort. In addition, nivolumab decreased the risk of cancer recurrence or death by 30% versus placebo.

Metastatic Disease

Cisplatin appears to be the agent with the greatest activity against urothelial carcinoma of the bladder; however, single-agent therapy response rates are only in the range of 10% to 30%. Traditionally, chemotherapy for bladder cancer included M-VAC. In the MD Anderson Cancer Center trial of M-VAC, a complete response rate of 35% and a partial response rate of 30% were observed. Other trials have documented similar response rates, with a median survival of approximately 1 year. Newer regimens using GC have demonstrated no significant difference in survival when compared with M-VAC, but adverse side effects and toxicity are decreased with the newer regimen, which is now used most commonly in this setting. Future management of metastatic bladder cancer is evolving rapidly with multiple promising trials currently assessing the role checkpoint inhibitors in metastatic bladder cancer.

Renal Cancer

Epidemiology and Etiology

Tumors of the renal and perirenal tissues comprise 3% of cancer incidence and mortality in the United States. Renal cell carcinoma (RCC) represents 85% of all renal parenchymal tumors and is the only renal tumor discussed in this chapter. In 2021, an estimated 76,080 people were diagnosed with malignancies of the kidney and renal pelvis, and close to 13,780 people died of this disease. From 1975 to 1995, both the incidence and mortality rates of RCC have increased. The upward trend in mortality rates suggests that the increased incidental diagnosis of early-stage asymptomatic tumors does not fully account for the overall increase in incidence. This rise in incidence is seen more significantly in African Americans. Males are affected twice as often as females. RCC most frequently occurs in the fifth to sixth decades of life.

Several risk factors have been identified to be associated with RCC. Case-control studies have found strong correlations with smoking and obesity. Hypertension, diabetes mellitus, occupational exposure (including cadmium, asbestos, and gasoline) and diuretic use have also been found to be associated with RCC; however, it is unclear whether this is a causal relationship. RCC can occur either sporadically or genetically. Hereditary RCC tends to occur at an earlier age of onset and tends to be bilateral and multifocal. A well-described familial syndrome is von Hippel–Lindau (VHL) disease, which is characterized by cerebellar hemangioblastoma, retinal angiomata, bilateral clear cell RCC, and islet cell tumors of the pancreas. Both sporadic and VHL disease types have a common genetic mechanism that includes loss of a region of chromosome 3p. Most of clear cell RCCs are believed to have loss of the VHL gene either through mutation, deletion, or silencing by methylation. Hereditary papillary RCC (papillary type 1) is an autosomal dominant syndrome associated with abnormalities of the *MET* gene on chromosome 7. Other genetic RCC syndromes include hereditary leiomyomatosis and RCC (papillary type 2) that is associated with mutations in the Krebs cycle enzyme fumarate hydratase, and Birt–Hogg–Dubé syndrome, which manifests as bilateral multifocal tumors with both chromophobe RCC and oncocytoma histology. RCC is also associated with polycystic kidney disease, tuberous sclerosis, and acquired renal cystic disease.

Pathology

Clear cell histology is the most common RCC subtype. Most RCCs originate in the proximal tubular cells of the kidney. The tumor is multifocal in 6.5% to 10% of cases, more commonly with papillary histology. The renal capsule and Gerota fascia surrounding the kidney typically limit local extension of the tumor. The tumor cells are typically rich in glycogen and lipid, giving the tumor a clear cell appearance microscopically and a characteristic yellow appearance grossly. Less common pathologies include papillary and chromophobe RCC. Unclassified RCC is a waste-basket classification for tumors that do not fit the criteria of the classically described histologies. Sarcomatoid dedifferentiation, once believed to be a separate histologic classification, is now recognized as a dedifferentiation pathway that can occur with any RCC histology, including clear cell, papillary, and chromophobe. Oncocytoma is a benign tumor with no malignant potential that can be problematic to differentiate from chromophobe RCC on needle biopsy: both are collectively referred to as oncocytic neoplasms when a definitive diagnosis cannot be reached on the biopsy specimen. Angiomyolipoma (AML) is a benign renal mass that consists of blood vessels, smooth muscle, and fat. It is mostly commonly asymptomatic, however AMLs have the potential to grow and spontaneously bleed. Masses over 4 cm are more likely to bleed and are often treated at or above this size. AMLs can often be diagnosed on CT imaging, where high-fat concentration is common and on kidney biopsy, positive staining for HMH-45 is pathognomonic for AML.

Clinical Presentation

RCC was traditionally called the "internist's tumor" because of its subtle presentation. Now more than 80% of clinically unsuspected tumors are found incidentally by abdominal imaging done for other reasons. Gross or microscopic hematuria, the most common presenting symptom, is present in some patients with RCC. The classic triad of hematuria, abdominal mass, and flank pain is now less frequently encountered. Paraneoplastic syndromes occur in 10% to 40% of cases and consist of fever, anemia, erythrocytosis, hypercalcemia, liver dysfunction (Stauffer syndrome), and hypertension. Other common symptoms include bone pain and central nervous system abnormalities, due to bone and brain metastases. Risk of metastases at presentation and risk of renal mass being RCC at presentation are strongly associated with tumor size.

Diagnosis

The workup of a patient with the preceding symptoms should include a history, physical examination, complete blood cell count, serum chemistry panel (including alkaline phosphatase and liver function tests), urinalysis, urine culture, chest x-ray, and a contrast-enhanced abdominal CT scan. In most cases, the CT scan will define the nature of the mass. If any of the studies obtained suggests tumor thrombus involvement of the renal vein or vena cava, an MRI or CT scan with three-dimensional reconstruction should be obtained to assess the extent of the tumor thrombus. In contrast to the management of other renal tumors, RCC may be treated surgically without preoperative histologic diagnosis of the tumor. The role of renal mass biopsy for patients who are surgical candidates, who have resectable localized tumors may be limited unless the radiographic characteristics of the mass suggest an etiology other than RCC, such as an abscess, lymphoma, urothelial carcinoma, or a metastasis from another malignant primary. Guidelines strongly recommend renal mass biopsy prior to ablation therapy or AS for localized RCC, or systemic therapy (without previous histopathology) for advanced or metastatic disease.

If a mass suggests RCC, a metastatic workup consisting of a chest radiograph, CT scan (if not already obtained), and liver function tests should be performed. The most common sites of metastases of RCC in decreasing order are the lung, bone, and regional lymph nodes. If the patient does not have an increased alkaline phosphatase level or skeletal pain, a bone scan is usually not required. An MRI scan of the brain can be performed if there is any suspicion of brain metastases, and should be performed in patients who have metastatic disease elsewhere.

Grading and Staging

The most widely used grading system for RCC is the WHO/ISUP system, which is based on nuclear and nucleolar morphology, rated on a scale of 1 to 4.

Management

Localized/Locally Advanced Renal Cell Carcinoma

To date, surgical excision remains the only proven effective treatment of localized RCC.

There are situations in which nephron-sparing surgery is indicated for patients with RCC when feasible. For example, in cases of cT1a tumors, partial nephrectomy is the standard of care and an alternative standard for cT1b renal masses especially when there is a need to preserve renal parenchyma. Partial nephrectomy is also indicated for bilateral tumor involvement, renal insufficiency, solitary kidney, and hereditary RCC such as VHL. In this procedure, the renal artery is temporarily occluded, the kidney cooled down, and a partial nephrectomy or wedge resection performed. Gross assessment of the surgical margins is typically evaluated intraoperatively to ensure adequacy of resection. Arterial blood flow is restored after sutured reconstruction of the resection bed or renorrhaphy and approximation of renal capsule; alternatively, perirenal fat or biodegradable homeostatic material is sutured to the defect to promote healing and hemostasis. Five-year cancer-specific survival rates after partial nephrectomy for patients with stage I or II disease are approximately 90% and 80%, respectively.

Currently, partial nephrectomy constitutes the standard of care for patients with localized renal tumors less than 4 cm in size. Nephron-sparing surgery and radical nephrectomy provide equally effective curative treatments for single, small, well-localized tumors; partial nephrectomy yields 5-year cancer-specific survival rates of 92% to 97%. The incidence of tumor recurrence within the renal remnant is reported to be from 0% to 6%. Recent data also demonstrate that performing partial nephrectomy on anatomically favorable tumors between 4 and 7 cm is feasible, and when carefully performed in centers of excellence, cancer-specific survival is equivalent to those treated with radical nephrectomy. More importantly, several investigators have recently reported that radical nephrectomy is associated with a higher rate of cardiovascular complications, chronic kidney disease, noncancer mortality, and overall mortality when compared to partial nephrectomy, emphasizing the role of nephron-preserving surgery whenever feasible.

The oncologic outcome of partial nephrectomy was compared to that of radical nephrectomy in a randomized noninferiority, multicenter, controlled trial (EORTC 30904) for 541 patients with small ($\leq$5 cm), solitary, T1–T2 N0 M0 suspected RCC. The study which was prematurely closed because of poor accrual, showed an intention-to-treat analysis of 10-year overall survival rates of 81.1% for radical nephrectomy and 75.7% for nephron-sparing surgery. With a hazard ratio of 1.50, the test for noninferiority was not significant ($P = .77$), and test for superiority was significant ($P = .03$). However, in RCC patients (clinically and pathologically eligible patients), the difference was even less pronounced (HR = 1.43 and HR = 1.34, respectively), and the trend in favor of radical nephrectomy was no longer significant ($P = .07$ and $P = .17$, respectively). The study concluded that both methods provided excellent oncologic results.

More recent advances in the surgical therapy of localized RCC have focused on minimally invasive strategies. Minimally invasive radical nephrectomy, performed either through pure laparoscopic, hand-assisted or robot-assisted approaches, has become the gold standard for the treatment of patients with localized/locally advanced RCC that is not amenable to nephron-sparing approaches. Pure laparoscopic partial nephrectomy is used in some centers, although renal reconstruction under constrains of warm ischemia times and increased risk of urologic complications have prevented this minimally invasive technique from being widely assimilated. In the last decade, robot-assisted laparoscopic partial nephrectomy has gained ground in the treatment of small renal tumors, as it is less technically challenging than the pure laparoscopic counterpart. More recent clinical research has focused on energy ablative strategies such as percutaneous cryotherapy or radiofrequency ablation as strategies to treat small (<4 cm) renal masses. These energy ablative strategies have recently reported encouraging long-term oncologic outcomes when compared to partial nephrectomy. These modalities are considered an option for patients refusing surgery or when surgical resection is contraindicated. Thermal ablative techniques for larger cT1b tumors however, should be reserved for those patients in which surgery is not an option. Furthermore, AS of renal masses less than 3 cm has emerged as an alternative management strategy in selected patients and the elderly with severe medical comorbidities who cannot undergo surgery. A recent meta-analysis of 10 studies of AS that included 331 patients with localized RCC demonstrated a metastatic progression rate of less than 2%, which is encouraging. However, the long-term results of such approaches are still pending.

In a radical nephrectomy, the kidney, ipsilateral adrenal gland (if involved), surrounding Gerota fascia and regional lymph nodes are all resected en bloc. Although no randomized study has proved its benefit over simple nephrectomy, radical nephrectomy has the theoretical advantage of removing the lymphatics within the perinephric fat. Up to 10% of patients can have evidence of regional lymphatic metastases without distant disease, although the incidence of occult nodal involvement is in the range of 3% to 5%. The 5-year survival rates for patients with positive lymph nodes range from 8% to 35%; however, patients with papillary histology and node metastases that undergo aggressive surgical resection can enjoy an extended progression-free and overall survival, in contrast to those patients with nodal metastases from clear cell histology. Extended lymphadenectomy has never been proven to be of benefit in patients who undergo radical nephrectomy for early-stage localized RCC, except in the presence of clinically positive lymph nodes, and many surgeons prefer a limited node dissection, which has limited morbidity, for prognostic information. There are clear data that all evidence of gross disease should be removed, if feasible, at the time of nephrectomy. However, results of the EORTC randomized phase 3 trial (30881) showed a low incidence (4.0%) of unsuspected lymph node metastasis preoperatively and there were no significant differences in overall survival, time to progression of disease, or progression-free survival between patients who underwent radical nephrectomy with or without a complete lymph node dissection. National consensus guidelines recommend regional lymph node dissection for patients with palpable disease or enlarged nodes identified on preoperative imaging.

The surgical approach to radical nephrectomy is determined by the size and location of the tumor and the surgeon's preference. A modified flank, midline, or subcostal (chevron) incision can be used. Large upper-pole tumors may be approached through a thoracoabdominal incision for greater exposure. Adrenalectomy is generally not indicated if the adrenal gland is not involved with malignancy on imaging or intraoperatively.

Approximately 15% to 20% of RCCs invade the renal vein, and 8% to 15% invade the inferior vena cava. RCC invasion of the renal vein usually does not pose a significant surgical problem. Vena caval involvement, however, may require additional extensive procedures to completely excise the tumor. Vena caval thrombi can be classified according to Mayo classification into five levels: level 0, thrombus is within the renal vein only; level I (renal), thrombus extending into the IVC but not more than 2 cm above the renal vein; level II (infrahepatic), thrombus extending into the IVC to more than 2 cm above the renal vein but not to the hepatic veins; level III (intrahepatic), thrombus extending into the IVC to above the hepatic veins but not to the diaphragm; and level IV, thrombus extending into the supradiaphragmatic IVC or right atrium. In cases with vena caval involvement, it is imperative that the surgeon be familiar with techniques of vascular surgery, and consideration should be given to consulting with a cardiothoracic surgeon, especially for level 3–4 thrombi. Cardiopulmonary bypass, deep hypothermic arrest, and venovenous bypass have been used in the resection of these locally advanced tumors that extend to the suprahepatic vena cava.

In patients with local/regional disease with high risk of recurrence and metastasis, multiple studies have shown benefit of adjuvant therapy after nephrectomy. The STRAC trial randomized 615 patients with high-risk local/regional RCC to adjuvant sunitinib or placebo. Sunitinib offered significantly improved disease-free survival compared to placebo (6.8 years vs. 5.6 years, $P = .03$). More recently, the preliminary results of KEYNOTE 564 have been reported which compared adjuvant pembrolizumab and placebo in 994 patients with high-risk local/regional RCC after nephrectomy. Adjuvant pembrolizumab also demonstrated significantly improved disease-free survival compared to placebo.

Metastatic Renal Cell Carcinoma

Approximately 40% to 50% of patients either present with or develop metastases during the course of the natural history of their disease. The median survival for patients with metastatic RCC is 12 months. Distant metastatic disease can be categorized as oligometastatic disease or bulky metastatic disease. Solitary lung metastases appear to be associated with better survival rates than metastases to other organ sites.

Cytotoxic chemotherapy has been largely ineffective in RCC; the highest objective response rate for single-agent therapy is only 16%. More recently, regimens with gemcitabine and capecitabine have shown significant activity in selected patients. Interleukin-2 (IL-2) has yielded durable response rates of 15% to 19% in various trials, primarily with the use of high-dose bolus intravenous regimens. Subcutaneous IL-2, either alone or in combination with interferon, is believed to be inferior to intravenous IL-2 regimens, but associated with significantly less toxicity. Until recently, IL-2 was the gold standard of therapy for patients with metastatic disease, but recent inroads into the understanding of the molecular pathways associated with renal cell carcinogenesis and progression have resulted in the development of specific molecular targeted therapies that have rapidly replaced IL-2 in the armamentarium of the oncologist. Since 2005, several drugs (bevacizumab, sunitinib, sorafenib, pazopanib, axitinib, cabozantinib, lenvatinib, temsirolimus, everolimus, nivolumab, pembrolizumab, avelumab) have been approved for the treatment of metastatic RCC. The usage of these drugs depends on histology, previous treatments received and failed, and patient risk stratification.

The CARMENA trial was a phase 3 trial that evaluated 450 intermediate- and poor-risk mRCC patients treated with cytoreductive nephrectomy (CN) and adjuvant sunitinib versus sunitinib alone. With a median follow-up of 50.9 months, median overall survival was 18.4 months with sunitinib alone versus 13.9 CN and sunitinib. While this trial has its limitations, it found that sunitinib alone is noninferior to CN plus sunitinib. Since the CARMENA trial was published, multiple trials have evaluated combination immunotherapy compared to sunitinib including pembrolizumab plus axitinib, cabozantinib plus nivolumab, levantinib plus pembrolizumab and ipilimumab plus nivolumab. These novel combination systemic therapy regimens are now the mainstay of treatment of metastatic RCC. The SURTIME trial was a randomized control trial that evaluated sunitinib prior to CN to sunitinib followed by CN in 99 patients with mRCC with clear cell subtype and a resectable primary tumor. With deferred CN, more patients received sunitinib and overall survival was improved. The trial suggests that pretreatment with sunitinib may help identify patients with inherent resistance to systemic therapy rendering CN to not be of benefit in those patients.

Testicular Cancer

Epidemiology and Etiology

Malignant tumors of the testis are rare. It has been reported that approximately 9,470 cases of testicular cancer were diagnosed in 2021, but only 440 men will die of this disease. Ninety-five percent of these tumors are of germ cell origin. Although testicular tumors can occur at any age, specific tumor types tend to occur at different ages. Choriocarcinomas tend to occur between 24 and 28 years of age, embryonal carcinomas from 26 to 34 years of age, seminomas from 32 to 42 years of age, and lymphomas and spermatocytic seminomas after the age of 50 years.

The most well-known etiologic factor in the development of testicular cancer is cryptorchidism. Between 3% and 11% of all cases of testis cancer occur in cryptorchid testes. Genetic factors may also play a significant role.

CIS (otherwise known as intratubular germ cell neoplasia) is a precursor of testicular germ cell cancer. A total of 5% to 6% of men with a unilateral germ cell tumor have CIS in the contralateral testis, and a germ cell tumor will develop in 50% of these men. Other men with a high risk of CIS are individuals with intersex, cryptorchidism, infertility, or an extragonadal germ cell tumor.

Clinical Presentation

Testicular cancer typically presents as a painless testicular mass and/or enlargement. Advanced disease can present as back pain, flank pain, or with systemic symptoms. The differential diagnosis includes varicocele, hydrocele, hematoma, epididymitis, orchitis, and inguinal hernia.

Diagnosis

Although the diagnosis is usually evident at physical examination to an experienced clinician, scrotal ultrasound should be performed to confirm the diagnosis, evaluate local extension and assess the contralateral testis. Any solid testicular mass is considered a testicular tumor until proven otherwise. Patients with testicular enlargement that is believed to be inflammatory in nature (epididymo-orchitis) must be re-examined after the infection has been treated to rule out the presence of an occult testicular mass. Once a testicular tumor is suspected, the patient's levels of the tumor markers alpha-fetoprotein (AFP), human chorionic gonadotropin (hCG), and lactate dehydrogenase (LDH) should be tested. Following this, the patient should undergo a radical inguinal orchiectomy. There is no role for fine-needle aspiration or Tru-cut biopsy in the workup of this disease.

Before or after radical orchiectomy, staging CT scans of the chest, abdomen, and pelvis as well as postorchiectomy serum tumor markers (obtained at least 4 weeks after surgery) should be obtained in all patients for risk stratification to direct subsequent treatment. Alternatively, a chest radiograph may be obtained in patients with a low risk of thoracic metastasis such as those with normal postorchiectomy tumor markers and a normal CT of the abdomen/pelvis. Elevated serum tumor markers should be followed postorchiectomy after allowing the appropriate time for each marker to return to baseline, if possible, for precise staging. This would be approximately 1 week for hCG and 5 weeks for AFP. Preoperative sperm banking must be discussed with patients who are interested in future fertility prior to undergoing therapeutic interventions that may reduce fertility potential such as retroperitoneal lymph node dissection (RPLND), radiation or chemotherapy.

Staging

The newest AJCC 8th edition staging has added pT1a (tumors less than 3 cm in size) and pT1b (tumors 3 cm or larger in size). Importantly the pT1a and pT1b subclassification only applies to pure seminoma. In terms of biologic behavior and therapy, testicular tumors can be categorized as seminomatous or nonseminomatous germ cell tumors (NSGCTs). Seminomas are radiation-sensitive and chemosensitive tumors that undergo lymphatic spread in an orderly fashion. In contrast, NSGCTs are minimally radiation sensitive and have a higher metastatic potential than seminomas.

Management

Seminomatous Germ Cell Tumors

After radical orchiectomy, the standard management options for stage I seminomas are either enrolment in AS (preferred for pT1–pT3 disease) which requires a highly compliant patient, or treatment with single-agent carboplatin chemotherapy or radiation therapy to the retroperitoneal nodes up to the level of the diaphragm (doses of ~20 Gy). The cancer-specific survival for stage I seminoma is 99% irrespective of treatment modality used. Stage II seminomas are treated with radiation therapy to the retroperitoneal nodes and ipsilateral pelvic nodes up to the level of the diaphragm (doses of 30 Gy for stage IIA to 36 Gy for low-volume stage IIB). The overall survival with radiation treatment in patients with stage II disease is almost 100%. Although 5% to 6% of patients with stage IIA disease have relapses, more than half of these respond successfully to salvage therapy. In contrast, cisplatin-based chemotherapy is the preferred treatment alternative for stage IIB seminoma.

Stage IIC and III diseases are usually treated with primary chemotherapy with bleomycin, etoposide, and cisplatin (BEP). Surgery is generally reserved for lymphatic disease (which is usually documented on post-chemotherapy PET/CT scans) that does not respond to chemotherapy or radiation therapy and is rarely performed in the setting of metastatic seminoma following radiation and/or chemotherapy. Using this approach, 5-year disease-free survival rates of 86% and 92% have been obtained for patients with stage IIB and III diseases, respectively.

Nonseminomatous Germ Cell Tumors

The management strategies for stage IA disease include surveillance and nerve-sparing RPLND. While these two options are considered for stage IB NSGCT, primary systemic chemotherapy is another option to reduce the risk of relapse in these patients. Overall, approximately 20% to 30% of patients with stage I disease who undergo surveillance experience relapse. Patients at high risk of relapse include those with lymphovascular invasion or predominant embryonal histology present in the primary tumor.

The recurrence rate after RPLND for low-volume stage II disease is less than 20%. Thus, both RPLND and primary systemic chemotherapy have been used to treat low-volume retroperitoneal disease. Survival rates of 97% or better have been associated with both forms of therapy. At the MD Anderson Cancer Center, patients with stage II disease are treated with primary chemotherapy, and RPLND is used to subsequently eradicate residual disease.

Because of the high recurrence rates associated with primary RPLND alone in patients with high-volume stage IIB, IIC, and III NSGCTs, primary systemic chemotherapy is the treatment of choice for this disease. RPLND is used to remove any residual disease that may be present after primary chemotherapy and to determine the need for further therapy. Recent experience with chemotherapy for advanced NSGCT at the MD Anderson Cancer Center has shown 5-year survival rates of 96% and 76% for low- and high-volume stage III disease, respectively.

Despite the relatively early age of onset of testicular cancer, this disease remains one of the most curable cancers. A majority of NSGCTs produce either AFP or β-hCG, rendering these markers helpful in monitoring the patient for treatment response and recurrent disease. RPLND can be performed in the primary setting (before chemotherapy, usually in stage I and IIA NSGCTs) with excellent sparing of the sympathetic nerves, and resulting preservation of ejaculatory function. RPLND in this setting is performed using modified templates (and not just simply a mass excision). For residual masses after chemotherapy (in the setting of normal markers), postchemotherapy RPLND is performed with the goal of removing any retroperitoneal lymph nodes, including any residual viable tumor or teratoma. Teratomas can be life-threatening, as they can grow very fast (growing teratoma syndrome), invade adjacent vital organs, degenerate into a sarcoma or carcinoma (somatic malignant transformation), and are resistant to chemotherapy and radiotherapy. Teratomas can only be cured by comprehensive and complete surgical excision. Typically, with postchemotherapy RPLND, a full bilateral template is performed, aiming to remove all retroperitoneal lymph nodes. Postchemotherapy RPLND is a technically challenging procedure that should only be done in experienced centers, as it is associated with higher complication rates, and could require resection of nearby involved organs (kidney, ureter, spleen, vena cava, colon) in as many as 25% of cases.

CASE SCENARIO

Case Scenario 1

Presentation

An asymptomatic 65-year-old man with a history of hypertension, hyperlipidemia, and no prior surgeries presents to the Urologist with an elevated PSA of 7.9 ng/mL that was identified on routine screening. He denies lower urinary tract symptoms and erectile dysfunction. He has a family history of low-risk prostate cancer in his brother who is living and is managed with active surveillance. On confirmatory test, his PSA is 8.1 ng/mL. DRE demonstrates a smooth 25-g prostate without nodules or concerning lesions. After extensive discussion, the patient wishes to proceed with a pre-biopsy MRI. The MRI demonstrates a PIRADS 4 lesion in the left peripheral zone of the prostate without evidence of extraprostatic extension, neurovascular bundle invasion, lymph node metastasis, or boney metastasis.

Confirmation of Diagnosis and Treatment

After a discussion of his MRI findings, the patient proceeds with an MRI-guided fusion biopsy. Using a combination of TRUS and fusion images from the MRI, 4 targeted cores are then obtained from the PIRADS 4 lesion in the left peripheral zone and 12 systematic cores are obtained. The biopsies reveal 3 of 4 targeted cores positive for Grade Group 3 prostate adenocarcinoma and no other cores positive. After further discussion of his new diagnosis of Prostate Cancer and his treatment options, the patient elects to proceed with a robot-assisted radical prostatectomy.

Surgical Approach—Key Steps

After insufflation of the abdomen, 4 robotic trocars are placed with an additional assistant port on the patients right for suction and clip placement. The robot is then docked, adhesions are taken down and the bladder is dropped to expose the pelvis. An extended pelvis lymph node dissection is carried out to include the obturator nodes, internal iliac nodes, external iliac nodes, common iliac nodes, and the pre sacral nodes. Care is taken to identify and preserve the obturator nerves bilaterally. The bilateral endopelvic fascia are incised and the deep venous complex is ligated with a Vicryl suture. The anterior and posterior bladder neck is then incised just proximal to the prostate with attention to ensure the ureteral orifices are not injured. The vas deferens and seminal vesicles are identified, and the vas is clipped and ligated. Judicious cautery should be used lateral to the seminal vesicles. The nerve bundles are then identified on the high lateral sides of the anterior prostate. The nerve bundles are meticulously dissected from the prostate without the use of electrocautery. The bilateral nerve dissections are continued caudally toward the apex of the prostate. The apex is then taken sharply and the urethra is incised with attention to maintain urethral length. The prostate is then placed in an endocatch bag and meticulous hemostasis is obtained. The anastomosis is then completed with an absorbable double-armed barbed suture. A new catheter is placed prior to completion of the anastomosis.

Postoperative Management

The patient is observed overnight and is afebrile with stable vital signs. Because his surgery and anastomosis were uncomplicated, the surgeon elected not to place a drain, however this practice is variable between providers. If a drain is placed, it is often removed on POD #1 unless there is a concern for urine leak. Labs are often not needed unless clinically indicated. The patient is ambulatory, tolerating PO diet and his catheter contains clear yellow urine. The patient is discharged to home with his catheter on POD #1 with 30 days of prophylactic lovenox. He is set up for a catheter removal and a voiding trial 7 to 10 days postoperatively.

His pathology returns Gleason 4+3 prostate cancer, negative surgical margins and 0 of 27 lymph nodes positive. He is set up for PSA check and clinic visit at 3 months, which demonstrates an undetectable PSA of <0.1 ng/mL.

Take Home Points

- Long-term outcomes for localized prostate cancer are excellent with appropriate management.
- 10-year data have demonstrated similar oncologic outcomes in localized prostate for both surgery and radiation.
- MRI has become a mainstay for pre-biopsy evaluation.
- Meticulous dissection and judicious use of electrocautery are imperative for preservation of potency and continence.

CASE SCENARIO 1 REVIEW

Case Scenario 1 Questions

1. At what age does the AUA recommend stopping annual PSA screening?

    A. 55 years old
    B. 60 years old
    C. 65 years old
    D. 70 years old

2. A PIRADS 4 lesion identified on MRI means:

    A. Grade Group 4 prostate cancer identified on MRI
    B. Prostate cancer is unlikely
    C. Low-risk prostate cancer is very likely
    D. Clinically significant prostate cancer is likely

3. What is this patient's AUA risk group:

    A. Low risk
    B. Unfavorable intermediate risk
    C. Favorable intermediate risk
    D. High risk

4. Which factor in this patient eliminates active surveillance as a guideline-based option?

    A. Age
    B. Grade group
    C. PSA
    D. Number of cores positive

5. Where on the prostate are the neurovascular bundles located?

    A. Anterior prostate
    B. Apex of the prostate
    C. Posterolateral prostate
    D. Medial prostate

Case Scenario 1 Answers

1. **The correct answer is D.** *Rationale:* The AUA currently recommends discontinuing annual PSA screening at the age of 70 years.

2. **The correct answer is D.** PIRADS 4 lesions correlate with likely presence of clinically significant prostate cancer.

3. **The correct answer is B.** *Rationale:* This patient's AUA risk group is unfavorable intermediate risk based on the Grade Group 3 disease. Risk groups can be seen in Table 20.1.

4. **The correct answer is B.** *Rationale:* This patient is not eligible for active surveillance because of his Grade Group which puts him in the unfavorable intermediate-risk group. Age does not impact risk stratifications and while life expectancy can help guide treatment decisions, age alone does not impact guideline-based eligibility for active surveillance. While PSA and number of cores positive can eliminate active surveillance as an option, in this man, neither his PSA or number of positive cores are high risk.

5. **The correct answer is C.** *Rationale:* The neurovascular bundle of the prostate runs in a posterior-lateral fashion of the prostate at 5 and 7 o'clock.

CASE SCENARIO

Case Scenario 2

Presentation

A 71-year-old man presents with new-onset gross hematuria and 2 years of lower urinary tract symptoms for which he has not previously sought evaluation. He has a past medical history of hyperlipidemia, hypertension, COPD, and GERD. He denies any prior surgeries. He has a 50 pack-year smoking history but quit smoking approximately 5 years ago. He owned and ran a dry-cleaning business for 50 years.

Initial Evaluation

With gross hematuria, the patient requires a formal hematuria evaluation to include a basic metabolic evaluation, a urinalysis, a cystoscopy, urine cytology, and upper tract imaging (CT Urogram is preferred), as recommended by the AUA guidelines. His renal function profile demonstrates a creatinine of 1.1 and eGFR of 70. Flexible office cystoscopy identifies a 5-cm mixed papillary and sessile bladder tumor along the posterior bladder wall concerning for invasive disease. His urine cytology is positive for high-grade malignant cells. His CT Urogram demonstrates no upper tract filling defects and a large posterior bladder wall filling defect consistent with the findings on the cystoscopy. There are no suspicious lymph nodes or concerns for T3 disease on CT.

Confirmation of Diagnosis

With a suspicious bladder tumor identified, the patient will require a transurethral resection of the bladder tumor (TURBT) and bimanual examination to obtain a pathologic diagnosis and to appropriately stage the patient. Under general anesthesia, a ridged cystoscope is placed in the bladder and formal pan-cystoscopy is performed. No additional lesions are identified. The patient's urethra is then gently and sequentially dilated to 30-French diameter to accommodate the resectoscope. Using an electrocautery loop, the tumor is resected systematically until the resection includes detrusor muscle. The resection site is then fulgurated for hemostasis and a catheter is placed. There is no evidence of perforation. Bimanual examination under anesthesia does not reveal any residual bladder mass or bladder wall fixation. The pathology reveals urothelial carcinoma invading into the muscularis propria.

Treatment Options

With a new diagnosis of muscle invasive bladder cancer, the patient returns for a visit with urology and medical oncology. Given the muscle invasion of his pathology (cT2), he will require additional treatment. The gold standard treatment would be a radical cystectomy with bilateral extended pelvic lymph node dissection. An extensive discussion with the patient regarding options of urinary diversion is had. Alternatives to radical cystectomy including trimodal therapy or partial cystectomy are also discussed, but the patient agrees that he would like to proceed with a radical cystectomy and an ileal conduit urinary diversion. In discussion with medical oncology, the option of neoadjuvant chemotherapy is discussed. Given the survival advantages associated with neoadjuvant chemotherapy, the patient elects to proceed with neoadjuvant gemcitabine and cisplatin. After four cycles of neoadjuvant chemotherapy, he is set to proceed with an open radical cystectomy with bilateral pelvic lymph node dissection and an ileal conduit diversion.

Surgical Approach—Key Steps

After being placed under general anesthesia, a midline incision is made with entry into the peritoneum in the standard fashion. The urachus is ligated and the space of Retzius is developed. At this point, the posterior peritoneum is incised to enable the development of the plane between the bladder and rectum which is carefully performed using blunt dissection. The ureters are dissected free to the level of the bladder and are ligated as they enter the bladder. Care is taken to prevent spillage of urine from the bladder. The pedicles of the bladder are then ligated with a bipolar thermal device. Care is taken to avoid the rectum laterally. Once mobilized, the urethra is ligated and the bladder and prostate are removed enbloc. With the bladder removed, a bilateral pelvic lymph node dissection is performed to include the obturator, internal iliac, external iliac, common iliac, and presacral lymph nodes bilaterally. With the lymph nodes removed, attention is turned to the urinary diversion. The terminal ileum and cecum are identified and marked 15 cm proximal to the ileal–cecal valve. Another proximal 15 cm is marked. While transilluminating the mesentery, the mesentery is divided with attention to preserve the blood supply of the conduit and the conduit is created. The bowel is then put back in continuity. The ureters are then anastomosed to the conduit in a Bricker refluxing fashion. Ureteral stents are then placed bilaterally. The conduit is then matured in the right lower quadrant of the abdomen where the patient was marked preoperatively by an experienced enterostomal therapist. A drain is placed in the left lower quadrant.

Postoperative Management

The patient is admitted for an expected hospital stay of 4 to 5 nights. While ERAS protocols vary, the patient is placed on a clear liquid diet on POD#1 and is advanced to a general diet when the patient has clinical signs of return of bowel function. Clinical deviation from this pathway is based on bowel function, patient hunger, nausea, and physical examination. On POD#4 the patient begins passing gas and is advanced to a general diet. The JP drain output is monitored daily to assess for increases in output which can be a sign of a urine leak. This patient has a mildly elevated 24-hour drain output of 1,000 cc and a JP creatine is checked. The JP creatinine returns consistent with serum which is reassuring that a urine leak is unlikely. The patient is encouraged to begin ambulation on POD#1, however he is at an increased risk for DVT and he wears sequential compression devices while in bed and he is given prophylactic lovenox for 30 days. Importantly, the enterostomal therapy team educates him on how to manage his conduit and the stoma appliance. Ultimately this patient meets criteria for discharge on POD#5 and his drain is removed. His stents are removed between week 1 and week 2.

His pathology returns urothelial carcinoma with microscopic perivesical fat invasion and 0 of 25 nodes positive. His pathologic stage is pT3aN0M0. He is at higher risk for recurrence with the perivesical fat invasion and elects to proceed with adjuvant nivolumab after meeting with medical oncology 6 weeks postoperatively.

Take Home Points

- Muscle invasive urothelial carcinoma of the bladder is an aggressive cancer that requires radical treatment often in combination with systemic therapies.
- For muscle invasive bladder cancer, radical cystectomy with pelvic lymph node dissection is the treatment of choice.
- Neoadjuvant cisplatin-based chemotherapy and adjuvant immunotherapy with nivolumab have been shown to improve survival outcomes.

CASE SCENARIO 2 REVIEW

Case Scenario 2 Questions

1. Substituting carboplatin instead of cisplatin in neoadjuvant regimens has been shown to:
   A. Increase the risk of complications and adverse events
   B. Offer similar oncologic benefit
   C. Offer significantly worse oncologic benefit
   D. Reduce the risk of nodal metastasis

2. A patient is found to have muscle invasive bladder cancer in the deep muscularis propria and 1 common iliac lymph node positive for cancer at the time of radical cystectomy with lymph node dissection. The evaluation and staging is otherwise negative for metastatic disease. What is the TNM stage?
   A. pT2bN3M0
   B. pT2bN1M0
   C. pT2bN2M0
   D. pT2aN2M0

3. In nonmuscle invasive bladder cancer, a single perioperative dose of mitomycin C or gemcitabine is given in patients with low- or intermediate-risk bladder cancer because:
   A. It reduces progression
   B. It reduces recurrences
   C. It promotes bladder healing
   D. It radiosensitizes residual tumor

4. When creating an ileal conduit, leaving at least 15 cm of terminal ileum is recommended because:
   A. It reduces the risk of vitamin B12 deficiency
   B. It reduces the risk of postoperative appendicitis
   C. It provides a more robust segment of bowel for the ileal conduit
   D. It allows the conduit to more easily reach the skin

5. Which of the following is an absolute contraindication to orthotopic urinary neobladder:
   A. Positive urethral surgical margin
   B. Prior BCG therapy
   C. Preoperative elevated PSA
   D. History of smoking greater than 50 pack-years

Case Scenario 2 Answers

1. **The correct answer is C.** *Rationale:* Carboplatin has been shown to provide inferior oncologic benefit compared to cisplatin. Current guidelines do not recommend using carboplatin as a neoadjuvant or adjuvant chemotherapy agent.

2. **The correct answer is A.** *Rationale:* The patients TNM stage is pT2bN3M0. His T stage is pT2b because it is muscle invasive into the deep layer of the muscularis propria. The N stage is N3, as any common iliac node is considered N3. He is M0 as his evaluation is negative for metastasis.

3. **The correct answer is B.** *Rationale:* A single perioperative dose of mitomycin C or gemcitabine is recommended within 24 hours of TURBT in patients with suspected low- or intermediate-risk bladder cancer because it has been shown to reduce the risk of recurrence. Despite this reduced risk of recurrence, it has not been shown to reduce the risk of progression.

4. **The correct answer is A.** *Rationale:* When creating an ileal conduit, it is important to mark 15 cm proximal to the ileal–cecal valve. Because the terminal ileum is important for bile salt and folate reabsorption, staying at least 15 cm proximal to the ileal–cecal valve reduces the risk of vitamin B12 deficiency. It does not impact the risk of appendicitis, nor does it provide a more robust segment of bowel for the ileal conduit. It would not improve the mobility of the conduit to reach the skin and in cases in which the conduit is unlikely to reach the skin, a turnbull stoma should be considered.

5. **The correct answer is A.** *Rationale:* A positive urethral margin and an uncorrectable urethral stricture are absolute contraindications to an orthotopic urinary neobladder. The remaining options are not contraindications to orthotopic neobladder.

Recommended Readings

Prostate Cancer

Adamy A, Yee DS, Matsushita K, et al. Role of prostate specific antigen and immediate confirmatory biopsy in predicting progression during active surveillance for low risk prostate cancer. *J Urol.* 2011;185: 477–482.

Ahmed S, Lindsey B, Davies J. Emerging minimally invasive techniques for treating localized prostate cancer. *BJU Int.* 2005;96:1230–1234.

Andriole GL, Bostwick DG, Brawley OW, et al. Effect of dutasteride on the risk of prostate cancer. *N Engl J Med.* 2010;362:1192–1202.

Beer TM, Armstrong AJ, Rathkopf DE, et al. Enzalutamide in metastatic prostate cancer before chemotherapy. *N Engl J Med.* 2014;371:424–433.

Berthold DR, Sternberg CN, Tannock IF. Management of advanced prostate cancer after first-line chemotherapy. *J Clin Oncol.* 2005;23:8247–8252.

Beyer D, Nath R, Butler W, et al. American Brachytherapy Society Recommendations for Clinical Implementation of NIST-1999 Standards for (103) Palladium Brachytherapy. The Clinical Research Committee of the American Brachytherapy Society. *Int J Radiat Oncol Biol Phys.* 2000;47:273–275.

Bill-Axelson A, Holmberg L, Ruutu M, et al. Radical prostatectomy versus watchful waiting in early prostate cancer. *N Engl J Med.* 2005;352:1977–1984.

Catalona WJ, Partin AW, Slawin KM, et al. Use of the percentage of free prostate-specific antigen to enhance differentiation of prostate cancer from benign prostatic disease: a prospective multicenter clinical trial. *JAMA.* 1998;279:1542–1547.

Catalona WJ, Richie JP, Ahmann FR, et al. Comparison of digital rectal examination and serum prostate specific antigen in the early detection of prostate cancer: results of a multicenter clinical trial of 6,630 men. *J Urol.* 1994;151:1283–1290.

Chen Y, Clegg NJ, Scher HI. Anti-androgens and androgen-depleting therapies in prostate cancer: new agents for an established target. *Lancet Oncol.* 2009;10:981–991.

Chybowski FM, Keller JJ, Bergstralh EJ, Oesterling JE. Predicting radionuclide bone scan findings in patients with newly diagnosed, untreated prostate cancer: prostate specific antigen is superior to all other clinical parameters. *J Urol.* 1991;145:313–318.

Cooner WH, Mosley BR, Rutherford CL, et al. Prostate cancer detection in a clinical urological practice by ultrasonography, digital rectal examination and prostate specific antigen. *J Urol.* 1990;143:1146–1152; discussion 1152–1154.

D'Amico AV, Manola J, Loffredo M, Renshaw AA, DellaCroce A, Kantoff PW. 6-month androgen suppression plus radiation therapy vs radiation therapy alone for patients with clinically localized prostate cancer: a randomized controlled trial. *JAMA.* 2004;292:821–827.

de Bono JS, Oudard S, Ozguroglu M, et al. Prednisone plus cabazitaxel or mitoxantrone for metastatic castration-resistant prostate cancer progressing after docetaxel treatment: a randomised open-label trial. *Lancet.* 2010;376:1147–1154.

Epstein JI, Walsh PC, Carmichael M, Brendler CB. Pathologic and clinical findings to predict tumor extent of nonpalpable (stage T1c) prostate cancer. *JAMA.* 1994;271:368–374.

Ferlay J, Soerjomataram I, Dikshit R, et al. Cancer incidence and mortality worldwide: sources, methods and major patterns in GLOBOCAN 2012. *Int J Cancer.* 2015;136:E359–E386.

Fizazi K, Scher HI, Miller K, et al. Effect of enzalutamide on time to first skeletal-related event, pain, and quality of life in men with castration-resistant prostate cancer: results from the randomised, phase 3 AFFIRM trial. *Lancet Oncol.* 2014;15:1147–1156.

Fizazi K, Scher HI, Molina A, et al. Abiraterone acetate for treatment of metastatic castration-resistant prostate cancer: final overall survival analysis of the COU-AA-301 randomised, double-blind, placebo-controlled phase 3 study. *Lancet Oncol.* 2012;13:983–992.

Hamdy FC, Donovan JL, Lane JA, et al. 10-year outcomes after monitoring, surgery, or radiotherapy for localized prostate cancer. *N Engl J Med.* 2016;375(15):1415–1424.

Higano CS, Schellhammer PF, Small EJ, et al. Integrated data from 2 randomized, double-blind, placebo-controlled, phase 3 trials of active cellular immunotherapy with sipuleucel-T in advanced prostate cancer. *Cancer.* 2009;115:3670–3679.

Hofman MS, Emmett L, Sandhu S, et al. [177Lu]Lu-PSMA-617 versus cabazitaxel in patients with metastatic castration-resistant prostate cancer (TheraP): a randomized, open-label, phase 2 trial. *Lancet.* 2021;397(10276):797–804.

James ND, Sydes MR, Clarke NW, et al. Addition of docetaxel, zoledronic acid, or both to first-line long-term hormone therapy in prostate cancer (STAMPEDE): survival results from an adaptive, multiarm, multistage, platform randomised controlled trial. *Lancet.* 2016;387:1163–1177.

Klotz L, Zhang L, Lam A, Nam R, Mamedov A, Loblaw A. Clinical results of long-term follow-up of a large, active surveillance cohort with localized prostate cancer. *J Clin Oncol.* 2010;28:126–131.

Laufer M, Denmeade SR, Sinibaldi VJ, Carducci MA, Eisenberger MA. Complete androgen blockade for prostate cancer: what went wrong? *J Urol.* 2000;164:3–9.

Lippman SM, Klein EA, Goodman PJ, et al. Effect of selenium and vitamin E on risk of prostate cancer and other cancers: the Selenium and Vitamin E Cancer Prevention Trial (SELECT). *JAMA.* 2009;301:39–51.

Lowrance WT, Eastham JA, Savage C, et al. Contemporary open and robotic radical prostatectomy practice patterns among urologists in the United States. *J Urol.* 2012;187 2087–2092.

Mohler JL, Armstrong AJ, Bahnson RR, et al. Prostate cancer, Version 1.2016. *J Natl Compr Canc Netw.* 2016;14:19–30.

Oesterling JE, Martin SK, Bergstralh EJ, Lowe FC. The use of prostate-specific antigen in staging patients with newly diagnosed prostate cancer. *JAMA.* 1993;269:57–60.

Parker WP, Davis BJ, Park SS, et al. Identification of site-specific recurrence following primary radiation therapy for prostate cancer using C-11 choline positron emission tomography/computed tomography: a nomogram for predicting extrapelvic disease. *Eur Urol.* 2017;71(3):340–348.

Parker C, Nilsson S, Heinrich D, et al. Alpha emitter radium-223 and survival in metastatic prostate cancer. *N Engl J Med.* 2013;369:213–223.

Ristau BT, Cahn D, Uzzo RG, Chapin BF, Smaldone MC. The role of radical prostatectomy in high-risk localized, node-positive and metastatic prostate cancer. *Future Oncol.* 2016;12:687–699.

Ryan CJ, Smith MR, de Bono JS, et al. Abiraterone in metastatic prostate cancer without previous chemotherapy. *N Engl J Med.* 2013;368:138–148.

Ryan CJ, Smith MR, Fizazi K, et al. Abiraterone acetate plus prednisone versus placebo plus prednisone in chemotherapy-naive men with metastatic castration-resistant prostate cancer (COU-AA-302): final overall survival analysis of a randomised, double-blind, placebo-controlled phase 3 study. *Lancet Oncol.* 2015;16:152–160,

Saad F, Gleason DM, Murray R, et al. Long-term efficacy of zoledronic acid for the prevention of skeletal complications in patients with metastatic hormone-refractory prostate cancer. *J Natl Cancer Inst.* 2004;96:879–882.

Sartor O, de Bono J, Chi KN, et al. Lutetium-177-PSMA-617 for metastatic castration-resistant prostate cancer. *N Engl J Med.* 2021 Jun 23;385:1091–1103.

Scardino PT, Frankel JM, Wheeler TM, et al. The prognostic significance of post-irradiation biopsy results in patients with prostatic cancer. *J Urol.* 1986;135:510–516.

Scher HI, Fizazi K, Saad F, et al. Increased survival with enzalutamide in prostate cancer after chemotherapy. *N Engl J Med.* 2012;367:1187–1197.

Schroder FH, Hugosson J, Roobol MJ, et al. Screening and prostate-cancer mortality in a randomized European study. *N Engl J Med.* 2009;360:1320–1328.

Siegel RL, Miller KD, Jemal A. Cancer statistics. *CA Cancer J Clin.* 2016;66:7–30.

Sweeney CJ, Chen YH, Carducci M, et al. Chemohormonal therapy in metastatic hormone-sensitive prostate cancer. *N Engl J Med.* 2015;373:737–746.

Tannock IF, de Wit R, Berry WR, et al. Docetaxel plus prednisone or mitoxantrone plus prednisone for advanced prostate cancer. *N Engl J Med.* 2004;351:1502–1512.

Thompson IM, Goodman PJ, Tangen CM, et al. The influence of finasteride on the development of prostate cancer. *N Engl J Med.* 2003;349:215–224.

Thompson IM Jr, Goodman PJ, Tangen CM, et al. Long-term survival of participants in the prostate cancer prevention trial. *N Engl J Med.* 2013;369(7):603–610.

Thompson I, Thrasher JB, Aus G, et al. Guideline for the management of clinically localized prostate cancer: 2007 update. *J Urol.* 2007;177:2106–2131.

Touijer KA, Mazzola CR, Sjoberg DD, Scardino PT, Eastham JA. Long-term outcomes of patients with lymph node metastasis treated with radical prostatectomy without adjuvant androgen-deprivation therapy. *Eur Urol.* 2014;65:20–25.

Vargas HA, Akin O, Afaq A, et al. Magnetic resonance imaging for predicting prostate biopsy findings in patients considered for active surveillance of clinically low risk prostate cancer. *J Urol.* 2012;188:1732–1738.

Yamoah K, Johnstone PA. Proton beam therapy: clinical utility and current status in prostate cancer. *Onco Targets Ther.* 2016;9:5721–5727.

Zincke H, Bergstralh EJ, Blute ML, et al. Radical prostatectomy for clinically localized prostate cancer: long-term results of 1,143 patients from a single institution. *J Clin Oncol.* 1994;12:2254–2263.

Bladder Cancer

Bajorin DF, Witjes JA, Gschwend JE, et al. Adjuvant nivolumab versus placebo in muscle-invasive urothelial carcinoma. *N Engl J Med.* 2021;384(22):2102–2114.

Cummings KB, Barone JG, Ward WS. Diagnosis and staging of bladder cancer. *Urol Clin North Am.* 1992;19:455–465.

Grossman HB, Gomella L, Fradet Y, et al. A phase III, multicenter comparison of hexaminolevulinate fluorescence cystoscopy and white light cystoscopy for the detection of superficial papillary lesions in patients with bladder cancer. *J Urol.* 2007;178:62–67.

Grossman HB, Natale RB, Tangen CM, et al. Neoadjuvant chemotherapy plus cystectomy compared with cystectomy alone for locally advanced bladder cancer. *N Engl J Med.* 2003;349:859–866.

Heney NM, Ahmed S, Flanagan MJ, et al. Superficial bladder cancer: progression and recurrence. *J Urol.* 1983;130:1083–1086.

Herr HW. Tumour progression and survival in patients with T1G3 bladder tumours: 15-year outcome. *Br J Urol.* 1997;80:762–765.

Herr HW. Transurethral resection of muscle-invasive bladder cancer: 10-year outcome. *J Clin Oncol.* 2001;19:89–93.

Kachnic LA, Kaufman DS, Heney NM, et al. Bladder preservation by combined modality therapy for invasive bladder cancer. *J Clin Oncol*. 1997;15:1022–1029.

Kirkali Z, Chan T, Manoharan M, et al. Bladder cancer: epidemiology, staging and grading, and diagnosis. *Urology*. 2005;66:4–34.

Lamm DL. Long-term results of intravesical therapy for superficial bladder cancer. *Urol Clin North Am*. 1992; 19:573–580.

Lamm DL, Blumenstein BA, Crissman JD, et al. Maintenance bacillus Calmette-Guerin immunotherapy for recurrent TA, T1 and carcinoma in situ transitional cell carcinoma of the bladder: a randomized Southwest Oncology Group Study. *J Urol*. 2000;163:1124–1129.

Logothetis CJ, Dexeus FH, Finn L, et al. A prospective randomized trial comparing MVAC and CISCA chemotherapy for patients with metastatic urothelial tumors. *J Clin Oncol*. 1990;8:1050–1055.

Logothetis CJ, Johnson DE, Chong C, et al. Adjuvant cyclophosphamide, doxorubicin, and cisplatin chemotherapy for bladder cancer: an update. *J Clin Oncol*. 1988;6:1590–1596.

Logothetis C, Swanson D, Amato R, et al. Optimal delivery of perioperative chemotherapy: preliminary results of a randomized, prospective, comparative trial of preoperative and postoperative chemotherapy for invasive bladder carcinoma. *J Urol*. 1996;155:1241–1245.

Parekh DJ, Reis IM, Castle EP, et al. Robot-assisted radical cystectomy versus open radical cystectomy in patients with bladder cancer (RAZOR): an open-label, randomized, phase 3, non-inferiority trial. *Lancet*. 2018;391(10139):2525–2536.

Pollack A, Zagars GK, Swanson DA. Muscle-invasive bladder cancer treated with external beam radiotherapy: prognostic factors. *Int J Radiat Oncol Biol Phys*. 1994;30:267–277.

Shipley WU, Kaufman DS, Zehr E, et al. Selective bladder preservation by combined modality protocol treatment: long-term outcomes of 190 patients with invasive bladder cancer. *Urology*. 2002;60:62–67; discussion 67–68.

Stein JP, Lieskovsky G, Cote R, et al. Radical cystectomy in the treatment of invasive bladder cancer: long-term results in 1,054 patients. *J Clin Oncol*. 2001;19:666–675.

Stockle M, Wellek S, Meyenburg W, et al. Radical cystectomy with or without adjuvant polychemotherapy for non-organ-confined transitional cell carcinoma of the urinary bladder: prognostic impact of lymph node involvement. *Urology*. 1996;48:868–875.

Sylvester RJ, Oosterlinck W, van der Meijden AP. A single immediate postoperative instillation of chemotherapy decreases the risk of recurrence in patients with stage Ta T1 bladder cancer: a meta-analysis of published results of randomized clinical trials. *J Urol*. 2004;171:2186–2190.

Sylvester RJ, van der MA, Lamm DL. Intravesical bacillus Calmette-Guerin reduces the risk of progression in patients with superficial bladder cancer: a meta-analysis of the published results of randomized clinical trials. *J Urol*. 2002;168:1964–1970.

Vogeli TA. The management of superficial transitional cell carcinoma of the bladder: a critical assessment of contemporary concepts and future perspectives. *BJU Int*. 2005;96:1171–1176.

Renal Cancer

Andrews JR, Atwell T, Schmit G, et al. Oncologic outcomes following partial nephrectomy and percutaneous ablation for cT1 renal masses. *Eur Urol*. 2019;76(2):244–251.

Bex A, Mulders P, Jewett M, et al. Comparison of immediate vs deferred cytoreductive nephrectomy in patients with synchronous metastatic renal cell carcinoma receiving sunitinib: The SURTIME Randomized Clinical Trial. *JAMA Oncol*. 2019;5(2):164–170.

Blom JH, van Poppel H, Marechal JM, et al. Radical nephrectomy with and without lymph-node dissection: final results of European Organization for Research and Treatment of Cancer (EORTC) randomized phase 3 trial 30881. *Eur Urol*. 2009;55:28–34.

Cohen HT, McGovern FJ. Renal-cell carcinoma. *N Engl J Med*. 2005;353:2477–2490.

Couillard DR, deVere White RW. Surgery of renal cell carcinoma. *Urol Clin North Am*. 1993;20:263–275.

Escudier B, Eisen T, Stadler WM, et al. Sorafenib in advanced clear-cell renal-cell carcinoma. *N Engl J Med*. 2007;356:125–134.

Escudier B, Pluzanska A, Koralewski P, et al. Bevacizumab plus interferon alfa-2a for treatment of metastatic renal cell carcinoma: a randomised, double-blind phase III trial. *Lancet*. 2007;370:2103–2111.

Flanigan RC, Salmon SE, Blumenstein BA, et al. Nephrectomy followed by interferon alfa-2b compared with interferon alfa-2b alone for metastatic renal-cell cancer. *N Engl J Med.* 2001;345:1655–1659.

Hudes G, Carducci M, Tomczak P, et al. Temsirolimus, interferon alfa, or both for advanced renal-cell carcinoma. *N Engl J Med.* 2007;356:2271–2281.

Kletscher BA, Qian J, Bostwick DG, Andrews PE, Zincke H. Prospective analysis of multifocality in renal cell carcinoma: influence of histological pattern, grade, number, size, volume and deoxyribonucleic acid ploidy. *J Urol.* 1995;153:904–906.

Lam JS, Belldegrun AS, Pantuck AJ. Long-term outcomes of the surgical management of renal cell carcinoma. *World J Urol.* 2006;24:255–266.

Méjean A, Ravaud A, Thezenas S, et al. Sunitinib alone or after nephrectomy in metastatic renal-cell carcinoma. *N Engl J Med.* 2018;379(5):417–427.

Mickisch GH, Garin A, van Poppel H, de Prijck L, Sylvester R; European Organisation for Research and Treatment of Cancer (EORTC) Genitourinary Group. Radical nephrectomy plus interferon-alfa-based immunotherapy compared with interferon alfa alone in metastatic renal-cell carcinoma: a randomised trial. *Lancet.* 2001;358:966–970.

Motzer RJ, Escudier B, McDermott DF, et al. Nivolumab versus everolimus in advanced renal-cell carcinoma. *N Engl J Med.* 2015;373:1803–1813.

Motzer RJ, Escudier B, Oudard S, et al. Efficacy of everolimus in advanced renal cell carcinoma: a double-blind, randomised, placebo-controlled phase III trial. *Lancet.* 2008;372:449–456.

Motzer RJ, Hutson TE, Tomczak P, et al. Sunitinib versus interferon alfa in metastatic renal-cell carcinoma. *N Engl J Med.* 2007;356:115–124.

Ravaud A, Motzer RJ, Pandha HS, et al. Adjuvant sunitinib in high-risk renal-cell carcinoma after nephrectomy. *N Engl J Med.* 2016;375(23):2246–2254.

Van Poppel H, Da Pozzo L, Albrecht W, et al. A prospective randomized EORTC intergroup phase study comparing the complications of elective nephron-sparing surgery and radical nephrectomy for low-stage renal cell carcinoma. *Eur Urol.* 2007;51:1606–1615.

Wirth MP. Immunotherapy for metastatic renal cell carcinoma. *Urol Clin North Am.* 1993;20:283–295.

Testis Cancer

Albers P, Albrecht W, Algaba F, et al. Guidelines on testicular cancer. *Eur Urol.* 2005;48:885–894.

Carver BS, Serio AM, Bajorin D, et al. Improved clinical outcome in recent years for men with metastatic non-seminomatous germ cell tumors. *J Clin Oncol.* 2007;25:5603–5608.

Carver BS, Sheinfeld J. Germ cell tumors of the testis. *Ann Surg Oncol.* 2005;12:871–880.

Carver BS, Sheinfeld J. Management of post-chemotherapy extra-retroperitoneal residual masses. *World J Urol.* 2009;27:489–492.

Feldman DR, Bosl GJ, Sheinfeld J, Motzer RJ. Medical treatment of advanced testicular cancer. *JAMA.* 2008;299:672–684.

Leão R, van Agthoven T, Figueiredo A, et al. Serum miRNA predicts viable disease after chemotherapy in patients with testicular nonseminoma germ cell tumor. *J Urol.* 2018;200(1):126–135.

Logothetis CJ. The case for relevant staging of germ cell tumors. *Cancer.* 1990;65:709–717.

Ray S, Pierorazio PM, Allaf ME. Primary and post-chemotherapy robotic retroperitoneal lymph node dissection for testicular cancer: a review. *Transl Androl Urol.* 2020;9(2):949–958.

Schmidberger H, Bamberg M, Meisner C, et al. Radiotherapy in stage IIA and IIB testicular seminoma with reduced portals: a prospective multicenter study. *Int J Radiat Oncol Biol Phys.* 1997;39:321–326.

Spiess PE, Brown GA, Liu P, et al. Predictors of outcome in patients undergoing postchemotherapy retroperitoneal lymph node dissection for testicular cancer. *Cancer.* 2006;107:1483–1490.

Spiess PE, Kassouf W, Brown GA, et al. Surgical management of growing teratoma syndrome: the M. D. Anderson Cancer Center experience. *J Urol.* 2007;177:1330–1334; discussion 1334.

Svatek RS, Spiess PE, Sundi D, et al. Long-term outcome for men with teratoma found at postchemotherapy retroperitoneal lymph node dissection. *Cancer.* 2009;115:1310–1317.

Wishnow KI, Johnson DE, Swanson DA, et al. Identifying patients with low-risk clinical stage I nonseminomatous testicular tumors who should be treated by surveillance. *Urology.* 1989;34:339–343.

INTRODUCTION

Surgical oncologists are often consulted by general obstetrician/gynecologists to assist in the management of patients with primary gynecologic malignancies. It is therefore important to understand the surgical staging procedures involved with each disease process (i.e., ovarian, fallopian tube, uterine, cervical, vulvar, and vaginal). This chapter reviews the basic principles of gynecologic oncology, with an emphasis on the appropriate management of these neoplasms when they are unexpectedly encountered during a surgical procedure that is being performed for a different medical indication. Emphasis is placed on diagnosis, staging, and surgical management.

Ovarian Cancer

Ovarian cancer has the highest mortality of gynecologic malignancies and is the second most common gynecologic malignancy in the United States. Every year approximately 21,400 new cases are diagnosed, and 13,700 women die from this disease. Ovarian cancers are heterogeneous, and subtypes are defined by histology. The most common, and "typical" subtype is epithelial ovarian cancer, which includes high-grade serous ovarian carcinoma. Because the majority of high-grade serous ovarian cancers originate in the fallopian tube, "ovarian cancer" often refers to all epithelial cancers that originate in the ovary, fallopian tube, or from primary peritoneal cancers. Other less common subtypes are germ cell tumors and sex cord stromal tumors.

Epithelial Ovarian Cancer

Incidence and Risk Factors

Epithelial ovarian cancer occurs in 1 in 70 women and constitutes 90% of all ovarian cancers. The median age at diagnosis is 63 years. Most epithelial ovarian cancers are sporadic, but approximately 15% to 20% of these cases are hereditary due to germline mutations. For instance, hereditary breast ovarian cancer syndrome demonstrates mutations in the BRCA-1 or BRCA-2 genes while Lynch syndrome, or hereditary nonpolyposis colorectal cancer, harbors mutations in DNA mismatch repair genes including MLH1, PMS2, MSH2, and MSH6. These are both known hereditary forms of ovarian cancer. Mutations in homologous recombination (HR) genes also cause a hereditary form of ovarian cancer. These genes include but are not limited to RAD51, ATM ATR, Faconi anemia, BARD1, BRIP1, PALB2, RB1, and NF1.

Factors believed to increase the risk of a woman developing epithelial ovarian cancer are increased age (peak age is 70 years), nulliparity, early menarche, late menopause, delayed childbearing, Ashkenazi Jewish descent, personal history of breast cancer, endometriosis, and pelvic inflammatory disease. Early studies suggested an association with fertility drugs (i.e., clomiphene and gonadotropin), but subsequent studies have not confirmed this link. Both tubal ligation and salpingectomy have demonstrated a protective effect against the development of epithelial ovarian cancer, as has the use of oral contraceptives for more than 5 years. Currently, studies demonstrating an association between genital exposure to talc-based powder and risk of ovarian cancer are inconsistent.

Pathology

Tumor subtypes are listed in Table 21.1. The most common subtype is high-grade serous epithelial ovarian carcinoma. Cases of synchronous appendiceal and ovarian mucinous tumors have also been reported, but because it is not unusual for appendiceal cancer to spread to the ovaries, it can be difficult to determine the true site of the primary disease. Endometrioid ovarian carcinomas have also been shown to have higher rates of concurrent endometrial carcinomas, though determining whether the tumors are separate primaries or represent metastatic disease can be difficult.

Routes of Spread and Sites of Metastasis

Because exfoliated cells tend to assume the circulatory path of the peritoneal fluid and implant along this path, the most common route of metastasis is by seeding. Epithelial ovarian cancer may also metastasize to the lymph nodes. Hematogenous spread is uncommon.

Histologic Subtype	Percentage Distribution
Serous	71–75
Mucinous	3
Endometrioid	8–11
Clear cell	10–12
Other (including transitional, carcinosarcoma, mixed, undifferentiated, unclassified)	2–4

TABLE 21.1 Percentage Distribution of Epithelial Ovarian Carcinomas by Histologic Subtype

Clinical Features

Symptoms The interval from onset of disease to diagnosis is often prolonged because of the lack of specific urinary and abdominal symptoms such as pelvic and abdominal pain, bloating, gastrointestinal symptoms, early satiety, and weight loss. The diagnosis is often not made until patients have disseminated disease, with more than 70% of cases presenting at stage III or IV. Patients with stage IV disease and malignant pleural effusions may present with a cough or shortness of breath. It is uncommon for ovarian cancer to be diagnosed by abnormal Papanicolaou (Pap) smear results.

Physical Findings An adnexal mass noted on routine pelvic examination and a palpable fluid wave are often found in patients with advanced-stage epithelial ovarian cancer. About 5% of patients with presumed ovarian cancer have another primary tumor that has metastasized to the ovary, though some estimates suggest up to 30% may be metastases from other sites. The most common primary cancers that metastasize to the ovary are breast, gastrointestinal tract, and other gynecologic cancers.

Pretreatment Workup

Careful physical examination, including pelvic examination with rectovaginal examination, is required. Pretreatment workup also includes clinical tests (e.g., complete blood cell count, serum glucose, blood urea nitrogen, creatinine, liver function, serum albumin, and CA-125 [which is elevated in approximately 80% of cases]), chest radiography, and mammography. Computed tomography (CT) analysis may help determine the extent of disease. Colonoscopy is useful in examining the colon and can be particularly helpful in distinguishing between a primary ovarian and primary colon cancer, which may present in the same way.

Staging

The surgical staging schema for epithelial ovarian cancer is outlined in Table 21.2.

Treatment

Traditionally, the initial step in treatment is surgical cytoreduction with appropriate intraoperative staging procedures, including abdominal and pelvic cytologic analysis (or collection of ascites), careful exploration of all abdominal and pelvic structures and surfaces, total abdominal hysterectomy and bilateral salpingo-oophorectomy (except in cases of concern about fertility or of early-stage disease), omentectomy, and selective pelvic and para-aortic lymph node sampling. In patients with a mucinous tumor, the appendix should be evaluated and removed if it is abnormal. Primary cytoreduction is a key component in advanced cases because survival is inversely correlated to the amount of residual tumor remaining. In the past, optimal tumor reductive surgery was defined as the diameter of the largest residual tumor implant being less than 1 cm. However, studies suggest significantly improved outcomes for optimal tumor reductive surgery to no visible residual disease.

For some patients, there may be a role for neoadjuvant (upfront) chemotherapy followed by an interval cytoreduction procedure. In patients with advanced cancer, neoadjuvant chemotherapy may be warranted for those with multiple medical comorbidities that preclude aggressive surgical debulking or extensive disease that cannot be optimally reduced (as determined by CT scan, laparotomy, or diagnostic laparoscopy). Multiple large, prospective phase 3 clinical trial have demonstrated that neoadjuvant chemotherapy followed by interval cytoreductive surgery does not have inferior survival outcomes compared to primary tumor reductive surgery followed by adjuvant chemotherapy in patients with stage IIIC and IV disease.

After surgical cytoreduction, patients should be treated with combination platinum- and taxane-based chemotherapy. Bevacizumab may also be considered in this setting. The addition of bevacizumab has been

Tumor Stage	Description
I	Tumor limited to the ovaries (or fallopian tubes)
IA	Tumor limited to one ovary (or fallopian tube), negative washings, no tumor on the external ovarian surfaces, intact capsule
IB	Tumor in both ovaries, negative washings, no tumor on the external surfaces, intact capsules
IC1	Tumor in one or both ovaries (or fallopian tubes), with intraoperative rupture or surgical spill
IC2	Tumor in one or both ovaries (or fallopian tubes), capsule rupture before surgery or tumor present on external ovarian surfaces
IC3	Tumor in one or both ovaries (or fallopian tubes), malignant ascites or malignant cells in peritoneal washings
II	Tumor involving one or both ovaries (or fallopian tubes) with pelvic extension; primary peritoneal cancer is considered at least stage II
IIA	Extension and/or metastases to the uterus and/or fallopian tubes (and/or ovaries)
IIB	Extension to other pelvic tissues
III	Tumor involving one or both ovaries (or fallopian tubes) with spread outside the pelvis and/or positive retroperitoneal lymph nodes; tumor limited to the true pelvis but with histologically proven malignant extension to the small bowel or omentum; superficial liver metastasis are included in stage III
IIIA1(i)	Extrapelvic spread that only involves retroperitoneal lymph nodes, ≤10 mm in size
IIIA1(ii)	Extrapelvic spread that only involves retroperitoneal lymph nodes, >10 mm in size
IIIA2	Macroscopic peritoneal involvement outside of the pelvis above the pelvic brim, with or without positive retroperitoneal lymph nodes
IIIB	Histologically confirmed implants of abdominal peritoneal surfaces ≤2 cm in diameter, with or without involvement of the retroperitoneal lymph nodes; includes extension to the capsule of liver or spleen
IIIC	Abdominal implants >2 cm in diameter with or without positive retroperitoneal or inguinal nodes; includes extension to the capsule of liver or spleen
IV	Tumor involving one or both ovaries (or fallopian tubes) with distant metastases; positive cytologic results from pleural effusion or pathologic confirmation of parenchymal liver metastases
IVA	Pleural effusion with positive cytology
IVB	Hepatic or splenic parenchymal metastasis, or metastasis to other organs outside of the abdomen; includes inguinal lymph nodes and lymph nodes outside of the abdomen

TABLE 21.2 Surgical Staging of Epithelial Ovarian Cancer or Fallopian Tube Cancer

associated with a progression-free survival benefit, though no overall survival benefit in optimally debulked patients has been demonstrated. After six to eight courses of chemotherapy, treatment decisions are based on the presence of persistent disease or the disease-free interval. Following treatment, imaging studies are now used to determine treatment response.

Following the completion of adjuvant treatment, maintenance therapy may be considered for patients to decrease risk of recurrence. For patients who received bevacizumab in the upfront setting, they may consider its use as maintenance therapy, with or without a PARP inhibitor such as olaparib or niraparib. Alternatively, for patients with a germline or somatic BRCA mutation, olaparib can be used alone. For those with HR deficiency, other PARP inhibitors like niraparib may be used.

Prognostic Factors

Disease diagnosed in an early stage is curable in 90% of women, but most women are diagnosed at an advanced stage. Furthermore, most women will relapse within 2 years. Patients who recur after 6 months of platinum-based chemotherapy demonstrate platinum-sensitivity; while recurrence in a shorter interval is considered to demonstrate platinum-resistance, and is a poor prognostic indicator.

In addition, other prognostic pathologic factors include tumor grade (low or high grade), histologic subtype, and DNA ploidy. Clinical factors of prognostic significance include surgicopathologic stage, extent of residual disease remaining after primary cytoreduction (Tables 21.3 and 21.4), volume of ascites, patient age, and patient performance status. Patients with poor performance status before treatment have significantly shorter survival than do patients with good performance status.

Recommended Surveillance

Patients should be followed every 2 to 4 months for the first 2 years, every 3 to 6 months for years 3 to 5 of surveillance, and then annually after 5 years. A physical examination with pelvic examination should be performed at each visit. The option of monitoring CA-125 levels should be discussed with the patient, particularly if this was initially elevated. As clinically indicated, a CT of the chest, abdomen and pelvis, +/− a PET component can be performed.

TABLE 21.3	Five-Year Survival Rates for Patients With High-Grade Epithelial Ovarian Cancer, by Tumor Stage and Amount of Residual Disease[a]

Tumor Stage	Survival (%) High Grade
I	90
IA	94
IB	92
IC	85
II	70
IIA	78
IIB	73
III	39
IIIA	59
IIIB	52
IIIC	39
IV	20

Prognosis Based on Residual Disease following Primary Cytoreductive Surgery

Amount of Residual Disease	Medial Overall Survival
Microscopic (residual disease)	70–86 months
Macroscopic (optimal debulking)	40–46 months
Macroscopic (suboptimal debulking)	39 months

[a]Based on prior staging system; most recent staging system was developed in 2014 so data are not yet mature.

Treatment of Recurrent Disease

The risk of recurrent disease for all women with epithelial ovarian carcinoma is 60%, but up to 85% in women with advanced stage disease. Patients with recurrence are stratified based on their time to recurrence from completion of platinum-based therapy, known as the platinum-free interval (PFI). Women who have a recurrence 6 months or longer after completion of platinum-based therapy, are considered to have "platinum-sensitive" disease, while women with a recurrence diagnosed less than 6 months after completion of platinum-based therapy have "platinum-resistant" disease. This designation will assist in determining the next chemotherapy option as well as providing prognostic information.

Women with platinum-sensitive recurrent disease that is oligometastatic may also be considered candidates for secondary cytoreductive surgery. Although many recent studies have been conducted to determine the utility of secondary cytoreductive surgery in recurrent ovarian carcinoma; the challenge remains in determining who are the optimal candidates for a second cytoreductive surgery, in order to optimize survival.

Borderline Tumors of the Ovary

Incidence and Risk Factors

Borderline tumors, otherwise known as ovarian tumors of low malignant potential (LMP), are ovarian lesions characterized by atypical epithelial proliferation but without stromal invasion. They constitute as many as 10% to 20% of epithelial ovarian malignancies. The highest incidence is among white women, and the median age at diagnosis is 40 to 50 years (approximately 10 to 20 years younger than that for epithelial ovarian cancer). No risk factors have been identified, and pregnancy and exogenous hormones do not appear to be protective. There is no apparent association with family history or BRCA gene mutations.

Pathology

The most common histologic subtypes of borderline tumors are serous and mucinous (Table 21.5), although rarely endometrioid, clear cell, or transitional cell tumors are present. Diagnosis requires the absence of frank

TABLE 21.4	Ten-Year Survival and Median Survival Rates for Low-Grade Ovarian Cancer by Tumor Stage

Stage	10-Year Survival (%)	Median Survival
I	92	123 months
II–IV	55	82–97 months

| TABLE 21.5 | Distribution of Borderline Ovarian Tumors, by Tumor Stage and Histologic Type |

Tumor Stage	Histologic Type	
	Serous (%)	Mucinous (%)
I	65	90
II	14	1–2
III	20	5–10
IV	1	1

stromal invasion. Distinct pathologic features that may be associated with a more aggressive disease course include micropapillary architecture, microinvasion, and invasive implants.

Clinical Features

Patients with borderline tumors, as well as those with epithelial ovarian cancers, present similarly. The most common symptoms are lower abdominal pain or discomfort, early satiety, dyspepsia, and a sense of abdominal enlargement. Borderline ovarian tumors can also be identified as an adnexal mass on routine pelvic examination. The CA-125 levels may be elevated in serous tumors.

Treatment

In contrast to patients with invasive epithelial ovarian cancer, the vast majority of patients with borderline ovarian tumors are diagnosed with early-stage disease. Recommended treatment for all patients is primary surgery; fertility-sparing procedures should be performed in patients with stage I disease who desire children in the future. The use of adjuvant chemotherapy in advanced disease is uncertain. Recent studies suggest that these tumors may be responsive to hormonal therapies. Typically, these tumors have an indolent clinical course and may recur after a long disease-free interval either as a borderline tumor or a low-grade serous cancer. Tumor stage is the most important predictor of survival (Table 21.6). Secondary cytoreduction can be considered in selected patients with recurrent disease.

Ovarian Germ Cell Tumors

Incidence and Risk Factors

Germ cell tumors are the second most common type of ovarian tumor. Among women 20 years of age or younger, up to 75% of ovarian tumors are of germ cell origin, and up to one-third of these are malignant. The mean age at diagnosis is 19 years; germ cell tumors rarely occur after the third decade of life. Sixty to 75% of cases are stage I at diagnosis.

Pathology

The histologic subtypes of germ cell tumors and their incidences are listed in Table 21.7.

Routes of Spread and Sites of Metastasis

Germ cell tumors have the same potential as epithelial ovarian tumors to metastasize.

Clinical Features

Germ cell malignancies grow rapidly and are often characterized by pain secondary to torsion, hemorrhage, or necrosis. They may also cause mass effects including bladder or rectal complaints, or menstrual abnormalities. Dysgerminomas account for up to 20% to 30% of malignant ovarian tumors diagnosed during pregnancy. Embryonal carcinomas may produce estrogen and cause precocious puberty.

| TABLE 21.6 | Five-Year Survival Rates for Patients With Borderline Ovarian Tumors, by Tumor Stage |

Tumor Stage	Survival Rate (%)
I	>95
II	77–98
III	74–96
IV	77

TABLE
21.7 Clinical Features of Ovarian Germ Cell Tumors, by Histologic Subtype

| Histologic Subtype | Incidence (%) | Tumor Markers | | | Other Notes |
		AFP	β-hCG	LDH	
Dysgerminoma	34–40	−	−	±	May be bilateral in 10–15% of cases
Endodermal sinus tumor	14–22	±	−	±	
Immature teratoma	20–36	±	−	±	
Embryonal carcinoma	1–4	±	±	−	
Choriocarcinoma	1–3	−	+	−	
Polyembryonal	1–3	±	±	−	
Mixed tumor	5–15	±	±	±	Clinical characteristics depend on components present

AFP, α-fetoprotein; β-hCG, beta subunit of human chorionic gonadotropin; LDH, lactic dehydrogenase; +, positive result; −, negative result; ±, positive/negative result.

Pretreatment Workup

Careful physical examination, including pelvic examination, is required. Other components of the pretreatment workup include clinical tests (e.g., complete blood cell count, serum glucose, blood urea nitrogen, creatinine, liver function, serum albumin) and chest radiography. Serum markers, including α-fetoprotein (AFP), β-human chorionic gonadotropin (β-hCG), and lactic dehydrogenase (LDH), should be measured (Table 21.7). Premenstrual women with an ovarian mass should undergo karyotyping because the incidence of dysgenic gonads is increased in patients with these tumors.

Staging

The surgical staging criteria are the same as those for epithelial ovarian cancer (Table 21.2).

Treatment

In general, surgery may be both diagnostic as well as therapeutic. The extent of surgery depends on the patient's desire for fertility preservation, as many patients are of childbearing age. For those who desire fertility-sparing surgery, staging includes unilateral salpingo-oophorectomy, peritoneal cytology, omentectomy, and selective biopsies of retroperitoneal lymph nodes and abdominal structures. Lymph node involvement varies by histology and is particularly rare in malignant teratomas.

For patients whose disease is inadequately staged, there are two options: surgical re-exploration and appropriate staging, or initiation of chemotherapy without re-exploration. In most cases, it is unnecessary to delay chemotherapy by re-exploration and staging because these tumors are highly chemosensitive.

Chemotherapy is recommended for all patients with germ cell tumors, although chemotherapy for those with stage I tumors does remain controversial. Chemotherapy should begin 7 to 10 days after surgical exploration because of the potential for rapid tumor growth. The first-line regimen is bleomycin, etoposide, and cisplatin administered for three or four cycles in 21-day intervals. Alternative therapies may include etoposide with carboplatin or etoposide with cisplatin. Radiotherapy may have a limited role in the treatment of dysgerminomas.

Prognostic Factors

The survival rates for individual ovarian germ cell tumor subtypes are listed in Table 21.8. Prognostic factors for immature teratomas include tumor grade, extent of disease at diagnosis, and amount of residual tumor. The tumor grade of immature teratomas is determined by the extent of immature tissue present. Older age has been associated with increased risk of recurrence in dysgerminomas. Tumor stage is also an important prognostic factor for all ovarian germ cell tumors (Table 21.9).

Recommended Surveillance

Patients should be followed up every 2 to 4 months for the first 2 years, and then annually. A physical examination with pelvic examination should be performed at each visit. Labs (e.g., CA-125, AFP, β-hCG, and LDH) should be checked if they were initially elevated. As clinically indicated, a CT of the chest, abdomen, and pelvis, +/− a PET/CT scan can be performed.

TABLE 21.8 Five-Year Survival Rates for Patients With Most Common Ovarian Germ Cell Tumors, by Histologic Subtype and Tumor Stage

Histologic Subtype and Tumor Stage or Grade	Survival Rate (%)
Dysgerminoma	
Overall	80–98
Stage I	90–95
Endodermal Sinus Tumor	
Overall	70
Stages I and II	75–95
Immature Teratoma	
Overall	90–100
Stage I	90–100

Sex Cord Stromal Tumors

Incidence and Risk Factors

Sex cord stromal tumors account for 5% to 8% of ovarian malignancies and up to 5% of childhood malignancies. Occurrence before menarche is often associated with precocious puberty.

Pathology

As their name suggests, these tumors are derived from sex cords or stroma. Derivatives include granulosa cells, theca cells, stromal cells, Sertoli cells, Leydig cells, and cells resembling embryonic precursors of these cell types.

Routes of Spread and Sites of Metastasis

The pattern and sites of metastatic spread are analogous to that of epithelial ovarian cancers.

Clinical Features

Fibromas and Fibrosarcomas Fibromas are the most common sex cord stromal tumors and constitute 4% of ovarian neoplasms. The mean age at diagnosis for fibromas is in the fifth decade of life. Ten percent of these lesions are bilateral. Symptoms include ascites especially in patients with tumors larger than 6 cm in diameter, increased abdominal girth, Meigs syndrome (right pleural effusion and ascites), and Gorlin syndrome with basal nevi. These tumors are primarily inert but may secrete small amounts of estrogen.

Granulosa Cell Tumors Granulosa cell tumors comprise 2% to 5% of ovarian malignancies and 90% of malignant sex cord stromal tumors. Adult-type tumors (90% to 95% of granulosa cell tumors) are characterized by secretion of excess estrogen. Patients may experience menstrual irregularities or postmenopausal bleeding. Five to 15% of patients present with an acute abdomen caused by tumor hemorrhage. Patients with juvenile-type granulosa cell tumors (5% to 10% of granulosa cell tumors) can also present with abnormal uterine bleeding and abdominal pain. Because granulosa cell tumors produce estrogen, coexisting endometrial pathologic processes occur in approximately 30% of patients. In rare cases, these tumors may produce testosterone and cause some virilizing features.

Thecomas Thecomas are rarer than granulosa cell tumors, but also produce estrogen. The mean age at diagnosis is around 50 years, and these tumors are rarely bilateral. Menstrual abnormalities and postmenopausal bleeding are the most common presenting symptoms. Most thecomas are benign in nature.

TABLE 21.9 Five-Year Survival Rates for Patients With Ovarian Germ Cell Tumors, by Tumor Stage

Tumor Stage	Survival Rate (%)
I	98
II	94
III	87
IV	69

Sertoli Cell Tumors The average age at diagnosis of Sertoli cell tumors is approximately 30 years, but these tumors can occur at any age. Sertoli cell tumors are unilateral. Patients more frequently have symptoms related to excess estrogen, though may exhibit signs of virilization. Rarely, hyperaldosteronemia manifested as hypertension and hyperkalemia may develop. Seventy percent of these tumors produce both estrogen and androgens, whereas 20% produce androgens alone.

Leydig Cell Tumors Leydig cell tumors occur at an average age of 50 to 70 years but can occur at any age. These tumors are often unilateral. Symptoms often include signs of virilization or postmenopausal bleeding due to a propensity to produce androgens and/or estrogen.

Sertoli–Leydig Cell Tumors Sertoli–Leydig cell tumors can occur at any age, but 75% occur before age 40. These tumors are rarely bilateral. Most of these tumors produce testosterone, and virilization may occur in up to 85% of patients.

Gynandroblastomas Gynandroblastomas are rare tumors with a mean age of diagnosis of 30 years. Histologically, both granulosa cell and Sertoli–Leydig cell components may be present in these tumors. Patients may experience estrogenic effects or virilization secondary to the hormone products of these tumors. These tumors may produce androgens or estrogen, or they may be inert.

Sex Cord Tumors with Annular Tubules The average age of patients with sex cord tumors with annular tubules is 25 to 35 years. These tumors may be associated with Peutz–Jeghers syndrome, and in these cases, 66% are bilateral and most produce estrogen. These tumors are also associated with endocervical adenocarcinomas.

Pretreatment Workup
Careful physical examination, including pelvic examination, is required. Other components of the pretreatment workup include clinical tests (e.g., complete blood cell count, serum glucose, blood urea nitrogen, creatinine, liver function, serum albumin, CA-125), chest radiography, and mammography. Evaluation of serum concentrations of estradiol, dehydroepiandrosterone, testosterone, 17-OH-progesterone, and hydrocortisone may be helpful in diagnosis. CT and ultrasonography should be performed to evaluate the adrenal glands and ovaries. Although imaging studies may be helpful, they do not often change the planned staging procedure. For women with abnormal uterine bleeding and a noted adnexal mass, endometrial sampling should be routinely performed.

Staging
The surgical staging criteria are the same as those for epithelial ovarian cancer (Table 21.2).

Treatment
Surgical staging is the same as for other ovarian malignancies, although lymph node metastasis is rare in these tumors. In addition, fertility preservation should be considered for young patients with tumors confined to the ovary. Thus, for those desiring fertility preservation, surgical staging of sex cord stromal tumors can be accomplished by unilateral salpingo-oophorectomy, peritoneal cytology, infracolic omentectomy, selective biopsies of nodes and abdominal structures, and appropriately targeted biopsies. If a hysterectomy is not performed at the time of surgery, dilatation and curettage and endocervical curettage should be performed to evaluate any coexistent pathologic processes.

Tumors of stromal origin (i.e., thecomas and fibromas) and Leydig cell tumors generally follow a benign course; surgery is the only treatment. Sertoli cell or granulosa cell tumors are generally of low malignant potential, tend to recur late, and rarely metastasize. Postoperative adjuvant therapy with bleomycin, etoposide, and cisplatin or other platinum-based chemotherapy should be considered in patients with disease greater than stage I or recurrent tumors, or higher-risk stage I tumors such as those with heterologous elements or that are poorly differentiated. Pelvic radiation therapy is controversial in this setting.

Prognostic Factors
Younger age and earlier stage are associated with better survival outcomes. Survival rates are described in Tables 21.10 and 21.11.

Recommended Surveillance
Patients should be followed up every 2 to 4 months for the first 2 years, then every 6 months following. A physical examination with pelvic examination should be performed at each visit. Current recommendations

TABLE 21.10   Five-Year Survival Rates for Patients With Sex Cord Stromal Tumors, by Histologic Subtype

Histologic Subtype	Survival Rate (%)
Granulosa cell tumor	
Stage I	90–100
Stage II–IV	30–80
Sertoli–Leydig	
Stage I	92
Stage II–IV	33

suggest that there is insufficient data to support routine use of serum tumor markers, but some clinicians will monitor labs at each visit if they were initially elevated. As clinically indicated, a CT of the chest, abdomen and pelvis, +/− a PET component can be performed.

Management of Incidental Cancers Found at Laparotomy

The finding of an unsuspected ovarian mass at the time of exploratory laparotomy or at laparotomy for an unrelated condition can pose a therapeutic dilemma to the surgeon. Appropriate treatment depends on several factors, including the patient's age, the size and consistency of the mass, possible bilaterality, and gross involvement of other structures. Informed consent is a key component to the decision-making. Unless there is a life-threatening situation, a hysterectomy and bilateral salpingo-oophorectomy should be performed only with proper informed consent, especially in women of childbearing age.

Ovarian Mass in Premenopausal Women: Functional Cysts

An unsuspected mass in a young patient is most likely benign. The most frequently found benign masses involving the adnexa are functional cysts, which are related to the process of ovulation. These cysts are significant because they cannot be easily distinguished from true neoplasms on clinical grounds alone. The corpus luteum, which is formed during ovulation, may become abnormally large if there is hemorrhage within it. A patient with a hemorrhagic corpus luteum may present with an acute abdomen, which necessitates surgery. Often the bleeding area may be over sewn without the need for removal of the cyst, fallopian tube, or ovary. Resolution of incidentally found simple cysts up to 5 cm can be evaluated with physical examination alone or in conjunction with pelvic ultrasonography.

Other Common Masses   Other common ovarian masses found in premenopausal women are listed in Table 21.12. Masses may be asymptomatic, but if large enough may cause abdominal or pelvic pain. Ovarian torsion may occur with ovarian masses, and commonly occurs in children, young women, and pregnant women. Severe acute abdominal pain is usually the initial symptom, and this condition constitutes a surgical emergency. If a patient is hemodynamically stable, a diagnostic laparoscopy should be considered.

Treatment

If ascites is present on opening of the abdomen, it should be evacuated and submitted for cytologic analysis. After careful inspection and palpation, if the ovarian mass appears to be confined to one ovary and malignancy is suspected, unilateral salpingo-oophorectomy is appropriate in most circumstances. If the mass is believed to be benign, ovarian cystectomy may be preferable. The ovarian capsule should be inspected for any evidence of rupture, adherence, or excrescence. Once removed, the ovarian specimen should be sent for

TABLE 21.11   Five-Year Survival Rates for All Patients With Sex Cord Stromal Tumors

Stage	Survival Rate (%)
I	95
II	78
III	65
IV	35

TABLE 12	Benign Ovarian Masses in Premenopausal Women		
	Symptoms	**Treatment**	**Other Notes**
Functional cyst	Usually asymptomatic	Conservative management, especially if <5 cm in diameter	Extremely common, can occur with normal ovulation and usually resolve spontaneously
Dermoid cyst	May be asymptomatic; if large may have pelvic pain, possibility of ovarian torsion	Cystectomy or unilateral oophorectomy with close inspection of the contralateral ovary; attempt to retain normal-appearing ovarian tissue	15% are bilateral
Cystadenoma	May be asymptomatic; if large may have pelvic pain, possibility of ovarian torsion	Unilateral oophorectomy (if other ovary appears normal)	Serous or mucinous histology
Endometrioma	Often have a history of pelvic pain related to endometriosis	Possible cystectomy or unilateral oophorectomy; attempt to retain normal-appearing ovarian tissue	Endometriotic lesions may be visible in the abdomen

frozen-section examination. If malignancy is diagnosed, surgical staging should be performed. This should include biopsies of the omentum, peritoneal surfaces of the pelvis and upper abdomen, and retroperitoneal lymph nodes (including both the para-aortic and the bilateral pelvic regions).

If the contralateral ovary appears normal, random biopsy or wedge resection is not indicated because it may interfere with future fertility due to peritoneal adhesions or ovarian failure. If the histologic diagnosis is questionable based on frozen-section results, it is always preferable to wait for permanent section results before proceeding with a hysterectomy and bilateral salpingo-oophorectomy in a young patient. General criteria for conservative management include young patients desiring future childbearing; patient and family consent and agreement to close follow-up; no evidence of dysgenetic gonads; any unilateral malignant germ cell, stromal, or borderline tumor; and stage IA invasive epithelial tumor.

Advances in assisted reproduction have greatly influenced intraoperative management decisions. Traditionally, if a bilateral salpingo-oophorectomy is indicated, a hysterectomy has also been performed. Current technology for donor oocyte transfer and hormonal support, however, allows a woman without ovaries to sustain a normal intrauterine pregnancy. Similarly, if the uterus and one tube and ovary are removed because of tumor involvement, current techniques allow for retrieval of oocytes from the patient's remaining ovary, in vitro fertilization with sperm from her partner, and implantation of the embryo into a surrogate.

Ovarian Mass in Postmenopausal Women The risk of an ovarian mass being malignant begins to increase at 40 years of age and rises steadily thereafter. Therefore, the finding of an unsuspected ovarian mass in a postmenopausal woman is more ominous. The most common malignant neoplasms in this age group are malignant epithelial tumors; germ cell and stromal cell tumors rarely occur. Benign lesions, such as epithelial cystadenomas and dermoid cysts, can still occur in this population, although they do so much less frequently than in younger patients. Treatment of an unanticipated ovarian mass in a postmenopausal patient includes salpingo-oophorectomy and further staging if the frozen section reveals a diagnosis of cancer. Appropriate staging biopsies should also be performed. A gynecologic oncologist should be consulted.

Laparoscopy for the Management of Ovarian Cancer

Laparoscopy has been widely used as the standard surgical approach for benign and suspicious adnexal masses. The role of laparoscopy in the treatment of ovarian cancer is less clear, but some studies have suggested that it can be used safely at the time of surgical staging for patients with early ovarian cancer. The role of laparoscopy in treating patients with advanced ovarian cancer still needs to be defined, although laparoscopic surgery is associated with significantly less morbidity than laparotomy.

Uterine Cancer

Cancers of the uterus are divided into three main categories: those arising from the endometrium (endometrial cancer), those arising from the myometrium or muscle layer (uterine sarcomas), and those associated with pregnancy (gestational trophoblastic disease).

Endometrial Cancer

Incidence and Risk Factors

Endometrial cancer is the most common malignancy of the female genital tract and the fourth most common cancer among women in the United States (following breast, lung, and colon cancers). Approximately 67,000 new cases are diagnosed annually and approximately 13,000 women die yearly from this disease. The median age at diagnosis is 63 years, although up to 25% of patients are premenopausal at the time of diagnosis. Approximately 3% of cases of endometrial cancer are hereditary. Lynch syndrome/hereditary nonpolyposis colorectal cancer is a hereditary cancer predisposition syndrome characterized by the development of multiple cancers, including endometrial, colorectal, and ovarian cancer. Other risk factors for endometrial cancer include obesity, nulliparity, early menarche, late menopause, unopposed estrogen therapy, history of polycystic ovarian syndrome, and chronic diseases such as diabetes mellitus and hypertension. Use of tamoxifen increases the risk of endometrial cancer due to its estrogenic effects on the uterus.

Pathology

Up to 90% of endometrial cancers are endometrioid adenocarcinomas (approximately 15% of these are grade 3 endometrioid), with the remaining being primarily papillary serous carcinomas, clear cell carcinomas, and carcinosarcomas (previously called malignant mixed mullerian tumors). The latter three histologic subtypes are more aggressive, accounting for a largely disproportionate number of the recurrences and deaths due to endometrial cancer.

Routes of Spread and Sites of Metastasis

Endometrial cancer metastasizes primarily by myometrial invasion and direct extension to adjacent structures, including the cervix, vagina, and adnexa. Lymphatic embolization and hematogenous dissemination can also occur.

Clinical Features

Patients commonly present complaining of abnormal uterine bleeding or postmenopausal bleeding; approximately 15% of patients with postmenopausal bleeding have uterine cancer. Patients may also experience pelvic pressure and pelvic pain. Other associated findings include abnormal vaginal discharge, heavy menses, intermenstrual bleeding, and, in some cases, an abnormal Pap smear result. The presence of atypical glandular cells on a Pap smear requires that an endometrial biopsy be performed to rule out malignancy.

Pretreatment Workup

Careful physical examination, including pelvic examination, is required. Pathologic confirmation of the disease by endometrial biopsy or dilatation and curettage is essential. Other components of the pretreatment workup include clinical tests (e.g., complete blood cell count, serum glucose, blood urea nitrogen, creatinine, and CA-125) and chest radiography. Diagnostic tests, including CT or magnetic resonance imaging (MRI) should be performed as indicated by symptom examination findings or preoperative histology evaluation.

Staging

The surgical staging schema for endometrial cancer is described in Table 21.13. The FIGO grading schema is based on both architecture and nuclear appearance (Table 21.14).

TABLE 21.13 Surgical Staging of Endometrial Cancer

Tumor Stage	Description
I	Tumor confined to the uterine corpus
IA	Tumor confined to the uterus, no or <½ myometrial invasion
IB	Tumor confined to the uterus, ≥½ myometrial invasion
II	Cervical stromal invasion, but not beyond uterus
III	Extension of the tumor outside the uterus but confined to the true pelvis or para-aortic area
IIIA	Tumor invades serosa or adnexa
IIIB	Vaginal and/or parametrial involvement
IIIC1	Pelvic node involvement
IIIC2	Para-aortic involvement
IV	Distant metastases or involvement of adjacent pelvic organs
IVA	Tumor invasion of the bowel or bladder mucosa
IVB	Distant metastases, including intra-abdominal and/or inguinal lymph nodes

Tumor Grade	Description
1	Well-preserved glandular morphology, <5% of the tumor has a nonsquamous or nonmorular solid growth pattern; nuclei are uniform round or oval with even distribution of chromatin and inconspicuous nucleoli
2	5–50% of the tumor has a nonsquamous or nonmorular solid growth pattern; nuclei are irregular and oval-shaped, with chromatin clumping and moderate-sized nucleoli
3	>50% of the tumor has a nonsquamous or nonmorular solid growth pattern; nuclei are large and pleomorphic with coarse chromatin and large irregular nucleoli

TABLE 21.14 International Federation of Gynecology and Obstetrics Grading of Endometrial Cancer

Treatment

Endometrial cancer is surgically staged, and in many instances, surgery alone may be curative for women with low-risk disease. Unless a patient has comorbidities that do not allow for surgical intervention, hysterectomy and bilateral salpingo-oophorectomy are the standard treatment for patients with endometrial cancer. Additional surgical staging biopsies, omentectomy, and lymph node assessment are also recommended in certain cases. A minimally invasive approach is most commonly used.

Low-risk patients with grade 1 or 2 endometrioid adenocarcinoma with myometrial invasion of <50% with a primary tumor diameter of <2 cm do not benefit from lymphadenectomy. Furthermore, if lymphadenectomy is performed in high-risk patients (i.e., those with high-grade tumors or deep myometrial invasion), a systematic clearance of lymph nodes in the pelvis and para-aortic regions is recommended.

Recent studies have demonstrated that sentinel lymph node mapping with ultrastaging may be considered for surgical staging to detect lymph node metastasis and help determine prognosis, instead of systemic lymphadenectomy due to the increased morbidity associated with a complete lymph node dissection. This is often performed using indocyanine green (ICG) injected into the uterine cervix. If mapping is unsuccessful, side-specific nodal dissection should be performed. In addition, any suspicious or grossly enlarged nodes should also be removed regardless of mapping.

Up to 25% of premenopausal patients with endometrial cancer have a synchronous or metastatic ovarian malignancy, so in young patients who want to preserve their ovarian function, the ovaries should be carefully inspected at the time of exploration.

After surgical management, adjuvant chemotherapy, radiation, or both may be indicated. For patients at risk for pelvic or vaginal cancer recurrence, whole pelvic radiotherapy and/or vaginal brachytherapy has been shown to decrease local recurrence. However, adjuvant radiation has not been shown to improve overall survival.

In those patients whose comorbidities preclude surgery, or those patients who desire future fertility, local or high-dose systemic progesterone treatment may be effective. Frequent surveillance with endometrial sampling is recommended in these patients. Estrogen antagonists, aromatase inhibitors, and progestational agents with a more tolerable side effect profile when compared to conventional chemotherapy, may have a role in the treatment of recurrent and advanced disease.

Prognostic Factors

Tumor stage is the most important prognostic variable for endometrial cancer (Table 21.15). Other prognostic factors are percentage of myometrial invasion, presence of lymphovascular space invasion, nuclear grade,

Tumor Stage	Survival Rate (%)
IA	88
IB	75
II	69
IIIA	58
IIIB	50
IIIC	47
IVA	17
IVB	15

TABLE 21.15 Five-Year Survival Rates for Patients With Endometrial Cancer, by Tumor Stage

histologic subtype, tumor size, patient age, hormone receptor status, and type of primary treatment used (surgery vs. radiation therapy).

Recommended Surveillance

Physical and pelvic examinations should be performed every 3 to 6 months in the first 2 to 3 years after diagnosis depending on risk status, every 6 months for up to year 5, and annually thereafter. Routine Pap smears and imaging during surveillance are not recommended as there is no evidence to show benefit in outcome. Imaging should be performed as clinically indicated. CA-125 may be monitored if initially elevated.

Uterine Sarcomas

Incidence and Risk Factors

Uterine sarcomas account for approximately 5% of uterine cancers. Most patients have no known risk factors. A small number of patients have a history of pelvic irradiation. Though exact rates vary, less than 1% of hysterectomies performed for benign indications contain an occult sarcoma.

Pathology

Uterine sarcomas arise from mesodermal derivatives that include uterine smooth muscle, endometrial stroma, and blood and lymphatic vessel walls. These account for less than 10% of all uterine cancers but often behave more aggressively than endometrial adenocarcinomas. The number of mitoses per 10 high-power fields, the degree of cytologic atypia, and the presence of coagulative necrosis are the most reliable predictors of biologic behavior. This disease is classified according to the type of elements involved (pure, only mesodermal elements present and mixed, both mesodermal and epithelial elements present) and whether malignant mesodermal elements are normally present in the uterus (homologous, only smooth muscle and stroma present and heterologous, striated muscle and cartilage present). The most common histologic subtypes are leiomyosarcomas (approximately 60%) and endometrial stromal sarcomas (up to 20%). Less common subtypes are adenosarcomas, pure heterologous sarcomas, and other variants.

Routes of Spread and Sites of Metastasis

Sarcomas demonstrate a propensity for early hematogenous dissemination and lymphatic spread. Metastasis is exhibited in one-third of patients.

Pretreatment Workup

Careful physical examination, including pelvic examination, is required. Clinical features of uterine sarcomas are listed in Table 21.16. Endometrial biopsy, dilatation and curettage, or both are essential to providing pathologic confirmation of disease. Other components of the pretreatment workup include clinical tests (e.g., complete blood cell count, serum glucose, blood urea nitrogen, creatinine, and liver function), and chest radiography. Diagnostic tests, including CT or MRI should be performed as indicated by symptoms examination findings, or preoperative histology evaluation.

TABLE 21.16 Clinical Features of Uterine Sarcomas and Basis for Pathologic Confirmation of the Disease, by Histologic Subtype

Histologic Subtype	Patient's Age	Signs and Symptoms	Other Notes
Endometrial Stromal Sarcoma	40–55 years	Vaginal bleeding Lower abdominal pain and/or pressure Enlarged uterus May be asymptomatic	Low grade most common, high grade and undifferentiated are less common Low grade tumors may be sensitive to hormones, and therefore, may benefit from oophorectomy.
Leiomyosarcoma	45–55 years	Vaginal bleeding Pelvic mass Lower abdominal pain and/or pressure	May be misdiagnosed as fibroids on imaging and only recognized on surgical pathology evaluation
Adenosarcoma	Average age is 58 years, but can premenopausal as well	Vaginal bleeding Uterine enlargement	Often relatively large, polypoid tumors, may be visible protruding from the cervix on examination

Tumor Stage	Description
Leiomyosarcoma and Endometrial Stromal Sarcoma	
I	Tumor limited to the uterus
IA	Tumor limited to uterus, size <5 cm
IB	Tumor limited to uterus, size >5 cm
II	Tumor extends outside the uterus, but within the pelvis
IIA	Tumor extends to adnexa
IIB	Tumor extends to other pelvic tissue
III	Tumor invades abdominal tissues
IIIA	Tumor invades abdominal tissues, one site
IIIB	Tumor invades abdominal tissues, more than one site
IIIC	Metastasis to pelvic and/or para-aortic lymph nodes
IV	Tumor invades bladder or rectum, or has distant metastasis
IVA	Tumor invades bladder and/or rectum
IVB	Distant metastasis
Adenosarcoma	
I	Tumor limited to the uterus
IA	Tumor limited to endometrium/endocervix but no myometrial invasion
IB	Tumor limited to the uterus, invasion to ≤½ myometrium
IC	Tumor limited to the uterus, invasion to >½ myometrium
II	Tumor extends outside the uterus, but within the pelvis
IIA	Tumor extends to adnexa
IIB	Tumor extends to other pelvic tissue
III	Tumor invades abdominal tissues
IIIA	Tumor invades abdominal tissues, one site
IIIB	Tumor invades abdominal tissues, more than one site
IIIC	Metastasis to pelvic and/or para-aortic lymph nodes
IV	Tumor invades bladder or rectum, or has distant metastasis
IVA	Tumor invades bladder and/or rectum
IVB	Distant metastasis

TABLE 21.17 Surgical Staging of Uterine Sarcomas

Staging

In 2009, FIGO defined surgical staging criteria specifically for uterine sarcomas in order to better reflect its clinical behavior (Table 21.17).

Treatment

Surgical excision is the only treatment of curative value. Pelvic radiation therapy has a role in local control of the tumor, but because of the propensity of uterine sarcomas for early hematogenous spread, this treatment does not affect the outcome. Leiomyosarcomas generally do not respond to radiation therapy. In early-stage leiomyosarcoma, adjuvant chemotherapy has not been shown to improve outcomes compared to surveillance. However, in advanced or recurrent leiomyosarcoma, the combination of gemcitabine and docetaxel or doxorubicin combinations are considered first-line therapy. Hormonal therapy is the treatment of choice for advanced or recurrent low-grade endometrial stromal sarcomas.

Prognostic Factors

The most important prognostic factor for uterine sarcomas is cell type and tumor stage. Recurrence rates are high in general for high-grade sarcomas, and although stage I leiomyosarcoma has a 5-year survival rate up to 76%, diagnosis at any other stage has 5-year survival rates that are much worse (Table 21.18). Endometrial

Tumor Stage	Survival Rate (%)
I	51–76
II	25–60
III	45
IV	29

TABLE 21.18 Five-Year Survival Rates for Uterine Leiomyosarcomas, by Tumor Stage

stromal sarcomas, when low grade, tend to be less aggressive and therefore have better survival outcomes. Sarcomatous overgrowth and deep myometrial invasion must be considered in cases of adenosarcoma because they adversely affect prognosis.

Recommended Surveillance

Physical and pelvic examinations should be performed every 3 to 6 months for 2 to 3 years after diagnosis, then every 6 to 12 months thereafter. CT imaging may also be considered for surveillance in high-grade sarcomas.

Gestational Trophoblastic Disease

Incidence and Risk Factors

Gestational trophoblastic disease is characterized by an abnormal proliferation of trophoblastic tissue; all forms develop in association with pregnancy. Because this disease is associated with a gestational event, the age of occurrence spans the entire reproductive spectrum. In the United States, hydatidiform moles occur in 1 in 1,000 to 2,000 pregnancies. Among complete hydatidiform moles, approximately 20% develop malignant sequelae, including invasive moles, placental site trophoblastic tumors, and gestational choriocarcinoma. Choriocarcinoma is estimated to occur in 1 in 20,000 to 40,000 pregnancies, with half following term gestations.

A number of well-established risk factors are positively associated with hydatidiform mole. These include age younger than 20 years or older than 40 years, previous molar pregnancy (women who have had one molar pregnancy have a 0.5% to 2.5% risk of a second occurrence, and women who have had two molar pregnancies have at least a 15% to 20% risk of a third occurrence), previous spontaneous abortion (the risk increases with each subsequent spontaneous abortion), and Asian race.

Pathology

Gestational trophoblastic disease is categorized as hydatidiform mole, invasive mole, placental site trophoblastic tumor, and choriocarcinoma. Nonmetastatic disease after molar evacuation may be hydatidiform (invasive) mole or choriocarcinoma. Gestational trophoblastic disease persisting after a nonmolar pregnancy is predominantly choriocarcinoma or, rarely, placental site trophoblastic tumor. Metastatic gestational trophoblastic disease diagnosed in the early months after molar evacuation may be hydatidiform mole or choriocarcinoma. When gestational trophoblastic disease is found remote from a gestational event, it is characteristically choriocarcinoma.

Routes of Spread and Sites of Metastasis

Malignant gestational trophoblastic disease spreads primarily by hematogenous route. The most frequent site of metastasis is in the lung (80%). Other common sites are the vagina (30%), brain (10%), liver (10%), and bowel, kidney, and spleen (less than 5% each).

Clinical Features

Hydatidiform Mole Vaginal bleeding, uterus size larger than expected for gestational age, and the presence of prominent theca lutein ovarian cysts are characteristic clinical features of hydatidiform mole. Features of partial and complete hydatidiform moles are listed in Table 21.19. Other associated findings include toxemia, hyperemesis, hyperthyroidism, and respiratory symptoms such as dyspnea and respiratory distress. Patients with partial moles may present in the same manner as those with missed or incomplete abortions: vaginal bleeding and the passage of tissue through the vagina.

Pretreatment Workup for Molar Pregnancy

Careful physical examination, including pelvic examination, is required. Other components of the pretreatment workup include clinical tests (e.g., complete blood cell count, serum glucose, blood urea nitrogen, creatinine, liver function, serum albumin, thyroid function tests, serum β-hCG) and chest radiography.

Malignant Gestational Trophoblastic Disease Malignant gestational trophoblastic disease can be categorized as nonmetastatic or locally invasive, or as metastatic. Clinically, patients are often diagnosed with malignant gestational trophoblastic disease when β-hCG levels fail to normalize during monitoring following molar pregnancy evacuation.

Metastatic Workup for Malignant or Persistent Gestational Trophoblastic Disease

Metastatic workup for malignant or persistent gestational trophoblastic disease consists of the tests described for molar pregnancy plus pelvic sonography; CT scan of the chest, abdomen and pelvis; and CT or MRI of the

TABLE 21.19	Classification of Hydatidiform Moles	

Feature	Complete Mole	Partial Mole
Hydatidiform swelling of villi	Diffuse	Focal
Trophoblast	Diffuse trophoblastic hyperplasia, variable atypia	Focal trophoblastic hyperplasia, mild atypia
Embryo	Absent	Present
Villous capillaries	Absent	Many fetal red blood cells
β-hCG concentration	Usually >50,000 mIU/mL, and may be >100,000 mIU/mL	Usually <100,000 mIU/mL
Proportion that progress to choriocarcinoma	15–20%	<5%
Karyotype	46XX (majority), 46XY (less common)	Usually triploid (69XXY most common)

Clinical Feature	Incidence of Malignant Gestational Trophoblastic Disease (%)
Delayed postmolar evacuation hemorrhage	75
Theca lutein cyst >5 cm	60
Acute pulmonary insufficiency after mole evacuation	58
Uterus large for gestational dates	63
Serum β-hCG concentration >2,000 mIU/mL during 4th week postevacuation	64
Second molar gestation	40
Maternal age >40 years	25

β-hCG, beta subunit of human chorionic gonadotropin.

brain. Metastatic lesions (e.g., a vaginal nodule) should not be biopsied because these lesions are very vascular and can result in significant bleeding.

Staging
The FIGO staging schema of gestational trophoblastic disease is outlined in Table 21.20.

Treatment
Molar Pregnancy Suction dilation and curettage is the standard treatment for molar pregnancy and is followed by close monitoring of the β-hCG antigen titer to normal. Hysterectomy may be performed if future fertility is not a concern. Prophylactic chemotherapy is not recommended.

Nonmetastatic Gestational Trophoblastic Disease (FIGO Stage I) If preserving fertility is not a consideration, a total hysterectomy can be offered. If preserving fertility is desirable, adjuvant single-agent chemotherapy with methotrexate or dactinomycin is the most common treatment choices. Chemotherapy should be continued until at least one cycle beyond normalization of the β-hCG antigen titer. If there is disease resistance (i.e., the β-hCG antigen titer increases or plateaus), the patient should be treated with an alternate single agent. If resistance persists, combination chemotherapy with EMA-CO (etoposide, methotrexate, dactinomycin, cyclophosphamide, and vincristine) should be administered.

TABLE 21.20	International Federation of Gynecology and Obstetrics Staging of Gestational Trophoblastic Disease

Tumor Stage	Description
I	Tumor confined to the uterine corpus
II	Metastasis to the pelvis and vagina
III	Metastasis to the lung
IV	Distant metastasis to the brain, liver, kidneys, or gastrointestinal tract

TABLE 21.21 Prognostic Indicators for Patients With Gestational Trophoblastic Disease, by World Health Organization Prognostic Index Score

	World Health Organization Prognostic Index Score			
Prognostic Indicator	0	1	2	4
Age (years)	<40	≥40		
Type of antecedent pregnancy	Hydatidiform mole	Abortion	Term	—
Interval between antecedent pregnancy and start of chemotherapy (months)	<4	4–6	7–12	>12
β-hCG concentration (mIU/mL)	$<10^3$	$10^3–10^4$	$10^4–10^5$	$>10^5$
Diameter of largest tumor (cm)	<3	≥3, <5	≥5	—
Site of metastasis	Lung, vagina, pelvis	Spleen, kidney	Gastrointestinal tract	Brain, liver
Number of metastases identified	0	1–4	5–8	>8
Prior chemotherapy			1 drug	≥2 drugs

β-hCG, beta subunit of human chorionic gonadotropin.
Low risk 0–6, high risk ≥7.

Metastatic Gestational Trophoblastic Disease (FIGO Stages II to IV): Low-Risk Disease (World Health Organization Risk Score 0 to 6) For initial treatment, patients generally receive single-agent therapy with methotrexate or dactinomycin. If there is disease resistance, the patient should be treated with an alternate single agent. If resistance persists, combination chemotherapy with EMA-CO should be administered. If there is resistance to EMA-CO, salvage therapy includes the combination of cisplatin, bleomycin, and etoposide, or the use of EMA-EP (etoposide, methotrexate, dactinomycin alternating with etoposide and cisplatin). Combinations with paclitaxel or ifosfamide have also shown some efficacy.

High-Risk Disease (World Health Organization Risk Score 7 or Higher) Combination chemotherapy is the treatment of choice. EMA-CO is the initial chemotherapeutic regimen, and EMA-EP or bleomycin, cisplatin, and etoposide regimens can be used as salvage treatment.

Special Considerations Patients with brain metastases may be treated with radiotherapy for local control and prophylaxis against hemorrhage. If this is not performed, intrathecal methotrexate use may be considered. Patients with residual solitary liver or lung lesions may be candidates for surgical resection.

Current studies are investigating the use of immune checkpoint inhibitors in the treatment of gestational trophoblastic disease, particularly in the resistant setting.

Prognostic Factors
Factors that may affect a patient's prognosis and response to treatment are outlined in Table 21.21. The cure rate for low-risk gestational trophoblastic disease is essentially 100%. The cure rates for high-risk metastatic disease are still 80% to 90% with appropriate treatment.

Recommended Surveillance
Surveillance is essentially the same for all cases of gestational trophoblastic disease, except for patients with stage IV disease, who require a longer period of surveillance. β-hCG antigen titers are measured weekly until the level is normal for 3 consecutive weeks and then measured monthly until the level is normal for 12 consecutive months. Patients with stage IV disease are typically followed for 12 to 24 months after normalization of β-hCG antigen titer values. Contraception is mandatory throughout the follow-up period.

Management of Incidental Uterine Masses Found at Laparotomy
The finding of an enlarged or abnormal uterus at the time of exploratory laparotomy or surgery for an unrelated condition can pose a therapeutic dilemma to the surgeon. Uterine fibroids, which are benign tumors of the uterus, are the most common cause of uterine enlargement. In most cases, immediate surgical intervention is unnecessary. Unless the situation is life-threatening, hysterectomy and bilateral salpingo-oophorectomy should be performed only after proper informed consent has been obtained, especially in women of childbearing age.

Laparoscopy for the Management of Endometrial Cancer
The use of minimally invasive surgery in the staging of endometrial cancers is now the preferred surgical approach. With this approach, a thorough inspection of the peritoneal cavity, peritoneal washings (only if

required by study protocols), and appropriate staging biopsies are still important. Laparoscopy has been compared with laparotomy for comprehensive surgical staging of endometrial cancer in multiple prospective trials, and has been found to be not only feasible and safe, but also associated with fewer complications and shorter hospital stays.

Cervical Cancer

Incidence and Risk Factors

Approximately 600,000 women worldwide develop cervical cancer each year. It is the most common cause of cancer-related death among women in underdeveloped countries, with roughly 340,000 deaths worldwide each year. In the United States, an estimated 14,500 new cases of cervical cancer and 4,000 deaths due to this disease occur annually.

Cervical cancer is a sexually transmitted disease. It was the first solid tumor to be linked to the human papillomavirus (HPV), specifically types 16 and 18, is associated with the development of this disease. Other risk factors include early age at first intercourse, multiple sexual partners, multiparity, smoking, and other behaviors associated with exposure to the HPV. Half of women with newly diagnosed invasive cervical cancer have not had adequate cervical cancer screening, and approximately 40% of newly diagnosed women have never had a Pap smear.

Pathology

Approximately 75% of cervical cancers are squamous cell carcinomas, and 25% are adenocarcinomas, including the less common adenosquamous subtype. Rare histologic subtypes include small cell tumors, sarcomas, lymphomas, and melanomas.

Routes of Spread and Sites of Metastasis

Cervical cancer spreads through various mechanisms. It can directly invade surrounding structures, including the parametria, the uterine corpus, and the vagina. Lymphatic spread commonly occurs in an orderly and predictable sequence involving the parametrial, pelvic, iliac, and finally para-aortic lymph nodes. Hematogenous metastases and intraperitoneal implantation can also occur.

Clinical Features

Symptoms   Discharge and abnormal bleeding, including postcoital, intermenstrual, menorrhagia, and postmenopausal bleeding are often the first signs of cervical cancer. Frequent voiding and pain on urination can also occur and may indicate advanced disease.

Physical Findings   Findings on examination vary depending on the site of the lesion (endocervix or ectocervix). Careful inspection and palpation, including bimanual and rectovaginal examinations, are required to determine the size and extent of the lesion.

Pretreatment Workup

Careful physical examination must be performed, including pelvic examination and biopsy of the lesion. Other components of the pretreatment workup include clinical tests (e.g., complete blood cell count, serum glucose, blood urea nitrogen, creatinine, liver function), and chest radiography.

Traditionally, cervical cancer was staged clinically, but current staging may now incorporate surgical and radiologic assessment. Pathology findings supersede other imaging or clinical findings.

Staging

The clinical staging scheme for cervical cancer is outlined in Table 21.22. The term microinvasive cervical cancer is sometimes used interchangeably with stage IA lesions. This diagnosis must be made from a cone biopsy or hysterectomy specimen.

Treatment

Stage IA1 without Lymphovascular Space Invasion   Lesions that qualify as microinvasive disease without LVSI may be treated conservatively with simple hysterectomy, or cervical conization in cases where patients desire future fertility, if margins are negative.

Stage IA1 with Lymphovascular Space Invasion or Stage IA2   For microinvasive lesions with LVSI or lesions that have stromal invasion > 3 mm but </= 5 mm standard of care options include radical surgery with lymph node dissection or radiation therapy. For those desiring fertility-sparing procedures, radical trachelectomy with lymph node assessment or cone biopsy with negative margins with lymph node assessment are considered acceptable alternatives. Lymph node assessments may consist of full pelvic lymphadenectomy or sentinel lymph node mapping with biopsy.

TABLE 21.22	Surgical Staging of Cervical Cancer

Tumor Stage	Description
I	Lesions generally confined to the cervix; uterine involvement is disregarded
IA	Preclinical cervical cancers diagnosed by microscopic analysis alone
IA1	Stromal invasion ≤3 mm deep
IA2	Stromal invasion >3 mm but ≤5 mm deep
IB	Lesions larger than stage IA lesions or >5 mm, limited to the cervix
IB1	Lesion ≤2 cm in greatest dimension with stromal invasion >5 mm
IB2	Lesions >2 cm and ≤4 cm in greatest dimension
IB3	Lesions >4 cm in greatest dimension
II	Extension beyond the cervix but not to the pelvic sidewall or the lower third of the vagina
IIA1	Involvement of the upper two-thirds of the vagina, without parametrial invasion, ≤4 cm in greatest dimension
IIA2	Involvement of the upper two-thirds of the vagina, without parametrial invasion, >4 cm in greatest dimension
IIB	With parametrial involvement
III	Extension to the pelvic wall with no cancer-free space between the tumor and the pelvic wall; tumor involving the lower third of the vagina; causes hydronephrosis or nonfunctioning kidney unless secondary to an unrelated cause; or involves pelvic and/or para-aortic lymph nodes
IIIA	Involvement of the lower third of the vagina; no extension to the pelvic sidewall
IIIB	Extension to the pelvic wall, hydronephrosis, or nonfunctioning kidney
IIIC	Involvement of pelvic and/or para-aortic lymph nodes (including micrometastases)
IIIC1	Pelvic lymph node metastasis only
IIIC2	Para-aortic lymph node metastasis
IV	Extension beyond the true pelvis or clinical involvement of the mucosa of the bladder or rectum
IVA	Spread to adjacent pelvic organs
IVB	Spread to distant organs

Stages IB1 and IB2 and IIA1 In locally advanced disease, surgery or chemosensitizing radiation therapy results in similar cure rates when patients are carefully selected. The standard surgical option for patients with tumors <4 cm is radical hysterectomy with pelvic lymph node dissection, but radical trachelectomy can be used in patients desiring future fertility. Again, sentinel lymph node biopsy may be used in the place of lymph node dissection. Nonsurgical management may include weekly chemotherapy and 45-Gy external-beam irradiation followed by brachytherapy. Among patients who undergo surgery, chemoradiation is used postoperatively in those believed to be at high risk for disease recurrence.

Stages IB3 to IVA Chemosensitizing radiation therapy is the treatment of choice for locally advanced disease. Surgery may be used as adjuvant therapy for patients with persistent central disease after radiation therapy.

Stage IVB Stage IVB disease is treated primarily with chemotherapy because the disease is disseminated. Chemotherapy regimens containing a platinum agent are most common, but regimens which include the combination of topotecan and paclitaxel can also be used. Bevacizumab with or without pembrolizumab is often used in combination with other regimens in this setting. Radiation therapy may be considered for local control and palliation of symptoms.

Recurrent Disease

Treatment of recurrent cervical cancer depends on the location of the disease and the type of primary treatment the patient received. Central recurrence may be managed with pelvic radiation therapy in patients treated with primary surgery alone. Pelvic exenteration can be considered in patients who have undergone prior radiation therapy. Patients who have unresectable disease or distant metastatic disease are treated with systemic chemotherapy. Chemotherapy options are similar to those used in metastatic disease. For tumors demonstrating PD-L1 positivity or MSI-H/dMMR tumors, pembrolizumab, an immune checkpoint inhibitor, may be considered.

Prognostic Factors

The most important prognostic factors for stage I disease include lymphovascular space involvement, tumor size, depth of invasion, and presence of lymph node metastases (Table 21.23). For patients with stage II to IV disease, tumor stage, presence of lymph node metastases, tumor volume, age, and the patient's performance status are key prognostic factors. The survival rates for patients with cervical cancer are shown in Table 21.24. Among patients who have recurrent cervical cancer, 75% of patients are diagnosed with their recurrent disease within 2 years, and 95% within 5 years.

Incidence of Cervical Cancer Lymph Node Metastasis (Surgically or Based on Imaging), by Tumor Stage

Tumor Stage	Incidence (%) as Indicated by Lymph Node Metastasis	
	Pelvic	Para-Aortic
I		
IA1	<1	<1
IA2	2–9	<1
IB	12–51	2–9
II		
IIA	27–50	11–21
IIB	39–54	10–21
III	50–68	11–25
IV	55–85	27–60

Recommended Surveillance

Physical and pelvic examinations should be performed every 3 to 6 months in the first 2 years after diagnosis depending on risk factors, every 6 to 12 months in years 3 to 5 depending on risk, and annually thereafter. A Pap smear should also be obtained annually, and imaging should only be used if a recurrence is suspected.

Surgical Approach to Cervix Cancer

Upon the adoption of minimally invasive surgical techniques for other gynecologic cancers such as endometrial cancer, laparoscopic techniques were also utilized for cervical cancer by the 2000s. Often these radical hysterectomies were performed either through conventional laparoscopy or robotic-assisted laparoscopy. However, recent prospective and retrospective studies have demonstrated that these minimally invasive radical hysterectomies have worse oncologic outcomes compared to laparotomy in cervical cancer patients. This includes a lower rate of disease-free survival, lower rate of overall survival, and higher rate of death from cervical cancer in the minimally invasive group compared to laparotomy. Thus, it is recommended that patients undergoing radical hysterectomy for cervical cancer have this performed via a laparotomy rather than a minimally invasive approach.

Vulvar Cancer

Incidence and Risk Factors

Vulvar cancer accounts for 3% to 5% of gynecologic malignancies. Almost 6,100 new cases are diagnosed annually with 1,500 deaths each year in the United States. The incidence of vulvar cancer tends to be bimodally distributed. Most cases are solitary lesions that occur in postmenopausal women, and the tumors are often associated with chronic vulvar dystrophy. Recently, a subset of tumors has been identified in a younger population; these tumors tend to be multifocal and are associated with HPV infection.

Five-Year Survival Rates for Patients With Cervical Cancer, by Tumor Stage and Histologic Subtype

Tumor Stage and Histologic Subtype	Survival Rate (%)
Stage I	
Squamous	69–93
Adenocarcinoma	68–84
Stage II	
Squamous	55–58
Adenocarcinoma	46
Stage III	
Squamous	31–34
Adenocarcinoma	20–30
Stage IV	
Squamous	6–17
Adenocarcinoma	8–9

The cause of vulvar cancer appears to be multifactorial. Risk factors include HPV infection, advanced age, low socioeconomic status, hypertension, diabetes mellitus, prior lower genital tract malignancy (e.g., cervical cancer), vulvar lichen sclerosis, and immunosuppression.

Pathology

Eighty percent of vulvar malignancies are squamous cell carcinomas, and up to 10% are malignant melanomas. Less common histologic subtypes include basal cell carcinomas, Bartholin gland carcinomas, Paget disease, and adenocarcinomas arising from sweat glands.

Routes of Spread and Sites of Metastasis

Vulvar cancer spreads by direct extension to the vagina, urethra, and rectum. Embolization to regional lymphatics (e.g., the groin) and hematogenous spread to distant sites can also occur.

Clinical Features

Symptoms Chronic pruritus, ulceration, and nodules on the vulva are the most common presenting symptoms of this disease.

Physical Findings Lesions may arise from the labia majora (30% to 50%), labia minora (20% to 30%), periclitoral area (10% to 20%), and perineum or posterior fourchette (10% to 15%). Multifocal lesions occur less frequently. Lesions may appear as a dominant mass, warty area, ulcerated area, or thickened white epithelium.

Diagnosis

Any suspicious area must undergo biopsy. A Keyes punch biopsy should be used, and lidocaine without epinephrine should be administered for anesthesia.

Pretreatment Workup

Careful physical examination, including pelvic examination and measurement of the lesion, is required. Other components of the pretreatment workup include clinical tests (e.g., complete blood cell count, serum glucose, blood urea nitrogen, creatinine, liver function), and chest radiography CT or MRI should be performed if indicated. PET/CT should be considered in patients with invasive melanoma.

Staging

In 2009, FIGO updated vulvar staging criteria to better reflect the clinical and prognostic factors related to this disease (Table 21.25). Of note, vulvar melanoma is staged via the melanoma staging system.

Treatment

Stage I Wide local excision should be performed if the lesion has less than 1 mm of invasion into the underlying tissue. Wide radical excision with a traditional 2-cm gross margin (measured with a ruler) and lymph node evaluation of the ipsilateral groin are appropriate for all other stage I lesions. Bilateral groin evaluation should be performed if the lesion is within 2 cm of the midline. Although in the past superficial groin dissections were used for lymph node evaluation, several prospective randomized trials have found sentinel lymph node evaluation to have excellent sensitivity and decreased morbidity. Sentinel lymph node biopsy is now used routinely

TABLE 21.25 Surgical Staging of Vulvar Cancer

Tumor Stage	Description
I	Tumor confined to the vulva
IA	Lesion ≤2 cm in size and stromal invasion ≤1 mm; negative nodes
IB	Lesion >2 cm in size and stromal invasion >1 mm; negative nodes
II	Tumor of any size with adjacent extension (lower 1/3 urethra, lower 1/3 vagina, anus); negative lymph nodes
III	Tumor of any size with or without adjacent extension, with positive inguinofemoral lymph nodes
IIIA1	1–2 lymph node metastases <5 mm
IIIA2	1 lymph node metastasis ≥5 mm
IIIB1	3 or more lymph nodes metastases each <5 mm
IIIB2	2 or more lymph node metastases ≥5 mm
IIIC	Positive node(s) with extracapsular spread
IV	Tumor invades other regional or distant structures
IVA	Fixed or ulcerated inguinofemoral lymph nodes
IVB	Any distant metastasis, including to the pelvic lymph nodes

in patients with a single tumor measuring less than 4 cm in diameter, with groin dissection performed in cases where sentinel lymph nodes are not identified. Adjuvant radiation therapy may be administered for higher-risk patients.

Stage II Wide radical excision and resection of bilateral inguinal nodes is the standard approach to stage II disease. The local recurrence rate is similar when the more conservative approach of radical wide excision is used instead of radical vulvectomy. Adjuvant radiation therapy may be indicated if high-risk features are present, including tumor-free margin of resection less than 8 mm, tumor thickness greater than 5 mm, or lymphovascular space invasion.

Stage III Treatment must be individualized for each patient with stage III disease. Options include surgery, radiation, and a combination of treatment modalities. A modified radical vulvectomy (or a radical wide local excision) with inguinal and femoral node dissection can be performed; pelvic and groin radiation therapy should be administered if positive groin nodes are found. Preoperative radiation therapy (with or without radiation-sensitizing chemotherapy) can be given to increase the operability of the lesion and decrease the extent of resection. Radical excision with bilateral superficial and deep groin node dissection can then be performed. Radiation therapy alone is an option if the patient is ineligible for radical surgery or the lesion appears to be inoperable based on location near vital structures.

Stage IV Treatment of stage IV disease must also be individualized. Options include radical vulvectomy with pelvic exenteration, radical vulvectomy followed by radiation therapy, preoperative radiation therapy (with or without radiation-sensitizing chemotherapy) followed by radical surgical excision, and radiation therapy (with or without radiation-sensitizing chemotherapy) and/or systemic chemotherapy if the patient is ineligible for surgery or the patient has distant metastatic disease.

Recurrent Disease

Treatment of recurrent disease depends on the site and extent of the recurrence. Options include radical wide excision with or without radiation therapy (depending on prior treatment and extent of recurrence), groin node debulking followed by radiation therapy (depending on prior treatment), systemic chemotherapy, and pelvic exenteration. Regional or distant metastasis is difficult to treat, and palliative therapy is often the only option.

Prognostic Factors

The prognostic factors for vulvar carcinoma are various. Inguinal node metastasis appears to be the single most important prognostic variable. Other factors include lymphovascular space invasion, tumor stage (Table 21.26), lesion size, lesion site, histologic grade, and depth of invasion.

Recommended Surveillance

Physical and pelvic examinations should be performed every 3 to 6 months in the first 2 years after diagnosis depending on risk factors, every 6 to 12 months in years 3 to 5 depending on risk, and annually thereafter. A cervical or vaginal Pap smear should be obtained as indicated and may include HPV testing and imaging should only be used if a recurrence is suspected.

Vaginal Cancer

Incidence and Risk Factors

Primary vaginal cancer represents 1% to 2% of malignancies of the female genital tract. The average age at diagnosis is 60 years. Most vaginal neoplasms represent metastases from another primary source.

Risk factors associated with vaginal cancer include history of HPV infection, chronic vaginal irritation, prior abnormal Pap smear result with cervical intraepithelial neoplasia, prior hysterectomy (59% of patients with primary vaginal cancer), prior treatment for cervical cancer, and in utero exposure to diethylstilbestrol

TABLE 21.26	Five-Year Survival Rates for Patients With Vulvar Cancer, by Tumor Stage

Tumor Stage	Survival Rate (%)
I	79–97
II	59–64
III	43–49
IV	13–24

during the first half of pregnancy. Diethylstilbestrol was used from 1940 to 1971 to prevent pregnancy complications such as threatened abortion and prematurity. Clear cell carcinoma of the vagina developed in approximately 1 in 1,000 women exposed to diethylstilbestrol in utero. Since this agent is no longer available, the incidence of this disease has dramatically declined.

Pathology
Approximately 80% to 90% of vaginal cancers are squamous cell neoplasms. Other histologic subtypes include adenocarcinoma (10%), sarcoma, melanoma, and clear cell carcinoma.

Routes of Spread and Sites of Metastasis
Vaginal cancer metastasizes via direct extension to adjacent structures. It can also spread through a well-established lymphatic drainage distribution. Lesions of the upper two-thirds of the vagina metastasize directly to pelvic lymph nodes, and lesions of the lower third of the vagina metastasize primarily to the inguinofemoral nodes and secondarily to pelvic nodes. Hematogenous spread is likely a late occurrence because, in most cases, the disease is confined primarily to the pelvis.

Clinical Features
Symptoms Painless vaginal bleeding and vaginal discharge are the primary symptoms associated with vaginal cancer. Bladder symptoms, tenesmus, and pelvic pain, which are usually indicative of locally advanced disease, are less commonly seen.

Physical Findings Lesions are located primarily in the upper third of the vagina, usually on the posterior wall. The appearance of lesions varies. Surface ulceration is usually not present, except in advanced cases. Visualization of lesions identified by Pap smear may require colposcopy.

Pretreatment Workup
Careful physical examination, including pelvic examination with colposcopy, is required unless the lesion is visible. Other components of the pretreatment workup include clinical tests (e.g., complete blood cell count, serum glucose, blood urea nitrogen, creatinine, and liver function), chest radiography and cystoscopy or proctoscopy, depending on the site and extent of the lesion. CT or MRI should be performed to determine the extent of the disease.

Staging
The clinical staging scheme for vaginal cancers is outlined in Table 21.27.

Treatment
Stage 0 Stage 0 disease may be treated by surgical excision, laser ablation, and, in some cases, topical 5-fluorouracil or imiquimod.

Stage I All stage I lesions (including lesions of the upper vaginal fornices) may be treated by surgical excision or with radiation therapy, usually using a combination of external beam and intracavitary or interstitial brachytherapy. Lesions of the upper vaginal fornices may be treated with radical hysterectomy and lymphadenectomy or with radiation therapy alone. For tumors larger than 2 cm, radiation therapy is often preferred due to difficulty achieving negative margins.

Stages II to IV External-beam radiation therapy and intracavitary or interstitial radiation therapy are used for stage II to stage IV disease. Concurrent radiosensitizing chemotherapy is often considered in the form of weekly cisplatin. Radiation to the groin lymph nodes may be indicated as well.

| TABLE 21.27 | Clinical Staging of Vaginal Cancer |

Tumor Stage	Description
0	Carcinoma in situ, intraepithelial carcinoma
I	Tumor limited to the vaginal wall
II	Tumor involving subvaginal tissue but not extending to the pelvic wall
III	Extension to the pelvic wall
IV	Extension beyond the true pelvis, or involvement of the bladder or rectal mucosa
IVA	Spread to adjacent organs and/or direct extension beyond the pelvis
IVB	Any distant metastasis

	Five-Year Survival Rates for Patients With Vaginal Cancer, by Tumor Stage

Tumor Stage	Survival Rate (%)
I	78–84
II	52–75
III/IV	36–58

Recurrent Disease

Treatment of recurrent vaginal cancer depends on the extent and location of the recurrence. Options include wide local excision, partial vaginectomy, and pelvic exenteration. Chemotherapy may be given for distant metastatic disease; however, the efficacy of chemotherapy is not well known.

Prognostic Factors

The most important prognostic factor for vaginal cancer is the tumor stage (Table 21.28).

Recommended Surveillance

Physical and pelvic examinations should be performed every 3 to 6 months in the first 2 years after diagnosis depending on risk factors, every 6 to 12 months in years 3 to 5 depending on risk, and annually thereafter. A Pap smear should also be obtained annually, and imaging should only be used if a recurrence is suspected.

CASE SCENARIO

Case Scenario 1: Acute Presentation of Pelvic Mass

Presentation

A 38-year-old G0 female presents to a local emergency department with acute onset of right-sided pelvic pain with associated nausea and vomiting. Her past medical history is relevant for hypertension, obesity (BMI 36), and tobacco use. She has no prior surgical history. Upon presentation, she has a temperature of 100.5° and mild tachycardia with heart rate of 108. Her abdominal examination demonstrates acute peritonitis. Labs return demonstrating a leukocytosis with a WBC of 18. Due to concern for possible appendicitis, a CT scan of her abdomen and pelvis are obtained demonstrating an enlarged appendix with associated stranding and inflammation in her right lower pelvis. Her adnexa could not be visualized on imaging.

She is consented to proceed to the OR urgently for a diagnostic laparoscopy and appendectomy due to concern for appendicitis. Urine pregnancy test is obtained and this is negative.

Patient was taken to the operating room. Laparoscopic exploration of her pelvis demonstrates an enlarged appendix, but no signs of appendicitis. However, her enlarged right ovary is torsed along the infundibulopelvic ligament and appears nonviable. The left ovary appears abnormal as well. The decision is made to remove the right ovary and fallopian tube, while keeping the left ovary and tube intact. To remove the ovary, the specimen was placed in a bag and removed after controlled aspiration.

Differential Diagnosis

Ovarian Tumor	Secondary Malignancy
Benign cyst (including hemorrhagic cyst, endometrioma, corpus luteum cyst, or tubo-ovarian abscess)	Appendiceal tumor
Borderline tumor of the ovary	Colorectal cancer
Malignant neoplasm of the ovary	Gastric cancer
	Pancreatic cancer
	Cholangiocarcinoma

Confirmation of Diagnosis and Treatment

Final pathology of the specimen demonstrates a high-grade serous carcinoma of the right ovary. She is subsequently referred to a gynecologic oncologist for further management. She was extensively counseled on her diagnosis and treatment moving forward including the utility of surgical staging, tumor reductive surgery, and adjuvant chemotherapy. Due to her premenopausal status, the risks and benefits of her undergoing a left salpingo-oophorectomy were discussed including risks associated with premature surgical menopause such as osteoporosis, heart disease, and cognitive function. After a thorough discussion, the patient decides to proceed with additional surgical staging including a left salpingo-oophorectomy and tumor reductive surgery.

Of note, a frozen pathology evaluation may have been performed during the time of surgical intervention; however, without adequate counseling about potential staging, additional surgical procedures should not be performed.

Surgical Approach—Key Steps

The patient proceeds to the operative room for staging and primary cytoreductive surgery. Her left ovary appears abnormal with nodularity, but upon abdominal and pelvic exploration, there are no other areas concerning for disease. She undergoes an exploratory laparotomy, total abdominal hysterectomy, left salpingo-oophorectomy, pelvic and para-aortic lymph node dissection, and omentectomy for an optimal cytoreduction to R0.

Postoperative Management

The patient's final pathology demonstrates a stage IIa high-grade serous ovarian carcinoma. She is recommended to undergo adjuvant chemotherapy with carboplatin and paclitaxel for six cycles. Genetic testing is performed, and she is noted to have a germline BRCA1 mutation, and she is counseled to discuss the risk of various cancers with the rest of her family. Although she has a BRCA1 mutation, because of her early-stage disease, she is not recommended to proceed with maintenance therapy.

Patient was followed every 3 months for the first 2 years, then every 6 months for year 3, and annually after 5 years with an examination. A CA-125 was collected on the patient, although this was never elevated.

Common Curve Balls

- Incidentally found pelvic or adnexal masses
- Bilateral salpingo-oophorectomy in premenopausal women with malignancy
- BRCA mutation

Take Home Points

- Unless a situation is life threatening, hysterectomy with bilateral salpingo-oophorectomy should only be performed after proper informed consent, especially in women of childbearing age.
- Controlled removal of specimens during surgery with care to avoid spillage or leakage of associated fluid is prudent.

CASE SCENARIO 1 REVIEW

Case Scenario 1 Questions

1. A 38 year-old woman is found to have an adnexal mass. Which tumor marker would be least helpful for diagnosis?

    A. CEA
    B. CA-125
    C. PSA
    D. AFP

2. A patient with a BRCA1 mutation has increased risk for all of the following malignancies except:

    A. Breast cancer
    B. Stomach cancer
    C. Pancreatic cancer
    D. Prostate cancer

Case Scenario 1 Answers

1. **The correct answer is C.** *Rationale:* Ca-125 is an unreliable tumor marker in a pre-menopausal women because it can fluctuate with menstruation.

2. **The correct answer is B.** *Rationale:* BRCA1 mutation is associated with breast cancer, pancreatic cancer, and prostate cancer in patients.

CASE SCENARIO

Case Scenario 2: Lynch Syndrome in Gynecology

Presentation

A 55-year-old G2P2 woman with Lynch syndrome and history of early-stage colorectal surgery status post hemicolectomy presents for routine screening. She reports one episode of vaginal spotting a few months ago, but none since. Her past medical history is otherwise notable for hypertension controlled on antihypertensives. She has had no other surgeries aside from her hemicolectomy.

Differential Diagnosis

Endometrial Atrophy
Vaginal atrophy
Endometrial polyp
Endometrial hyperplasia
Endometrial adenocarcinoma

Confirmation of Diagnosis and Treatment

During her clinic visit, the patient undergoes an endometrial biopsy. Pathology report returns demonstrating a grade 2 endometrioid adenocarcinoma of the endometrium.

She is recommended to proceed with additional imaging to assess for metastatic disease including CT of her chest abdomen and pelvis, which showed no evidence of distant disease. She is counseled on management and is recommended to undergo surgical intervention.

Surgical Approach—Key Steps

The patient was recommended to undergo surgical staging for her endometrial adenocarcinoma. This was performed laparoscopically. She underwent a total laparoscopic hysterectomy, bilateral salpingo-oophorectomy, sentinel lymph node mapping, and biopsy. Sentinel lymph node mapping was achieved on both hemi-pelvises. Ultrastaging was performed for pathologic assessment of the sentinel lymph nodes.

Postoperative Management

Patient is discharged from the hospital on the day of surgery from her minimally invasive procedure. Final pathology returns with stage IA grade 2 endometrioid endometrial adenocarcinoma of the endometrium with less than 50% myometrial invasion, tumor size of 1.5 cm, lymphovascular space invasion present, and negative sentinel lymph nodes. She was recommended to proceed with vaginal brachytherapy to reduce her risk of recurrence at the vaginal cuff.

She was then followed every 3 months for the first 2 years and then every 6 months for up to year 5, then annual with physical examinations.

Common Curve Balls

- Lynch syndrome
- Isolated tumor cells and micrometastasis of the sentinel lymph nodes

Take Home Points

- Lynch patients are at increased risk for endometrial adenocarcinoma.
- Surgical staging should include hysterectomy, bilateral salpingo-oophorectomy, and lymph node assessment, such as with sentinel lymph node mapping and biopsy.
- For premenopausal women, a discussion should be had regarding the risks and benefits of bilateral salpingo-oophorectomy.
- In addition, in patients with Lynch syndrome the increased risk of ovarian cancer with Lynch syndrome should also be considered in the discussion of bilateral salpingo-oophorectomy.
- Prognostic factors in endometrial cancer include percentage of myometrial invasion, presence of lymphovascular space invasion, histology, tumor size, and age. These factors are considered when determining adjuvant therapy.

CASE SCENARIO 2 REVIEW

Case Scenario 2 Questions

1. For patients with grade 1 endometrioid adenocarcinoma and no myometrial invasion seen on imaging, what is another option for management aside from surgery?

   A. Observation
   B. Copper-based IUD
   C. Progestin-based IUD
   D. Methotrexate

2. For endometrial carcinoma patients with serous, clear cell, or carcinosarcoma histologies, what additional sampling should be taken to assess staging?

   A. Omental biopsy
   B. Peritoneal biopsies
   C. Bladder peritoneal biopsy
   D. No additional biopsies necessary for these histologies

3. Isolated tumor cells found on sentinel lymph node biopsy would upstage a patient and be considered for adjuvant therapy.

   A. True
   B. False

Case Scenario 2 Answers

1. **The correct answer is C.** *Rationale:* Progestin-based IUDs can be used as an alternative treatment option in grade 1 endometrioid adenocarcinomas with no myometrial invasion, particularly for those desiring fertility preservation.

2. **The correct answer is A.** *Rationale:* Omental biopsies are commonly performed for these histologies given their propensity for metastasis to the omentum.

3. **The correct answer is B.** *Rationale:* Currently, the presence of isolated tumor cells do not change the stage for patients. There is currently insufficient evidence to suggest change in treatment based on the presence of isolated tumor cells.

Recommended Readings

Burger RA, Brady MF, Bookman MA. Incorporation of bevacizumab in the primary treatment of ovarian cancer. *N Engl J Med.* 2011; 365:2473–2483.

Chung HC, Ros W, Delord JP, et al. Efficacy and safety of pembrolizumab in previously treated advanced cervical cancer: results from the Phase II KEYNOTE-158 Study. *J Clin Oncol.* 2019;37:1470–1478.

Clamp AR, James EC, McNeish IA, et al. Weekly dose-dense chemotherapy in first-line epithelial ovarian, fallopian tube, or primary peritoneal carcinoma treatment (ICON 8): primary progression free survival analysis results from a GCIG phase 3 randomised controlled trial. *Lancet.* 2019;394:2084–2095.

Cohen PA, Jhingran A, Oaknin A, et al. Cervical cancer. *Lancet.* 2019;393:169–182.

de Boer SM, Powell ME, Mileshkin L, et al. Adjuvant chemoradiotherapy versus radiotherapy alone for women with high-risk endometrial cancer (PORTEC-3): final results of an international, open-label, multicenter, randomized, phase 3 trial. *Lancet Oncol.* 2018;3:295–309.

Gershenson DM. Management of borderline ovarian tumors. *Best Pract Res Clin Obstet Gynaecol.* 2017;41:49–59.

Hacker NF, Eifel PJ, van der Velden J. Cancer of the vulva. *Int J Gynaecol Obstet.* 2015;131:S76–S83.

Harter P, Sehouli J, Lorusso D, et al. A randomized trial of lymphadenectomy in patients with advanced ovarian neoplasms. *N Engl J Med.* 2019;380:822-832.

Kehoe S, Hook J, Nankivell M, et al. Primary chemotherapy versus primary surgery for newly diagnosed advanced ovarian cancer (CHORUS): an open-label, randomised, controlled, non-inferiority trial. *Lancet.* 2015;386:249–257.

Keys HM, Roberts JA, Brunetto VL, et al. A phase III trial of surgery with or without adjunctive external pelvic radiation therapy in intermediate risk endometrial adenocarcinoma: A Gynecologic Oncology Group study. *Gynecol Oncol.* 2004;92:744–751.

Lu KH, Broaddus RR. Endometrial cancer. *N Engl J Med.* 2020;382:2053-2064.

Mariani A, Dowdy SC, Cliby WA, et al. Prospective assessment of lymphatic dissemination in endometrial cancer: a paradigm shift in surgical staging. *Gynecol. Oncol.* 2008;109:11–18.

Matulonis UA, Sood AK, Fallowfield L, et al. Ovarian cancer. *Nat Rev Dis Primers.* 2016;2:1–22.

Moore DH, Blessing JA, McQuellon RP, et al. Phase III study of cisplatin with or without paclitaxel in stage IVB, recurrent, or persistent squamous cell carcinoma of the cervix: a gynecologic oncology group study. *J Clin Oncol.* 2004;22:3113–3119.

Moore K, Colombo N, Scambia G, et al. Maintenance olaparib in patients with newly diagnosed advanced ovarian cancer. *N. Engl J Med.* 2018;379:2495–2505.

Nout RA, Smit VT, Putter H, et al. Vaginal brachytherapy versus pelvic external beam radiotherapy for patients with endometrial cancer of high-intermediate risk (PORTEC-2): An open-label, non-inferiority, randomised trial. *Lancet.* 2010;375:816–823.

Nout RA, van de Poll-Franse LV, Lybeert ML, et al. Long-term outcome and quality of life of patients with endometrial carcinoma treated with or without pelvic radiotherapy in the postoperative radiation therapy in endometrial carcinoma 1 (PORTEC-1) trial. *J Clin Oncol.* 2011;29:1692–1700.

Pujade-Lauraine E, Hilpert F, Weber B, et al. Bevacizumab combined with chemotherapy for platinum-resistant recurrent ovarian cancer: The AURELIA open-label randomized phase III trial. *J Clin Oncol.* 2014;32:1302–1308.

Ramirez PT, Frumovitz M, Pareja R, et al. Minimally invasive versus abdominal radical hysterectomy for cervical cancer. *N Engl J Med.* 2018;379:1895–1904.

Rose PG, Bundy BN, Watkins EB, et al. Concurrent cisplatin-based radiotherapy and chemotherapy for locally advanced cervical cancer. *N Engl J Med.* 1999; 340:1144–1153.

Rossi EC, Kowalski LD, Scalici J, et al. A comparison of sentinel lymph node biopsy to lymphadenectomy for endometrial cancer staging (FIRES trial): a multicenter, prospective, cohort study. *Lancet Oncol.* 2017;18:384–392.

Seckl MJ, Sebire NJ, Berkowitz RS. Gestational trophoblastic disease. *Lancet.* 2010; 376:717–729.

Shi T, Zhu J, Feng Y, et al. Secondary cytoreduction followed by chemotherapy versus chemotherapy alone in platinum-sensitive relapsed ovarian cancer (SOC-1): a multicenter, open-label, randomized, phase 3 trial. *Lancet Oncol.* 2021; 22:439–449.

Tewari KS, Sill MW, Long HJ, et al. Improved survival with bevacizumab in advanced cervical cancer. *N Engl J Med.* 2014;370:734–743.

Thomas G, Dembo A, Fyles A, et al. Concurrent chemoradiation in advanced cervical cancer. *Gynecol Oncol.* 1990;38:446–451.

Walker JL, Piedmont MR, Spirtos NM, et al. Laparoscopy compared with laparotomy for comprehensive surgical staging of uterine cancer: Gynecologic Oncology Group study LAP2. *J Clin Oncol.* 2009;27:5331–5336.

Neurosurgical Malignancies: Treating Tumors of Brain and Spine and Their Effects on the Nervous System

Ian E. McCutcheon and Chibawanye I. Ene

INTRODUCTION

The interplay of neurosurgery with other disciplines in the broader field of surgical oncology leads to frequent instances of neurosurgical treatment in patients whose tumors originated outside the central nervous system. Tumors also originate within the brain or spine and require neurosurgical care. To many oncologists the nervous system remains an arcane, poorly understood area yet it is one with profound implications on patient outcome. Neurosurgical oncologists aim to cure or palliate tumors when possible, but even more so to preserve function at the highest possible level and for the longest period of time. It is a technically demanding discipline very much concerned with maintaining the functions that make life worthwhile. This chapter will provide an overview of fundamental clinical scenarios and basic tumor types relevant to the practice of neurosurgical oncology in a cancer center.

Clinical Evaluation

Neurologic Examination

All encounters with patients suspected of harboring some form of neurologic disease must perforce begin with an interview and neurologic examination. All too often this portion of the physical examination is skipped or notated scantily or not at all in the chart, yet a good history and intelligently focused neurologic examination will yield 90% of the elements needed to make clinical decisions for a tumor affecting the neuraxis. Ultimately the interpretation of such information depends on a sound working knowledge of the anatomy of the nervous system. The 10 subsystems (cerebral cortex, pyramidal tracts, basal ganglia, brainstem, cranial nerves, cerebellum, spinal cord, nerve roots, peripheral and autonomic nerves, and muscle) each cause different changes on neurologic examination that allow accuracy in anatomical localization.

Questions to Ask

First, *is the patient conscious?* The classic way of measuring consciousness is by grading eye movements, verbalization, and motor function on the Glasgow Coma Scale (GCS), in which perfect wakefulness and function result in a score of 15 and complete coma without even reflex movements yields a score of 3 (Table 22.1). Note that even a dead person has a score of 3, and prognosis is very poor in a living patient with this low a GCS.

TABLE 22.1 Glasgow Coma Scale

		Score
Eye opening	Spontaneously	4
	To speech	3
	To pain	2
	None	1
Verbal response	Oriented	5
	Confused	4
	Inappropriate	3
	Incomprehensible	2
	None	1
Motor response	Obeys commands	6
	Localizes to pain	5
	Withdraws from pain	4
	Flexion to pain	3
	Extension to pain	2
	None	1

The scale measures whether such responses occur spontaneously or only after varying degrees of stimulation. Even patients in deep coma will preserve flexor or (in the worst case) extensor motor responses to such deep painful stimuli as a sternal rub. In the relatively awake patient, speech function can be assessed by noting speech patterns during conversation, but subtle patterns of dysphasia may elude the observer unless they address pointed questions to the patient. In most patients the speech areas reside in the brain's left hemisphere. However, because speech function arises only in the *right* hemisphere in 15% of left-handed subjects, this generalization is not absolute. Depending on which part of the speech network is affected by a lesion, patients can show difficulties with expressing words (Broca's area), with naming objects (uncinate fasciculus), with reading (posterior parasylvian), or with understanding spoken phrases (Wernicke's area). In addition, speech may be impaired from a motor perspective if the cranial nerves subserving coordination of tongue, throat muscles, and vocal cords are impaired.

Is the patient weakened or paralyzed in one or more limbs? Even in a comatose patient, differential degrees of withdrawal to painful stimuli can uncover a weakness. In the awake patient, a simple request to pull or push against resistance provided by the examiner, and made for each of the four limbs, can uncover various patterns of weakness. These include a hemiparesis (weakness of one side of the body), quadriparesis (weakness in all four limbs and implying a lesion of the cervical spinal cord or brain), or paraparesis (weakness of both legs, implying a spinal lesion above the lumbosacral junction). In an oncology patient the possibility of tumor affecting neural elements at the appropriate location in the nervous system must be considered before other diagnoses common in the nononcologic population (stroke, trauma, etc.).

Does the patient have a myelopathy? This term implies a disorder of the spinal cord as opposed to the brain, and ruling myelopathy in or out is done in any patient who complains of sensory or motor symptoms that could have arisen from such a spinal lesion. The delicacy of the spinal cord in the face of extrinsic (or for that matter, intrinsic) compression means that such compression cannot be allowed to persist for long before permanent deficits ensue. Myelopathy is detected by examining: (1) reflexes at the knees and elbow (quadriceps and biceps reflexes, respectively), (2) muscle tone, and (3) response of the toes to plantar stimulation, that is, the Babinski response. When myelopathy is present, reflexes and tone are increased, clonus is present, and the plantar response is extensor.

Can the patient see? Four of the 12 cranial nerves are used for seeing (optic nerve, cranial nerve II), eye movement (cranial nerves III, IV, and VI), or eyelid opening (cranial nerve III). Eye movements should be checked because they give an indicator of the function of the brainstem, where the nuclei of these cranial nerves reside, and because increases in intracranial pressure (ICP) can affect ocular motility most commonly by causing a sixth nerve palsy in which lateral movement (abduction) of one or both eyes is impaired. In addition, increases in ICP can cause papilledema visible on fundoscopy. Perfect vision requires the integrity of a system that extends from the retina through the optic nerves, chiasm, and tracts back through the geniculate body of the thalamus, and thence through the optic radiations to the calcarine cortex in the occipital lobes. If the patient passes a good visual examination then malfunction of a significant portion of the brain has been excluded.

Can the patient swallow? This aspect of the neurologic examination is often overlooked, but the ability to swallow is critically important to good outcome for any patient undergoing surgery for a tumor. Patients with impairment of the gag reflex or with pharyngeal dysmotility are harder to wean safely off ventilatory assistance, are more prone to aspiration and its consequences, and often cannot achieve oral intake sufficient to maintain the good nutrition needed for postsurgical healing. Decisions about gastrostomy or about transnasal tube feeding should be made early in patients in whom such issues have been discovered.

Finally, *can the patient walk?* Walking is a complex function that needs inputs from sensory systems, proprioceptive processing systems, and motor systems to prevent falls. Tumors in the cerebellum, which acts as a computer processing and modulating proprioceptive inputs and motor outputs, cause ataxia. Intrinsic disease within nerves (e.g., diabetic neuropathy) can reduce sensory input and cause a patient to stumble more easily. When seeing a patient with a recent history of stumbling or falling, the surgical oncologist should examine for signs of incipient myelopathy indicating an impending spinal cord compression. As the window of therapeutic opportunity in such cases is small (within 24 hours from loss of ambulation), a decline in the ability to walk can be a vitally important clue, and demands prompt investigation.

Increased Intracranial Pressure

Basic Principles

The cranium in man is a rigid structure. Its contents include the brain, blood (arterial and venous), and cerebrospinal fluid (CSF). Because intracranial volume is constant, when an intracranial mass is introduced compensation first occurs through a reciprocal decrease in the volume of venous blood and CSF. This concept, known as the Monro–Kellie doctrine, is most applicable in adults. Children younger than the age of skull suture fusion will show cranial expansion when high ICP is chronic; the doctrine assumes a rigid skull. CSF volume increases with age due to brain atrophy.

When compensatory mechanisms have been exhausted, minute changes in volume produce precipitous increases in pressure. The pressure–volume curve reflects very small increases in pressure when an expanding mass begins in the intracranial compartment. ICP rises more precipitously as compensation allowed by egress of CSF and venous blood disappears. When ICP overcomes arterial pressure, perfusion ceases and brain death occurs.

The blood–brain barrier (BBB) is formed by linked astrocytic foot processes along the adventitial surfaces of cerebral endothelial cells. It prevents many substances carried in the blood from reaching the brain, and protects neural tissue from potentially toxic materials. It also regulates the flow of biologically active molecules into the brain. Lipid-soluble substances can usually penetrate more effectively than amino acids and sugars, which are transported across the endothelium by specific carrier-mediated mechanisms. When the barrier is disrupted, plasma components cross into the brain and cause vasogenic edema. Relative disruption of the BBB by intracranial tumors causes local edema around the tumor leading to neurologic malfunction in the edematous zone. In addition, the BBB prevents most chemotherapy agents from penetrating into the brain and has stymied the development of effective medical treatments for brain tumors. In the past 40 years only four drugs have been approved by the FDA for brain tumor therapy: *bis-chloronitrosourea (BCNU)*, now little used, but which has the advantage of lipid solubility; its cognate alkylating agent *CCNU*, which is given orally; *temozolomide* (TMZ), also given by mouth and having a low side-effect profile; and *Avastin*, an antiangiogenic monoclonal antibody whose efficacy in extending survival is controversial. Polycarbonate wafer impregnated with BCNU (Gliadel) has been separately approved for treatment of glioblastoma and is placed during surgery along the walls of the surgical resection cavity. It provides a modest increase in survival through slow diffusion of the drug locally into potential sites of microscopic invasion in the edematous peritumoral brain.

Cerebral edema is treated with steroids (usually dexamethasone) and in more refractory cases with osmotic agents such as mannitol, urea, or hypertonic saline. Use of steroids is routine after resection of intracranial or spinal tumors as a way of reducing the flare-up of edema commonly seen after intraoperative tumor manipulation. Tumors that produce copious amounts of vascular endothelial growth factor (VEGF) give the most extensive edema; a classic example is metastasis from renal cell carcinoma. Since dexamethasone could suppress the immune system, bevacizumab (Avastin), an anti-VEGF monoclonal antibody is sometimes used as an alternative to dexamethasone to reduce edema especially in patients receiving immunotherapy.

Cerebral blood flow is determined most significantly by the cerebral perfusion pressure (CPP), defined as the difference between the incoming mean arterial pressure (MAP: calculated from the systolic blood pressure [SBP] and diastolic blood pressure [DBP]), and the opposing ICP.

Because the heart spends twice as much time in diastole as in systole, the formulae are:

$$CPP = MAP - ICP$$
$$MAP = [SBP + 2\,(DBP)]/3$$

As ICP rises, CPP decreases. Under physiologic conditions several factors regulate cerebral blood flow: systemic blood pressure, pCO_2 and pH in the arterial blood, and pO_2. Autoregulation maintains blood flow to the brain at a constant level over a wide range of MAP. When MAP is low, cerebral arterioles dilate to allow adequate flow. Increased systemic blood pressure causes arterioles to constrict for the same purpose. At MAP <50 mm Hg perfusion is inadequate; with MAP >150 the autoregulatory system fails and cerebral blood flow increases, leading to vasogenic edema, hypertensive encephalopathy, and dangerous elevations in ICP.

Arterial pCO_2 is the most potent stimulus for dilation of cerebral arterioles. As pCO_2 decreases from 80 to 15 mm Hg, cerebral blood flow decreases. Since it diminishes cerebral blood flow and blood volume, hyperventilation can be used to treat increased ICP. A patient with decreased level of consciousness (GCS ≤9) from increased ICP is typically intubated for airway protection and prevention of aspiration, but also for hyperventilation to a pCO_2 of 28 mm Hg. Such patients are maintained normoxic or slightly hyperoxic. As hypoxia causes cerebral arteriolar dilation, maintaining good oxygenation helps dampen increases in ICP. Brain tissue oxygen partial pressure ($PbtO_2$) can be measured using an intraparenchymal probe (LICOX). Although this is typically used in trauma, $PbtO_2$ probe readings have allowed for better understanding of the relationship between autoregulation, ICP, and brain tissue oxygenation.

The normal ICP is 10 to 15 mm Hg (13 to 20 cm H_2O) in an awake patient. Causes of raised ICP are given in Table 22.2. Increased ICP harms the brain in two ways. First, ischemia can occur when CPP reaches critically

Common Causes of Increased Intracranial Pressure (ICP)	
Pathologic Process	**Examples**
Localized masses	Hematomas: epidural, subdural, intracerebral
	Neoplasms: gliomas, meningiomas, metastases
	Abscesses
	Focal edema: from trauma, infarction, tumor
Obstruction of CSF pathway	Obstructive hydrocephalus
	Communicating hydrocephalus
Obstruction of major venous sinus	Depressed skull fracture over sinus
	Thrombosis from dehydration or oral contraceptive use
Diffuse brain edema	Encephalitis, meningitis
	Diffuse head injury
	Subarachnoid hemorrhage
	Water intoxication
	Lead poisoning causing encephalopathy
Idiopathic	Pseudotumor cerebri

low levels and can lead to stroke. Second, focal masses (e.g., tumors or hematomas) cause distortion of the brain which if profound enough causes compression of brainstem structures vital to life. Herniation of the cerebellar tonsils through the foramen magnum, or the midbrain and aqueduct of Sylvius through the tentorial incisura, further elevate ICP by blocking CSF pathways. Increases in ICP are better tolerated when shift of brain structures is absent. When ICP is increased slowly and chronically by generalized syndromes such as pseudotumor cerebri (a little-understood condition labeled variously as a disorder of CSF absorption, a structural defect in venous sinuses, or a product of morbid obesity), neurologic dysfunction may be absent or limited to specific cranial neuropathies.

Herniation occurs when the brain moves within the cranial cavity relative to the edge of dural folds intended to prevent its movement. The four main types of brain herniation are:

1. *Cingulate herniation*, in which pressure is greater in one hemisphere than the other, leading to shift of the cingulate gyrus beneath the falx.
2. *Uncal herniation*, which is the most clinically dramatic and most common herniation syndrome. It occurs when a lesion in the middle cranial fossa (temporal lobe) expands the uncus, the most inferomedial structure of the temporal lobe, and displaces it against the peduncle of the midbrain. Uncal herniation gives a clinical syndrome of progressively impaired consciousness, dilation of the ipsilateral pupil ("blown pupil"), and contralateral hemiplegia. Disturbance of consciousness comes from disturbance of the reticular activating system in the midbrain, pupillary dilation from compression of the oculomotor nerve and its parasympathetic pupillary constrictors, and hemiplegia from the compression of the corticospinal tract above its decussation.
3. *Central transtentorial herniation*, which is caused by hemispheric lesions in the frontal or parietal areas of the brain. Here the diencephalon and midbrain shift down through the tentorial incisura. The clinical syndrome is more difficult to recognize than that of uncal herniation and may include small reactive pupils, obtundation, loss of vertical gaze, and Cheyne–Stokes respiration.
4. *Tonsillar herniation* is caused by expansion of a posterior fossa mass. The cerebellar tonsils move through the foramen magnum into the upper spinal canal and compress the dorsolateral medulla and upper cervical cord. This leads to hypertension, cardiorespiratory impairment, neurogenic hyperventilation, and impaired swallowing and consciousness. Ultimately death occurs due to cardiac and respiratory instability.

Symptoms of increased ICP include headache, worse in the early morning due to a rise of pCO_2 from hypoventilation during sleep and increased venous pressure from the recumbent position. However, headache is not a specific symptom and it is perfectly possible to have increased ICP without headache. The combination of headache and vomiting is suggestive, and accompanying neurologic signs such as papilledema and cranial neuropathies are further confirmatory. The speed of onset of the increase in ICP influences symptoms as well. More chronic or slowly progressive rises in pressure are less likely to cause obtundation or pronounced neurologic decline.

Monitoring ICP

Continuous monitoring of ICP is important in patients whose neurologic examination and radiologic studies support the suspicion of increased pressure. Controlling such pressure rises significantly reduces morbidity and mortality in neurosurgical patients. Although the most common indicators for such monitoring are closed head injury and subarachnoid hemorrhage, patients in the oncology setting may require it in a number of circumstances including: after posterior fossa surgery (to determine whether preexisting hydrocephalus has cleared); when brain injury has led to coma and thus abrogated use of the neurologic examination as an index of brain function; or when an intracranial hemorrhage caused by chemotherapy-induced thrombocytopenia leaves the patient at risk for hydrocephalus or further bleeding, with decisions about shunting or clot evacuation assisted by ICP measurement over time.

The most effective method of measuring ICP is through placement of a ventriculostomy drainage catheter. This is inserted through a frontal burr hole made either at the bedside or in the operating room. The catheter is tunneled a short distance to prevent infection, and exits the scalp through a separate stab incision. It is connected to a pressure transducer and a drainage system. The catheter can be used to measure pressure but also to drain CSF to treat ICP increases when it exceeds a prespecified limit. This limit is set by raising or lowering the loop of the drain, which provides resistance to CSF egress. For example, when the loop is set at 10 cm above the external auditory meatus (the typical "zero" point), no drainage occurs unless CSF pressure exceeds 10 cm of H_2O.

Treatment of Increased ICP

The first order of business in ICP treatment is always to address the cause directly. If the increased pressure results from the presence of an intracranial mass such as a tumor or clot, the mass should be promptly removed. Such surgery restores ICP to normal more effectively than any other measure. However, the clinical situation is often complex with other causes of increased ICP at play such as hydrocephalus or cerebral edema. The main methods for ICP control (other than direct surgery) are:

1. *Ventricular drainage.* This can be maintained for 10 to 14 days before catheter change is recommended to reduce the risk of ventriculitis or meningitis. Antibiotic-coated catheters are now standard and keep the rate of infection low.

2. *Mannitol.* The usual dose is 0.25 g/kg IV q4–6h. It is given in small boluses, and an increase in serum osmolality of as little as 10 mOsm/mL can be enough to reduce cerebral edema significantly. Mannitol also improves perfusion by reducing blood viscosity. It is effective for 48 to 72 hours, but its use is not recommended beyond that time frame. In emergent situations, mannitol is the preferred agent because unlike hypertonic saline, mannitol can be administered through a peripheral IV line.

3. *Hypertonic saline.* This has been used increasingly in the past 10 years, and studies have shown that it is as effective as mannitol. It is available as concentrations of 2%, 3%, and 23.4%. Hypertonic saline at 2% to 3% can be used to slowly correct hyponatremia to levels >145 mEq/L which increases serum osmolality and draws edema away from brain tissue. Although in emergent situations both 2% and 3% saline can be administered via a peripheral IV line, some prefer that 3% saline be administered via a peripherally inserted central catheter (PICC) or 18-gauge large-bore IV line to prevent irritation of surrounding tissue. More concentrated (23.4%) hypertonic saline is administered as a 30-mL bolus in emergent situations to reduce edema. Unlike mannitol, however, it must be administered via a central line. It is also important not to correct serum sodium levels by more than 0.5 mEq/L/hr or more than 12 mEq/L/day to avoid central pontine myelinolysis, a phenomenon of acute demyelination of white matter tracts traversing the pons.

4. *Hyperventilation.* This requires intubation, and in a patient above the level of coma it also requires paralysis and sedation. Hyperventilation should be moderate with end-tidal pCO_2 lowered to 28 to 32 mm Hg. Reducing pCO_2 below that level will compromise cerebral blood flow and compound the ischemia already produced by increased ICP.

5. *Loop diuretics* (furosemide; Lasix). These are sometimes used as an adjunct to mannitol, but are not dependable when used alone for the reduction of ICP.

6. *Steroids.* Dexamethasone is given at a loading dose of 10 mg IV followed by 4 to 8 mg q6h. It should be tapered over 7 to 10 days once its therapeutic effect has been achieved. Other steroids (hydrocortisone or methylprednisolone) are not used, as they are insufficiently potent or have inconsistent metabolism that impairs their effectiveness.

7. *Barbiturate coma.* Short-acting barbiturates to induce coma are a last resort in managing increased ICP. These agents reduce cerebral metabolism and cerebral blood flow; the most commonly used is thiopental

(loading dose, 3 to 10 mg/kg IV over 10 minutes; maintenance dose, 1 to 2 mg/kg/hr). Serum levels are checked and should be maintained at 3 to 4 mg/L. Patients in barbiturate coma need intensive monitoring and may require vasopressors to counteract arterial hypotension. Spectral EEG monitoring confirms burst suppression.

8. *Normothermia.* It is important to maintain normothermia in a critically ill patient who is intubated. While cooling blankets can counter fevers in some patients, these blankets may also cause shivering which contributes to elevated ICP. Shivering increases energy expenditure by skeletal muscles and brain tissue oxygen demand/metabolism. Therefore, it is critical to prevent shivering by using a forced-air warming system such as a Bair Hugger and/or magnesium sulfate infusion, or (in intubated patients) by applying neuromuscular blockade, dexmedetomidine (Precedex), or propofol.

Seizures

Seizures in the tumor patient are caused by cortical irritation provoked by brain tumor (either primary or metastatic), intracranial bleeding (usually subdural), electrolyte abnormality (in sodium, calcium, or magnesium), infections such as meningitis or encephalitis, or head trauma after a fall. As they are most easily corrected, metabolic causes should always be eliminated, but radiologic investigation is usually needed as well. Seizures should be controlled because they are distressing to the patient and their family, but also because the hypermetabolic effects of active epilepsy can impair function in an already compromised brain around a tumor, or in a zone of cerebral edema. Seizures can be focal or general, simple or complex, and occur with or without loss of contact with surroundings. A seizure can also be "subclinical," a situation in which no externally visible seizure activity is present but abnormal electrical activity within the brain is causing a neurologic deficit such as obtundation, speech arrest, or focal weakness. A patient with a chronic seizure disorder need not be scanned every time a new seizure is noted. However, a patient with no history of seizures should undergo scanning by computed tomography (CT) or magnetic resonance imaging (MRI) to examine the brain for bleeding, edema, or increased ICP needing intervention. Subclinical seizures should be considered as a cause for any new deficits associated with stable imaging of the brain. The seizure itself can usually be suppressed by levetiracetam (Keppra) or the older drugs, phenytoin (Dilantin) or valproic acid (Depakote). Occasionally seizures will be refractory and will require more than one drug, particularly in patients with status epilepticus requiring intubation and intravenous barbiturates. The most common cause of new-onset seizure in a previously healthy adult is not tumor but stroke. Nevertheless, brain tumors yield seizures as a presenting symptom in 20% to 30% of cases. After surgery, the seizure tendency does not decrease for ≥2 weeks after an offending mass lesion has been resected. If a patient has had seizures prior to surgery and is on anticonvulsants to control them, we continue the drug therapy for 3 to 6 months after surgery before attempting a taper in those who have been seizure-free and shown no regrowth of tumor. After an uncomplicated craniotomy without prior history of seizure, we do not routinely use anticonvulsants after surgery. For those with complicated cases involving significant brain trauma in epileptogenic zones like the temporal lobe or motor cortex, anticonvulsant prophylaxis after surgery is used by surgeon preference.

Myelopathy

Myelopathy refers to the clinical syndrome caused by dysfunction of the spinal cord, but does not specify where in the spinal cord such dysfunction has arisen. Syndromes differ depending on the spinal level, as lesions in the cervical cord can produce weakness and sensory loss in all four limbs, whereas lumbar lesions produce such loss only in the legs because of their location well below the exit point of the nerves supplying the arms. The spinal cord also influences bladder and bowel function and, in the neck, it gives rise to the phrenic nerve (C3–5) controlling diaphragmatic excursion. The most common reason for myelopathy in an oncology practice is extrinsic compression of the spinal cord by a metastatic tumor within a vertebral body or pedicle immediately adjacent to the cord. Such patients commonly present with an ascending sensory loss that begins in the feet and can ascend no higher than the level of the lesion itself. In addition, they often show weakness more likely affecting the legs and impairing the ability to walk. They also can complain of bladder and sometimes bowel incontinence. The key to successful treatment of a compressive myelopathy is early intervention *before* loss of the ability to walk. A patient who has been bed-bound for more than 24 hours is unlikely to benefit from a decompressive operation. Indeed, the first symptom is often not a neurologic dysfunction at all, but back pain caused by compression of nerve roots or by local instability due to bony collapse or ligamentous disruption. Any patient with a history of cancer who presents with back pain should have an MRI of the symptomatic spinal region to rule out spinal involvement by tumor. Certainly, an aging population can contain patients with cancer who also have coincident degenerative disease of the spine with spondylosis, disc protrusion, and osteophyte formation causing a typical degenerative pain syndrome. However, it is never wise to assume the absence of neoplasm in a patient with a history of systemic cancer, and MRI will also help in diagnosing nontumor pathologies.

Radiologic Assessment

Imaging for tumors of the brain and spine has evolved significantly during the past 20 years and now depends heavily on computerized scans of various types to diagnose lesions, select which are appropriate for surgery, and provide data helpful in planning operative strategies.

Computed Tomography

CT is a vital component of oncologic diagnosis for sites in the chest, abdomen, and pelvis. However, its utility in diagnosing brain lesions has diminished somewhat with the advent of the more anatomically detailed images provided by MRI. When oncologists suspect intracranial tumor, they often order CT almost by reflex, but MRI will generally be needed whether the CT finding is positive or negative. As the cost differential is not great, the exposure to ionizing radiation is eliminated, and the sensitivity is greater, we recommend using MRI rather than CT as the first-line scanning modality for patients being screened for intracranial or spinal tumor. The advantages of MRI include the anatomical detail that it provides, the multiplanar capacity that permits three-dimensional visualization, the sensitive depiction of the extent of edema, and the ability of MRI to show subtle lesions through the hypersensitive FLAIR sequence usually included in such scans.

CT remains useful in limited areas. First, it is much quicker to obtain than an MRI, thus it should be used for any patient in whom urgent imaging is needed. In a postoperative patient in whom concern has arisen over the possibility of a clot in the resection cavity, CT is typically requested. Second, the scanner is more open and allows easier access to an unstable patient than the closed tube of an MRI, so CT is favored for very sick patients in the ICU for whom constant nursing access is necessary. Third, the depiction of bone is better on CT than MRI, thus a tumor of the spine, skull vault, or skull base usually requires a CT as part of the radiologic workup. It can also be used to detect calcification in tumor as a way of narrowing the differential diagnosis. Examples of this include meningiomas and craniopharyngiomas, both benign tumors that often calcify. Fourth, CT angiography has supplanted digital subtraction angiography as a mode of screening for intracranial aneurysm or other vascular malformations. Formal angiography is still required for patients with vascular lesions who require surgical or endovascular intervention, but CT angiography is an excellent way of deciding whether a patient with an intracerebral hematoma of the temporal lobe and a history of cancer has an aneurysm or a metastatic tumor as the inciting cause of the bleed. Finally, some patients with pacemakers, with metallic fragments in the brain or orbit from prior traumatic injury, or with ferromagnetic aneurysm clips placed before the early 1990s, may not be able to undergo MRI safely and thus a CT may be required.

In the spine, depiction of bony anatomy can be done with great precision by CT using reconstructed sagittal and coronal, as well as axial views. Three-dimensional reconstruction of the spine in patients with complex bony defects, particularly those who have had prior surgery, can be a very valuable tool in planning further surgery.

Magnetic Resonance Imaging

MRI is the most useful radiographic modality in neurosurgical oncology. Frequently used sequences for imaging tumors of the brain include T1-weighted spin-echo before and after injection of gadolinium contrast agent; T2-weighted spin-echo or fast-spin echo sequences; and FLAIR images. Fat suppression can be used as needed to enhance image clarity. Standard depiction of tumors occurs on T1 pre- and postcontrast sequences, with T2 sequences useful for showing edema, cyst, or tumor water content. FLAIR sequences bring out subtle abnormalities that can be missed on other less sensitive images. In addition, diffusion-weighted images show areas of diminished perfusion indicative of stroke, and diffusion tensor imaging can be used for mapping fiber tracts such as the corticospinal tract, arcuate fasciculus, inferior fronto-occipital fasciculus (IFOF), and frontal aslant tract, the localization of which can enhance safety during surgery. Functional MRI is now commonly used for patients in whom preoperative mapping of speech areas is desirable. Such patients include those with a tumor near Broca's or Wernicke's area, or the left-handed patient in whom localization of speech to the left hemisphere is not guaranteed. Motor mapping can also be done on functional imaging, but is less often requested because intraoperative methods of motor mapping are easy to apply and highly accurate.

MRI spectroscopy has been advocated as a method of distinguishing one tumor type from another by virtue of the varied metabolic spectra produced by tumors in vivo. This is a controversial area, and we do not routinely use spectroscopy for that purpose. Its main utility is in distinguishing tumor from posttreatment effect in patients who have undergone prior radiotherapy or chemotherapy. Even in that group, however, the sensitivity and specificity are imperfect and biopsy may be needed to make that distinction. The classic tumor signature is an increase in the choline/creatinine ratio (and decrease in N-acetyl aspartate [NAA]) over that of normal brain. This pattern is based on the principle that the choline metabolite increases during membrane turnover; thus, highly proliferative tumors have significantly higher levels of choline relative to nontumor tissue in the vicinity. On the other hand, NAA is a metabolite typically associated with normal neurons and axons. Consequently, a highly proliferative neoplasm such as a glioma will displace or destroy normal neurons and therefore suppress the NAA metabolic peak.

In the larger world of oncology, combining CT with positron emission tomography (PET) is commonly done for metastatic surveys. This is not particularly helpful for brain imaging because of the diffuse hypermetabolism exhibited by the brain on such images. However, PET/CT can detect metastatic deposits in the spine and pinpoint areas that should undergo MRI for anatomic delineation. In addition, such imaging is quite useful in assessing tumors of peripheral nerves as it can depict formerly benign tumors undergoing dedifferentiation to an "atypical" or intermediate state, and ultimately to full-blown malignancy, an absolute indication for surgical resection.

Primary Tumors of Central Nervous System

Brain

Primary brain tumors arise in most cases from neuroglial cells, and fall into an umbrella category, the gliomas. These make up 50% to 65% of intracranial tumors in most series. Their pathology, locations, and prognosis are diverse. Annually in the United States 20,000 new cases of malignant primary brain tumors are detected, and gliomas form >90% of these. The median age at diagnosis is the mid- to late 50s, but such tumors can occur in childhood and the incidence of the most malignant form (glioblastoma) increases in the elderly. Rare familial syndromes have been identified; for example, the Li–Fraumeni and Turcot syndromes link gliomas with other nonneural cancers, but most gliomas are sporadic and lack specific risk factors. Basic types are listed in Table 22.3.

Histologic Classification

Since the initial attempts at histologic classification of gliomas by Cushing and others in the 1920s and 1930s, the multiplicity of definitions has muddied the literature tremendously. Both three- and four-tiered systems have been suggested, but the current WHO classification contains four grades for astrocytomas. Grade I lesions, which include the subependymal giant cell astrocytomas and pilocytic astrocytomas, are uncommonly seen; grade II lesions are the classical "low-grade" astrocytomas. The uniformly invasive group of anaplastic astrocytomas (grade III) represents the first level of malignancy, and glioblastomas and gliosarcomas are classified in grade IV.

Molecular Classification

With the current and growing emphasis on genomic analysis, several molecular alterations can be used as distinguishing characteristics beyond the traditional grading schemes that rely on histology alone. This focus on molecular signature is driven by the significant impact molecular alterations (especially *IDH1* mutations) have been shown to have on survival. Therefore, it is important to know specific mutational status when counseling patients about their prognosis and options for treatment. In the sections below, we describe the histologic criteria and molecular signatures required to diagnose specific types of brain tumors.

Astrocytic Tumors

Pilocytic Astrocytomas These WHO grade I tumors commonly affect patients in the second decade of life and do not invade adjacent brain tissue, nor do they usually undergo malignant degeneration. The majority (two-thirds) occur in the cerebellum, 30% in the optic nerves, chiasm, and hypothalamus, and the rest in the cerebral hemispheres. The treatment for these is surgery, and complete removal is generally curative. Although some have advocated using radiotherapy and chemotherapy at recurrence, this methodology is controversial, and reoperation is often advocated in that circumstance. Such tumors in the cerebellum or cerebral hemisphere are typically resectable with minor or no morbidity. However, those termed "optic gliomas," typically seen in patients with neurofibromatosis type 1 (NF1), are much less amenable to surgery without compromise of vision. Typically, such patients are observed and followed conservatively, and treated with radiotherapy should they progress. From a molecular standpoint, pilocytic astrocytomas have been shown to harbor $BRAF^{V600E}$ mutation (9%) and/or KIAA1549-BRAF fusions (60% to 80%). Targeting these alterations remains an ongoing area of clinical investigation in pilocytic astrocytoma.

Familial Syndromes Predisposing to Gliomagenesis

	Gene	Chromosome	CNS Tumor	CNS Tumor Risk	Tumors Outside CNS	Systemic Tumor Risk
Li–Fraumeni syndrome	*TP53*	17p13.1	Astrocytoma Medulloblastoma Choroid plexus carcinoma	14%	Breast carcinoma Adrenal cortical carcinoma Soft tissue sarcoma	Men: 70%/Women: 100%
Neurofibromatosis type 1	*NF1*	17q11.2	Pilocytic astrocytoma Astrocytoma	10% 1%	Neurofibroma Malignant peripheral nerve sheath tumor Gastrointestinal stromal tumor Pheochromocytoma Leukemia	>97% 10% 15% 4% Rare
Nevoid basal cell carcinoma syndrome (Gorlin syndrome)	*PTCH1 SUFU*	9q22.3 10q24.3	Medulloblastoma	<2% (PTCH1) 30–40% (SUFU)		
Turcot syndrome type 1	*MLH1* *MSH2* *PMS2* *MSH6*	3p21.3 2p21 7p22.2 2p16	Astrocytoma	53%	Colorectal carcinoma Hematologic cancers	100%
Turcot syndrome type 2	*APC*	5q31	Medulloblastoma	<1%	Familial adenomatous polyposis	100%
Tuberous sclerosis	*TSC1 TSC2*	9p34 16p13.3	Subependymal giant cell astrocytoma	10–15%	Hamartomas (skin, retina, heart, lung, kidney)	>90%

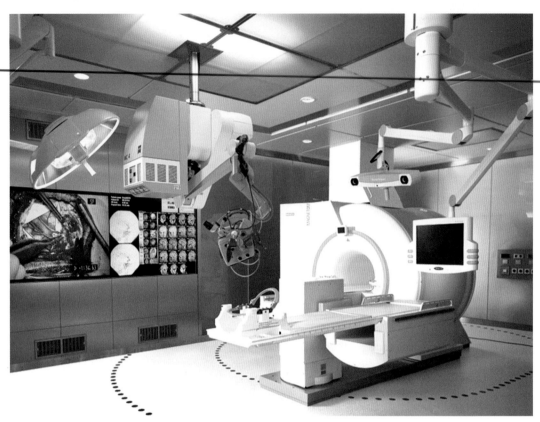

FIGURE 22.1 The intraoperative MRI is located within a magnetically shielded room with integrated components allowing efficiency of workflow. The patient lies on a bed outside the 5-Gauss line for surgery, then is covered to maintain sterility and rotated into the MRI scanner for imaging at intervals during the operation.

Low-Grade Astrocytomas The low-grade (grade II) astrocytomas make up 10% to 25% of gliomas in most series and are usually detected in the fourth or fifth decade life. Such tumors grow slowly and often present with seizures or are incidentally found. They do not show well on CT in many cases, and MRI is a more reliable modality for comparative imaging over time. Traditionally these tumors have been managed conservatively, but in the past decade a growing consensus has arisen in the literature over the desirability of resection prior to malignant transformation. The mean time from detection to such transformation is 8 years, at which point they become much more aggressive and have a significant likelihood of killing the patient. Because mitosis is so sparse in such tumors, chemotherapy and radiotherapy each have not been particularly effective in controlling them long term. However, a study by Buckner et al. (2016) showed that patients receiving both modalities survive longer than do those receiving radiotherapy alone; debate continues over which chemotherapy is most appropriate in this population. Patients with such tumors may be reluctant to undergo surgical resection because of their lack of symptoms, but we do advocate early removal to as complete a degree as possible given local functional anatomy. Enhancing completeness of resection in these relatively subtle lesions is facilitated greatly by intraoperative MRI (Fig. 22.1). We achieve a significant improvement in radiographically complete resection with such technology relative to historical controls, and a concomitant increase in survival.

Anaplastic Astrocytoma These tumors occur in a slightly older age group (usually the fifth or sixth decade of life) either de novo or as a result of malignant degeneration within a low-grade astrocytoma. They form 10% to 15% of the gliomas and commonly present in the cerebral hemispheres with seizures and focal neurologic deficits. These tumors, unlike the low-grade tumors, frequently show contrast enhancement on MRI and have more surrounding edema, mass effect, and rapidity of growth. Age and preoperative functional status are prognostic, but the goal of treatment is not to cure but to extend life and maintain function. Current standard treatment consists of surgical resection followed by radiotherapy and then chemotherapy with TMZ. A variety of chemotherapy regimens have been tried in the past, but most have been unsuccessful in prolonging life by more than a few months. Most of these tumors will recur eventually as glioblastomas. The median survival is

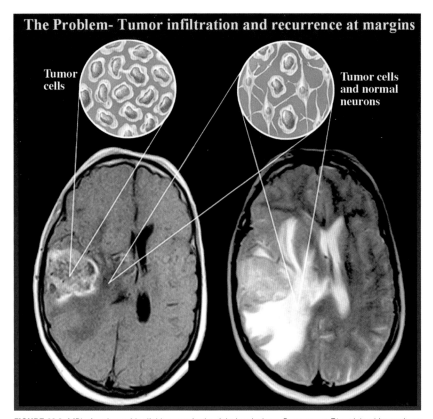

FIGURE 22.2 MRI of patient with glioblastoma in the right hemisphere. Postcontrast T1-weighted image is on the left side of the panel, and T2-weighted image shows edema on the right. Even when gross total removal of contrast-enhancing portions is achieved, the margins remain with infiltrating tumor cells that cannot be controlled by surgery.

3 years with about 20% surviving 5 years. From a molecular standpoint, these tumors are typically *IDH1* mutant and also possess an *ATRX* mutation, both of which confer a more favorable prognosis. In fact, astrocytoma grading is no longer histologically driven as *CDKN2A/B* homozygous deletion in an *IDH1* mutant astrocytoma is automatically assigned as a WHO grade 4 diffuse astrocytoma, even in the absence of microvascular proliferation or necrosis.

Glioblastoma   This is the most common intrinsic brain tumor and forms half of gliomas in most series. It usually occurs in the sixth or seventh decade, but can arise at any age. The common location is the cerebral hemisphere with occasional tumors in the corpus callosum giving rise to the classic "butterfly glioma" pattern that extends into both hemispheres from its central point of origin. Personality change and headache are common, but seizures are only sometimes seen. Glioblastoma is much less common in the posterior fossa and very rare in the spinal cord.

Such tumors have a heterogeneous pattern of enhancement with typically a centrally necrotic area that is relatively hypointense on MRI (Fig. 22.2). The edges are indistinct and such tumors may cross the midline. They have significant perilesional edema in many instances. The histology is characterized by vascular proliferation, frequent mitotic figures, hypercellularity, and necrosis, the last of which is the hallmark of these tumors.

Glioblastomas are the most aggressive brain tumors. Their treatment should be aggressive as well, and include a meaningful attempt at radical surgical resection followed by whole-brain radiotherapy and chemotherapy in patients able to tolerate it. Lacroix et al. showed at M D Anderson Cancer Center (MDACC) that the greatest positive influence on survival occurs after resection of ≥98% of the contrast-enhancing portion of the lesion. However, increasing benefit was seen at all percentages of resection above 90%. Thus, if resection is to be done, it makes little sense to remove less than 90% of these tumors, and the ideal approach is complete radiographic removal. Since these tumors have an infiltrating edge and have been shown through biopsy of theoretically unaffected brain to have infiltrating cells as far as 4 cm from the radiographic edge of the tumor, the "gross total" resection is by no means total. For this reason, adjunctive therapies must be used to make a more meaningful impact on this disease. In the realm of chemotherapy, the most studied drugs are the nitrosoureas (BCNU and its analog CCNU) which give a 10% increase in 18-month survival and little change in median survival. With TMZ and newer multidrug combinations, the median survival in our institution is 21 months, and possibly longer for patients harboring tumors with MGMT promoter hypermethylation, an epigenetic state that makes tumors more sensitive to TMZ. This is significantly better than the 9 to 12 months of survival quoted in most textbooks, but still far too short for the patient struck by this tumor in the peak of life, as many are.

Innovative approaches include biologically based therapies such as immunotherapy and gene therapy. Weller et al. reported that glioblastomas positive for the EGF receptor variant III (EGFRvIII, found in 35% to 40% of glioblastomas) treated with rindopepimut, a conjugated EGFRvIII-specific peptide (also known as CDX-110 and PEPvIII), show significant prolongation of survival to 20 months. Nonetheless, all tumors eventually recurred, possibly from non-EGFRvIII expressing clonal expansion. Lang et al. conducted a phase 1 study at MDACC using the Delta 24 oncolytic virus, given through intraparenchymal injection of the tumor or of the edges of its resection cavity, and showed safety and clinical efficacy against recurrent glioblastoma. Kunwar et al. used convection-enhanced delivery to infuse IL-13-PE38QQR (IL-13 linked to pseudomonas exotoxin) into the brain's interstitial space in patients with glioblastoma, but without significant added benefit. Given that this approach combined a new mode of delivery with a new therapeutic agent, it is hard to tell whether the agent would be effective if delivered by other means, or whether the mode of delivery would work with a differently targeted agent.

The 5-year survival for glioblastoma is <15% and recurrence occurs within 2 to 3 cm of the original resection margin in 80% of patients. The remaining patients also show recurrence, but farther afield within the brain, and even in the opposite hemisphere. Metastasis to extraneural sites is vanishingly rare. Occasional patients are seen with gliomatosis, that is, a multifocal involvement of more than one lobe of the brain, or with leptomeningeal dissemination. Because many patients with systemic cancer are elderly, and glioblastoma tends to be a disease of older patients, it is not infrequent to find a glioblastoma arising in a patient being treated for a second cancer, so it is important for general oncologists to recognize its manifestations, implications, and modes of therapy.

The most recent WHO CNS tumor classification now reserves the diagnosis of glioblastoma WHO grade 4 for an astrocytoma that is *IDH1* wild-type and also possesses either an EGFR alteration or *TERT* promoter mutation, and either chromosome 7 gain or chromosome 10 loss. This specific designation is now applied because *IDH1* wild-type astrocytomas are different clinically from *IDH1* mutant astrocytomas, with the *IDH1* mutation associated with a better prognosis. *IDH1* mutant astrocytomas with *CDKN2A/B* alterations, however, have a very poor prognosis mirroring that of *IDH1* wild-type glioblastoma. These *IDH1* mutant astrocytomas with *CDKN2A/B* alterations are not called "glioblastoma" but instead are now called diffuse astrocytoma WHO grade 4.

Oligodendrogliomas

These tumors form 10% to 15% of gliomas and typically involve the cerebral hemispheres, with involvement of the thalamus, brainstem, and cerebellum much less likely. They present in the fifth or sixth decade, frequently with seizures although headache and focal deficit may also occur. They are more likely to be calcified than are the astrocytomas, indicative of their slower pace of growth. The majority present as grade II lesions, but the occasional anaplastic tumor arises de novo as a grade 3 lesion. The classic histologic finding is a perinuclear halo known as a "fried egg" appearance which is caused by shrinkage of the cellular components during exposure to formalin.

Cairncross et al. have shown that chromosomal analysis further differentiates a subgroup of oligodendrogliomas forming 60% to 70% of the whole, with deletions of chromosome 1p, 19q, or both. Those tumors with such deletions are more sensitive to chemotherapy (prototypically, procarbazine, CCNU, and vincristine), radiotherapy, or both. Median survival is affected by the presence or absence of these chromosomal alterations: it is 3 to 5 years for patients with tumors without loss of heterozygosity, and 10 to 12 years for those with loss of heterozygosity. Therapy for oligodendrogliomas mirrors that for astrocytomas, with surgery followed by radiotherapy and chemotherapy used in most cases. Chemotherapy is overall more effective in oligodendrogliomas than astrocytomas. Based on the most recent WHO CNS classification, chromosomal 1p/19q codeletion is now required for the diagnosis of oligodendroglioma. In the past, a mixed oligo-astrocytic was recognized, but the WHO CNS classification no longer includes this mixed tumor as a unique category. Most oligodendrogliomas are *IDH1* mutant, and carry a more favorable prognosis relative to *IDH1* wild-type tumors. Furthermore, *IDH1* mutant oligodendrogliomas have a more favorable prognosis relative to *IDH1* mutant astrocytomas, indicating that an astrocytic lineage/histology confers aggressive behavior. Molecular features also distinguish oligodendrogliomas from tumors of astrocytic lineage as 1p/19q codeletion in oligodendrogliomas is mutually exclusive from the ATRX mutations typically found in astrocytomas. Such molecular distinctions will be increasingly important in personalizing therapeutic choices of the drugs most likely to work in the tumors most likely to respond.

Metastatic Brain Tumors

Between 20% and 40% of patients with systemic cancer develop brain metastasis. Such tumors can be extra-axial (involving the dura and subdural space, or leptomeninges and subarachnoid space), but usually occur within the brain parenchyma. MRI confirms that two-thirds of such patients have more than one metastasis in the brain, and that the classic solitary metastasis is uncommon. As with other tumor types, available methods for treating brain metastases include surgery, focused or diffuse irradiation, or chemotherapy.

The true incidence of brain metastasis is unknown. CT underrepresents the number of metastases in many patients and is insufficiently sensitive to use as a screening study. MRI is the imaging modality of choice as it can show not only subtle lesions but also leptomeningeal disease, the presence of which greatly impacts prognosis and mode of treatment. Brain metastases are the most common intracranial tumors in adults. Their incidence has risen because of increased detection by MRI and because of longer survival from more effective systemic therapies. The biology and thus the nuances of surgical treatment differ among the various histologies, so brain metastasis cannot be considered as a single disease. Only 1% to 2% of ovarian and prostate cancers spread to the brain, but at least half of melanomas do so, when other systemic metastases are present. The most common histologic type of brain metastasis is carcinoma of the lung (40% to 60% of large clinical series), followed by those derived from breast cancers (15% to 20%) and melanoma (10% to 20%). Colorectal and renal cell carcinomas account for 5% to 10% each. These five sources yield most cerebral metastases. Melanoma has the highest propensity to spread to the brain but is less represented than lung cancer because of the much greater incidence of the latter in the general population. In children with systemic cancer, the incidence of intracerebral metastasis is <5% and arises mainly from neuroblastoma, Wilms tumor, and sarcoma (especially rhabdomyosarcoma).

Two-thirds of patients with brain metastasis present with neurologic decline, usually focal deficits or impairment of cognitive function. Many asymptomatic patients actually have disordered cognition unrecognized by external observers. Increase in ICP through edema or blockage of CSF pathways can combine with local ischemia to give localized cerebral dysfunction. In 20% to 30% of patients seizures occur, more often in those with multiple metastases. Two histologies are particularly prone to intratumoral bleeding: melanoma and choriocarcinoma in which the bleeding rates are 45% and 95%, respectively. On MRI a large amount of edema around a recent hematoma (<6 hours old) suggests but does not confirm a tumor beneath the hematoma. Metastases can produce cysts, especially carcinomas of the breast and adenocarcinomas of the lung, but other histologies can also provoke them.

Radiology

MRI is the most sensitive test, and thus should be used for surveillance whenever possible. Most metastases are hypo- to isointense on T1-weighted images and hyperintense on T2-weighted images. Hemorrhage may be suggested by the presence of a hemosiderin ring hypointense on T2-weighted images along the tumor margin, or by hyperintensity on precontrast T1-weighted images. Some small tumors may fail to enhance due to relative preservation of the BBB, but can still be detected on FLAIR sequences.

These tumors are classically located at the junction between gray and white matter. However, they can grow anywhere in the brain. As radiologic diagnosis is sometimes inexact, presumed metastases meeting the above criteria may turn out to be other tumor types when resected. Patchell et al. (1990) reported that 11% of patients thought to have a single brain metastasis actually had other pathology. Multiple brain lesions in patients without a history of cancer represent metastasis in only 15% of cases. Spinal tap is the only other diagnostic test sometimes helpful in workup of such patients, and can unmask the occasional case of cysticercosis misdiagnosed as metastasis. If cytologic analysis is positive for malignant cells in CSF, the patient has leptomeningeal dissemination of tumor and may benefit from intrathecal instillation of chemotherapy. This is usually done through an Ommaya reservoir, a silastic chamber placed beneath the scalp in the frontal area with a ventriculostomy tube leading into the frontal horn of the lateral ventricle. As the ventricles are the site of origin for CSF, this places the drug at the beginning point of the pathways of CSF flow, which are thus able to carry it widely through the subarachnoid space.

Life expectancy of patients with brain metastasis depends more on the status of their systemic disease than the status of their brain metastasis (which can usually be controlled); however, patients with leptomeningeal dissemination of tumor have the worst prognosis with a median survival of 3 months. They are at risk for hydrocephalus and survival can be prolonged by shunting, but their prognosis remains poor even with aggressive multimodality therapy including intrathecal chemotherapy and radiotherapy.

Unknown Primary Tumors

One-third of patients with symptomatic brain metastases have no systemic cancer previously diagnosed. Such patients should undergo metastatic workup to screen the most likely primary sites (lung, breast, kidney, colon, and skin). Lung cancer is the culprit in 70% of these patients. Thus, chest x-ray, mammography (in women), and a skin survey should be obtained. CT of the chest, abdomen, and pelvis, or PET-CT, should also be done. In the absence of any accessible extracranial tumor, stereotactic biopsy or (more often) open resection of the cerebral tumor should be done to confirm diagnosis prior to treatment. The source of an unknown primary brain metastasis remains occult in 15% of patients despite extensive investigation.

Treatment

The management of brain metastasis is both complex and controversial. It includes surgery, stereotactic radiotherapy, whole-brain radiotherapy, and chemotherapy. Patients with edema on MRI receive steroids to suppress it. Clinical improvement is generally noted within 12 hours of beginning steroid therapy in 70% to 80% of cases, but the peak effect may be delayed for up to a week. After surgery a steroid taper is instituted over 1 to 2 weeks. We reserve anticonvulsants for patients with a known seizure history.

Single Brain Metastasis

The median survival for patients without treatment is 6 weeks. Adding steroids improves this to 3 months, and external beam (whole-brain) radiotherapy improves survival to 4 to 6 months. Randomized clinical trials comparing surgery + radiotherapy with radiotherapy alone suggest a significant benefit from surgery on overall survival and quality of life (Table 22.4). If systemic disease is not controlled, however, the benefits of controlling brain metastasis are eroded.

The variables to be considered when selecting patients with a single metastasis for surgery are: (1) the overall clinical status, (2) the surgical accessibility of the tumor, (3) its size, and (4) its radiosensitivity. Patients with absent or controlled systemic disease and no leptomeningeal dissemination of tumor derive the most significant benefit from the removal of brain metastasis. Obviously distinguishing "controlled" from "uncontrolled" systemic disease can be somewhat arbitrary. We usually look for expected survival of ≥4 months in patients being considered for surgery, while advanced age, poor medical condition, and Karnofsky Performance Scale (KPS) <70 argue against surgery.

Ultimately brain metastasis is a multifocal or even a diffuse process. Focal treatments such as surgery or radiosurgery can suppress the disease, but eliminating it may require whole-brain irradiation to treat microscopic foci unseen on MRI as well as small tumor fragments left at sites of resection. However, standard

TABLE 22.4	Randomized Trials Comparing (Surgery + Postop Radiotherapy) Versus (Radiotherapy Alone)		
	Patchell et al. (1990)	**Vecht et al. (1993)**	**Mintz et al. (1996)**
No. of patients	48	63	84
Inclusion criteria	>17 years old	>17 years old	<80 years old
	Single lesion	Single lesion	Single lesion
	KPS >60	Functional level at least 2	KPS >40
	Lesion surgically accessible	Life expectancy >6 months	Lesion surgically accessible
	No LMD	No LMD	No LMD
	Very radiosensitive tumor excluded	No SCLC or lymphoma	No SCLC, lymphoma, or non-melanoma skin cancer
Disseminated cancer	38%	32%	45%
Imaging	MRI	CT	CT
Histologic proof in radiotherapy group	Yes	No	Occasional
Radiotherapy regimen	36 Gy/12 fractions	40 Gy/20 fractions (b.i.d.)	30 Gy/10 fractions
Overall survival (weeks)	Surgery better	Surgery better	No difference
Surgery	40	40	24
Radiotherapy	15	24	24

LMD, leptomeningeal disease; SCLC, small cell carcinoma of lung; CT, computed tomography; MRI, magnetic resonance imaging; KPS, Karnofsky performance scale.

radiotherapy is less effective than radiosurgery for radiographically evident tumors because the fractional dose in the former must be lowered to prevent toxicity to normal brain. Standard whole-brain radiotherapy uses 10 fractions of 3 Gy each for a total dose of 30 Gy. Radiosurgery applies a single fraction of 15 to 18 Gy with highly conformal dosimetry at each target site. Given the delayed cognitive dysfunction associated with WBRT, however, SRS is now favored even for patients with 10 to 15 lesions with a cumulative tumor volume <15 cm³.

Surgery Versus Radiosurgery: The Conundrum

The basic dilemma for most patients with brain metastasis is whether to treat with surgery or use focused methods of stereotactic irradiation to target the lesion(s) (Fig. 22.3). Attempts at randomized trials have not been wholly successful due to the difficulty of convincing patients to enroll. Many patients have a bias favoring stereotactic radiosurgery (SRS) as it has the benefit of avoiding a surgical incision, anesthesia, and a hospital stay of several days with recovery over several weeks. Radiosurgery procedures are done in a single day and require little to no posttreatment recovery. They do require placement of a head frame with resulting moderate discomfort, but most patients tolerate this well; in some, frameless stereotactic irradiation is now done when less eloquent locations permit less tightly conformal targeting of the metastases they contain. Retrospective comparison implies a similar outcome between surgery and stereotactic irradiation but is unreliable because of selection bias. Prospective comparison has suggested that resection yields lower rates of local recurrence than does radiosurgery, but their relative effects on survival are less clear. Advantages and disadvantages of radiosurgery are shown in Table 22.5. At MDACC we now treat five patients with radiosurgery for each one treated surgically.

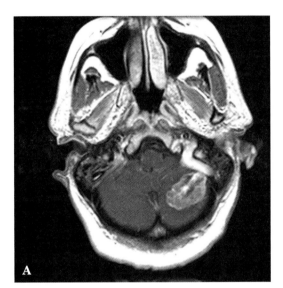

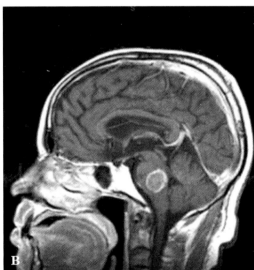

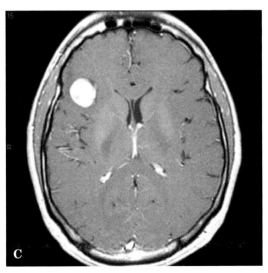

FIGURE 22.3 A: MRI showing metastasis from carcinoma of colon in left cerebellar hemisphere. This patient should have surgery, because the lesion's size puts it slightly above the 3 cm limit for stereotactic radiosurgery, and its location in the posterior fossa means that brainstem should be protected from the possibility of edema postirradiation. **B:** This metastatic carcinoma of unknown primary sits within the brainstem, a site that is unsafe for surgery. It should be treated with stereotactic radiosurgery. **C:** This small metastasis from renal cell carcinoma sits in the right frontal lobe. This area is safe for both surgery and radiosurgery, and this patient can be assigned either treatment, with little advantage to be gained from choosing one over the other.

TABLE 22.5	Advantages Versus Disadvantages of Stereotactic Radiosurgery

Advantages
  No incision
  Treats surgically inaccessible lesions
  More easily tolerated by physiologically compromised patient
  Short hospital stay (usually 1 day)
Disadvantages
  Poor targeting for tumors >3 cm in diameter
  Tumor persists on scans, so must be followed to prove success
  No tissue diagnosis
  Persistent edema or radionecrosis may require surgical removal of tumor
  Cannot be used on targets within 5 mm of optic nerve/chiasm/tract without significant dose modification

Drawbacks to radiosurgery remain. Even when local control of a tumor is achieved, patients with significant peritumoral edema may remain steroid-dependent for 3 months or even longer. Many tumors show temporary mild enlargement and intensification of enhancement during the first 1 to 2 months after radiosurgery. Persistence of edema, development of necrosis exerting mass effect, or frank tumor growth after radiosurgery imply treatment failure, and are all indications for resection. With both surgery and radiosurgery, local rates of control of 85% to 95% are achieved, which are similar for various histologies; and median survivals range from 8 to 13 months depending on histology. The so-called "radioresistant" tumors such as melanoma, renal cell carcinoma, and soft tissue sarcomas do respond to radiosurgery because of the high doses used, but local rates of control are still lower than in carcinomas of the lung and breast.

Recent comparisons of patients operated by en bloc resection versus piecemeal removal have shown that en bloc resection yields better local control and a lower rate of subsequent leptomeningeal dissemination. Clearly surgical technique is important in metastasis removal. Tumors that are soft and friable, necrotic, cystic, or hemorrhagic are particularly difficult to remove cleanly, and in such cases strong consideration should be given to subsequent adjuvant radiotherapy either as a stereotactic boost to the operative cavity or by whole-brain mode.

The morbidity after radiosurgery is comparable to that seen after surgery. In each the local recurrence rate is 5% to 15%. Hemorrhage and seizures can occur after either. Worsening of cerebral edema is rare after resection of a metastasis; most postsurgical patients improve neurologically and can stop steroids within 1 to 2 weeks. Steroid tapers tend to take longer after radiosurgery, and flaring of cerebral edema due to pseudoprogression or postirradiation necrosis occurs in 2% to 3% of targeted tumors. The 30-day postoperative mortality is 2% to 3% in major centers with an overall morbidity of 10% to 15%.

We recommend surgery to patients with a single, accessible metastasis causing marked mass effect and neurologic decline. When systemic disease is controlled the brain metastasis can usually be removed without inciting or worsening neurologic deficits, and surgery is a good option. However, locations in deep portions of the brain or in/near eloquent areas may shift the balance in favor of radiosurgery. Very large tumors respond best to surgery. Radiosurgery is the preferred treatment for tumors <2.5 cm in diameter, especially in patients whose age or medical condition renders them imperfect candidates for surgery or whose tumors are located in areas of relatively higher surgical risk.

Patient preference is a major driving factor in making the choice between surgery and radiosurgery. The perception of radiosurgery as noninvasive often trumps the therapeutic benefits of surgery in the minds of patients and physicians alike.

Radiotherapy After Surgery
Whole-brain irradiation is often given after surgical resection of brain metastases to reduce local recurrence and eliminate occult micrometastases. The conventional dosing scheme is 30 Gy/10 fractions. Such smaller fraction sizes give a decreased risk of neurotoxicity, but this regimen does not eliminate the long-term cognitive effects of irradiating the entire brain. Given the longer survivals now achieved by multimodality or personalized treatment regimens for various cancers with a propensity for brain metastasis, such delayed toxicity (which usually takes at least 18 months to develop) has been seen more often recently, and is very difficult to treat.

Patchell et al. (1998) described a randomized trial assigning surgical patients to postoperative observation versus radiotherapy. The study was limited to patients with a single, completely resected brain metastasis, and the radiotherapy consisted of 50.4 Gy in 28 fractions, a significantly longer course of treatment than is given in most centers to patients with brain metastasis. This regimen lowered the local rate of recurrence from 46%

to 10% and the appearance of brain metastasis at new sites from 37% to 14%. Differences in overall survival and functionally independent survival were not statistically significant. This study is flawed in that a local recurrence rate of 46% is higher than that expected with surgery alone, thus conclusions about the efficacy of whole-brain irradiation in controlling local recurrence are muddied. It does appear to reduce formation of new brain metastases, which suggests that micrometastases are indeed present in many patients.

In the past, whole-brain radiotherapy (WBRT) after surgical removal was considered standard, in part because of the perceived need to eliminate such putative micrometastases. Brown et al. compared the efficacy and safety of WBRT versus SRS after surgery for brain metastasis. Although their trial found that both were clinically equivalent at preventing local recurrence, WBRT was associated with higher rates of cognitive dysfunction relative to SRS. As a prospective clinical trial comparing surgery alone to surgery with adjuvant SRS showed that the combination was better at preventing local recurrence, most neurosurgeons now favor this latter approach for managing up to three resectable brain metastases. The question of whether neoadjuvant SRS confers different outcomes from adjuvant SRS remains unresolved and is the basis of an ongoing prospective clinical trial here at MDACC.

Multiple Metastases

A nihilistic attitude is maintained by many neurosurgeons toward patients with multiple brain metastases. However, studies from our institution have shown through retrospective and case-control analysis that multiple surgical resections via one or more simultaneous craniotomies are both safe and effective. In the case-control study by Bindal et al., survival of patients undergoing complete resection of up to three metastases was significantly better than that of patients in whom one or more tumors were left unresected; and it was similar to survival after removal of a single metastasis, without increase in morbidity or mortality. Surgery should definitely be considered for a single, dominant, surgically accessible metastatic tumor causing mass effect and neurologic compromise, regardless of the presence of smaller and less dangerous tumors elsewhere in the brain. When a cluster of tumors can be removed through a single craniotomy, this too may be beneficial in preserving neurologic function. In many large centers (including ours) local therapy (with or without subsequent whole-brain irradiation) is offered for multiple metastases in patients with controlled systemic disease, KPS >70, and life expectancy of at least 3 to 4 months. Argument continues over the ideal cut-off number for brain metastases above which focal therapy should not be offered. In one typical clinical scenario, lesions >2.5 cm in diameter are resected and the remainder, especially those that are surgically inaccessible, are treated with radiosurgery. When all tumors are <3 cm in diameter, focal therapy should be offered for all tumors, since treating some but not others yields little benefit.

Given the association of WBRT and cognitive dysfunction, several studies have assessed the efficacy of SRS for treating up to 10 to 15 lesions (<15 cc^3 total volume) within the brain and found that it is just as effective at preventing local recurrence without the cognitive dysfunction associated with WBRT. Therefore, for many patients with 10 lesions (still with <15 cc^3 total volume), it is conceivable that each of those lesions could receive SRS with similar outcome to WBRT. AT MDACC, we currently follow that policy of treating up to 10 separate brain metastases with SRS in order to minimize the negative cognitive impact of WBRT without jeopardizing positive outcomes for survival and maintenance of neurologic function.

Chemotherapy

Chemotherapy has not been very successful in controlling cerebral metastases. The BBB provides a pharmacologic sanctuary for metastatic lesions. Occasional responses by chemosensitive solid tumors such as breast cancer or nonseminomatous germ cell tumors of the testis belie the sturdiness of the barrier, and 10% of melanoma brain metastases will respond to TMZ given systemically. New targeted agents given systemically also yield imperfect control of brain metastases, but some produce dramatic shrinkage of these lesions. Some targeted agents (such as osimertinib for adenocarcinoma of lung with specific EGF receptor mutations), or immune checkpoint inhibitors (such as nivolumab and ipilimumab) for melanoma have yielded better control of brain metastases than has traditional cytotoxic chemotherapy. Because steroids reduce the efficacy of checkpoint inhibitors, that category of immune activators is best reserved for patients with small, asymptomatic tumors provoking little or no brain edema. In general, however, chemotherapy for brain metastasis gives little improvement in survival or quality of life, and is usually a last resort after other therapies have failed.

Small Cell Carcinoma: A Special Case

Randomized prospective trials have shown that prophylactic whole-brain radiotherapy reduces the incidence of brain metastasis in patients with small cell carcinoma of the lung, a histology exquisitely sensitive to irradiation. Enthusiasm for this technique is tempered by concern over its effects on cognitive function in patients who survive longer than a year. In addition, radiation necrosis can occur idiosyncratically beyond 9 months from radiation delivery. Neurologic toxicity can be limited by keeping fractions small and by withholding concurrent chemotherapy. The current consensus holds that prophylactic whole-brain irradiation confers a survival advantage of 5% at 3 years and a reduction in the incidence of brain metastasis by 25%, and is thus considered standard treatment for patients with this disease who are in complete remission after initial treatment. The situation for patients who have not achieved complete remission is less clear.

Surgical Technique for Brain Metastasis
Ideally resection is done en bloc when removal of a circumferential 5-mm margin of brain is not limited by nearby functional areas. When it is so limited, or when tumors are friable or cystic, a careful piecemeal technique must be used. When intratumoral hemorrhage eliminates the en bloc option, the blood should be carefully drained from the tumor pocket and not allowed to spill and produce seeding that leads to early recurrence. In addition, the wall of any associated cyst should be excised along with the tumor. The more friable tumors (melanoma, nonseminomatous germ cell tumors, and some lung cancers) should be isolated with cottonoids prior to resection to avoid tumor escape into the subdural space.

Because the risk of local recurrence after resection ranges from 10% to 30%, in 2017 we completed a randomized trial comparing surgery alone with surgery followed by radiosurgery to the margins of the operative cavity. That study showed a significant benefit to using adjuvant radiosurgery, so it has become standard practice at MDACC (when cavity size permits).

General Principles of Intracranial Surgery
In the majority of cases the goal of surgery is resection, either to the maximum possible degree or to a more limited degree for the purposes of decompression and open biopsy. When tumors present in locations preventing safe resection, or the use of prior therapy has raised the possibility of the lesion's representing treatment effect rather than tumor, stereotactic biopsy may be chosen over open resection.

Stereotactic biopsy involves the placement of a biopsy needle under image guidance into a radiologically specified target within a brain lesion. This can be done using a frame-based system or with frameless technology. The latter is now used for almost all cases. A suction-aspiration method is used that pulls small portions of the lesion into the side window at the needle tip, where they are trapped in an inner sleeve that is removed to extract the specimen. Such biopsy is therefore not useful for achieving meaningful resection; if resection is the goal, a craniotomy should be done instead.

To enable frameless stereotactic biopsy, either of two methods can be employed. In one, small fiducial markers are placed on the surface of the patient's scalp at multiple points. A scan (usually an MRI) is then performed prior to surgery, and the patient comes to the operating room with the markers still in place. The patient is registered to the system by localizing each of the external markers with a reflective wand whose position is determined by the workstation through an infrared detector. This process registers the patient's head into the three-dimensional space predicted by the scan; similar infrared detection is then used on the biopsy needle itself, which effectively becomes the localizing probe. Frameless systems are subject to slightly more error than frame-based systems, and thus should not be chosen for brainstem biopsies, but their accuracy is quite sufficient for biopsy in supratentorial locations.

It is important to recognize that the heterogeneity of gliomas may lead to sampling error if biopsy is not taken from several points within the lesion. The main risk of stereotactic biopsy is the induction of bleeding at the biopsy site. Most such hematomas are clinically insignificant, but in 1% of patients a craniotomy must be done to relieve pressure from an expanding clot.

The advantage of surgical resection is that it is more likely to overcome the intratumoral heterogeneity (and thus give a more accurate pathologic diagnosis) and of course, it does achieve physical removal of tumor with elimination of mass effect, reduction of ICP, and improvement in neurologic impairment. Intraoperative mapping of cortical function allows the resection of tumors even when located in or near so-called "eloquent" areas, that is, those containing important functions such as speech or motor control. It is our routine practice to perform cortical mapping in any patient whose tumor is suspected by radiographic criteria of being within 2 cm of the motor strip, Broca's area, or Wernicke's area.

In patients in whom tumor is intimately involved with speech areas, we perform craniotomy awake with anesthesia induced through a laryngeal mask airway during the opening and closing phases of the operation. The anesthesiologist removes the airway (and fully awakens the patient) for the core portion of the procedure when speech mapping and then tumor resection are performed. This is made possible by an extensive scalp block placed after the patient is asleep and lasting for a number of hours beyond completion of the procedure. Speech mapping is done in areas near tumor suggested by preoperative functional MRI as containing speech function (Fig. 22.4). Mapping proceeds as the surgeon applies a low-voltage electrical

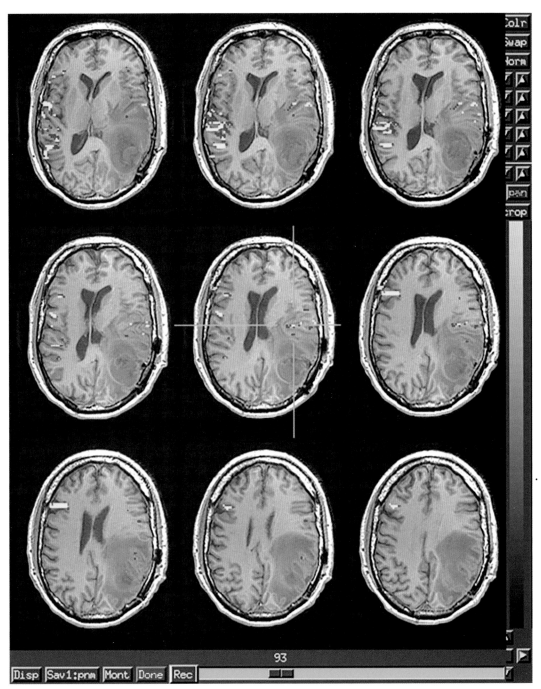

FIGURE 22.4 Functional MRI (fMRI) acquired before surgery and imported into BrainLab neuronavigational workstation. It shows a glioblastoma in the left posterior temporal area with peritumoral edema. The fMRI is obtained while the patient speaks and listens to recorded sentences in a standardized way that follows established paradigms for expressive and receptive speech. The red and yellow pixels anterior to the tumor were acquired during such speech testing, and indicate foci of increased blood flow which correlate with increased neuronal activity. In this way, the patient's cortical speech areas (both Broca's and Wernicke's area) can be mapped noninvasively. In this patient, the more pronounced cluster of foci of increased blood flow suggests that the tumor began as a low-grade astrocytoma and that, during its long period of slow growth prior to transformation, receptive speech switched from the left to the right hemisphere. Such remodeling is possible due to brain plasticity; in this patient, once intraoperative speech mapping done while he is awake confirms the accuracy of the cortical localization predicted by the fMRI, the tumor can be removed without injury to speech function because of such plasticity.

stimulus to the cortical surface at sites being tested while the patient carries on a conversation or names objects shown on cards. Interruption of speech by the electrical stimulus denotes active function at the site touched. In this way, the completeness of resection can be enhanced while reducing the risk of neurologic injury to maximal degree.

The mortality rate from craniotomy in large series is 1% to 2%. Surgical morbidity includes increased neurologic deficit (8% to 11%), hemorrhage at the operative site (4% to 5%, although no more than 1% require reopening and evacuation), and wound infection (1% to 2%). Medical complications such as deep vein thrombosis, myocardial infarction, and pneumonia occur in 3% to 9%. It is worth noting that venous Doppler studies of patients with glioblastoma before surgery have shown deep venous thrombosis in the legs of 30% to 40% of patients. Thus, the postoperative finding of such thrombosis may simply imply an ongoing hypercoagulable state that predated the surgery. In glioma surgery and in particular when resecting malignant gliomas, the added risk of an aggressive resection is less than the risk of leaving tumor behind and thereby provoking an ongoing edematous reaction within the residual tumor. Such edema causes worsening of pre-existing deficits and responds only slowly to osmotic diuresis and steroids. In accessible brain tumors, the main constraint on resection is the presence of nearby eloquent brain that cannot be breached without causing a functional decline in the patient.

The use of computer-assisted navigational techniques is optional for most brain tumor cases, but can be quite helpful in minimizing the size of the craniotomy opening and in identifying the extent of the lesion (Fig. 22.5). When such stereotactic navigation is used, four stages are followed: image acquisition, registration, planning, and intraoperative navigation. Typically the images are acquired before the operation after fiducial markers have been placed on the skin of the anterior half of the head. It is also possible to forego fiducial markers altogether and use instead an array of points on the surface of the patient's head, which are used to reconstruct the surface contours within the three-dimensional workspace of the workstation. The images acquired by either technique are transferred to the intraoperative computer workstation, and can be overlaid on imaging data from functional MRI or tractography to identify anatomic boundaries constraining resection as mentioned above, and thus reduce the risk of neurologic injury. When the patient is placed into final position in the operating room, registration is done to synchronize the patient's fiducial array with the array depicted in the previously acquired images. From that point on the surgeon can check the position of any point within the head in three dimensions relative to the tumor or to anatomical landmarks with accuracy of 1 to 2 mm. This accuracy diminishes, however, as the operation proceeds due to brain shift caused by hyperventilation, CSF loss, and tumor removal. Thus, we generally also use intraoperative ultrasound for real-time imaging, as it is cheaper, provides immediate feedback, and is not subject to the vicissitudes of brain shift.

Hydrocephalus

Hydrocephalus is an accumulation of CSF within the head (generally, the ventricles) leading to a rise in ICP that when high enough will compromise brain function. It can be "noncommunicating" when the CSF pathways are blocked somewhere along their course, or "communicating" when the blockage is at the final point of the pathway, that is, the arachnoid granulations near the superior sagittal sinus, where CSF is absorbed into the venous system. Patients with cancer develop hydrocephalus for any of several reasons:

1. Tumor may be located in the brain near the ventricular system, against which it produces mass effect sufficient to trap the upstream portion and cause it to balloon.
2. Leptomeningeal disease, defined as tumor cells in the subarachnoid space where CSF flow occurs, can clog the absorptive pathways or cause radiographically occult blockage at points of narrowing along the CSF pathways, for example, the aqueduct of Sylvius.
3. The effects of treatment may cause hydrocephalus. The likeliest scenario occurs after whole-brain radiotherapy with formation of scarring either in the ventricles or on the arachnoid granulations that interfere with CSF absorption or flow. Radiotherapy may additionally alter brain compliance and thereby magnify the effects of pathway blockage by shifting the pressure–volume curve.

Treatment

Medical therapies for hydrocephalus reduce CSF production to mitigate rises in pressure. The drugs generally used are Diamox (a carbonic anhydrase inhibitor) and dexamethasone. Both reduce the rate of CSF production but do not increase its absorption, and are temporizing measures useful while preparing a more definitive plan of action. The most direct way of treating hydrocephalus is to remove any mass that causes obstruction. In many patients, however, no such mass exists, and placement of a shunt is the appropriate treatment.

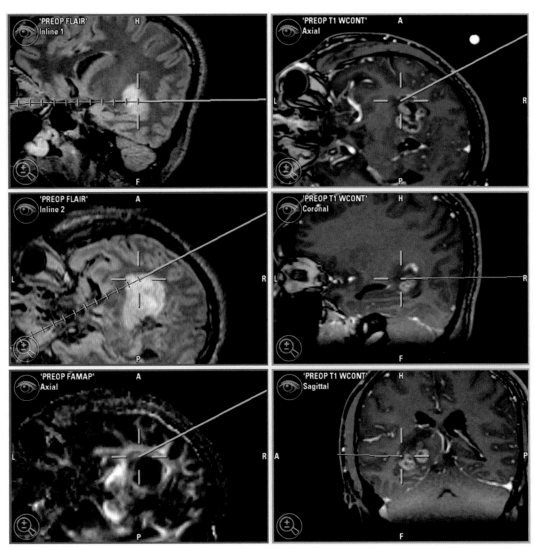

FIGURE 22.5 MRI acquired before surgery and imported into BrainLab neuronavigational workstation. It shows a glioblastoma in the deep posterior right temporal area, localized by wand guidance that will allow optimal creation of the craniotomy opening and of the transcerebral corridor needed to expose the tumor.

A ventriculostomy is in effect a temporary shunt that diverts CSF out of the ventricle into an external collecting system. This may be placed to record CSF pressures to show whether a shunt is needed, and if so, to help in selecting its valve strength. Indwelling shunts offer a more permanent solution, usually in the form of a ventriculoperitoneal system that runs from the lateral ventricle up through a burr hole into the subgaleal space over the cranium, and thence behind the ear and through the subcutaneous space of the neck, anterior chest, and abdominal wall to a point where it penetrates the peritoneum to deposit CSF into the peritoneal cavity. There the large surface area facilitates efficient CSF absorption. Shunts contain a valve usually located either at the burr hole where the shunt emerges or further downstream above or behind the ear. The valve allows the shunt to provide a set resistance to flow. This mechanism shuts off flow through the shunt when the ICP falls to the desired level, and opens the shunt when the ICP rises above it.

Patients sometimes require instillation of intraventricular chemotherapy for leptomeningeal carcinomatosis with concomitant hydrocephalus. Such treatment would be ineffective in the presence of a standard shunt, which would immediately flush it from the ventricles. In such cases, we place a shunt with an "on-off" valve that allows the shunt to be closed or opened by external pressure on the valve. Just before chemotherapy is instilled into the ventricular system through an in-line Ommaya reservoir, the shunt is closed. It is reopened after a suitable interval (usually 3 to 5 hours later) to relieve built-up CSF pressure and carry the patient safely until the next treatment. As these patients are usually quite shunt-dependent, longer periods of occlusion are unsafe.

Once an indwelling shunt has been placed, it is expected to function for the remainder of the patient's life. However, later problems do arise including shunt blockage, infection, or shift in the dynamics of the hydrocephalus that require valve renewal at a different level of resistance. When a shunt is blocked or infected, reoperation is needed to unblock it or remove it. Shunt infection is particularly troublesome as the ongoing hydrocephalus requires "externalization" of the shunt, meaning it is replaced by an external ventriculostomy catheter alone that must then be reinstalled as an indwelling system in a third procedure done only after the infection has cleared. To avoid the necessity for repeat operations done to change out the valve, systems have been developed with adjustable valves in which the setting can be changed by application of a magnetic wand external to the skin overlying the valve. The wand can increase or decrease the valve's resistance depending on the clinical need. The problem with their use in the cancer setting is that patients with tumor require frequent MRIs, and even during scans of the limbs or torso, such systems can be affected by the magnetic field of the scanner. They must be interrogated, and if necessary reset, after any MRI. Each company's system uses a different wand device, and the lack of a universal wand makes it hard for patients to transfer care to hospitals that use a system other than the one originally placed. We try to avoid using such systems for these reasons.

In some patients endoscopic third ventriculostomy serves as a substitute for an indwelling shunt. In this procedure an endoscope is inserted through a frontal burr hole and advanced under stereotactic guidance through the lateral ventricle, foramen of Munro, and into the third ventricle. There the surgeon can see the ventricular floor and create an opening that allows egress of CSF into the subarachnoid space, whence it can be absorbed. This technique is not universally applicable, but it can help patients with hydrocephalus caused by aqueductal stenosis or other compressive etiologies within the posterior fossa. It is not useful in patients with noncommunicating hydrocephalus as the success of the procedure depends on patency of absorptive pathways that are nonfunctional in this scenario.

Spinal Tumors

Tumors in the spine form a significant part of neurosurgical oncology and are subcategorized by their anatomic localization. They are either intradural or extradural, with extradural implying an intraosseous location within one or more vertebrae. Intradural tumors are further subdivided into those within the spinal cord, denoted as intramedullary, and those within the space between dura and spinal cord, denoted as intradural/extramedullary. The latter tend to arise from nerve roots or from the dura itself and are usually schwannomas or meningiomas.

Intradural Tumors

Intramedullary Tumors

These form 4% to 10% of all CNS tumors. From their location inside the spinal cord they can affect neurologic function in a variety of ways depending on their precise site of origin and pattern of growth within that very small space. As always, the rate of growth has relevance to the way symptoms develop. Tumors of the cord create symptoms by direct compression of adjacent neural pathways. Because sensory and motor tracts are packed tightly together, either or both can be affected by such compression. In addition, highly vascular tumors in the cord can create neurologic dysfunction by a steal phenomenon, and tumors of any vascularity may provoke formation of a syrinx, that is, a cyst that extends within the cord above or below the tumor, sometimes for great distances. Almost all spinal cord tumors (about 98%) fall within one of three categories, to which we will confine this discussion.

Ependymomas and Astrocytomas

Ependymomas are the most common intramedullary tumor in adults and make up 60% to 65% of such lesions. They are generally discrete with a distinct interface with the cord and little tendency to invade. Although the histologic appearance of ependymomas of the cord is similar to that of cerebral ependymomas, their behavior is quite different. Cord ependymomas are much less likely to produce metastases by CSF spread, and rarely convert to malignant forms. Ependymomas of the cord tend to enhance on MRI and grow slowly with an insidious clinical onset (Fig. 22.6). The exception to this comes when they hemorrhage (6% to 8%), in which case a sudden worsening occurs, often associated with neuropathic pain. They can occur anywhere along the cord although they are somewhat more common in the cervical region. The tanycytic variant of intramedullary ependymomas is associated with NF1, and such tumors are usually (although not invariably) indolent and asymptomatic, and can be managed conservatively.

Astrocytomas arising in the spinal cord, such as ependymomas, show a different biology from that of their cousins in the brain. Those in the cord are more likely to be well differentiated. Indeed, 90% of them fall into

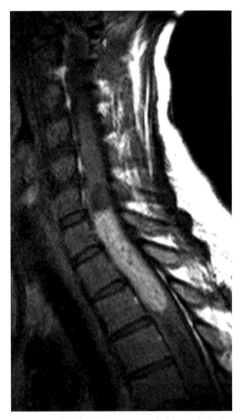

FIGURE 22.6 MRI (sagittal, postcontrast) of the cervical spine showing a well-defined enhancing tumor within the cord, consistent with ependymoma. Note the syrinx both rostral and caudal to the tumor. This patient presented with quadriparesis and recovered significantly after total removal of the tumor.

this category as either pilocytic astrocytomas or diffusely infiltrating (but benign) lesions. The infiltrating variety have pure tumor at the heart of the mass, but tend to mingle with normal cord at their periphery and thus are difficult to remove in a truly complete fashion. Pilocytic astrocytomas, similar to those in the brain, are quite discrete and can be removed completely. The main difficulty is identifying the interface with an accuracy sufficient to prevent resection of slivers of normal cord along with the tumor. Only 10% of the intramedullary astrocytomas are malignant and those are overwhelmingly anaplastic in grade. True glioblastomas of the cord occur, but at the minute incidence of 1/15 million people/year.

Astrocytic tumors are more common in children in the spinal cord than are ependymomas (the reverse is true for adults) and 5-year survival varies between 60% and 85% with a 10-year survival of 55%. The mortality may reflect the fallout of profound neurologic deficits imposed by the tumor or transformation to more malignant forms.

The primary mode of therapy for these tumors is surgical removal via laminectomy, dural opening, and myelotomy. Complete resection is achieved in our hands in >90% of ependymomas and is much less likely in astrocytomas. Even with use of intraoperative neurophysiologic monitoring techniques such as somatosensory-evoked potentials and motor-evoked potentials, about half of patients develop new deficits immediately after surgery; these deficits are transient in all but 10% of those operated on. As the most important influence on the postoperative neurologic status is the preoperative status, patients should ideally be operated before they show neurologic decline. Those with longstanding deficits rarely improve after resection, even when tumor removal is complete. A recurrence rate of 5% to 10% over 5 years is typical and radiotherapy should not be used in ependymomas of the cord unless (1) gross total resection cannot be achieved despite valiant efforts to do so, or (2) an unresectable remnant shows signs of growth while under surveillance by MRI. There is no current role for chemotherapy in the treatment of the benign forms of ependymomas and astrocytomas of the spinal cord, but in anaplastic variants of both those tumor types, chemotherapy and radiotherapy may provide some palliative benefit.

As it has been difficult to assign prognosis to ependymomas based solely on histopathologic diagnosis, more standardized molecular criteria with clinical utility are needed. To date, based on DNA methylation profiling of intracranial and spinal ependymomas, 9 molecular subgroups of ependymomas have been identified. These include three location-specific categories: supratentorial (balanced genome, YAP1, and RELA-driven); posterior fossa (balanced genome, Group A, and Group B); and spinal (balanced genome, NF2-driven, and myxopapillary).

Hemangioblastoma The third most common category of spinal cord tumor (10%) is the hemangioblastoma. These tumors grow slowly and form 5% to 8% of intramedullary tumors. They often provoke syrinx formation that can be quite extensive (in some cases, even occupying the entire cord), and have a characteristic orange or reddish color due to their extreme vascularity and their content of lipid-laden cells. When a cyst is present, it is often the dominant portion of the mass and the source of compression on the cord. However, even a small hemangioblastoma can provoke a significant expansion of the coronal venous plexus through arteriovenous shunting causing venous hypertension that can itself affect cord function.

These tumors can be solitary or multiple, with multiple hemangioblastomas always denoting von Hippel–Lindau disease (VHL), a genetic tumor syndrome in which renal cell carcinoma, pheochromocytoma, pancreatic islet cell tumor, and hemangioblastoma of the brain are also seen. Thus, patients with one hemangioblastoma should undergo MRI of the entire craniospinal axis to search for others. Eighty percent of patients with hemangioblastoma have VHL, while the remainder represent sporadic cases without a germ-line mutation.

When the hemangioblastoma is removed, care should be taken to interrupt the arterial supply before occluding the dominant draining vein. It can be difficult to sort out which vessel belongs in which category, so a preoperative spinal angiogram may be useful. However, we have found that the discomfort and risk to the patient with angiography outweigh the benefits, and that we can usually tell by direct inspection which vessels are arterial. The tumor is removed by entering its interface with the cord, preferably within the associated syrinx. If no syrinx is present, the surgeon adheres intimately to the tumor capsule and carefully dissects and incises the tumor's attachments to the cord at the pial surface. Once the tumor is freed from the pia it will tend to extrude slightly from the cord, and the remaining attachments can be divided without difficulty. If the draining vein is taken prematurely, the tumor will swell while still tethered in place, and the potential for damage to the cord is significant in this scenario. Piecemeal removal is sometimes necessary, but will provoke significant bleeding from the tumor as it remains perfused by small branches of the anterior spinal artery that can only be cauterized and divided after the deepest part of the tumor has been isolated. Thus, en bloc resection is recommended for most hemangioblastomas.

Patients who have extensive syrinx show excellent resolution of the cystic changes in the cord if tumor removal is complete. The cord generally continues to show some minor gliotic changes, but the syrinx will resolve during the 3 months after surgery.

We have found that resection of multiple hemangioblastomas is quite feasible and safe, although tumors located in the anterolateral quadrant pose more risk as the manipulation required to extract them is greater unless a truly lateral approach is taken. However, this is rarely done in intradural surgery to avoid both spinal destabilization and breach of the lateral corticospinal tract.

Metastatic Tumors Metastasis confined within the spinal cord is unusual. Such tumors make up no more than 2% of all cord tumors and are most commonly seen in patients with carcinomas of the breast or lung. Renal cell carcinoma and melanoma also metastasize to the spinal cord with some regularity. The majority of such patients do not undergo surgery because the cord metastasis generally appears during the late stages of the disease when the patient is already somewhat debilitated. As patients with systemic metastasis are living longer, metastasis to the spinal cord is becoming more common, but we still rarely perform surgery on these patients. At MDACC we have operated on intramedullary metastasis because of diagnostic uncertainty or because the patient was in relatively good medical and neurologic condition and preservation of function was sought through surgical decompression. Such tumors usually have an incompletely defined plane with the cord and can therefore be debulked, but not cured, by surgery. Postoperative radiotherapy is typically used, but leptomeningeal dissemination still occurs in 30% of our patient cohort after surgery. No patient with pre-existing leptomeningeal metastasis underwent surgery; it is a contraindication due to the relatively short survival of such patients. In our experience, the median survival after surgery was 5 months, but it is possible to maintain good function during extended survival for up to 4 years.

Intradural/Extramedullary Tumors

These are tumors that occur inside the dura but outside the spinal cord, and thus usually arise from nerve roots or from the dura/arachnoid interface. They are mainly meningiomas of dural/arachnoidal origin or schwannomas arising from nerve roots. Each of these tumor types shows excellent delineation from the cord and can be resected completely. The tendency of the schwannoma to arise from a sensory root generally means that the root can be cut with minimal loss of function, as transfer of that function may already have occurred to adjacent sensory roots or because enough anatomic overlap already exists to prevent a deficit. Some schwannomas extend transdurally into the intervertebral foramen and can be chased there, while others form a "dumbbell" tumor which necessitates resection outside the spine as well as within the spinal canal and intervertebral foramen. Schwannomas have a globular appearance on MRI with a sharp border and moderate enhancement. The presence of a dumbbell picture confirms the diagnosis of schwannoma when it is present. Meningiomas have a different appearance in that they tend to show a tapering, sloping defect with gradual narrowing of the subarachnoid space up to the point of contact between cord and tumor at both its rostral and caudal ends. They tend to be low grade and often calcify. The presence of calcification in a tumor in this compartment is pathognomonic for meningioma. The meningiomas are intimately apposed to the dura into which they may even invade; thus a complete resection may entail dural removal as well.

Metastasis can also be found within the intradural/extramedullary space, usually as drop metastasis from a tumor in the posterior fossa. Almost all patients with this rare phenomenon have known systemic metastasis to other sites, and the diagnosis is not difficult by MRI as the tumor will have an ill-defined and fuzzy border quite different from the typical meningioma or schwannoma. Even so, some patients undergo surgery due to diagnostic confusion; meningiomas and schwannomas are quite curable, so if there is any room for belief that they belong in the differential diagnosis, an operation is indicated. As with intramedullary metastases, metastasis within the intradural/extramedullary space is not curable, but can be debulked. Although this is best regarded as a focal form of leptomeningeal dissemination, the life expectancy of these patients may exceed that of patients with more classically diffuse leptomeningeal spread, so surgery may actually provide benefit in carefully selected cases.

The general surgical approach for intradural/extramedullary tumors is similar to that used for the intramedullary tumors (laminectomy and durotomy), but no myelotomy is necessary. Intraoperative ultrasound localizes tumors nicely in both these categories. In patients who are at risk for swan neck deformity due to tumor impairment of nerves to the paraspinal muscles or because of multiple levels of root involvement, a laminoplasty may be more desirable than a laminectomy to allow better maintenance of spinal stability. However, we have not been impressed by the efficacy of laminoplasty in preventing kyphosis, and tend to avoid it for that reason, and because it fosters earlier onset of recurrent myelopathy in the event of subsequent regrowth of tumor.

Tumors of the Osseous (Extradural) Spine

Patients with tumors within the vertebra present with pain or neurologic deficit, patterns that depend on the level of spine involvement, the degree of root compression, and the degree of mechanical spinal instability. Surgery is more intended to help with diagnosis, palliation, and restoration of spinal stability rather than to achieve oncologic cure, although for primary tumors of the spine cure is a desirable objective. Just as with brain tumors, the multidisciplinary approach is crucial for optimal management of extradural spinal tumors.

Diagnostic Tests

Testing begins with plain x-rays which are inexpensive and easy to obtain, and the results may be diagnostic of tumor. AP and lateral x-rays of the entire spine are also useful in assessing spinal alignment and stability, and can be used to predict the quality of bone strength to be encountered during surgery. The classic findings on x-ray of a spinal bony tumor are loss of pedicle definition (metastases have a heavy predilection for the vertebral pedicle), compression fracture, or destruction of one or more vertebrae with disc preservation; all these features suggest a malignant lesion. However, plain films show an abnormality in only 60% to 80% of patients who have neurologic deficits due to spinal cord compression, and thus merely begin a radiologic investigation of this problem.

Much more useful are MRI and CT in delineating the extent of tumor and the degree of spinal stability. Although MRI provides optimal visualization of epidural compression and paraspinal soft tissue involvement, CT gives better insight into the degree of bony destruction. When metastasis is suspected the entire spine should be imaged to determine the presence of multiple coincident lesions. When MRI is contraindicated (e.g., by presence of a pacemaker) or when images are obscured by artifact (e.g., by prior rod and screw placement) CT myelography can give good imaging of bony anatomy and neural constituents. CT-guided needle biopsy is performed when no prior malignancy exists and pathologic diagnosis is needed. Three-dimensional reconstruction of the CT is quite useful for surgical planning, particularly in those patients who have undergone

TABLE 22.6	Bilsky Epidural Disease Grading Scale

Bilsky Grade	Description
0	No epidural disease
1a	Epidural impinging the thecal sac but without deformation
1b	Epidural disease deforming the thecal sac but not the spinal cord
1c	Epidural disease deforming the thecal sac and spinal cord contact
2	Epidural spinal cord compression with CSF visible
3	Epidural spinal cord compression and no CSF visible

prior operation in the same region. In those with potential need for spinal instrumentation and pedicle screw placement to correct pre-existing mechanical instability (or instability created by the bone removal necessary to resect the spinal tumor), CT is superior to MRI for providing accurate measurement of pedicle dimensions.

MRI is the key to studying spinal tumors completely and accurately. The degree of spinal cord compression is readily disclosed on T2-weighted images, and fat suppression techniques are quite useful in eliminating overshadowing from epidural or paraspinal fat. The Bilsky scoring system categorizes the degree of impingement by an extradural tumor on the spinal cord, as shown by MRI (Table 22.6). MRI is also the most sensitive and specific modality for distinguishing spinal metastases from osteoporotic compression fractures, common among patients with cancer. Osteoporotic fractures are most often seen in the thoracic spine, do not involve the pedicle, and on T1-weighted images lack signal change. Pathologic fractures (i.e., those caused by tumor disruption of bone structure) tend to have a homogeneous signal on T1-weighted images and often involve the pedicle. Radionuclide bone scanning is sensitive but not very specific in detecting metastatic spinal disease. It relies on osteoblastic bone deposition to detect tumor, so rapidly progressive tumors may not be well seen by this technique. It is also relatively insensitive to myelomas limited to the bone marrow. Furthermore, osteomyelitis, hemangiomas, fractures, and even degenerative spondylosis can show as increased uptake on bone scan.

Primary Bone Tumors

Such tumors are not common, as <10% of all primary tumors of bone involve the spine. They present with symptoms that include night pain, pain at rest (either in the back or as a radicular component), or neurologic deficit. The course can be insidious with relatively nonspecific complaints. Once a lesion is suspected, CT or MRI will typically identify its location and offer clues to its cell type of origin.

Hemangioma

These vascular lesions are found more commonly in females than males, and are solitary two-thirds of the time. They tend to be located in the lower thoracic or upper lumbar spine and have a characteristic honeycomb appearance on plain films due to linear reactive calcification around the radiolucent vascular tissue. Most are confined to their vertebral body and pose no particular clinical issue. Only occasionally do they cause compression of the cord due to extension of the vascular tissue into the epidural space. Pain alone is not an indication for surgery and only those patients in whom neurologic symptoms have occurred are operated on. Asymptomatic lesions can generally be ignored until pain or neurologic deficits develop. Complete resection is possible and surgery is the mainstay of treatment.

Aneurysmal Bone Cyst

These lesions occur most often in children and are uncommon in patients over 30 years of age. They tend to involve the posterior vertebral elements more than the anterior elements, and the lumbar vertebrae more than other levels. These are benign lesions but can be proliferative and lytic, and occasionally expand rapidly. When they spill into the canal they can cause neurologic compromise. Surgical resection is the favored treatment, sometimes after preoperative embolization. Incomplete resection leads to a high rate of recurrence, but complete resection generally gives long term cure. Radiotherapy is relatively ineffective.

Osteoblastic Lesions

These benign tumors of the spine occur more often in males and are categorized either as osteoid osteomas or as osteoblastomas. The distinction is purely made on the basis of size, with osteoid osteomas being <1.5 cm in diameter. Any young patient with back or neck pain, scoliosis, or radicular pain should be considered for such a lesion. X-rays show a dense sclerotic rim of reactive bone around a small central nidus. They have intense radionuclide uptake on bone scan. The pain caused by these lesions can be treated with nonsteroidal anti-in-flammatory agents and occasionally the osteoid osteomas will spontaneously resolve. If pain is an ongoing issue and no resolution has occurred, surgical excision can be performed and if complete, will successfully eliminate the lesion. Osteoblastomas are more likely to come to surgery because of their larger size. Complete tumor removal by en bloc resection is curative. Intralesional debulking is more likely to lead to incomplete resection and thus carries a higher risk of recurrence.

Osteochondroma

These tumors are the most frequently encountered benign lesions of the bone. They consist of cartilage-cov-ered cortical bone with underlying medullary bone. The osteochondroma is formed when the cartilaginous cap undergoes calcification. These are most commonly seen in males in the third decade of life. They also tend to affect the posterior elements including the pedicle. They have a predilection for the cervical spine. The best diagnostic test for them is a CT scan as they show less radionuclide uptake on bone scan than do other lesions such as osteoid osteoma. They tend to increase in size during adolescence and sometimes into adulthood. Malignant transformation is rare and surgical removal is the treatment of choice.

Giant Cell Tumor

These tumors are uncommon, locally aggressive, and occur more often in females. The most frequent spinal location is the sacrum but they can occur anywhere in the spine and usually involve a single vertebra in which an expansile mass has formed. They transform to a malignant state in 10% of cases and then can metastasize. Interestingly, the "giant cells" are not the neoplastic element of the tumor; rather this is usually the other cell component, traditionally believed to be the stromal cells. Thus this tumor is misnamed. The best resection of such lesions is done en bloc as recurrence is more common after intralesional curettage. When found in the sacrum, a sacrectomy (partial or total) with sacrifice of neural elements may be necessary to achieve cure. These tumors are quite vascular and preoperative embolization is useful. They may benefit as well from radiotherapy after a subtotal resection. Neoadjuvant treatment with denosumab can shrink giant cell tumors and make complete resection easier and more secure.

Plasmacytoma

These are the most common malignant lesions of the adult spine. Malignant proliferation of the plasma cells occurs in the bone marrow, spleen, and lymphoid tissues. A few patients have a solitary plasmacytoma but multiple plasmacytomas (called "multiple myeloma") are far more common. Such patients have infiltration of bone marrow by plasma cells with resulting reduction in immunoglobulin levels. However, with solitary plasmacytomas serum protein electrophoresis is normal because the bone marrow is largely functional. Bone in patients with multiple myeloma generally has a poor quality and thus aggressive resections necessitating vertebral reconstruction and instrumentation affixed to adjacent segments are not ideal. The treatment of choice is thus vertebroplasty for pain control and possibly radiotherapy thereafter for tumor control. Half of patients with solitary plasmacytoma progress to multiple myeloma within 5 years (and usually within 3 years), so patients with solitary disease should be followed closely to detect distant recurrence. Combination che-motherapy is often used for multiple myeloma, and sometimes stem cell transplant, especially if progression is apparent.

Chordoma

These tumors arise from remnants of the embryonic notochord and tend to be indolent but locally progres-sive; they can sometimes metastasize. Fifty percent of chordomas occur in the sacrum, 40% in the clivus, and the rest in mobile regions of the spine. The 5-year survival rate ranges from 50% to 75% and the 10-year survival rate is about 50%. En bloc resection is the best currently available intervention for chordoma. For tumors of the sacrococcygeal spine, ventral, dorsal, or combined surgical approaches may be needed together with nerve sacrifice and sometimes resection of adjacent bowel leading to colostomy. Such cases are always done in conjunction with both neurosurgeon and colorectal surgeon, and often with a plastic surgeon as well. There are no current indications for using chemotherapy to manage chordomas, but radiotherapy may have a role. It has been suggested that proton beam irradiation may be especially useful in treating clival chordomas in which an incomplete resection has been done due to the inability to perform en bloc resection in this difficult anatomical area. Resection of clival chordomas requires special skull base techniques, a subject beyond the scope of this chapter but often involving an endoscopic approach through the sinonasal cavities or nasophar-ynx, with good results when this is followed by proton beam radiotherapy.

Ewing Sarcoma

These tumors are most common in the first two decades of life and occur more often in males. More than half of these involve the sacrum. Plain x-ray shows a lytic lesion with a sclerotic rim. Treatment often starts with chemotherapy with surgery reserved for those patients with an incomplete response or if decompression of the spinal canal is desirable. Radical resection may be necessary here, just as with chordoma

Osteosarcoma

These are seen occasionally in the spine either as primary tumors or as metastases from sites of origin in the appendicular skeleton. Osteosarcomas can be primary in young adults, or in older patients they may be secondary lesions arising as a result of radiotherapy to bone. En bloc resection is now advocated followed by radiotherapy and aggressive chemotherapy. Although occasional long-term survival is seen, patients generally die of this disease through widespread metastasis.

Chondrosarcoma

Such tumors are typically indolent and show multiple local recurrences over long periods of time before they switch to a metastatic mode. They are more common in men and have a poor prognosis despite their slow pace of growth. They are quite resistant to radiotherapy and chemotherapy, and thus complete (en bloc) resection is the ideal goal of an operation done for this tumor type.

Spinal Metastasis

From 5% to 10% of patients with all types of cancer combined develop symptomatic spinal metastasis at some point during the course of their disease. In one-fifth of patients with involvement of the vertebral column by metastasis, frank spinal cord compression ultimately occurs (Fig. 22.7). The thoracic spine is the most common location for spinal metastasis, with the lumbar spine yielding 20% of cases and the cervical spine 10%. Over half of cases arise from carcinomas of breast, lung, and prostate, due to the fact that these cancers are relatively common and (in the case of breast and prostate cancer) because of their tendency to metastasize to bones throughout the skeleton. Since pain is the most common symptom, back pain in a patient with known cancer should be assumed to be caused by metastasis until proven otherwise. The pain can be mechanical due to spinal instability from bony destruction or radicular due to nerve root irritation. Pain that worsens with movement and improves when the patient lies down denotes mechanical instability, and suggests that stabilizing instrumentation should be part of any operation done. Although spinal metastasis usually presents with pain before myelopathy, a complete neurologic examination is important to detect the latter in any patient suspected of having this condition.

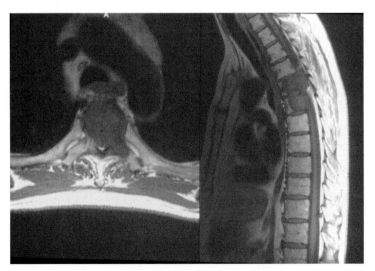

FIGURE 22.7 MRI (T1-weighted) of thoracic spine of patient with metastatic renal cell carcinoma. The images show (**left**) an axial view at the site of maximum epidural compression. The vertebral body, pedicle, and lamina are involved and the cord is severely effaced. (**Right**) Sagittal view shows tumor in two contiguous vertebral segments (T2 and T3) with the epidural compression caused at T2. Both segments must be resected for long-term local control. This patient requires an operation done by transpedicular approach with reconstruction and posterior instrumentation by a rod-and-screw construct.

The oncologist's weapons for treating metastatic spinal disease include chemotherapy, radiotherapy, and surgery. The most important factor affecting prognosis is the patient's ability to walk when treatment starts. Surgery is palliative in patients with metastatic disease to the spine. The clinical goals should focus on reduction of pain, preservation of neurologic function, and restoration of mobility while maintaining sphincter control. Loss of such control predicts a poor outcome. The debate over the relative efficacy of radiotherapy versus surgery is complex and continues today. However, a patient in relatively good shape from the medical and oncologic perspective with a reasonable life expectancy overall (>6 months) should be considered for surgery if spinal metastasis endangers neurologic function but has not yet eroded it. In addition, pain of instability (axial loading pain) will be helped more by resection and stabilization than by radiotherapy, which controls the tumor but leaves the mechanical instability in place. The goal of surgery is to provide decompression of the spinal cord and nerve roots and/or to stabilize the spinal column. Radiotherapy is a good modality, however, for treating radiosensitive spinal tumors or those causing minimal or no neurologic deficits. We have found that SRS for spinal metastases can be quite effective in suppressing focal deposits of disease with good safety to the nearby cord, and that it shortens the time of treatment significantly without compromising effectiveness. Radiosurgical delivery requires five or fewer sessions, while standard external beam irradiation is given in 10 fractions to a total dose of 30 to 40 Gy.

Metastatic breast cancer is typically radiosensitive and also can respond to hormonal therapy, cytotoxic chemotherapy, or both. Thus, in breast cancer cases (and in particular those with multiple spinal lesions) surgical intervention is limited. Spinal involvement from a lung cancer can result from direct extension of a tumor from the chest wall to the nearby spine, or may develop from hematogenous routes. Superior sulcus tumors in particular can involve the spine and require intricate cooperation between thoracic surgeon and neurosurgeon for ideal resection of the lung, chest wall, spinal, and occasionally neural components, with reconstruction of the chest wall needed in many cases. Because of its high degree of radiosensitivity, small cell carcinoma rarely needs surgery. Prostate cancer also responds more often than not to palliative efforts without surgery and is sensitive to radiotherapy at least for a time. Its spinal involvement tends to be multifocal, and thus surgical cases must be carefully chosen. The role of surgery in prostate cancer tends to focus on correction of spinal instability, control of intractable pain caused by a focal lesion, or prevention of neurologic decline.

The non–small cell carcinomas of the lung (squamous cell carcinoma and adenocarcinoma) can metastasize to the spine and are somewhat resistant to radiotherapy. Although surgery can be considered for such patients, they often have poor pulmonary function in which case a transthoracic approach is less desirable. Transpedicular approaches through a midline posterior incision are preferred for them or indeed for any patient with a significant burden of lung metastasis compromising pulmonary mechanics. The more concentrated dosing allowed by stereotactic delivery of radiotherapy to the spine may yield better control than that achieved by standard radiotherapy. Renal cell carcinomas also resist radiotherapy and the systemic disease varies significantly in its clinical behavior. In many patients the pace of the disease is relatively indolent even when lung or other metastases are present. Renal cell carcinoma thus lends itself to surgery, but it is quite vascular and preoperative embolization is often helpful in limiting intraoperative hemorrhage. The key to resection of a renal cell carcinoma from the spine is a quick removal after a careful and comprehensive isolation of the tumor and as much devascularization as possible prior to tumor entry. Such tumors must usually be removed in piecemeal fashion and bleed significantly during that removal. When the tumor has been removed completely or almost so, the bleeding slows and stops, or at least becomes much more responsive to the usual topical control measures.

Indications for Spinal Surgery

Because patients with vertebral column tumors usually have a life expectancy limited to 1 to 2 years, and may have multiple sites of disease when the tumor is metastatic, oncologic cure is not the usual goal of an operation. The benefits must be balanced against the risks of a major procedure and the time needed for recuperation, usually 4 to 8 weeks. A patient with 3 to 4 months of predicted survival would not be a good candidate for such an operation as it would consume half his remaining life span in recovery time. Thus, the goals of surgery are dictated by the patient's life expectancy, functional (including neurologic) status, tumor type, chance for oncologic cure, degree and type of pain, degree and duration of compression of spinal cord or nerve roots, and the need to restore spinal stability.

The classic indication for surgery is rapid neurologic decline due to epidural compression of the spinal cord caused by a radioresistant tumor. Spinal instability is a commonly cited reason as well, but there is no uniformly accepted definition of that phrase. Commonly used definitions include disruption of two of the three bony columns of the thoracolumbar spine (although this does not apply to the cervical spine, whose structure is different); kyphotic deformity >20 degrees; or loss of >50% of vertebral body height in any portion

SINS Component	Score
Location	
Junctional (occiput-C2, C7–12, T11-L1, L5–51)	3
Mobile spine (C3–C6, L2–L4)	2
Semirigid (T3–T10)	1
Rigid (52–55)	0
Pain	
Yes	3
Occasional pain but not mechanical	1
Pain-free lesion	0
Bone Lesion	
Lytic	2
Mixed lytic/blastic	1
Blastic	0
Radiographic Spinal Alignment	
Subluxation/translation present	4
De novo deformity (kyphosis/scoliosis)	2
Normal alignment	0
Vertebral Body Collapse	
>50% collapse	3
<50% collapse	2
No collapse with >50% body involved	1
None of the above	0
Posterolateral Involvement of Spinal Elements	
Bilateral	3
Unilateral	1
None of the above	0

TABLE 22.7 Spinal Instability Neoplastic Score (SINS)[a]

[a]Scores of 13 to 18 suggest mechanical instability, and surgery may be considered for scores ≥7.

of the spine. If patients meet one or more of these criteria and have a well-defined syndrome of axial loading pain, then surgery is a reasonable consideration as vertebral resection and reconstruction with appropriate anterior and/or posterior instrumentation may give excellent pain relief long term. Spinal stability in oncology patients can also be quantified by calculating a spinal instability neoplasm score (SINS), with points assigned for which spinal segment the tumor occupies, whether pain improves when the patient lies down, the nature (lytic or blastic) of the lesion, disruptions of spinal alignment, the degree of vertebral body collapse, and the extent to which posterolateral spinal elements are involved. Scores of 13 to 18 suggest instability and surgery may be considered for scores ≥7 (Table 22.7). In addition to stabilization of mechanically unstable spinal segments, restoration of sagittal balance (allowing correction to comfortable, erect, energy-efficient posture) in patients with kyphotic deformity, significantly improves the quality of life.

Overall the aims of spinal surgery are four in number. These include: (1) decompression of the spinal cord to improve or maintain neurologic status, (2) decompression of nerve roots to reduce radicular pain, (3) stabilization of the spine to reduce the pain of instability, and (4) correction of kyphotic or scoliotic deformities impairing sagittal/coronal balance, or loss of vertebral height, that add to the patient's pain burden.

Surgical Adjuncts

Embolization done prior to surgery (within 24 hours) can reduce blood loss during operations and may be useful for hypervascular metastases such as renal cell carcinoma and thyroid carcinoma. Bleeding from thyroid carcinoma is the most profound and difficult to stop of any metastasis, and such tumors should be approached surgically with great caution and with an adequate supply of blood readily available. Embolization requires spinal angiography which carries risk and some discomfort to the patient. The embolization itself can cause spinal cord infarction and complete paralysis should the injection be done too proximally within the vascular tree. This procedure should only be performed by interventional neuroradiologists expert in its application.

Blood loss during resection of spinal metastases ranges from minimal to extreme. If large blood loss is expected, transfusion should begin as soon as tumor resection starts to avoid having to play "catch-up" and to prevent hemodynamic instability. Patients who have received multiple transfusions will take longer to recover and may be in the hospital for several weeks after the surgery. We do not advocate the use of cell savers out of concern that they may recirculate malignant cells into the bloodstream. Cryocoagulation of the tumor in situ can be very effective in stopping intractable bleeding, but the cord must be excluded from the zone of freezing.

We routinely perform intraoperative monitoring of somatosensory-evoked potentials and motor-evoked potentials, which give immediate feedback on the integrity of neural pathways in the dorsal and ventral portions of the spinal cord, respectively. When motor-evoked potentials are used, anesthesia techniques must be modified to exclude paralytic agents.

Fluoroscopy is useful for localizing vertebral levels early in surgery. It also helps to ensure good screw placement during spinal fixation, with avoidance of pedicle breach or penetration of the vertebral endplate or cortex by a misdirected or overly long screw.

Surgical Techniques

Extradural spinal metastases can be approached from an anterior, posterior, or combined direction. The choice of approach is determined by tumor location (vertebral body vs. posterior elements), the spinal level, the extent of the tumor, and the degree of patient debility. When tumors involve only the posterior spine and laminae, decompression is done through a posterior laminectomy approach. However, it is more common to see the compression along the anterior aspect of the thecal sac, in which case effective decompression can be achieved either via an anterior/anterolateral or a posterolateral (transpedicular or costotransversectomy) approach. When the dural sac is surrounded by tumor from all directions, resection proceeds either by the posterolateral transpedicular method or by combined anterior and posterior approaches.

The anterior approach is awkward at the highest cervical and thoracic levels (C1, C2, and T1–T3) and the lowest lumbar and sacral segments (L5 and below). Access to the upper cervical spine can be done through a transoral or mandibular splitting approach but these are technically difficult procedures and in the context of malignant disease may be unrealistic for palliation. The high thoracic segments can be reached by performing a sternal split with reflection of the first and second ribs laterally. The heart and great vessels limit caudal exposure as does the natural spinal curve. We have preferred to approach tumors in these locations purely from a posterior transpedicular direction. The lumbosacral junction can be reached from the front without great difficulty, but stabilization at this level is difficult and requires complex posteriorly placed lumbopelvic rod constructs and bone grafts; thus such operations are always done as combined anterior–posterior cases. Sacral reconstruction is essentially impossible although replacement of the L5 vertebral body can be performed.

Spinal stabilization is needed after any anterior corpectomy and after most (but not all) posterolateral decompressions. When two or more vertebral body segments have been removed, anterior fixation alone is usually insufficient for long-term stability and supplementation with posterior rods and screws is helpful. The current posterior instrumentation systems are highly developed and allow stabilization anywhere from the occipitocervical area to the lumbar spine. Lumbopelvic fixation remains a difficult area in which the perfect construct has not yet been achieved.

Patient debility plays an important role in selecting surgical approaches. Many patients have undergone previous radiotherapy, and surgery performed through an irradiated field carries a higher risk of wound complications. Thus, plastic surgical assistance can be quite helpful for wound closure in such patients.

In patients whose debility or overall physiologic impairment make wound healing problematic, laser interstitial thermal therapy (LITT) is an alternative to open spinal surgery. This involves stereotactic placement of a thermal probe into a tumor targeted for ablation (Fig. 22.8). Under real-time thermal imaging in an intraoperative MRI suite, the lesion is heated to >45 degrees to induce cell death and tumor shrinkage. At MDACC we have used this method to achieve not only tumor control but also decompression of spinal cord distorted by adjacent tumor. In addition, new minimally invasive methods for placing spinal instrumentation are gaining ground in spinal oncology, and allow spinal stability to be restored by percutaneous screw and rod placement, without lengthy incisions requiring prolonged convalescent times and pain due to paraspinal muscle trauma. Such techniques have promoted postoperative mobility and recovery in the select group of patients in whom they can be used effectively.

Vertebral replacement can be done with autologous or allograft bone cut to appropriate size, methylmethacrylate, or an expandable titanium alloy cage. We use expandable cages for the majority of our vertebrectomy patients as they permit adjustment in situ which can restore lost vertebral body height without drilling into the adjacent vertebral bodies, as must be done to anchor a methylmethacrylate strut graft. However, a number of patients still

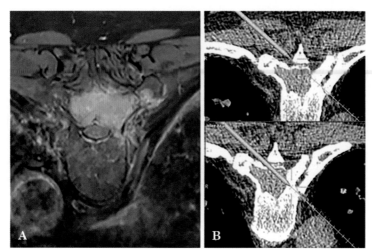

FIGURE 22.8 Laser interstitial thermal therapy. **A:** Renal cell carcinoma of spine in posterior elements of T9 with incipient cord compression, as shown in MRI (T1-weighted, postcontrast, axial). **B:** Thermal probe placement on cognate CT slices through the same tumor. The tumor will be heated at this safe location to avoid thermal damage to the nearby spinal cord.

receive methylmethacrylate grafts when expandable cages will not fit the bony defect or when the corridor of access to the vertebrectomy site is offset and prevents placement of the tools necessary for cage expansion. We are least likely to use a bone graft because long-term fusion is not generally necessary in a patient population whose life expectancy rarely extends beyond 2 to 3 years, and in which strenuous physical activity is not common.

Multidisciplinary cooperation between surgical services is frequently necessary in performing these operations. It is routine to engage the services of a thoracic surgeon for anterolateral approaches to the thoracic spine needing thoracotomy or a thoracoabdominal approach for spinal tumors near the diaphragm. Retroperitoneal or transabdominal approaches require the services of a general surgeon, and complex neck approaches from an anterolateral or posterolateral angle may benefit greatly from help by a head and neck surgeon. Although brain operations are exclusively the province of the neurosurgeon, spinal procedures can involve any of these named services as well as plastic surgery when significant tissue loss has occurred that compromises wound closure, or when the effects of prior treatment make wound healing tenuous.

Cervical Spine

High cervical (C1 and C2) vertebral tumors can be approached transorally with or without transmandibular modification, depending on the degree of rostral extension of the tumor. This approach is destabilizing and mandates posterior occipitocervical fixation as part of the procedure. Tumors in the anterior portion of the subaxial cervical spine can be approached through the anterolateral neck along the edge of the sternocleidomastoid muscle. This provides excellent exposure but puts the function of the recurrent laryngeal nerve at risk through potential stretch injury. To avoid postoperative hoarseness, retractors should be relaxed at 30-minute intervals throughout the case. En bloc resection in the cervical spine is challenging and usually not possible due to the anatomic constraints imposed by the vertebral artery, nerve roots, and spinal dura.

Thoracic Spine

Tumors in the T1 vertebral body that do not extend laterally can be approached through an incision in the low anterolateral neck, but many cannot be well exposed without sternal split (trapdoor approach). Thoracic vertebral tumors with a lateral paraspinal extension require posterolateral thoracotomy from the side of greatest tumor bulk. Transpedicular vertebrectomy is useful for tumors in this region but will usually not clear the disease as effectively as the transthoracic approach. Because the transpedicular method is facilitated by bilateral transection of nerve roots it is usually not used at T1, where the roots may be important for hand function.

Thoracolumbar Spine

Direct exposure of a thoracolumbar (T10–L1) vertebral tumor requires a thoracoabdominal approach in which a portion of the diaphragmatic crus is divided to uncover the spine not only over the tumor site, but also over adjacent levels needed for fixation of an anterior plate-and-screw construct. The side of the approach is decided by the location of the tumor within the vertebral body; those extending equally to both sides are approached from the left to avoid the liver. En bloc resection of tumors in the thoracic, thoracoabdominal, and lumbar spine is challenging but is being used more as surgeons become familiar with this special technique.

Lumbar Spine

For vertebral tumors below L1 a retroperitoneal approach is favored. Transpedicular vertebrectomy in this region is difficult because of the larger size of the vertebral body and the obstruction by nerve roots that cannot be transected as they control leg strength and sensation. L4 and L5 are often best approached from an anterior direction because of obstruction of direct lateral access by the ilium, the extent of which varies from patient to patient.

Sacrum

Tumors in the distal sacrum (S3 and below) can be approached solely from the back, usually without need for reconstruction, stabilization, or sacrifice of bowel or bladder function. Maintenance of such function requires that both S2 nerve roots be kept intact as well as one S3 nerve root. High sacral tumors (S1 and S2) require complete sacrectomy. This is a technically challenging and usually staged procedure with a total surgical time exceeding 24 hours and using the talents of multiple surgical services. Rehabilitation after total sacrectomy takes at least 3 months and the hospital stay is lengthy.

Postoperative Radiotherapy

Although en bloc resections are now being done in selected cases, most patients undergo removal of spinal metastasis by intralesional debulking. Although removal may appear complete both at the time of surgery and on postoperative imaging, microscopic disease almost invariably remains. Therefore, postoperative radiotherapy is given in most patients who have not previously undergone irradiation of the site. When used before surgery, radiotherapy is associated with infection and other problems of wound healing in one-third of patients. However, newer intensity-modulated methods and stereotactic radiosurgical techniques may allow tumor control without imposing such regional tissue compromise.

Laser Interstitial Thermal Therapy

In some patients who are poor surgical candidates but still need reduction in the size of an extradural tumor before going on to radiotherapy, LITT offers a way to decrease tumor volume without the stress and rigor of an open resection. In this methodology, a laser-emitting probe is inserted into the tumor under image guidance. The heat emitted from the probe tip ablates and shrinks the tumor, providing decompression of the spinal cord and adjacent nerves. The size and shape of the area of ablation can be controlled by using different probe windows, depths, and rotational angles; the intralesional temperature is monitored in real time by intraoperative MRI thermography. Patients so treated can proceed to radiotherapy without the delay for healing that a surgical incision would impose. As our clinical experience with LITT grows, we are determining with more precision which patients will gain maximum benefit from its application. This new approach, pioneered at MDACC, causes sufficient tumor shrinkage to decompress the spinal cord in some patients and achieves durable responses in many. It is particularly useful in elderly or frail patients.

Tumors of Peripheral Nerve

Tumors may arise on peripheral nerves anywhere that peripheral nerves go. Such tumors can be found anywhere in the extremities, trunk, soft tissues of neck and scalp, or on the skin surface. Most are benign and are identified either as neurofibromas or schwannomas. Solitary tumors such as those often found in the paraspinal region are typically schwannomas. Multiple such tumors confer a syndromic diagnosis of either neurofibromatosis or schwannomatosis, depending on tumor histology.

Neurofibromas can be either solitary (intraneural), diffuse (cutaneous), or plexiform (involving several nerve branches). Solitary neurofibromas are the most commonly encountered benign tumors of peripheral nerve. They are slow growing and relatively circumscribed lesions that cause pain, and less often sensory loss or weakness when they grow to large size. Solitary neurofibromas are not linked to a genetic disorder, but multiple neurofibromas indicate the presence of NF1, caused by loss of function of the *NF1* tumor suppressor gene on chromosome 17. Diffuse neurofibromas occur on the skin and in subcutaneous tissue of children and adolescents, and often are associated with NF1. Plexiform neurofibromas are pathognomonic for NF1 and appear as a fusiform and often quite large expansion of nerves in the extremities, face, or trunk. They can affect the brachial plexus or the lumbosacral plexus. When superficial they can cause cosmetic deformity to a distressing degree, and when a limb is affected, substantial expansion can compromise venous return and limb function.

Schwannomas are benign and slowly growing, well-encapsulated tumors composed of neoplastic Schwann cells in a collagenous matrix. They are the second most common tumor involving peripheral nerves and

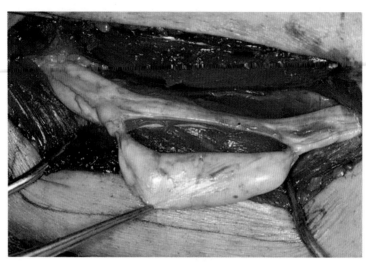

FIGURE 22.9 Intraoperative view of neurofibroma after its separation from the tibial nerve. The entering and exiting fascicles remain connected to the tumor, but are divided at this point to free the tumor. This approach allows preservation of most of the nerve, which courses around the tumor outside its capsule and remains connected and functional. This patient has NF1 and suffered no deficit from the tumor removal.

usually occur in patients between 30 and 60 years of age. Twenty percent are found along the median, ulnar, or radial nerves. These tend to cause a mild (or no) neurologic deficit, but pain can be a significant component of the clinical presentation. The classic distinction between neurofibromas and schwannomas holds that schwannomas are likely to arise from a small number of fascicles within the nerve, whereas neurofibromas arise more diffusely in the nerve and thus are more difficult to tease out surgically without nerve sacrifice.

In our experience both schwannomas and neurofibromas can usually be resected without sacrifice of nerve function by performing an intracapsular shelling out of the tumor (Fig. 22.9). Since these tumors are almost always histologically benign, any small remnants left behind in the approach rarely re-establish themselves to form recurrent tumor. Often the tumor arises from only one or two fascicles of the several hundred that make up the nerve, with most of the nerve bypassing the tumor albeit by following a somewhat distorted course. Although neurofibromas sometimes arise from a larger number of fascicles, many of them grow from four feeding fascicles or fewer. Thus, they too can be usually be resected in similar subcapsular fashion with similar likelihood of preserving nerve function. Some neurofibromas do run diffusely through the nerve as per the classical description, but the majority do not. Therefore, identity of a tumor as a neurofibroma should not preclude an attempt at resection as the nature of the tumor's origin and its resectability can only be determined at the time of surgical exposure.

Mutation of the *NF1* gene provokes the formation of neurofibromas. However, the alterations imposed by this syndrome are not limited to the induction of nerve sheath tumors. Patients are prone to have optic gliomas and frequently have short stature, neuropsychological abnormalities, a higher incidence of mental retardation, and dysplasia in the axial and appendicular skeleton as well as the skull. They have a higher incidence of intracranial glioma, usually astrocytoma, and of gastrointestinal stromal tumors and carcinomas of the breast. The diagnostic criteria for NF1 (and for neurofibromatosis type 2 [NF2], a separate disease with an entirely different tumor profile) are given in Table 22.8.

NF2 is a separate, much less common, and somewhat misnamed condition caused by a completely different gene defect on chromosome 22. Patients with this disease do not get neurofibromas at all, but schwannomas that largely affect cranial and spinal nerves. They are also susceptible to the development of multiple cranial or spinal meningiomas and have some risk of developing intracranial glioma. The pathognomonic lesion of NF2 is a bilateral vestibular schwannoma leading to loss of hearing.

The malignant form of each of these tumors is termed *malignant peripheral nerve sheath tumor* (MPNST) as a general descriptor. Although most schwannomas do not transform to a malignant tumor, melanotic schwannomas have a 10% chance of such transformation. For patients with NF1, the chance of developing an MPNST over the course of their lifetime is 10%. Such tumors are highly aggressive, invade locally, and can metastasize. Chemotherapy is ineffective, radiotherapy is palliative, and the main hope for treatment is early detection with a radical surgical removal. Two-thirds of MPNSTs arise from neurofibromas, usually in a patient with NF1. The 5-year survival rate is 15% to 20% in this category. Sporadic MPNSTs not associated with

NF1 have a somewhat better survival rate with a 5-year survival rate of 50%. It is possible to acquire an MPNST after exposure of the nerve to external beam irradiation. The treatment of these tumors, whatever their origin, is surgery and this can be performed either as radical amputation of the involved limb, sparing of the limb with transection of the involved nerve, or selective resection with nerve-sparing analogous to that performed for benign nerve sheath tumors. Although it is logical to suggest more radical strategies given the malignancy of this tumor type, we have had success in occasional patients treated with intracapsular resection because the MPNST may occupy only the core of the benign neurofibroma in which it arose, and which has maintained benign histology around its periphery. Using this strategy, we have achieved recurrence-free survival exceeding 10 years in some patients. Thus, we do advocate using this approach to give the patient at least a chance of retention of function, and save more aggressive resection for a second operation done for local recurrence.

In the past 5 years the classical categories of NF1 and NF2 have been joined by a third category, schwannomatosis. This occurs in patients with mutation of the *INI1* gene located on chromosome 22q at a separate locus from the *NF2* gene. Such patients have multiple schwannomas in peripheral, spinal, and cranial nerves. About one-third have segmental schwannomatosis limited to a single region of the body. Bilateral vestibular schwannomas have not yet been described in this disease, but unilateral involvement of the vestibular complex has been noted in a few patients. Schwannomatosis is not associated with learning disability and cannot be diagnosed without first ruling out the presence of a mutation in the *NF2* gene. Such patients present with pain syndromes which are quite amenable to relief by surgical resection (with nerve sparing, as above) of the offending tumor or tumors. The diagnostic criteria for schwannomatosis are based either on clinical criteria, or on molecular criteria combined with clinical criteria (Table 22.8).

TABLE 22.8   Diagnostic Criteria for NF1 and NF2

Neurofibromatosis Type 1
Patient has two or more of the following:
    Six or more café-au-lait spots
        >1.5 cm in post-puberty
        >0.5 before puberty
    Two or more neurofibromas of any type or at least one plexiform neurofibroma
    Freckling in axilla or groin
    Optic glioma
    Two or more Lisch nodules (hamartomas of iris)
    One or more distinctive bone lesions, e.g., sphenoid dysplasia or thinning of cortex of long bone
    One or more first-degree relatives with NF1

Neurofibromatosis Type 2
Confirmed NF2 has:
    Bilateral vestibular schwannomas
    Or
    Family history of NF2
    plus
    unilateral vestibular schwannoma at age <30 years or one or more of the following:
        Glioma
        Schwannoma
        Juvenile posterior subcapsular cortical opacities (in eye)

Schwanommatosis (Clinical Criteria or Molecular Combined With Clinical Criteria)
Clinical Criteria
Either of the following:
• Two or more nonintradermal schwannomas (at least one biopsy-confirmed) AND no evidence of bilateral vestibular schwannomas by high-quality MRI examination and detailed study of internal auditory canal (with and without gadolinium and with slices ≤3 mm) Note: Presence of a unilateral vestibular schwannoma or meningioma(s) does not exclude the diagnosis.
    or
• One pathologically confirmed schwannoma, unilateral vestibular schwannoma, or intracranial meningioma AND an affected first-degree relative with confirmed schwannomatosis

Combined Molecular and Clinical Criteria
Either of the following:
• A germline pathogenic mutation of either *SMARCB1* or *LZTR1* AND one pathologically confirmed schwannoma or meningioma
    or
• Two or more tumors (schwannoma, meningioma) each with 22q loss of heterozygosity and each with a different somatic pathogenic mutation of *NF2* AND two or more pathologically confirmed schwannomas or meningiomas AND none of the exclusion criteria
• The 22q deletions should have different breakpoints indicative of independent events

CHAPTER REVIEW

Questions

1. What is the most common overall cause of new-onset seizures in adults?

   A. Tumor
   B. Infection
   C. Electrolyte abnormality
   D. Stroke
   E. Head trauma

2. Brain tumors that frequently have calcifications seen on CT scan include:

   A. Meningiomas
   B. Astrocytomas
   C. Craniopharyngiomas
   D. Glioblastoma
   E. A and C

3. Cerebral perfusion pressure (SPP) is regulated by all of the below, except:

   A. Systemic blood pressure
   B. Arterial pCO_2
   C. Electrolyte abnormalities
   D. pO_2
   E. pH

4. The most common tumors that metastasize to the brain are:

   A. Melanoma
   B. Lung
   C. Breast
   D. Prostate
   E. Colorectal

5. The two histologic types of metastasis that are most likely to develop intracranial bleeding are:

   A. Colorectal and lung
   B. Melanoma and choriocarcinoma
   C. Choriocarcinoma and lung
   D. Lung and melanoma

Answers

1. **The correct answer is D.** *Rationale:* Overall, stroke is responsible for 25% to 40% of new-onset seizures, followed by metabolic causes (15% to 25%) and idiopathic causes (15% to 20%). Focal seizures are most commonly due to stroke (42%), infection (27%), and tumors (15%). Generalized seizures are most commonly due to idiopathic causes (34%), metabolic causes (20%), and infection (17%). Seizures occur 20% to 30% of the time as the presenting symptom in a patient with a brain tumor.

2. **The correct answer is E.** *Rationale:* Meningiomas and craniopharyngioma are both benign tumors that often contain calcifications. CT scan can help to narrow the differential diagnosis if calcifications are seen in the tumor.

3. **The correct answer is C.** *Rationale:* Arterial pCO_2 is the most potent stimulus for dilation of cerebral arterioles. Under physiologic conditions several factors regulate cerebral blood flow: systemic blood pressure, pCO_2 and pH in the arterial blood, and pO_2. Autoregulation maintains blood flow to the brain at a constant level over a wide range of MAP. When MAP is low, cerebral arterioles dilate to allow adequate flow. Increased systemic blood pressure causes arterioles to constrict for the same purpose. At MAP <50 mm Hg perfusion is inadequate; with MAP >150 the autoregulatory system fails and cerebral blood flow increases, leading to vasogenic edema, hypertensive encephalopathy, and dangerous elevations in ICP.

4. **The correct answer is B.** *Rationale:* Only 1% to 2% of ovarian and prostate cancers spread to the brain, but at least half of melanomas do when other systemic metastases are present. The most common histologic type of brain metastasis is carcinoma of the lung (40% to 60% of large clinical series), followed

by those derived from breast cancers (15% to 20%) and melanoma (10% to 20%). Colorectal and renal cell carcinomas account for 5% to 10% each. These five sources yield most cerebral metastases.

5. **The correct answer is B.** *Rationale:* Two histologies are particularly prone to intratumoral bleeding: melanoma and choriocarcinoma in which the bleeding rates are 45% and 95%, respectively.

Recommended Readings

Beiko J, Suki D, Hess KR, et al. IDH1 mutant malignant astrocytomas are more amenable to surgical resection and have a survival benefit associated with maximal surgical resection. *Neuro Oncol.* 2014;16:81–91.

Bilsky MH, Laufer I, Fourney DR, et al. Reliability analysis of the epidural spinal cord compression scale. *J Neurosurg Spine.* 2010;13:324–328.

Bindal RK, Sawaya R, Leavens ME, Lee JJ. Surgical treatment of multiple brain metastases. *J Neurosurg.* 1993;79:210–216.

Bolton WD, Rice DC, Goodyear A, et al. Superior sulcus tumors with vertebral body involvement: a multimodality approach. *J Thoracic Cardiovasc Surg.* 2009;137:1379–1387.

Brown PD, Ballman KV, Cerhan JH, et al. Postoperative stereotactic radiosurgery compared with whole brain radiotherapy for resected metastatic brain disease (NCCTG N107C/CEC·3): a multicentre, randomised, controlled, phase 3 trial. *Lancet Oncol.* 2017; 18: 1049–1060.

Buckner JC, Shaw EG, Pugh SL, et al. Radiation plus procarbazine, CCNU, and vincristine in low grade glioma. *N Engl J Med.* 2016;374:1344–1355.

Cairncross JG, Ueki K, Zlatescu MC, et al. Specific genetic predictors of chemotherapeutic response and survival in patients with anaplastic oligodendrogliomas. *J Natl Cancer Inst.* 1998;90:1473–1479.

Chi GH, Sciubba DM, Rhines LD, et al. Surgery for primary vertebral tumors: en bloc vs. intralesional resection. *Neurosurg Clin North Am.* 2008;19:111–117.

de Groot JF, Kim AH, Prabhu S, et al. Efficacy of laser interstitial thermal therapy (LITT) for newly diagnosed and recurrent IDH wild-type glioblastoma. *Neuro Oncol Adv.* 2022;4(1):vdac040. doi: 10.1093/noajnl/vdac040.

Dirks PB. Cancer: stem cells and brain tumors. *Nature.* 2006;444:687–688.

Dunn-Pinio AM, Vlahovic G. Immunotherapy approaches in the treatment of malignant brain tumors. *Cancer.* 2017;123:734–750.

Fisher CG, DiPaola CP, Ryken TC, et al. A novel classification system for spinal instability in neoplastic disease: an evidence-based approach and expert consensus from the Spine Oncology Study Group. *Spine.* 2010;35:E1221–E1229.

Fourney DR, Abi-Said D, Rhines LD, et al. Simultaneous anterior-posterior approach to the thoracic and lumbar spine for the radical resection of tumors followed by reconstruction and stabilization. *J Neurosurg.* 2001;94:232–244.

Fourney DR, Rhines LD, Hentschel SJ, et al. En bloc resection of primary sacral tumors: classification of surgical approaches and outcome. *J Neurosurg Spine.* 2005;3:111–122.

Garces-Ambrossi GL, McGirt MJ, et al. Factors associated with progression-free survival and long-term neurological outcome after resection of intramedullary spinal cord tumors: analysis of 101 consecutive cases. *J Neurosurg Spine.* 2009;11:591–599.

Goldberg SB, Schalper KA, Gettinger SN, et al. Pembrolizumab for management of patients with NSCLC and brain metastases: long-term results and biomarker analysis from a non-randomised, open-label, phase 2 trial. *Lancet Oncol.* 2020;21:655–663.

Hanbali F, Fourney DR, Marmor E, et al. Spinal cord ependymoma: radical resection and outcome. *Neurosurgery.* 2002;51:1162–1174.

Hansen-Algenstaedt N, Kwan MK, Algenstaedt P, et al. Comparison between minimally invasive surgery and conventional open surgery for patients with spinal metastasis: a prospective propensity score-matched study. *Spine.* 2017;42:789–797.

Hatiboglu MA, Weinberg JS, Suki D, et al. Impact of intraoperative high-field magnetic resonance imaging guidance on glioma surgery: a prospective volumetric analysis. *Neurosurgery.* 2009;64:1073–1081.

Hawkins C, Walker E, Mohamed N, et al. BRAF-KIAA1549 fusion predicts better clinical outcome in pediatric low-grade astrocytoma. *Clin Cancer Res.* 2011;17:4790–4798.

Hegi ME, Diserens AC, Gorlia T, et al. MGMT gene silencing and benefit from temozolomide in glioblastoma. *New Engl J Med.* 2005;352:997–1003.

Ho JC, Tang, C, Deegan BJ, et al. The use of spine stereotactic radiosurgery for oligometastatic disease. *J Neurosurg Spine.* 2016;25:239–247.

Holman PJ, Suki D, McCutcheon IE, Wolinsky JP, Rhines LD, Gokaslan ZL. Surgical management of metastatic disease of the lumbar spine: experience with 139 patients. *J Neurosurg Spine.* 2005;2:550–563.

Huse JT, Aldape KD. The evolving role of molecular markers in the diagnosis and management of diffuse glioma. *Clin Cancer Res.* 2014;20:5601–5611.

Jackson RJ, Fuller GN, Abi-Said D, et al. Limitations of stereotactic biopsy in the initial management of gliomas. *Neuro Oncol.* 2001;3:193–200.

Jackson RJ, Loh SC, Gokaslan Z. Metastatic renal cell carcinoma of the spine: surgical treatment and results. *J Neurosurg.* 2001;94:18–24.

Jiang H, Gomez-Manzano C, Lang FF, Alemany R, Fueyo J. Oncolytic adenovirus: preclinical and clinical studies in patients with human malignant gliomas. *Curr Gene Ther.* 2009;9:422–427.

Kehrer-Sawatzki H, Farschtschi S, Mautner VF, Cooper DN. The molecular pathogenesis of schwannomatosis, a paradigm for the co-involvement of multiple tumour suppressor genes in tumorigenesis. *Hum Genet.* 2017;136:129–148.

Kim SS, McCutcheon IE, Suki D, et al. Awake craniotomy for brain tumors near eloquent cortex: correlation of intraoperative cortical mapping with neurological outcomes in 309 consecutive patients. *Neurosurgery.* 2009;64:836–846.

Kim AH, Tatter S, Rao G, et al. Laser ablation of abnormal neurological tissue using robotic NeuroBlate system (LAANTERN): 12-month outcomes and quality of life after brain tumor ablation. *Neurosurgery.* 2020;87:E338–E346.

Knoll MA, Oermann EK, Yang AI, et al. Survival of patients with multiple intracranial metastases treated with stereotactic radiosurgery: does the number of tumors matter? *Am J Clin Oncol.* 2018;41:425–431.

Kunwar S, Chang S, Westphal M, et al. Phase III randomized trial of CED of IL13-PE38QQR vs Gliadel wafers for recurrent glioblastoma. *Neuro Oncol.* 2010;12:871–881.

Lacroix M, Abi-Said D, Fourney DF, et al. A multivariate analysis of 416 patients with glioblastoma multiforme: prognosis, extent of resection, and survival. *J Neurosurg.* 2001;95:190–198.

Lang FF, Conrad C, Gomez-Manzano C, et al. Phase I study of DNX-2401 (Delta-24-RGD) oncolytic adenovirus: replication and immunotherapeutic effects in recurrent malignant glioma. *J Clin Oncol.* 2018;36:1419–1427.

Louis DN, Perry A, Reifenberger G, et al. The 2016 World Health Organization classification of tumors of the central nervous system: a summary. *Acta Neuropathol.* 2016;131:803–820.

Louis DN, Perry A, Wesseling P, et al. The 2021 WHO classification of tumors of the central nervous system: a summary, *Neuro Oncol.* 2021;23:1231–1251.

MacCollin M, Chiocca EA, Evans DG, et al. Diagnostic criteria for schwannomatosis. *Neurology* 2005;64:1838–1845.

Mack F, Baumert BG, Schäfer N, et al. Therapy of leptomeningeal metastasis in solid tumors. *Cancer Treat Rev.* 2016;43:83–91.

Mahajan A, Ahmed S, McAleer MF, et al. Post-operative stereotactic radiosurgery versus observation for completely resected brain metastases: a single-centre, randomised, controlled, phase 3 trial. *Lancet Oncol.* 2017;18:1040–1048. Erratum in: Lancet Oncol. 2017;18(8):e433. Erratum in: Lancet Oncol. 2017;18(9):e510.

Maldaun MV, Khawja SN, Levine NB, et al. Awake craniotomy for gliomas in a high-field intraoperative magnetic resonance imaging suite: analysis of 42 cases. *J Neurosurg.* 2014;121:810–817.

Molinaro AM, Hervey-Jumper S, Morshed RA, et al. Association of maximal extent of resection of contrast-enhanced and non-contrast-enhanced tumor with survival within molecular subgroups of patients with newly diagnosed glioblastoma. *JAMA Oncol.* 2020;6:495–503. Erratum in: JAMA Oncol. 2020;6(3):444.

Muldoon LL, Soussain C, Jahnke K, et al. Chemotherapy delivery issues in central nervous system malignancy: a reality check. *J Clin Oncol.* 2007;25:2295–2305.

Ostrow KL, Bergner AL, Blakeley J, et al. Creation of an international registry to support discovery in schwannomatosis. *Am J Med Genet A.* 2016;173:407–413.

Pajtler KW, Witt H, Sill M, et al. Molecular classification of ependymal tumors across all CNS compartments, histopathological grades, and age groups. *Cancer Cell.* 2015;27:728–743.

Patchell RA, Tibbs PA, Regine WF, et al. Postoperative radiotherapy in the treatment of single metastases to the brain: a randomized trial. *JAMA.* 1998;280:1485–1489.

Patchell RA, Tibbs PA, Regine WF, et al. Direct decompressive surgical resection in the treatment of spinal cord compression caused by metastatic cancer: a randomised trial. *Lancet.* 2005;366:643–648.

Patchell RA, Tibbs PA, Walsh JW, et al. A randomized trial of surgery in the treatment of single metastases to the brain. *N Engl J Med.* 1990;322:494–500.

Patel AJ, Suki D, Hatiboglu MA, et al. Factors influencing the risk of local recurrence after resection of a single brain metastasis. *J Neurosurg.* 2010;113:181–189.

Plotkin SR, Blakeley JO, Evans DG, et al. Update from the 2011 international schwannomatosis workshop: from genetics to diagnostic criteria. *Am J Med Genet. A* 2013;161A:405–416.

Prabhu SS, Gasco J, Tummala S, Weinberg JS, Rao G. Intraoperative magnetic resonance imaging-guided tractography with integrated monopolar subcortical functional mapping for resection of brain tumors. *J Neurosurg.* 2011;114:719–726.

Rao G, Chang GJ, Suk I, Gokaslan Z, Rhines LD. Midsacral amputation for en bloc resection of hordoma. *Neurosurgery.* 2010;66(suppl 3):41–44.

Rao G, Suki D, Charkrabarti I, et al. Surgical management of primary and metastatic sarcoma of the mobile spine. *J Neurosurg Spine.* 2008;9:120–128.

Sampson JH, Archer GE, Mitchell DA, et al. An epidermal growth factor receptor variant III-targeted vaccine is safe and immunogenic in patients with glioblastoma multiforme. *Mol Cancer Ther.* 2009;8:2773–2779.

Schindler G, Capper D, Meyer J, et al. Analysis of BRAF V600E mutation in 1,320 nervous system tumors reveals high mutation frequencies in pleomorphic xanthoastrocytoma, ganglioglioma and extra-cerebellar pilocytic astrocytoma. *Acta Neuropathol.* 2011;121:397–405.

Smith MJ, Bowers NL, Bulman M, et al. Revisiting neurofibromatosis type 2 diagnostic criteria to exclude LZTR1-related schwannomatosis. *Neurology.* 2017;88:87–92.

Smith JS, Chang EF, Lamborn KR, et al. Role of extent of resection in the long-term outcome of low grade hemispheric gliomas. *J Clin Oncol.* 2008;26:1338–1345.

Stupp R, Hegi ME, Mason WP, et al. Effects of radiotherapy with concomitant and adjuvant temozolomide versus radiotherapy alone on survival in glioblastoma in a randomised phase III study: 5-year analysis of the EORTC-NCIC trial. *Lancet.* 2009;10:459–466.

Suki D, Hatiboglu MA, Patel AJ, et al. Comparative risk of leptomeningeal dissemination of cancer after surgery or stereotactic radiosurgery for a single supratentorial solid tumor metastasis. *Neurosurgery.* 2010;64:664–676.

Tatsui CE, Lee SH, Amini B, et al. Spinal laser interstitial thermal therapy: a novel alternative to surgery for metastatic epidural spinal cord compression. *Neurosurgery.* 2016;79(suppl 1):S73–S82.

Tawbi HA, Forsyth PA, Algazi A, et al. Combined nivolumab and ipilimumab in melanoma metastatic to the brain. *N Engl J Med.* 2018;379:722–730.

Tawbi HA, Forsyth PA, Hodi FS, et al. Long-term outcomes of patients with active melanoma brain metastases treated with combination nivolumab plus ipilimumab (CheckMate 204): final results of an open-label, multicentre, phase 2 study. *Lancet Oncol.* 2021;22:1692–1704.

Traylor JI, Patel R, Muir M, et al. Laser interstitial thermal therapy for glioblastoma: a single-center experience. *World Neurosurg.* 2021;149:e244-e252.

Weller M, Butowski N, Tran DD, et al. Rindopepimut with temozolomide for patients with newly diagnosed, EGFRvIII-expressing glioblastoma (ACT IV): a randomised, double-blind, international phase 3 trial. *Lancet Oncol.* 2017;18:1373–1385

Weller M, Kaulich K, Hentschel B, et al. Assessment and prognostic significance of the epidermal growth factor receptor VIII mutation in glioblastoma patients treated with concurrent and adjuvant temozolomide radiochemotherapy. *Int J Cancer.* 2014;134:2437–2447.

Williams BJ, Fox BD, Sciubba DM, et al. Surgical management of prostate cancer metastatic to the spine. *J Neurosurg Spine.* 2009;10:414–422.

Yamamoto M, Serizawa T, Shuto T, et al. Stereotactic radiosurgery for patients with multiple brain metastases (JLGK0901): a multi-institutional prospective observational study. *Lancet Oncol.* 2014;15:387–395.

Yu J, Deshmukh H, Gutmann RJ, Emnett RJ, Rodriguez FJ, Watson MA, Nagarajan R, Gutmann DH. Alterations of BRAF and HIPK2 loci predominate in sporadic pilocytic astrocytoma. *Neurology.* 2009;73:1526–1531.

INTRODUCTION

Cancer of unknown primary (CUP) comprises 1% to 2% of the global cancer burden. This enigmatic process is defined as any metastatic tumor for which all standard investigations have failed to identify a primary site. As diagnostic studies have improved the prevalence of CUP has declined, but the majority of primaries are only identified post-mortem. Surgeons are often asked to evaluate patients with CUP to obtain tissue for diagnostic studies or to treat isolated or clinically symptomatic metastases.

In this chapter we define the entity of CUP in the modern era of precision medicine, discuss the role of the surgeon in the care of this unique population and introduce chemotherapeutic and more novel immunotherapeutic treatment options.

Definition of the Entity

Despite the beguiling simplicity of the concept, our understanding of CUP as an entity is lacking. The prevailing hypotheses suggest that either a microscopic primary exists intact throughout the disease process but is unable to be identified, or that angiogenic incompetence of the primary results in its involution after seeding metastatic cells elsewhere. With the advent of new molecular assessments and improved radiologic examinations in the last three decades, the incidence of CUP has declined from 3% to 5% of all malignancies to the current incidence of 1% to 2%. However, there are still a significant number of patients for whom primary processes are never identified despite spending their last year of life performing exhaustive diagnostic testing.

CUP is comprised of a heterogeneous group of histologic subtypes, including adenocarcinoma (60%, typically poorly differentiated), squamous cell cancer (5%) and carcinoma or other undifferentiated neoplasms (35%). The median survival for all patients with CUP is 6 to 9 months, regardless of treatment options. Separately, the literature now differentiates patients with "favorable" and "unfavorable" subsets with regard to clinicopathologic prognosis (Table 23.1). The favorable subset is defined by a group of patients whose tumors have clinical or histologic characteristics allowing providers to link treatment to a targeted tissue type (e.g., breast, ovarian, head and neck squamous cell, cervical, anal) and therefore have an expectation of better response and overall survival. The median survival for this group is 11 to 13 months. For patients with poorly differentiated CUPs or those that cannot be assigned to a putative tissue type (80% to 85% of patients with CUP), the prognosis is very poor, driving clinicians to seek targetable mutations and other routes to generate more effective treatment plans.

Two schools of thought govern the care of patients with CUP. Many clinicians focus on aggressively seeking the tissue of origin to guide therapy, running often lengthy diagnostic workups that may or may not be revealing. The alternative "tissue agnostic" approach suggests using tumor marker positivity to direct targeted therapy, regardless of tissue type. As targeted therapy becomes more mainstream for known tumor types, the

TABLE 23.1 Favorable and Unfavorable Clinicopathologic Subsets of Cancer of Unknown Primary (CUP)

Favorable Subsets	Unfavorable Subsets
Poorly differentiated carcinoma with midline nodal distribution	Adenocarcinoma metastatic to the liver or other organs
Poorly differentiated neuroendocrine carcinoma	Malignant ascites from a nonpapillary adenocarcinoma
Squamous cell carcinoma involving the cervical lymph nodes	Multiple cerebral metastases of any type
Single small metastasis, any type	Multiple lung/pleural metastases from adenocarcinoma
Isolated inguinal lymphadenopathy from squamous carcinoma	Multiple metastatic bone lesions from adenocarcinoma
Men with blastic bone lesions from adenocarcinoma with elevated serum prostate-specific antigen	
Women with papillary adenocarcinoma of peritoneal cavity	
Women with adenocarcinoma involving only axillary lymph nodes	

Adapted from Pentheroudakis G, Greco FA, Pavlidis N. Molecular assignment of tissue of origin in cancer of unknown primary may not predict response to therapy or outcome: a systematic literature review. *Cancer Treat Rev.* 2009;35:221–227, with permission from Elsevier.

utility of these medications for CUP patients will expand, hopefully improving the relatively dire prognosis of this elusive disease process.

The Role of the Surgeon

Surgeons interact with patients with CUP at many stages, from diagnosis to palliation. Frequently, the amount of tissue required to complete immunohistochemistry studies, cytogenetic analysis, and molecular profiling exceeds what can be obtained on core needle biopsy. Surgeons can provide more tissue for pathologic evaluation by performing excisional biopsy of lymph nodes or peritoneal nodules. Patients with a single site of disease and no evidence of distant metastases are even candidates for curative resection. Determining which patients should undergo resection and for what indication can be challenging. The response to any neoadjuvant chemotherapy or immunotherapy, patient performance status and the implications for patient quality of life must be carefully considered before proceeding to the operating room.

General Workup

History and Physical

A thorough oncologic history including personal history of cancers or resection of benign growths can reveal potential sources of latent metastases. A minority of patients with CUP (10%) have a history of an antecedent cancer. A family history of cancer can likewise guide the investigation toward familial syndromes or genetic testing.

The physical examination should be complete, with particular care taken in areas of suspicion. For example, isolated cervical lymphadenopathy demands an examination of the oropharynx, hypopharynx, nasopharynx and larynx, typically aided with an indirect fiberoptic laryngoscopy. The thyroid gland should be examined for enlargement or asymmetry and all nodal basins should be palpated.

A careful breast examination for both women and men should be performed, as well as a bimanual pelvic examination for females and testicular and prostate examinations for men. A digital rectal examination and thorough skin examination of lower extremities should be performed, including perianal skin, particularly for isolated inguinal nodal masses.

Biopsy and Pathologic Evaluation

Often one of the first steps in caring for patients with CUP is obtaining a fine needle aspiration biopsy of the most accessible lesion to attempt to determine the tissue of origin. Historical details should be communicated clearly to the pathologist to help guide their review. Simple light microscopy with hematoxylin and eosin staining is often sufficient to determine the cellular type. Previously, electron microscopy was used to evaluate for particular signs of melanoma or lymphoma, however, immunohistochemical staining has largely replaced that methodology.

Laboratory Studies, Serum Markers

All patients should have routine laboratory evaluation, including complete blood cell count, chemistry studies, and liver function tests, as well as fecal occult blood testing for those with anemia or history of blood in stool. Beyond these basic tests, clinical laboratory studies are of marginal value. Serum tumor markers for standard oncologic processes should be obtained, including CEA, CA19-9, CA 15-3, CA125, PSA and AFP, β-hCG if pertinent based on patient and tumor characteristics, although many markers can be overexpressed in a nonspecific fashion and may not guide treatment. Evaluating human papillomavirus (HPV) status by PCR can aid in prognostication for patients with squamous type CUP, as patients with HPV+ tumors often have a better outcome. Tumor markers can be helpful in trending progress on treatment. Table 23.2 lists several common tumor markers and their roles in clinical evaluation with CUP.

Imaging

Radiographic evaluation should be focused on delineating the extent of disease, as well as on potentially identifying a primary lesion. A CT scan of the chest, abdomen and pelvis with intravenous contrast is essential to the baseline workup of these patients. Mammography for females is indicated. For younger women or those with dense breasts, MRI is an important alternative, identifying otherwise occult breast tumors in 75% of patients. Females with isolated axillary lymphadenopathy and adenocarcinoma features on pathology fall into the favorable subset of CUP patients and often have a much better prognosis than the overall cohort. Identifying a lesion on breast imaging can dramatically change therapy, in that a negative breast MRI predicts a low yield at mastectomy and may drive clinicians to pursue nonoperative therapies including chemotherapy, breast radiation, and watchful waiting.

A Stepwise Approach to Utilizing Immunohistochemistry in the Diagnosis of CUP

Immunohistochemical Marker[a]	Potential Cancer Type
Step 1: detects broad types of cancer	
Pan-cytokeratin and/or EMA	Carcinoma
CLA and/or CD45RB and EMA⁻	Lymphoma
Vimentin, desmin, S100, αSMA, myoDl, CD34, KIT, and/or CD99	Sarcoma
S100, HMB45 and/or Melan-A	Melanoma
Step 2: detects broad types of carcinoma	
PAS, CK7 and/or CK20	Adenocarcinoma
CK5, CK6 and/or p63	SCC
Chromogranin, synaptophysin, PGP9.5 and/or CD56	Neuroendocrine carcinoma
PLAP, OCT4, AFP, and/or hCG	Germ-cell carcinoma
Step 3: categorizes carcinomas into subgroups according to CK7 and CK20 expression	
CK7⁺ and CK20⁺	Ovarian mucinous or pancreatic adenocarcinoma, urothelial carcinoma or cholangiocarcinoma
CK7⁺ and CK20⁻	Lung adenocarcinoma, cholangiocarcinoma, or breast, thyroid, endometrial, ovarian, cervical, salivary gland, or pancreatic carcinoma
CK7⁻ and CK20⁺	Colorectal or Merkel cell carcinoma
CK7⁻ and CK20⁻	SCC or hepatocellular, renal cell, prostate, small-cell lung or head and neck carcinoma
Step 4: suggests potential origin of adenocarcinoma	
ER, GCDFP-15, and/or mammaglobulin (CK7⁺ and CK20⁻)	Breast carcinoma
CA-125, mesothelin, WT 1 and/or ER (CK7⁺ and CK20⁻)	Ovarian cancer (serous papillary)
CA-125 and/or ER (CK7⁺ and CK20⁻)	Endometrial carcinoma
PSA and/or PAP (CK7⁻ and CK20⁻)	Prostate carcinoma
CDX2 and/or CEA (CK7⁻ and CK20⁺)	Colon carcinoma
CA-125 and/or mesothelin (CK7⁺ and CK20±)	Pancreatic adenocarcinoma
Hep Par-1, AFR, polyclonal CEA, CD10 and/or CD13 (CK7⁻ and CK20⁻)	Hepatocellular carcinoma
TTF1 (CK7⁺ and CK20⁻)	Non–small-cell lung cancer (lung adenocarcinoma)
CD10 (CK7⁻ and CK20⁻)	Renal cell carcinoma
TTF1 and/or thyroglobulin (CK7⁺ and CK20⁻)	Thyroid carcinoma

αSMA, α-smooth muscle actin; AFP, α-fetoprotein; CA-125; cancer antigen 125; CDX2, caudal type homeobox 2; CEA. carcinoembryonic antigen; CK, cytokeratin; CLA, cutaneous lymphocyte-associated antigen; CUP, cancer of unknown primary; EMA, epithelial membrane antigen; ER, estrogen receptor; GCDFP-15, gross cystic disease fluid protein 15; hCC, human chorionic gonadotropin; Hep Par-1, hepatocyte-specific antigen; myoD1, myoblast determination protein 1; OCT4, octamer-binding transcription factor 4; PAP; prostatic acid phosphatase; PAS, periodic acid Schiff; PGP9.5, protein gene product 9.5; PLAP, placental alkaline phosphatase; PSA, prostate-specific antigen; SCC, squamous-cell carcinoma; TTF1, thyroid transcription factor 1; WT1, Wilms tumor protein.
[a]Potential cancer type designation is determined by positivity for marker, unless otherwise indicated.
Reprinted by permission from Springer: Rassy E, Pavlidis N. Progress in refining the clinical management of cancer of unknown primary in the molecular era. *Nat Rev Clin Oncol.* 2020;17:541–554.

Positron emission tomography (PET) is controversial for the initial evaluation of all CUP patients. For those with squamous cell histology and isolated head/neck lymphadenopathy (cervical CUP), it is particularly useful. If an occult primary or further sites of disease can be identified, radiation therapy can be better targeted, decreasing complications and also allowing for improved prognostication and surveillance. In a review of 16 studies, Rusthoven et al. found that PET scan has a sensitivity of 88% in the cervical CUP population and PET scans allowed for the identification of 25% more primary tumors and 27% more regional or distant metastases than were found on conventional workup including panendoscopy. PET is also beneficial in the subset of CUP patients with primarily osseous disease, as it can be used to both identify the extent of disease and in surveillance for response to therapy.

Further Location-Specific Workup
Patients with cervical CUP with suspicion for head and neck squamous origin have a better prognosis than all-comers with CUP. The neck comprises more than 25 nodal basins, and common sites of metastases can

guide localization of an occult primary. A CT of the head, neck and chest with intravenous contrast will provide complete staging information. The base of the tongue, pyriform sinus and nasopharynx routinely harbor occult disease and some recommend random biopsy of these areas for diagnostic purposes. In addition, for those with a truly occult primary, bilateral tonsillectomy is indicated and can yield a small cancer in the deep crypts.

Axillary adenopathy histologically consistent with adenocarcinoma should prompt evaluation for lung, gastrointestinal, and genitourinary tumors. In females, the concern for occult breast tumors is at the top of the differential. As discussed earlier, bilateral breasts should be examined and thoroughly imaged, including MRI. The specimen should be studied for ER, PR and Her-2/neu status, in addition to GATA-3, mammoglobulin and TRPS1 to optimize chances of a primary diagnosis.

Immunohistochemistry

Immunohistochemical analysis has become routine, with a broad range of markers available to assist in diagnosis. Thyroid transcription factor (TTF-1) and cytokeratins 7 and 20 are commonly used, as the combination of these three markers can delineate between primary lung tumors and metastatic adenocarcinoma. This can be particularly useful in the setting of metastatic pleural effusion. No single marker is 100% specific, and many of the tests can even increase confusion when taken into context with radiographic findings, so it is imperative to appreciate the groupings that together can improve sensitivity and specificity in the proper cellular context.

Breast markers are particularly pertinent for patients presenting with adenocarcinoma found in axillary lymphadenopathy. Estrogen receptor (ER), progesterone receptor (PR), Her-2/neu and gross cystic disease fibrous protein should be checked in this group. Isolated liver metastases can present a diagnostic challenge, distinguishing cholangiocarcinoma from adenocarcinoma and hepatocellular carcinoma and thus markers can be used in a directed fashion in these CUP cases. Hep-par-1 is a hepatocellular carcinoma marker and CK-19 can be useful in cholangiocarcinoma. Neuron-specific enolase and chromogranin are useful for neuroendocrine cancers.

Molecular Profiling

It is presently possible to use epigenetic or transcriptomic classification and DNA or RNA sequencing to describe both potential tumor tissue type and biomarkers, allowing for guided therapies. The tissue from CUP lesions does not necessarily have the same genetic signature as the primary lesion does (or did), likely reflecting the difference in biology and behavior of these aggressive clones. A variety of specific gene mutations or levels of protein expressions have been studied in CUP patients, with some of the relationships offering prognostic implications and treatment direction. For instance, in 54% of patients, higher levels of MAPK phosphorylation (>40% of cells) are associated with a much worse overall survival than those with lower levels of phosphor-MAPK, related to chemotherapy responsiveness (9 months vs. 17 months, $P = .016$). Expression of $3p21^{CIP1}$ correlates with CUP subtype and is associated with favorable survival.

Molecular signatures can be ascertained from CUP specimens using quantitative real-time PCR, microarray analysis or microRNA profiling and compared to banks of known molecular profiles for common cancer types. The degree of similarity between the unknown and known cancer types can facilitate prediction of the primary tumor type, with accuracy ranging 54% to 98% in studies compared to clinicopathologic criteria. This would allow tissue-directed chemotherapy treatment.

Even more interesting is the use of next-generation sequencing, in that it allows physicians to compare the CUP tumors to typical sets of mutations that occur in specific types of known tumors, but more importantly, it can identify targetable mutations and allow for directed therapy, without necessarily identifying a tumor type at all. As new drugs are approved in a tissue-agnostic fashion that target specific genomic alterations, some patients with CUP stand to benefit from targeted therapies.

Treatment and Management of Specific Clinicopathologic Subgroups

In general, the 15% to 20% of patients who have a constellation of findings that suggest a specific tissue of origin can be treated with chemotherapy targeting the putative primary tumor type and have a better overall survival. However, the majority of patients with disseminated disease who do not have a tissue type have a much poorer response to chemotherapy and therefore, a worse prognosis. Adolescents and younger adults tend to have better survival than the overall group, in part, due to the fact that they are more likely to have squamous (29% vs. 10%) or neuroendocrine type (39% vs. 5%) CUP.

For cervical CUP, a radical neck dissection and postoperative radiation is indicated. Chemotherapy is advised for N2-3 disease. The survival for patients with squamous cervical CUP ranges from 32% to 55% at 5 years, with a local control rate of 75% to 85%. For metastatic adenocarcinoma, the survival is significantly lower. Both lymphadenectomy and radiation therapy are less effective, with local recurrence essentially 100% and 5-year survival 0% to 10%.

For patients with a positive left supraclavicular node (Virchow's node), the differential widens to include metastatic adenocarcinoma from abdominal origin. One retrospective study reviewed 152 FNA biopsy samples of clinically positive supraclavicular nodes, comparing sites of primary tumor when the mass was in the right compared to the left supraclavicular node. Sixteen of 19 primary pelvic tumors metastasized to the left supraclavicular node and 100% (6 of 6) primary abdominal malignancies metastasized to the left supraclavicular node. However, thoracic, breast, and head and neck malignancies did not differ in patterns of metastasis to the right and left supraclavicular nodes. On the basis of this study, the search for the primary tumor should be focused on the abdomen and pelvis in patients who present with adenocarcinoma in a left-sided supraclavicular (Virchow's) node. Front line chemotherapy based on histology is the treatment of choice, as involvement of this node in adenocarcinoma is often a marker of aggressive biology.

In patients with axillary lymph node adenocarcinoma, the presumptive diagnosis of breast cancer in females implies better prognosis when compared to other patients with CUP. Treatment for this condition has evolved immensely of late, with several accepted initial approaches: mastectomy with axillary dissection, observation, neoadjuvant chemotherapy (of particular consideration in triple negative subtypes) or locoregional radiation therapy alone. A retrospective review shows that mastectomy patients with occult tumors had primaries found in the mastectomy specimen in 50% to 65% of cases. Observation of the breast along with axillary dissection can result in recurrence in the breast (anywhere from 25% to 75% of cases), which requires further treatment. The third approach, using locoregional radiation therapy alone, has been shown to decrease local recurrence rate. At the MD Anderson Cancer Center, patients treated with axillary dissection alone were found to have a recurrence rate of 65% at 10 years, while the combination of axillary dissection and regional radiation including the breast reduces the recurrence rate to 25%. In terms of overall survival, this treatment was no different than those who had undergone mastectomy for the same stage of disease. For those who continue on to adjuvant chemotherapy after axillary dissection and radiation, the survival rate is increased from 60% to 85% at 10 years. Selective ER blockade is indicated for ER or PR positive tumors.

Patients with hepatic CUP make up 30% to 40% of the "unfavorable" subset, having a median overall survival of 1 to 7 months and a 1-year survival of 5% to 12%. Peritoneal lesions carry a similarly poor prognosis. Empiric treatment with platinum agents, gemcitabine, 5FU, leucovorin, or capecitabine in a variety of combinations is the standard-of-care. However, as genotyping becomes more readily available, targeting of specific mutations in these tumors may allow for improved survival over the generic chemotherapy available presently. In patients with disease confined to the liver, that appears to be resectable, there may be a role for surgery.

A few patients with CUP present with isolated inguinal adenopathy, many of whom may have squamous cell carcinomas presumed to arise from the pelvis, anus, or genitourinary tract. A thorough workup and examination to search for primary lesions is indicated, as these patients may be candidates for multimodality curative therapy to possibly include radiation, surgery and chemotherapy, even with spread to regional lymph nodes.

The choice of systemic therapy has evolved with the utility of more sophisticated diagnostic tools. As molecular classification based on gene mutations and protein expression improves, more patients will move from the unfavorable to the favorable subset with better targeted therapies available. For example, following identification of renal-cell carcinoma gene signatures, patients with renal-cell–like CUP responded very well to tyrosine kinase inhibition, whereas they had poor response to standard-of-care empiric chemotherapy. Patients with an IHC suggestive of a colon profile (CK20+, CK7-, and CDX2+) may respond to established chemotherapy regimens for colorectal cancer and have an improved overall survival. Nonrandomized prospective studies have been completed demonstrating better overall survival for all patients who received tumor type-specific therapy after primary type prediction (overall survival 12.5 to 13.6 months vs. 6 to 9 months). One study used a 92-gene quantitative real-time PCR classifier and the other a DNA-methylation microarray classifier, identifying CUP types consistent with pancreatic, breast, cholangio, colorectal and urothelial origin among others. Clinically relevant "druggable" genetic mutations have been reported in 85% to 96% of CUP patients, of which 13% to 64% can be targeted using FDA-approved techniques. This includes use of tyrosine kinase inhibitors, immune modulators, and agents targeted at BRAF and HER2 mutations.

In addition, as the role of immunotherapy expands across the oncologic landscape, it may play a role in certain patients with CUP. For example, PD-1 is expressed in 63% of masses, PD-L1 in 21%, and 1.8% demonstrate microsatellite instability (MSI-H). For these patients, plus those with a high tumor mutational burden (TMB-H), treatment with immune checkpoint inhibitors could offer substantial benefit for patients with ambiguous CUP tumors and an otherwise very poor prognosis.

Conclusion

For patients with CUP, curative therapy remains elusive and perhaps unrealistic. As surgeons, we must appreciate our role in diagnosis, workup, and palliation of CUP. However, as progress continues in the identification of new targetable mutations, we must advocate for this group of patients to ensure they are included in trials of agents that can offer them the possibility of therapeutic benefit. Treatment of CUP is the epitome of personalized medicine, and as such, these patients should be managed by a multidisciplinary team, focusing on improving both survival and quality of life.

CASE SCENARIO

Case Scenario 1

Presentation

A 60-year-old Caucasian male presents to your clinic with an enlarged right axillary lymph node that he palpated in the shower. The node is nontender, somewhat mobile, but firm. He has no known history of any medical problems. He has no surgical history except removal of a skin lesion from his posterior shoulder when he was 22 years old. He was told the lesion was "just a mole" when it was removed, and no pathology information is available.

Additional Workup

A full history reveals he was adopted and is unsure of his family history with regard to cancers. He does drink 2 beers daily but has no other drug use history. His sun exposure history is minimal—he lives in a cold climate and has never had a peeling sunburn. On physical examination, he is overweight with BMI 32. He has no other suspicious skin lesions including on his extremities and nail beds. His prior mole excision scar was unremarkable with no surrounding pigmentation. You do note a small firm density in the subareolar region of his right nipple. He states he has never noticed this in the past.

He has baseline labs that demonstrate a normal CBC, normal liver function, and normal creatinine. He is sent for bilateral mammogram, FNA of the palpable lymph node, axillary ultrasound, as well has core needle biopsy of the right breast lesion. The mammogram reveals a cluster of calcifications in the right breast just under the areola, approximately 1.5 cm in size. His breast biopsy returns as ductal carcinoma in situ. His lymph node biopsy demonstrates invasive ductal carcinoma, and there are no other suspicious lymph nodes on right axillary ultrasound. Tissue from the lymph node is estrogen and progesterone receptor positive, HER2/*neu* negative.

Approach to Treatment

At the time of his axillary node biopsy, a clip should be placed to facilitate localization during surgical resection. His case is concerning for primary invasive ductal carcinoma with metastasis to the right axillary nodal basin, despite his biopsy revealing only DCIS in the breast. He should undergo further imaging for possible extrathoracic spread including CT of the chest, abdomen, and pelvis as well as a bone scan. If those are negative for spread outside of the breast and axilla, he should undergo simple mastectomy with sentinel lymph node biopsy using blue dye and technetium for mapping. At the time of his sentinel node resection, the grossly positive node should also be removed using localization techniques if necessary (magnetic seed can be placed preoperatively if the node is challenging to palpate).

His risk of further nodal spread is >10%, and axillary lymph node dissection should be considered, particularly if the sentinel nodes are positive. Depending on the Ki-67 index, tumor grade and size of the metastatic disease in the lymph nodes, he could also be a candidate for chest wall and regional lymphatic radiation if axillary dissection is not performed.

Next Steps and Surveillance

The patient should have genetic testing for BRCA, as he could be at higher risk for subsequent cancers in the future. If he is BRCA positive, he should undergo high-risk screening, including biannual clinical examinations and bilateral mammograms alternating with breast MRI every 6 months. He may consider risk-reducing prophylactic contralateral mastectomy. He will require hormone therapy (tamoxifen).

Take Home Points

- A broad differential is required in treating cancer of unknown origin. Although this case was highly suspicious for melanoma, a thorough history and physical helped to diagnose the underlying malignancy.
- Biopsy of the lymph node is critical. Without a clear primary to target, core needle biopsy may confer more information than an FNA, where tissue is limited.

CASE SCENARIO 1 REVIEW

Case Scenario 1 Questions

1. What factors put this patient at higher risk of male breast cancer?

   A. Alcohol use
   B. Obesity
   C. Age >50 years
   D. Caucasian race
   E. A–C are risk factors

2. If the patient had a prior diagnosis of melanoma that was resected, not just a mole, how would that change your management?

   A. It would not, I would still proceed with full history and physical examination first.
   B. I would request a biopsy of the node before evaluating the patient.
   C. I would order a workup associated with metastatic melanoma including chest x-ray and LDH levels before evaluating the patient.
   D. I would refer the patient directly to medical oncology first.

3. What is the patient's risk of testing positive for BRCA2 given his diagnosis of breast cancer?

   A. 85%
   B. 74%
   C. 50%
   D. 22%
   E. 14%

4. What is the lifetime risk of breast cancer for males? For males with BRCA1? For males with BRCA2?

   A. 0.1%, 15%, 99%
   B. 1%, 15%, 99%
   C. 0.1%, 1%, 7%
   D. 1%, 7%, 15%
   E. None of the above

Case Scenario 1 Answers

1. **The correct answer is E.** *Rationale:* Alcohol use, obesity and older age are risk factors for male breast cancer. Family history of breast cancer, particularly BRCA+, is a prominent risk factor. In addition, history of exposure to estrogen therapy, radiation exposure to the chest, Klinefelter syndrome or history of testicular surgery/orchiectomy all increase the risk of male breast cancer. Race is not associated with an increased risk.

2. **The correct answer is A.** *Rationale:* Workup for any new mass should always begin with a full history and physical examination.

3. **The correct answer is E.** *Rationale:* Up to 14% of males diagnosed with breast cancers are found to have BRCA2 positivity.

4. **The correct answer is C.** *Rationale:* The lifetime risk of breast cancer in males is 0.1%, increasing 10-fold to 1% for those with known BRCA1 mutation, and between 7% and 8% for those with BRCA2 mutation.

CASE SCENARIO

Case Scenario 2

Presentation

A 29-year-old male is seen by his primary care physician for a lump in his left neck, just below his ear. He just noticed the lump following a particularly bad head cold—describing he had "swollen glands" but this one lump did not seem to resolve as the rest did. He has no other medical problems. He had a laparoscopic appendectomy as a child, but no other surgical history. He has no family history of cancers, no history of exposure to ionizing radiation. He does not smoke or chew tobacco.

Additional Workup

A full history and physical examination are performed. He has a single firm, small, left-sided level II lymph node that is nontender to palpation. His thyroid gland is small with no palpable nodularity. A complete oral examination is negative for any suspicious lesions. An indirect fiberoscopic examination of the larynx and pharynx are unrevealing. His tonsils and adenoids are intact with no obvious lesions.

He is sent for basic laboratory tests which are unrevealing. An ultrasound of his left neck lymph basins is performed with only one suspicious node demonstrated. An FNA is performed that is unrevealing—only necrotic and inflammatory cells are found. He returns for a core needle biopsy under ultrasound guidance, as well as a thyroid ultrasound which is unrevealing. The core needle biopsy is sent for pathologic evaluation including a variety of tumor markers and is found to be squamous cell in nature with positive HPV PCR.

A CT of the head, neck and chest is performed with no visible lesions noted aside from his single left neck node. PET-CT is pursued with no FDG-avid lesions aside from the palpable lymph node. He is taken to the OR for a more complete endoscopy and random biopsies of his base of tongue, nasopharynx, and oral mucosa are performed. A tonsillectomy and adenoidectomy are also performed with no suspicious lesions on final pathology.

Approach to Treatment

Unfortunately, no primary lesion was able to be identified, so further management will include either radiotherapy or radical lymphadenectomy of the left neck, or both. He would be a candidate for radiation therapy of the left neck nodal basins, however, given his age, absent comorbidities and palpable disease, a selective lymphadenectomy would be indicated (minimum 18 nodes). As his PET/CT was negative for other sites of disease, he would not require further chemotherapy. If he had a large burden of positive nodes during the dissection or extranodal extension, adjuvant high-dose cisplatin chemotherapy or lower-dose cisplatin chemotherapy with adjuvant radiation to the nodal basin would be recommended. If the patient had already undergone resection of the affected node and did not have a proper lymphadenectomy, radiation therapy would be indicated.

Next Steps and Surveillance

Follow-up and surveillance require a 3-month postoperative PET-CT, then PET-CT every 4 to 6 months for 3 years. Any suspicious mass should undergo biopsy, and recurrence would necessitate further chemotherapy or radiation, depending on the location.

Take Home Points

- Squamous cell CUP has the best outcomes of any CUP because local surgical and radiotherapy for the involved mass can significantly prolong survival.
- In addition, in the head and neck, multiple diagnostic modalities can be used, including panendoscopy and PET-CT to identify a primary lesion, further increasing survival rates if the primary is able to be treated surgically or with radiation.

CASE SCENARIO 2 REVIEW

Case Scenario 2 Questions

1. What other historical information would have been helpful in this case?
   - A. Alcohol and other drug use history
   - B. Social history including sexual activity
   - C. Dietary habits
   - D. History of anabolic steroid use
   - E. None of the above

2. What is the expected survival for patients with squamous cell CUP following treatment of their local disease?
   - A. 30–55% at 3 years
   - B. 20–40% at 3 years
   - C. 30–55% at 5 years
   - D. 80–90% at 3 years
   - E. 80–90% at 5 years

3. If this patient had a lateral neck node positive for adenocarcinoma, what would the expected 5-year survival be?
   - A. Same as squamous cell
   - B. Worse than squamous cell
   - C. Better than squamous cell

Case Scenario 2 Answers

1. **The correct answer is B.** *Rationale:* Social history including sexual activity is a standard feature of a "full history and physical." In this particular case, risk factors for contracting oral HPV through sexual activity would have been helpful. In addition, immunization history for the HPV vaccine would have been relevant, although rates of immunization for young males have been historically low secondary to misconception of the utility for males by the general public. The HPV vaccine series is recommended for males age as early as age 9 to prevent HPV and associated cancers, not limited to oropharyngeal, anal, penile, and rectal cancers, as well as cancers in female sexual partners related to HPV transmission including cancer of the cervix, vulva, and vagina. The CDC recommends HPV vaccination for males and females under the age of 26 and for high-risk groups through age 45.

2. **The correct answer is C.** *Rationale:* The survival for patients with squamous cell CUP after control of the identifiable disease (not necessarily the primary lesion) is much greater than all comers with CUP and nonsquamous type, however, it is still relatively poor with 30% to 55% survival at 5 years.

3. **The correct answer is B.** *Rationale:* Worse than squamous cell. Survival at 5 years for head and neck adenocarcinoma CUP is 0% to 10%, with nearly 100% recurrence after local control.

Recommended Readings

Pentheroudakis G, Greco FA, Pavlidis N. Molecular assignment of tissue of origin in cancer of unknown primary may not predict response to therapy or outcome: a systematic literature review. *Cancer Treatment Reviews.* 2009;35:221–227.

Aboulkheyr H, Mahdizadeh H, Hedayati Asl A, Totonchi M. Genomic alterations and possible druggable mutations in carcinoma of unknown primary (CUP). *Nature Portfolio Scientific Reports.* 2021;11:15112.

Olivier T, Fernandez E, Labidi-Galy I, et al. Redefining cancer of unknown primary: is precision medicine really shifting the paradigm? *Cancer Treatment Reviews.* 2021;97:102204.

Hayashi H, Kurata T, Takiguchi T, et al. Randomized Phase II Trial comparing site-specific treatment based on gene expression profiling with carboplatin and paclitaxel for patients with cancer of unknown primary site. *Journal of Clinical Oncology.* 2019;37:570–579.

Kodaira M, Yonemori K, Shimoi T, et al. Prognostic impact of presumed breast or ovarian cancer among patients with unfavorable-subset cancer of unknown primary site. *BMC Cancer.* 2018;18:176.

Surgical Emergencies and Palliative Interventions in Cancer Patients

Allison N. Martin and Brian D. Badgwell

INTRODUCTION

Oncologic emergencies have been defined as "an acute condition that is caused by cancer or the treatment of cancer and that requires intervention as soon as possible to avoid mortality or severe permanent morbidity." Cancer patients are at increased risk of developing emergent conditions due to malnutrition, immunosuppression, limited physiologic reserve, and side effects of treatment. Emergent conditions impacting cancer patients could be the presenting sign of previously undiagnosed cancers or can arise years after the patient has completed therapy. Tumors can create emergent conditions through local or systemic effects. Targeted therapies and medications used to manage side effects of systemic therapy can increase the risk of oncologic emergency in some cases.

Surgical consultation for oncologic emergencies generally occurs in a complex clinical scenario, requiring a rapid gathering of information of the patients' previous treatment and oncologic history and at least an attempt at gathering multidisciplinary input. Such situations require physician to physician interaction and may often occur in the middle of the night or in the emergency room when the primary oncology or treatment team is unavailable. Surgeons should not hesitate to contact the "off-service" physician that may be best informed of the patient's treatment history and current prognosis. Patients must first be rapidly evaluated for hemodynamic stability. A quick assessment, similar to the Advanced Trauma Life Support evaluation of trauma patients, can be utilized to evaluate the airway, vital signs, and neurologic status.

For the purposes of this chapter, the spectrum of oncologic emergencies will be categorized into primarily surgical or medical problems, with emphasis on the surgical emergencies and particularly on intra-abdominal conditions. Patients experiencing surgical oncologic emergencies have a high risk of mortality. A prospective registry study by Bosscher et al. identified several examination or laboratory features, including low handgrip strength, poor performance status, elevated serum lactate dehydrogenase level, and low serum albumin level that are associated with an increased risk of 90-day mortality in this population. As almost half of all cancers diagnosed are not amenable to cure, the distinction between a surgical oncologic emergencies and an indication for nonoperative palliative care is sometimes challenging to make. Therefore, this chapter will also include a summary on emergent palliative surgical conditions.

Surgical Oncologic Emergencies

Bowel Obstruction

Bowel obstruction is a frequent cause for surgical consultation in the general population and cancer patients are no exception. As many cancer patients have had previous abdominal surgery, bowel obstruction can be due to adhesions or associated with incisional hernias. Such patients are treated according to commonly accepted surgical principles. In patients with a history of cancer, however, the cause of obstruction may be malignant, either from primary tumors, metastases, or peritoneal carcinomatosis.

The general approach to a patient with a bowel obstruction is to obtain a history focused on determining the type of obstruction and whether the obstruction represents a partial or complete obstruction. Obstructions can be classified according to location such as gastric outlet obstruction (GOO), small bowel obstruction (SBO), or large bowel obstruction (LBO). Furthermore, obstruction etiology should be considered, such as mechanical (adhesive, hernia, malignant, or intrinsic/extrinsic compression) or nonmechanical (pseudo-obstruction). Recent chemotherapy and treatment history is of critical importance in evaluating the risk/benefit ratio of potential surgical intervention. Physical examination should begin by assessing the hemodynamic status of the patient. An abdominal examination is performed to determine the severity of symptoms and to evaluate for the presence of hernias, particularly investigating the possibility of underlying strangulation. During the evaluation, the need for a nasogastric tube decompression, Foley catheter placement, aggressive intravenous fluid resuscitation, and electrolyte replacement should be addressed. These decisions may be influenced by physical examination and laboratory findings. The goal of management should be to perform any indicated surgical intervention prior to the development of bowel ischemia; however, physical examination findings on presentation of fever, tachycardia, and leukocytosis suggest that ischemia or perforation may have already occurred. Initial imaging typically includes an acute abdominal series (chest, supine abdomen, and upright abdomen plain films) to evaluate for the presence of intraperitoneal free air and to determine the severity of the obstruction. CT imaging can be useful in determining etiology, severity, and site of obstruction. A gastrograffin enema or sigmoidoscopy may be required to evaluate distal obstruction.

Malignant Bowel Obstruction

Malignant bowel obstruction (MBO) is defined as "the blockage of the small or large intestine in a patient with advanced cancer" and represents up to half of all palliative surgical consultations. Although it is understood that this definition applies to blockage caused by tumor, in many patients it is not evident on imaging if the obstruction is due to direct tumor involvement. Bowel obstruction in patients with a history of cancer may be due to benign causes in up to a third of patients. Regardless of the cause, indicators of adverse outcome present at the time of initial evaluation upon which to base treatment decisions have not been firmly established. There is a paucity of prospective research and are no evidence-based algorithms upon which to base treatment decisions for MBO. Current treatment patterns are based on retrospective reviews that outline the considerable morbidity and mortality associated with surgical intervention. As outlined in a review by Ripamonti et al., the operative mortality for surgery in patients with MBO ranges from 9% to 40% with morbidity rates of 9% to 90%. Until recently, there were very few resources on patient-reported outcome measures such as symptom severity for patients with MBO. A recent study conducted at The University of Texas MD Anderson Cancer Center attempted to validate a 24-item questionnaire—the MD Anderson Symptom Inventory (MDASI)—in patients with gastrointestinal obstruction (MDASI-GIO). The survey was found to be a valid measure of patient symptom severity and functional impact. This tool will be useful in both studying MBO management and creating guidelines for management in the future.

MBO rarely requires immediate operative intervention, which allows time for an appropriate evaluation and imaging. CT scans can be very helpful in identifying factors associated with poor outcomes following surgery, such as carcinomatosis and ascites. Advanced age, hypoalbuminemia, and diminished performance status are also adverse predictors of outcome. Although it is difficult to delineate absolute contraindications to surgery for MBO, areas of significant concern include previous abdominal surgery which found diffuse metastatic cancer, known intra-abdominal carcinomatosis, imaging suggesting a motility disorder, ascites which rapidly recurs after drainage, extra-abdominal metastases which cause symptoms that are difficult to control, and previous radiotherapy to the abdomen or pelvis. Surgery is rarely successful and the risk of postoperative morbidity is considerable in patients with both carcinomatosis and ascites. Patients who are not candidates for surgery may benefit from corticosteroids, antiemetics, octreotide, analgesics, or venting gastrostomy tube placement to control obstructive symptoms. A 2021 update to the Multinational Association of Supportive Care in Cancer (MASCC) guidelines for medical management of MBO identified octreotide as standard of care for nonoperable cases.

Gastric Outlet Obstruction

With reported 30-day mortality rates of up to 30% for palliative gastrojejunostomy in patients with malignant GOO, patients should be selected carefully and considered for endoscopic stent placement, although this option is heavily dependent on availability and experience. Limited data from randomized trials, prospective observational, and retrospective studies comparing endoscopic stent placement to gastrojejunostomy demonstrate increased cost effectiveness, decreased length of stay, and decreased time to toleration of liquid diet with stent placement but an increased rate of recurrent obstructive symptoms when compared to surgical intervention. Some authors have recommended attempting stent placement in patients with a relatively short life expectancy and pursuing gastrojejunostomy in those with a longer life expectancy (>6 months).

Small Bowel Obstruction

Small bowel represents two-thirds of all MBOs, although in approximately 20% of cases, both small and large bowel are involved. Surgery remains an important consideration in these patients, as stents are difficult to place downstream of the proximal small bowel. Surgery may involve an enteric bypass procedure or resection. Determining the need for operation can be difficult, as not all partial bowel obstructions in patients with a history of cancer are due to direct tumor involvement and partial obstructions may resolve with conservative therapy.

Large Bowel Obstruction

A significant advancement in the treatment of malignant LBO has been endoscopic, self-expanding metallic stents. A recent systematic review by Watt et al. found that although the evidence-based quality of the studies

Treatment	Gastric Outlet Obstruction (%)	Small Bowel Obstruction (%)	Large Bowel Obstruction (%)
Surgery	44	25	57
Interventional radiology or endoscopic procedure	34	24	18
Nonoperative or nonprocedural	22	52	25

Treatment Strategies for Patients with Gastrointestinal Obstruction, Stratified by Site of Obstruction[a]

[a]Patients with suspected bowel obstruction were referred for palliative surgical consultation and stratified according to site of obstruction, as above. Surgery was more commonly performed in patients with large bowel obstruction and gastric outlet obstruction. Endoscopic/interventional radiology procedures were more frequently performed in patients with gastric outlet obstruction, while nonoperative or nonprocedural management was recommended most often in patients with small bowel obstruction.
Adapted from Badgwell BD, Contreras C, Askew R, Krouse R, Feig B, Cormier JN. Radiographic and clinical factors associated with improved outcomes in advanced cancer patients with bowel obstruction. *J Palliat Med.* 2011;14(9):990–996.

was generally low, expandable stents demonstrated a lower rate of serious adverse events and hospital stay with similar mortality to open surgery.

A review of patients with advanced cancer and gastrointestinal (GI) obstruction at The University of Texas MD Anderson Cancer Center reported a median overall survival of 3.5 months, highlighting the need for careful patient selection to identify patients that will experience symptom improvement from surgery and regain meaningful quality of life prior to death from disease progression. Table 24.1 demonstrates the treatment strategies for this group of patients, stratified by anatomic site of location: GOO, SBO, and LBO. In this series, 24% of patients with GOO, 23% with SBO, and 8% with LBO were treated with venting gastrostomy tube placement. Venting gastrostomy tubes are an option for poor surgical candidates, allowing for nasogastric tube removal and discharge home with hospice. However, in patients with a competent ileocecal valve, venting gastrostomy tube will not alleviate obstruction in the large intestine and those patients are still at risk for colonic distension and perforation. Rather than an algorithmic approach, patients with MBO require multifaceted, individualized decision-making that incorporates the many variables important in treatment selection, as illustrated in Figure 24.1.

Bowel Perforation

Cancer patients may be at increased risk of bowel perforation due to side effects of chemotherapy, immunotherapy, radiation, immunosuppression, steroid administration, or direct tumor invasion. Cancer patients are at risk of iatrogenic bowel perforation as endoscopic and interventional radiology procedures are commonly used in diagnosis, surveillance, and treatment. Bowel perforation may be caused by conditions that are unrelated to oncologic disease or treatment, such as diverticulitis, peptic ulcer disease, or appendicitis. Outside of any recent cancer treatment, these patients are usually treated with the same prompt intervention as noncancer patients, including surgical management or nonoperative management.

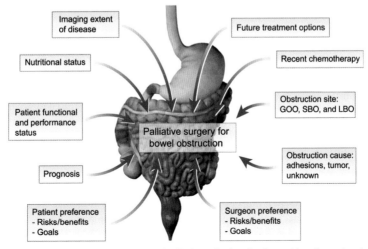

FIGURE 24.1 Multifaceted approach required in the evaluation of patients with malignant bowel obstruction.

The majority of cancer patients with bowel perforation have advanced or incurable disease. Therefore, in addition to clinical presentation, factors such as prognosis, symptom burden, treatment history, and patient and family desires play an important part in decision-making and management. Although the majority of patients can be managed with surgery, comfort care and nonoperative management are options in these complex clinical scenarios.

Approximately 2% of colorectal cancers present with perforation. Perforation may occur as a direct result of transmural invasion of the bowel wall or, less frequently, as a result of distal obstruction leading to proximal bowel dilation. Perforated colorectal cancers are associated with both increased local and systemic recurrence. Operative mortality rates in these cases approach 20%, much higher than rates for resection of non-perforated cancers.

Chemotherapy-associated bowel perforation following bevacizumab treatment deserves mention. Bevacizumab, a humanized monoclonal antibody to vascular endothelial cell growth factor, has demonstrated efficacy in combination with chemotherapy for patients with metastatic colorectal cancer and lung cancer. It is presently being studied and utilized in a wide variety of malignancies. The incidence of spontaneous bowel perforation in patients receiving bevacizumab is 1% to 2%, but the event rate appears to vary across cancer types. Although infrequent, bevacizumab-associated bowel perforation is associated with a 30-day mortality rate of 13% to 50%. Concerns regarding emergency surgery in the setting of recent bevacizumab administration include wound-healing difficulties and bleeding. Given the concerns over increased postoperative complications, most surgeons wait for 6 weeks after bevacizumab administration prior to proceeding with elective surgery. Consideration should be given to the need for stoma creation in patients with bevacizumab-associated bowel perforation requiring both emergent or elective operations.

Cholecystitis

Patients with immunosuppression, malnutrition, and those receiving systemic therapy may be at increased risk for acalculous cholecystitis. Other causes for cholecystitis in the cancer population include hepatic artery embolization and biliary stent placement. Cancer patients may have intra-abdominal fluid or malignant ascites that complicates interpretation of pericholecystic fluid or gallbladder wall thickening on ultrasound or CT imaging. Hepatobiliary scintigraphy may be required to confirm the diagnosis of cholecystitis. Treatment for cancer patients may be atypical in that not all patients can undergo a prompt laparoscopic cholecystectomy due to treatment issues such as recent chemotherapy, immunosuppression, neutropenia, malnutrition, comorbidities, and stage of disease or prognosis. With these concerns in mind, some patients are best treated with a percutaneous cholecystostomy tube to prevent delaying treatment or performance of an operation with risk of conversion to an open procedure that may not be appropriate in the context of poor oncologic prognosis. Subsequent laparoscopic cholecystectomy and cholecystostomy tube removal has been described with low conversion rates.

Biliary Obstruction

Patients rarely present with biliary obstruction and cholangitis but treatment in this situation focuses on endoscopic drainage and antibiotics. The vast majority of patients with malignant sources of biliary obstruction have a diagnosis of pancreatic cancer. Stable patients with potentially resectable causes of biliary obstruction are described elsewhere; unresectable patients may benefit from endoscopic, percutaneous, or surgical bypass procedures. In general, endoscopic or percutaneous methods offer less initial morbidity but decreased durability of palliation. Surgical methods, conversely, have more up-front morbidity with a longer durability of palliation. The best approach remains a matter of debate and is also dependent on available adjuncts at individual institutions. Biliary obstruction from metastatic disease present in the porta hepatis can be associated with a wide variety of cancers and often represents a condition with a very poor prognosis and prohibitive surgical mortality and morbidity. Endoscopic or percutaneous biliary stent placement best accomplishes drainage and therefore subsequent consideration can be given to radiation therapy with or without chemotherapy.

Neutropenia and Abdominal Pain

Neutropenia is a frequent toxic result of chemotherapy. Abdominal pain in neutropenic patients has a broad differential with significant associated mortality for which surgeons are frequently asked to evaluate in consultation. Surgeons asked to assist in diagnosing and managing this scenario must consider the broad list of general surgical conditions that can cause abdominal pain, in addition to conditions unique to the neutropenic patient. Neutropenic enterocolitis is one such entity and has been referred to as neutropenic enteropathy, agranulocytic colitis, or typhlitis (if the disease is confined to the cecum). In a recent series of 60 neutropenic patients presenting with abdominal pain at The University of Texas MD Anderson Cancer Center, neutropenic enterocolitis was found in 28%, SBO in 12%, and the cause remained uncertain in 35% of patients. Less frequent conditions included *Clostridium difficile* colitis, diverticulitis, appendicitis, cholecystitis, colonic pseudo-obstruction, and splenic rupture. Thirty- and 90-day mortality rates for all patients in this series was 30% and 52%, respectively, and likely reflects oncologic disease severity and frequent comorbidities present in this patient population. Surgical intervention was performed in 15%, with attempts made to delay surgery until resolution of neutropenia when possible.

The clinical and pathologic criteria for diagnosing neutropenic enterocolitis have not been firmly established. A commonly accepted clinical diagnostic triad is neutropenia (defined as neutrophil count of <1,000 cells/μL), abdominal pain, and bowel wall thickening on imaging. In patients with diarrhea, it is important to rule out *C. difficile* colitis. Surgery is reserved for perforation, sepsis, or progression of disease and worsening of overall condition felt to be attributable to the enterocolitis.

The mortality rate associated with surgery in patients with neutropenia has been well established with early reports documenting mortality rates of 41% to 57%. More recent reports reflect attempts to delay surgery to allow for resolution of neutropenia and demonstrate improved survival rates, which also may be attributable to improved critical care, antibiotics, colony stimulating factors, and white blood cell transfusions. There are no formal recommendations for medical treatment of neutropenia associated with intra-abdominal sepsis and many clinicians rely on recommendations from the Infectious Diseases Society of America (IDSA) for febrile neutropenia. These guidelines were last updated in 2010 and propose monotherapy with an anti-pseudomonal β-lactam agent, a carbapenem or piperacillin-tazobactam with the addition of an aminoglycoside, fluoroquinolone, and/or vancomycin for patients with signs of complications or for patients with a history or suspicion of antimicrobial resistance. However, the majority of patients in our series were treated with vancomycin for suspicion of gram-positive infection in patients with severe sepsis and metronidazole was often added for coverage of anaerobic species, such as *Clostridium*, which are often involved in neutropenic enterocolitis. The use of antifungal agents is not established but can be considered in patients that remain febrile or shows signs of infection concomitantly with neutropenia for ≥5 days based on IDSA recommendations.

Hemorrhage

GI bleeding in cancer patients is commonly found to arise from benign causes such as peptic ulcer disease and gastritis. Primary tumors are rarely a source of brisk, uncontrollable hemorrhage. Gastric lymphoma patients receiving systemic chemotherapy are a population at high risk of GI bleeding with reported rates of up to 11%. Metastatic tumors to the GI tract, such as melanoma, can be a source of bleeding but also are more commonly associated with a chronic, relatively slow rate of blood loss. The management approach is that of standard surgical principles. After stabilization in the intensive care unit if necessary, initial diagnostic approaches are based on clinical signs indicating an upper or lower GI source. Endoscopic control of malignant upper GI bleeding is often successful and allows for elective surgical intervention. Postoperative mortality in patients undergoing surgery for bleeding gastric cancer approaches 10% and therefore consideration should be given to a second endoscopy prior to surgery, based on hemodynamic stability. For signs of lower GI bleeding, the initial diagnostic procedure is endoscopy, allowing for hemorrhage control followed by an elective surgical procedure if indicated. Tagged red blood cell scans and angiography are adjunctive maneuvers that may be useful for localization of hemorrhage prior to either endoscopic control or interventional angioembolization.

Anorectal Infections

Anorectal infections in noncancer patients are rarely a source of major morbidity or mortality and are typically treated with prompt incision and drainage, either at bedside with local anesthesia or under general anesthetic conditions in an operating room. Anorectal infections in patients with cancer receiving systemic therapy with or without associated neutropenia, however, can be a significant and potentially lethal condition. Reports from the 1970s describing anorectal infections in immunosuppressed cancer patients documented mortality rates as high as 50%. The authors of these early reports noted that many anorectal infections in the immunosuppressed cancer population were ulcerative without associated abscess formation and recommended caution in proceeding with surgical intervention. A recent study from the National Cancer Institute, demonstrating a selective surgical approach, found that surgery was required in 37% of patients and there were no deaths associated with anorectal infections. In a recent study from The University of Texas MD Anderson Cancer Center, 100 patients with anorectal infections underwent surgical oncology consultation and 58% were treated with operative intervention. Identification of an abscess and erythema on physical examination were most commonly associated with surgical intervention. The frequency of necrotizing soft tissue infection in this study was low (2%) but was associated with the only infection-related mortality in the cohort (1%).

Palliative Aspects of Surgical Oncologic Emergencies

The definition of palliative surgery has many minor variations but is generally defined as any procedure that is performed to reduce symptoms or improve quality of life in a patient with an advanced or incurable malignancy. Palliative surgical procedures were reported to account for 13% of all operations at a major U.S. cancer center and up to 21% of all operations performed by surgical oncologists. A recent report attempted to determine the percentage of inpatients undergoing surgical evaluation at a cancer center that met the criteria for palliative evaluation. In this study, 40% of all inpatient surgical oncology evaluations were requested for symptom palliation in patients with advanced or incurable malignancies. GI obstruction was the most common reason for consultation (43%) while wound complications/infection and GI bleeding accounted for 10% and 8%, respectively. Almost half of the patients had received systemic therapy within 6 weeks preceding the request for surgical palliative consultation. Palliative surgical procedures were performed in 27% of patients, with a 90-day morbidity and mortality rate of 40% and 7%. The median overall survival of all patients undergoing palliative surgical evaluation was only 2.9 months, again highlighting the need for careful patient selection based on disease prognosis.

Palliative surgical consultation is arguably the most complex and time-consuming category of surgical consultation and evaluation. Although the majority of patients deemed suitable for surgery will experience symptom improvement, roughly a quarter of patients will develop recurrent symptoms and another quarter will develop new symptoms requiring evaluation during short-term follow-up. There are many approaches to palliative surgery consultation such as the palliative triangle technique, traditional risk–benefit discussion, and utilizing questions aimed to identify patient's goals and trade-offs they are willing to make in pursuit of their goals. One example of a risk–benefit-based approach is outlined in Figure 24.2. The first step in this approach is to thoroughly review the history and previous imaging, in addition to discussing the family dynamics with the assigned nurse prior to entering the room. Next, an empathic statement, such as an apology for meeting the patient in such circumstances, can acknowledge the difficulty that these patients experience in transitioning from a therapeutic to palliative management strategy. When asking about prognosis, it is important to not state a prognosis that significantly differs from the patient's understanding of their prognosis. Silence from the physician during at least a few periods of the consultation can be crucial to allow the patient the opportunity to express their understanding of their symptoms, prognosis, and goals. Several visits may be required to proceed through this approach, particularly in situations where surgical intervention is not an option.

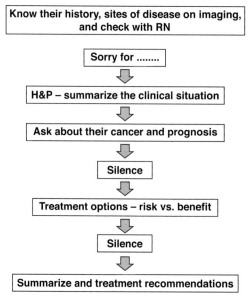

FIGURE 24.2 Example of a risk–benefit-based approach to palliative surgical consultation.

Further studies are needed to better characterize patients with surgical oncologic emergencies requiring inpatient evaluation and identify indicators of adverse surgical outcome based on specific symptom clusters such as MBO or GI hemorrhage. These studies would be strengthened by inclusion of patient-reported outcomes and symptom improvement data, comorbidity indices, performance status, and large study populations through multi-institutional collaboration.

Medical Oncologic Emergencies

Superior Vena Cava Syndrome

Superior vena cava obstruction can result from invasion, fibrosis, thrombosis, or external compression by a malignancy. Lung cancer is the leading cause in 65% to 85%, while lymphoma, breast cancer, and thymic cancer are other relatively common malignant causes. In the majority of cases, there is time to obtain a histologic diagnosis to guide therapy. Clinical presentation includes dyspnea, cough, headache, venous engorgement of the face, neck and chest wall, cyanosis, and worsening of symptoms when patient bends forward or assumes supine position. Symptoms typically develop slowly and progress over a few weeks. CT angiography is the initial test of choice and can differentiate venous thrombosis from external compression as well as guide image-directed biopsy. CT can also detect other emergent conditions, such as spinal cord compression, pericardial metastases, and impending airway obstruction. Diuretics, head elevation, steroids, intubation, and radiation therapy may be required to stabilize the patient and mitigate symptoms until definitive treatment can be pursued. Vena caval stents have been described in severe cases as temporizing measures during an ongoing workup. Further treatment includes tumor-specific therapy or thrombolysis. Removal of any pre-existing venous catheters is required.

Spinal Cord Compression

The majority of patients with spinal cord compression present with back pain that may be exacerbated by movement, recumbency, coughing, sneezing, or straining. Progressive symptoms include weakness, numbness, urinary retention, and constipation. MRI is the current diagnostic study of choice. Treatments may involve steroids, radiotherapy, systemic therapy, or surgery.

Pericardial Tamponade

Signs and symptoms of pericardial tamponade can include chest pain, dyspnea, tachycardia, distant heart sounds, jugular venous distention, pulsus paradoxus, and hypotension. Electrocardiogram may demonstrate a low-voltage rhythm, but echocardiography is the most useful test for diagnosing and evaluating the hemodynamic severity of a pericardial effusion. Pericardiocentesis can be performed under echocardiographic monitoring with placement of a drainage catheter and subsequent sclerosing agent if indicated. Surgical treatment generally consists of subxiphoid pericardiotomy, however, if a previous subxiphoid approach has been performed, a transthoracic pleuropericardial window may be the preferred option. Radiotherapy can also be administered, particularly in patients with malignant effusions secondary to lymphoma.

Paraneoplastic Crises

Hypercalcemia

Common cancer etiologies for hypercalcemia include breast, lung, kidney, and multiple myeloma and are often seen in association with bone metastases. Elevated parathyroid hormone (PTH) levels in association with hypophosphatemia indicate ectopic PTH secretion. Hypercalcemia secondary to malignancy may be accompanied by elevated or normal serum phosphate. Hypercalcemia may cause changes on ECG, first with shortening of the QT interval and arrhythmias that can progress to bradycardia, prolonged PR interval, and widened T waves. Symptomatic patients and those with a serum calcium >12 mg/dL require prompt treatment. Aggressive intravenous hydration with isotonic fluids followed by loop diuretics is the initial treatment. Calcitonin may also be administered as an adjunctive measure in the acute setting. Bisphosphonates can reduce bone resorption from metastatic disease but require 3 to 4 weeks to take effect. Plicamycin is also an effective inhibitor of bone resorption that can take effect within 6 to 48 hours but has associated toxicities such as thrombocytopenia, hypotension, and hepatic and renal insufficiency. Gallium nitrate is another effective inhibitor of bone resorption with a main side effect of nephrotoxicity.

Hyponatremia and Syndrome of Inappropriate Anti-Diuretic Hormone (SIADH)

SIADH can result in mental status changes, nausea, headaches, seizures, coma, and ultimately death. Small cell lung cancer is a commonly associated malignancy, but SIADH may be present with prostate, adrenal, esophagus, pancreas, colon, and head and neck cancers. Pseudohyponatremia is due to hyperproteinemia, hyperglycemia, or hyperlipidemia. Chemotherapy such as vincristine and cyclophosphamide are also associated with hyponatremia. SIADH findings include a low BUN, hypouricemia, and hypophosphatemia. Treatment for SIADH is etiology specific. For example, small cell lung cancer–associated SIADH may be treated with appropriate chemotherapy while SIADH resulting from brain metastases may improve with the use of corticosteroids and radiation therapy. Treatment otherwise consists of water restriction to 500 to 1,000 mL/day to correct sodium levels over several days. Further treatment can involve demeclocycline, an ADH antagonist. Severe hyponatremia can be treated with 3% hypertonic saline infusion with IV furosemide, although the rate of correction should be limited to 0.5 to 1.0 mEq/hr to minimize the risk of neurologic toxicity.

Hypoglycemia

Symptoms of hypoglycemia may include weakness, dizziness, and confusion that can progress to seizures and coma. There are many nonmalignant causes but insulinomas, adrenocortical tumors, hepatomas, sarcomas (fibrosarcoma, neurofibrosarcoma, and hemangiopericytoma), and mesotheliomas are associated with the development of hypoglycemia. Resection or enucleation is of these masses is performed, when possible, and alleviates the associated electrolyte abnormalities. For unresectable or multifocal insulin-secreting tumors, somatostatin analogs, diazoxide, radiation, diet modification, corticosteroids, glucagon, and growth hormone may be of benefit for symptomatic relief.

Tumor Lysis Syndrome

Tumor lysis syndrome is manifested by hyperuricemia, hyperkalemia, hyperphosphatemia, and hypocalcemia resulting from rapid cell lysis during cytotoxic therapy. Acute renal failure is caused by renal tubule accumulation of uric acid and calcium phosphate. Tumor lysis syndrome most often occurs in the setting of induction chemotherapy for lymphoma and leukemia but may occur in other cancer types following radiation, hormonal, or ablative therapy. Preventive measures include intravenous hydration, alkalinization of the urine, and allopurinol administration before or at the time of chemotherapy initiation. Treatment of tumor lysis syndrome involves aggressive correction of electrolyte abnormalities, particularly hyperkalemia. Hemodialysis may be required.

Central Venous Catheter Sepsis

Intravenous antibiotic therapy for catheter-associated infections has been reported with success rates of up to 80%. However, catheter removal is indicated for patients with persistent blood cultures, neutropenia, signs of systemic infection, and a history of vascular grafts or implanted prostheses.

CASE SCENARIO

Case Scenario 1

Presentation

A 54-year-old previously healthy man is referred to you with an existing diagnosis of gastric adenocarcinoma. He underwent an upper endoscopy at an outside hospital and was diagnosed with a tumor of the lesser curvature of the stomach, 5 cm proximal to the pylorus. However, he lost his insurance and presents 18 months following his initial diagnosis with worsening bloating with ingestion of solid foods. He has lost 30 lb over the previous 6 months. He undergoes a staging workup with PET-CT of the chest, abdomen, and pelvis, which shows a near occlusion of the pylorus, proximal circumferential thickening of the gastric wall, associated perigastric lymphadenopathy, and concern for direct invasion of the pancreas.

Take Home Points

- Patients with gastric outlet obstruction and a life expectancy of greater than 6 months are best managed with a surgical gastrojejunostomy.
- A life expectancy of <6 months is an indication for endoscopic stenting.
- Venting gastrostomy is an option for patients who are not operative or endoscopic stent candidates.

CASE SCENARIO 1 REVIEW

Case Scenario 1 Questions

1. The patient in Case Scenario 1 is admitted and receives IV rehydration and correction of electrolytes, as well as nasogastric decompression and bowel rest. What is the next best step for relief of his symptoms of bloating and oral intolerance?

   A. Endoscopic bypass
   B. Diagnostic laparoscopy
   C. Surgical gastrojejunostomy
   D. Palliative chemotherapy and/or chemoradiation

2. What would the best treatment option be for a 75-year-old patient in a nursing home, presenting with bloating and weight loss, with evidence of omental caking and diffuse peritoneal enhancement on imaging?

   A. Surgical gastrojejunostomy
   B. Endoscopic stenting
   C. Immediate chemotherapy
   D. Hospice referral

Case Scenario 1 Answers

1. **The correct answer is C.** *Rationale:* The patient has clinical symptoms and imaging findings consistent with a malignant gastric outlet obstruction. Given his young age and otherwise good health, his life expectancy is likely to exceed 6 months, longer than the anticipated durability of an endoscopic stent. Although endoscopic interventions could be considered if his life expectancy were shorter, endoscopic stenting would be a better initial option than a more technically challenging endoscopic bypass procedure. Simultaneous referral for medical and radiation oncology evaluation for chemotherapeutic and radiation options should be performed, as downstaging is possible in a patient with no definitive evidence of distant metastases.

2. **The correct answer is B.** *Rationale:* While the patient would benefit from a comprehensive discussion of palliative options including potential hospice care, endoscopic stenting has been shown to be beneficial for symptom management for patients with gastric outlet obstruction who have a limited life expectancy and/or decreased functional status.

CASE SCENARIO

Case Scenario 2

Presentation

A 45-year-old woman with recently diagnosed acute myelogenous leukemia admitted to undergo induction chemotherapy begins to complain of severe pain with defecation on day 2 of therapy. She is also febrile to 38.5° C. A comprehensive blood count with differential notes a white blood cell count of 0.2 K/uL with an absolute neutrophil count of 0.6 K/uL. Her platelet count is 17 K/uL. A surgical consult is obtained, and physical examination is notable for a 2-cm diameter area of tenderness at the anal verge with surrounding erythema. The patient is unable to tolerate digital rectal examination because of pain. A CT scan of the pelvis demonstrates soft tissue stranding in the perianal region, but no obvious fluid collection.

Take Home Points

- Patients with depressed cell counts secondary to chemotherapy with suspicion of perianal abscess on physical examination should be evaluated with cross-sectional imaging (either abdominal/pelvic CT scan or pelvic MRI) to evaluate for a drainable fluid collection.
- A perianal fluid collection that is not improving with intravenous antibiotics warrants drainage, preferably with percutaneous drain placement to avoid a wound from open drainage.

CASE SCENARIO 2 REVIEW

Case Scenario 2 Questions

1. What is the best option for initial management?

   A. Bedside incision and drainage
   B. Intravenous antibiotics
   C. Operative incision and drainage
   D. Warm compresses and narcotic pain medications

2. The patient in Case Scenario 2 is started on meropenem. Three days later, she continues to experience low-grade fevers and develops perianal fluctuance and intermittent foul-smelling drainage. Repeat imaging demonstrates a 3.5-cm fluid collection in the area of prior induration noted on her first CT scan. What is the next best step in management?

   A. Image-guided drain placement
   B. Operative incision and drainage
   C. Pelvic MRI
   D. Referral to infectious disease specialists for alternative antibiotics

Case Scenario 2 Answers

1. **The correct answer is B.** *Rationale:* As there is no drainable fluid collection, an interventional procedure is not indicated for treatment of this patient's symptoms. The presence of cellulitis, particularly in a neutropenic patient, is an indication for antibiotics and symptoms should be monitored closely for progression.

2. **The correct answer is A.** *Rationale:* In a patient with a normal absolute neutrophil and platelet count, the next step would likely be operative incision and drainage. The patient in Case Scenario 2 would be at high risk for a complication with an open drainage, such as a chronic wound or fistula, therefore a consultation to interventional radiology is warranted for percutaneous drain placement. Continuing the same antibiotic regimen alone is unlikely to result in improvement in symptoms. The CT scan adequately diagnosed the abscess, therefore pelvic MRI is not necessary.

CASE SCENARIO

Case Scenario 3

Presentation

A 48-year-old woman with metastatic breast cancer limited to the chest wall and vertebrae is treated with a combination of radiation and chemotherapy including bevacizumab (Avastin). She experiences remarkable tumor regression, but suddenly develops progressive mid-abdominal pain, fevers, and severe fatigue. She is brought to the emergency room by her husband and is found to be tympanitic. She is tachycardic with a heart rate of 114 beats per minute and her blood pressure is 76/45 mmHg. Plain abdominal x-ray is unremarkable. She has a leukocytosis with a white blood cell count of 15K. A CT scan obtained of her abdomen/pelvis demonstrates a bowel perforation in the distal small bowel suggested by oral contrast leakage.

Take Home Points

- Bevacizumab-associated spontaneous bowel perforation in unstable patients should be managed surgically with bowel resection or diverting ostomy depending on the degree of contamination and sepsis.
- When used as part of a neoadjuvant regimen, bevacizumab should be routinely held for at least 6 weeks prior to any elective operation.

CASE SCENARIO 3 REVIEW

Case Scenario 3 Question

1. What is the next best step in her management?
   A. Nonoperative management with IV antibiotics
   B. Serial abdominal examinations with cessation of chemotherapy
   C. Palliative care consult
   D. Bowel resection

Case Scenario 3 Answer

1. **The correct answer is D.** *Rationale:* Patients with bevacizumab-associated bowel perforation who are unstable require urgent operative intervention. The patient should receive an IV fluid bolus and initiation of broad-spectrum antibiotics prior to being taken promptly to the operating room. For patients who present without significant delay and have small bowel perforation without significant spillage, resection, and primary anastomosis is indicated. For colonic perforation in unstable patients, a diverting ostomy may be performed. Observation of without operation is inappropriate in an unstable patient with obvious perforation, despite treatment with bevacizumab and the anticipated postoperative complications, unless a large volume of intra-abdominal metastatic disease is known. In that case, a palliative approach without operative intervention would be appropriate.

Recommended Readings

Badgwell BD, Camp ER, Feig B, et al. Management of bevacizumab-associated bowel perforation: a case series and review of the literature. *Ann Oncol.* 2008;19(3):577–582.

Badgwell BD, Chang GJ, Rodriguez-Bigas MA, et al. Management and outcomes of anorectal infection in the cancer patient. *Ann Surg Oncol.* 2009;16(10):2752–2758.

Badgwell BD, Contreras C, Askew R, Krouse R, Feig B, Cormier JN. Radiographic and clinical factors associated with improved outcomes in advanced cancer patients with bowel obstruction. *J Palliat Med.* 2011;14(9): 990–996.

Badgwell BD, Cormier JN, Wray CJ, et al. Challenges in surgical management of abdominal pain in the neutropenic cancer patient. *Ann Surg.* 2008;248(1):104–109.

Badgwell B, Feig BW, Ross MI, Mansfield PF, Wen S, Chang GJ. Pneumoperitoneum in the cancer patient. *Ann Surg Oncol.* 2007;14(11):3141–3147.

Badgwell BD, Smith K, Liu P, Bruera E, Curley SA, Cormier JN. Indicators of surgery and survival in oncology inpatients requiring surgical evaluation for palliation. *Support Care Cancer.* 2009;17(6):727–734.

Badgwell B, Williams LA, Chen TH, Cleeland C, Mendoza T. Development and validation of a patient-reported outcome measure for gastrointestinal obstruction in the setting of advanced malignancy. *Ann Surg.* 2021. doi: 10.1097/SLA.0000000000004752. Epub ahead of print.

Bliss LA, Eskander MF, Kent TS, et al. Early surgical bypass versus endoscopic stent placement in pancreatic cancer. *HPB (Oxford).* 2016;18(8):671–677.

Bosscher MR, Bastiaannet E, van Leeuwen BL, Hoekstra HJ. Factors associated with short-term mortality after surgical oncologic emergencies. *Ann Surg Oncol.* 2016;23(6):1803–1814.

Davis M, Hui D, Davies A, et al. Medical management of malignant bowel obstruction in patients with advanced cancer: 2021 MASCC guideline update. *Support Care Cancer.* 2021;29:8089–8096

Freifeld AG, Bow EJ, Sepkowitz KA, et al. Clinical practice guideline for the use of antimicrobial agents in neutropenic patients with cancer: 2010 update by the Infectious Diseases Society of America. *Clin Infect Dis.* 2011;52(4):e56–e93.

Glenn J, Funkhouser WK, Schneider PS. Acute illnesses necessitating urgent abdominal surgery in neutropenic cancer patients: description of 14 cases and review of the literature. *Surgery.* 1989;105(6):778–789.

Helton W, Fisichella P. Intestinal obstruction. In: Souba W, ed. *American College of Surgeons, Principles & Practice.* Web MD Professional Publishing; 2007:514–533.

Krouse RS. The international conference on malignant bowel obstruction: a meeting of the minds to advance palliative care research. *J Pain Symptom Manage.* 2007;34(1 Suppl):S1–S6.

Krouse RS, Nelson RA, Farrell BR, et al. Surgical palliation at a cancer center: incidence and outcomes. *Arch Surg.* 2001;136(7):773–778.

Lehrnbecher T, Marshall D, Gao C, Chanock SJ. A second look at anorectal infections in cancer patients in a large cancer institute: the success of early intervention with antibiotics and surgery. *Infection.* 2002;30(5):272–276.

McCahill LE, Krouse R, Chu D, et al. Indications and use of palliative surgery-results of Society of Surgical Oncology survey. *Ann Surg Oncol.* 2002;9(1):104–112.

Miner TJ, Brennan MF, Jacques DP. A prospective, symptom related, outcomes analysis of 1022 palliative procedures for advanced cancer. *Ann Surg.* 2004;240(4):719–726; discussion 726–727.

Ripamonti C, Twycross R, Baines M, et al. Clinical-practice recommendations for the management of bowel obstruction in patients with end-stage cancer. *Support Care Cancer.* 2001;9(4):223–233.

Saillard C, Zafrani L, Darmon M, et al. The prognostic impact of abdominal surgery in cancer patients with neutropenic enterocolitis: a systematic review and meta-analysis, on behalf the Groupe de Recherche en Réanimation Respiratoire du patient d'Onco-Hématologie (GRRR-OH). *Ann Intensive Care.* 2018;8(1):47.

Watt AM, Faragher IG, Griffin TT, Rieger NA, Maddern GJ. Self-expanding metallic stents for relieving malignant colorectal obstruction: a systematic review. *Ann Surg* 2007;246(1):24–30.

Yeung SJ, Escalante C. Oncologic emergencies. In: *Cancer Medicine.* 8th ed. BC Decker Inc; 2010.

Principles of Radiation Oncology

Michael K. Rooney, Shalini Moningi, Christopher Crane, and Prajnan Das

INTRODUCTION

Radiation oncology is the practice of using focused high-energy electromagnetic radiation to treat oncologic diseases. Radiation can be delivered in a variety of forms, each having different physical characteristics that offer unique advantages in individual patients. The total radiation dose and its fractionation vary, depending on the clinical goals of each patient's overall treatment plan. In general, radiation therapy can be used as either the definitive treatment of localized disease or for palliation of symptoms (e.g., pain or bleeding). More recently, radiation therapy has also emerged as an effective treatment approach for oligometastatic disease. It can be given concurrently with chemotherapy, as neoadjuvant, as adjuvant therapy, or as primary therapy for a wide range of malignancies with potential resultant superior patient outcomes.

Basic Radiobiology and Principles of Fractionation

Radiation kills tumor cells by irreversibly damaging their DNA. Tissues and organs have known dose and volume tolerances to late radiation injury that must be respected to avoid permanent late toxicity. Therefore, the total radiation dose and the delivery technique are chosen in an effort to balance efficacy and a patient's risk of developing acute and late complications from radiation treatment. Some organs such as the liver, lungs, and kidneys can tolerate large tissue-ablative doses to small tissue volumes without disruption of function. In addition, larger volumes of these organs can safely receive lower doses of radiation without impairing function. Other organs, such as the spinal cord and gastrointestinal tract, cannot tolerate tissue-ablative doses delivered to one part of the organ without functional consequences. In these structures, the *maximum radiation dose* is the dose above which late injury is caused to any part of the organ.

Fractionation

Fractionation is the process of dividing the total radiation dose into smaller, equal doses that are delivered over time. Fractionation exploits the inherent biologic differences between normal cells and tumor cells to maximize tumor cell death while minimizing normal cell damage. Standard radiation dose fractions range from 1.8 to 2 Gray (Gy). *Hypofractionation* refers to the delivery of larger doses per fraction of radiation (>2 Gy) over a shorter overall time. *Accelerated fractionation* refers to the delivery of standard fraction sizes given in a shorter overall time, often twice daily. Four radiobiologic cellular processes—repair, repopulation, redistribution, and reoxygenation—dictate the optimization of fractionation.

The Four R's: Repair, Repopulation, Redistribution, and Reoxygenation

All cells have the ability to *repair* some of the DNA damage caused by radiation. Normal cells can repair sublethal DNA damage much more effectively than tumor cells can, however this superior cell-repair ability is generally lost with increasing doses per fraction as the mounting double-stranded DNA damage from higher doses overwhelms the cells' ability to repair it. Fractionation of radiation into smaller doses exploits the repair capacity differences between tumor cells and normal cells and facilitates increased normal cellular repair while maintaining tumor cell death. *Repopulation* refers to the ability of tumor cells to repopulate during a course of radiation treatment, which can happen if the time to deliver the full course of radiation is too long. Shortening the period between radiation doses may increase the probability of killing all tumor clonogenic cells. *Redistribution* refers to the distribution of tumor cells in different stages of the cell cycle. In each phase of the cell cycle, a cell has a different sensitivity to radiation. *Reoxygenation* is the process in which hypoxic, radioresistant tumor cells become increasingly radiosensitive as they are exposed to oxygen with subsequent radiation fractions. Oxygen stabilizes radiation-produced free radicals, which leads to ionization, DNA strand breaks, and ultimately cell death in tumors. When a tumor reaches a diameter of 3 to 5 mm, it outgrows its blood supply and develops hypoxic areas that are radioresistant. When the tumor is irradiated, oxygenated (and thus radiosensitive) cells on the periphery of the tumor die, causing the tumor to shrink and allowing oxygen to diffuse to formerly hypoxic areas, reducing treatment resistance.

591

Basic Radiation Physics

Radiation can be delivered externally via low- or high-energy beams or internally via implanted radiation sources. The method of preferred radiation delivery depends on the type and location of the tumor, as well as the patient's overall health. Radiation is most commonly delivered with high-energy electromagnetic radiation (x-rays or photons) that penetrates tissues to varying degrees, depending on the energy of the beams. In general, beams with energies between 6 and 18 MV are used. The decision to use one type of beam versus another depends on the distance of the lesion from the skin's surface. In general, lesions closer to the surface of the skin are treated with lower-energy photons.

External-Beam Radiation Therapy (EBRT)

As the name implies, EBRT is delivered from an external source, typically a linear accelerator. When receiving treatment, a patient is immobilized on a treatment table while multiple radiation beams are stereotaxically targeted at various angles, converging on the treatment volume. External beam radiation can be delivered in the form of photons, electrons, or protons. Photon beams (x-rays or gamma rays) penetrate the body, irradiating both the tumor and the normal tissue. Electrons are subatomic negatively charged particles that only partially penetrate the body, depositing their energy at a depth that is dependent on the initial energy of the beam. Electron beams can be used to treat tumors typically within 6 cm of the surface of the skin. Protons are positively charged particles that provide no exit dose beyond the target, allowing sparing of normal tissue.

This difference in dose distribution between photon and proton radiation has led to increased interest in the use of proton therapy, particularly in regions where toxicity avoidance is a priority. For example, protons are beneficial in pediatric patients by reducing the dose to normal growing pediatric tissues and therefore reducing long-term toxicity, such as the risk of developing secondary malignancies. At the time of this writing, determination of the clinical advantages of using protons over photons is an area of active investigation. A large body of retrospective research suggests a benefit of proton therapy in certain settings but ongoing randomized clinical trials in various cancer sites, including head and neck, breast, prostate, pediatric CNS, esophageal and thoracic, will clarify the clinical benefits of proton therapy. Early results have alluded to lower toxicity profiles with the use of protons in these disease sites.

Brachytherapy

In contrast to EBRT, brachytherapy is the practice of directly delivering radiation by placing radioactive sources near the tumor or tumor bed. Brachytherapy offers advantages over external beam radiation because it can be used to deliver very high doses of radiation directly to the tumor while sparing surrounding normal tissues. Accurate placement of the source using an applicator positioned directly on the tumor or tumor bed allows for the most conformal of therapies. In general, the level of radiation diminishes with the square of the distance from the radioactive source. Common uses of brachytherapy with curative intent include temporary cesium placement for cervical cancer, temporary iridium-192 placement for a variety of tumors, permanent iodine-125 seed implantation for prostate cancer, and permanent gold-198 seed implantation for various malignancies.

Source activity, dose rate, and source-to-tumor exposure time are all considered when planning therapy and help dictate the modality used. High-dose rate (HDR) and pulse-dose rate (PDR) brachytherapy are commonly used for gynecologic malignancies including cervical, vaginal, and endometrial cancers. Low-dose rate brachytherapy is commonly used for prostate cancer. Indications for brachytherapy include locally contained, small-volume disease that can be accessed by an applicator device.

Intraoperative Radiation Therapy (IORT)

IORT is defined as radiation that is delivered to the tumor or tumor bed during surgery. There are many benefits to IORT including increased local control, ability to deliver higher doses of radiation, and increased delivery of radiation to the region of interest with minimal dose to surrounding tissue. IORT is usually used in conjunction with preoperative EBRT. It is a helpful technique for gastrointestinal malignancies, such as recurrent or locally advanced colorectal cancers.

IORT can be delivered as intraoperative electron radiation therapy or as HDR-IORT. Intraoperative electron radiation therapy uses electron, and HDR-IORT uses HDR brachytherapy delivered through catheters. Both techniques deliver a high dose to the tumor region and minimize the dose to the surrounding normal tissue.

Treatment Techniques

In modern radiation oncology practice, radiographic imaging is used to plan treatment that targets tumors while physically avoiding normal tissues to the greatest extent possible. *Radiation treatment planning* or *dosimetry* involves the creation of an optimized virtual treatment plan. Three-dimensional (3D) computed

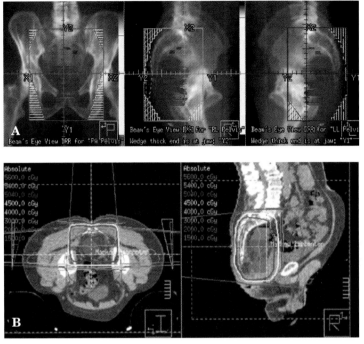

FIGURE 25.1 Three-dimensional plan for treatment fields (**A**) and dosimetry (**B**) for a patient receiving neoadjuvant chemoradiation. The lines surrounding the treatment volume in (**B**) represent the dose levels delivered to the planned volume and surrounding tissues.

tomography (CT) or magnetic resonance (MR) images are used to design radiation fields and dose calculations, and blocking is used to block normal tissue structures (Fig. 25.1). A dose–volume histogram (Fig. 25.2) graphically represents the treated volumes of the tumor and the regional target that receives various doses (Fig. 25.1). The dose–volume histogram, along with visual inspection of the plan, are used to assess target coverage and dose to organs at risk (OARs) during plan evaluation.

3D Conformal Radiotherapy (3D-CRT)

Conventional radiotherapy delivers radiation in rectangular-shaped fields with additional tools such as blocks and wedges to modulate treatment dose. This form of radiation therapy is delivered by using beams that are conformed to the shape to the area of interest (e.g., tumor, nodal stations) in hopes of minimizing the radiation dose to surrounding healthy tissue. This is often termed *forward planning*, referring to the process of targeting

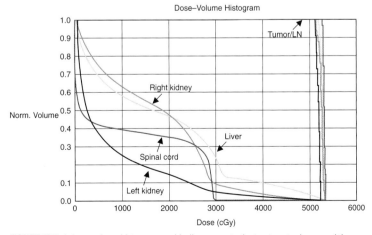

FIGURE 25.2 A dose–volume histogram graphically represents the treatment volumes and the various radiation doses received. Dose–volume histograms enable radiation oncologists to objectively assess the safety of a radiation treatment plan and the adequacy of organ coverage.

beams at the area of interest. Conventional radiotherapy is commonly used to treat cervical cancer, rectal cancer, and breast cancer.

Intensity-Modulated Radiation Therapy (IMRT) and Volumetric-Modulated Arc Therapy (VMAT)

IMRT allows for the delivery of radiation consisting of variable intensities delivered through multiple beam angles. In contrast to 3D-CRT, IMRT requires *inverse planning*, which involves initial delineation of structures (target volume, organs at risk, etc.), and subsequent use of a computer algorithm to optimize beam position and intensity to meet dose distribution goals. This further helps reduce toxicity to surrounding tissues and maximizes dose delivery to the region of interest. IMRT is commonly used in head and neck, esophageal, pancreatic, and anal malignancies.

VMAT is a type of IMRT in which a single or multiple beams are given in a volumetric arc around the patient, with a large number of beam directions delivered through the arc trajectories.

Stereotactic Radiosurgery

Stereotactic radiosurgery (SRS) uses radiation beams aimed at specific targets in the head and spine regions. A multidisciplinary approach is critical, with the involvement of neurosurgery, radiation oncology, and medical oncology, in order to accurately and safely treat these intracranial and intraspinal tumors. A Gamma Knife is a machine used to deliver SRS that uses multiple cobalt-60 sources of radiation to deliver beams in a noncoplanar fashion, resulting in less dose to surrounding normal brain tissue.

Stereotactic Body Radiation Therapy (SBRT)

SBRT is similar in nature to SRS in that it delivers highly conformal ablative doses of radiation with a limited number of fractions, typically defined as 5 fractions or less. SBRT is commonly used in thoracic and gastrointestinal malignancies and metastases. IMRT (Fig. 25.3) and SBRT deliver a radiation dose that conforms more precisely to the tumor than does a radiation dose delivered with conventional means. At the time of this writing, there is increasing interest in expanding the use of SBRT or other hypofractionated regiments in various disease sites, including prostate cancer and breast cancer. There will likely be continued increases in the adoption of hypofractionated radiotherapy in the future.

Image-Guided Radiation Therapy

In image-guided radiation therapy, imaging studies are used to verify that the radiation delivered during treatment is in accordance with the radiation delivery that was planned with use of the patient's initial CT scans. It enables a more accurate setup in the delivery of treatment by ensuring that the tumor is not missed. Other reasons for using image-guided radiation therapy are to prevent day-to-day setup uncertainty, to accurately position the patient over the course of treatment, to adjust for organ motion during treatment such as that due to gastric emptying or filling, and to account for tumor shrinkage out of the planned field of radiation, which may occur with radiosensitive tumors such as lymphoma and anal cancer. Daily cone-beam CT studies (a limited CT scan obtained on the treatment machine immediately before treatment) are commonly used to guide radiation therapy.

Chemoradiation

Radiotherapy has been delivered concurrently with chemotherapy (often termed chemoradiation) since the 1980s to treat rectal cancer patients. While the precise mechanisms are not fully understood, the addition of

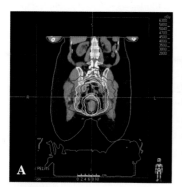
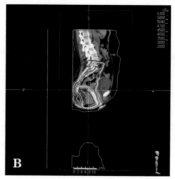
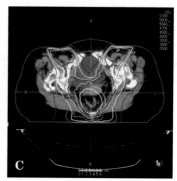

FIGURE 25.3 Volumetric-modulated arc therapy (VMAT) and intensity-modulated radiation therapy (IMRT) allow for optimal sparing of normal tissues and for the possibility of improved local tumor control with use of higher radiation doses. VMAT for anal cancer is one of the best uses for this therapy. Dosimetry in the coronal (**A**), sagittal (**B**), and axial (**C**) planes for a typical VMAT plan are shown.

chemotherapy act to sensitize the tumor cells to the toxic effects of radiation while having less-to-no effect on surrounding normal tissue. Radiotherapy in the treatment of rectal cancers has served as a model for other gastrointestinal sites. In virtually every tumor site where combined modality approaches are standard (e.g., head and neck cancer, gastrointestinal cancers), chemoradiation contributes to locoregional disease control by eradicating microscopic disease or by reducing disease recurrence in regional lymph nodes. For most tumor sites, the patients who benefit the most are those with T3 or T4 tumors, lymph node involvement, or microscopically close or positive surgical margins.

Preoperative chemoradiation has been shown to be more effective and less toxic than postoperative chemoradiation for many patients, likely because with the former, the chemotherapy is delivered with an intact blood supply, and hypoxia-related chemoradiation resistance is avoided. In the specific setting of gastrointestinal irradiation, preoperative chemoradiation results in less acute toxicity than postoperative chemoradiation due to the greater ability of the preoperative procedure to avoid gastrointestinal mucosal irradiation. After gastrointestinal surgery, the small bowel is fixed in the tumor bed and/or the gastrointestinal tract anastomosis will have to be irradiated, which increases the risk of mucosal or anastomotic injury. In contrast, with preoperative chemoradiation, the irradiated gastrointestinal tract with the targeted tumor is removed during surgery, and healthy bowel is used in the reconstruction, considerably lowering the possibility of late radiation injury to these structures. The assertion that preoperative chemoradiation offered advantages over postoperative chemoradiation was controversial until the question was successfully tested in a randomized phase III trial in rectal cancer patients (Sauer et al.). Patients who received preoperative chemoradiation had improved sphincter preservation, better local tumor control, and lower rates of acute and late toxicities (such as anastomotic strictures and chronic diarrhea) than did patients who received postoperative chemoradiation.

Preoperative chemoradiation also offers unique advantages in patients with poor performance status, high operative risk, or high risk of distant metastasis. Most compelling is that preoperative chemoradiation offers the ability to treat virtually all patients who present with localized, resectable cancer with therapy that immediately addresses the limitations of curability—namely, micrometastatic disease. In contrast, delayed recovery from surgery can prevent the timely initiation of postoperative chemoradiation (optimally within 6 to 8 weeks after surgery), thus limiting its efficacy and enabling residual microscopic clonogenic cells to repopulate to gross residual disease. An additional benefit of preoperative chemoradiation is that it facilitates patient selection for complex surgeries that have a significant risk of morbidity or mortality by identifying patients who would not do well with surgery.

Indications for Radiotherapy

Radiation therapy is a versatile treatment modality that has been used effectively in a number of clinical contexts, ranging from the treatment of benign diseases, localized cancers, palliation of symptoms, and, most recently, in the treatment of oligometastatic cancers.

Benign Conditions

Although radiotherapy has been used less commonly for benign conditions in the last few decades, likely owing to increased efforts to avoid long-term side effects of radiation, there are still many benign diseased that are effectively treated with radiotherapy. For example, keloids, heterotopic ossification, gynecomastia, Dupuytren contraction, and various conditions of the central nervous system including arteriovenous malformation and trigeminal neuralgia have been effectively treated with various forms of radiation. More recently, there has also been growing interest in using radiation for the treatment of cardiac arrhythmia refractory to medication or traditional ablative approaches.

Localized Cancer

Radiation therapy has been used extensively in the treatment of localized cancers throughout a large variety of anatomic sites. Radiotherapy may be used in the neoadjuvant setting, for example per the RAPIDO protocol for the high-risk locally advanced rectal cancer, or in the adjuvant setting such as the Stupp protocol for the treatment of glioblastoma. Furthermore, radiotherapy can be used in the definitive setting, either alone or as part of a multimodality treatment approach. For example, chemoradiation can be used to definitively treat locally advanced pancreas cancer, prostate cancer, or various cancers of the head and neck.

Oligometastatic Cancer

In recent years, there has been growing interest in the use of radiotherapy for cancer that has spread past the local site of origin but with only limited metastatic sites. This state of limited spread is termed "oligometastases." Historically, radiation was rarely used for curative treatment of metastatic cancer, even with limited distant disease, as it is fundamentally a local therapy. However, randomized clinical trials, such as the SABR-COMET trial (Palma et al.) and MD Anderson Phase II trial (Gomez et al.) provide encouraging early evidence that radiotherapy can be used to improve outcomes, including progression-free and possibly overall survival, for patients with oligometastatic disease. While the precise definition of oligometastases remains unclear (how many lesions, role of histology, etc.), this represents an exciting avenue for increasing use of curative radiotherapy. Many ongoing clinical trials will be important in clarifying the role of ablative radiotherapy in treating oligometastatic cancers.

Palliative of Symptoms

Radiotherapy is commonly used for palliation of malignancy-associated symptoms. Likely the most common clinical situation requiring palliative radiotherapy is painful metastasis, often involving bone. These can be treated with short courses of EBRT, typically less than 10 fractions, with recent evidence suggesting that even one-fraction regimens provide equivalent pain control. Other common clinical situations requiring palliative radiotherapy are symptomatic brain metastases and bleeding related to invasive tumors.

Radiation Side Effects

In normal tissues, radiation reactions are classified as either acute reactions or late reactions. Acute radiation reactions are due to the temporary depletion of rapidly dividing cells. Common acute radiation reactions include skin desquamation, nausea, diarrhea, and reduced blood cell counts. After an acute radiation reaction, progenitor cells repopulate the tissue, and the effects of the acute reaction resolve. In contrast, late radiation reactions, which can include severe fibrosis, transverse myelitis of the spinal cord, blindness, and pulmonary fibrosis, are caused by microvasculature damage or the depletion of terminally differentiated cells. These late reactions are much less likely to resolve.

Radiation Safety

Time, distance, and shielding should be considered in order to protect health care personnel and patients from radioactive sources. Specifically, the following should be noted.

1. Health care personnel should minimize the amount of time they spend in close proximity to radiation sources.
2. Since the level of radioactivity falls off with the square of the distance to the radiation source, maximizing one's distance from the source diminishes one's exposure to radiation. Radioactive sources should never be touched directly.
3. Shielding is an important aspect of radiation protection. All linear accelerators, CT scanners, and x-ray tubes are shielded in lead- and/or concrete-encased rooms; thus, exposure to radiation for most hospital personnel is minimal. However, shielding is much more of a challenge for personnel who work more directly with radiation sources. In general, lead aprons are effective protection against low-energy radiation sources such as traditional diagnostic and fluoroscopic x-rays.

Multidisciplinary Approach

Multidisciplinary clinics (MDCs) are becoming increasingly prevalent in the management of oncologic disease. MDCs establish a common forum for specialists in radiation oncology, medical oncology, surgery, radiology, pathology, palliative/supportive care, nutrition, and social work to discuss patient cases and formulate a coherent, organized management plan. The practice model of MDCs has been shown to increase the accuracy of initial staging and improve survival for patients with breast, ovarian, and pancreatic cancers. Moreover, the multidisciplinary approach reduces time to treatment and patient anxiety, increases patient exposure to support services and resources, improves overall patient satisfaction, and increases enrollment into clinical trials.

Summary

Radiotherapy is a versatile treatment modality that can be used in a myriad of clinical scenarios, ranging from treatment of benign diseases to definitive treatment of localized cancers to treatment of oligometastatic cancers. The choice of radiation modality and treatment planning technique is based on the goal of achieving the optimal dose distribution. Typically, complex treatment plans are needed when the tumor is located near critical structures such as the spinal cord and bowel. Newer technologies such as proton therapy, IMRT, SRS, SBRT, and image-guided radiation therapy have enhanced our ability to give higher radiation doses to targets while reducing normal tissue exposure.

CASE SCENARIO

Case Scenario 1: Radiotherapy for Rectal Adenocarcinoma

Presentation

A 68-year-old woman presents to the clinic with rectal bleeding for 3 months. Digital rectal examination did not identify any lesions but a sigmoidoscopy was performed and revealed a lesion 8 cm from the anal verge. A biopsy was obtained and pathologic evaluation showed moderately differentiated adenocarcinoma. Computed tomography of the chest, abdomen, and pelvis identified a 4-cm rectal mass with two enlarged perirectal lymph nodes suspicious for metastatic involvement. MRI of the pelvis was consistent with a stage T3c N1 lesion with extramural vascular invasion (EMVI) and no invasion of the mesorectal fascia (MRF). There was no evidence of distant metastatic disease.

Treatment Paradigm

At MDACC, the typical treatment approach for locally advanced rectal cancer at the time of this writing is total neoadjuvant therapy per the RAPIDO trial protocol. This entails short course radiotherapy (25 Gy in 5 fractions) followed by chemotherapy and subsequent surgical resection.

Radiotherapy: Key Steps

- After the decision is made to proceed with radiotherapy, the first step in treatment planning is a simulation. The patient is brought to the radiotherapy department and imaging (typically CT) is obtained with the patient in the treatment position, which may involve custom or generic immobilization devices.
- Using images obtained at simulation, the treating radiation oncologist delineates the treatment target volume and potential organs at risk in three-dimensional space using treatment planning software.
- A team of specialists works with the radiation oncologist to develop an optimal treatment plan to optimize dose coverage of the target volumes while minimizing dose to organs at risk.
- Once a final treatment plan is created, it undergoes quality assurance with a multidisciplinary team of physicians and physicists.
- After final approval of the plan, the patient is ready to initiate treatment.

CASE SCENARIO 1 REVIEW

Questions

1. Radiation therapy for the treatment of rectal cancer can be delivered with 3D conformal radiation therapy (3DCRT) or with intensity-modulated radiotherapy (IMRT). Which of the following most accurately describes differences between 3DCRT and IMRT?

    A. 3DCRT is used to deliver higher doses of radiation
    B. 3DCRT typically spares normal tissues more than IMRT
    C. 3DCRT typically involves forward treatment planning whereas IMRT typically involves reverse treatment planning
    D. IMRT uses a different type of radiation compared to 3DCRT

2. In patients with locally advanced rectal cancer at high risk of local recurrence following surgical resection, which of the following radiotherapy techniques may be considered at the time of surgery to decrease risk of local recurrence?

    A. Proton therapy
    B. Gamma Knife
    C. Intraoperative radiation therapy (IORT)
    D. Stereotactic body radiation therapy (SBRT)

3. Which of the following does NOT represent a potential indication for radiotherapy in patients with rectal cancer?

    A. Neoadjuvant radiotherapy prior to resection
    B. Stereotactic body radiotherapy (SBRT) for oligometastatic disease sites
    C. Palliation of painful bone metastases
    D. Palliation of small bowel obstruction from peritoneal disease

4. Suppose this patient develops symptoms of dizziness 3 years after completing definitive treatment. She is evaluated in the Emergency Center and a brain MRI is obtained, which identifies a single 1.5-cm metastasis in the pons. Which of the following radiation therapy techniques represents the optimal treatment option?

   A. Stereotactic radiosurgery (e.g., Gamma Knife)
   B. Hippocampal-sparing whole brain radiotherapy
   C. Brachytherapy
   D. Proton therapy

5. Which of the following is an expected acute side effect of pelvic radiation therapy for rectal cancer?

   A. Chest pain
   B. Diarrhea
   C. Dyspnea
   D. Nerve damage

Answers

1. **The correct answer is C.** *Rationale:* IMRT generally delivers higher doses of radiation in more precise locations due to coning of the energy beams. This coming requires revers treatment planning, delineating the structures then optimizing beam strength and position to achieve the desired dose distribution.

2. **The correct answer is C.** *Rationale:* IORT can be used at the time of surgery to deliver energy directly to the tumor bed. The advantages over other adjuvant radiation is the ability for the surgeon to move any other organs, including the body wall, away from the radiation field.

3. **The correct answer is D.** *Rationale:* Radiation therapy can be used in a variety of ways to treat rectal cancer patients. However, due to toxicity and resultant complications, radiation therapy cannot be used to treat peritoneal disease on the small bowel.

4. **The correct answer is A.** *Rationale:* Gamma Knife has the advantages of high accuracy and minimizing dose delivery to surrounding tissue, ideal for application to brain metastasis.

5. **The correct answer is B.** *Rationale:* The toxic effects of radiation on the bowel cause difficulty with nutrient and bile absorption. This may cause diarrhea, bowel incontinence, and intolerance to certain foods. Radiation enteritis can present in an early or delayed manner, and is related to the cumulative dose of radiation received.

Recommended Readings

Bahadoer RR, Dijkstra EA, van Etten B, et al. Short-course radiotherapy followed by chemotherapy before total mesorectal excision (TME) versus preoperative chemoradiotherapy, TME, and optional adjuvant chemotherapy in locally advanced rectal cancer (RAPIDO): a randomised, open-label, phase 3 trial. *Lancet Oncol.* 2021;22(1):29–42. doi:10.1016/S1470-2045(20)30555-6

Frank SJ, Blanchard P, Lee JJ, et al. Comparing intensity-modulated proton therapy with intensity-modulated photon therapy for oropharyngeal cancer: the journey from clinical trial concept to activation. *Semin Radiat Oncol.* 2018;28(2):108–113. doi:10.1016/j.semradonc.2017.12.002

Gomez DR, Tang C, Zhang J, et al. Local consolidative therapy vs. maintenance therapy or observation for patients with oligometastatic non-small cell lung cancer: long-term results of a multi-institutional, phase ii, randomized study . *J Clin Oncol.* 2019;37(18):1558–1565. doi:10.1200/JCO.19.00201

Kachnic LA, Winter K, Myerson RJ, et al. Long term outcomes of NRG Oncology/RTOG 0529: a phase ii evaluation of dose-painted intensity modulated radiation therapy (DP-IMRT) in combination with 5-fluorouracil and mitomycin-c for the reduction of acute morbidity in anal canal cancer. *Int J Radiat Oncol Biol Phys.* 2021;112(1):146–157, S0360-3016(21)02647-X. doi:10.1016/j.ijrobp.2021.08.008

Lin SH, Hobbs BP, Verma V, et al. Randomized phase IIb trial of proton beam therapy versus intensity-modulated radiation therapy for locally advanced esophageal cancer. *J Clin Oncol Off J Am Soc Clin Oncol.* 2020;38(14):1569–1579. doi:10.1200/JCO.19.02503

Nguyen Q-N, Chun SG, Chow E, et al. Single-fraction stereotactic vs conventional multifraction radiotherapy for pain relief in patients with predominantly nonspine bone metastases: a randomized phase 2 trial. *JAMA Oncol*. 2019;5(6):872–878. doi:10.1001/jamaoncol.2019.0192

Palma DA, Olson R, Harrow S, et al. Stereotactic ablative radiotherapy versus standard of care palliative treatment in patients with oligometastatic cancers (SABR-COMET): a randomised, phase 2, open-label trial. *The Lancet*. 2019;393(10185):2051–2058. doi:10.1016/S0140-6736(18)32487-5

Stupp R, Mason WP, van den Bent MJ, et al. Radiotherapy plus concomitant and adjuvant temozolomide for glioblastoma. *N Engl J Med*. 2005;352(10):987–996. doi:10.1056/NEJMoa043330

Willett CG, Czito BG, Tyler DS. Intraoperative radiation therapy. *J Clin Oncol Off J Am Soc Clin Oncol*. 2007;25(8):971–977. doi:10.1200/JCO.2006.10.0255

Reconstructive Surgery in Cancer Patients

Margaret S. Roubaud, Donald P. Baumann, Mark T. Villa, Geoffrey L. Robb, and Matthew M. Hanasono

In cancer patients who have undergone extirpative surgery, the goal of reconstructive surgery is to restore form and function. This goal is best accomplished by replacing the resected tissue—bone, skin, fat, etc.—with similar tissue. Reconstructive options vary from simple to complex based on the needs of the wound and patient. Simple procedures include primary closure, local tissue rearrangement, and skin grafting. More complex procedures include the use of pedicled flaps or microvascular free flaps. The ability to perform complete oncologic resections has increased with our ability to perform reconstructive surgery more safely and reliably with decreased morbidity.

General Principles of Reconstructive Surgery

To select the appropriate reconstructive technique, it is critical to evaluate physiologic status of the patient. A patient with multiple comorbidities and/or poor nutrition may not be able to tolerate a lengthy procedure and therefore consideration should be made to treat with a more conservative reconstruction. In contrast, a patient with adequate physiologic reserve may be best served by a more technically complicated procedure, such as microsurgical reconstruction, when it provides the optimal restoration of both form and function.

In addition to wound closure and maintenance of function, an important goal of reconstructive surgery is aesthetic restoration. While most people may immediately associate aesthetics with cosmetic surgery, aesthetics in the cancer patient focuses on the restoration of one's prior appearance. Many patients that present to the reconstructive surgeon have significant body image concerns and anxiety about their ability to interact with others, especially their loved ones, in the future. The goal of the reconstructive surgeon is to not only heal wounds, but allow patients to return to their lives feeling whole. It is not acceptable to close a wound that radically deforms the patient, if alternatives exist.

The timing of reconstruction is most often dictated by the status of the tumor and oncologic treatment. Reconstruction can be performed in an immediate or delayed fashion. Immediate reconstruction is considered when a patient needs restoration of a vital structure, such as the pharynx or abdominal wall, and when their physiologic reserve allows extended time under anesthesia. When immediate reconstruction is performed, tissue planes are readily accessible and the wound bed has little or no fibrotic tissue. In contrast, when the reconstruction is delayed, scar tissue, fibrosis, and wound contracture can inhibit optimal aesthetic and functional outcomes. However, delayed reconstruction may be necessary when margins are not clear, as in permanent section evaluation for melanoma, or when the patient requires significant postoperative radiation that will damage the reconstruction, such as in breast reconstruction.

Reconstructive Techniques

The core principle of the reconstructive algorithm is to progress from simple to more complex reconstructions based on the specific wound requirements. This is referred to as the reconstructive ladder. The primary goal is to close a wound with tissue that will be tension-free and obliterate any dead-space. Ideally, it should be durable and functional if possible. In general, primary closure is the simplest and lowest rung of the ladder. Skin grafts may be considered next. When these alternatives are insufficient, local tissue rearrangement or flaps can be used to close more complex wounds. Finally, microsurgical techniques may be required to transfer free autologous tissue from one area of the body to another when local options are not available. In addition, when reconstruction is not immediately necessary, local tissue may also be expanded to cover a defect.

Skin grafts contain epidermis and variable amounts of dermis. A partial-thickness skin graft includes superficial dermis, whereas a full-thickness graft includes the entire dermis. Skin grafts require a vascularized bed for ingrowth, such as granulated tissue, fascia, muscle, or periosteum. Because full-thickness skin grafts contract less than split-thickness skin grafts, full-thickness grafts are preferable in regions where wound bed contraction is not desirable. For example, they are frequently used on the face, where wound bed contraction near the eyelids, nose, or mouth would compromise aesthetic and/or functional outcome. Aesthetic outcomes are inferior to those of local or free-tissue flap options in many instances due to minimal tissue thickness and color match.

Local tissue rearrangement and locoregional flaps enable surgeons to reconstruct wounds with similar tissue from a nearby location. The tissue that is moved is called a flap. Random local flaps are the basis of local tissue rearrangement. Local flaps are usually comprised of adjacent skin and subcutaneous tissue that are based on a subdermal plexus vascular supply. By definition, random flaps do not have a distinct, named blood vessel as their vascular supply. They are generally limited in size with 3:1 length to width ratio. In contrast, pedicled flaps are based on named blood vessels, including an arterial and venous pedicle. These flaps can be moved as far as their vascular pedicle will allow and may not necessarily be from an immediately adjacent location, hence, they are considered regional flaps. An example is the latissimus dorsi flap, which may be rotated from the posterior trunk to the anterior trunk. A pedicled flap may be very small or large depending on the area perfused by the pedicle blood vessels. For example, a nasolabial flap is a small flap based on the angular artery, a branch of the facial artery, and is approximately 4×1.5 cm because it is a small blood vessel encompassing a limited vascular territory. In contrast, a latissimus dorsi muscle pedicled flap can be as large as 30×40 cm. Pedicled flaps can be cutaneous, fasciocutaneous (deep muscle fascia with overlying skin), muscular, myocutaneous (muscle with skin), osseous, or osteocutaneous (bone with overlying skin). These multiple options enable the reconstructive surgeon to repair defects with tissue that is similar to the resected tissue.

Microvascular free flaps are tissues with a pedicle blood supply from a distant region of the body that is ligated and then transferred to a defect. They are called "free flaps" because they become free of their native vascular origin and require reanastomosis for perfusion. Vascular anastomoses between the flap's donor (pedicle) vessels and recipient vessels within or near the defect are performed under magnification provided by a microscope or high-powered surgical loupes. The decision to use a particular flap is based on the requirements for replacing missing skin, adipose tissue, fascia, muscle, and/or bone. The primary advantage of microvascular free tissue transfer is that tissue of a quality similar to that of the resected tissue can be moved from a remote part of the body, enabling optimal aesthetic and functional outcomes. Drawbacks of free tissue transfer are related to donor site morbidity, the potential for long operative times, and possible complications with the vascular anastomoses. However, when performed with appropriate technique and efficiency, free flaps are highly reliable and often the best choice for reconstruction for both form and function.

Tissue expansion is a process in which an inflatable prosthetic implant with a silicone shell is used to expand local and regional tissues. In breast reconstruction, they are used to stretch or expand the remaining mastectomy skin for future implant placement. In other defects, the skin is expanded so that it can eventually be advanced into the wound for coverage in a delayed fashion. The inflatable implant is inserted at the time of tumor extirpation or during a second procedure. At subsequent office visits, saline is injected through an integrated or remote port to gradually expand the implant. Once the tissue has been sufficiently expanded, the expander is removed and the tissue is used for wound coverage or as an implant pocket, in the case of breast reconstruction. Risks of tissue expansion include implant exposure, infection, and pain related to serial expansions.

Head and Neck Reconstruction

The goals of reconstruction in the head and neck include preservation of speech, swallowing, and masticatory function, maintaining an airway while preventing aspiration and velopharyngeal insufficiency, supporting the orbit, and maintaining the appearance of the face. Coverage of the facial bones, dura and brain, as well as the neurovascular structures of the neck may also be indications for reconstructive surgery. Each region of the head and neck has specific reconstructive needs and defects are usually best reconstructed as separate subunits. With a few notable exceptions described below, microvascular free flaps are usually associated with superior outcomes and the preferred reconstructive method for most patients undergoing all but the most limited resections.

Scalp and Calvarium

The scalp, including the forehead, is a well-vascularized region composed of five layers that can be remembers using the mnemonic *SCALP*: *S*kin, sub*C*utaneous tissue, galea *A*poneurosis (a dense fibrous connective tissue layer interspersed between the frontalis, occipitalis, and temporalis muscles that fuses with the temporoparietal fascia at the temporal crest), *L*oose areolar tissue, and *P*ericranium (the periosteum coving the calvarial bones).

The reconstructive method of choice depends on surface area and depth of the wound. If the pericranium remains intact, one option is to allow the wound to heal by secondary intention or resurface the wound with a split- or full-thickness skin graft. Skin grafting results in an area of alopecia that may be noticeable in patients who are not bald.

Because the scalp is poorly distensible, only very small full-thickness wounds can be closed primarily, even with wide undermining in the loose areolar plane deep to the galea aponeurotica. Scoring the galea at right angles to the direction of advancement decreases wound tension and may allow primary closure of wounds up to 3 cm wide. Care needs to be taken not to injure the blood vessels they lie above the galea, which could compromise the viability of the scalp.

Defects greater than 3 cm but less than 6 cm can generally be reconstructed with one or more rotation flaps. Larger defects can be closed with rotation flaps and skin grafting of the flap donor site, provided there is intact pericranium. Such scalping flaps may result in a cosmetically unfavorable bald spot if the skin grafted donor site is noticeable in a patient with an otherwise full head of hair. The base of each rotation flap should contain an intact named blood vessel (i.e., supraorbital, supratrochlear, superficial temporal, post auricular, or occipital) to serve as an axial blood supply. In some cases, wounds approaching 50% of the scalp surface area can be closed with a scalping flap or skin grafted, if the periosteum is intact. Then, tissue expansion of the hair bearing scalp can be performed so that the skin-grafted area can be removed. The risks of tissue expansion include exposure of the expansion device, infection, and decreased hair density inherent to the expansion process. Irradiation is a relative contraindication to tissue expansion due to the high rate of exposure of the expansion device and poor expansion of radiated tissue.

Defects larger than about 6 cm, or even smaller defects in irradiated scalps, usually require microvascular free flap reconstruction. The scalp can usually be reconstructed with thin cutaneous or fasciocutaneous free flaps, such as the anterolateral thigh (ALT) free flap, or a muscle flap, such as the latissimus dorsi muscle free flap, covered with a skin graft. For the largest defects, the latissimus dorsi muscle free flap is considered the flap of choice due to its large surface area, often sufficient to resurface the entire scalp. The superficial temporal blood vessels are the preferred recipient blood vessels for free flap reconstruction but may not be available due to ligation during prior surgeries. In such cases, vein grafting may be needed to reach recipient blood vessels in the neck.

Occasionally, skin cancers of the scalp can invade the underlying bone necessitating removal of the outer-table or full-thickness calvarium. The repair of such defects requires autologous bone grafts such as split-calvarial grafts or prosthetic materials such as titanium mesh or methyl methacrylate in addition to free flaps. Well-vascularized coverage over grafts and implants is mandatory. As long there is not gross contamination, simultaneous scalp and calvarial reconstruction is usually safe and reliable. In the setting of infected bone or prosthetic, scalp reconstruction followed by delayed cranioplasty is usually recommended.

Face

Facial reconstruction is divided into specific units, each with its own anatomy and function: cheek, eyelids, nose, lips, and neck. Each region must be considered independently and collectively when defects cross facial zone boundaries.

Cheek

Small defects of the facial skin can often be closed primarily after an elliptical incision. Such an incision should be made in the direction of the facial skin-tension lines. If the wound cannot be closed primarily without significant distortion of the face, the next option is a local tissue flap based on a random blood supply. Moderate medial cheek defects, up to 5 cm, require fasciocutaneous rotation flaps based on the cervicofacial vessels. The greater the amount of rotation needed, the greater the risk for ectropion of the lower eyelid as a complication. Full-thickness skin grafts can be used instead of local flaps or in addition to local flaps as long as bone or neurovascular structures are not exposed, but may be prone to contraction. The best skin graft donor site for facial reconstruction is the region above the clavicle or the preauricular or postauricular skin, because of the good color and texture match to the rest of the facial skin. Skin grafts are avoided when postoperative radiation therapy is planned due to concerns for graft loss or contracture. When a wound cannot be covered with local tissue, reconstruction with cutaneous or fasciocutaneous free flaps, such as the ALT or parascapular free flaps, may be necessary.

Nose

The nose consists of nine aesthetic subunits: the dorsum, two sidewalls, the tip, the columella, two soft-triangles, and two alae. The adage to replace "like with like" is critical in this anatomical region, and, therefore, local and regional flaps are the mainstay of nasal reconstruction. A possible exception is use of full-thickness skin grafts on the dorsum of the nose, where the native skin tends to be thin and contracture is unlikely to distort the shape of the nose. Nasal defects involving <50% of an aesthetic subunit can be reconstructed with a local flap and the remaining subunit can be retained. However, the entire subunit should be reconstructed if the defect involves ≥50% of a subunit. Local flaps such as bilobed flaps can be used to reconstruct defects of the nasal sidewall and dorsum. The paramedian forehead flap, based on the supratrochlear artery, is the workhorse flap for most sizable defects, larger than about 1.5 cm in diameter up to the entire exterior nasal skin, because of its excellent color and texture match to nasal skin. A secondary choice is the nasolabial flap, based on the angular artery, which can also be used to reconstruct defects in the lower nasal elements due to its thickness. Full-thickness defects of the nose comprise the external skin, cartilage, and nasal lining, and all three layers must be considered in repair. The nasal lining often can be reconstructed with local flaps obtained from the nasal mucosa. Cartilaginous structures can be reconstructed using cartilage grafts from the rib or ear. The paramedian forehead flap is preferred for external skin coverage in full-thickness defects.

Lip

The vermilion–cutaneous junction, the border between the red of the lip and surrounding skin, is a distinct anatomical line that requires meticulous reconstruction. Asymmetries at the vermillion–cutaneous junction of greater than 1 mm will lead to visible irregularities in a reconstructed lip.

Defects less than one-third the width of the lower or upper lip are generally repaired with wedge resection and multilayered primary closure. For larger defects, a local flap, must be considered. Lip switch flaps, also known as Abbé-Estlander flaps, are pedicled flaps transferred from the opposite lip that are based on the labial branch of the facial artery. Lip switch flaps are used to repair defects that are between one and two-thirds the width of the lip.

Defects larger than on half to two-thirds the width of the lip require bilateral rotation or advancement flaps, which recruit larger segments of tissue from adjacent cheek tissue. One such flap is the Karapandzic advancement flap, a neurovascular flap that preserves the elements of the facial nerve branches to the orbicularis oris. The use of advancement flaps can reduce the oral aperture, resulting in microstomia. Total lip defects are usually reconstructed with a free radial forearm flap suspended by a palmaris longus tendon graft to support the reconstructed lip and maintain lip height.

Ear

The outer ear is composed of skin closely adherent to an underlying cartilaginous framework. The surface anatomy of the ear consists of the helix, anti-helix, concha, tragus, and lobule.

Small defects in the skin of the helical rim can be repaired with excision of a triangular wedge and direct approximation. If the defect is small but direct approximation cannot be performed, the remaining helix can be reconstructed with local chondrocutaneous flaps; in this instance, the remaining helical rim is dissected off the scapha and advanced. Large defects of the helical rim can be covered with a postauricular skin flap over a cartilage graft from the concha of the same or the contralateral ear to maintain shape. This is a staged procedure in which division of the base of the flap and completion of the flap inset are performed about 3 weeks after the initial transposition of the flap. A skin graft is usually applied to the denuded mastoid or temporal region at the flap donor site.

Large auricular defects with missing cartilaginous components can be reconstructed using cartilage grafts from the ribs. These grafts can be sculpted to conform to the missing helical rim and require coverage with a pedicled temporoparietal fascia flap based on the superficial temporal artery. Alloplastic frameworks, such as those composed of high-density polyethylene, can also be used to repair cartilaginous defects in the ear, obviating the need for donor cartilage. Alloplastic implants also require coverage with vascularized tissue such as a temporoparietal fascia flap. Alternately, substantial auriculectomy defects may be addressed with a maxillofacial prosthesis attached with adhesives or osseointegrated titanium implants embedded in the adjacent temporal bone.

Oral Cavity

The oral cavity includes the anterior tongue, floor of the mouth, alveolar ridges, retromolar trigone, hard palate, and buccal mucosa. Resection of oral tumors can result in both functional and aesthetic defects in the face and mouth. Defects involving any of these structures can compromise speech, chewing, swallowing, and breathing.

The thin, pliable fasciocutaneous forearm free flaps, based on either the radial or ulnar artery, are excellent options for reconstructing mucosal defects of the floor of the mouth and buccal area without creating bulk that can interfere with function. They are pliable and do not restrict tongue movement or mouth opening, which are important for speech and diet. The lateral arm flap, which is supplied by the posterior radial collateral vessels, and the ALT flap may also be appropriate choices provided the patient has minimal subcutaneous fat in these areas. For full-thickness buccal mucosa-cheek defects, the radial or ulnar forearm free flaps or other fasciocutaneous flaps of appropriate thickness can be folded in on themselves to provide an internal and external lining.

Very small tongue defects may be skin grafted or allowed to heal secondarily. Free flaps should be consid ered for any defect in which contracture may limit tongue movement, which could impair speech, deglutition, or oral hygiene by inhibiting the sweeping function of the tongue used to clear food debris from the oral cavity. Partial glossectomy and hemi-glossectomy defects are best reconstructed with a thin, pliable free flap, such as the radial or ulnar forearm fasciocutaneous free flaps (Fig. 26.1). Total and near-total glossectomies require bulky flaps to help prevent aspiration by directing food, liquids, and saliva away from the larynx and down the lateral pharynx into the esophagus. In most patients, the rectus abdominis myocutaneous free flap or the ALT free flap, including a portion of the vastus lateralis muscle, can provide adequate bulk for reconstructing total and near-total tongue defects. Prior to the advent of free flap reconstruction, many total glossectomy patients required laryngectomy to avoid chronic aspiration. In recent years, the majority of patients can avoid laryngectomy, and up to half are able to sustain themselves partially or completely without feeding tube supplementation.

Mandible

The mandible plays a key role in mastication and giving shape to the lower third of the face, as well as deglutition, articulation, and stabilizing the airway based on its support and interaction with the tongue. Functional losses and aesthetic deformity depend on the size and location of the mandibular defect. Defects in the posterior body or ramus of the mandible are generally better tolerated than defects in the anterior mandible, which are associated with significant deformity and loss of function. Malocclusion may develop as a result of a shift in the position of the mandible following mandibulectomy. Mandibular reconstruction following surgery optimally preserves mastication, speech, swallowing, and airway integrity. It restores lower facial aesthetics and enables subsequent dental reconstruction.

In mandibulectomy defect repair, the functional and aesthetic results obtained with microvascular tissue transfer are superior to those obtained with nonvascularized bone grafts or pedicled tissue transfers. Small segmental mandibulectomy defects (less than 5 cm) may be reconstructed with nonvascularized grafts and metal plates when adjuvant radiation is not planned, but such defects are rare following cancer resections. In most patients, mandibulectomy defects involve a large segment of the bony mandible, the internal oral lining,

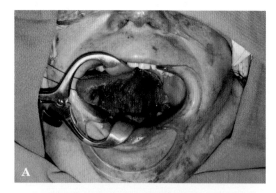
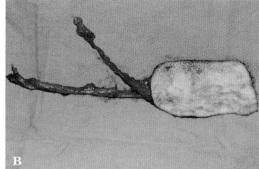
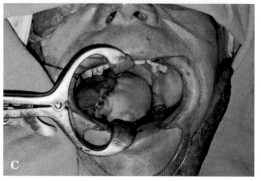

FIGURE 26.1 A left hemiglossectomy defect (**A**) is reconstructed with a radial forearm free flap (**B**), which is a thin, pliable fasciocutaneous flap that is well suited to resurfacing the tongue without restricting its movement. Completed reconstruction (**C**).

and the external skin. Free flap reconstruction provides sufficient bony and soft tissue coverage with a reliable vascular supply. Vascularized bone free flaps have high bone union rates because the flaps heal by primary bone healing, similar to how fractures heal. In contrast, nonvascularized bone grafts heal by osteoconduction.

The mainstay of mandibular reconstruction is the fibula osteocutaneous free flap. This flap provides up to 20 cm of bone. Because of its rich periosteal blood supply, osteotomies can be made to contour the bone such that it takes on the shape of the resected mandible without devascularization. In addition, a skin paddle can be harvested to provide soft-tissue coverage. Functionally, harvest of the central fibula is well tolerated as long as 5 cm of proximal and distal fibula are preserved in situ for tibial stability. The length and caliber of the pedicle vessels are sufficiently large to be anastomosed to vessels in the neck.

The fibula flap is based on the peroneal artery and vein; therefore, its use requires that either the anterior or the posterior tibial vessels adequately perfuse the distal lower limb. An angiogram may be required to confirm this before harvest. Secondary flap sources for mandible reconstruction include the iliac, scapular, and radial bone free flaps.

Pharynx

The goal of pharyngoesophageal reconstruction is to restore swallowing and speech. Reconstruction of the pharynx and proximal esophagus is challenging. Most patients who require reconstruction also receive radiation therapy which complicates reconstructive efforts.

Traditional methods of pharyngeal and esophageal reconstruction, including the use of tubed deltopectoral pedicled flaps, have given way to immediate reconstruction with jejunal segment, radial forearm, or ALT free flaps. Pharyngeal and esophageal reconstruction with the ALT free flap has been shown to result in a better voice restoration with a tracheoesophageal prosthesis (TEP) than reconstruction with the jejunal free flap, which results in a wet voice. In addition, swallowing after the jejunal flap is often interrupted by disordered peristalsis within the flap. Harvest of a jejunal flap requires laparotomy and bowel anastomosis adding the potential for greater morbidity in the setting of a complication. ALT free flaps and jejunal free flaps have similar rates of stricture formation and fistula formation. Both options are superior to nonmicrovascular alternatives.

Breast Reconstruction

The treatment for breast cancer involves multiple modalities, including surgery (resectional and reconstructive), systemic therapy (chemotherapy and/or hormonal therapy), and radiation therapy. From a reconstructive standpoint, one must consider the amount of breast parenchyma removed (mastectomy vs. partial mastectomy), the amount of skin remaining after surgical resection (skin-sparing vs. traditional mastectomy), whether radiation may be required or has already been given, and the use and timing of systemic therapy.

Each type of breast reconstruction has its advantages and disadvantages. Some women desire no reconstruction at all. There is no one approach to breast reconstruction that is appropriate in all patients. Some aspects to consider in helping a patient choose the right reconstructive option include: (a) the patient's desires and expectations, (b) the treatment that they have undergone and still have to undergo, (c) their willingness to undergo surgery, and (d) their overall prognosis. Although, there are certain instances in which a single-stage reconstruction may be possible, breast reconstruction generally is a process that entails multiple surgical procedures over the course of 4 to 12 months. These procedures include the initial breast reconstruction, any subsequent operations for achieving breast symmetry, and nipple reconstruction.

When counseling patients on reconstructive options it is important to remember that the primary focus of treatment is the cancer. Reconstruction is important, but it is a secondary goal. Women can often feel overwhelmed by all of the treatment options, not only in treating their cancer but also in the reconstruction. It is important to remember that every patient has different expectations for their body following treatment for breast cancer. Counseling patients on all options for reconstruction and then allowing patients to make their own decisions, leads to highest long-term satisfactions rates posttreatment for breast cancer. It is additionally important to give patients a realistic idea of what to expect after reconstruction.

Timing Considerations for Breast Reconstruction

An important aspect to discuss with patients is the timing of breast reconstruction. This is based not only on the patient's wishes but also on the characteristics of the disease. Immediate reconstruction takes place at the time of the breast cancer surgery. Delayed reconstruction takes place after the treatment for the cancer is complete (Fig. 26.2). Immediate reconstruction results in the best aesthetic outcomes if postmastectomy radiation therapy is not needed. Delayed reconstruction is preferred if postmastectomy radiation therapy is

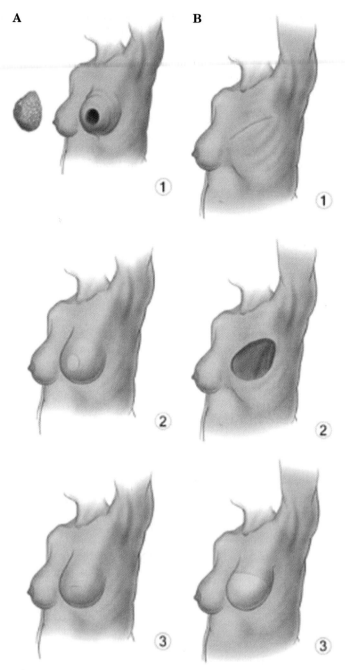

FIGURE 26.2 Immediate reconstruction (**A**) is performed at the time of the breast cancer surgery. Delayed reconstruction (**B**) is performed after the patient has completed breast cancer treatment.

required, as it avoids potential radiation delivery problems and generally results in a superior aesthetic outcome. Unfortunately this is often not known until the surgical pathology returns well after the surgery is over.

At MD Anderson Cancer Center, the "delayed-immediate protocol" is commonly used to answer this conundrum. The protocol is designed to preserve the breast skin envelope for an optimal aesthetic outcome, while considering the possibility that a patient may need to receive adjuvant radiation therapy.

Delayed-immediate breast reconstruction is a two-staged approach. In the first stage, after a skin-sparing mastectomy is performed, a tissue expander is placed until it is known whether or not adjuvant radiation therapy is necessary. If radiation is not required, then patients undergo more immediate reconstruction, usually within weeks of their initial operation, with an implant or autologous tissue.

If radiation is required, then the tissue expander remains in place during radiation and delayed reconstruction is performed after the oncologic treatment is finished. Typically, after radiation, breast reconstruction is performed with autologous tissue from the abdomen, back, or thigh to avoid the increased complications associated with implants in a radiated field. In general, patients require 6 to 12 months for the chest wall to recover before delayed radiation can commence.

Reconstruction after Partial Mastectomy

In a partial mastectomy, only the portion of the breast that contains the cancer is removed, and the remainder of the breast tissue is left in place. This is performed with the expectation that adjuvant radiation will be required to complete treatment. For some, reconstruction is not required because little or no skin and only a portion of breast tissue are removed during a partial mastectomy. When larger amounts of tissue are removed, the remaining breast tissue can be "rearranged" subcutaneously to fill the defect. The skin envelope can be adjusted in a mastopexy or breast lift technique. Collectively, these techniques are referred to as oncoplastic breast reconstruction. If the remaining breast tissue volume is insufficient, additional tissue may be brought to the breast, usually a pedicled or free flap from the back or the abdomen. Immediate reconstruction is preferred in patients who undergo partial mastectomy rather than to performed delayed reconstruction within an irradiated field. Autologous fat grafting may be beneficial following the completion of cancer therapy to correct any residual volume deficits or contour deformities that remain.

Reconstruction After Mastectomy

The majority of breast reconstructions are performed using (1) tissue expanders and implants, (2) latissimus dorsi myocutaneous flaps and implants, or (3) abdominal tissue-based pedicled and free flaps. A staged reconstruction consisting of tissue expansion followed by permanent implant placement is the most common method of breast reconstruction in the United States (Fig. 26.3).

Implant-Based Reconstruction

Implant-based breast reconstruction generally begins with tissue expansion, when an expander is placed under the pectoralis major muscle at the time of mastectomy. The overlying incisions are allowed to heal, and

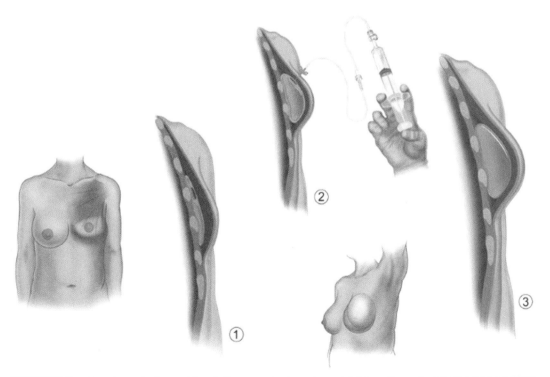

FIGURE 26.3 Staged breast reconstruction consisting of a tissue expander place submuscularly followed by permanent implant placement. (**1**) The tissue expander is placed under the muscle followed by serial expansion, (**2**) the tissue expander is replaced with a permanent implant, and (**3**) the unlabeled images reflect pre- and postreconstruction states.

then saline solution is injected into the expander weekly or every other week until the desired final volume is achieved. After the patient has completed and recovered from all oncologic treatment, a second-stage operation is performed to remove the tissue expander and place the permanent breast implant. Recently, select patients with ideal tissue vascularity and laxity, including patients undergoing nipple-sparing mastectomy, have been reconstructed without tissue expansion and with immediate placement of a permanent breast implant. Early outcomes from direct-to-implant patients are promising with respect to complication rates and acceptable aesthetic results. This technique is not recommended in patients who will require radiation.

The advantages of implant-based reconstruction are that it is simple, requires less operating room time than reconstruction with flaps, and is suitable for women who are not able to undergo reconstruction utilizing autologous tissue flaps. The disadvantages of implant-based reconstruction include the potential for infection, capsular contracture, and implant rupture; in addition, young patients may need to undergo implant replacement several times over the course of their lives. Implant-based reconstruction is a poor choice for patients who have received radiation therapy, as it is associated with significantly higher risk of seroma formation, infection, capsular contracture, and implant extrusion.

Another type of implant-based reconstruction employs a latissimus dorsi myocutaneous pedicled flap over an implant (Fig. 26.4). The latissimus dorsi is a broad, fan-shaped muscle that originates on the back and inserts into the humerus. Because most women do not have enough tissue volume on their backs for complete breast reconstruction, the latissimus dorsi flap is rarely used alone to reconstruct the breast. Instead, the latissimus dorsi muscle with some of the overlying skin is rotated anteriorly to the chest to cover an implant, facilitate closure of the mastectomy defect, and give the reconstructed breast a more natural contour. The implants used in reconstruction with a latissimus dorsi muscle flap are generally the same as those used after tissue expansion.

The primary advantage of using the latissimus dorsi flap is that it is highly vascularized, generally resists infection, and can protect an implant against extrusion and capsular contracture. Therefore, it can be used

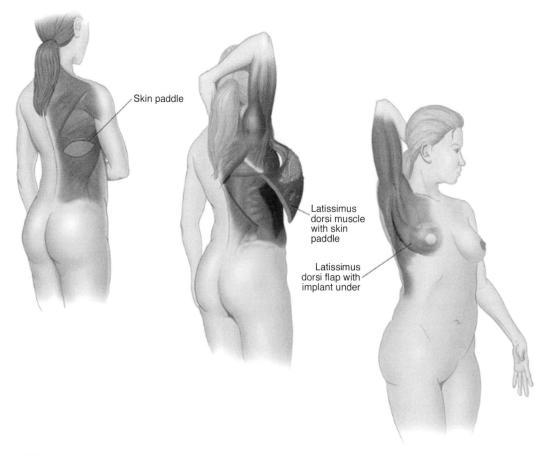

FIGURE 26.4 The latissimus dorsi muscle flap with skin component (myocutaneous flap). The flap comprising the latissimus dorsi muscle and some of the overlying skin is rotated anteriorly to the chest. An implant can be placed under this flap for appropriate volume reconstruction.

as an adjunct in radiated patients to allow implant-based reconstruction. In some patients, the skin paddle can provide sufficient tissue to cover the implant without the need for tissue expansion, and thus a staged approach may not be required. The drawbacks of using the latissimus dorsi flap include longer surgery and recovery times than with implant-only reconstructive surgery, a scar on the back, and potential arm adduction weakness following surgery. Regardless, the approach is a viable option for women who are thin and thus are not candidates for an abdominal flap.

Autologous Tissue Reconstruction

In autologous tissue reconstruction, the patient's own skin, fat, and muscle are transferred from one area of the body to the chest to reconstruct one or both breast mounds, usually without the need for a supplemental prosthesis or implant. Autologous reconstruction can be performed as a pedicled flap or a free flap. The most common donor site is the abdomen.

Transverse Rectus Abdominis Myocutaneous Flap

A classic transverse rectus abdominis myocutaneous (TRAM) flap includes the skin and subcutaneous tissue located between the pubic bone and the umbilicus and the rectus abdominis muscle. The flap can be isolated on either the superior epigastric vessels (pedicled TRAM flap) or the deep inferior epigastric vessels (free TRAM flap), as they travel through the rectus muscle.

When used as a pedicled flap, a tunnel is created in the subcutaneous tissue between the abdomen and breast cavities, and the flap is passed through this tunnel and rotated into the breast cavity. When used as a free flap, the superior and deep inferior epigastric vessels are divided when the flap is harvested, and then the deep inferior epigastrics are reanastomosed to recipient blood vessels in the chest (internal mammary or thoracodorsal vessels) under an operating microscope (Fig. 26.5). The free TRAM avoids several pitfalls of the pedicled TRAM, including an iatrogenic bulge in the upper abdomen and improved fat survival due to better perfusion.

While these TRAM techniques are originally described as taking the entire width of the rectus abdominis muscle, as time has progressed, efforts to take less and less muscle have resulted in several refinements including the muscle-sparing TRAM flap, in which only a small amount of muscle is taken with the blood supply, the deep inferior epigastric artery perforator (DIEP) flap, in which the blood supply is dissected out completely and no muscle is taken with the flap, and the superficial inferior epigastric artery (SIEA) flap (Fig. 26.6).

Other Flaps

Autologous tissue flaps for breast reconstruction can also be harvested from other sites, including the buttocks or thighs (Fig. 26.7). These flaps are reserved for patients in whom the abdomen is not available as a donor site. Overall, breast reconstruction with autologous tissue produces the best long-term results. However, these procedures are of greater magnitude, associated with longer operative and recovery times, and have a small (<2% in most high-volume centers) risk of failure.

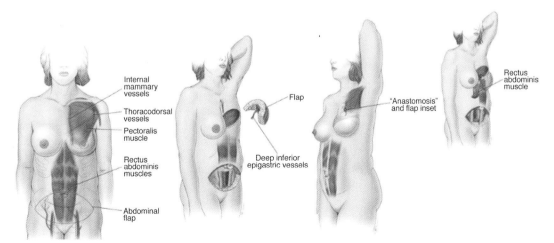

FIGURE 26.5 The free transverse rectus abdominis myocutaneous flap. This flap is based on the deep inferior epigastric vessels. In breast reconstruction with a free transverse rectus abdominis myocutaneous flap, the deep inferior epigastric vessels are divided at the time of flap harvest and then reattached to recipient vessels (e.g., internal mammary vessels) in the chest under an operating microscope.

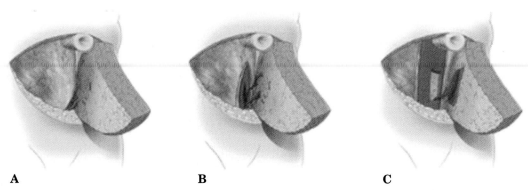

A   **B**   **C**

FIGURE 26.6 (A) The superficial inferior epigastric artery (SIEA) flap is based on blood vessels that run under the skin and whose harvest does not require dissection into the rectus abdominis fascia or muscle. **(B)** The deep inferior epigastric artery perforator (DIEP) flap is based on a dissection of the blood vessels that pass through the rectus abdominis muscle; no muscle or fascia is taken when the flap is harvested. **(C)** In breast reconstruction with a muscle-sparing transverse rectus abdominis myocutaneous flap, only a small amount of rectus muscle is taken with the deep inferior epigastric vessels.

Nipple and Areola Reconstruction

Nipple–areolar reconstruction, if desired, is performed as a separate procedure after the reconstructed breast has attained its final shape and position. Nipple position on the breast mound is determined based on symmetry with the contralateral breast, and a three-dimensional nipple is constructed with a local skin flap, usually from the breast itself (Fig. 26.8). After the reconstructed nipple has had the opportunity to heal, a new areola is tattooed around the reconstructed nipple with medical grade pigments.

Reconstruction of the Trunk

The chest and abdominal wall account for roughly one-third of the entire surface area of the human adult body. Surgical defects in the trunk can expose or compromise critical anatomical structures. In addition, there are dynamic structures that must be able to move and flex with the patient. When possible, oncologic cutaneous defects of the trunk are repaired with wide undermining of the adjacent subcutaneous tissue and local tissue advancement. However, when neoplasm resection creates full-thickness defects of the abdominal or chest wall, pedicled or free flaps may be required.

Thorax

Aside from isolated skin cancers, thoracic reconstruction must account for involved pleural cavity, skeletal support (ribs and sternum), and soft-tissue coverage of the chest and axilla. Forming an airtight seal at the time of wound closure is crucial to preserving the intrathoracic negative pressure gradient. Skeletal stabilization with prosthetic materials is used to reduce the risk of paradoxical chest wall motion (flail chest) when resections involve four or more rib segments or span more than 6 cm in diameter. Exceptions to this rule include posterior resections underneath the scapula.

The majority of chest wall defects can be reconstructed with local or regional myocutaneous flaps. Muscle coverage is especially important if there is exposed hardware or prosthetic material. On the anterior chest, the pectoralis major flap is an excellent option for sternal coverage, either as a pedicled flap based on the thoracoacromial vessels or as a turnover flap based on the internal mammary perforator vessels. In addition, if the mammary vessels are intact, the rectus muscles may be used as rotational flaps for larger defects. Occasionally, the omentum is used when other options are not available. Options for axillary coverage include the pectoralis major and latissimus dorsi flaps. On the posterior thorax, the paraspinous muscles are frequently transposed to cover the spine. Alternatively, the trapezius muscle may be isolated on its vascular pedicle and used to cover the upper spine and cervical region. The latissimus dorsi muscle may also be mobilized on it primary thoracodorsal pedicle or on secondary lumbar perforators as a turnover flap.

Rarely, a free tissue transfer is needed to close oncologic resections of the thorax. In these instances, local options are unavailable due to radiation damage, pedicle ligation, previous use, or insufficient volume. Free tissue options are then tailored on the exact needs of the defect and may include bone, muscle, and soft tissue.

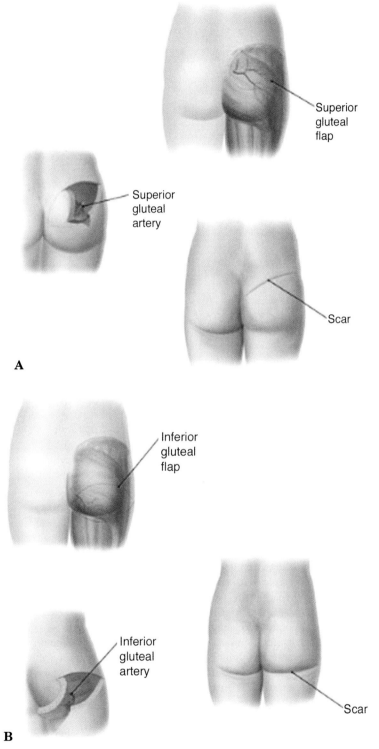

FIGURE 26.7 Other flap options for breast reconstruction include the superior gluteal artery perforator flap (**A**) and the inferior gluteal artery perforator (**B**) flap.

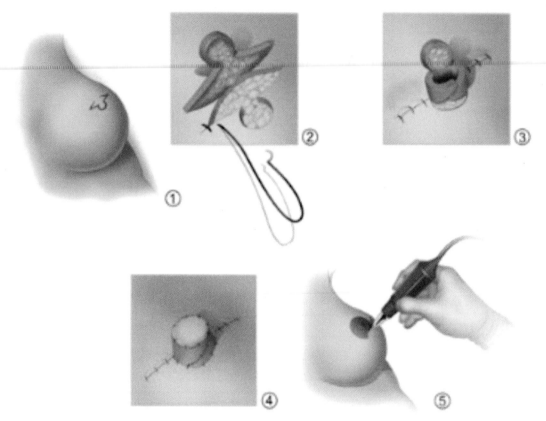

FIGURE 26.8 Local tissue flaps on the reconstructed breast mound are used to reconstruct the nipple (1). A local skin flap is reflected up and folded to reconstruct a three-dimensional nipple (2–4). Areola pigmentation is performed once the reconstructed nipple has healed (5).

Abdomen

Most cutaneous defects that result from oncologic surgery in the abdomen can be closed primarily because of the laxity of the skin and subcutaneous tissue in the region. Laterally, the abdominal wall has abundant segmental blood supply from the intercostal vessels and medially it has axial blood supply from the epigastric vessels. In a virgin abdomen, this allows wide undermining and advancement of cutaneous flaps.

If the defect involves the fascia of the abdominal wall, the goal of reconstruction is to restore the integrity and continuity of the abdominal wall. When there is a paucity of fascia, component separation is often employed. This technique often allows primary closure of the rectus muscle and fascia in the midline while preserving their neurovascular bundles. Laterally, the oblique and transversus muscles are left intact so the entire abdominal wall maintains dynamic contractility. Less commonly, fascial grafts can be taken from tensor fascia lata in the thigh. However, vascularized tissue will always perform better than a graft. A pedicled ALT flap can recruit both fascia and cutaneous elements when other options are scarce.

In the oncologic patient, adjuvant treatment can decrease abdominal wall strength and healing potential. Often, mesh is used to reinforce abdominal repairs that otherwise would have a high rate of hernia. Acellular dermal matrix, a bioprosthetic mesh usually derived from porcine or bovine sources, is often used in an underlay fashion to provide wound strength. Prosthetic meshes can be considered in a clean field. Underlay and retro-rectus techniques have better long-term outcomes than a bridged repair.

Perineum

Perineal reconstruction presents a unique challenge. The perineum is important for sitting, hip mobility, sexual function, pregnancy, and bowel and bladder motility. Perineal skin and fatty tissue are very sensitive to pressure and touch and are durable, elastic, and weight-bearing. In addition, the perineal skin is soft, pigmented, and hair bearing, which makes it challenging to match with distant tissue. The reconstructive discussion and postoperative care is also challenged by strong emotions which may be tied to this area.

Superficial surgical defects of the perineum can be repaired with split-thickness skin grafts if the wound base is healthy and no vital structures are exposed. Split-thickness skin grafts are especially useful if the status of excision margins is uncertain or the risk of local recurrence is high, as they can be excised and repeated if further resection is required. However, in this dependent area, skin grafts can have a higher risk of failure because of fluid collection below the graft and shear.

Local flaps are commonly employed in perineal reconstruction. If the perineum has previously been radiated, or groin dissection has occurred, the area will be prone to seromas, wound dehiscence, and infection. Local flaps bring in healthy tissue to combat this. Small skin defects in the perineum can be repaired with a local rotation flap, such as a rhomboid skin flap. The V to Y random pattern local flap is often used for vulvo-perineal reconstruction. Larger defects may require pedicled flaps such as a posterior thigh fasciocutaneous flap or muscle flaps such as a pedicled gracilis flap.

The pedicled vertical rectus abdominis musculocutaneous (VRAM) flap is a workhorse flap for reconstruction of abdominoperineal resections and pelvic exenterations. The rectus muscle is elevated on the deep inferior epigastric vessels with a vertical skin island. The flap is then passed through the pelvic inlet. The muscle can be used for pelvic dead space and the cutaneous portion lines the neoperineum or creates a neovagina. The flap is extremely durable and allows patients to return to baseline activities within weeks. Other alternatives include the pedicled omental flap, gracilis flap, or profunda artery perforator flap.

Reconstruction in the Extremities

Multimodality therapy has expanded the indications for limb salvage in patients with cancers of the extremities. Limb salvage, however, must not be performed at the expense of an oncologically adequate resection. In addition, preserving a limb that is nonfunctional, insensate, or painful provides no benefit over amputation. Indications for amputation after extirpative surgery include: major neurovascular compromise, significant loss of muscle bulk causing a nonfunctional limb, infection or fractures that compromise reconstruction and delay adjuvant therapy, poor nutrition, serious medical conditions, and a lack of patient motivation or compliance with rehabilitation.

Defects from surgery for soft tissue and bony neoplasms, such as sarcomas, generally require reconstruction with pedicled or free flaps. While neoadjuvant radiation therapy can often decrease tumor size and facilitates limb salvage, it also may hinder wound healing and necessitate a nonirradiated tissue flap closure to provide coverage of neurovascular structures, tendons, bone, and endoprostheses.

In limb reconstruction, bony defects can be repaired with prosthetics, allografts, bone grafts, or vascularized bone flaps. Bones may also be temporarily shortened and plated, with bone lengthening procedures such as bone transport, employed later in the patients' treatment algorithm. Free and pedicled muscle flaps not only provide well-vascularized wound coverage but can also be neurotized to provide functional muscle. Tendons transfers may be performed to allow functioning muscle bellies to take over the function of resected ones. Microsurgical techniques can be used to repair or graft damaged nerves, thereby restoring motor and sensory functions. However, because nerve regeneration occurs at a rate no faster than 1 mm/day, some muscle end plates may die before reinnervation occurs. If reinnervation is expected to take more than 12 to 18 months, some patients may be better served with tendon transfers or amputation.

At a minimum, functional upper limb reconstruction should provide a stable shoulder joint, restore elbow flexion, median nerve sensibility, and prehensile grip. Functional lower limb reconstruction should provide at least stable hip and knee joints, moderate knee flexion, and tibial nerve sensation. This allows the patient to feed and clothe themselves and ambulate with assistive devices. Ultimately, if a limb is amputated, fillet of digit or fillet of arm or leg flaps, can be used as tissue transfers to cover open wounds. In this operation, the uninvolved soft tissue portions of the distal limb are isolated on the neurovascular structures, with the bone removed, and transferred as a pedicle or free flap.

Proximal Arm, Elbow, and Forearm

Proximal arm wounds can be covered with local flaps from the trunk and cervical region. Common flaps include the pectoralis major flap or pedicled latissimus dorsi flap. These flaps can be used to repair defects in the shoulder, axilla, and upper arm. The pedicled latissimus dorsi muscle flap can also be used as a functional muscle transfer to restore elbow flexion or extension in many patients. A common indication for a fillet-of-arm flap is the forequarter amputation, which includes amputation at the shoulder joint for tumors involving the brachial plexus and axillary vessels.

Soft tissue defects in the elbow and forearm can be reconstructed with a pedicled reverse radial forearm or an ulnar forearm flap. Due to the paucity of muscle bellies in the distal forearm, other local options are scarce. If critical elements are exposed, a free-tissue transfer should be considered. Neurotized latissimus dorsi or gracilis muscle is frequently used for functional muscle belly reconstruction. If bone is required, free vascularized grafts from the fibula or scapula are options.

Hand

The hand is one of the most specialized and ergonomically efficient structures in the body. Comprised mostly of bone, tendon, nerves, and skin, the hand is a compact structure with unparalleled motor and sensory function. Because the hand is crucial to the functions of everyday life, a baseline functional assessment should be performed before any tumor excision.

The comprehensive review of hand reconstruction is outside the limits of this text and is a subspeciality of its own. However, certain principles apply throughout. For example, glabrous skin on the palm and fingers is highly specialized and should be repaired by primary closure whenever possible. Skin grafts from the contralateral palm or plantar foot may be the best match if this is not possible. Some sensation, especially at the fingertips, is better preserved by secondary healing than replacement with an alternate tissue. The skin of the dorsum of the hand is thin with moderate laxity and may be replaced with similar tissue from another area, such as the groin.

As a general principle, digit length should be preserved to the greatest extent possible during oncologic resection. This allows proper function of the extensor and flexor tendons, which function like a pulley system and require a fine balance. The tendons of the hand are surrounded in vascularized paratendon and every effort should be made not to strip them of this covering, as it can lead to necrosis or rupture. If they are stripped by tumor resection, they should be covered by vascularized tissue, including a free flap if necessary. Bone grafts can be used to replace phalangeal and metacarpal resections. When amputation is necessary, it is generally performed through the most distant joint possible.

When neural structures are involved, primary nerve repair or a nerve graft may be used to preserve adequate function. Epineurial or interfascicular repairs are typically performed depending on the nerve and location. Small sensory branches can be spared from the extremities and make useful grafts. A commonly harvested nerve is the sural nerve from the lower leg.

Lower Extremity

Oncologic extirpation in the lower extremity can result in defects of the groin, thigh, knee, lower leg, and foot. The most common tumor in the lower extremity is sarcoma.

When defects occur in the groin or thigh, many times they can be closed by pedicled flaps. The most common flaps in this region are a pedicled rectus abdominis myocutaneous flap or an ALT flap. After groin dissection, the proximal femoral vessels are often exposed and the neighboring sartorius muscle can be transposed for coverage. With massive defects of the thigh, free tissue transfers can be performed and the femoral and deep femoral vessels are usually good recipients. End-to-side anastomoses are commonly performed in the lower extremity to preserve blood flow to the distal limb.

In the knee and leg, many defects are associated with osteotomies associated with tumor resection. Bony defects in the distal femur and proximal tibia are usually reconstructed with an allograft or endoprosthesis. Soft tissue coverage of defects in the knee and proximal one-third of the lower leg can be achieved with pedicled gastrocnemius muscle flaps. The medial or lateral heads of the gastrocnemius can be separated and used as individual pedicled muscle flaps, or both heads can be used to provide more coverage. If both heads of the gastrocnemius muscle are to be used for reconstruction, the soleus muscle must be preserved to provide plantar flexion of the foot. Alternatively, when soft tissue coverage is required in the middle third of the leg, the soleus muscle is used as it has better reach in this area.

In comparison to the more proximal thigh and leg, reconstructing the distal third of the leg with local or regional muscle flaps is not usually possible because of the sparse amount of local tissues available. In the distal third of the leg, most muscle bellies have become tendinous and tightly fixed to the bone. In general, all but the smallest wounds in this region must be repaired with free fasciocutaneous, or myocutaneous free flaps. Three sets of vessels are present in the lower leg, the anterior tibial, posterior tibial, and peroneal vessels. Any of these can be suitable for free flap anastomosis. The lower leg and foot can survive off a single vessel, if necessary, although it is preferable to leave at least two systems intact.

Foot

Like the hand, the foot is extremely specialized. It bears the entire weight of the body and therefore must have extremely durable coverage. In addition, it must have fine sensation to protect against frequent trauma and infection. Because of this, sacrifice of the tibial nerve during tumor extirpation and subsequent rendering of the plantar foot insensate, makes it imperative that the patient clearly understands this risk and that amputation may the safer, more prudent alternative.

Similar to the hand, very small oncologic resections are best repaired with primary closure or secondary healing. Small defects are repaired with skin grafts and local flaps. Due to the paucity of muscle and soft tissue in the lower leg, there are few local flaps available for foot reconstruction. The reverse sural artery rotation flap can repair small defects at the heel or malleolus. The medial plantar artery flap includes the glabrous skin of the instep and can be moved short distances from the non–weight-bearing area of the foot to the weight-bearing surface. However, both these flaps are limited in their reach.

When defects reach over 5 cm, they must be reconstructed with a free flap. Smaller but durable muscles such as the gracilis or serratus anterior can be used and then covered with a skin graft. Fasciocutaneous flaps such as the radial forearm flap are also used for foot reconstruction and can be designed to include sensory innervation. Insensate muscle and fasciocutaneous flaps are susceptible to pressure ulceration and so they must be vigilantly monitored for the breakdown of skin and soft tissue. Care must be taken when planning free flaps for the foot, as bulky flaps are usually unfavorable for ambulation and may necessitate special orthotic footwear and/or revision surgery.

New Advancements

As with most areas of surgery, the field of Plastic and Reconstructive Surgery is constantly evolving to improve patient outcomes and quality of life in patients with cancer. With this in mind, two developing areas warrant additional description.

Surgical Management of Chronic Pain and the Amputee

Chronic residual limb pain and phantom limb pain are debilitating outcomes following oncologic amputation. In general, 10% to 76% of amputees report residual limb pain and up to 85% report phantom limb pain. Due to this, many amputees suffer not only from the initial insult of amputation, but also develop chronic consequences.

Neuromas are masses of disorganized axons that form after a nerve is ligated and send painful and distressing signals to the brain. This can result in phantom pain as the neural efferent-afferent loop is disrupted from the amputated limb to the brain. Fortunately, in the past decade, there have been emerging and promising microsurgical treatments for the treatment of postamputation pain. Dumanian and Valerio pioneered work in the surgical technique of Targeted Muscle Reinnervation (TMR), which coapts mixed major nerves (those that contain motor and sensory fibers) to available motor nerves in the surrounding tissue using microsurgical sutures in the epineurium. Trophic stimulus from the cut recipient motor nerves encourages regenerative and physiologic healing of the amputated major mixed nerves. Cederna and colleagues have published their novel work with Regenerative Peripheral Nerve Interfaces (RPNIs) which use free autologous muscle wrapped around the proximal amputated nerve to provide trophic regenerative stimulus. Both techniques give the amputated proximal nerve a target for regeneration and encourage the nerve to heal as opposed to more conventional methods which consist of burying or crushing the amputated nerve fascicles.

TMR and RPNI were initially developed for the control of myoelectric prosthetics. Myoelectric prosthetics function by detecting EMG signals on remaining muscle of the amputee and translating these signals into multiple coordinated movements on a highly specialized prosthetic. TMR and RPNI surgical nerve transfers were designed to create specific muscle sites in the amputee that these prosthetics could detect. Fortuitously, treated patients were found to have less pain after their neuromas were resected and the nerves coapted to healthy remaining motor nerves. While TMR and RPNI remain highly important for developing myoelectric prosthetics, these techniques are most broadly applicable for pain control. Myoelectric prosthetics remain cost-prohibitive for most patients and require a heavy battery; therefore, they require further technologic advancement in order to be useful to a wider population of patients.

Lymphedema and Treatment Options

Oncologic lymphedema is the buildup of fluid within the interstitial tissues of the body. It occurs due to the disruption of normal lymph channels and lymph nodal basins after nodal dissection or radiation. The protein and lipid-dense fluid stagnates and causes fibrotic scarring within the affected area. As scar matures, the lymphedema advances and becomes irreversible.

Traditional lymphedema treatments have centered on compression garments and manual decompression, in the form of massage, to move stagnant fluid from the affected area and prevent scar formation. This is considered complete decongestive therapy (CDT) and starts with a reductive and then maintenance phase.

The maintenance phase is lifelong and requires strict compliance. For patients with uncontrolled, irreversible lymphedema, the only previous surgical treatments were surgical or liposuction-assisted debulking, which reduced the volume of scarred tissue but did not treat the pathology.

More recently, supermicrosurgery has developed to allow microsurgeons to anastomose vessels as small as 0.3 to 0.8 mm in diameter, including lymph channels. Using supermicrosurgical techniques, lymphovenous (LVB) bypasses are performed which divert lymph fluid from lymph channels into nearby veins for an alternate drainage pathway. This technique is highly dependent on the presence of healthy lymph channels and small caliber veins remaining after the tumor is extirpated and may be performed prophylactically in some settings.

As an alternative, some microsurgeons are performing autologous lymph node transfers, in which a group of lymph nodes is harvested within a small flap with a pedicle artery and vein. An example of this is the harvest of a portion of the omentum with identified lymph nodes. The affected extremity undergoes scar release and then the omental flap pedicle vessels are anastomosed to available vessels in the extremity. The vascularized nodes then survive and begin a process of inosculation and the formation of new draining lymph channels.

Both lymphovenous bypass and lymph node transfer are currently undergoing trials to determine the optimal indications, timing, and postoperative care. They offer emerging and promising surgical treatments for an otherwise devastating extirpative side effect.

Summary

Reconstruction for oncologic defects requires attention to both aesthetic and functional requirements. These defects can be routinely and safely reconstructed using multidisciplinary and systematic approaches that maintain oncologic principles. The ultimate goal of reconstructive surgery is a healed wound with minimal patient morbidity.

CASE SCENARIO

Case Scenario 1: Consult for Breast Reconstruction

Presentation

A 45-year-old female presented to the breast oncology center with a palpable mass in the central right breast 3.2 cm in largest dimension, located 2 cm from the nipple. Biopsy shows IDC with associated DCIS spanning an area of 4.5 cm on MRI. On immunohistochemical analysis the tumor is found to be ER+, PR+, HER2+. On ultrasound there are 2 lymph nodes that appear suspicious, and biopsy of one node shows the presence of metastatic mammary carcinoma. Genetic testing reveals a BRCA1 mutation. There was no evidence of metastatic disease outside the axilla. The patient received preoperative chemotherapy with dual anti-HER2 therapy with an excellent response; the mass decreased to 2.5 cm and the lymph nodes showed a significant response, currently appearing normal in architecture. The breast surgical oncology service is recommending that the patient undergo a skin-sparing right mastectomy with targeted axillary node dissection. The patient wants to be considered for a nipple-sparing mastectomy; a prophylactic mastectomy is indicated on the contralateral (left) breast in view of the BRCA1 mutation. She is sent to you for reconstructive options. Her BMI is 28 and she is otherwise healthy. She reports that her current bra size is 36C.

Potential Reconstructive Options

- Immediate reconstruction with autologous tissue
- Immediate reconstruction with autologous tissue and implant
- Delayed-immediate reconstruction
- Prophylactic/skin-sparing/nipple-sparing contralateral mastectomy

These options, including their potential risks (both oncologic and technical) are discussed with the patient in detail. After this extensive discussion the patient wishes to be considered for bilateral nipple-sparing/skin-sparing mastectomies with immediate reconstruction, if possible. As the patient had 2 lymph nodes radiographically positive for metastatic disease, there is a possibility depending on the final pathology, that postmastectomy radiation therapy will be recommended.

Common Curve Balls

- The role for postmastectomy radiation is often dependent on the final pathology of the breast and nodal specimens, especially in a patient that receives neoadjuvant systemic treatment for biopsy-documented positive axillary lymph nodes. An immediate reconstruction can potentially interfere with the delivery of radiation and/or be affected by radiation changes. Therefore, immediate reconstruction is not recommended in this particular patient. However, a tissue expander may be placed to maintain the breast skin envelope until the final pathology is determined. This is called delayed-immediate reconstruction and is used to preserve the cosmetic benefit of the natural breast skin envelope.

■ A nipple-sparing procedure cannot be guaranteed when the tumor is in the central quadrant of the breast within 2 cm of the nipple/areolar complex. Frozen section analysis of the margins on the nipple areolar complex must be performed at the time of surgery, to minimize the risk of a positive margin.

■ Contralateral prophylactic mastectomy is indicated due to the BRCA1 status; however, because of the need to delay breast reconstruction until final pathology is determined and the oncologic treatment plan is finalized, it may be beneficial to delay the contralateral mastectomy until there is a definitive decision on the role for radiation therapy. This has two potential benefits:

1. It limits the chance of adjuvant therapy being delayed due to a complication on the side of the prophylactic mastectomy, such as infection or dehiscence.
2. It may optimize the cosmetic outcome of the prophylactic mastectomy by limiting side effects of radiation.

The patient is taken to the operating room and a nipple-sparing, skin-sparing mastectomy and a targeted lymph node dissection is performed. Frozen section analysis of the nipple/areolar complex shows that there are tumor cells present at the deep margin of the nipple/areolar complex and the breast surgical oncologist determines that the nipple/areolar complex needs to be excised in order to provide adequate local control. In addition, the sentinel lymph node is also found to have evidence of metastatic disease on frozen section analysis and therefore, the breast surgical oncologist performs a completion axillary dissection. The extirpative portion of the surgery is completed, and you proceed to the operating room to perform the reconstruction. At this juncture, you are informed by the breast surgical oncologist that there is a possibility that the patient may require postmastectomy radiation therapy based on the size of the tumor on presentation and depending on how many lymph nodes remain positive on final pathology. The breast surgical oncologist requests your opinion regarding whether it is appropriate to proceed with the contralateral prophylactic mastectomy.

At this time your reconstructive options are:

■ Proceed with the prophylactic contralateral mastectomy and place bilateral tissue expanders.
■ Delay the prophylactic contralateral mastectomy and proceed with immediate reconstruction with autologous tissue on the cancer mastectomy side.
■ Delay the prophylactic contralateral mastectomy and proceed with placement of a tissue expander only on the cancer mastectomy side.

The most conservative course of action is to delay the prophylactic mastectomy to prevent unnecessary complication which could delay/interfere with her oncologic treatment. It is reasonable to proceed with tissue expander placement to preserve the mastectomy pocket on the cancer side, to allow for delayed-immediate reconstruction. One exception to this rule may be considered in healthy women with very large breast size. In that specific scenario, it may be reasonable to proceed with the prophylactic mastectomy to limit severe aesthetic deformity or back pain that can result from unbalanced weight on the chest wall. This should be discussed well in advance with the patient and their risk for complication must be low. This is not indicated in this patient.

The final pathology reveals the tumor to be 3 cm in greatest dimension and there are 3 lymph nodes with histologic evidence of metastatic disease. In view of this report the patient is recommended to have postmastectomy radiation therapy in addition to a year of adjuvant anti-HER2 therapy.

Reconstructive Recommendations

It is necessary to delay the final breast reconstruction until the patient has received postmastectomy radiation treatment. This is called delayed–delayed reconstruction. The patient may receive reconstruction 6 to 12 months after radiation is complete, to limit the complication risk from a radiated chest wall. In addition, the patient will be receiving adjuvant anti-HER2 therapy. After multidisciplinary discussion, it is recommended that the anti-HER2 therapy can be held at the 6-month treatment time point in order to complete the reconstruction.

Reconstructive options at this time are:

- Prophylactic contralateral skin-sparing mastectomy and immediate bilateral reconstruction with implants.
- Prophylactic contralateral skin-sparing mastectomy and immediate bilateral reconstruction with combined implant and rotated/pedicled autologous tissue (latissimus dorsi flap).
- Prophylactic contralateral skin-sparing mastectomy and immediate bilateral reconstruction with free autologous tissue.

The placement of implants into a radiated field is possible, but generally fraught with complications. Capsular contracture around the implant, increased risk of infection, and malposition are common complications. For this reason, on the radiated side, it is strongly recommended that the patient undergo autologous reconstruction.

In regard to autologous reconstruction, both a pedicled latissimus dorsi flap with implant and a free abdominal-based flap are reasonable options. A pedicled latissimus dorsi flap will cover the implant and shield it from most of the radiation effects, although capsular contracture can still happen. However, it is a great option for women who do not have sufficient excess tissue for a free flap. In contrast, a purely autologous reconstruction, such as a free flap from the abdomen, eliminates the risks associated with implants. It also provides a more natural feeling breast that will age with the patient. In a patient with sufficient abdominal tissue, such as multiparous women with a reasonable BMI, this option is the most favorable. In addition, studies have shown that women who underwent autologous reconstruction have better outcomes with less revision surgeries in the long-term.

On the prophylactic side, the patient may receive an implant or autologous flap. In general, the cosmetic outcome will be more favorable if both sides are reconstructed in similar manner, although the plastic surgeon may be able to create an excellent outcome with a mixture of techniques.

The single most important factor in patient reconstructive satisfaction is early and clear communication between clinician and patient. Listening to the patient's desires, while clearly explaining the necessary steps in reconstruction, is paramount to a happy patient. Breast reconstruction may be a 1- to 2-year journey for some women. It is important to communicate why it may take this extended time, which is often for both a patient's oncologic safety and improved cosmetic outcome. Breast reconstruction is one of the few areas that a breast cancer patient can potentially regain some choice over their breast cancer treatment options. It is empowering to the patient to know that they will ultimately determine which option is best for them, as long as oncologic safety is followed.

CASE SCENARIO 1 REVIEW

Questions

1. A patient has a basal cell cancer removed from the nose. What is the advantage of using a full thickness skin graft versus a split thickness skin graft?

    A. Decreased contraction
    B. Ease of harvest
    C. Better sensation
    D. No difference
    E. None of the above

2. A patient has breast cancer requiring mastectomy. She would like autologous reconstruction. What is the difference between a pedicled and free flap?

    A. A pedicle flap does not take skin and muscle
    B. A pedicle flap cannot be used in radiated patients
    C. A free flap requires a microvascular anastomosis and a pedicled flap does not
    D. A free flap requires delayed reconstruction
    E. A pedicle flap is usually smaller

3. A patient presents with an invasive squamous cell carcinoma of the scalp that results in a defect 6 × 7 cm. What is the best form of reconstruction?

    A. Split-thickness skin graft
    B. Full-thickness skin graft

C. Rotational scalp flap
D. Free flap
E. None of the above

4. The free fibula flap is a workhorse flap for microvascular bone reconstruction. Which artery supplies the free fibula?

   A. Anterior tibial artery
   B. Peroneal artery
   C. Posterior tibial artery
   D. Descending branch of the lateral circumflex femoral artery
   E. Sural artery

5. A breast cancer patient will require a mastectomy and likely adjuvant radiation. When is the best time to perform breast reconstruction?

   A. Immediately
   B. Delayed

6. A very thin breast cancer patient desires breast reconstruction. She previously underwent a mastectomy and radiation. She does not have enough abdominal tissue for autologous reconstruction. The patient strongly prefers to use an implant. Can this be safely offered to the patient? Choose the correct answer.

   A. No, implants should never be used in a radiated field
   B. Yes, if the implant is placed under the pectoralis muscle
   C. Yes, if the implant is completely covered with muscle, including the harvest and use of a rotational latissimus dorsi muscle
   D. All of the above
   E. None of the above

7. When is skeletal stabilization required after resection of thoracic wall tumors?

   A. When more than two ribs are resected
   B. When four or more ribs are resected
   C. When any posterior ribs are resected
   D. When there is a cavity greater than 6 cm in diameter
   E. B and D

8. What are the advantages of component separation when closing abdominal wall defects?

   A. The rectus muscles are medialized
   B. The oblique and transversus remain innervated
   C. Continuity of the abdominal wall musculature is restored
   D. Decreased need for "bridging" meshes and, if needed, complete coverage of biologic or synthetic mesh
   E. All of the above

9. A 30-year-old female presents with a lower extremity soft tissue sarcoma. Resection results in the exposure of the proximal tibia. What reconstructive method is preferred?

   A. Soleus flap
   B. Gastrocnemius flap
   C. Full-thickness skin graft
   D. Free flap
   E. All of the above

10. A 60-year-old make requires a forequarter amputation for axillary sarcoma. His chest wall tissue is ulcerated and his axillary vasculature will be sacrificed with the resection. What reconstruction provides the most coverage with the least donor site morbidity?

    A. Anterolateral thigh flap
    B. Latissimus dorsi flap
    C. Fillet of arm flap
    D. Split thickness skin graft
    E. All of the above

Answers

1. **The correct answer is A.** *Rationale:* Because full-thickness skin grafts contract less than split-thickness skin grafts, full thickness grafts are preferable in regions where wound bed contraction is not desirable.

2. **The correct answer is C.** *Rationale:* Microvascular free flaps are tissues with a blood supply from a distant region of the body that is ligated and then transferred to a defect. They are called "free flaps" because they become free of their native vascular origin and require reanastomosis for perfusion.

3. **The correct answer is D.** *Rationale:* Scalp defects larger than about 6 cm, or even smaller defects in irradiated scalps, usually require microvascular free flap reconstruction. The scalp can usually be reconstructed with thin cutaneous or fasciocutaneous free flaps, such as the anterolateral thigh (ALT) free flap, or a muscle flap, such as the latissimus dorsi muscle free flap, covered with a skin graft.

4. **The correct answer is B.** *Rationale:* The fibula flap is based on the peroneal artery and vein; therefore, its use requires that either the anterior or the posterior tibial vessels adequately perfuse the distal lower limb. An angiogram may be required to confirm this before harvest. Secondary flap sources for mandible reconstruction include the iliac, scapular, and radial bone free flaps. The descending branch of the lateral circumflex femoral artery is the blood supply for the anterolateral thigh (ALT) free flap. The sural artery is the blood supply for the medial sural artery perforator (MSAP) free flap.

5. **The correct answer is B.** *Rationale:* Immediate breast reconstruction results in the best aesthetic outcomes if postmastectomy radiation therapy is not needed. However, if postmastectomy radiation therapy is required, delayed reconstruction is preferred as it avoids potential radiation delivery problems and generally results in a superior aesthetic outcome.

6. **The correct answer is C.** *Rationale:* When used in combination with an implant, the primary advantage of using the latissimus dorsi flap is that it is a highly vascularized and generally resists infection and protects an implant against extrusion and capsular contracture. Therefore, it can be used as an adjunct in radiated patients to allow implant-based reconstruction. However, patients must be warned complications, especially contracture, can still occur.

7. **The correct answer is E.** *Rationale:* Skeletal stabilization with prosthetic materials is used to reduce the risk of paradoxical chest wall motion (flail chest) when resections involve four or more rib segments or span more than 6 cm in diameter. Exceptions to this rule include posterior resections underneath the scapula.

8. **The correct answer is E.** *Rationale:* If a defect involves the fascia of the abdominal wall, the goal of reconstruction is to restore the integrity and continuity of the abdominal wall. When there is a paucity of fascia, component separation, in which the layers of the abdominal wall fascia and muscle are separated to increase medialization of the rectus components, is often employed. This technique often allows primary closure of the rectus muscle and fascia in the midline while preserving their neurovascular bundles. Laterally, the oblique and transversus muscles are left intact so the entire abdominal wall maintains dynamic contractility.

9. **The correct answer is B.** *Rationale:* Soft-tissue coverage of defects in the knee and proximal one-third of the lower leg can be achieved with pedicled gastrocnemius muscle flaps. The medial or lateral heads of the gastrocnemius can be separated and used as individual pedicled muscle flaps, or both heads can be used to provide more coverage. If both heads of the gastrocnemius muscle are to be used for reconstruction, the soleus muscle must be preserved to provide plantar flexion of the foot.

10. **The correct answer is C.** *Rationale:* A common indication for a fillet-of-arm flap is the forequarter amputation, which includes amputation at the shoulder joint for tumors involving the brachial plexus and axillary vessels. In this operation, the uninvolved soft tissue portions of the distal limb are isolated on the neurovascular structures, with the bone removed, and transferred as a free flap. There is no donor site morbidity because the arm is amputated.

Recommended Readings

Head and Neck Reconstruction

Burget GC, Menick FJ. Nasal reconstruction: seeking a fourth dimension. *Plast Reconstr Surg*. 1986;78:145–157.

Chang EI, Yu P, Skoracki RJ, Liu J, Hanasono MM. Comprehensive analysis of functional outcomes and survival after microvascular reconstruction of glossectomy defects. *Ann Surg Oncol*. 2015;22:3061–3069.

Chao AH, Yu P, Skoracki RJ, DeMonte F, Hanasono MM. Microsurgical reconstruction of composite scalp and calvarial defects in patients with cancer: a 10-year experience. *Head Neck*. 2012; 34, 12:1759–1764.

Hanasono MM, Matros E, Disa JJ. Important aspects of head and neck reconstruction. *Plast Reconstr Surg*. 2014;134:968e–980e.

Hanasono MM, Silva AK, Skoracki RJ, et al. Skull base reconstruction: an updated approach. *Plast Reconstr Surg*. 2011;128:675–686.

Hanasono MM, Silva AK, Yu P, Skoracki RJ. A comprehensive algorithm for oncologic maxillary reconstruction. *Plast Reconstr Surg*. 2013;131:47–60.

Hanasono MM, Weinstock YE, Yu P. Reconstruction of extensive head and neck defects with multiple simultaneous free flaps. *Plast Reconstr Surg*. 2008;122:1739–1746.

Lee EI, Chao AH, Skoracki RJ, Yu P, DeMonte F, Hanasono MM. Outcomes of calvarial reconstruction in cancer patients. *Plast Reconstr Surg*. 2014;133:675–682.

Menick FJ. Nasal reconstruction. *Plast Reconstr Surg*. 2010;125:138e–150e.

Yu P, Hanasono MM, Skoracki RJ, et al. Pharyngoesophageal reconstruction with the anterolateral thigh flap after total laryngopharyngectomy. *Cancer*. 2010;116(7):1718–1724.

Yu P, Lewin JS, Reece GP, Robb GL. Comparison of clinical and functional outcomes and hospital costs following pharyngoesophageal reconstruction with the anterolateral thigh free flap versus the jejunal flap. *Plast Reconstr Surg*. 2006;117(3):968–974.

Breast Reconstruction

Alderman A, Gutowski K, Ahuja A, Gray D, Postmastectomy ExpanderImplant Breast Reconstruction Guideline Work Group. ASPS Clinical Practice Guideline Summary on Breast Reconstruction with Expanders and Implants. *Plast Reconstr Surg*. 2014;134:648–655e.

Baumann DP, Crosby MA, Selber JC, et al. Optimal timing of delayed free lower abdominal flap breast reconstruction after postmastectomy radiation therapy. *Plast. Reconstr Surg*. 2011;127:1100–1106.

Kroll SS, Schusterman MA, Reece GP, et al. Choice of flap and incidence of free flap success. *Plast Reconstr Surg*. 1996;98:459–463.

Kronowitz SJ. Immediate versus delayed reconstruction. *Clin Plast Surg*. 2007;34(1): 39–50.

Kronowitz SJ. Delayed-immediate breast reconstruction: technical and timing considerations. *Plast Reconstr Surg*. 2010;125(2):463–474.

Kronowitz SJ, Kuerer HM. Advances and surgical decision-making for breast reconstruction. *Cancer*. 2006;107:893–907.

Kronowitz SJ, Kuerer HM, Buchholz TA, Valero V, Hunt KK. A management algorithm and practical oncoplastic surgical techniques for repairing partial mastectomy defects. *Plast Reconstr Surg*. 2008;122(6):1631–1647.

Momoh AO, Ahmed R, Kelley BP, et al. A systematic review of complications of implant-based breast reconstruction with prereconstruction and postreconstruction radiotherapy. *Ann Surg Oncol*. 2014:21:118–124.

Trunk and Perineum Reconstruction

Althubaiti G, Butler CE. Abdominal wall and chest wall reconstruction. *Plast Reconstr Surg*. 2014;133:688e–698e.

Arnold PG, Pairolero PC. Chest wall reconstruction: an account of 500 consecutive patients. *Plastic Reconstr Surg*. 1996;98:804–810.

Booth JH, Garvey PB, Baumann DP, et al. Primary fascial closure with mesh reinforcement is superior to bridged mesh repair for abdominal wall reconstruction. *J Am Coll Surg*. 2013:217(6):999–1009.

Buchel EW, Finical S, Johnson C. Pelvic reconstruction using vertical rectus abdominis musculocutaneous flaps. *Ann Plast Surg*. 2004;52:22–26.

Butler CE, Gündeslioglu AO, Rodriguez-Bigas MA. Outcomes of immediate vertical rectus abdominis myocutaneous flap reconstruction for irradiated abdominoperineal resection defects. *J Am Coll Surg*. 2008;206(4):694–703.

Chang RR, Mehrara BJ, Hu QY, Disa JJ, Cordeiro PG. Reconstruction of complex oncologic chest wall defects: a 10-year experience. *Plastic Reconstr Surg*. 2004;52:471–479.

Garvey PB, Rhines LD, Dong W, Chang DW. Immediate soft-tissue reconstruction for complex defects of the spine following surgery for spinal neoplasms. *Plast Reconstr Surg*. 2010;125(5):1460–1466.

McCraw JB, Papp C, Ye Z, Huang V, McMellin A. Reconstruction of the perineum after tumor surgery. *Surg Oncol Clin N Am*. 1997;6:177–189.

Extremity Reconstruction

Barwick WJ, Goldberg JA, Scully SP, Harrelson JM. Vascularized tissue transfer for closure of irradiated wounds after soft tissue sarcoma resection. *Ann Surg*. 1992;216:591–595.

Bosse MJ, MacKenzie EJ, Kellam JF, et al. An analysis of outcomes of reconstruction or amputation of leg-threatening injuries. *NEJM*. 2002; 347-1924-1931.

Brennan MF. Management of extremity soft-tissue sarcoma. *Am J Surg*. 1989;158:71–78.

Cordeiro PG, Neves RI, Hidalgo DA. The role of free tissue transfer following oncologic resection in the lower extremity. *Ann Plast Surg*. 1994;33:9–16.

Hidalgo DA, Carrasquillo IM. The treatment of lower extremity sarcomas with wide excision, radiotherapy, and free-flap reconstruction. *Plast Reconstr Surg*. 1992;89:96–101.

Reece GP, Schusterman MA, Pollock RE, et al. Immediate versus delayed free-tissue transfer salvage of the lower extremity in soft tissue sarcoma patients. *Ann Surg Oncol*. 1994;1:11–17.

Robb GL, Reece GP. Lower extremity reconstruction. In: Schusterman MA, ed. *Microsurgical Reconstruction of the Cancer Patient*. Lippincott-Raven; 1997:289–322.

Ver Halen JP, Yu P, Skoracki DW, Chang DW. Reconstruction of massive oncologic defects using free fillet flaps. *Plast Reconstr Surg*. 2010;125:913–922.

New Advancements
TMR and RPNI

Dumanian GA, Potter BK, Mioton LM, et al. Targeted muscle reinnervation treats neuroma and phantom pain in major limb amputees: a randomized clinical trial. *Ann Surg*. 2019;270:238.

Kubiak CA, Kemp SW, Cederna PS, Kung TA. Prophylactic regenerative peripheral nerve interfaces to prevent postamputation pain. *Plast Reconstr Surg*. 2019;144:421e.

Mioton LM, Dumanian GA. Targeted muscle reinnervation and prosthetic rehabilitation after limb loss. *J Surg Oncol*. 2018;118(807):18.

Valerio IL, Dumanian GA, Jordan SW, et al. Preemptive treatment of phantom and residual limb pain with targeted muscle reinnervation at the time of major limb amputation. *J Am Coll Surg*. 2019;228:217.

Lymphedema

Allen RJ, Cheng MH. Lymphedema surgery: patient selection and an overview of surgical techniques. *J Surg Oncol*. 2016;113:923.

Garza R 3rd, Skoracki R, Hock K, Povoski SP. A comprehensive overview on the surgical management of secondary lymphedema of the upper and lower extremities related to prior oncologic therapies. *BMC Cancer*. 2017;5:468.

Ito R and Suami H. Overview of lymph node transfer for lymphedema treatment. *Plast Reconstr Surg*. 2014;134:548.

Rodriguez JR, Fuse Y, Yamamoto T. Microsurgical strategies for prophylaxis of cancer-related extremity lymphedema: a comprehensive review of the literature. *J Reconstr Microsurg*. 2020;36:471.

INDEX

Note: Page number followed by f and t indicates figure and table respectively.